Conceptual Review of

Preventive & Social Medicine (PSM)

Exclusive Section on Epidemiology, Research Methodology & Biostatistics

Covering 2600+ MCQs with Explanations, 100+ IBQs & 500+ Colored Illustrations/Images

3rd Edition

Mukhmohit Singh
MBBS, MD (Community Medicine) PGDHS
Gold Sp Award (2012) ERS

Ex Assistant Professor
Community Medicine and Public Health
Preventive Medicine and Public Health Specialist

Formerly
Epidemiologist – IDSP, UT Administration, Chandigarh
Research Officer, PGIMER, Chandigarh

Member
Indian Public Health Association
Indian Association of Preventive and Social Medicine
Research Society for Study of Diabetes
European Respiratory Society

Editor
Shveta Saini
MBBS, MD (Community Medicine)

Ex Assistant Professor
Community Medicine and Public Health
Preventive Medicine and Public Health Specialist

Member
Indian Public Health Association
Indian Association of Preventive and Social Medicine

Foreword
Ashok K Bhardwaj
Murali Mohan Reddy

CBS
Dedicated to Education

CBS Publishers & Distributors Pvt Ltd
• New Delhi • Bengaluru • Chennai • Kochi • Kolkata • Mumbai
• Hyderabad • Nagpur • Patna • Pune • Vijayawada

Conceptual Review of
Preventive & Social Medicine (PSM)

DISCLAIMER

This book contains questions based on important topics frequently asked in previous years National Level PG Entrance Examinations & State Level Examinations in India. Often repeated topics and sub-topics have been included for students' benefit. We do not claim that these questions are exact or similar to questions asked in any recent examinations in India. If any such similarity is found, it is purely coincidental and by chance.

ISBN: 978-81-945783-2-1

Third Edition: 2020

Published by **Satish Kumar Jain** and produced by **Varun Jain** for

CBS Publishers & Distributors Pvt Ltd

4819/XI Prahlad Street, 24 Ansari Road, Daryaganj, New Delhi 110 002, India.

Ph: +91-11-23289259, 23266861, 23266867 Website: www.cbspd.com

Fax: 011-23243014

e-mail: delhi@cbspd.com; cbspubs@airtelmail.in.

Corporate Office: 204 FIE, Industrial Area, Patparganj, Delhi 110 092

Ph: +91-11-4934 4934 Fax: 4934 4935

e-mail: feedback@cbspd.com; bhupesharora@cbspd.com

Branches

- **Bengaluru:** Seema House 2975, 17th Cross, K.R. Road Banasankari 2nd Stage, Bengaluru 560 070, Karnataka
  Ph: +91-80-26771678/79 Fax: +91-80-26771680 e-mail: bangalore@cbspd.com
- **Chennai:** 7, Subbaraya Street, Shenoy Nagar, Chennai 600 030, Tamil Nadu
  Ph: +91-44-26680620, 26681266 Fax: +91-44-42032115 e-mail: chennai@cbspd.com
- **Kochi:** 68/1534, 35, 36-Power House Road, Opp. KSEB, Cochin-682018, Kochi, Kerala
  Ph: +91-484-4059061-65 Fax: +91-484-4059065 e-mail: kochi@cbspd.com
- **Kolkata:** 6/B, Ground Floor, Rameswar Shaw Road, Kolkata-700 014, West Bengal
  Ph: +91-33-22891126, 22891127, 22891128 e-mail: kolkata@cbspd.com
- **Mumbai:** 83-C, Dr E Moses Road, Worli, Mumbai-400018, Maharashtra
  Ph: +91-22-24902340/41 Fax: +91-22-24902342 e-mail: mumbai@cbspd.com

Representatives

- **Hyderabad** +91-9885175004
- **Patna** +91-9334159340
- **Pune** +91-9623451994
- **Vijayawada** +91-9000660880

Printed at:

From the Publisher's Desk

Dear Readers,

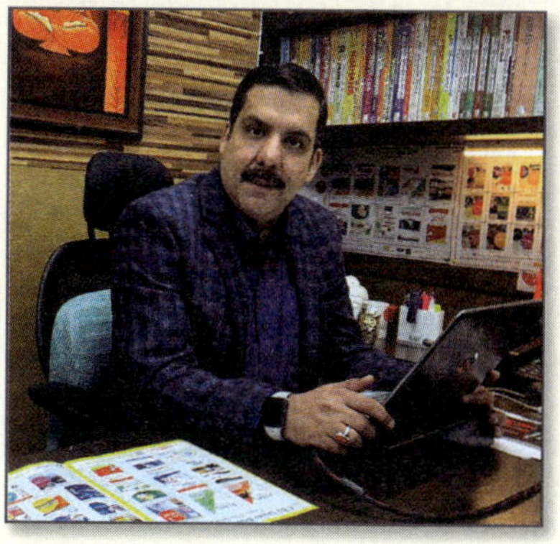

I extend my warm welcome and convey my heartfelt thanks for appreciating the CBS Exam Books for another successful year. It has been an amazing journey so far and I am highly grateful for your support and cooperation to help us achieve various milestones in this whole span of time. The mission with which we started in the year 2015 was to bring nothing but the best of everything to our target audience and today I can proudly say that we have maintained that standard and are committed to continue the same in future as well.

Every single title under the banner of CBS Exam Books has been developed and nurtured like an infant. The authors and our entire team work day and night to bring the best in everything for you. Be it content, presentation, social media contests and offers, we strive to meet your expectations with every passing year. Your trust has motivated us to maintain and upgrade ourselves during this period. I am extremely thankful to all our authors who are the real pillars of the complete series of CBS Exam Books. The contributions of our esteemed authors have laid the foundations of CBS Exam Books.

At this juncture, I can recall these lines by Drake,

"Sometimes it's the journey that teaches you a lot about your destination".

We have grown and changed with the passage of time to upgrade our ways of providing our readers with maximum benefits and help them manage their time and efforts in effective manner. Previous year was the year of great achievements. Let me show you a glimpse of our successful journey:

- Most of the titles of CBS Exam Books received wide acceptance and recognition by the readers of proving their usefulness and supremacy. To mention a few, SARP Anatomy, CRISP, Surgery Sixer, Complete Review of Pathology, Conceptual Review of Pharmacology, SOCH, Forensic Medicine, Complete Review of Medicine, Conceptual Review of PSM, MICRONS, My PGMEE Notes, AIIMS MedEasy, and PRIMEs. With your constant support and our consistent efforts, I am sure that we will together witness an exponential acceptance of all CBS Exam Books in coming future as well.
- The presence of CBS Exam Books has broadened through our various social media platforms. We have received great appreciation for our regular Facebook activities such as online test series, giveaways, scientific content for knowledge enhancement, authors' live sessions, and various contests, like Bid 2 Win, Fastest Finger First, Book Fair and Facebook Community Awards. Join us on all these platforms to avail and enjoy our exciting offers and benefits.

A book is incomplete if it does not have the right readers. We value you and your feedback. Please share your feedback and suggestions directly with me at **bhupesharora@cbspd.com.** We promise to deliver in our books, what you desire to see.

I would like to sum up with these eternal lines of Robert Frost:

Woods are lovely dark and deep,
But I have promises to keep.
And miles to go before I sleep,
And miles to go before I sleep!
Wishing you success in all your endeavors!

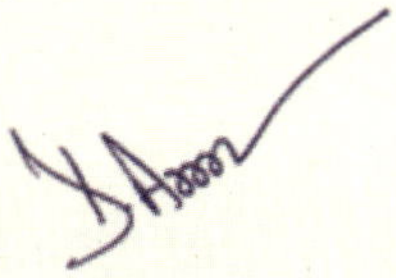

Bhupesh Arora
Vice President – Publishing & Marketing
(PGMEE and Nursing Division)
Email: bhupesharora@cbspd.com
Mobile: (+91) 9555590180

Foreword

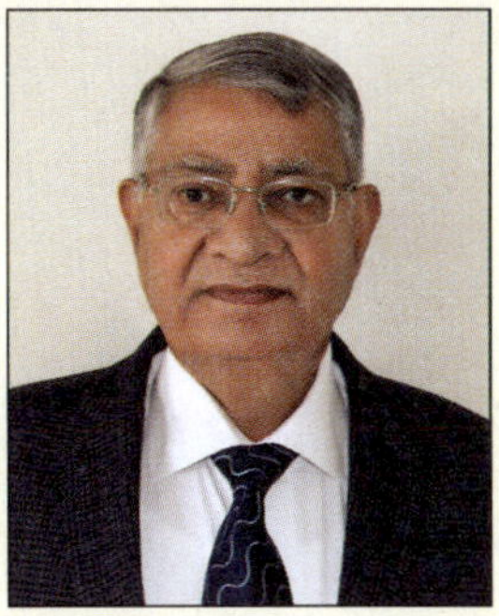

It is indeed a great opportunity for me to write the foreword of the book—"Conceptual Review of PSM" written by Dr Mukhmohit Singh and edited by Dr Shveta Saini for the benefit of the PG aspirants.

I have known the authors for last 8 years and have found them an asset to the entire fraternity of Medical Science, particularly to the public health services, in the field of academics, scientific research and teaching. Their passion to work, innovate and envision to provide the best is a unique feature, reflecting in the manuscript of this book.

This book will provide a very good platform for UG students and PG aspirants for taking up the daunting task of solving MCQs pertaining to Preventive & Social Medicine/Community Medicine.

Dr Ashok K Bhardwaj
Professor & Head
Department of Community Medicine
Dr Radhakrishnan Government Medical College
Hamirpur, Himachal Pradesh

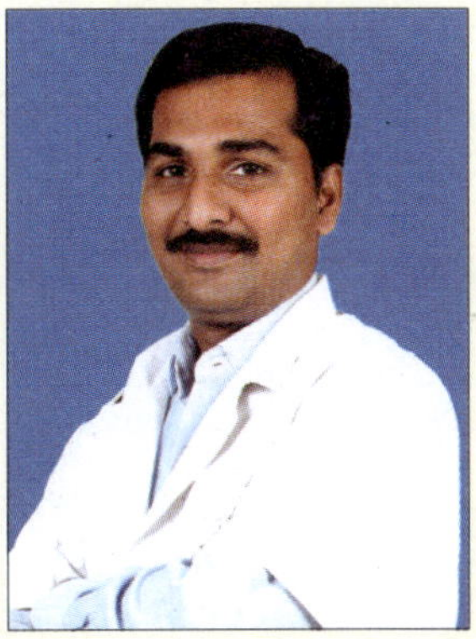

It gives me immense pleasure that Dr Mukhmohit Singh and Dr Shveta Saini, have endeavored to bring out a book on "Conceptual Review of PSM". At the outset, I would like to compliment them for the same.

Public health and community medicine is an ever changing concept and involves tremendous efforts in understanding the basics, which have been reflected in this book. The deepness on concepts and clarity is essential for any student of medicine, which shall carry a long way in the practice and art of preventing ailments and healing humans.

The updates, recent guidelines, protocols and policies by the international and national health care organizations are well organized in the book to give the reader "most of the information in one book".

I acknowledge and appreciate the perseverance and dedication shown by both the experts led by Dr Mukhmohit Singh and congratulate them for commendable and superlative effort.

I recommend and forward this book to my juniors and colleagues aspiring for higher studies entrance or licensing examinations.

Professor Dr Murali Mohan Reddy
MD, Community Medicine (PGI, Chandigarh)
MSc, Epidemiology (University of London)
Founder and CEO, Evidencian Research Associates, Bangalore

Preface

Where the mind is without fear and head is held high,
Where the knowledge is free and not broken into fragments,
Where the mind is led forward by thee into ever widening thought and action...

Adopted from poem by Sri Rabindranath Tagore

Dear students,

It is a matter of pride and pleasure to present the updated 3rd edition of the book, "Conceptual Review of Preventive and Social Medicine".

For us, medicine is about science and science is about exploration, understanding, concepts and innovation, and we are a firm believer that medicine and science cannot be crammed, but always understood.

The basic foundation of this book lies in the fact that concepts should be presented in the simplest manner not just for learning but for retention in long-term memory and as the name goes – Conceptual understanding.

A new approach to the book is to provide the reader with a summary of complete Community Medicine in the form of annexures and recent updates. For students who have already covered the theory part of the subject and wish to revise and update the latest changes and innovations, can take maximum benefit from the updated section of PSM Annexures in the book. A new topic of *Tribal Health in India* is also included in the annexures list in the book.

The book is divided into 3 Sections:

Section A: Medical Research

Section B: Preventive Medicine

Section C: Public Health

Each section has been divided into chapters. Each chapter is presented with a chapter outline, which will help the students revise and mark the topics which require in-depth understanding from their perspective.

Community Medicine has many non-conventional topics of medical sciences as Epidemiology, Biostatistics and Research Methodologies which are sometimes challenging for us as well as the students. So, we have tried to provide ample illustrations, diagrams and flow charts to create a sustained interest in the topic and understand the basics of statistical analysis, null hypothesis, probability values and other advance statistical terms.

As readers, we value your feedback. We also know how important this publication is for many students across country and abroad. Although, all the efforts have been put in for providing an error free manuscript and maintaining the quality of content, some lapses can't be denied.

For any query, difference of opinion or suggestions, please feel free to write to me at dr_mukhmohit5@hotmail.com or contact me on Facebook@mukhmohitdr

All contributions will be duly acknowledged.

Subscribe to our Student Support for Recent advances and updates in PSM

YouTube channel – "Dr.Mukhmohit Singh's Community Medicine Simplified"

Telegram: https://t.me/mukhmohit01

Facebook@mukhmohitdr

A brand-new website for updating the content, revision of frequently asked topics and recent advances in community medicine is available at

www.mukhmohit.com and **www.psmsimplified.com**

Sincerely,

Mukhmohit Singh
Shveta Saini

Acknowledgements

Our humble thanks to our students, teachers and mentors.

We would like to thank our parents to show us the righteous path and support us in all our endeavours. We would also like to express our immense gratitude to our children for providing all possible support in preparation of this manuscript. The time used for writing this book shall be reflected in the time saved by students while preparing for exams using this book.

The motivation for understanding the field concepts in field work, providing elementary health care and understanding public health to core was nurtured by our respected teachers. We would like to express our thanks to our respected mentors (Prof.) Dr Jagjeet Singh, (Prof.) Dr Ashok Bhardwaj, (Prof.) Dr Anshu Mittal, (Prof.) Dr Rambha Pathak and (Prof.) Dr Anu Bhardwaj for teaching us the fundamentals of Community Medicine.

We are immensely thankful to Dr G Dewan, Director Health Services, UT Chandigarh, for his support and continuous motivation for writing of the manuscript.

We shall fail in duty if we forget to acknowledge of the relentless efforts of Mr Harpreet Singh and Mr Rakinder Singh for providing the much appreciated student helpline centers and management of all data relating to ever changing guidelines, protocols and recent advances. They have been the phenomenal pillars of the team "PSM-Simplified".

We are extending our special thanks to **Mr Satish Kumar Jain** (*Chairman*) and **Mr Varun Jain** (*Managing Director*), M/s CBS Publishers and Distributors Pvt Ltd for their wholehearted support in publication of this book. I have no words to describe the role, efforts, inputs and initiatives undertaken by **Mr Bhupesh Arora** (*Vice President - Publishing & Marketing, PGMEE and Nursing Division*) for helping and motivating us.

We sincerely thank the entire CBS team for bringing out the book with utmost care and attractive presentation. We would like to thank Dr Mrinalini Bakshi (Editorial Head & Content Strategist) for her editorial support and Ms Nitasha Arora (Production Head & Content Strategist), Dr Anju Dhir (Project Manager & Senior Scientific Coordinator), Mr Shivendu Bhushan Pandey (Senior Editor), Mr Ashutosh Pathak (Senior Proof Reader) and all the production team members Mr Chaman Lal, Mr Prakash Gaur, Mr Phool Kumar, Mr Bunty Kashyap, Ms Tahira Parveen, Ms Manorama Gupta, Ms Babita Verma, Mr Chander Mani, Mr Raju Sharma, Mr Manoj Chaudhary, Mr Vikram Chaudhary, Mr Manoj Malakar, Mr Arun Kumar and Mr Rahul Negi for devoting laborious hours in designing and typesetting of the book.

Contents

AIIMS New Pattern 2019 Model Questions

Annexures

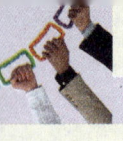

SECTION A: MEDICAL RESEARCH

SECTION B: PREVENTIVE MEDICINE

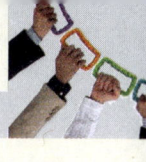

SECTION C: PUBLIC HEALTH

Contents

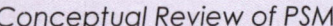

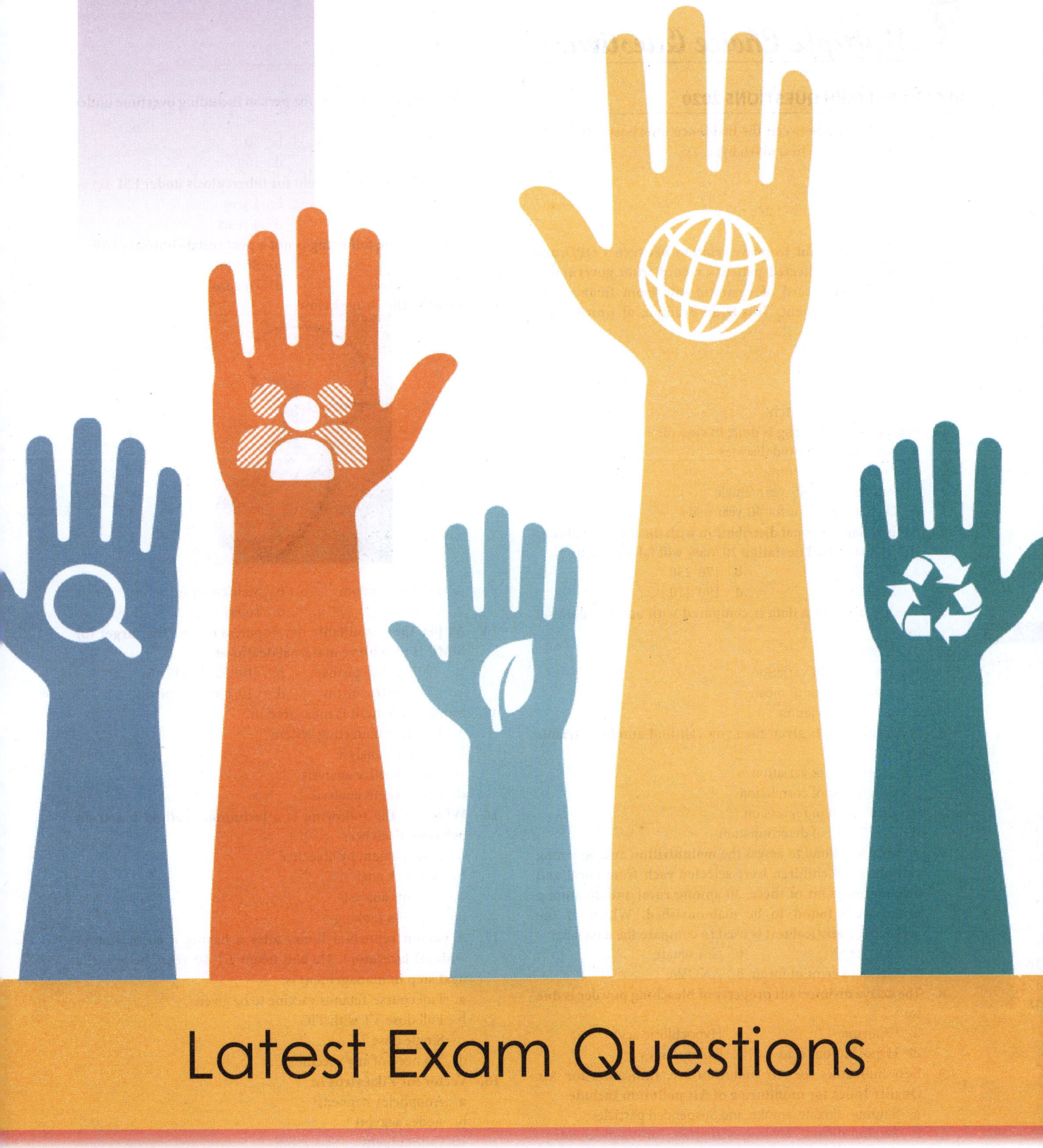

Latest Exam Questions

- Recent Pattern Questions 2020
- AIIMS November 2019
- JIPMER May 2019
- PGI May 2019

Multiple Choice Questions

RECENT PATTERN QUESTIONS 2020

1. **The difference between the incidence in exposed and non-exposed group is best given by:**
   a. Relative risk
   b. Attributable risk
   c. Population attributable risk
   d. Odds ratio
2. **A researcher want to prove relation between COPD and smoking. He collected patient's record from government hospital and record of cigarette sale from finance and taxation department. This is an example of which study design:**
   a. Cross sectional
   b. Posological study
   c. Ecological study
   d. Operations research
3. **Prospective screening is done in case of:**
   a. Neonate for thyroid diseases
   b. Immigrant screening
   c. Pap smear for 45-year female
   d. Diabetes mellitus for 40-year male
4. **A study had a normal distribution with the median value as 200 and standard deviation 20. 68% will fall between:**
   a. 160-240 b. 170-230
   c. 180-220 d. 190-210
5. **The variation in a data is compared with another data set by:**
   a. Variance
   b. Coefficient of variation
   c. Standard error of mean
   d. Standard deviation
6. **If one variable is given then you can find another variable by:**
   a. Coefficient of variation
   b. Coefficient of correlation
   c. Coefficient of regression
   d. Coefficient of determination
7. **A study was done to assess the malnutrition among young children. 100 children were selected each from rural and urban areas. Out of these, 30 among rural and 20 among urban were found to be malnourished. Which of the following statistical test is used to compare the data sets?**
   a. Paired t test b. Chi square
   c. Standard error of mean d. ANOVA
8. **The active disinfectant property of bleaching powder is due to:**
   a. Chlorine b. Hypochloric acid
   c. Hypochlorous acid d. Chloramines
9. **Best indicators for Air pollution are: Indicators for Air Quality Index for monitoring of Air pollution Include:**
   a. Sulphur dioxide, smoke, and Suspended particles
   b. Sulphur dioxide, Hydrogen sulphide, carbon monoxide
   c. Carbon dioxide, hydrogen sulphide, lead
   d. Sulphur dioxide, Lead and particulate matter
10. **Maximum work hours for person including overtime under the Factories Act:**
    a. 48 b. 50
    c. 60 d. 100
11. **Extended sickness benefit for tuberculosis under ESI Act is:**
    a. 91 days b. 1 year
    c. 2 years d. 4 years
12. **Which of the following is not a post coital contraceptive:**
    a. Cut 200 b. Ru 486
    c. Estrogens d. Danazol
13. **Identify the image below:**

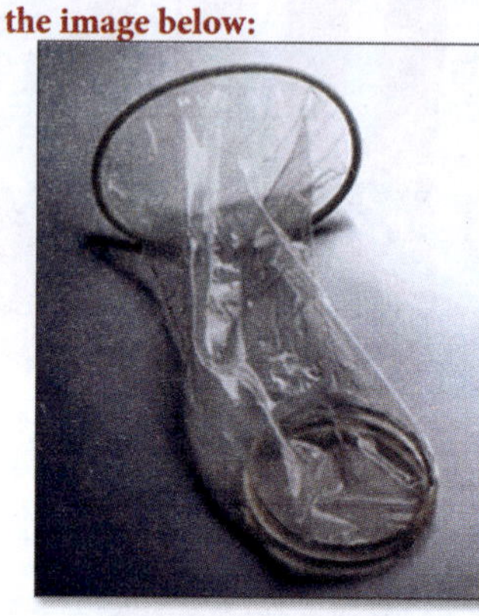

    a. Female condom b. Male condom
    c. Chaaya d. Today
14. **As per the sustainable development goals. The target for MMR is to achieve maternal deaths of:**
    a. <70/Lac live births b. <100/lac live births
    c. <7/1000 live births d. <10/1000 live births
15. **Monetary benefit is measured in:**
    a. Program budgeting system
    b. Network analysis
    c. Cost effective analysis
    d. Cost benefit analysis
16. **Which of the following is a technique/method based on behaviour sciences**
    a. Management by objective
    b. Network analysis
    c. Systems analysis
    d. Decision making
17. **A person reports 4 hours after a having a clean wound without laceration. He had taken TT 10 years before. the next step in management is:**
    a. Full course Tetanus vaccine to be given
    b. Full dose TT with TIG
    c. Single dose TT
    d. No need of any vaccine
18. **Vector for Zika virus is:**
    a. Anopheles stephensi
    b. Aedes aegypti
    c. Culex pipens
    d. Phelebotomus papatasi

Ans.

1. b
2. c
3. b
4. c
5. b
6. c
7. b
8. c
9. a
10. c
11. c
12. d
13. a
14. a
15. d
16. a
17. c
18. b

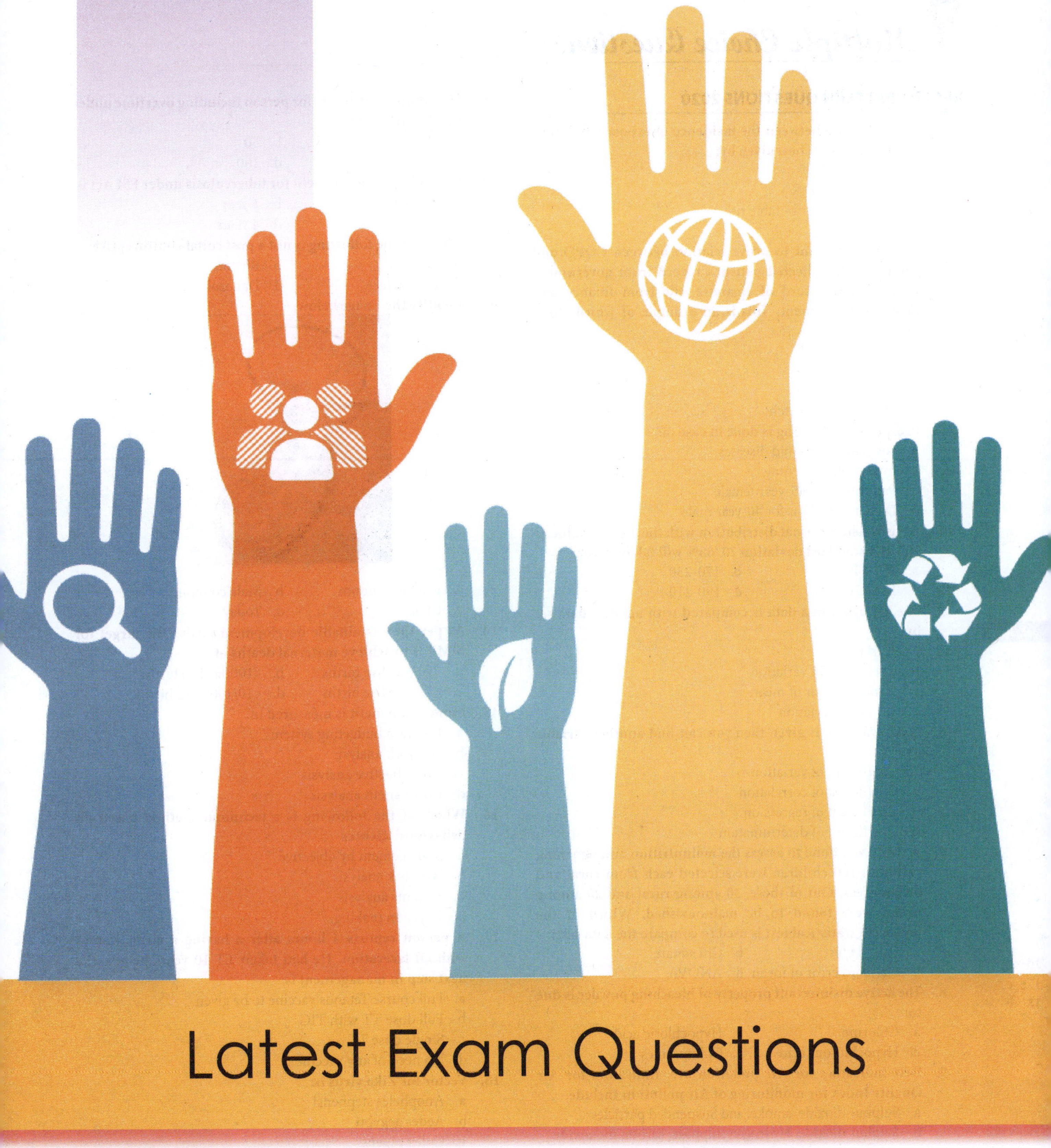

Latest Exam Questions

- Recent Pattern Questions 2020
- AIIMS November 2019
- JIPMER May 2019
- PGI May 2019

Multiple Choice Questions

RECENT PATTERN QUESTIONS 2020

1. The difference between the incidence in exposed and non-exposed group is best given by:
a. Relative risk
b. Attributable risk
c. Population attributable risk
d. Odds ratio

2. A researcher want to prove relation between COPD and smoking. He collected patient's record from government hospital and record of cigarette sale from finance and taxation department. This is an example of which study design:
a. Cross sectional
b. Posological study
c. Ecological study
d. Operations research

3. Prospective screening is done in case of:
a. Neonate for thyroid diseases
b. Immigrant screening
c. Pap smear for 45-year female
d. Diabetes mellitus for 40-year male

4. A study had a normal distribution with the median value as 200 and standard deviation 20. 68% will fall between:
a. 160-240 b. 170-230
c. 180-220 d. 190-210

5. The variation in a data is compared with another data set by:
a. Variance
b. Coefficient of variation
c. Standard error of mean
d. Standard deviation

6. If one variable is given then you can find another variable by:
a. Coefficient of variation
b. Coefficient of correlation
c. Coefficient of regression
d. Coefficient of determination

7. A study was done to assess the malnutrition among young children. 100 children were selected each from rural and urban areas. Out of these, 30 among rural and 20 among urban were found to be malnourished. Which of the following statistical test is used to compare the data sets?
a. Paired t test b. Chi square
c. Standard error of mean d. ANOVA

8. The active disinfectant property of bleaching powder is due to:
a. Chlorine b. Hypochloric acid
c. Hypochlorous acid d. Chloramines

9. Best indicators for Air pollution are: Indicators for Air Quality Index for monitoring of Air pollution Include:
a. Sulphur dioxide, smoke, and Suspended particles
b. Sulphur dioxide, Hydrogen sulphide, carbon monoxide
c. Carbon dioxide, hydrogen sulphide, lead
d. Sulphur dioxide, Lead and particulate matter

10. Maximum work hours for person including overtime under the Factories Act:
a. 48 b. 50
c. 60 d. 100

11. Extended sickness benefit for tuberculosis under ESI Act is:
a. 91 days b. 1 year
c. 2 years d. 4 years

12. Which of the following is not a post coital contraceptive:
a. Cut 200 b. Ru 486
c. Estrogens d. Danazol

13. Identify the image below:

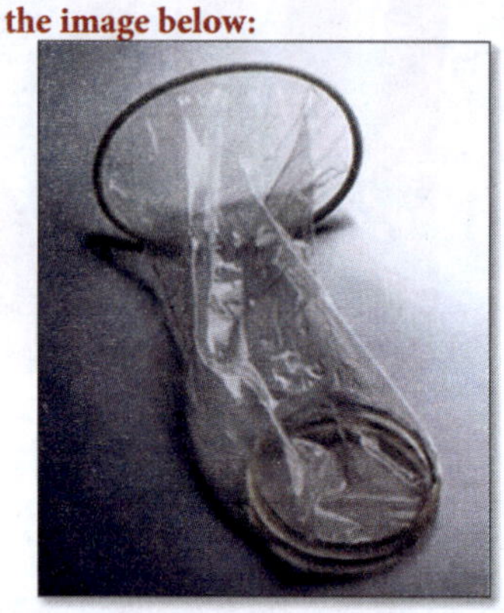

a. Female condom b. Male condom
c. Chaaya d. Today

14. As per the sustainable development goals. The target for MMR is to achieve maternal deaths of:
a. <70/Lac live births b. <100/lac live births
c. <7/1000 live births d. <10/1000 live births

15. Monetary benefit is measured in:
a. Program budgeting system
b. Network analysis
c. Cost effective analysis
d. Cost benefit analysis

16. Which of the following is a technique/method based on behaviour sciences
a. Management by objective
b. Network analysis
c. Systems analysis
d. Decision making

17. A person reports 4 hours after a having a clean wound without laceration. He had taken TT 10 years before. the next step in management is:
a. Full course Tetanus vaccine to be given
b. Full dose TT with TIG
c. Single dose TT
d. No need of any vaccine

18. Vector for Zika virus is:
a. Anopheles stephensi
b. Aedes aegypti
c. Culex pipens
d. Phelebotomus papatasi

Ans.
1. b
2. c
3. b
4. c
5. b
6. c
7. b
8. c
9. a
10. c
11. c
12. d
13. a
14. a
15. d
16. a
17. c
18. b

19. An image with diphtheria patient is shown. The patient reports to have another 3 year old sibling at home, who is fully immunized as per the immunization schedule. What is the best measure to prevent diphtheria in the sibling of the diphtheria case child.

a. Give diphtheria toxoid booster
b. Give full course of DPT vaccine
c. Give prophylactic erythromycin
d. Nothing is required to be done

20. Recent Influenza Pandemic was due to:

a. H1N1
b. H5N1
c. H7N7
d. H3N2

21. All of the following are correct for JE EXCEPT:

a. Humans are reservoirs
b. Main vector is Culex tritaeniorhynchus
c. Birds are maintenance hosts
d. It has seasonal transmission

22. A 3-year-old child presents to PHC with fever. He had chest indrawing and Respiratory rate of 38 per minute. The next step in management is:

a. Give antipyretics only
b. Not an emergency, give oral antibiotics and follow up
c. Refer urgently to a tertiary care centre
d. Give antibiotics and refer to a tertiary care centre

23. What is MONICA project:

a. Multinational MONItoring of trends and determinants in CArdiovascular disease
b. MOther, Newborn, Child, Adolescent Project
c. Monitoring of Non Invasive Cardiac Accident
d. Management of Novel CoronA virus infections

24. Mission Indradhanush is for:

a. Non-communicable diseases
b. Universal immunization
c. Family planning
d. Safe water and sanitation

25. Blood bags are discarded in:

a. Yellow category
b. Red category
c. Blue category
d. Blue category

26. Vaccine to be given after disaster

a. Mass vaccination against typhoid
b. Mass vaccination against cholera
c. Vaccination against Tetanus, typhoid and cholera to health workers
d. Mass vaccination against tetanus

27. Which among these is a type A bioterrorism agent:

a. Nipah virus
b. Coxiella brunetti
c. Clostridium perfringes
d. B anthracis

28. Liquid chemical waste is discarded in:

a. Yellow category
b. Red category
c. Blue category
d. Black category

AIIMS NOVEMBER 2019

29. A study is to be designed to understand the correct technique for injection by a health care professional. The best way to assess will be:

a. In depth interview with the patient
b. Using CCTV
c. In depth interview with the health care professional
d. Questionnaire based with checklist

30. Which of the following is not a primary prevention?

a. Giving pentavalent vaccine to children
b. Health education about hand washing
c. Addition of iron to wheat flour
d. Ribavirin to close contact of meningitis patient

31. Hand washing steps (Arrange sequentially):

A. Back of hand
B. Back of fingers
C. Fingernails
D. Palm to palm

The options are:

a. A → B → D → C
b. B → D → A → C
c. A → B → C → D
d. D → A → B → C

32. Assertion: Malathion used in dengue control as anti-adult in ULV fogging
Reasoning: Malathion has residual effect as an insecticide

a. Both Assertion and Reasons are independently true/correct statements and the Reason is the correct explanation for the Assertion
b. Both Assertion and Reasons are independently true/correct statements, but the Reason is not the correct explanation for the Assertion
c. Assertion is independently a true/correct statement, but the Reasons is independently a false/incorrect statement
d. Assertion is independently a false/incorrect statement, but the Reasons is independently a true/correct statement
e. Both Assertion and Reasons are independently false/incorrect statements

33. Multiple options correct:
Causes of Death may be assessed by

a. Medical death certificate
b. Census
c. Death reporting
d. SRS
1. If a, b, c are correct
2. If a and c are correct
3. If b and d are correct
4. If all four (a, b, c, & d) are correct

34. Assertion: Lead poisoning produces eosinophilia
Reason: Lead inhibits ALA dehydratase in heme synthesis

a. Both Assertion and Reasons are independently true/correct statements and the Reason is the correct explanation for the Assertion
b. Both Assertion and Reasons are independently true/correct statements, but the Reason is not the correct explanation for the Assertion
c. Assertion is independently a true/correct statement, but the Reasons is independently a false/incorrect statement
d. Assertion is independently a false/incorrect statement, but the Reasons is independently a true/correct statement
e. Both Assertion and Reasons are independently false/incorrect statements

Ans.

19. c
20. a
21. a
22. b
23. a
24. b
25. a
26. c
27. d
28. a
29. d
30. b
31. d
32. a
33. 2
34. d

35. Assertion: Typhoid vaccine is used in endemic areas in disaster management
Reasoning: Vaccine is cost-effective way to deal with disease prevention in endemic area
a. Both Assertion and Reasons are independently true/correct statements and the Reason is the correct explanation for the Assertion
b. Both Assertion and Reasons are independently true/correct statements, but the Reason is not the correct explanation for the Assertion
c. Assertion is independently a true/correct statement, but the Reasons is independently a false/incorrect statement
d. Assertion is independently a false/incorrect statement, but the Reasons is independently a true/correct statement
e. Both Assertion and Reasons are independently false/incorrect statements

36. Which of the following is not true about influenza?
a. Virus shedding is present before symptoms begins
b. Secondary attack rate is 5-15%
c. Aquatic birds act as reservoir
d. 1-5 years is the highest risk group

37. A 5-year-old boy presents to emergency with bleeding wound from bite of his pet dog which was fully vaccinated. He previously had complete anti rabies immunization on December 2018. The next course of management is:
a. No ARV required
b. Single site 2 doses - days 0 and 3
c. Single site 4 doses – 0,3,7,28 days
d. RIG and 4 dose regime

38. Dengue hemorrhagic fever discharge criteria is:
a. After 24 hours fever controlled on paracetamol
b. After return of appetite
c. Urine output 200ml/day
d. 24 hrs after control of shock

39. Indicator for vector burden on humans in malaria is:
a. Man biting rate
b. Inoculation rate
c. slide positivity rate
d. Human blood index

40. Intensified malaria control under the national framework for malaria elimination is defined as:
a. States with API ≥ 1
b. Zero incidence of malaria
c. No longer a health problem
d. 3 consecutive years no local transmission in the state

41. Which of the following is true regarding new management protocol for Paucibacillary leprosy?
a. 2 drug combination for 6 months
b. 3 drug combination for 6 months
c. 2 drug combination for 12 months
d. 3 drug combination for 12 months

42. Mass drug administration done for all except:
a. Filariasis
b. Worm infestation
c. Vit A
d. Scabies

43. Pneumococcal vaccine will be most beneficial for which of the following groups:
a. Cystic fibrosis patient
b. Sickle cell anemia
c. Recurrent otitis and sinusitis
d. Child less than 2 years

44. What is the Numerator in perinatal mortality rate?
a. Still birth more than 500 grams
b. Still births after 28 weeks
c. Post neonatal death <2500 grams
d. Neonatal deaths up till 28 days

45. Match the following with color coded bins:

Waste material	Color coded bins
1. Expired medicine	a. Red
2. Catheter	b. Yellow
3. Discarded lab report form	c. Blue
4. Antibiotic bottle	d. Green
e. Black	

JIPMER MAY 2019

46. In a prospective study, 1200 patients were randomly selected to study the effect of a new drug. The drug will be given for 5 years and its association with cataract will be studied. What type of study is this?
a. Case control study
b. Cohort study
c. Randomized clinical trial
d. Cross sectional study

47. Which of the following option is true about ROC curve:
a. It is a method of evaluating the quality or performance of screening tests
b. It is plotted as test sensitivity as x coordinate versus its 1 – false positive rate as the y coordinate
c. A perfect test has an area under the ROC curve of 1
d. A decrease in sensitivity results in decrease in specificity

48. A total of 130 patients were screened for disc prolapse by CT scan and confirmation of the disease was made by discectomy operation. Out of 56 patients who screened positive in CT scan, 46 were confirmed for disease in operation and the rest 74 patients who were screened negative in CT scan, only 40 patients were confirmed negative for the disease in operation. Calculate the positive and negative likelihood ratio.
a. 2.875 and 0.531
b. 6.07 and 1.12
c. 1.12 and 6.07
d. 0.531 and 2.875

49. What happens to sample size when range of allowable error is doubled?
a. Reduced to 1/4
b. Reduced to 1/2
c. Sample size does not depend on acceptable error
d. Cannot to be calculated

50. Rejection of Null hypothesis which was true in reality will commit which type of error?
a. Type II error
b. Type I error
c. Both
d. None

51. Human developmental index includes all except:
a. Adult literacy
b. Per capita income
c. Life expectancy
d. Infant mortality rate

52. Median incubation period means:
a. Time for 50% cases to occur
b. Time between primary case and secondary case
c. Time between onset of infection and period of maximum infectivity
d. Median of several incubation period

Ans.
35. d
36. d
37. b
38. b
39. d
40. a
41. b
42. c
43. b
44. b
45. 1(b), 2(a), 3(e), 4(c)
46. c
47. c
48. a
49. a
50. b
51. d
52. a

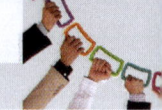

53. Allowed amount of chlorine in drinking water:
a. 2 ppm
b. 0.5 ppm
c. 1.5 ppm
d. 4 ppm

54. What is saturation index?
a. It is used to assess the quality of air by measuring concentration of pollutants
b. It is used to assess the quality of water by estimating hardness, total dissolved solids, alkalinity and PH
c. It is used to assess the quality of soil that whether it is good for growing crops
d. It is used to assess the quality of milk by estimating the bacterial count in it

55. To prevent recurrent diarrhoeal attacks, which of the following is effective public health measure:
a. Hand scrub with alcohol-based antiseptics is superior to hand washing with soap and water
b. Hand washing should be done only with clean water
c. Hand washing with hot water is superior than cold water
d. Antiseptic detergents are better than alcohol-based hand rubs

PGI MAY 2019

56. Confounding can be minimized or corrected by:
a. Matching
b. Randomization
c. Stratification
d. Multivariate regression analysis
e. Blinding

57. Which of the following statement(s) is/are true about Operational research:
a. Help in increasing efficiency of a program
b. Useful for decision-making
c. Use mathematical methods
d. Non-scientific approach
e. Optimizes resource allocation

58. Global reference list for 100 core health indicators include(s):
a. Still birth rate
b. Neglected tropical diseases
c. Tribal health
d. Asthma and COPD
e. Substance abuse

59. Which of the following is/are included in seven priority areas of National Health Policy (2017):
a. Emphasis on make in India initiative for invasive cardiac instruments
b. Yatri Suraksha- preventing deaths due to rail and road traffic accidents
c. Nirbhaya Nari-action against gender violence
d. Reduced stress and improved safety in the work place
e. Better screening of genetic diseases

60. In the Integrated Disease Surveillance Programmed (IDSP), which of the following condition is/are included under "Fever without localized signs":
a. Measles
b. Japanese Encephalitis
c. Typhoid
d. Hepatitis
e. Leptospirosis

61. True statement(s) about Elephantiasis:
a. Most commonly occurs due to lymphatic filariasis
b. Equally common in upper and lower limb
c. Graded compression stockings are used to control limb swelling
d. Chyluria is the most common presenting feature
e. Commonly seen in workers in volcanic areas, working with bare foot

62. True statement(s) regarding lymphatic filariasis elimination programme:
a. National Filaria Control Programme was started in 1962
b. Aim for elimination by 2020
c. Objectives included control through anti-larval measures
d. Source reduction was the part of control strategy
e. Home-based management of lymphedema cases included for elimination strategy

63. Vaccine(s) which should not administer in children with severe egg allergy:
a. Influenza vaccine
b. Rabies vaccine
c. Measles vaccine
d. Yellow fever vaccine
e. Rubella

64. Live vaccines is/are contraindicated in which of the following case(s)
a. Pregnancy in third trimester
b. Tuberculosis
c. Allergy to the vaccine adjuvant
d. Active acute infection
e. Immunodeficiency

Ans.
53. b
54. b
55. a
56. a, b, c, d
57. a, b, c, e
58. a, b, e
59. b, c, d
60. a, b, c
61. a, c, e
62. b, c, d, e
63. a, d
64. a, c, e

Answers with Explanations

RECENT PATTERN QUESTIONS 2020

1. Ans. (b) Attributable risk

Ref: K. Park 25th edition. Pg. 86

For more detail, refer to theory section: Interpretation of Observational Studies, Chapter – Epidemiology, (page 8)

The relative risk is Risk ratio = $\frac{\textit{Incidence exposed}}{\textit{Incidence among nonexposed}}$

Risk difference (attributable risk) = *Incidence – exposed Incidence nonexposed*

Attributable risk Proportion = $\frac{\textit{Incidence exposed – Incidence nonexposed}}{\textit{Incidence exposed}}$

2. Ans. (c) Ecological study design

Ref: K. Park 25th edition. Pg. 70

For more detail, refer to theory section: Ecological Studies, Chapter – Epidemiology, (page 8)

- Use population as unit of analysis
- Data maybe used from different third party sources
- Use database from entire population to compare frequency of a particular disease/attribute

3. Ans. (b) Immigrant Screening

Ref: K. Park 25th ed. p 149

For more detail, refer to theory section: Screening, Chapter - Principles of Screening for Disease, (page 56)

Prospective screening (or predictive/presumptive) screening is done for primary prevention of disease events and to stop spread of infections to population. Example for this could be testing of food handlers for contagious diseases, immigrant screening, HIV screening for blood donations, screening of streptococcal infections to prevent rheumatic fever.

Prescriptive screening is 'case detection'.

4. Ans. (c) 180-220

For more detail, refer to theory section: Inferential stats, Chapter - Biostatistics, (page 94)

As the median value is 200 and the standard deviation is 20, the normal distribution is:

68% of the population will have values between — median +/– 1 SD = 220 +/– 20 = 180–220

95% of the population will have values between — median +/– 2 SD = 220 +/– 40 = 160–240

68% of the population will have values between — median +/– 3 SD = 220 +/– 60 = 140–260

Note: In the MCQ, as the data shows a normal distribution, the median will be equal to mean and the mode.

5. Ans. (b) Coefficient of variation

Ref: Fundamentals of Biostatistics, 8th ed. p. 22

For more detail, refer to theory section: Measures of Dispersion, Chapter - Biostatistics, (page 90)

Coefficient of Variation (CV):

- It is the ratio between the standard deviation and the mean
- Formula: Coefficient of variation (CV) = SD/mean × 100
- Interpretation: The higher the coefficient of variation, the greater is the level of dispersion around the mean and conversely — the lower the coefficient of variation, the more precise is the data
- Use: It is frequently used to compare and evaluate relative risks.

Variance	Is the square of SD. It tells about the standard deviation
Coefficient of variation	It may help by comparing the variations in the data set
Standard error of mean	It is to compare the means of the data sets, which have different sample size, central tendency and standard deviations
Standard deviation	It is the deviation of values from the mean

6. Ans. (c) Coefficient of regression

Ref: K. Park 25th ed. p 916

For more detail, refer to theory section: Regression, Chapter - Biostatistics, (page 103)

Regression Analysis

- Regression analysis is a mathematical model to describe the effect of ≥1 independent variable on a dependent variable
- Linear regression describes effect of one independent variable on a dependent variable.
- Multiple linear regression describes effect of two or more independent variable on a dependent variable.
- Nonlinear regression involves more complex mathematical forms, including logarithmic functions.
- Logistic regression describes effect of multiple independent (Qualitative, Quantitative or Mixed) variable on dichotomous qualitative variable.
- Regression coefficient is average change in dependent variable for each unit of independent variable.

7. Ans. (b) Chi square test

For more detail, refer to theory section: Tests of significance, chapter - Biostatistics, (page 98)

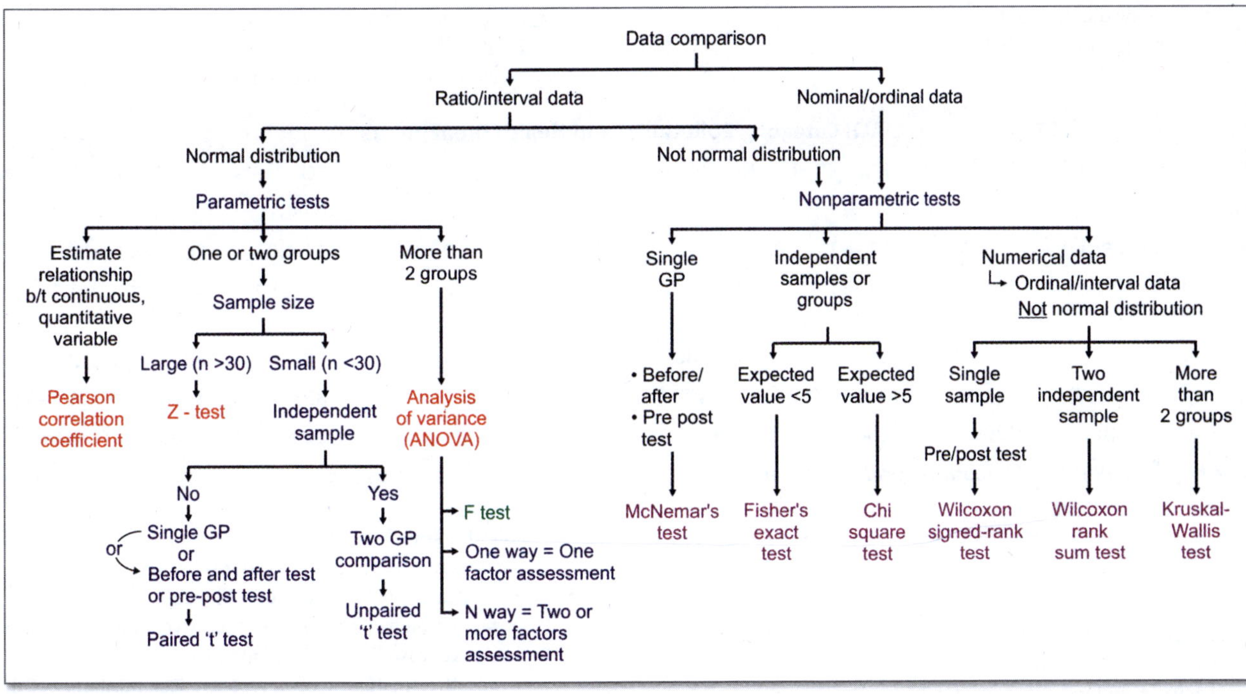

Table 1: Parametric and nonparametric test for qualitative data

Testing groups – situation	Parametric test	Nonparametric test
Testing association between two qualitative variables		Chi square test
Comparison of two **independent groups**	t-test for independent samples	Wilcoxon rank sum test
Comparison of data between **paired observations** (usually single group – before and after)	t-test for paired observation	Wilcoxon rank sign test
Comparison of several groups **(three or more groups)**	ANOVA	Kruskal-Wallis test
Assessment of relationship between two variables	Pearson correlation for linear relation	Spearman rank correlation

Table 2: Tests used in various number of groups

Between one group	Paired t-test	McNemar's test
Between two groups	Unpaired t-test	Chi square test
Between 3 or more groups	ANOVA	Kruskal-Wallis test

8. Ans. (c) Hypochlorous acid

Ref: CRPSM 2nd ed. p 261

For more detail, refer to theory section: Disinfection of Water, Chapter – Environment and Related National Health Program, (page 272)

Disinfection of Water

Chlorination

- Kills bacteria, but does not kill spores/certain virus (e.g., polio, hepatitis) except in high doses.[Q]
- Disinfecting action of chlorine is mainly due to hypochlorous acid.[Q] (at a pH of around 7).
- Minimum recommended concentration of free chlorine is 0.5 mg/L for one hour.[Q]
- Free residual chlorine provides a margin of safety against subsequent microbial contamination during storage and distribution - *Residual Effect*

Must Remember

- Chlorine demand - Horrock's apparatus
- Chlorine estimation - chloroscope (orthotolidine test)

9. Ans. (a) Sulphur dioxide, Smoke, and Suspended particles

Ref: K. Park 25th ed. p 796

http://aqicn.org/map/india/
https://pib.gov.in/newsite/PrintRelease.aspx?relid=110654

Note: There could be different variants of this MCQ. If the MCQ mentions for Air Quality Index – which takes into account multiple indicators, it would include following:

- Particulate matter (less than 2.5 micrometre and 10 micrometre – $PM_{2.5}$ and PM_{10})
- Nitrogen dioxide (NO_2)

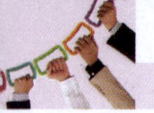

- Sulphur dioxide (SO_2)
- Carbon monoxide (CO)
- Ozone (O_3)
- Ammonia (NH_3)
- Lead (Pb)

Source: The World Air Quality Project, US

AQI Category, Pollutants, and Health Breakpoints								
AQI Category (Range)	PM_{10} 24–hr	$PM_{2.5}$ 24–hr	NO_2 24–hr	O_3 8–hr	CO 8–hr (mg/m^3)	SO_2 24–hr	NH_3 24–hr	Pb 24– hr
Good (0–50)	0–50	0–30	0–40	0–50	0–1.0	0–40	0–200	0–0.5
Satisfactory (51–100)	51–100	31–60	41–80	51–100	1.1–2.0	41–80	201–400	0.5–1.0
Moderately polluted (101–200)	101–250	61–90	81–180	101–168	2.1–10	81–380	401–800	1.1–2.0
Poor (201–300)	251–350	91–120	181–280	169–208	10–17	381–800	801–1200	2.1–3.0
Very poor (301–400)	351–430	121–250	281–400	209–748*	17–34	801–1600	1200–1800	3.1–3.5
Severe (401–500)	430+	250+	400+	748+*	34+	1600+	1800+	3.5+
One hourly monitoring (for mathematical calculations only)								

10. Ans. (c) 60 hours

Ref: K. Park 25th ed. p 876

For more detail, refer to theory section: Acts and Legislations, Chapter – Occupational Health, (page 358)

Factories Act permits work for 48 hours per week with 2 hours overtime every day.

Making it approximately 60 hours of maximum work as per the Factories Act of India

11. Ans. (c) 2 years

Ref: K. Park 25th ed. p 878

For more detail, refer to theory section: ESI Act, Chapter – Occupational Health, (page 359)

Remember:

Under ESI Act - sickness benefit – 91 days extended sickness benefit – 2 years

12. Ans. (d) Danazol

Ref: K. Park 25th ed. p 552

For more on formation refer to theory section: Methods of Contraception, chapter – Demography and Family Planning (page 399)

https://www.medicines.org.uk/emc/product/4380/smpc

Post coital contraception:

Recommended within 72 hours of unprotected intercourse.

- IUD – copper containing device within 5 days
- Hormonal Levonorgestrel 1.5 mg
  - Levonorgestrel 0.75 mg in two doses (first within 72 hours and another after 12 hours of first dose)
  - Two oral contraceptive pills containing 50 mcg of ethinyl estradiol with 72 hours and another after 12 hours of first dose
  - 4 tablets OCPs with 30–35 mcg Ethinyl estradiol within 72 hrs and another after 12 hours
  - Mifepristone 10 mg once within 72 hours

Danazol capsules are recommended for the treatment of:

- Endometriosis. To control pain, pelvic tenderness and other associated symptoms and to resolve or reduce the extent of endometriotic foci. Danazol capsules may be used as sole therapy, in preparation for or following surgery or in patients not responding to other treatments.
  - Dysfunctional uterine bleeding presenting as menorrhagia. To control excessive blood loss and to control associated dysmenorrhea.
  - For the treatment of severe cyclical mastalgia with or without nodularity (fibrocystic disease) unresponsive to counselling or simple analgesics. To reduce pain, tenderness and nodularity.
  - For the control of benign, multiple or recurrent breast cysts in conjunction with aspiration.
  - Severe symptomatic gynecomastia, both idiopathic as well as drug induced, to reduce the size of the breast and to control associated pain and tenderness.
  - Preoperative thinning of the endometrium prior to hysteroscopic endometrial ablation.

13. Ans. (a) Female condom

Ref: K. Park 25th ed. p 546

For more detail refer to theory section, Contraception, chapter – Demography and Family Planning (page 401)

14. Ans. (a) <70/Lac live births

Ref: K. Park 25th ed. p 522

Goal 5: Improve maternal health

Goal 6: Combat HIV/AIDS, malaria, and other diseases

Target 6A: Have halted by 2015 and begun to reverse the spread of HIV/AIDS

Target 6B: Achieve, by 2010, universal access to treatment for HIV/AIDS for all those who need it

Target 6C: Have halted by 2015 and begun to reverse the incidence of malaria and other major diseases

Goal 7: Ensure environmental sustainability

Target 7A: Integrate the principles of sustainable development into country policies and programs; reverse loss of environmental resources

Target 7B: Reduce biodiversity loss, achieving by 2010, a significant reduction in the rate of loss

Target 7C: Halved by 2015, the proportion of the population without sustainable access to safe drinking water and basic sanitation

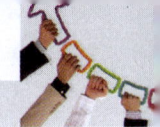

Goal 8: Develop a global partnership for development

Sustainable Development Goals (2015–2030)

Survive – thrive and transform health

Important points to remember:

- Reduce global maternal mortality to less than 70 per 100,000 live births
- Reduce newborn mortality to at least as low as 12 per 1,000 live births in every country
- Reduce under-five mortality to at least as low as 25 per 1,000 live births in every country
- End epidemics of HIV, tuberculosis, malaria, neglected tropical diseases and other communicable diseases
- Reduce by one third premature mortality from noncommunicable diseases and promote mental health and well-being.

15. Ans. (d) Cost Benefit Analysis

Ref: K. Park 25th ed. p 934

Management Techniques

Input Output Analysis

How much of each "Input" is needed to produce a unit amount of each "Output".

Cost-benefit Analysis: Economic benefits of any program are compared with cost of that program.

Drawback: Benefits in health field as a result of a particular program cannot always be expressed in monetary means.

Cost-effective Analysis: Here, benefit is expressed in terms of results achieved, e.g., number of lives saved and number of days free from disease.

16. Ans. (a) Management by objectives

Ref: K. Park 25th ed. p 934

The methods based on behaviour sciences include

- Organisational design
- Personal management
- Management by objectives
- Information systems
- Communication

The Quantitative methods include:

- Cost benefit analysis
- Cost effective analysis
- Input output analysis
- Network analysis as pert and CPM
- Planning programming budgeting systems
- Decision making

17. Ans. (c) Single dose TT

Ref: K. Park 25th ed. p 796

Prevention of Traumatic Tetanus

Patient category		Wound category	
		Clean, non penetrating wound	**Any other wound**
Category A	Has complete course of TT vaccine or booster dose within 5years	Nothing required	Nothing required
Category B	Has complete course of TT vaccine or booster dose more than 5 years ago but within 10 years	TT 1 dose	TT 1 dose
Category C	Has complete course of TT vaccine or booster dose more than 10 years ago	TT 1 dose	TT 1 dose + human TIG
Category D	Unknown status	TT complete course	TT complete course + Human TIG

18. Ans. (b) Aedes aegypti

Ref: K. Park 25th ed. p 301

Zika Virus

- **Causative agent:** Flavivirus (known to circulate in Africa, the Americas, Asia and the Pacific)
- First identified in Uganda in1947
- First large outbreak of disease was reported from island of Yap in 2007. Currently, 22 countries and territories in America have reported local transmission of Zika virus.
- **Reservoir:** Unknown
- **Incubation period:** Not clear, likely to be few days.
- **Vector:** Aedes mosquitoes
  - Also, vertical transmission is a possibility.
- **Symptoms:** Mild fever, maculopapular skin rash (exanthema), conjunctivitis, muscle and joint pain, malaise, headache. Symptoms last for about 2–7 days. Only one in four infected people develop symptoms of disease. Clustering of cases of microcephaly (Vertical transmission).

19. Ans. (c) Give prophylactic erythromycin

Ref: K. Park 25th ed. p 174

https://www.cdc.gov/diphtheria/downloads/close-contacts.pdf (updated 2014)

Note: Both D (as per PARK, 25ed) and C (as per WHO/CDC guidelines) may be the correct answer.

This is purely personal opinion that C > D, keeping in mind the public health issues and impact of preventive measures in our country.

As per the national immunization protocol, each child receives DPT booster at 16-24 months, and then at 5 years. Now as the child in the MCQ is 3 years old and is immunized till date, the child must have received the DPT booster injection just within last 2 years. Hence the child is protected and probably no added immune-prevention or vaccination is recommended, but chemoprophylaxis with antibiotics may be recommended in such cases.

Let us look at the CDC/WHO update and summary of guidelines (May 2014):

- Culture all close contacts, regardless of their immunization status.
- After culture, all contacts should receive antibiotic prophylaxis (Benzathine Penicillin G or oral erythromycin)
- Inadequately immunized contacts should receive DTaP/DT/Td/Tdap boosters.
- If fewer than three doses of diphtheria toxoid have been given, or vaccination history is unknown, an immediate dose of diphtheria toxoid should be given and the primary series completed according to the current schedule.
- If more than 5 years have elapsed since administration of diphtheria toxoid - containing vaccine, a booster dose should be given.
- If the most recent dose was given last 5 years, no booster is required

Summary of WHO/CDC Diphtheria Case Management Protocol

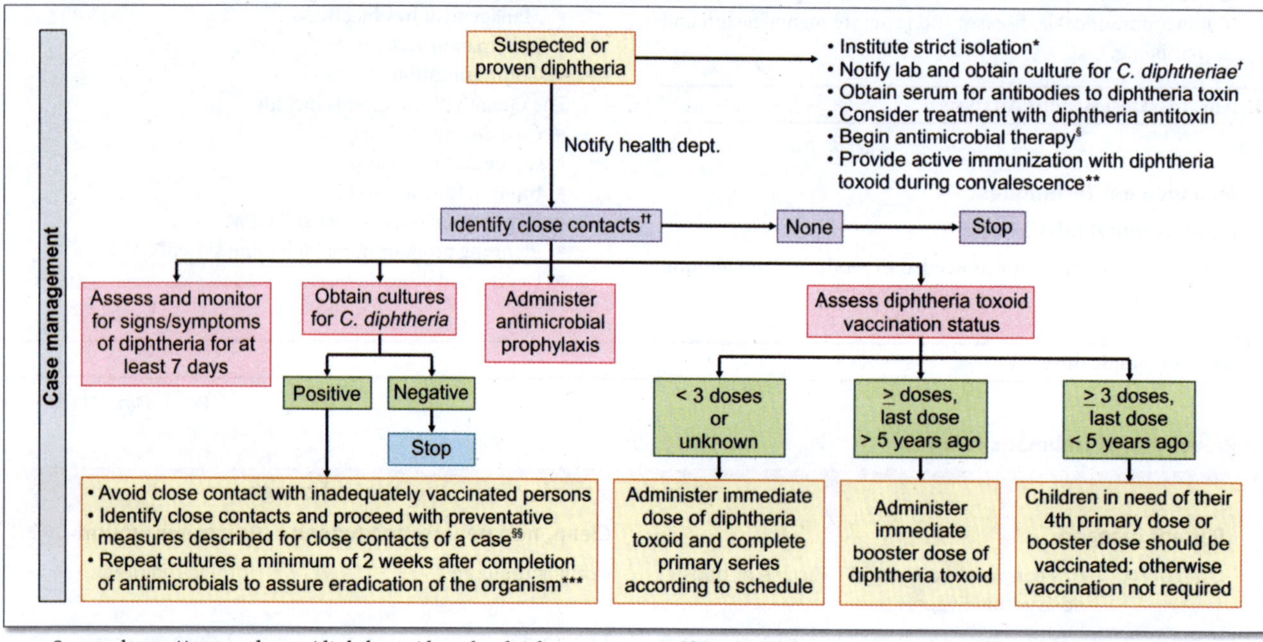

Source: https://www.cdc.gov/diphtheria/downloads/close-contacts.pdf (may 2014)

Ref: K Park, 25th ed., p. 174 – summary is as follows.

Primary immunization or booster dose received within 2 years	No further action is required
Primary immunization or booster dose received more than 2 years	Booster dose of diphtheria toxoid
All Non immunized close contacts	Prophylactic penicillin or erythromycin 1000-2000 IU of Diphtheria antitoxin Diphtheria immunization

Therefore, to give antibiotic or not depends on the guidelines followed. For exam set-up, it is recommended to follow the CDC/WHO guidelines as they are updated and may not be challenged until specific guidelines are issued by NHM or MoHFW

20. Ans. (a) H1N1

Ref: K. Park 25th ed. p 171

H1N1 – Swine flu – caused the major flu Pandemic (1918 and 2009)

H5N1 – Avian influenza. may cause sporadic outbreaks or epidemics. It is associated with high mortality.

21. Ans. (a) Humans are reservoirs

Ref: K. Park 25th ed. p 312

Humans are dead end host and the reservoirs are pig and birds. The disease is transmitted to man by the bite of infected mosquitoes. Man is an incidental "dead-end" host. Man to man transmission has not so far been recorded.

Pigs are considered as amplifying host, while some species of birds such as pond herons; cattle egrets and poultry/ducks maybe the maintenance host for JE virus

- Pig → mosquito → pig
- Ardied bird → mosquito → ardied bird
- Pig – Amplifying host
- Ardied birds – maintenance host
- **Mosquito:** Predominantly – C. tritaeniorhynchus, C. vishnui are implicated as vector for JE

High Yield Points

Man is an incidental dead end host

Clinical Features

- Prodromal stage: 1-6 days – Lethargy, fever and GI complaints
- Acute encephalitic stage: Fever is high, focal CNS signs, convulsions, raised ICP, speech, gait, hemi/quadriplagia, altered sensorium
- Late and sequel stage: Inflammation subsides, CNS signs tend to regress,
- Case fatality – approx. 20-40%

Good to Remember

Ardied birds: long legged birds, for example, herons and egrets.

Pls note: Culex quinquefasciatus is NOT the main vector for JE.

It is a vector for bancroftian filariasis, West Nile fever, Western equine encephalitis

22. Ans. (b) Not an emergency, give oral antibiotics and follow up

Ref: WHO Revised WHO Classification and treatment of childhood pneumonia at health facilities. 2014.

https://apps.who.int/iris/bitstream/handle/10665/137319/9789241507813_eng.pdf;jsessionid=68B5D3B52D484E5ABDAA841475E0894F?sequence=1

Recommendation 1

- Children with fast breathing pneumonia with no chest indrawing or general danger sign should be treated with oral amoxicillin: At least 40 mg/kg/dose twice daily (80 mg/kg/day) for five days.
- In areas with low HIV prevalence, give amoxicillin for three days.
- Children with fast-breathing pneumonia who fail on first-line treatment with amoxicillin should have the option of referral to a facility where there is appropriate second-line treatment.

Recommendation 2

- Children age 2–59 months with chest indrawing pneumonia should be treated with oral amoxicillin: At least 40 mg/kg/dose twice daily for five days.

Recommendation 3

- Children aged 2–59 months with severe pneumonia should be treated with parenteral ampicillin (or penicillin) and gentamicin as a first-line treatment.
    - Ampicillin: 50 mg/kg, or benzyl penicillin: 50,000 units per kg IM/IV every 6 hours for at least five days
    - Gentamicin: 7.5 mg/kg IM/IV once a day for at least five days
- Ceftriaxone should be used as a second-line treatment in children with severe pneumonia having failed on the first-line treatment.

Recommendation 4

- Ampicillin (or penicillin when ampicillin is not available) plus gentamicin or ceftriaxone are recommended as a first-line antibiotic regimen for HIV-infected and - exposed infants and for children under 5 years of age with chest indrawing pneumonia or severe pneumonia.
- For HIV-infected and - exposed infants and for children with chest indrawing pneumonia or severe pneumonia, who do not respond to treatment with ampicillin or penicillin plus gentamicin, ceftriaxone alone is recommended for use as second-line treatment.

Recommendation 5

- Empiric cotrimoxazole treatment for suspected *Pneumocystis Jirovecii* (previously *Pneumocystis carinii*) pneumonia (PCP) is recommended as an additional treatment for HIV-infected and -exposed infants aged from 2 months up to 1 year with chest indrawing or severe pneumonia.
- Empirical cotrimoxazole treatment for *Pneumocystis Jirovecii* pneumonia (PCP) is not recommended for HIV-infected and -exposed children over 1 year of age with chest indrawing or severe pneumonia.

23. Ans. (a) Multinational MONItoring of trends and determinants in CArdiovascular disease

Ref: K. Park 25th ed. p 397

MONICA is an Acronym for "Multinational **MONI**toring of trends and determinants in **CA**rdiovascular disease"

A World Health Organization Working Group developed a major international collaborative study with the objective of measuring over 10 years, and in many different populations, the trends in, and determinants of, cardiovascular disease. Specifically, the program focuses on trends in event rates for validated fatal and non-fatal coronary heart attacks and strokes, and on trends in cardiovascular risk factors (blood pressure, cigarette smoking and serum cholesterol) in men and women aged 25-64 in the same defined communities.

24. Ans. (b) Universal immunization

For more detail, refer to theory section: Mission Indradhanush, Chapter - Immunization and Vaccine, (page 742)

Nothing to explain. It's a direct question!

The Ministry of Health and Family Welfare has launched "Mission Indradhanush", depicting seven colors of the rainbow, in December 2014, to fully immunize 90% of children who are either unvaccinated or partially vaccinated; those that have not been covered during the rounds of routine immunization for various reasons, by 2018.

The intensified mission Indradhanush started in 2018, aims to immunize all children in selected high risk states and districts. It involves intensive preparation, implementation and integration of sessions into regular immunization microplans. The focus is on urban slum areas and districts with slowest progress and completion of due-list of beneficiaries on the basis of head count surveys.

25. Ans. (a) Yellow category

Ref: K. Park 25th ed. p 452

Remember:

White category–Needles, scalpel, syringe with fixed needle, LP needle, suture needle, sharps

Blue category–Broken glass, empty vial, metallic body implants

Red category–Foley's catheter, urine bag, RT, i/v bottles, gloves, syringe without needle, vacutainer

Yellow category

- Anatomical, animal, placenta, fetus, soiled waste, discarded linen, beddings
- Microbiological, blood bags, lab waste, expired medicines
- Cytotoxic drugs–Yellow category (special mention – CYTOTOXIC waste)
- Infectious liquid waste, body secretions, liquid chemical waste from lab, disinfectants, X-ray film liquid

26. Ans. (c) Vaccination against tetanus, typhoid and cholera to health workers

Source:

- https://www.who.int/immunization/sage/meetings/2012/april/2_SAGE_WGVHE_SG1__Lit_Review_CaseStudies.pdf
- https://www.cdc.gov/disasters/immunizations.html
- https://www.cdc.gov/disasters/disease/responderimmun.html

Remarks:

We will mark the option with vaccine for health workers, as only such is indicated. There is NO recommendation for any vaccine for general population or mass vaccination until there's a specific disease outbreak.

Only the ongoing National Immunization Schedule should be ensured to cover universal immunization with specific focus on Measles and OPV vaccines.

Explanation:

The major concern for anyone exposed to unsanitary conditions is that they should be up to date with tetanus-containing vaccine, because if they are injured (as is common in disaster settings), the injury is likely to be contaminated. Routinely recommended vaccines are recommended for evacuees, just like they are for everyone else.

Cholera and typhoid vaccine do not have any evidence for mass vaccination due to low level of exposure and prevention. Tetanus and HepB vaccine are required for health care providers and first responders.

Any other vaccine is also given to high risk individuals depending on the type, magnitude and impact of the disaster.

27. Ans. (d) B Anthracis

Ref:

For more detail, refer to theory section: Biological weapons, Chapter International Health Agencies, (page 854)

28. Ans. (a) Yellow category

Ref: K. Park 25th ed. p 853

For more detail, refer to theory section: Biomedical Waste, Chapter – Hospital Waste Management, (page 879)

S. No	Category	Type of waste	Color and type of container
1.	Yellow	▪ Human anatomical waste ▪ Animal anatomical waste ▪ Soiled waste ▪ Discarded or expired medicine ▪ Microbiology, biotechnology and other clinical laboratory waste ▪ Chemical waste ▪ Chemical liquid waste	Yellow colored nonchlorinated plastic bags (having thickness equal to more than 50 m) or containers 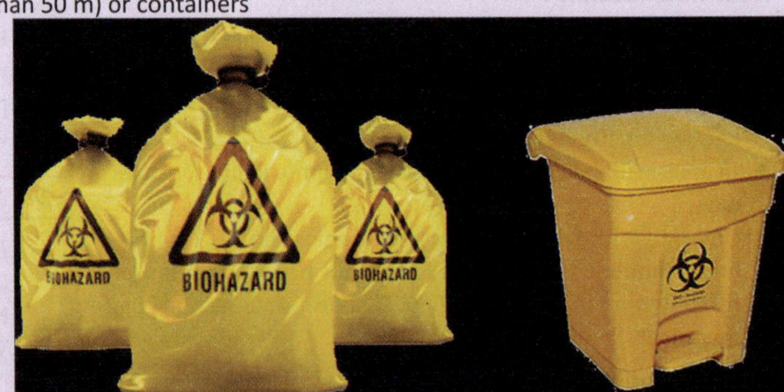 **Note** ▪ Chemical liquid waste such as spent hypo of X-ray should be stored in yellow container and sold to recycler authorized by SPCD/PCC ▪ Infected secretions, aspired body fluids etc. from laboratory should be disinfected before mixing with other wastewater from hospital ▪ Liquid chemical wastes should be pretreated/neutralized before mixing with other wastewater from hospital.

Note: Chemical waste is categorized into the yellow category. The hazardous chemical and cytotoxic waste is yellow category with special sign of "CYTOTOXIC" waste. Other liquid wastes as body secretions are categorized into the yellow category of biomedical waste guidelines, 2016

AIIMS NOVEMBER 2019

29. Ans. (d) Questionnaire based with checklist

Option	Discussion
In depth interview with the patient	Not a very good modality, as the patient may be biased towards health care professional or maybe influenced by subjective feeling towards injection process
Using CCTV	Not very good, as costly, and not proper visualization. Maybe subjective to positioning and environmental factors
In depth interview with the health care professional	Not reliable, prone to subject and interviewer bias
Questionnaire based with checklist	Better method for analysis of technique or at least may also have a small element of influencing the HCP towards proper technique and its evaluation process as well

HCP = health care professional

30. Ans. (b) Health education about hand washing

Ref: K. Park 25th ed. p 48

For more detail, refer to theory section: Concept of prevention, Chapter – Evolution and Concepts in Community Medicine, (page 151)

Option	Discussion
A. Giving pentavalent vaccine to children	Primary prevention
B. Health education about hand washing	Usually primordial prevention
C. Addition of iron to wheat flour	Specific protection and primary prevention
D. Ribavirin to close contact of meningitis patient	Chemoprophylaxis and primary prevention

31. Ans. (d) D → A → B → C

Ref: For more detail, refer to theory section: Infection control protocol, Chapter – Basics of Infection, (page 192)

Hand Hygiene: Why, How & When? online resource:
https://www.who.int/gpsc/5may/Hand_Hygiene_Why_How_and_When_Brochure.pdf
https://www.cdc.gov/handwashing/when-how-handwashing.html

Duration of the entire procedure: 40–60 second

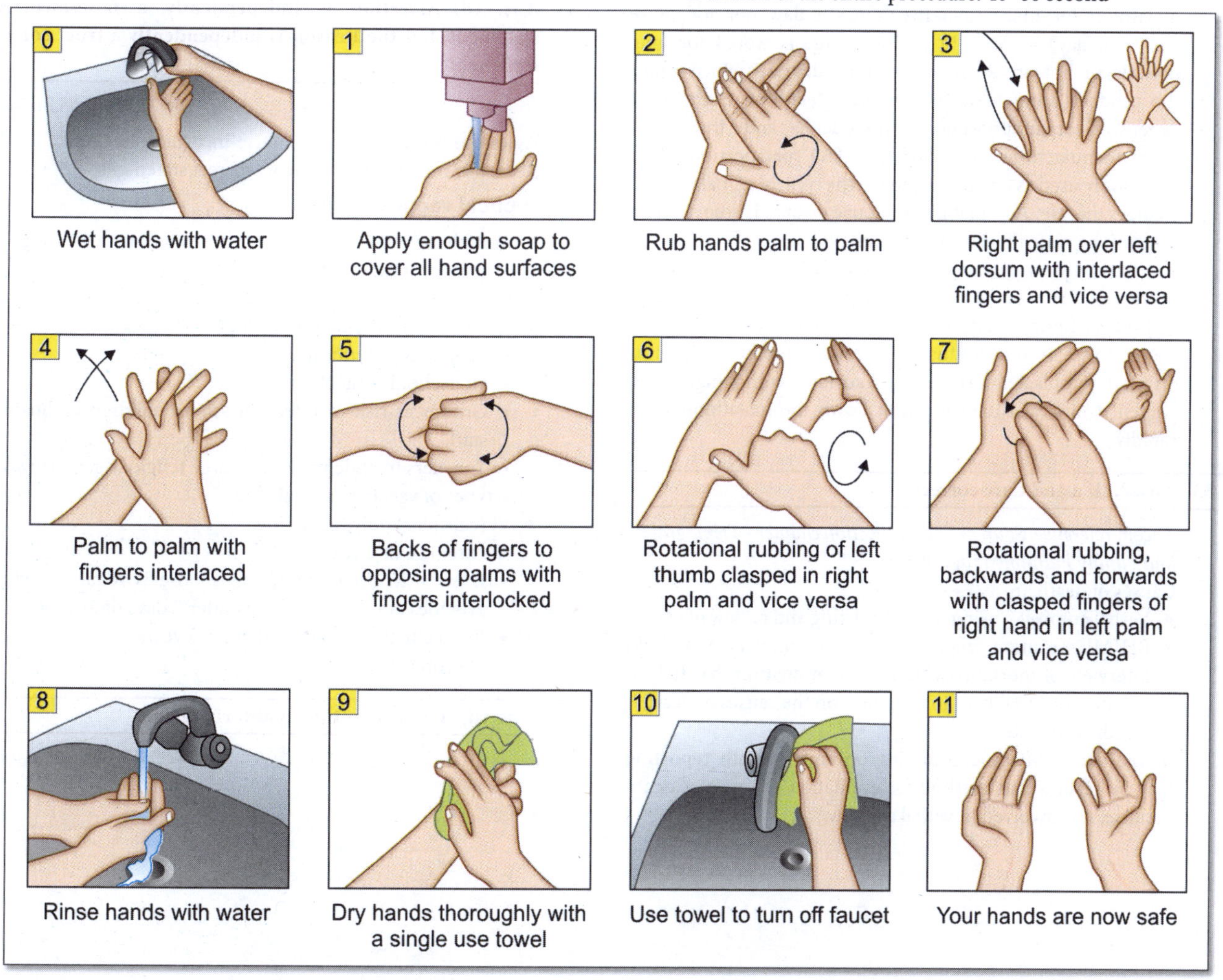
0 Wet hands with water
1 Apply enough soap to cover all hand surfaces
2 Rub hands palm to palm
3 Right palm over left dorsum with interlaced fingers and vice versa
4 Palm to palm with fingers interlaced
5 Backs of fingers to opposing palms with fingers interlocked
6 Rotational rubbing of left thumb clasped in right palm and vice versa
7 Rotational rubbing, backwards and forwards with clasped fingers of right hand in left palm and vice versa
8 Rinse hands with water
9 Dry hands thoroughly with a single use towel
10 Use towel to turn off faucet
11 Your hands are now safe

32. Ans. (a) Both Assertion and Reasons are independently true/correct statements and the Reason is the correct explanation for the Assertion

Ref: K. Park 25th ed. p 833

Both Assertion and Reasons are independently true/correct statements and the Reason is the correct explanation for the Assertion

Source:

https://www.who.int/water_sanitation_health/resources/vector357to384.pdf

ULV Fogging is ultra-low volume fogging. Most extensively used insecticides are malathion and fenitrothion

Most residual sprays are – DDT, lindane, Malathion, OMS 33 widely used space spray is Pyrethrum or pyrethrum extracts/ pyrethroids.

Malathion

This has become one of the most commonly used residual insecticides, following the development of resistance to DDT in many countries. It is classified as slightly hazardous. The absorption of particles by spray workers through inhalation, inagestion or contact with the skin reduces the activity of the enzyme cholinesterase in the nervous tissue. Signs of severe poisoning are muscle twitching and weakness followed by fits and convulsions. Spray personnel should not work with malathion for more than five hours a day, nor for more than five days a week. If the insecticide is stored for long periods in hot areas, impurities may develop which make the product more toxic to humans. Malathion is the least expensive organophosphorus insecticide and the safest when manufactured according to WHO specifications. It is commonly used as a residual spray in the control of malaria and changes disease. Acceptability to house owners is sometimes a problem because of its unpleasant smell.

Commonly available formulations: 50% water-dispersible powder and 50% emulsifiable concentrate.

Dosage: Residual effectiveness: At the higher dose it may last up to six months on thatch or wood but only 1–3 months on mud and plaster surfaces. Mud surfaces with a high alkali content (minerals) tend to break down the malathion most rapidly.

33. Ans. 2. If a and c are correct

Theory reference: Source of data collection chapter – Demography and Family Planning (page 396)

Causes of death are assessed by:

- Verbal autopsy – using death reporting and review of causes
- RHIME (routine, representative, re-sampled household interview of mortality with medical evaluation) has helped enhance the quality of information on the causes of death
- Death certificate

In the above MCQ, considering option C, death reporting may be regarded as method for evaluation of cause of death because, it is involved in verbal autopsy.

*Note: SRS (sample registration system) provides reliable estimates for the MMR, CBR, IMR… and some reports may also mention RHIME for understanding causes of maternal mortality (which is through an indirect activity and hence, we do not mark SRS in the MCQ stated above)

34. Ans. (d) Assertion is independently a false/incorrect statement, but the Reasons is independently a true/correct statement

Ref: K. Park 25th ed. p 869

For more detail, refer to theory section: Plumbism Chapter – Occupational Health, (page 353)

Assertion is independently a false/incorrect statement, but the Reasons is independently a true/correct statement

Lead inhibits TWO enzymes:

- Ferrochelatase
- ALA dehydratase

Hence: Protoporphyrin and ALA levels may be raised in lead toxicity – Plumbism

Laboratory: Lead toxicity causes a hypochromic microcytic anemia and basophilic stippling of red blood cells. Lead is a surface-acting poison and may produce increased RBC fragility and acute hemolytic anemia. Lead toxicity is not known to lead to eosinophilia.

35. Ans. (d) Assertion is independently a false/incorrect statement, but the Reason is independently a true/ correct statement

Ref: K. Park 25th ed. p 260

Assertion is independently a false/incorrect statement, but the Reason is independently a true/correct statement

Typhoid vaccine features:

- Complementary approach to prevention, with highest benefit for money spent
- Decrease incidence and seriousness of infection
- Special recommendation for high risk cases as:
  - People in endemic areas
  - Household contacts
  - Groups at risk of infection school children or hospital staff
  - Travelers to endemic zones, large religious gatherings

Two types of vaccine are available:

- Vi (capsular) polysaccharide
  - After age of 2 years
  - Dose – 25 microgram, single dose is required, which provides effective immunity after 7 days of injection
  - Revaccination is required every 3 years
- Ty21a (oral, live) vaccine

36. Ans. (d) 1-5 years is the highest risk group

Ref: K. Park 25th ed. p 170

Option	Discussion
Virus shedding is present before symptoms begins	Yes, the period of infectivity is from 1-2 days before and 1-2 days after onset of symptoms
Secondary attack rate is 5-15%	Yes, Park Textbook: The attack rates are 5-10 % for adults and 20-30% for children Other sources: Source: WHO influenza review of literature... https://www.who.int/influenza/preparedness/pandemic/PIRM_update_052017.pdf https://academic.oup.com/cid/article/50/11/1462/505636 Keeping in view different reviews of literature... the attack rates are 5-10 % for adults and 20-30% for children. some studies have shown low attack rates of 5% and maximum even upto 70%, so this option may or may not be true... but is NOT the false one...!
Aquatic birds act as reservoir	Major reservoirs are animals and birds, especially the aquatic birds... (source WHO Fact sheet on Influenza)
1-5 years is the highest risk group	No, influenza affects all age groups and gender. Certain high-risk groups are there which includes infants and children under 18 months (or under 2 years) Source: 1. NICD, influenza guidelines, April 2018, 2. https://www.cdc.gov/flu/highrisk/index.htm

So, technically speaking, the High-risk groups for severe influenza infection are:

- Infants and young children < 2 years
- Pregnant females
- Persons with preexisting COPD
- Persons with preexisting cardiac disease
- Persons with preexisting metabolic syndrome and/or morbid obesity
- Persons with preexisting renal, liver, neurological or immunosuppressive disease
- Children receiving chronic aspirin therapy
- Person age > 65 years

This is a doubtful MCQ… keeping in view the given options… 1-5 years is the best possible answer.

37. Ans. (b) Single site 2 doses - days 0 and 3

Option B – 2 doses 0,3 with wound washing-

Ref: K. Park 25th ed. p 305

Now, in this MCQ, the options and the MCQ statement may have some element of recall error, but anyways, let's learn the concept using the above recalled options only.

On review of literature, a few previous guidelines do mention as NO PEP required, if the dog is properly vaccinated and the efficacy of the vaccine is confirmed by laboratory evidence. But the recent WHO 2018 position does not have a mention on the same.

Basically the previous immunization status of animal should not necessarily be the deciding factor for ARV in India... This information is particularly true where pet animal laws are strictly adhered and regulated as in developed countries.

This is a point of discussion as far as Indian settings are concerned.

In my personal perception: **The main factor for consideration is the case fatality rate of rabies and risk involved on the background of knowledge of sporadic rabies cases (and some areas as rabies endemic) in our country.**

MCQ Discussion:

- Considering 2 chances of animal bites within 5 years of age of child (as mentioned in MCQ)– is scary..! This animal should be strictly observed and sent for examination if possible. Also search that why this child got bitten by dogs every now and then…!!
- Although the child has taken immunization last year, and now AGAIN an animal bite practically should give you some reasonable thoughts about giving ARV.

38. Ans. (b) After return of appetite

Ref: K. Park 25th ed. p ???

National Guidelines for Clinical Management of Dengue Fever, NVBDCP, MoHFW

Criteria for discharge of patients

- Absence of fever for at least 24 hours without the use of anti-fever therapy
- No respiratory distress from pleural effusion or ascites
- Platelet count > 50 000/mm3
- Return of appetite
- Good urine output
- Minimum of 2 to 3 days after recovery from shock
- Visible clinical improvement

39. Ans. (d) Human blood index

Ref: K. Park 25th ed. p 287

Vector burden for humans may be denoted by the term – anthrophilism

Human blood index	It is the proportion of freshly fed female Anopheline mosquitoes whose stomach contains human blood. It indicates the degree of anthrophilism
Sporozoite rate	It is the percentage of female anopheles with sporozoites in their salivary glands.
Mosquito density:	It is usually expressed as the number of mosquitoes per man-hour-catch.
Man-biting rate (biting density)	It is defined as the average incidence of anopheline bites per day per person. It is determined by standardized vector cache on human bait.
Inoculation rate:	The man-biting rate multiplied by the infective sporozoite rate is called the inoculation rate.

Remember:

- **Pre eradication era Malariometric Indicators** -parameters are based on clinical diagnosis (Spleen Rate, Average enlarged spleen, Parasite rate, Parasite density index, Infant parasite rate and proportional case rate).

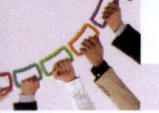

- **Eradication era Malariometric Indicators** - Parameters are based on microscopic diagnosis of malaria
  - Annual parasite incidence,
  - Annual blood examination rate
  - Annual falciparum incidence
  - Slide positivity rate
  - Slide falciparum rate
- **Vector Indices** are:
  - Human blood index, sporozoite rate, mosquito density
  - Man biting rate and inoculation rate

Indicator	High yield Point to remember
Spleen rate	Endemicity of malaria in a community
Infant parasite rate	The most sensitive index of recent transmission of malaria in a locality
Annual parasite incidence	Sophisticated measure of malaria incidence and burden of disease in a community
Annual Blood Examination Rate	Index of operational efficiency
Human Blood Index	Indicates the degree of anthrophilism

40. Ans. (a) States with API ≥ 1

Ref: K. Park 25th ed. p 447

The objectives of the national framework for malaria elimination are:

- By 2022, by all 26 states that were in categories 1,2 in year 2014
  - Interrupt transmission of malaria
  - Zero indigenous cases
- By 2024 → Incidence of malaria to be less than 1 per 1000 population in all states in India
- By 2027 → Indigenous transmission to be interrupted in all states in India
- By 2030 → Malaria to be eliminated and re-establishment prevented

Technically the NVBDCP divides the country into 4 categories based on the malaria burden:

Category	Definition	Naming
Category 0	Zero indigenous cases of malaria	Prevention of re-establishment phase
Category 1	Sates with API < 1and all districts with API <1	Elimination phase
Category 2	Sates with API < 1and few districts with API >1	Pre-elimination phase
Category 3	States with API ≥ 1	Intensified Control Phase

Option	Discussion
A. States with API ≥ 1	Yes, this is the technically right definition for intensified malaria control in an area.
B. Zero incidence of malaria	No, the incidence is to be reduced to less than 1/1000 cases by 2024
C. No longer a health problem	This has already been accomplished
D. 3 consecutive years no local transmission in the state	Probably, may be correct, but the criteria of 3 years is not true for malaria control. NVBDCP just provides fixed years for achieving the targets in districts and states in India

41. Ans. (b) 3 Drug combination for 6 months

Reference: Guidelines for the Diagnosis, Treatment and Prevention of Leprosy, WHO 2018

Revised WHO recommended Leprosy treatment regime:

42. Ans. (c) Vit A

Ref:

1. DK de Souza, PC Dorlo. *Safe mass drug administration for neglected tropical diseases.* Lancet, vol 6 (10) ; Oct 2018
2. Lymphatic filariais - manua lof elimination program, WHO, 2011

Mass drug administration: It is a term used for administration of drug to en-mass to control a particular disease. It is generally given for mass treatment of some disease

Mass drug administration for neglected tropical diseases gained particular prominence in the 1990s. Diseases such as onchocerciasis, lymphatic filariasis, trachoma, schistosomiasis, and soil-transmitted helminths are amenable to mass treatment and control as a result of the availability of safe and affordable drugs. MDA has also been tried for trachoma and scabies in various review of literature.

Vitamin A prophylaxis is a program by MoHFW for providing specific protection for vit A as cause of blindness in a specified category of 6 m to 59 months age group children in India the Program is being implemented using the ICDS facility and primary health care system of our country.

43. Ans. (b) Sickle cell anemia

Ref: K. Park 25th ed. p 186

For more detail, refer to theory section: Pneumococcal Vaccine, Chapter – Immunization and Vaccine, (page 748)

Indications of PPV are:

- Chronic cardiac disease
- Chronic lung disease and/or liver kidney
- Sickle cell disease
- Post splenectomy
- DM, alcoholism, malignancy, organ transplants (immune-suppressive condition)

In-detail Indications for PPV

The Advisory Committee on immunization practices (ACIP) and WHO recommendations are:

- PPV23 is NOT recommended for healthy adults aged 19–64 years
- PPV23 is recommended for:
  - Chronic heart disease, such as heart failure and cardiomyopathy (excluding hypertension alone)
  - Chronic lung disease, such as asthma and chronic obstructive pulmonary disease
  - Chronic liver disease
  - Poorly controlled diabetes mellitus
  - Current cigarette smoking
  - Alcohol use disorder
- Chronic renal disease – probably because of hypogammaglobulinemia, there is increased risk of invasive pneumococcal disease, especially people suffering from protein loosing nephropathies, nephrotic syndrome.
- Persons at risk of meningitis – Vaccination with both PCV13 and PPSV23 is indicated for individuals who are at increased risk of meningitis as:
  - Due to structural abnormalities that allow communication with the subarachnoid space e.g., CSF leaks or cochlear implant placements
  - Persons who previously had pneumococcal meningitis
- Impaired splenic function:
  - Anatomic asplenia or congenital hyposplenism
  - Sickle cell disease or other hemoglobinopathy
  - Functional asplenia or hyposplenism
- Immunosuppressive state:
  - HIV infection, organ transplant, immunodeficiency syndrome
  - Generalized malignancy or hematologic malignancy
- On case to case basis for age >65 years

44. Ans. (b) Still births after 28 weeks

Ref: Park's Textbook of PSM 25th ed. p 618

For more detail, refer to theory section: Perinatal Mortality Rate, Chapter - Preventive Pediatrics, (page 800)

Formula for perinatal mortality rate:

$$\textit{Perinatal mortality rate} = \frac{\textit{(Late fetal deaths (28 weeks gestation or more) + early neonatal deaths (within 7 days of life) in one year}}{\textit{Live births + late fetal deaths}}$$

Note: There is a difference in the denominator (and NOT in numerator) for developed countries and that given by WHO (more for countries with less established vital recording systems)

The WHO definition, which suits the less developed recording systems, takes into account ONLY Live births in the denominator

45. Ans. (1) b, (2) a, (3) e, (4) c

Ref: K. Park 25th ed. p 853

For more detail, refer to theory section: Biomedical Waste, Chapter – Hospital Waste Management, (page 878)

For updates/video sessions @Youtube channel – mukhmohit's community medicine simplified

JIPMER MAY 2019

46. Ans. (c) Randomized clinical trial

Ref: K. Park 25th edition. Pg. 92

For more detail, refer to theory section: Randomized Controlled Trials, Chapter – Epidemiology, (page 12)

It is a clear example of randomized clinical trial. As we are giving a drug and assessment of the outcome (cataract) is done, thus the study is not observational study. All other options in the MCQ above (case control, cohort, cross sectional study) are types of observational studies.

Some examples of clinical trials include – trial of beta blockers for CVD morbidity in AMI patients, trial of Folic acid supplementation for anemia cases and so on.

47. Ans. (c) A perfect test has an area under the ROC curve of 1

For more detail, refer to theory section: ROC curve, Chapter - Screening of Disease, (page 61)

The receiver operator characteristic curve (ROC) is constructed between the 'Sensitivity' and 'False positive' results. The area under curve of 1 indicates a perfect test. The area under the curve should be ranging from 0.6-1.

48. Ans. (a) 2.875 and 0.531

Let us make the Table,

Black font – data provided in MCQ

Red Font – data derived from values given

	Dis +ve	Dis -ve	TOTAL
Test +ve	46 (TP)	**10 (FP)**	56
Test -ve	**34 (FN)**	40 (TN)	74
TOTAL	**80**	**50**	130

TP = True positive, TN = True Negative, FP = False positive, FN = False Negative

So let us calculate the values.

$$\text{Sensitivity} = \frac{TP}{TP + FN} = \frac{46}{46 + 34} = 57.5\%$$

$$\text{Specificity} = \frac{TN}{TP + FP} = \frac{40}{40 + 10} = 80\%$$

So,

100–Sn% = 100–57.5 = 42.5 and

100–Sp% = 100–80 = 20

So, the Likelihood ratios are given by:

$$\text{Likelihood ratio for a Positive test} = \frac{\textit{Sensitivity}}{\textit{100 – specificty}} = \frac{57.5}{20} = 2.875$$

$$\text{Likelihood ratio for a Negative test} = \frac{\textit{100 – Sensitivity}}{\textit{specificty}} = \frac{42.5}{80} = 0.53125$$

49. Ans. (a) Reduced to 1/4

For more detail, refer to theory section: Sample size, Chapter Biostatistics, (page 104)

Sample size is given by the formula = $\frac{4PQ}{L_2}$

where, P = Prevalence, Q = 100 – Prevalence %, L = allowable error.

Hence, we can see that the denominator in the formula is squared. So, if the allowable error is doubled, it will decrease the sample size by 1/4th

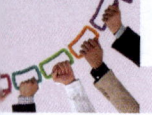

50. Ans. (b) Type I error

For more detail, refer to theory section: Inferential stats, Chapter Biostatistics, (page 98)

Remember:

If null hypothesis was **TRUE** and by mistake **Rejected** — Type 1 Error

If null hypothesis was **FALSE** and by mistake **Accepted** — Type 2 Error

51. Ans. (d) Infant mortality rate

Ref: K. Park 25th ed. p 17

For more detail, refer to theory section: HDI, chapter – Evolution and Concepts in Community Medicine, (page 152)

The HDI is human development index. It is a geometric mean which includes:

- Longevity - Life expectancy at 1 year
- Knowledge – Mean years of schooling and expected years of schooling
- Income – Gross net income per capita in purchasing power of parity

The HDI for India is 0.647, with 129 rank.

52. Ans. (a) Time for 50% cases to occur

Ref: K. Park 25th ed. p 107

Median is the middle value after arranging data in ascending or descending order. The Median incubation period will be the average incubation period for 50% of the cases to occur.

The time between primary and secondary case is known as serial interval.

Time between onset of infection and period of maximum infectivity is known as generation time.

53. Ans. (b) 0.5 ppm

Ref: K. Park 25th ed. p 775

The amount of free chorine in a sample of drinking water should always be more than 0.5 ppm

54. Ans. (b) It is used to assess the quality of water by estimating hardness, total dissolved solids, alkalinity and PH

The saturation Index (SI) is a tool to check for water quality – in terms of corrosiveness or scale forming.

The ideal SI is around zero (-0.3 to +0.3)

If the SI is below (-) 0.3 – indicates corrosive water

If the SI is above (+) 0.3 – indicates scaling water

The SI incorporates the five balance factors - pH, total alkalinity, calcium hardness, temperature, and total dissolved solids

55. Ans. (a) Hand scrub with alcohol-based antiseptics is superior to hand washing with soap and water

Recent data from review of literature shows (with low to moderate evidence) that alcohols have excellent in vitro germicidal activity against Gram-positive and Gram-negative vegetative bacteria (including multidrug-resistant pathogens such as MRSA and VRE), Mycobacterium tuberculosis, and a variety of fungi. The alcohol-based rubs also have in vivo activity against a number of non-enveloped viruses (e.g. rotavirus, adenovirus, rhinovirus, hepatitis A and enteroviruses).

PGI MAY 2019

56. Ans. (a) Matching, (b) Randomization, (c) Stratification, (d) Multivariate regression analysis

For more detail, refer to theory section: Bias and Confounding, Chapter - Epidemiology, (page 19)

Blinding is a technique for control of bias.

57. Ans. (a) Help in increasing efficiency of a program, (b) Useful for decision-making, (c) Use mathematical methods, (e) Optimizes resource allocation

For more detail, refer to theory section: Chapter - Epidemiology, (page 17)

Operations (aka operational) research is a method for research and enhancement of the system of the health care service, delivery or any program.

It is a scientific method to improve upon the existing system of the health program and betterment of the health of the population.

58. Ans. (a) Still birth rate, (b) Neglected tropical diseases, (e) Substance abuse

Ref: K. Park 25th ed. p 30

For more detail, refer to theory section: Global reference list, Chapter - Evolution and Concepts in Community Medicine, (page 155)

The global reference list is a set of 100 indicators relating to broad four categories as

1. Health status indicators—Mortality, fertility and morbidity of various diseases
2. Risk factor indicators as nutrition, environment and other diseases
3. Service coverage indicators for maternal and child health, newborn care, adolescent health, immunization, and other diseases of public health importance as malaria, TB, HIV, neglected tropical diseases, mental health
4. Health system indicators for quality of health care, service utilization, access to health care and governmental policy indicators including budgeting and implementation indicators.

A few diseases like asthma, COPD and rheumatic fever are not directly under the global reference list. Similarly, tribal health is presently not included into the reference list.

59. Ans. (b) Yatri Suraksha- preventing deaths due to rail and road traffic accidents, (c) Nirbhaya Nari-action against gender violence, (d) Reduced stress and improved safety in the work place

Source:

National Health policy, 2017. MoHFW, Govt of India. Page 6

The policy identifies coordinated action on seven priority areas for improving the environment for health and health of citizens (*Swasth Nagrik Abhiyan*)

- The *Swachh Bharat Abhiyan*
    - Balanced, healthy diets and regular exercises.

- Addressing tobacco, alcohol and substance abuse
- *Yatri Suraksha* – Preventing deaths due to rail and road traffic accidents
  - *Nirbhaya Nari* –action against gender violence
  - Reduced stress and improved safety in the work place
- Reducing indoor and outdoor air pollution

60. Ans. (a) Measles, (b) Japanese Encephalitis, (c) Typhoid

Ref: K. Park 25th ed. p 514

Page 90, IDSP module for state and district surveillance officers.

Syndrome under surveillance	Disease of interest
Fever with & without localizing signs	Malaria, Typhoid, JE, Dengue, Measles
Cough more than 3 weeks	Tuberculosis
Acute Flaccid Paralysis	Polio
Diarrhea	Cholera
Jaundice	Hepatitis, Leptospirosis, Dengue, Malaria, Yellow fever
Unusual Syndromes	Anthrax, Plague, Emerging epidemics

61. Ans. (a) Most commonly occurs due to lymphatic filariasis, (c) Graded compression stockings are used to control limb swelling, (e) Commonly seen in workers in volcanic areas, working with bare foot

Ref: K. Park 25th ed. p 298

Must remember points:

- Lymphedema (or Elephantiasis) is usually by filariasis but may also be caused by obstruction following other infections as TB, tumor, surgery or irradiations
- Elephantiasis may affect – legs > scrotum > arms > penis > vulva > breast
- Chyluria prevalence is low
- W. bancrofti may lead to genital involvement (rare with Burgian filariasis)
- Most commonly used investigation to diagnose - thick film of peripheral blood smear
- Most sensitive investigation – membrane filtration concentration method

62. Ans. (b) Aim for elimination by 2020, (c) Objectives included control through anti-larval measures, (d) Source reduction was the part of control strategy, (e) Home-based management of lymphedema cases included for elimination strategy

Ref: K. Park 25th ed. p 452

Theory reference: Malaria, Chapter – Communicable diseases and related program (page 567)

The National filariasis control program was started in 1955-57, which was later incorporated with the NVBDCP - National vector borne disease control program in 2004. It aims to eliminate LF by 2020 (previous target was elimination by 2017)

The program envisages to combat lymphatic filariasis using multiple strategies as chemoprophylaxis (using DEC and albendazole with/or without Ivermectin) vector control, mass drug administration and home-based management of cases with follow ups.

63. Ans. (a) Influenza vaccine, (d) Yellow fever vaccine

Ref: K. Park 25th ed. p 131

Theory reference: Vaccines for Influenza, Chapter 13, (page 514)

Theory reference: Immunization Contraindications, Chapter Immunization and Vaccine, (page 754)

Vaccine contraindicated in severe egg allergy is yellow fever and influenza vaccine.

Remember that:

- Influenza also has non-egg-based vaccine type, which may be given to patients with egg allergy.
- Measles and MMR may be given to egg allergy patients with caution.

64. Ans. (a) Pregnancy in third trimester, (c) Allergy to the vaccine adjuvant, (e) Immunodeficiency

Ref: K. Park 25th ed. p 131

Theory reference: Immunization Contraindications, Chapter - Immunization and Vaccine (page 754)

Live vaccines will be contraindicated in case of:

- Pregnancy
- Severe immunodeficiency

Any vaccine will be contraindicated in case of history of allergy or anaphylaxis to any specific vaccine or its component.

Tuberculosis and active acute infection (unless very serious or severe) is generally not a contraindication for vaccine administration.

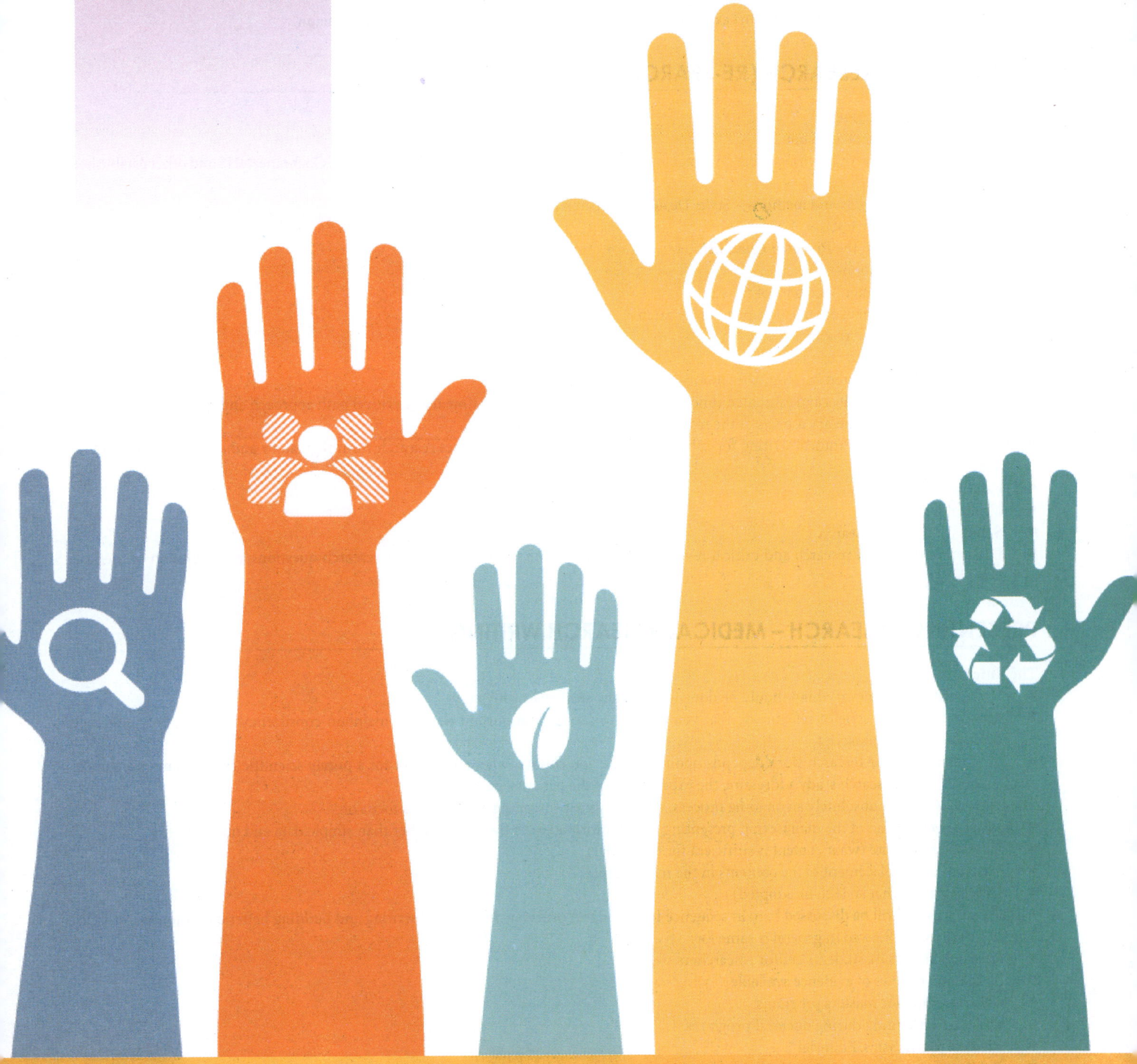

Latest Updates

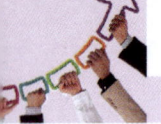

MEDICAL RESEARCH WRITING

The rule of Thumb is:

"If you can't explain something simply, you don't understand it well enough"

CONDUCTING RESEARCH (RE-SEARCH)

A few steps to be adopted are:

- Formulate the research question
- Review the literature/research available on same/similar topic from all sources as Medline, PubMed, Cochrane, NHS and other established sources.
- Plan for gross materials and methods – Style, Design of research to be conducted
- Conduct a feasibility test
- ***R**eassess, **R**econfirm the **Research Checklist**:*
    - Research question
    - Style, study design, outcome of the study
    - Data management & Statistical plan for research
    - Feasibility of the research
    - Ethical issues and clearance
    - Validated, pre-tested questionnaire, informed consent
    - Sequence of activites and estimated time for the research – evaluate the time using critical path approach and PERT methods
    - Funding and monetary aspects of the research
- Plan and prepare for Protocol writing for submission and permission to conduct research from regulatory authorities and/or funding agencies
- Conduct the research
- Medical writing
- Submission of the research
- Dissemination of the research and critical review of the research for formulating further research questions and evolution of medical knowledge

PRESENTING RESEARCH – MEDICAL RESEARCH WRITING

The **Rule** is:

- In scientific writing everything should be done to avoid any suspense or mystery
- Irrespective of the style of referencing that you choose to use, it is important that you maintain consistency by using only one style throughout the manuscript.
- The quality of your research work depends upon the topic you choose, whether you opt for a purely scientific experiment or a clinical trial or a social research study addressing the experiences of the patients, etc.

The research writing is absolutely an ongoing process, which is time consuming and requires focus on

- What to write (plan of the manuscript, presenting useful information to the reader rather than simple data and numbers)
- How much to write (what content is sufficient for the reader)
- When to write (placement of the contents in the manuscript)
- How to write (what style to be adopted)

All the components will be discussed here in sequence to provide an overview for medical writing and building better communication skills.
The structure to be followed in general is same for:

- Research articles by students and/or researchers
- Systematic reviews of evidence available
- Thesis writing for masters programs
- Dissertation writing during doctoral programs
- Medical journalisms/Editorial
- Publications and presentations
- Regulatory documents, formulating standard protocols/Guidelines for Medical Education

(All the variants of medical writing will be referred to as *manuscript* for further reading)

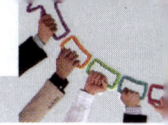

A step-by-step approach for medical research writing, dissertation writing in general is as follows:

Step 1: Title

Start your manuscript with a suitable 'Title'

- Use: Attract readers interested in this field of study
- The title is an introduction to the content of the manuscript. An ideal title should be within 65 characters (5-15 words), without any abbreviations and grammatical mistakes, and not contain stop words like 'a', 'an', 'the', 'of', 'but', etc.
- A good title should contain:
  - The purpose of the research (topic of research)
  - The type of research method (study design)
  - Geographical/Temporal scope of the study (defined area or time of study)

Step 2: Introduction

Next, write your manuscript 'Introduction'

- Use: It tells the readers why you conducted the particular study.
- Essential components on introduction are:
  - Why this study is undertaken – what problems the author is trying to address
  - What has already been done in the field, what were the gaps, and how you fill those gaps with your study?
- The end of introduction usually contains a statement for "Aims and Objectives" of the research. It is a brief statement describing the study outcomes, how the work contributes to better understanding of the disease condition or research topic or unanswered questions

Step 3: Review of Literature (RoL)

This is usually the most time and effort consuming section.

- Use: RoL represents the literature that provides background information on your topic and shows a correspondence between those writings and your research question.
- RoL is essential for research writing as it:
  - Explains the background of research on a topic.
  - Demonstrates why a topic is significant to a subject area.
  - Discovers relationships between research studies/ideas.
  - Identifies major themes, concepts, and researchers on a topic.
  - Identifies critical gaps and points of disagreement.
  - Discusses further research questions that logically come out of the previous studies.

The research articles to be cited may be placed in the manuscript according to

- Temporal distribution: Chronologically sequencing of articles by event/trend/publishing of the article – usually adopted and accepted method
- Geographical distribution – Studies from various parts of world are listed followed by studies from specific continent/country or region specific researches.
- Based on methodology adopted by different researches.

Usual accepted and most followed way is using a chronological sequence of all previous researches with subclassifying the literature based on geographical and methodology distribution

Step 4: Material and Methods (M&M)

This section follows after Introduction.

- **Use:**
  - To enable the readers to evaluate the study design. Nothing should be kept as 'presumed' The author should try to write every detail of the methods used to conduct the study
  - To allow the reader/researcher to replicate the study using same methodology for future researches.
- **The outlay** of "*materials and methods*" is
  - Setting—the environmental conditions in which you conducted your research
  - Sample—what materials were used in research and details about the participants in the study.
    - Type of study
    - Sample size calculation, sampling methodology used for collecting data
    - Inclusion and exclusion criteria – what factors were considered to include or exclude any participant in the study
  - **Measurement tools**—Discrete, elaborate description of all variable and methods used should be done. It may include all or some of the following:
    - Details about the methods and equipment used to measure the outcomes of the study. Include description of the instruments, devices used (manufacturer, quality control, year, and other specific descriptions) if any

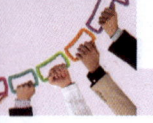

- Specifying the critical variables for that type of work, for example, how long the samples were incubated, how many minutes subjects were allowed to work on a task, or what strain of laboratory media was used or any other details.
- Questionnaire used for establishing a condition, the source, reliability, consistency and validity of the questionnaire.
- **Independent and Dependent variables**—what were the factors you controlled or changed during the experiment and what you measured as the outcome
- **Statistical plan for research**—elaborate on the tests of significance used, measures for confidence limits, cut off for power of study, allowable statistical error in interpretation of the research, software used during analysis of the study

Step 5: Results and Observations

- **Use:** To present the data, useful and meaningful interpretation of the data
- A good research writing should include presentation using appropriate Text, Tables, figure, graphs and other statistical presentation methods
- **The general rule is**—the results represented as tables or graphs should contain:
  - Title—describing the table/graph
  - Number (separate for tables and graphs/presentations)
  - Table should have header for columns and rows
  - Data presented should always show the units of data measured
  - Legend for the graphs, curves or other statistical presentations
  - Graph, curves should be readable and understandable
  - Data Labels on graphs, curves indicating the data value and format (absolute number or percentage)
  - The tables should be presented as variables in rows/columns with row total and column total on sides
  - Statistical analysis tables (summary tables) should contain the cut-off for p-values, with the confidence limits set for the research

Step 5: Discussion

It is the most crucial step where you include the '**Discussion**' of your results. An ideal discussion should include:

- The principal findings of your study
- Strengths and weaknesses of your study in relation to other studies in the field
- A take-home message for the clinicians and policymakers
- Questions that your study can't answer to propagate further research

Step 6: Follow the Discussion with the 'Limitations of your Study'

Step 7: References

At the end of your thesis, include your 'References'. Track all your references so you don't miss out on anyone.

Common Terms

A **bibliography** is a list of sources that the writer recommends for further reading.
A '**works cited list**' or a '**reference list**' is a list of sources that were included in the author's writing.

Referencing, Citation Styles

The most commonly used referencing and citation styles are as follows:

Vancouver Style

The Vancouver Style is formally known as Recommendations for the Conduct, Reporting, Editing and Publication of Scholarly Work in Medical Journals (ICMJE Recommendations). It was developed in Vancouver in 1978 by editors of medical journals and well over 1,000 medical journals (including ICMJE members BMJ, CMAJ, JAMA & NEJM) use this style

On the references page

- The last page of your paper is entitled references.
  - References are single spaced, with double-spacing between references.
- **Numbering:** List all references in order by number, not alphabetically.
  - Each reference is listed once only, since the same number is used throughout the paper.
- **Authors:**
  - List each author's last name followed by a space and then initials without any periods; there is a comma and space between authors and a period at the end of the last author.

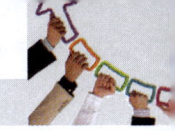

- If the number of authors exceeds six, give the first six followed by "et al."
- For edited books, place the editors' names in the author position and follow the last editor with a comma and the word editor (or editors). For edited books with chapters written by individual authors, list the authors of the chapter first, then the chapter title, followed by "In:", the editors' names, and the book title.

▪ **Title:** Capitalize the first letter of the first word in the title. The rest of the title is in lower-case, with the exception of proper names. Do not underline the title; do not use italics. If there is an edition for a book, it appears after the title, abbreviated and followed by a period, for example: 8th ed.

▪ **Publication information:**
- **Books**: After the title (and edition if applicable), place a period and space, then enter the city. Give the year of publication followed by a period. If no date of publication can be found, but the publication contains a date of copyright, use the date of copyright preceded by the letter "c", e.g. c2015.
- **Journals**: List the abbreviated journal title, place a period and a space, year, (and abbreviated month and day if applicable), semi-colon, volume, issue number in parentheses, colon, page range, and a period.

▪ **Online sources:**
- Include the same information and style as for print sources
- Add the retrieval information for location by the reader of the manuscript
  - Place word [Internet] in square brackets after the book title or abbreviated journal title
  - Indicate date of retrieval, preceded by the word "cited", in square brackets after the date of publication
  - Add retrieval information at the end of the citation using the full URL.
  - If a DOI exists, it is optional to add it after the retrieval information

Example

▪ Mukhmohit S et al, COPD - Prevalence and risk study among females of rural area, District Ambala, Haryana, India. JEMDS. Apr 2014;3(16):4183-4191

▪ Edward Seferian, Bekele Afessa. Demographic and clinical variation of adult intensive care unit utilization from a geographically defined population. Crit Care Med. 2006 Aug;34(8):2113-9. PubMed PMID: 16763514

▪ Eat right [Internet]. Chicago: Academy of Nutrition and Dietetics; c2016 [cited 01 May 2019]. Available from: https://www.eatright.org/.

▪ Nipah Virus [Internet] World Health Organisation. May 2018 [cited 01 May 2019]. Available from: https://www.who.int/news-room/fact-sheets/detail/nipah-virus

Some other Referencing Styles are:

▪ **APA (American Psychological Association)**
- Usually used for social sciences – for citing work from newspapers, articles, media, interviews and books
- APA format structure:
  - Author, A. (Year of Publication). Title of work. Publisher City, State: Publisher

▪ **MLA:**
- MLA format is often used for literature, language, liberal arts, and other humanities subjects.
- It has separate section for bibliography and work cited

▪ **Harvard style**
- AGPS (Australian) style
- Usually used for legal documentations, citations, precedence and rulebook formulations

Step 8: Abstract

Purpose: To provide a brief summary of the paper. This is a crucial component of research article writing. After reading the title, the reader usually reads the abstract and will decide if they wish to read the rest of the research article. commonly the abstract is structured for 150-300 words

Content: The abstract is written as a mini-article, i.e., it contains the following information in this order:

▪ **Introduction:** A few sentences to provide background information on the problem investigated
▪ **Methods:** Methodology and tools used during research
▪ **Results:** The major results presented in the paper; provide quantitative information when possible.
▪ **Discussion:** The authors' interpretation of the results presented
▪ **Final summary:** The major conclusions and implication of the research. It should be understandable for a general readership and provide the use of research.

Principles for a good abstract:

▪ Give a brief background information about the topic
▪ State the importance of the problem and what is unknown about it
▪ Clearly state the objectives of your study
▪ A brief selected review of literature. Do not include duplicity of results or well known facts and results
▪ **Selected high yield information should be given in abstract for a very precise and to-the-point information.**

• In the uncommon [illegible] where [illegible] exceeds [illegible] list the first [illegible] followed by [illegible].
• Editors: [illegible] editors [illegible] the authors [illegible] list the editor with a comma [illegible] editor(s) [illegible] for edited books with chapters written by individual authors, list the authors of the chapter first, then the chapter title, followed by "In" and the editor [illegible] of the book [illegible].
4. Title: Capitalise the first letter of the first word in the title [illegible] with the exception of proper nouns. Do not [illegible] the title [illegible] italics [illegible] title, [illegible] followed by a period. For example [illegible].
5. Publication information:
• Books: [illegible] place and publisher [illegible] a period [illegible] then the [illegible]. Give the year of publication followed by a period. If the date of publication cannot be found, but the [illegible] a date [illegible] use the [illegible] [illegible]
• Journals: List the abbreviated journal title [illegible] a space, volume number [illegible] issue number in brackets [illegible] colon, then page numbers [illegible].
6. Online sources:
• [illegible] the same information [illegible]
• Add the [illegible] [illegible]:
  • [illegible] [illegible] after [illegible]
  • Include date [illegible] preceded by the word "[illegible]" [illegible] for the date of publication.
  • [illegible]
  • [illegible]

Example

• [illegible] et al. [illegible] [illegible] 2013 [illegible]
• [illegible] [illegible] 2017 [illegible]
• [illegible] [illegible] Organization [illegible] [illegible]
• [illegible] [illegible]

Some other Referencing Styles are

• APA (American Psychological Association):
  • [illegible]
  • APA format reference:
    • Author, A. (Year of publication). Title of work. Publisher [illegible].
• MLA format [illegible] [illegible] Works [illegible].
  • [illegible] bibliography [illegible] work cited.
• Harvard style
• [illegible] style
  • [illegible] [illegible] or [illegible]

Step 8: Abstract

Purpose: [illegible] summary of the paper [illegible] research paper [illegible] [illegible] should [illegible] the [illegible] of the research [illegible].

Content: The abstract [illegible] following information [illegible]:
• Introduction: A few [illegible] [illegible]
• Methods: [illegible] tools used in research.
• Results: The major results [illegible].
• Discussion: The importance [illegible].
• Final summary: [illegible] [illegible] research.

Principles for a good abstract:
• [illegible]
• [illegible]
• [illegible]
• A [illegible] [illegible] results.
• Selected [illegible] information should be given [illegible] [illegible] information.

AIIMS New Pattern 2019 Model Questions

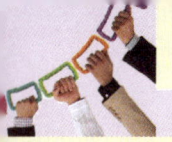

MULTIPLE TRUE/FALSE TYPE

Each question shall have a stem followed by five alternatives/statements and every alternative/statement will have to be marked as either True or False.

Correct answer: +1/5 for each alternative/statement and

Incorrect answer: –1/5 for each alternative/statement

1. **A researcher develops a new test for diagnosis of dengue (dg-test). When added to blood, the characteristic color change is noticed in presence of Dengue antigen. The test results are as shown below:**
   Total tested were 200, out of which 100 were with known dengue fever and 100 cases of established non-dengue causes of fever Dengue test was found to be positive in 91 out of established dengue cases and in 12 of the established non-dengue cases. Which of the following statement is true
   a. The sensitivity of the test was about 91%
   b. The specificity of the test was about 12%
   c. The false negative rate was about 9%
   d. The predictive value of a positive result cannot be determined from the above
   e. The predictive value of a negative result cannot be determined from the above

Ans: True options: A, C; False options: B, D, E

	Dengue	No dengue
Dg-Test +	91 (TP)	12 (FP)
Dg-test negative	9 (FN)	88 (TN)
Total	100	100

So we can calculate:

Sensitivity	= 91/100 = 91%
Specificity	= 88/100 = 88%
False negative error rate	= 9/100 = 9%
False positive error rate	= 12/100 = 12%
Positive predictive value	= 91/103 = 88%
Negative predicative Value	= 88/97 = 91%

So, the answer is:

a. The sensitivity of the test was about 91%	T	Yes correct
b. The specificity of the test was about 12%	F	No, the specificity is 88%
c. The false negative rate was about 9%	T	Yes correct
d. The predictive value of a positive result cannot be determined from the above	F	No, we can calculate PPV as TP/TP + FP
e. The predictive value of a negative result cannot be determined from the above	F	No, we can calculate NPV as TN/TN + FN

2. **Which of the following is False about chicken pox?**
   a. Cause by Human alpha herpes virus 3
   b. Secondary attack rate is 90%
   c. Transmitted by droplet infection
   d. Incubation period 7-21 days
   e. Period of communicability of chicken pox is 2 weeks and 4 weeks after onset of rash

Ans. True options: A, B, C, D; False option: E

a. Cause by Human alpha herpes virus 3	True	Yes, correct
b. Secondary attack rate is 90%	True	Yes, correct
c. Transmitted by droplet infection	True	Yes, correct
d. Incubation period 7-21 days	True	Yes, correct
Period of communicability of chicken pox is 2 weeks and 4 weeks after onset of rash	False	Period of communicability is 1-2 days before and 4-5 days after rash

3. **A 39-year-old female is diagnosed with varicella infection in the 2nd trimester. The physician should be concerned for which of the following defects in congenital varicella syndrome, if it occurs**
   a. Cardiac defects
   b. Cutaneous scar
   c. Microcephaly
   d. Hydrocephalus
   e. Atrophied limbs

Ans. True options: B, C, E; False options: A, D

a. Cardiac defects	F	No, it is not known to involve the heart
b. Cutaneous scar	T	Yes correct
c. Microcephaly	T	Yes correct, along with other CNS disorders as cerebro-cortical atrophy
d. Hydrocephalus	F	No, there's no evidence of hydrocephalus
e. Atrophied limbs	T	Yes correct

Features of congenital varicella syndrome include:

cutaneous scars	atrophied limbs	microcephaly
low birth weight	cataract	microphthalmia
chorioretinitis	deafness	cerebrocortical atrophy

4. **Natural prevention of cancers are/is**
   a. Nitrosamines
   b. Ascorbic acid
   c. Beta carotene
   d. Vitamin D
   e. α -Tocopherol

Ans. True options: C. Beta carotene; (D) Vitamin -D; (E) α-tocopherol; False options: A, B

- The following agents may have role in prevention of cancers:
  - Beta carotenes
  - Tocopherol
  - Retinol, (isotretinoin)
  - Selenium
  - Calcium (colon Ca)
  - Isoflavones (breast Ca)
  - Drugs — Tamoxifen, Raloxifene (breast Ca), NSAID (Ca colon), Finasteride (prostate Ca)
- Vit. D induces bile acid break down in vitro and may have role in protection against colon cancer.

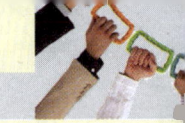

- Calcium appears to bind bile acids in bowel lumen; inhibiting bile acid induced mucosal damage and perhaps carcinogenesis.
- Nitrosamines are present in food preservative. It may contribute to the induction of gastric carcinoma

5. Which is not true regarding measles?

a. Only source of infection is a case
b. Subclinical measles not known
c. Incubation period 2–4 weeks
d. More severe in malnourished
e. Immunity after vaccination is short lasting

Ans. True options: A, B, D; False options: C, E

a. Only source of infection is a case	T	Yes correct
b. Subclinical measles not known	T	Yes correct
c. Incubation period 12-4 weeks	F	No, it is ranging from 10-14 days
d. More severe in malnourished	T	Yes correct
e. Period of communicability 4 days before and 2.5 days after rash	F	It is 4 days before and 4 days after rash

6. During post-measles states there may be:

a. Growth retardation, weight loss
b. Pyogenic infection, reactivation of tuberculosis
c. Cancrum oris
d. Diarrhoea
e. Pneumonia

Ans. True options: A, B, C, D, E; False options:

a. Growth retardation, weight loss	T	Yes correct
b. Pyogenic infection, reactivation of tuberculosis	T	Yes correct
c. Cancrum oris	T	Yes correct
d. Diarrhoea	T	Yes correct , Most frequent associated feature
e. Pneumonia	T	Yes correct, Most common cause of death in measles

7. There have been 3 cases of mumps from 2 different schools, but from within your area in April 2019. Regarding the Epidemiology of mumps, which of the following statement are true/false:

a. Disease more severe in children <5 years
b. Secondary attack rate 86%
c. Mumps is important cause for sensorineural hearing loss especially in young children
d. There are no subclinical cases
e. Period of maximum infectivity is just before and at onset of parotitis

Ans. True Options: B, C, E; False options: A, D

a. Disease more severe in children <5 years	F	No it is most frequent in age 5-9 years (early school years – kindergarten years)
b. Secondary attack rate 86%	T	Yes correct
c. Mumps is important cause for sensorineural hearing loss especially in young children	T	Yes correct. approx. 5 per 100,000 mumps cases may develop a permanent sensorineural hearing loss
d. There are no subclinical cases	F	No, around 30-40% of all mumps cases are clinically inapparent – subclinical infections
e. Period of maximum infectivity is just before and at onset of parotitis	T	Yes correct

8. Under revised RNTCP 2018-19 guidelines, which of following is true:

a. Sputum culture using solid culture is done for all cases from vulnerable high-risk population
b. TB patients with Rifampicin resistant strains maybe put on MDR regime
c. Revised regime for previously treated TB category is 2 HRZES + 1 HRZE + 4 HRE
d. Bedaquiline has been approved for all rifampicin resistant TB cases
e. CBNAAT is the investigation of choice for diagnosing TB in HIV cases

Ans. True Options: B, E; False options: A, C, D

Sputum culture using solid culture is done for all cases from vulnerable high-risk population	F	No, as per revised guidelines, CBNAAT is done for all vulnerable population, high risk groups and further First line – Line probe assay is done to asses for INH resistance pattern as well
TB patients with Rifampicin resistant strains maybe put on MDR regime	T	Yes, correct. RR-TB and MDR-TB are given shorter MDR regime or a MDR–conventional regime
Revised regime for previously treated TB category is 2 HRZES + 1 HRZE + 4 HRE	F	No, for both category I and category II – the new revised treatment plan is: 2HRZE + 4HRE

Contd...

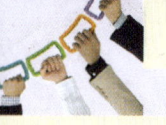

Bedaquiline has been approved for all rifampicin resistant TB cases	F	No, Bedaquiline and Delamanid are reserved drugs for XDR or polydrug resistant strains with unique criteria for initiation of these drugs as: The following patients are eligible for Bedaquiline • MDR TB with resistance to all FQs • MDR TB with resistance to all SLIs • XDR-TB ▪ All FQ and All SLI resistant ▪ All FQ and any SLI resistant ▪ Any FQ and all SLI resistant ▪ Any FQ and Any SLI resistant • Treatment failure of Cat IV –MDR • Treatment failure for XDR TB
CBNAAT is the investigation of choice for diagnosing TB in HIV cases	T	Yes correct. Usually in HIV-TB coinfection, the patients are more likely to develop sputum negative TB and no or negligible X-ray changes. The preferred investigation is CBNAAT

9. Which of following is correct for composition of the adult Fixed dose combination tablets:

a. INH 75 mg
b. Ethambutol 275 mg
c. Rifampicin 400 mg
d. Pyrazinamide 150 mg
e. Rifampicin 300 mg

Ans. True Options: A, B; False options: C, D, E

The correct combination of drugs in the fixed dose combination package is:
HRZE = 75/150/400/275

10. Mark true/false for the following options:

a. The end game strategy for NPSP includes complete cessation of OPV vaccine for community in future
b. The apex laboratory for polio virus isolation is in NIV, Pune
c. Highest chance of VDPV are because of wild polio virus – type 3
d. OPV should not be used during epidemic or outbreaks
e. The fractional dose of IPV is given at 6 and 14 weeks as intradermal injection

Ans. True Options: A, B, E; False options: C, D

The end game strategy for NPSP includes complete cessation of OPV vaccine in future	T	Yes, correct. The risk of Vaccine related and derived virus are major threat to polio eradication.
The apex laboratory for polio virus isolation is in NIV, Pune	T	Yes correct
Highest chance of VDPV are because of wild polio virus – type 3	F	No, Vaccine derived polio virus is mostly from type 2 Vaccine associated paralytic polio is usually seen from type 3
OPV should not be used during epidemic or outbreaks	F	No, OPV can be and should be given during outbreaks, to stop the chain of transmission
The fractional dose of IPV is given at 6 and 14 weeks as intradermal injection	T	Yes correct

11. Mark the following statements as True or False:

a. Pneumococcal conjugate vaccine is given as 0.5 mL SC, in right arm
b. Rota virus is given as 5 drops, oral
c. Hepatitis B vaccine is recombinant vaccine based on HBV core antigen
d. Pentavalent is given as 0.5 mL i/m in anterolateral thigh (LEFT)
e. JE vaccine is given as 0.5 mL SC in left upper arm

Ans. True Options: B, D, E; False options: A, C

Pneumococcal conjugate vaccine is given as 0.5 mL SC, in right arm	F	No, PCV vaccine is given as IM injection in the Antero-lateral Thigh (ALT) – right side
Rota virus is given as 5 drops, oral	T	Yes correct
Hepatitis B vaccine is recombinant vaccine based on HBV core antigen	F	HBV vaccine is recombinant vaccine based on the HBs Ag
Pentavalent is given as 0.5 mL i/m in anterolateral thigh (LEFT)	T	Yes correct
JE vaccine is given as 0.5 mL SC in left upper arm	T	Yes correct

12. Which of the following are true statements, while discussing maternal and infant care problems with health care professionals from international funding agency

a. Preterm causes comprise 44% of all causes of neonatal deaths in India
b. Child death rate is number of deaths aged 1-4 years per 1000 children in same age group
c. RHIME is an advanced form of verbal autopsy
d. Maternal mortality rate is the number of maternal deaths in a given period per 100,000 women of reproductive age group during the same time period
e. 30% of all infant deaths occur within first month of life

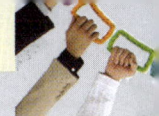

Ans. True Options: A, B, C, D; False options: E

Preterm causes comprise 44% of all causes of neonatal deaths	T	Yes, correct. preterm causes (44%) and intrapartum causes (19%) are the major causes for neonatal deaths in India
Child death rate is number of deaths aged 1-4 years per 1000 children in same age group	T	Yes correct
RHIME is an advanced form of verbal autopsy	T	Yes correct. RHIME is representative, Re-sampled, Routine Household Interview of mortality with Medical Evaluation
Maternal mortality rate is the number of maternal deaths in a given period per 100,000 women of reproductive age group during the same time period	T	Yes correct
30% of all infant deaths occur within first month of life	F	No, 61% of all infant deaths occur within the first month of life.

13. Regarding nutrition and health, mark the following statement as true and false:

a. Maize is a significant source of fat and lysine
b. Fat should be <10% of the total energy in diet
c. Weighing of cooked food is the most widely accepted measure for dietary intake
d. Heart rate is a good indicator for functional assessment of iron levels
e. Massive dose of 17 Lac IU of Vitamin A is given to all children till 5 years in 6 monthly divided doses

Ans. True Options: D, E; False options: A, B, C

Comment:

Maize is a significant source of fat and lysine	F	No, maize is rich in fat but deficient in tryptophan and lysine
Fat should be <10% of the total energy in diet	F	No, fat intake should be 10-30% of the dietary energy. Ideal fat intake is 20% of the dietary energy
Weighing of cooked food is the most widely accepted measure for dietary intake	F	No, weighing of raw or uncooked food I most widely accepted. Weighing of cooked foods is in fact, not practically possible and will be unacceptable by most communities
Heart rate is a good indicator for functional assessment of iron levels	T	Yes, correct
Massive dose of 17 Lac IU of Vitamin A is given to all children till 5 years in 6 monthly divided doses	T	Yes correct. The first dose is given as 100,00 IU at 9 months and subsequently 200,000 IU every six months is given till 5 years of age under the National Vit A deficiency prophylaxis program

Contd...

14. Filariasis has been a key focus area under the WHO's list of neglected tropical diseases in India. Which of the following are true and false regarding the technical component of the national program under NVBDCP

a. Triple drug regime including DEC, praziquantel and albendazole is launched in India
b. The filarial endemicity rate is the percentage of persons examined showing Mf in blood or disease manifestations of both
c. The intensity of infection as public health problem is given by the Microfilarial density rate
d. Membrane filtration method is the most sensitive method for estimation of the low density microfilaremia
e. Amphotericin B is the drug of choice for severe Acute-Dermato-Lymphangio-Adenitis (ADLA)

Ans. True Options: B, C, D; False options: A, E

Comment:

Triple drug regime including DEC, praziquantel and albendazole is launched in India	F	No, the triple drug regime constitutes – DEC + Albendazole + Ivermectin (not praziquantel)
The filarial endemicity rate is the percentage of persons examined showing Mf in blood or disease manifestations of both	T	Yes, correct, see explanation below
The intensity of infection as public health problem is given by the Microfilarial density rate	T	Yes, correct, see explanation below
Membrane filtration method is the most sensitive method for estimation of the low density microfilaremia	T	Yes correct. The thick slide preparation is the most commonly used, but the most sensitive method for detecting low density microfilaremia is by concentration techniques
Amphotericin B is the drug of choice for severe Acute-Dermato-Lymphangio-Adenitis (ADLA)	F	No, triple drug regime is the current choice of drugs for filariasis. for ADLA – I/V Benzyl Penicillin or I/V erythromycin is drug of choice

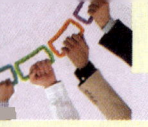

Assessment of Filaria Control Programs:

Clinical parameters:

a. Incidence of acute manifestations – Epididymo-orchitis, adenolymphangitis
b. Prevalence of chronic manifestations – elephantiasis, hydrocele and others

Parasitological parameters:

a. Microfilaria rate: %ages of population with Mf in the peripheral blood
b. Filarial endemicity rate: %of persons showing microfilaria in blood or clinical symptoms or both
c. Microfilarial density: It is the number of Mf per unit volume of blood in the samples from individual persons. it indicates intensity of infection
d. Average infestation rate: It is the average number of Mf per positive slide, made from 20 cu.mm of blood. It indicates prevalence of microfilaria in population

Entomological surveillance

a. Vector density per man hour
b. Percentage of mosquitos positive for all stages of development
c. Infectivity rate: Percentage of mosquito positive for stage III (infective stage) of larva
d. Annual biting rate

15. State which of the following is true or false:

a. Early diagnosis is a part of secondary prevention
b. Immunization with yellow fever vaccine is a typical example for primordial prevention
c. Rabies post-exposure prophylaxis is a typical example for primary prevention
d. Public health programs target the whole population and decrease the risk factors to prevent disease is an example for primordial prevention
e. Screening for breast cancer using mammography is a typical example for primary prevention

Ans. True Options: A, C, D; False options: B, E

Comment:

Early diagnosis is a part of secondary prevention	T	Yes, correct
Immunization with yellow fever vaccine is a typical example for primordial prevention	F	No, immunization is specific protection and a typical example to prevent the disease – hence a primary prevention
Rabies post-exposure prophylaxis is a typical example for primary prevention	T	Rabies vaccination – prevents the disease in case of dog bite (which is a risk factor) – a primary prevention
National Vitamin A Prophylaxis programs target the whole population and decrease the risk factors to prevent disease is an example for primary prevention	T	Yes correct. Preventing the disease is primary prevention
Screening for breast cancer using mammography is a typical example for primary prevention	F	Screening for breast cancer is a type of secondary prevention where early diagnosis is done to prevent any long term sequel or complications due to breast cancer

MATCH THE FOLLOWING TYPE

Each question shall have two columns with four items in one column (A) that need to be matched appropriately with the best alternative available in the next column (B).

Correct answer: +1/4 for each alternative and Incorrect answer: −1/4 for each alternative

16. Match list I (Name of vaccine) with list II (Type of vaccine) and select the correct answer using the codes given below the lists:

Column A - Name of vaccine	Column B - Type of vaccine
A. Fractional IPV	1. Polyvalent vaccine
B. bOPV	2. Conjugate vaccine
C. Measles vaccine	3. Toxoids vaccine
D. Td	4. Live vaccine
	5. Recombinant
	6. Killed vaccine

Ans. A6, B4, C4, D3

17. Match the following:

Column A - Activities	Column B - Levels of preventions
A. Yellow fever vaccine for students attending conference in Africa	1. Primordial prevention
B. Screening for hypertension	2. Primary level prevention
C. Surgical intervention for claw hand in leprosy	3. Secondary level prevention
D. Preventing emergence of overweight to prevent coronary artery disease	4. Tertiary level prevention
E. Providing dark goggles for welders in factory	
F. Providing condoms to commercial sex workers	

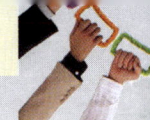

Ans. A2, B3, C4, D1, E2, F2

18. Match list I (Diseases) with list II (Toxins) and select the correct answer using the codes given below the lists:

List I (Diseases) List II (Toxins)

Column A – Diseases	Column B - Toxins
A. Epidemic dropsy	1. Ergot alkaloid
B. Neurolathyrism	2. Pyrrolizidine alkaloid
C. Hepatic carcinoma	3. Sanguinarine
D. Endemic ascites	4. Avidin
	5. Aflatoxins
	6. Beta-oxalyl amino alanine

Ans. A3, B6, C5, D2

19. Match list I (Antitubercular drugs) with list II (adverse effects)

Column A – Drugs	Column B – Adverse effects
A. Ethambutol	1. Hepatotoxicity, hyperuricemia
B. Rifampicin	2. Retrobulbar neuritis
C. Pyrazinamide	3. Nystagmus, vestibular damage
D. Streptomycin	4. Alopecia
	5. Joint pains
	6. Thrombocytopenia, hepatotoxicity and nephrotoxicity

Ans. A2, B6, C1, D3

20. Match column A with Colum B

Column A – Vector	Column B – Disease transmitted
A. Culex mosquito	1. Relapsing fever
B. Sand fly	2. Yellow fever
C. Aedes mosquito	3. Chagas disease
D. Head louse	4. Japanese encephalitis
	5. Kala-azar
	6. Malaria

Ans. A4, B5, C2, D1

Ref: Park 25ed, pg 832, 835, 837

Remember:

Mosquito borne disease

Types of mosquito	Disease
• Anopheles	Malaria Filaria (not in India)
• Culex	Bancroftian filariasis Japanese encephalitis West Nile fever Viral arthritis (epidemic/polyarthritis)
• Aedes	Yellow fever (not in India) Dengue Dengue haemorrhagic fever Chikungunya fever Chikungunya haemorrhagic fever Rift valley fever Filaria (not in India)
• Mansonoides	Malayan (Brugian) filariasis Chikungunya fever

Louse borne disease

Disease	Causative agent
• Epidemic typhus	Rickettssia prowazeki
• Relapsing fever	Borrelia recurrentis
• Trench fever	Rickettssia equintana
• Dermatitis	Due to scratching and secondary infection

Sand fly borne disease

Species	Diseases carried
Phlebotomus argentipes	Kala-azar
Phlebotomus papatasi	Sandfly fever
	Oriental sore
Phlebotomus sergenti	Oriental sore
S. punjabensis	Sandfly fever

21. Match the milestone for Maternal and child health program in India

Column A – National program	Column B – Year of program implementation
a. CSSM	1. 1952
b. NRHM	2. 1992
c. RMNCH+A	3. 1997
d. INAP	4. 2005
	5. 2013
	6. 2014-15

Ans. A2, B4, C5, D6

Ref: Park, 25th ed Pg 481

1992 – CSSM (child survival and safe motherhood program)
2005 – NRHM (national rural health mission)
2013 – RMNCH+A (Reproductive, maternal, neonatal, child health + adolescent)
2014 – INAP (India newborn action plan)

22. Match the following pathogens with the characteristic respiratory illness caused

Column A – Pathogen	Column B – Disease caused
a. Resp. syncytial virus	1. Atypical pneumonia
b. Rhinovirus	2. Acute epiglottitis

Contd...

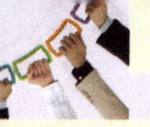

Column A – Pathogen	Column B – Disease caused
c. H influenza type B	3. Severe Bronchiolitis and pneumonia
d. Mycoplasma pneumonia	4. Lung Abscess
	5. Common cold
	6. Farmers lung disease

Ans. **A3, B5, C2, D1**

Ref: Park 25th ed. Pg 181

23. Match column A with Colum B for the demographic indicators and the definitions

Column A – Definition	Column B – Demographic indicator
a. Total number of daughters female would bear during her entire life assuming the current fertility and mortality trends	1. General fertility rate
b. Total number of children per 1000 women in reproductive age group	2. General marital fertility rate
c. Average number of children born to a married woman if she experiences the current fertility pattern throughout her reproductive span	3. Crude birth rate
d. Average number of girls that would be born to a woman if she experiences the current fertility pattern throughout her reproductive span assuming no mortality	4. Net reproduction rate
	5. Gross reproduction rate
	6. Total marital fertility rate

Ans. **A4, B1, C6, D5**

Ref: Park 25th ed, 540

24. Match column A with Colum B for the research scenario and the statistical measure to be used

Column A – Research scenario	Column B – Statistical measure
a. Survival analysis	1. Independent sample t-test
b. Comparing two groups with non-parametric data	2. Kolmogorov smirnov analysis
c. Check for level of agreement between groups	3. Wilcoxan rank sum test
d. Comparing independent groups with ordinal, qualitative data	4. Chi square test
	5. Kaplan Meier curve
	6. Kappa statistical analysis

Ans. **A5, B4, C6, D3**

Comment:

Statistical measure	Used for:
Independent sample t-test	Comparing two independent groups with parametric (Quantitative) data
Kolmogorov smirnov analysis	For assessment of the data distribution – to check for normal distribution in the data
Wilcoxan rank sum test	Used to compare independent groups with ordinal (non-parametric) data
Chi square test	Used to compare two (or maybe more) groups with non-parametric (qualitative) data
Kaplan Meier curve	Used for survival analysis
Kappa statistical analysis	To compare the levels of agreement between independent groups

25. Match column A with Colum B for social groups and definition of groups

Column A – Definition	Column B – Social groups
a. The group of people are under a leader and they follow without emotions or questions	1. Family
b. A group of families living together in an undefined geographical space	2. Mob
c. A group of people with common interest with a leader, who forces the members into action with emotional element	3. Band
d. Group of people come together temporarily with a common interest	4. Herd
	5. Village
	6. Crowd

Ans. **A4, B3, C2, D6**

Ref: Park 25th ed, pg 738

Village: A small collection of people permanently settled in a defined geographical area

26. Match column A with Colum B for the various types of government in modern societies

Column A – Political organisation	Column B – Definition
a. Socialistic	1. Head of state is chief or kingship
b. Democracy	2. Country is ruled by a family group
c. Oligarchy	3. The ruler is in absolute power
d. Monarchy	4. The production and wealth of nation are controlled by the state led by an authority

Contd...

Column A – Political organisation	Column B – Definition
	5. The leader is an officiating member representing another political organisation
	6. Government by the people, of the people

Ans. A4, B6, C2, D1

Ref: Park 25th ed, pg 738

Examples:

Democracy – India, US, Canada
Autocracy - ruler is in absolute power – Jordan, Ethiopia
Monarchy – UK, Nepal
Socialistic - China, Poland
Oligarchy - Thailand, Cambodia, Saudi Arabia

27. Match column A with Colum B for the various types Rickettsial diseases

Column A – Disease	Column B – Rickettsial organisms
a. Epidemic typhus	1. R. conorii
b. Murine Typhus	2. R. akari
c. Scrub Typhus	3. R. prowazekii
d. Indian Tick Typhus	4. R. rickettsii
	5. R. typhi
	6. R. tsutsugamushi

Ans. A3, B5, C6, D1

Ref: Park 25ed, pg 327

28. Match column A with Colum B for the various types management principles

Column A – Detail of activity	Column B – Management principle
a. A detailed management principle for analysis of sequence of events to be undertaken	1. Critical path method
b. A management principle for inventory control and stock management	2. PERT (Program evaluation and review technique)
c. Social benefits of a program in terms of output/results achieved	3. Cost benefit Analysis
d. Grouping of activities into smaller program objectives for better budgetary allocation decisions	4. FIFO (First-in, First out) principle
	5. Planning, programming budgeting System
	6. Cost effective analysis

Ans. A2, B4, C6, D5

Ref: Park 25th ed, pg 934

Network analysis: Branch deals with proper planning, drafting, testing, implementation and execution of a series of activities oriented towards a common goal. It is a graphic plan of all events to be completed in order to reach an end objective.

Critical Path method: It is a strategic quantitative method for network analysis. ***Keyword***: takes into account most time taking activity and allows to analyse activity as per time consumed.

PERT (Program evaluation and review technique): It is a management technique which makes possible more detailed planning and more comprehensive supervision.

Cost-Benefit Analysis: Economic benefits of any program are compared with cost of that program.

Drawback: Benefits in health field as a result of a particular program can't always be expressed in monetary means.

Cost-Effective Analysis: Here, benefit is expressed in terms of results achieved e.g. no. of lives saved & no. of days free from disease.

Planning Programming Budgeting System (PPBS): It calls for grouping of activities into programs related to each objective, so as to help decision makers to allocate resources efficiently.

Zero Budget Approach: Starting from a Zero Base of no funds for a program, every rupee is sanctioned, even for ongoing program.

29. Match the following:

Mosquito	Breeding place
a. Anopheles	1. Water with Aquatic vegetation
b. Culex	2. Cool, damp places
c. Aedes	3. Artificial collection of water
d. Mansonia	4. Clean, stagnant water
	5. Polluted, long standing water
	6. Faeces, sewage

Ans. A4, B5, C3, D1

SEQUENTIAL ARRANGEMENT TYPE

Each question shall have a list of items that need to be arranged sequentially or in order as indicated

Correct answer (full sequence correct): +01, Incorrect Answer (Sequence incorrect): –01

30. Consider the following stages:

1. Low stationary
2. Late expanding
3. Early expanding
4. Declining

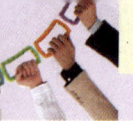

Arrange the stages according to the demographic gap. The stage with highest demographic gap to the stage with least demographic gap

Ans. 3 > 2 > 1 > 4

31. Arrange the phases of the operations research in ascending order, with the first activity to the last activity
1. Analysis of data
2. Formulation of problem
3. Choosing optimal solution
4. Implementing solution

Ans: 2 > 1 > 3 > 4

Ref: Park 25th ed, pg 753

Comment:

Phases in Operational Research
- Formulation of problem
- Collection of data
- Analysis of data
- Deriving solution
- Choosing optimal solution
- Testing of solution
- Implementing solution

32. Arrange the following in sequence for protein indicators with maximum usefulness for the public health program:
1. Protein efficiency ratio
2. Protein digestibility coefficient amino acid score
3. Net protein Utilization
4. Digestible indispensable amino acid score best indicator first and the least important indicator as last

Ans. 4 > 2 > 3 > 1

33. Arrange the following research designs in order of highest level of evidence of causality to the lowest level of evidence.
1. Case control study designs
2. Case series
3. Meta-analysis
4. Multifactorial study designs

Ans. 3 > 4 > 1 > 2

The order for hierarchy of evidence for establishment of causal risk factors is:
- Descriptive study designs - case study/case series – <u>most basic study designs</u>
- Analytical study designs
  - Cross sectional study
  - Case control study
  - Cohort study
- Clinical trials
  - Single group, quasi experimental trials
  - Randomised clinical trials
  - Multi-factorial clinical trials
- Evidence-based medicine designs
  - Systematic reviews
  - Meta-analysis - <u>best study to asses for causation</u>

34. Arrange the following steps from start of interview to finish of interview:
1. Encouragement
2. Recording
3. Securing rapport
4. Probe questions

Ans. 3 > 4 > 1 > 2

Ref: Park 25th ed, pg 751

The sequence of steps for conducting an interview are:
- Establishing contact
- Starting an interview
- Securing rapport
- Recall
- Probe questions
- Encouragement
- Guiding interview
- Recording
- Closing interview
- Report

35. Arrange the following as per incubation period, with the shortest incubation period to the longest incubation period
1. Cholera
2. Hepatitis A
3. Scrub typhus
4. Yellow fever

Ans. 1 > 4 > 3 > 2

Ref: Park 25ed, 241, 253, 327

Disease	**Incubation period (average)**
Cholera	1-2 days
Yellow fever	3-6 days
Scrub typhus	10-12 days
Hepatitis A	10-50 days

36. Arrange the following as leading cause of death for children in 1-4 years age group:
1. Congenital anomalies
2. Diarrhoeal diseases
3. Respiratory infections, pneumonia
4. Accidents and other injuries

Ans: 2 > 3 > 4 > 1

The leading cause of death in 1-4 years age groups are:
- Diarrhoeal diseases
- Respiratory infections
- Malnutrition
- Infectious diseases – as measles, pertussis
- Other febrile illness
- Accidents and injuries

37. Arrange the following steps from first to last step in a rapid sand water filtration system.
1. Sedimentation
2. Rapid mixing
3. Coagulation
4. Filtration

Ans: 3 > 2 > 1 > 4

Ref: Park 25th ed, pg 773

Steps for water filtration are:
- Coagulation – first step. water is mixed with chemical coagulant (as Alum)
- Rapid mixing – violent agitation in the mixing chamber
- Flocculation – slow and gentle mixing for 30 mins in flocculation chamber
- Sedimentation – the coagulated water is allowed to rest for 2-6 hours and the sediment is removed before subjecting to water sand filter
- Filtration – water is subjected to rapid sand filter room

38. Arrange the vaccines to be kept in an ILR with first - the vaccines at top followed by vaccines to be kept at bottom of ILR

1. Rota virus vaccine
2. OPV vaccine
3. Measles vaccine
4. Pentavalent vaccine

Ans. 2 > 3 > 1 > 4

The vaccine sensitivity

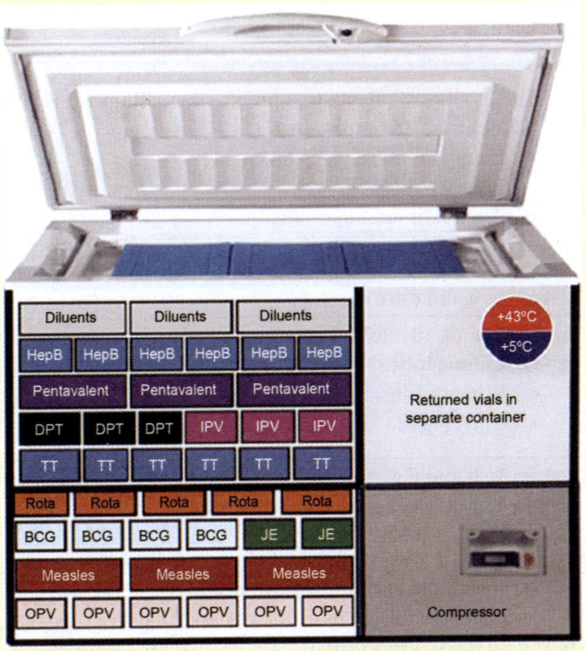

39. Arrange the following as per year of target achievement under the national health policy 2017

1. IMR < 28
2. Increase life expectancy to 70 years
3. Lymphatic filariasis elimination
4. Swachh Bharat mission

Ans. 3 > 1 > 4 > 2

Lymphatic filariasis and kala-azar elimination	2017
Leprosy elimination	2018
IMR < 28	2019
Safe water and sanitation to all (swach bharat mission)	2020
Life expectancy	2025

40. Consider the following developmental milestones and put in chronological sequence (from earliest to latest)

1. First words
2. Crawling
3. Begins to explore
4. Ability to smile

Ans. 4 > 2 > 1 > 3

Ref: Park 25th ed, pg 597

The correct chronological order (from the earliest to the latest) of these milestones is:

1. Ability to smile	6-8 weeks
2. Crawling	9-10 months
3. Begins to explore	18-21 months
4. First words	10-11 months

MULTIPLE COMPLETION TYPE

Each question/statement shall have four alternatives/statements of which one or more may be correct and need to be marked using the following key:

1. If a, b, c are correct
2. If a and c are correct
3. If b and d are correct
4. If all four (a, b, c, & d) are correct

Correct answer: +01 and Incorrect answer: −1/4

41. Tobacco smoking during pregnancy leads to:

a. Low-birthweight baby
b. Placental insufficiency
c. Stillbirth
d. Cephalopelvic disproportion

Ans. 1. a, b, c are correct

- A smoking women has increased carbon monoxide level, which can affect fetal and maternal Hb. Pregnant women who smoke are at risk for small infants (by an average of 250 g), growth-retarded infants, or both, with increased prenatal mortality. The vasoconstriction action of nicotine causes reduced perfusion of the placenta.
- Maternal complications of pregnancy associated with cigarette smoking:
  - Premature rupture of membrane,
  - Abruptio placentae and placenta previa,
  - Spontaneous abortion,
  - Preterm delivery,
  - Perinatal mortality;
  - Small for gestational age,
  - Infant respiratory distress syndrome,
  - Sudden infant death syndrome.

42. Which of the following should be stored in a deep freezer in order to preserve their potency?

a. BCG vaccine
b. Oral polio vaccine
c. Measles vaccine
d. DPT vaccine

Ans. 1. a, b, c are correct

DPT should never be frozen

43. Consider the following statements regarding poliomyelitis:

a. It is primarily an infection of alimentary tract but may affect the central nervous system in some cases
b. Most cases of VAPP are due to mutations in the extra OPV doses
c. It occurs sporadically, endemically, or in epidemic form
d. It occurs mostly in the age group of 5 to 10 years

Which of the above statements are correct?

AIIMS New Pattern 2019 Model Questions

Ans. 2. a and c are correct

Explanation:

- Poliomyelitis is primarily an infection of the human alimentary tract, but virus may infect the central nervous system in a very small (about 1%) percentage.
- Poliomyelitis can occur sporadically, endemically, or epidemically.
- In India, polio is essentially a disease of infancy and childhood. About 50% cases are reported in infancy. The most vulnerable age is between 6 months and 3 years.
- The VDPV poses threat for polio and is due to mutations. (Usually due to type 2 wild polio virus)

44. Consider the following measures:

a. Triple scan for fetal anomalies
b. Prevention of consanguineous marriages
c. Avoidance of teratogenic drugs
d. Avoiding late marriage

The measures which fit in with the primary level prevention of genetic disorders include:

Ans. 3. b and d are correct

45. Consider the following statements:
Symposium method of health education is characterized by:

a. Series of speeches on a selected topic
b. Presentation of different aspects of a topic by 3 or 4 experts
c. Chairperson making a comprehensive summary at the end of the session
d. Extensive Discussion among the symposium members

Which of the above statements are correct?

Ans. 1. a, b, c are correct

46. Consider the following statements: Vitamin A administration reduces the

a. Severity and mortality due to measles
b. Kolpik's spots appear on buccal. Mucosa on 3rd day of appearance of rash
c. Diarrhoea are the most common complications following measles
d. Children with measles infection should also be actively immunized to protect against future episodes

Which of these statements is/are true with regard to measles?

Ans. 2. a and c both are correct

47. Consider the following statements:
Tuberculosis in HIV-positive individuals is characterized by more:

1. Frequent negative sputum smears.
2. False-Negative tuberculin test result.
3. Extrapulmonary tuberculosis.
4. X-ray usually is not conclusive and show non-specific changes

Cavitating lesions in lungs as shown by chest X-ray which of the statements given above are correct?

Ans. 4. All options are correct

48. Which of the following are 'health care utilization indicators:

a. Proportion of children Fully immunized
b. Couple protection rate
c. Average length of stay
d. Bed turnover ratio

Ans. 4. All are utilization indicators

Ref: Park 25th ed. pg 27

The health care utilization indicators are:

a. Proportion of children Fully immunized
b. Proportion of ANC in pregnant females
c. Couple protection rate
d. Bed occupancy rates
e. Average length of stay
f. Bed turnover ratio

49. Which of the following disease is Louse borne:

a. Epidemic typhus
b. Relapsing fever
c. Trench fever
d. KFD

Ans. 1. a, b, c, are correct

Ref: Park 25th ed. pg 837

50. The yellow category, under the Biomedical waste Guidelines, 2016, contains:

a. Empty Blood transfusion bags
b. Empty Urine bags
c. Animal tissue and excreta
d. Discarded syringes

Ans. 2. a and c are correct

51. Which of the following food products have a medium Glycaemic index

a. Whole grains
b. Basmati rice
c. Corn flakes
d. Sucrose

Ans. 3. b and d are correct

Ref: Park 25th ed. pg 671

52. Which of the following are prevalence criteria for xeropthalmia as public health problem

a. Night blindness more than 1% in high risk population (6 months to 6 years)
b. Bitot spots more than 0.5% in high risk population (6 months to 6 years)
c. Corneal ulcers in more than 0.05% in high risk population (6 months to 6 years)
d. Low S. Retinol (less than 10 mcg/dL) in more than 5% in high risk population (6 months to 6 years)

Ans. 4. All are correct options

Ref: Park 25th ed. pg 673

53. Effective air temperature includes

a. Air humidity
b. Air movement
c. Cooling power of air
d. Radiant heat

Ans. 1. a, b, c, are correct

Ref: Park 25th ed. pg 792

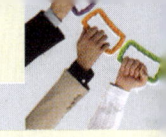

54. A study was conducted for assessment of haemoglobin levels in two villages. The study revealed a mean Hb 10.56 ± 1.5 gm% in village A and 11.2 ± 0.9 gm% in village B. The data was statistically compared and analysed using an unpaired t-test and the p-value was found to be 0.4 with 95% confidence limits. This may be interpreted as:

a. Both the village population have a non-significant variation between the haemoglobin levels
b. The p-value 0.4 denotes a negative association and that village B has better Hb levels compared to Village A
c. The analysis show that both the villages belong to the same population and that there is no difference between the Hb Levels
d. The data cannot be compared as different age groups could be a possibility

Ans. 2. a and c are correct statements

Ref: Park 25th ed. pg 914

REASON ASSERTION TYPE

Each question shall have two statements: Assertion (A) and Reason (B) connected by the term "because". The appropriate answer should be marked using the following key:

a. Both Assertion and Reasons are independently true/correct statements and the Reason is the correct explanation for the Assertion
b. Both Assertion and Reasons are independently true/correct statements, but the Reason is not the correct explanation for the Assertion
c. Assertion is independently a true/correct statement, but the Reasons is independently a false/incorrect statement
d. Assertion is independently a false/incorrect statement, but the Reasons is independently a true/correct statement
e. Both Assertion and Reasons are independently false/incorrect statements

In the above question Statement (A) is the Assertion and Statement (B) is the Reason that explains the Assertion (Statement A)
Correct answer: +01 and Incorrect answer: –1/4

55. Assertion (A): Foreign body aspiration usually lodges in right lower lobe.
Reason (R): The right lower lobe bronchus is in line with trachea.

Ans. (c) A is true but R is false

56. Assertion (A): Glucose is an important component of Oral Rehydration Solution (WHO)
Reason (R): Glucose provides calories for the child rendered weak by diarrhea.

Ans. (c) A is true but R is false

Explanation:
Oral fluid therapy is based on the observation that glucose given orally enhances the intestinal absorption of salt and water and is capable of correcting the electrolyte and water deficit. The inclusion of tri sodium citrate in place of sodium bicarbonate: (i) made the product more stable and (ii) use of ORS citrate results less stool output.

57. Assertion (A): Iron-deficiency anemia is more common in prolonged cow's milk fed babies.
Reason (R): Cow's milk has high phytates impairing absorption of iron.

Ans. (c) A is true but R is false

Explanation:
Cow's milk is a poor source of iron. Cow's milk allergy may cause occult gastrointestinal bleeding. Breast milk is relatively better source of iron. Hb level may remain normal in babies fed exclusively on breast for 5 to 6 months. Phytates, phosphates, calcium, salts (oxalates carbonates), milk, and egg in the diet inhibit iron absorption.

58. Assertion (A): While breastfeeding her child, a mother requires 150 g of green leafy vegetables per day.
Reason (R): Lactation requires 500 to 1,000 calories extra per day as compared to a non-pregnant adult female.

Ans. (b) Both A and R is true but R is NOT a correct explanation of A

RDA of green leafy vegetable
Adult man and child 1 to 3 years—40 g
Child (>4 years) and woman (heavy work)—50 g
Woman (moderate and sedentary)— 100 g
A healthy mother will produce about 500—800 ml milk/day to feed her infant with about 500 kcal/day. This requires about 600 kcal/day for the mother. For this, store of about 5 kg fat during pregnancy is essential to make up any nutritional deficit during lactation.

59. Assertion (A): Pulse polio immunization (PPI) requires all children being administered OPV at the same time.
Reason (R): It is easier to cover all the children at one point of time.

Ans. (b) Both A and R is true but R is NOT a correct explanation of A

PPIs are when oral polio vaccine is given to children up to 5 years of age in the country on a single day regardless to previous immunizations (PPIs are extra doses with supplement) as two rounds, 4 to 6 weeks apart during low transmission season of polio.

60. Assertion (A): Guinea worm disease has been eradicated from India.
Reason (R): Last case of guinea worm disease was reported from Rajasthan in July, 1996.

Ans. (a) Both A and R are true and R is the correct explanation of A

National Guinea Eradication Programme (1984): As zero cases were reported since August 1996, the International Commission for Certification of Dracunculiasis Eradication recommended that India is free of dracunculiasis transmission in February 2000.
In India, last reported case was in July, 1996. On 3 years completion of zero incidence, India was declared free of guinea worm disease.

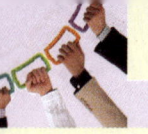

61. Assertion (A): In tetanus, herd immunity does not protect the individual.
Reason (R): Tetanus vaccine is a toxoid vaccine.

Ans. (b) Both A and R are individually true but R is not the correct explanation of A

62. Assertion (A): India is in the late expanding phase of the demographic cycle.
Reason (R): Birth rate in India is declining rapidly.

Ans. (b) Both A and R are individually true but R is not the correct explanation of A

63. Assertion (A): Use of soap water and disinfectants should be avoided in flushing where septic tank is used.
Reason (R); In India, septic tanks are designed to allow a retention period of 24 hours.

Ans. (b) Both A and R is individually true but R is not the correct explanation of A

Explanation:

Some important points regarding septic tank:

- Capacity: 20–30 gallon or 2.5–5 Cu ft per person
- Minimum capacity: 500 gallon
- Length: 2 × breadth
- Depth: 1.5–2 m (5–7 ft)
- Liquid depth: 1.2 m (4 ft)
- Air space: Minimum 30 cm (12 inches)
- Bottom shape: Sloping toward inlet end
- Retention period: 24 hours
- Digestion: Two stages—1st is anaerobic in septic tank proper and 2nd stage is aerobic, outside the tank is subsoil.

64. Assertion (A): BCG vaccination is capable of converting lepromin test from negative to positive.
Reason (R): Lepromin test is not a diagnostic test.

Ans. (a) Both A and R are individually true and R is the correct explanation of A

Lepromin test is not a diagnostic test.
The two disadvantages are:

- Falsely Positive result in healthy
- Falsely Negative result in lepromatous and near-lepromatous cases.

Key points regarding lepromin test:

Test is done by injecting 1 mL of lepromin into inner aspect of forearm.

Reaction to be read in 48 hours (early) and 21 days Late

65. Assertion: Bias are systematic errors arising from the study
Reason: Bias are mostly because of sampling variations

Codes:

a. Both A and R are true and R is the correct explanation of A
b. Both A and R are true but R is NOT a correct explanation of A
c. A is true but R is false
d. A is false but R is true

Ans. (c) A is true but R is false

66. Assertion: India is seen to have a demographic dividend
Reason: Late expanding stage will have a higher number of economically productive population and the dependency ratios start decreasing trend

Codes:

a. Both A and R are true and R is the correct explanation of A
b. Both A and R are true but R is NOT a correct explanation of A
c. A is true but R is false
d. A is false but R is true

Ans. (a) Both A and R are true and R is the correct explanation of A

67. Assertion: Hookworm infections are endemic in India, south Asia, tropical Africa
Reason: The hookworms live in damp, sandy and friable soil with decaying vegetation.

Codes:

a. Both A and R are true and R is the correct explanation of A
b. Both A and R are true but R is NOT a correct explanation of A
c. A is true but R is false
d. A is false but R is true

Ans. (a) Both A and R are true, and R is the correct explanation of A

68. Assertion: Cholera vaccine is not used as mass vaccination for prevention of cholera under national health program
Reason: Cholera has many types of carrier including healthy carrier, which are major reservoirs and sources of infection to the community

Codes:

a. Both A and R are true, and R is the correct explanation of A
b. Both A and R are true, but R is NOT a correct explanation of A
c. A is true but R is false
d. A is false but R is true

Ans. (b) Both A and R are true, but R is NOT a correct explanation of A

69. Assertion: Human milk has adequate source of iron till 6 months of life in a child
Reason: Human milk has highest lactose content

Codes:

a. Both A and R are true, and R is the correct explanation of A
b. Both A and R are true, but R is NOT a correct explanation of A
c. A is true but R is false
d. A is false but R is true

Ans. (b) Both A and R are true, but R is NOT a correct explanation of A

Most Recent Questions 2019

(Includes AIIMS May 2019 and Recent Question 2019)

1. **Study design of choice for testing circadian variation of fat content in expressed breast milk of mothers of preterm infant:** ***(AIIMS May 2019)***
   a. Case control b. Prospective cohort
   c. Ecological Study d. Cross sectional
2. **Confounding is removed by all except** ***(AIIMS May 2019)***
   a. Matching b. Randomization
   c. Restriction d. Blinding
3. **Cross product ratio is calculated in which study:** ***(Recent Question 2019)***
   a. Case control study b. Cohort study
   c. Cross sectional study d. Ecological study
4. **Confounding factor is defined as:** ***(Recent Question 2019)***
   a. Factor associated with both the exposure and the disease & is distributed unequally in study and control groups
   b. Factor associated with exposure only & is distributed unequally in study and control groups.
   c. Factor associated with both the exposure and the disease & is distributed equally in study and control groups
   d. Factor associated with the disease & is distributed equally in study and control groups
5. **Probability of a person with positive test result having the disease is given by:** ***(Recent Question 2019)***
   a. Sensitivity b. Specificity
   c. Positive predictive value d. Negative predictive value
6. **In a study with a new treatment, there were reported 36 deaths/ treatment failures out of sample of 120. With a new treatment, 26 treatment failures were reported from a sample size of 130. How many patients should be treated to avert 1 death?** ***(AIIMS May 2019)***
   a. 100 b. 10
   c. 250 d. 160
7. **A study was done to assess the risk factors for Breast cancer in 100 females from urban cities. A statistical graph and analysis is shown below.** ***(AIIMS May 2019)***

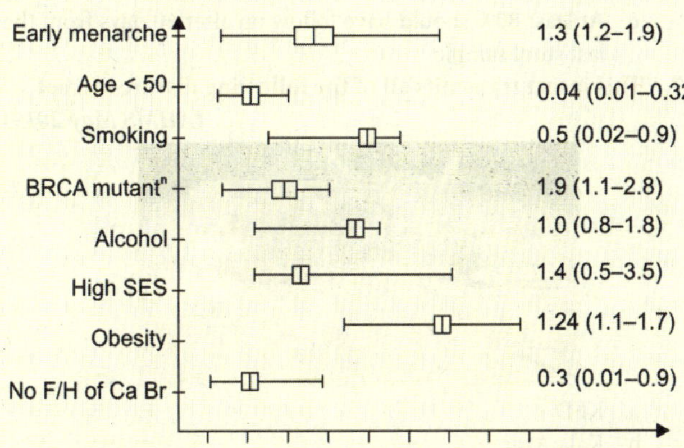

How many risk factors may be ascertained from the statistical analysis of the research
   a. 3 b. 4
   c. 5 d. 6

8. **Look at the image below find the correct corresponding option** ***(AIIMS May 2019)***

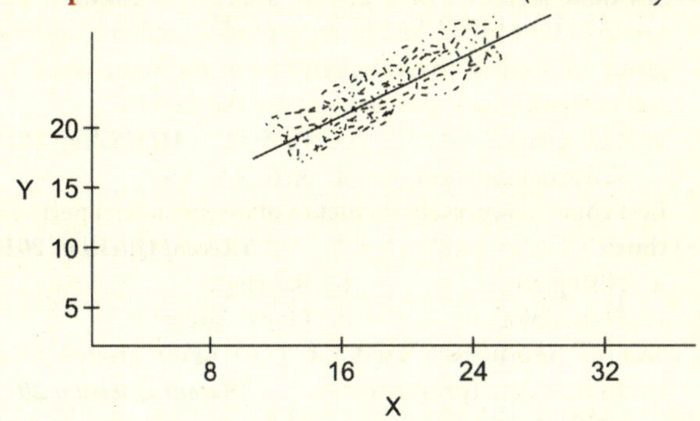

   a. y = 10 + x b. x = 10 + y
   c. y = 11 + 2x d. x = 11 + 2y
9. **The bone mineral density along with gestational age is plotted from two different researches. Which of the following is true for the relation between BMD and gestational age** ***(AIIMS May 2019)***

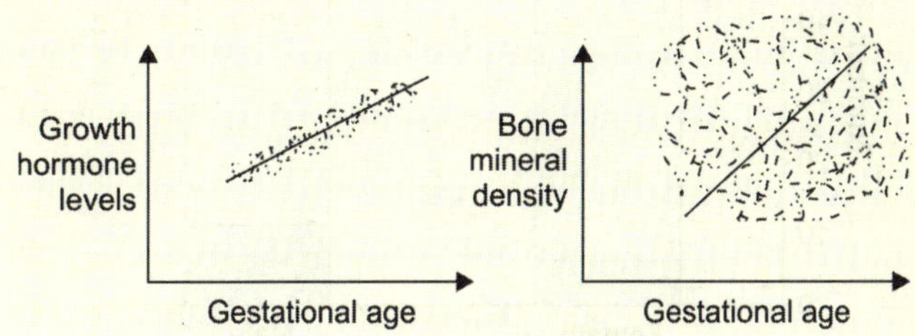

   a. Strength of relation is same in A and B
   b. Strength of relation is more in A than in B
   c. Strength of relation is more in B than in A
   d. Variation in variables is more with A than with B
10. **A study was conducted to assess the effect of an intervention for certain disease. The p-values for two similar researches A and B with 95% confidence limits, was found to be 0.02 and 0.001 respectively using test 'x' and 'y' with a control group. Based on preliminary analysis, the results may be interpreted as:** ***(AIIMS May 2019)***
   a. Study A is more precise than Study B and the population size in study A is higher than Study B
   b. Study B is more precise than Study A and the population size in study B is higher than study B
   c. Both study A and B show a significant variation and both interventions have similar statistical significance
   d. Both 'x' and 'y' show a significant variation, but study-B is more significant than Study-A
   e. Data is not sufficient to compare the investigations

   Which of the following options are correct?
   a. If a, b, c are correct
   b. If a and c are correct
   c. If b and d are correct
   d. If all four (a, b, c, & d) are correct

Ans.

1. b
2. d
3. a
4. a
5. c
6. b
7. a
8. c
9. b
10. c

11. A study was conducted on two different sample. The sample A had the mean value 110 ± 11 while the sample B had mean value of 18 ± 3. which of the following statement is correct: *(AIIMS May 2019)*
a. Sample A more than Sample B
b. Sample B more than Sample A
c. Variation in sample B is approximately 4 times that in sample A
d. It cannot be ascertained from information provided

12. Seasonal variation of a disease studied in children in a group in June to July and in august to September in another group of similar characteristics from the same area. The test of significance used to compare the data is: *(AIIMS May 2019)*
a. Chi square b. Paired t
c. Wilcoxan rank test d. ANOVA

13. Best chart to represent incidence of disease over a period of time: *(Recent Question 2019)*
a. Histogram b. Bar chart
c. Scatter plot d. Line diagram

14. Test of significance used for 2 or more groups using qualitative data (proportions): *(Recent Question 2019)*
a. ANOVA b. Chi-square test
c. Fischer's test d. Paired T test

15. Identify the graph *(Recent Question 2019)*

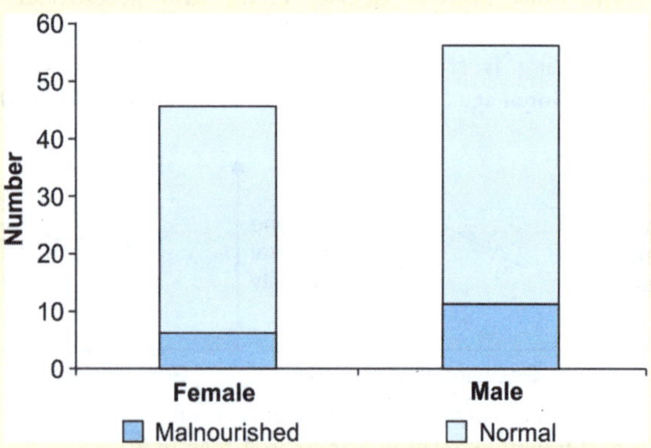

a. Histogram b. Simple bar chart
c. Multiple bar chart d. Component bar chart

16. Test of significance used for 2 independent means is: *(Recent Question 2019)*
a. Paired t test
b. Unpaired t test
c. ANOVA
d. Chi-square test

17. In a normal curve what is the area that comes under 1 standard deviation: *(Recent Question 2019)*
a. 50%
b. 68%
c. 95%
d. 100%

18. Permanent Hardness of water is not due to: *(Recent Question 2019)*
a. Calcium Sulfate
b. Calcium Chloride
c. Magnesium Nitrates
d. Magnesium Bicarbonate

19. Chlorine disinfection of water is due to which ions? *(Recent Question 2019)*
a. Hypochlorite ions
b. Hydrogen ions
c. Hypochlorous acid
d. Hydrochloric acid

20. Under the water supply program, which of the following statement is false: *(Recent Question 2019)*
a. At least 1 hand pump (safe water spot) for 250 population
b. At least 40 liters PCD in rural area
c. At least 140 L in urban areas with sewage
d. It is a problem village, if there is no safe water within 1 km

21. Which engineered water purification system is the most effective for elimination of *cryptosporidium parvum*? *(Recent Question 2019)*
a. Flocculation b. Disinfection
c. Boiling d. Filtration

22. How much land is required for a population of 10000, to have a deep trench: *(Recent Question 2019)*
a. 1 acre b. 2 acre
c. 3 acre d. 5 acre

23. In a town of 20,000 population, total 456 births were there in a year out of which 56 were dead born. The total deaths were 247 out of which 56 deaths were within first 28 days of life and another 34 had died after 28 days and before completing the first birthday. Calculate the infant mortality rate of the area. *(AIIMS May 2019)*
a. 225 b. 197
c. 392 d. 344

24. Regarding functions of ASHA, all are true except? *(AIIMS May 2019)*
a. Malaria Slide preparation
b. Facilitate Immunization
c. Accompany pregnant females to hospital
d. Spread awareness about contraception

25. Which of the following comes under concurrent list: *(Recent Question 2019)*
a. International immigration for quarantine
b. Prevention of communicable diseases
c. Mines and oilfield workers rules
d. Establishment and maintenance of drug standards

26. State which of the following statements is true: *(AIIMS May 2019)*
a. Surveillance only till 5 years of age
b. Sample collected for suspected AFP even after 15 years
c. At least one case of non-polio AFP should be detected annually per 100000 population
d. Stool specimen should reach the laboratory within 72 hours
e. At least 80% should have follow up after 60 days from the last stool sample

27. This insect transmits all of the following diseases except *(AIIMS May 2019)*

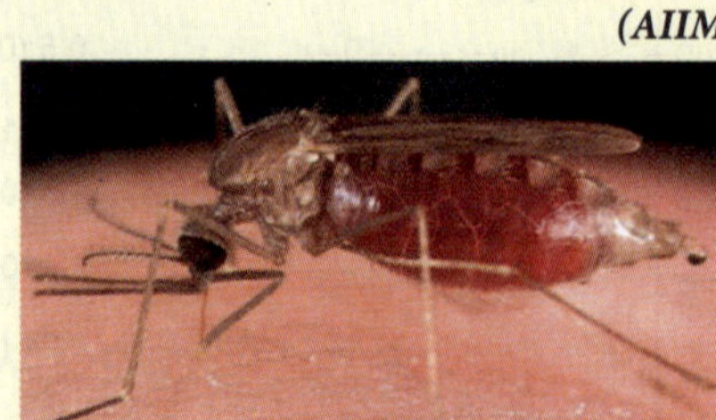

a. KFD
b. Kala Azar
c. babesiosis
d. Chandipura encephalitis
e. Oriental sore

Ans.

11. b
12. a
13. d
14. b
15. d
16. b
17. b
18. c
19. c
20. d
21. d
22. a
23. a
24. a
25. b
26. c,d
27. a

28. What is the sequence for removal of the personal protective equipment? *(Sequential arrangement type; AIIMS May 2019)*
a. Facemask b. Gloves
c. Eyewear d. Apron

29. Which of the following disease with bird, arthropod and human chain: *(Recent Question 2019)*
a. Japanese encephalitis b. Plague
c. Malaria d. Onchocerciasis

30. Drug of choice for Diphtheria carriers is: *(Recent Question 2019)*
a. Penicillin b. Erythromycin
c. Amoxycillin d. Tetracycline

31. Which of the following not an epidemiological indicator for malaria: *(Recent Question 2019)*
a. Annual blood examination rate
b. Annual parasite incidence
c. Annual parasite index
d. Annual falciparum incidence

32. Dose of diphtheria antitoxin is: *(Recent Question 2019)*
a. 1000-5000 IU b. 20000-1000000 IU
c. 1000-2000 IU d. None

33. Which among the following not a personal protective equipment? *(Recent Question 2019)*
a. Goggles b. Face shield
c. Gloves d. Lab coat

34. According to Commission on chronic illness (1957) chronic illness was defined as impairment with: *(AIIMS May 2019)*
a. Of more than 3 months duration
b. With residual disability
c. With irreversible pathological alteration
d. With significant impairment

35. Mw vaccine is made from: *(AIIMS May 2019)*
a. M. Bovis b. M. Welchii
c. M. indicus pranii d. M. Tuberculosis

36. Which of the vaccine strain changed every year: *(Recent Question 2019)*
a. Measles b. Mumps
c. Polio d. Influenza

37. Program for increasing quality of labor room care: *(AIIMS May 2019)*
a. LaQshya program
b. Janani Shishu suraksha karyakram
c. Ayushman bharat scheme
d. PM Surakshit Matritva Abhiyan

38. Under RMNCH program peripheral level of planning is done at: *(Recent Question 2019)*
a. Anganwadi b. Subcenter
c. District level d. PHC level

39. Vaccine contraindicated in pregnancy: *(Recent Question 2019)*
a. Rabies b. Hep A
c. Hep B d. Varicella

40. To call it as fast breathing in a child of 6 months of age, the respiratory rate should be more than: *(Recent Question 2019)*
a. 40 b. 50
c. 60 d. 30

41. A 2-year-old boy with Vitamin A deficiency is treated with: *(Recent Question 2019)*
a. 1 lakh IU on days 0,1,6
b. 2 Lakh IU on days 0,1,6
c. 2 lakh IU on days 0,1,14
d. 1 lakh IU on days 0,1,14

42. Based on WHO criteria, severe acute malnutrition is defined as: *(Recent Question 2019)*
a. Weight for age < 2 standard deviation
b. Weight for age < 3 standard deviation
c. Weight for age < 1 standard deviation
d. Weight for height < 1 standard deviation

43. Biomedical waste management in Match the following: *(AIIMS May 2019)*

Correct Match is

a. Yellow	1. Glassware
b. Red	2. Scalpel
c. Blue	3. Cytotoxic waste
d. White	4. Gloves
	5. Syringe Wrapper

44. Which immunization is useful in post-disaster relief phase: *(AIIMS May 2019)*
a. Measles b. Typhoid
c. Cholera d. Polio

45. Following disaster green colour of triage used for which patients: *(Recent Question 2019)*
a. Dead b. Medium priority
c. High priority d. Ambulatory

Ans.
28. d, b, c, a
29. a
30. b
31. c
32. b
33. b
34. a
35. c
36. d
37. a
38. c
39. d
40. b
41. c
42. b
43. a-3, b-4, c-1, d-2
44. a
45. d

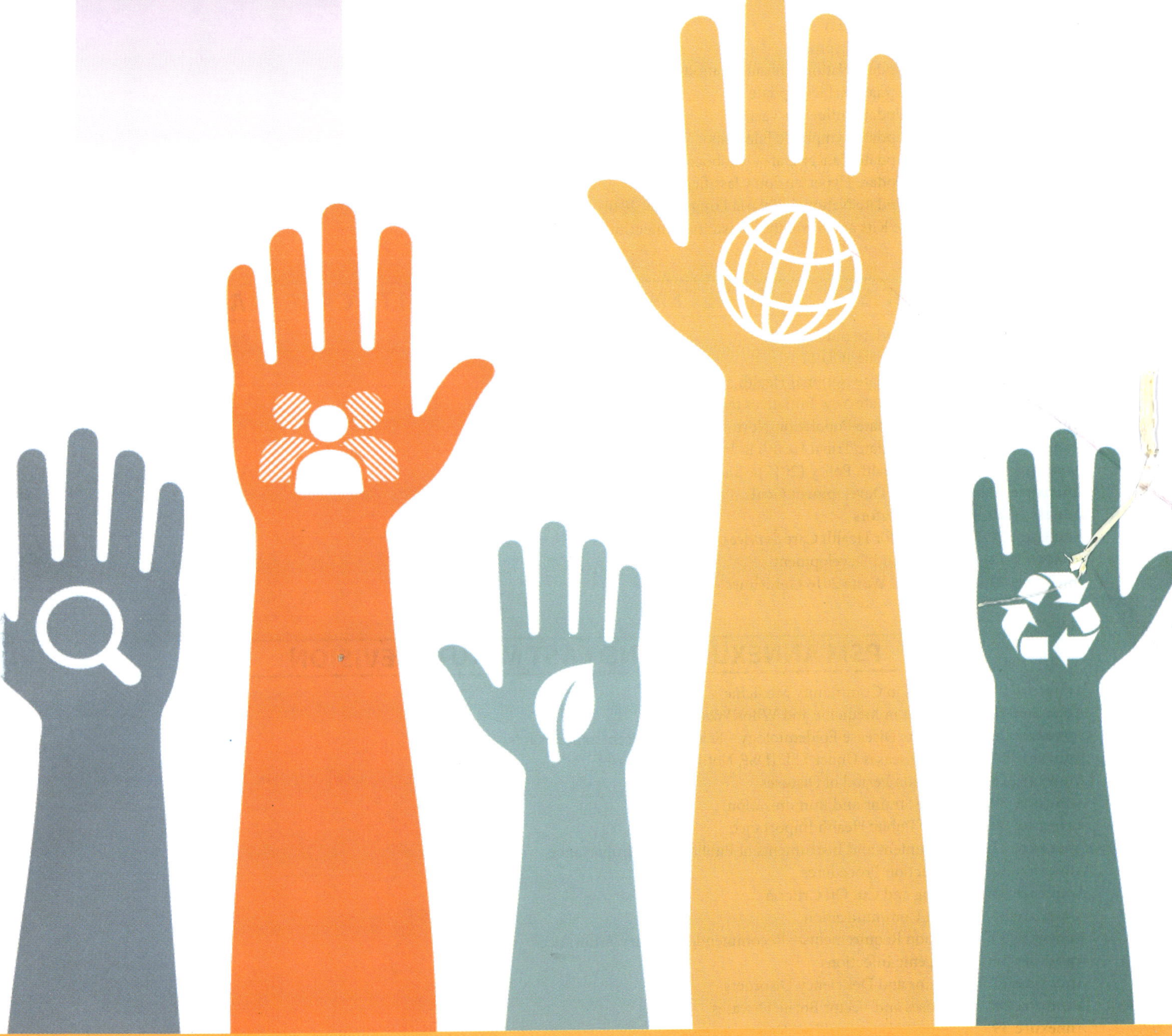

Annexures

LIST OF ANNEXURES

DISEASE GUIDELINES—RECENT UPDATE

INDIA STATISTICS AND RECENT CHANGES IN HEALTH CARE PLANNING

PSM ANNEXURES AND LAST MINUTE REVISION

DISEASE GUIDELINES—RECENT UPDATE

ANNEXURE 1: 2018-19 UPDATE RNTCP

- Diagnostic algorithm for adult population
- Diagnostic algorithm for pediatric population
- Diagnostic algorithm for extra-pulmonary TB
- Diagnostic algorithm for Drug resistant TB (DRTB)
- Treatment for drug sensitive TB
- Treatment regime for H-Mono/poly drug resistance
- Treatment for Multidrug resistance/Rifampicin resistance
- Eligibility criteria for Bedaquiline/Delamanid
- Newer initiative in RNTCP

DIAGNOSTIC ALGORITHM FOR ADULT POPULATION

Diagnostic Algorithm for Pulmonary TB

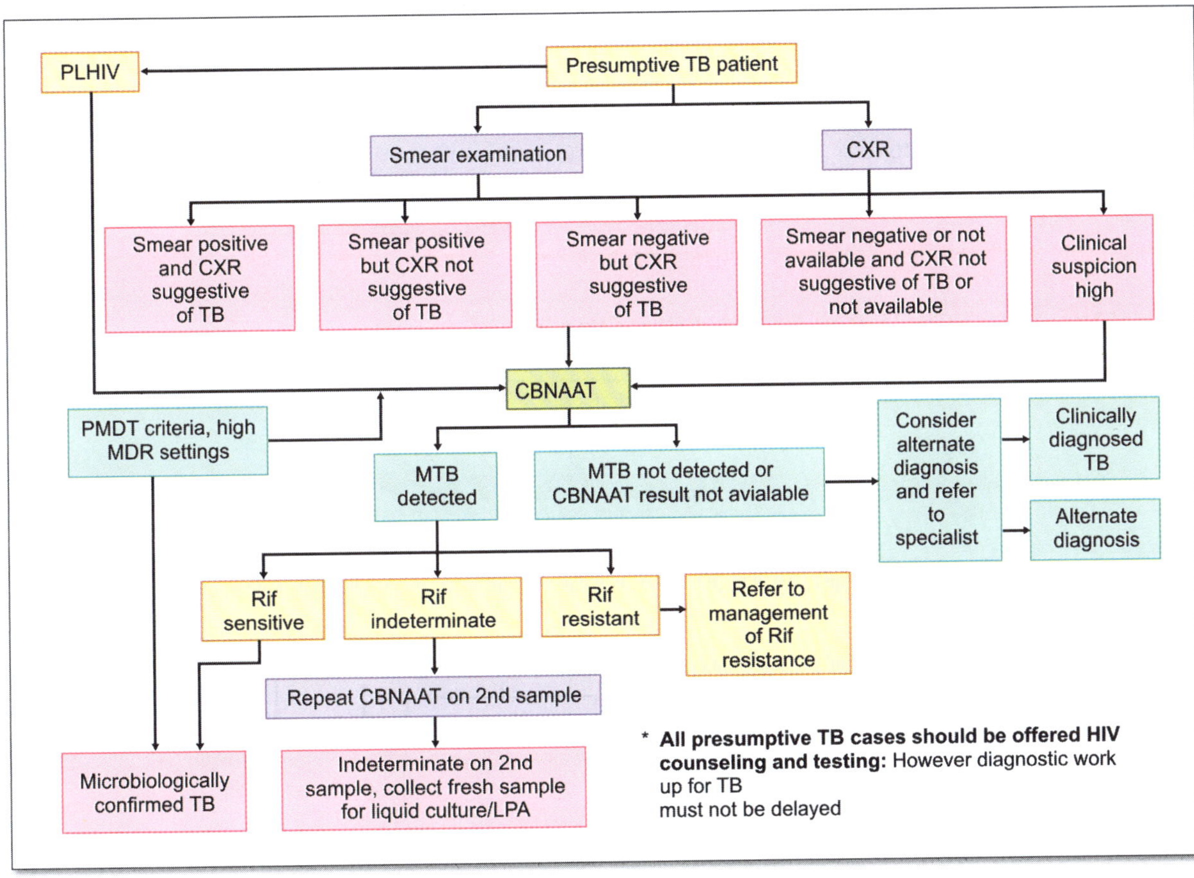

DIAGNOSTIC ALGORITHM FOR PEDIATRIC POPULATION

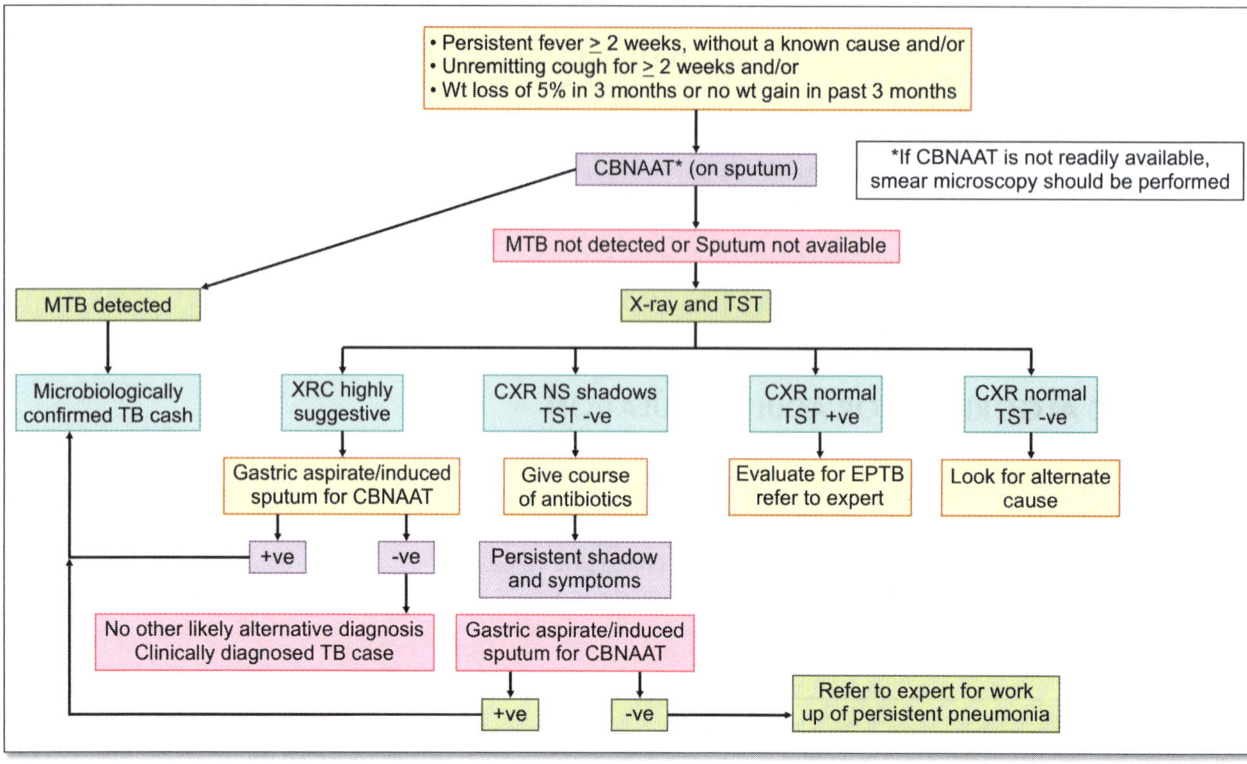

DIAGNOSTIC ALGORITHM FOR EXTRA-PULMONARY TB

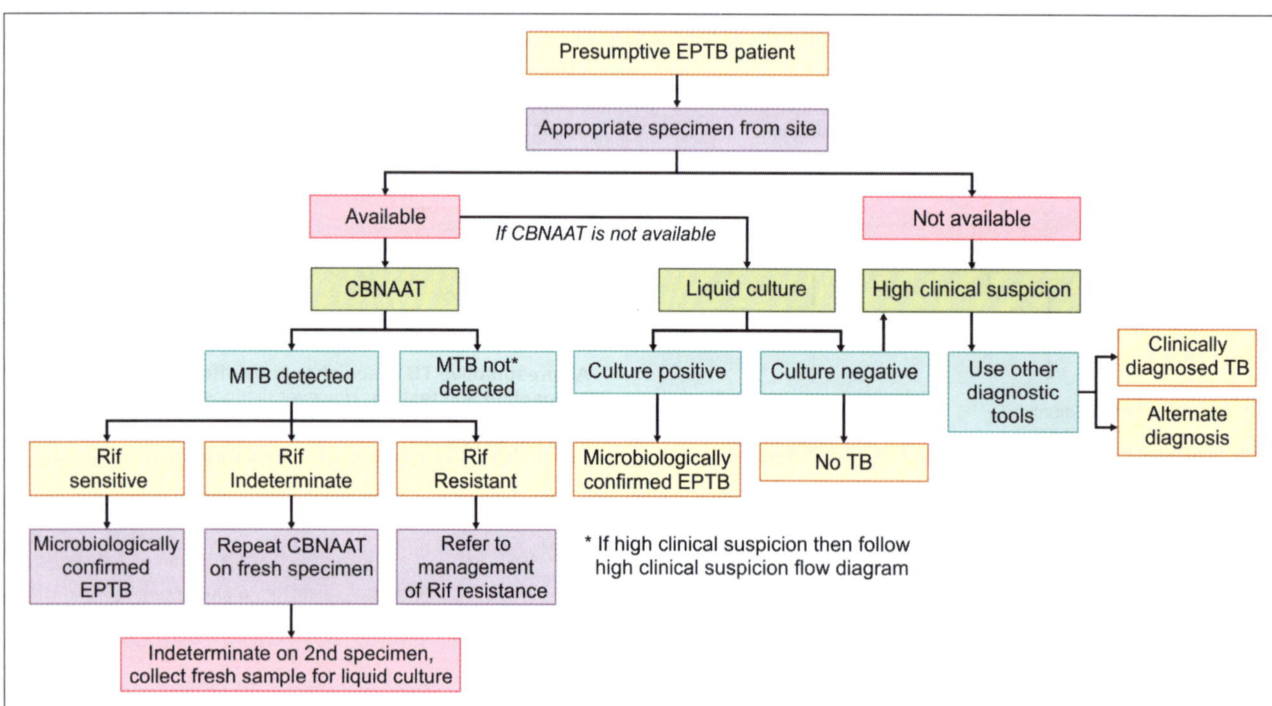

DIAGNOSTIC ALGORITHM FOR DRUG RESISTANT TB (DRTB)

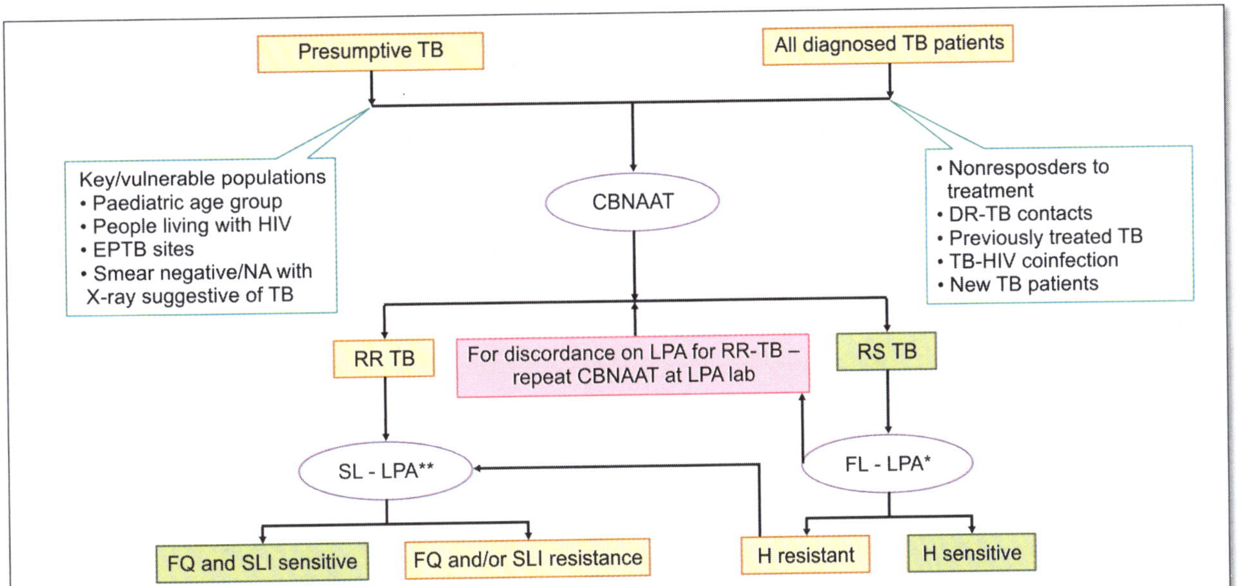

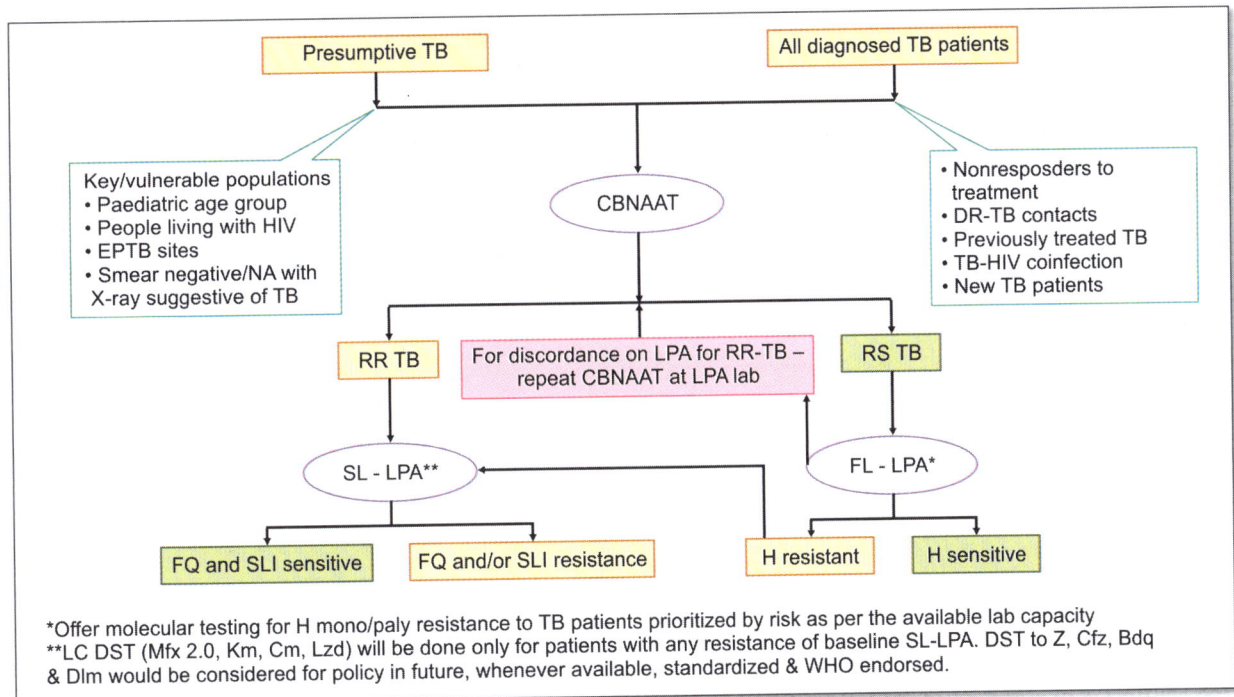

*Offer molecular testing for H mono/paly resistance to TB patients prioritized by risk as per the available lab capacity
**LC DST (Mfx 2.0, Km, Cm, Lzd) will be done only for patients with any resistance of baseline SL-LPA. DST to Z, Cfz, Bdq & Dlm would be considered for policy in future, whenever available, standardized & WHO endorsed.

TREATMENT FOR DRUG SENSITIVE TB – FIRST LINE REGIME

First line regime – 2 (HRZE) + 4 (HRE)

For

- New TB cases and
- Previously treated TB cases

Daily FDC Regimen–Revised May 2019, with New Weight Bands for TB Treatment

For Adults

Table 1: FDC schedule for adults, new and previously treated TB

Weight category	Number of tablets					
	Intensive phase			Continuation phase		
	HRZE (4 FDC) 75/150/275/400 mg per tab	Doses in IP	Number of strips	HRE (3 FDC) 75/150/275 mg per tab	Doses in IP	Number of strips
25–34 kg	2	56 doses	4 x 28	2	112 doses	8 x 28
35–49 kg	3	56 doses	6 x 28	3	112 doses	12 x 28
50–64 kg	4	56 doses	8 x 28	4	112 doses	16 x 28
65–75 kg	5	56 doses	10 x 28	5	112 doses	20 x 28
>75 kg*	6	56 doses	12 x 28	6	112 doses	24 x 28

*Weight more than 75 kg, maybe treated with 5 dose regime if not tolerating 6 doses

- Tab pyridoxine for Alcoholics, Malnourished persons, Pregnant and lactating women, Patients with chronic renal failure, diabetes, HIV infection
- No prolongation of the intensive phase, sample must be sent for FL-LPA (First line - line probe assay)

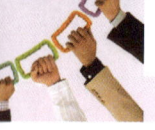

For Pediatric Population

Table 2: FDC schedule for age <18 years (pediatric), new and previously treated TB

Weight category	Number of tablets							
	Intensive phase				Continuation phase			
	HRZ (3 FDC) 50/75/150 mg per tab	E 100 mg	Doses in IP	3 FDC strips + Tablets for E	HR (2 FDC) 50/75 mg	E 100 mg	Doses in CP	2 FDC strips + E** in tablets
4–7 kg	2	1	56 doses	2 x 28 s + E – 56	1	1	112 doses	4 x 28 s + E – 112
8–11 kg	3	2	56 doses	4 x 28 s + E – 112	2	2	112 doses	8 x 28 s + E – 224
12–15 kg	4	3	56 doses	6 x 28 s + E – 168	3	3	112 doses	12 x 28 s + E – 336
16–24 kg	5	4	56 doses	8 x 28 s + E – 224	4	4	112 doses	16 x 28 s + E – 448
25–29 Kg	3 + 1 A*	3	56 doses	6 x 28 s + E – 168 + A – 56	3 + 1 A*	3	112 doses	12 x 28 s + E – 336 + A – 112
30–39 Kg	2 + 2 A*	2	56 doses	4 x 28 s + E – 168 + A – 56	2 + 2 A*	2	112 doses	8 x 28 s + E – 224 + A – 224

*A = Adult dose
**E = Ethambutol

TREATMENT REGIME FOR H-MONO/POLY DRUG RESISTANCE

Regime plan for H mono/poly DR-TB (R susceptible H resistant TB & DST of SEZ not known): 6 months of Levofloxacin, Rifampicin, Ethambutol, Pyrazinamide

TREATMENT FOR MULTIDRUG RESISTANCE/RIFAMPICIN RESISTANCE

Resistance Pattern	Regimen Class	Intensive Phase	Continuation Phase
Shorter MDR-TB Regimen			
R resistant + H sensitive/unknown Or MDR -TB	Shorter MDR-TB Regimen	(4-6) Mfx^h Km* Eto Cfz Z H^h E	(5) Mfx^h Cfz Z E
Regimen for MDR/RR-TB			
R resistant + H sensitive/unknown Or MDR -TB	Conventional MDR-TB Regimen	(6-9) Lfx Km Eto Cs Z E	(18) Lfx Eto Cs E

*If the intensive phase is prolonged, the injectable agent is only given three times a week in the extended intensive phase.

ELIGIBILITY CRITERIA FOR BEDAQUILINE/DELAMANID

Bedaquiline or Delamanid is indicated in MDR-TB patients not eligible for the newly WHO-recommended shorter regimen. These may include:

- MDR/RR-TB patients with resistance to any/all Fluoroquinolones OR to any/all Second Line Injectables
- XDR-TB patients
- Mixed pattern resistant TB patients
- Treatment failures of MDR-TB + FQ/SLI resistance OR XDR-TB
- MDR/RR-TB patients with extensive pulmonary lesions, advanced disease and others deemed at higher baseline risk for poor outcomes

NEWER INITIATIVE IN RNTCP

- Use of NIKSHAY software for patient notification, treatment and compliance
- 99 DOTS (software and SMS reminder based - for patient compliance)
- Nikshay Poshan Yojana – ₹500 per month for TB patients

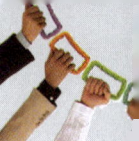

- Airborne infection control – as airborne infection control Kits for patients
- Direct benefit transfer scheme to the TB patients
- Fortnight clinical review of all TB cases by medical officer
- DOTS provider honorarium
  - For drug sensitive TB – INR 1000
  - For drug resistant TB – INR 5000
- Involvement of private practitioners, NGOs
- Treatment availability:
  - First line regime – at all DOTS centers
  - DRTB regimes - at all DOTS Plus sites and district level DRTB DOTS centers

ANNEXURE 2: 2018–19 UPDATE HIV

NEWER INITIATIVES IN HIV/NACO

- NACO has adopted the 'TREAT ALL STRATEGY' – Treat HIV for ANY CD4 count
- 90-90-90 strategy - SDG targets for NACO and HIV control

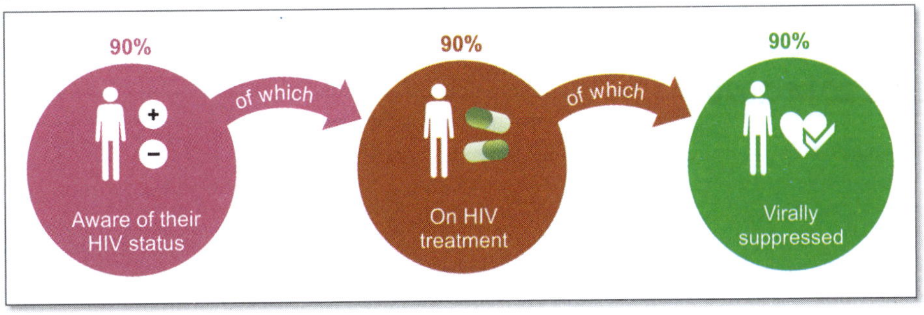

- For monitoring of response and patient prognosis – PCR and viral load replication test is the best investigation
- For initiation of ART in Infants, the Investigation of choice is: HIV DNA rtPCR test

DISTRICT CATEGORIZATION BASED ON PREVALENCE OF HIV IN ANC AND IN HRG'S (HIGH RISK GROUPS)

Table 3: NACO district categorization based on prevalence of HIV in ANC females and high risk groups (HRG)

District categorization	Prevalence in antenatal women (Last 3 year)	Prevalence in high risk groups
A	>1%	—
B	<1%	>5% (Any HRG)
C	<1%	<5% (All HRG with known hot spots/STD clinic)
D	<1%	<5% (All HRG /STD clinic, No known hot spot*)

*Hot spots—Aggregation of migrants, truckers, factory workers

- State categorization based on prevalence of HIV in ANC and in HRG's

Table 4: HIV Prevalence in adult Population in India

Groups	Criteria	States/UT
I: High Prevalence States	HIV infection >5% in high-risk group and ≥1% in antenatal women.	Maharashtra, Tamil Nadu, Karnataka, Andhra Pradesh, Manipur, and Nagaland
II: Moderate Prevalence States	HIV infection >5% high risk groups but <1% in antenatal women	Gujarat, Goa, and Puducherry
III: Low Prevalence States	HIV infection <5% in high risk groups and <1% in antenatal women	Remaining states

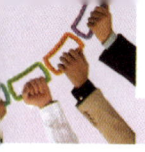

UNDER TRIAL HIV VACCINE

HIV Vaccines

Promising results are from: Ankara vaccine, rAAV vaccine

- **Recombinant subunit vaccines** stimulate antibodies to HIV by mimicking proteins on the surface of HIV. A range of HIV proteins has been produced as potential vaccines for HIV
- **Peptide vaccine:** A vaccine containing the V3 sequences from several strains of HIV has been used in animals and produced antibodies able to neutralize several laboratory-adapted virus strains. Peptide vaccines have been tested in HIV-positive patients, with some antibody and cellular immune responses against HIV
- **DNA vaccine:** After injection, the host's cells effectively make the vaccine themselves by expressing the HIV genes
- **Recombinant vector vaccines** are most often used for vaccines that attempt to stimulate cellular immunity, as the vaccine acts more literally like an infection than vaccines which simply contain proteins or DNA. These are made by incorporating fragments of HIV into the shells of viruses that can infect cells but cause no or few symptoms, such as the canarypox viruses or adenoviruses. Example: Ankara vaccine
- **Replicons** have the same physical properties as viruses and viral vectors, including the ability to enter cells of specific kinds, but they have the advantage of not reproducing after entering the human cell, so there is little or no immune response to the carrier virus. The replicon systems for HIV vaccines are based on Venezuelan equine encephalitis (VEE), Semliki forest virus (SFV), and adeno-associated virus (AAV). All three have shown some success in animal studies.

Live vaccines and inactivated have not been able to provide successful prevention from AIDS, rather showed a risk for development of HIV in later times.

NACO PROJECTS 2014-2020

- The **condom social marketing programme** (CSMP): aims to promote safer sex.
- **Project sunrise**: Responsible for the expansion of HIV interventions in north eastern states with a focus on key affected populations, particularly people who inject drugs.
- **Project NIRANTAR**: This three-year project began in 2014 and focuses on building the capacity of civil society organizations working with key affected populations in the states of Chhattisgarh, Madhya Pradesh and Odisha. Its main aim is to improve access to HIV prevention, care and treatment services, including social protection schemes, in an enabling environment.
- **Link Worker Scheme**: It involves highly motivated and trained community members, responsible for establishing links between the community on one hand and information, commodities and services on the other.

PREVENTION OF MOTHER TO CHILD TRANSMISSION OF HIV

Drug of Choice: Nevirapine

Infant age	Daily dosing
Birth* to 6 weeks ▪ Birth weight 2000–2500 g ▪ Birth weight > 2500 g	 10 mg (1 mL) once daily 15 mg (1.5 mL) once daily
>6 weeks – up to 6 months#	20 mg (2 mL) once daily
>6 months – up to 9 months#	30 mg (3 mL) once daily
>9 months – until breast feeding ends	40 mg (4 mL) once daily

**Infants weighting <2000 g; the suggested starting dose is 2 mg/kg once daily*
#NVP dose for older infants is provided in a stinting where HIV exposure is identified during infancy the mother is breastfeeding and the infant is either HIV infected or the status is yet to be detriment

In case of prior exposure to Nevirapine or in HIV-2 exposure, the alternate drug of choice is Zidovudine

Table 5: Dose of Zidovudine for infants of Nevirapine exposed mothers/Women infected with HIV-2

Infant birth weight	AZT daily dosage in mg	AZT daily dosage in ml	Duration
<2000 g	5 mg/dose twice daily	0.5 ml twice daily	6 weeks
2000–2500 g	10 mg/does twice daily	1 ml twice daily	6 weeks
>2500 g	15 mg/does twice daily	1.5 ml twice daily	6 weeks

ART FOR ADULTS

ART Regimen	Recommended For
Tenofovir + Lamivudine + Efavirenz	First line ART Regimen for: All ARV naive patients except those with ▪ Known renal disease (or) ▪ HIV-2 or HIV-1 & 2 infection (or) ▪ Women with single dose Nevirapine exposure in past pregnancy
Abacavir + Lamivudine + Efavirenz	First line ART Regimen for: All patients with known renal disease
Tenofovir + Lamivudine + Lopinavir/Ritonavir	First line ART regimen for: ▪ All women with single dose Nevirapine exposure in a past pregnancy; ▪ All confirmed HIV-2 or HIV- 1 & HIV-2 co-Infection

ART FOR PREGNANT FEMALES

Target population	Drug regimen	Remark
Pregnant and breastfeeding Women with HIV (ART Naive/"Not-already" receiving ART)	TDF + 3TC + EFV	FDC of TDF (300 mg) + 3TC (300 mg) + EFV (600 mg)- To be given 2 hours after low-fat or fat-free dinner
Pregnant and breastfeeding Women with HIV already receiving ART	The same ART regimen has to be continued	E.g. If they are already on AZT + 3TC + NVP/EFV, continue the same regimen
ART regimen for pregnant women having prior exposure to NNRTI for PPTCT	TDF + 3TC and LPV/r	FDC of TDF (300 mg) + 3TC (300 mg) -- 1-tab OD and FDC of LPV (200 mg)/r (50 mg) - 2-tab BD

ART FOR CHILDREN

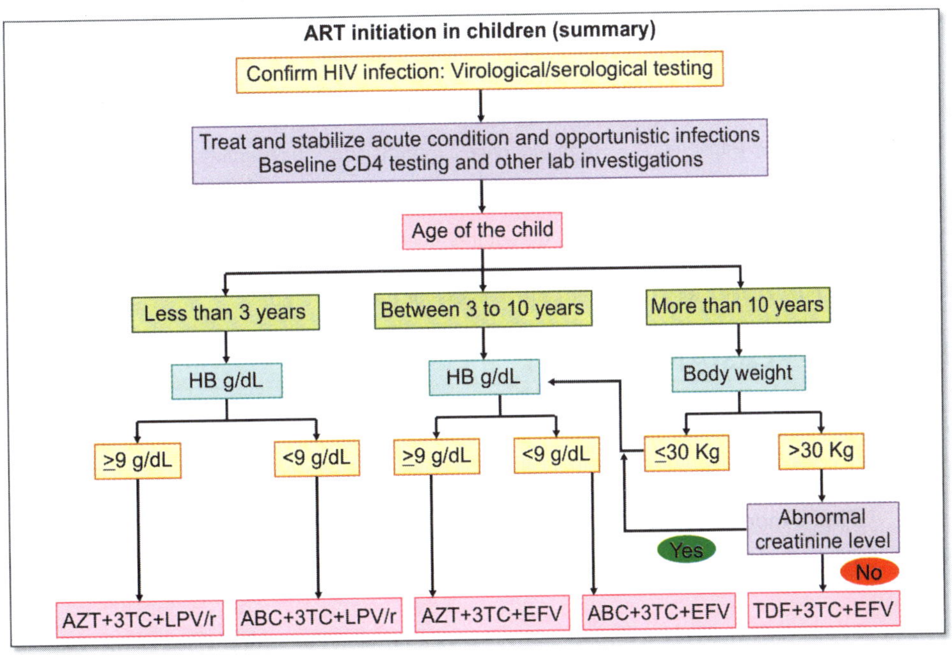

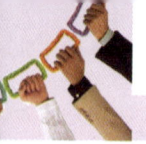

POST EXPOSURE PROPHYLAXIS GUIDELINES

Dosages of drugs for PEP for Adults	Recommendations for PEP	Duration
Tenofovir (300) + Lamivudine (300)- One tablet once daily	One tablet immediately within 2 hours of accidental exposure either at day or night time	Next day one tablet once a day, continue for 4 weeks
Lopinavir (200) + Ritonavir (50)-Two FDC tablets twice daily	Two tablets immediately within 2 hours of accidental exposure either at day or night time	Next day two tablets twice daily, continue for 4 weeks
If Lopinavir/ritonavir is not available or cannot be used, Tenofovir (300) + Lamivudine (300) + Efavirenz (600) may be given 2 hours after dinner before going to bed daily for four weeks		

COTRIMOXAZOLE PREVENTIVE THERAPY

- **START CPT:** when CD4 < 350/mm^3
- **Dose:** One double strength tablet – 800 SMZ + 160 mg TMP
- **STOP CPT:** CD4>350 on two occasions six months apart AND
  Ascending trend of CD4 AND
  Not in WHO stage 3,4

ANNEXURE 3: 2018–19 UPDATE LEPROSY

TREATMENT FOR DRUG SENSITIVE LEPROSY

Table 6: Recommended treatment regimens

Age group	Drug	Dosage and frequency	Duration	
			MB	PB
Adult	Rifampicin	600 mg once a month	12 months	6 months
	Clofazimine	300 mg once a months and 50 mg daily		
	Dapsone	100 mg daily		
Children (10–14 years)	Rifampicin	450 mg once a month	12 months	6 months
	Clofazimine	150 mg once a month, 50 mg daily		
	Dapsone	50 mg daily		
Children <10 years old or <40 kg	Rifampicin	10–mg/kg once month	12 months	6 months
	Dapsone	6 mg/kg once a months and 1 mg/kg daily		
	Clofazimine	2 mg/kg daily		

Note: The treatment for children with body weight below 40 kg requires single formulation medications since no MDT combination blister packs are available. For children between 20 and 40 kg, it would be possible to follow the instructions of the Operational Manual, Global Leprosy Strategy 2016–2020 on how to partly use (MB-Child) blister packs for treatment (60).

TREATMENT FOR DRUG RESISTANT LEPROSY

Table 7: Recommended regimens for drug-resistant leprosy

Resistance type	Treatment	
	First 6 months (daily)	Next 18 months (daily)
Rifampicin resistance	Ofloxacin 400 mg* + minocycline 100 mg + clofazimine 50 mg	Ofloxacin 400 mg* OR minocycline 100 mg + clofazimine 50 mg
	Ofloxacin 400 mg* + minocycline 500 mg + clofazimine 50 mg	Ofloxacin 400 mg* + clofazimine 50 mg
Rifampicin and ofloxacin resistance	Clarithromycin 500 mg + minocycline 100 mg + clofazimine 50 mg	Clarithromycin 500 mg OR minocycline 100 mg + clofazimine 50 mg

**Ofloxacin 400 mg can be replaced by levofloxacin 500 mg OR moxifloxacin 400 mg*

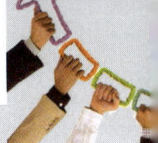

PROPHYLAXIS OF LEPROSY

The DOC is SDR – Single dose rifampicin

Table 8: Rifampicin dose for single-dose rifampicin (SDR)

Age/weight	Rifampicin single dose
15 years and above	600 mg
10–14 years	450 mg
Children 6–9 years (weight ≥ 20 kg)	300 mg
Children <20 kg (≥2 years)	10–15 mg/kg

ANNEXURE 4: 2018–19 UPDATE NATIONAL IMMUNIZATION SCHEDULE

UIP SCHEDULE AFTER INTRODUCTION OF TD VACCINE

Age	Vaccination schedule after Td introduction
At birth	BCG, OPV-zero dose, Hep B-birth dose
6 weeks	OPV-1, Pentavalent-1, Rota-1*, fiPV-1, PCV-1*
10 weeks	OPV-2, Pentavalent-2, Rota-2*
14 weeks	OPV-3, Pentavalent-3, Rota-3*, fiPV-2, PCV-2*
9 months	Measles-1/MR-1, Vit A, JE-1*, PCV-B*
16–24 months	DPT first booster dose, OPV-booster dose, Measles-2/ MR-2, JE-2*
5–6 years	DPT second booster dose
10 & 16 years	Td
For pregnant woman	Td: early in pregnancy Td-2: 4 weeks after Td-1 Td-B; If pregnancy occur within 3 years of last pregnancy and 2 Td doses received

NEWER VACCINES ADDED IN NATIONAL IMMUNIZATION SCHEDULE

- Pentavalent vaccine
- Rotavirus vaccine
- Bivalent OPV (bOPV) vaccine
- f-IPV (fractional IPV)
- Pneumococcal conjugate vaccine
- JE Live vaccine
- Td vaccine (replace TT Vaccine)
- MR Vaccine (replace Measles vaccine)

ANNEXURE 5: 2018–19 RABIES UPDATE

Category I – touching or feeding animals with licks on intact skin
Category II – nibbling of uncovered skin, minor scratch or abrasions without bleeding
Category III – single or multiple bites or scratches, contamination of mucous membrane.

WHO POSITION PAPER ON RABIES (2018)

	Category 1	Category 2	Category 3
No previous immunization	Wound wash	Wound wash	Wound wash
	No PEP required	ID - 2 site – 0, 3, 7 IM – 1 site – 0, 3, 7, 28 IM 2 site day 0 + 1 site IM 7, 21 RIG is NOT indicated	ID - 2 site – 0, 3, 7 IM – 1 site – 0, 3, 7, 28 IM 2 site day 0 + 1 site IM 7, 21 RIG is recommended

Contd...

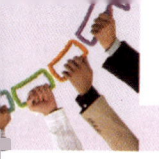

	Category 1	Category 2	Category 3
Previously immunized individuals of all ages (*Vaccine is NOT given if PEP received within <3 months previously)	Wound wash No PEP required	Wound Wash + vaccine* ID – 1 site 0, 3 ID – 4 site day 0 IM – 1 site day 0, 3 RIG is NOT indicated	Wound Wash + vaccine* ID – 1 site 0, 3 ID – 4 site day 0 IM – 1 site day 0, 3 RIG is NOT indicated
Compiled by Dr Mukhmohit Singh, MD			

SUMMARY

The current WHO recommendations are:

- ONE week; 2 site; ID regime; Institut pasteur du cambodge regime; 2–2–2–0–0
- Two week; 1 site; IM regime; 4 dose; ESSEN regime; 1–1–1–1–0
- Three week; IM regime; 5 dose; ZAGREB regime; 2–0–1–0–1
- Four Week; ID regime; 8 dose; Thai Red Cross regime; 2–2–2–0–2

  Pre-Exposure Prophylaxis:
  ID – 2 site 0, 7
  IM – 1 site 0, 7

Special Considerations

- If the doses are delayed, they should be resumed, not restarted.
- In case of complete vaccination < 3 months, repeat vaccine is not required.
- In case of time lapse is more than > 3 months, repeat vaccine maybe administered as required.
- RIG is not required to be repeated till 1 year of age.
- RIG - IM injection at a distant site is NO longer recommended
- NO contraindication for ID or IM vaccine with chloroquine or hydroxychloroquine
- Vaccine may be given to PREGNANT females

Wound Wash

- At least 15 minutes with soap and generous water. Iodine based or viricidal agents may be applied on wound
- Wounds which require suture – should have loose sutures
- RIG for category III wounds

Rabies Immunoglobulin (RIG)

- As soon as possible but not beyond 7 days of exposure
- hRIG – 20 IU per kg body weight; eRIG – 40 IU per kg body weight
- Infiltrate in wound as much as possible, remaining at IM site distant from the wound

  hRIG = Human Rabies Immunoglobulin; eRIG = Equine Rabies Immunoglobulin

ANNEXURE 6: 2018–19 UPDATE INFLUENZA VACCINE

FLU – INACTIVATED VACCINE

- **Egg based quadrivalent vaccines** for use in the 2019 southern hemisphere influenza season contain the following:
  - A/Michigan/45/2015 (H1N1)pdm09-like virus;
  - A/Switzerland/8060/2017 (H3N2)-like virus
  - B/Colorado/06/2017-like virus (B/Victoria/2/87 lineage)
  - B/Phuket/3073/2013-like virus (B/Yamagata/16/88 lineage).
- **Egg based trivalent vaccines** for use in the 2019 southern hemisphere influenza season contain the following:
  - A/Michigan/45/2015 (H1N1)pdm09-like virus;
  - A/Switzerland/8060/2017 (H3N2)-like virus; and
  - B/Colorado/06/2017-like virus (B/Victoria/2/87 lineage).
- **Non Egg Based Vaccine**
  - A/Singapore/INFIMH-16-0019/2016-like virus (H3N2 component) along with other vaccine components

    Route: Single dose I'm injection – upper arm

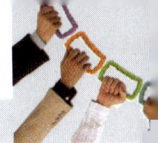

FLU LIVE ATTENUATED VACCINE (FLAV)– VIA NASAL SPRAY

FLAV Contraindications

- Immunocompromised patients
- Pregnant women
- Individuals who have taken an influenza antiviral medication within the previous 48 hours
- Adults aged ≥50 years
  Note: Vaccines are associated with higher risk of GBS

Indications

The influenza vaccine is recommended only for the category of 'high-risk children'.
This category contains the following:

- Chronic cardiac, pulmonary (excluding asthma)
- Hematologic and Renal (including nephrotic syndrome) condition
- Chronic liver diseases
- Congenital or acquired immunodeficiency (including HIV infection)
- Children on long term salicylates therapy

WHO suggests the following groups for vaccination according to their order of priority:

- Pregnant women
- Individuals aged more than 6 months with one of the several chronic medical conditions;
- Healthy young adults between age 15–49 years
- Healthy children
- Healthy adults between age 49–65 years
- Healthy adults aged more than 65 years

NEW DRUG Approved by FDA for Influenza

Baloxavir marboxil is a novel **oral selective inhibitor of influenza cap-dependent endonuclease** that blocks influenza proliferation by inhibiting the initiation of mRNA synthesis.
FDA approved Baloxavir in october, 2018 for the treatment of acute uncomplicated influenza (flu) in patients 12 years of age and older who have been symptomatic for no more than 48 hours.

ANNEXURE 7: 2018–19 UPDATE LYMPHATIC FILARIASIS

LYMPHATIC FILARIASIS

Treatment: triple drug regime: DEC + Albendazole + Ivermectin
Chemoprophylaxis: DEC + Albendazole

- Five to 6 rounds of annual MDA[Q] are required to interrupt transmission of LF.
- Each round of MDA should be 'effective' i.e. at least 65% treatment coverage[Q] should be accomplished.
- After MDA, the evidence of interruption of transmission is generated through implementation of the first transmission assessment survey (TSA 1) among children of 6–7 years age[Q] in each district.
- It the number of infected children found in TAS 1 is less than the threshold number (which is approximately 2% Ag or Ab prevalence[Q]), then the MDA is stopped.
- After stopping the MDA, post-MDA surveillance is initiated. This consists of two more rounds of TAS (TAS 2 and TAS 3).
- Simultaneously, the chronic disease burden should be estimated in all endemic districts, plans for delivery of care to chronic patients developed and each chronic patient provided minimum package of care.
- When all districts in a country complete TAS 3 successfully and minimum package of care is delivered to all patients with chronic disease, the country is deemed to have eliminated LF.
- Then the country prepares LF elimination dossier for validation of elimination of LF.

ANNEXURE 8: 2018–19 UPDATE CANCER DATA—GLOBOCON 2018

Incidence of cancer, 2018, INDIA – STATS summary
Source: GLOBOCON 2018

Male (%age among male cancers)	Female (%age among female cancers)	Both (%age among all cancers)
Lip oral cavity	Breast (27.7%)	Breast (14%)
Lung	Ca cervix (17%)	Lip oral cavity (10.5%)
Stomach	Ovary (6%)	Ca cervix (8.5%)
Colorectum	Lip oral cavity	Lung Ca
Esophagus	Colorectum	Stomach Ca

ANNEXURE 9: 2018–19 UPDATE HYPERTENSION CLASSIFICATION

ESC – European society of cardiology
ESH – European society of hypertension

SEVERITY GRADING OF HYPERTENSION 2018 UPDATE

Table 9: Classification of office blood pressure[a] and definitions of hypertension grade[b]

Category	Systolic (mm Hg)		Diastolic (mm Hg)
Optimal	<120	and	<80
Normal	120–129	and/or	80–84
High normal	130–139	and/or	85–89
Grade 1 hypertension	140–159	and/or	90–99
Grade 2 hypertension	160–179	and/or	100–109
Grade 3 hypertension	≥180	and/or	≥110
Isolated systolic hypertension[b]	≥140	and	<90

BP = Blood pressure; SBP = systolic blood pressure
a BP category is defined according to seated clinic BP and by the highest level or BP, whether systolic or diastolic
b Isolate systolic hypertension is graded 1, 2, or 3 according to SBP value in the ranges indicated
The same classification is used for all ages from 16 years

ANNEXURE 10: 2018–19 UPDATE NATIONAL MALARIA DRUG POLICY 2014

- Treatment for Pl. vivax infections
  - Chloroquine 25 mg/kg body weight divided in three days
    - 10 mg/kg body weight on day 1
    - 10 mg/kg body weight on day 2
    - 5 mg/kg body weight on day 3
  - Primaquine 0.25 mg/kg body weight for 14 days
- Treatment for plasmodium falciparum infections - For all states (except North eastern states)
- Artemisinin based combination therapy – (ACT-SP)
  - Artesunate 4 mg/kg body weight daily for 3 days
  - Sulfadoxine 25 mg/kg BW on day 1
  - Pyrimethamine 1.25 mg/kg BW on day 1
  - Primaquine 0.75 mg/kg BW on day 2

Dose Schedule for ACT-SP Regime with Color Coded Blister for Different Age Categories

Age group (years)	1st day		2nd day		3rd day
	AS	SP	AS	PQ	AS
0–1* Pink blister	1 (25 mg)	1 (250 + 12.5 mg)	1 (25 mg)	Nil	1 25 (mg)

Contd...

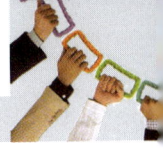

Age group (years)	1st day		2nd day		3rd day
1–4 Yellow blister	1 (50 mg)	1 (500 + 25 mg each)	1 (50 mg)	1 (7.5 mg base)	1 (50 mg)
5–8 Green blister	1 (100 mg)	1 (750 + 37.5 mg each)	1 (100 mg)	2 (7.5 mg base each)	1 (100 mg)
9–14 Red blister	1 (150 mg)	2 (500 + 25 mg each)	1 (150 mg)	4 (7.5 mg base each)	1 (150 mg)
15 & above White blister	1 (200 mg)	2 (750 + 37.5 mg each)	1 (200 mg)	6 (7.5 mg base each)	1 (200 mg)
* SP is not to be prescribed for children <5 months of age and should be treated with alternate ACT * ACT-AL is not to be prescribed for children weighing less than 5 kg.					

- Treatment for plasmodium falciparum infections - For North eastern states (NES)
  - ACT – Artemisinin based combination therapy – ACT-AL
    - Artemether 20 mg for 3 days
    - Lumefantrine 120 mg for 3 days

Based on kg body weight:

Co–formulated tablet ACT-AL	5–14 kg (>5 months to <3 years)	15–24 kg (>3 to 8 years)	25–34 kg (>9 to 14 years)	>34 kg (>14 years)
Total dose of ACT-AL	20 mg/120 mg twice daily for 3 days	40 mg/240 mg twice daily for 3 days	60 mg/360 mg twice daily for 3 days	80 mg/480 mg twice dily for 3 days
Pack size				
No. of tablets in the packing	6	12	18	24
Give	1 tablet twice daily for 3 days	2 tablets twice daily for 3 days	3 tablets twice daily for 3 days	4 tablets twice daily for 3 days
Colour of the pack	Yellow	Green	Red	White

- Treatment for mixed infections
  - In NES
    - ACT-AL for 3 days
    - Primaquine 0.25 mg/kg BW for 14 days
  - In all other states
    - ACT-SP for 3 days
    - Primaquine 0.25 mg/kg BW for 14 days

Treatment Considerations

- Avoid starting treatment empty stomach
- Dose to be repeated if vomiting occurs within 15 minutes of first dose
- To report back to malaria clinic if no improvement in 24 hours
- Consider sever malaria if any of the following signs are present
  - Impaired consciousness/coma
  - Repeated generalized convulsions
  - Renal failure (Serum creatinine > 3 mg/dL)
  - Jaundice (Serum Bilirubin >3 mg/dL)
  - Severe anaemia (Hb <5 g/dL)
  - Pulmonary edema/acute respiratory distress syndrome
  - Hypoglycaemia (Plasma glucose <40 mg/dL)
  - Metabolic acidosis
  - Circulatory collapse/shock (Systolic BP <80 mm Hg, <50 mm Hg in children)
  - Abnormal bleeding and disseminated intravascular coagulation
  - Haemoglobinuria

- Hyperthermia (Temperature >106°F or 42°C)
- Hyperparasitemia (<5% parasitized RBCs in low endemic and >10% in hyperendemic areas)

- **Treatment for severe malaria**

Initial management	Follow up treatment
20 mg quinine salt/kg BW (iv infusion or divided IM injection) and maintenance dose 10 mg/kg 8 hourly	Quinine 10 mg/kg TDS with doxycycline 100 mg OD x 7 days
Artesunate 2.4 mg/kg IV or IM then at 12 hours and then at 24 hrs	Full course oral ACT In NES – ACT AL x 3 days + PQ on day 2 In other states ACT SP x 3 days + PQ on day 2
Artemether 3.2 mg/kg IM and then 1.6 mg/kg per day	
Arteether 150 mg daily IM for 3 days (contraindicated in children)	

- **Malariometric Indicators**

$$API = \frac{\text{No. of blood smears found positive for malaria parasite}}{\text{No. of blood smears examined}} \times 1000$$

$$ABER = \frac{\text{No. of blood smears collected during the year}}{\text{Population covered under surveillance}} \times 100$$

$$MBER = \frac{\text{No. of blood smears collected during the months}}{\text{Population covered under surveillance}} \times 100$$

$$SPR = \frac{\text{No. of blood smears found positive for malaria parasite}}{\text{No. of blood smears examined}} \times 100$$

API = Annual parasite incidence
ABER = Annual blood examination rate
MBER = Monthly blood examination rate
SPR = Slide positivity rate
Impact indicator : API
Operational indicator : ABER
Outbreak Indicator : SPR
Evaluation of malaria control program : Infant parasite incidence

ANNEXURE 11: SYNDROMIC KITS AND SEXUALLY TRANSMITTED DISEASES

Features	Syphilis	Chancroid	Lymphogranuloma venerum	Donovanosis	Herpes genitalis
Agent	T. pallidum	Haemophilus ducreyi	Chlamydia trachomatis (L_1, L_2, L_3)	Calymmatobacterium granulomatis	Herpes simplex
Incubation period	9–90 days	1–7 days	3 days – 6 weeks	1–4 weeks	2–7 days
Early lesions	Superficial/deep seated papule	Excavated pustule	Superficial/deep seated papule or pustule	Elevated papule	Superficial vesicle
Edges	Sharply, demarcated, elevated, round or oval	Undermined, ragged, sloughed or irregular	Elevated, round or oval	Elevated, irregular serpiginous	Erythematous
Base	Smooth, non purulent, non-vascular	Purulent, bleeds easily	Variable, Non-vascular	Red, velvety bleeds easily with exuberant granulation tissue	Serous erythematous, non vascular
Induration	Firm	Soft	Firm	Firm	None
Pain	Uncommon	Very tender	Variable	Uncommon	Frequently tender
Lymphadenopathy	Firm, non tender, shotty, bilateral	Tender, loculated, suppurated, unilateral	Tender, loculated, suppurated unilateral	Pseudobuboes	Bilateral firm tender lymph nodes

Contd...

Features	Syphilis	Chancroid	Lymphogranuloma venerum	Donovanosis	Herpes genitalis
Diagnosis	Dark field microscopy; serodiagnosis	Gram staining	Demonstration of LGV as elementary and inclusion bodies; frie's test	Histopathological of biopsy; staining with Giemsa stain, wright's stain, silver stain, Leishman stain	Tzanck smear; culture
Treatment	Benzathine/Procaine/ Aqueous benzyl penicillin	Azithromycin (or) Erythromycin; Ceftriaxone; Ciprofloxacin	Doxycycline (or) Tetracycline; Erythromycin	Doxycycline (or) Tetracycline; Erythromycin	Acyclovir

SYNDROMIC KITS

Clinical condition	Kit to be prescribed	Drugs included	Image
Urethral or anorectal or cervical discharge	KIT 1: Grey	Tab azithromycin 1 g (1 tab) Tab cefixime 400 mg (1 tab)	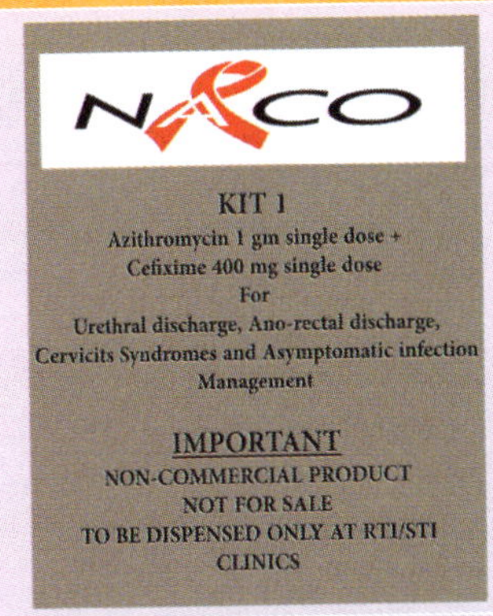
Vaginal discharge (vaginitis)	KIT 2: Green	Tab secnidazole 1 g (2 tab) Tab fluconazole 150 mg (1 tab)	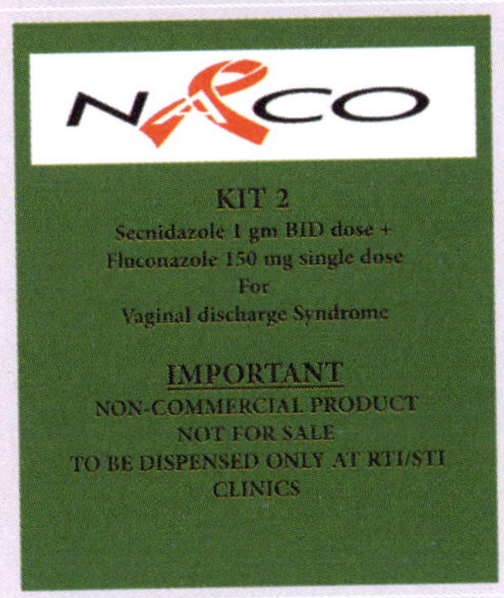
Genital ulcer diseases (nonherpetic)	KIT 3: White	Inj. benzathine penicillin 2.4 MU (1 vial) + tab Azithromycin 1 g (Kit also contains 10 mL disposable syringe + 21 gauge needle + 1 vial of 10 mL sterile water	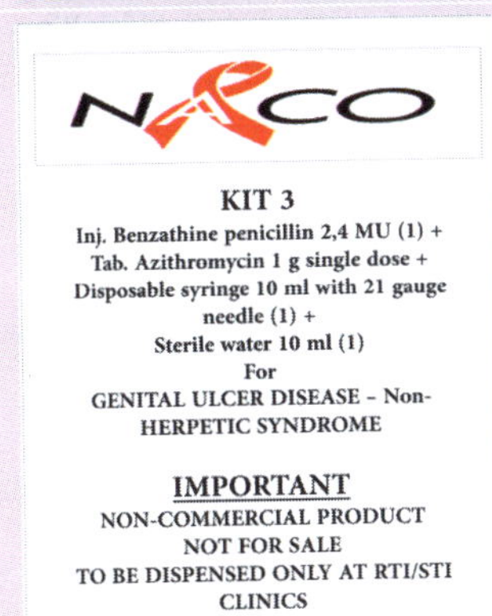

Contd...

Clinical condition	Kit to be prescribed	Drugs included	Image
Genital ulcer disease (nonherpetic) in patient allergic to penicillin	KIT 4: Blue	Tab doxycycline 100 mg (1 tab BD for 15 days) Tab azithromycin 1 g × 1 tab	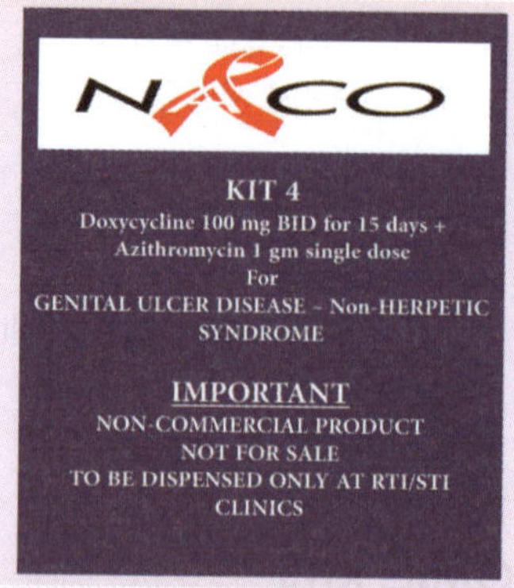
Genital ulcer disease	KIT 5: Red	Tab acyclovir 400 mg × 1 tab TDS × 7 days	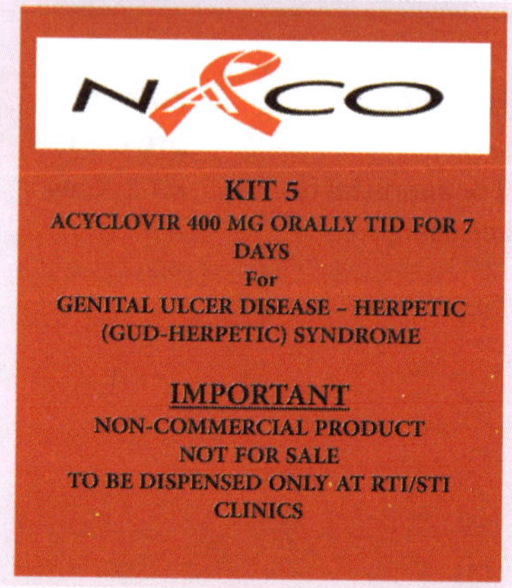
Lower abdominal pain (pelvic inflammatory disease)	KIT 6: Yellow	Tab cefixime 400 mg × 1 tab Tab metronidazole 400 mg × (1 BD 14 day) Tab doxycycline 100 mg (1 BD 14 days)	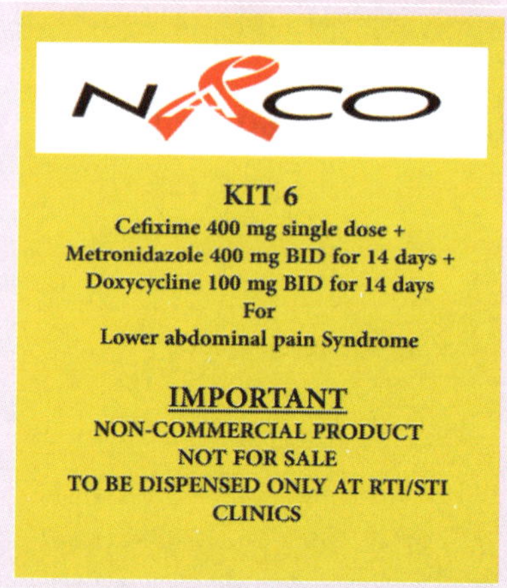
Inguinal Bubo	KIT 7: Black	Tab doxycycline 100 mg (1 BD × 21 days) Tab azithromycin 1 g × 1 tab	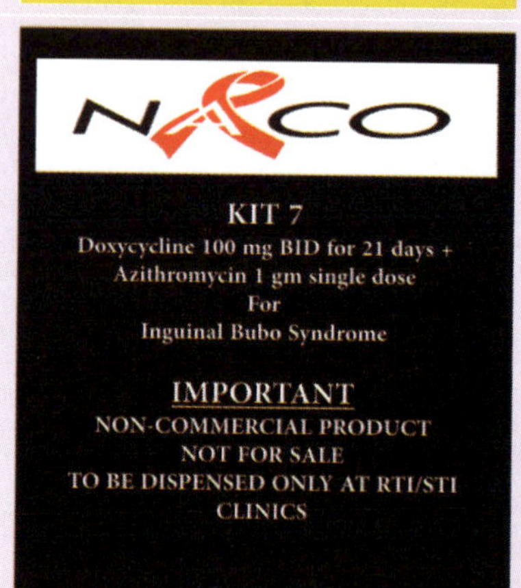

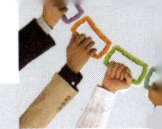

INDIA STATISTICS AND RECENT CHANGES IN HEALTH CARE PLANNING

ANNEXURE 12: 2018–19 UPDATE INDIA PROFILE

Indicator	Data	Source
Population (2016)	1329 million (17.5% of World population) most populated state - UP	Census 2011
Urban population (2011)	377.1 million (31.8%)	Census 2011
Rural population	833.1 million (68.8%)	Census 2011
Annual growth rate (2011)	1.19%	Institute of population studies, NFHS 4
Decadal growth rate (2011)	17.64% Highest in India –Dadra and N. Haveli, Lowest- Nagaland	Census 2011
Total dependency ratio	52.2	Census 2011
Young age dependency ratio Old age dependency ratio	43.6 8.6	Census 2011
Life expectancy at birth (2015)	Overall: 67.5 years Male = 67, Female = 70 Highest in world- Japan (Male = 80, Female = 86) and Switzerland (Male = 81, Female = 85)	Census 2011
Literacy rate (2011) (Age more than 15 and can read and write)	71.2%	Census 2011
Population <15 years	27.0	SRS 2016-18
Population >60 years	8.3	SRS 2016-18
CBR – crude birth rate	20.4	SRS 2016-18
GFR – general fertility rate	74.4	SRS 2016-18
CDR- crude death rate	6.4	SRS 2016-18
IMR – infant mortality rate	34	SRS 2016-18
IMR Madhya Pradesh	47 (Max)	SRS 2016-18
IMR Kerala	10 (Minimum)	SRS 2016-18
U5MR – under five mortality rate	39	SRS 2016-18
NNMR – neonatal mortality rate	24	SRS 2016-18
ENNMR – early neonatal mortality rate	18	SRS 2016-18
LNNMR – late neonatal mortality rate	5	SRS 2016-18
PNNMR – post neonatal mortality rate	11	SRS 2016-18
PNMR – perinatal mortality rate	23	SRS 2016-18
SBR – still birth rate	4/1000 births	SRS 2016-18
MMR – maternal mortality ratio	130	SRS 2018
Maternal mortality rate	8.8	SRS 2018
Lifetime mortality risk	0.3%	SRS 2018
Sex ratio adults	991	NFHS 4
Sex ratio at birth	919	NFHS 4
Registered births	79.7	NFHS 4
Female literacy (15-49 years)	68.4	NFHS 4
Male literacy (15-49 years)	85.7	NFHS 4

Contd...

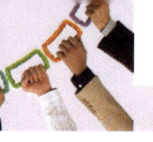

Indicator	Data	Source
TFR – total fertility rate	2.2	NFHS 4
Any contraceptive method used 15-49 years	53.5	NFHS 4
ANC first Trimester	58.6	NFHS 4
Institutional births	78.9	NFHS 4
Fully immunized children 12-23 months	62%	NFHS 4
Diarrhea prevalence in U5	9.2	NFHS 4
ARI in U5 (acute respiratory illness in under five)	2.7	NFHS 4
EBF – exclusive breast feeding	54.9	NFHS 4
Stunting in U5	38.4	NFHS 4
Wasting in U5	21	NFHS 4
Underweight for age in U5	35.8	NFHS 4
Overweight in 15-49 years males	18.9	NFHS 4
Overweight in 15-49 yrs females	20.6	NFHS 4
Anemia U5	58.6	NFHS 4
Anemia females 15-49 yrs	53.1	NFHS 4
Tobacco prevalence in females	6.8	NFHS 4
Tobacco in males	44.5	NFHS 4
Alcohol in males	29.2	NFHS 4
HDI in India	0.64	UN – 2017
Disease morbidity		
TB incidence	211/100,000 population	RNTCP 2018
Cause specific death rate TB	32/100,000 population	RNTCP 2018
HIV-TB coinfection incidence	6.6 per 100,000 population	RNTCP 2018
HIV Prevalence (15-49 years)	0.2%	NACO 2018
Diabetes prevalence	8%	ICMR 2018
COPD prevalence	17%	ICMR 2017
Hypertension prevalence	25%	Nature 2018

ANNEXURE 13: 2018–19 UPDATE ICD 11

SALIENT FEATURES OF ICD 11 CLASSIFICATION

- 3 volumes
- Arabic numbered chapter
- 4 categories with 2 subcategories first character of the chapter correlates to the chapter number
- 26 chapters
- Terminal letter 'Y' is reserved for the residual category 'other specified' and the terminal letter 'Z' is reserved for the residual category 'unspecified'

CHAPTERS IN ICD 11

ICD-11 Mortality and Morbidity Statistics

- Certain infectious or parasitic diseases
- Neoplasms
- Diseases of the blood or blood-forming organs

- Diseases of the immune system
- Endocrine, nutritional or metabolic diseases
- Mental, behavioural or neurodevelopmental disorders
- Sleep-wake disorders
- Diseases of the nervous system
- Diseases of the visual system
- Diseases of the ear or mastoid process
- Diseases of the circulatory system
- Diseases of the respiratory system
- Diseases of the digestive system
- Diseases of the skin
- Diseases of the musculoskeletal system or connective tissue
- Diseases of the genitourinary system
- Conditions related to sexual health
- Pregnancy, childbirth or the puerperium
- Certain conditions originating in the perinatal period
- Developmental anomalies
- Symptoms, signs or clinical findings, not elsewhere classified
- Injury, poisoning or certain other consequences of external causes
- External causes of morbidity or mortality
- Factors influencing health status or contact with health services
- Codes for special purposes
- Traditional medicine conditions—Module I
- Supplementary section of functioning assessment
- Extension codes

ANNEXURE 14: 2018–19 UPDATE NATIONAL HEALTH MISSION ORGANIZATION

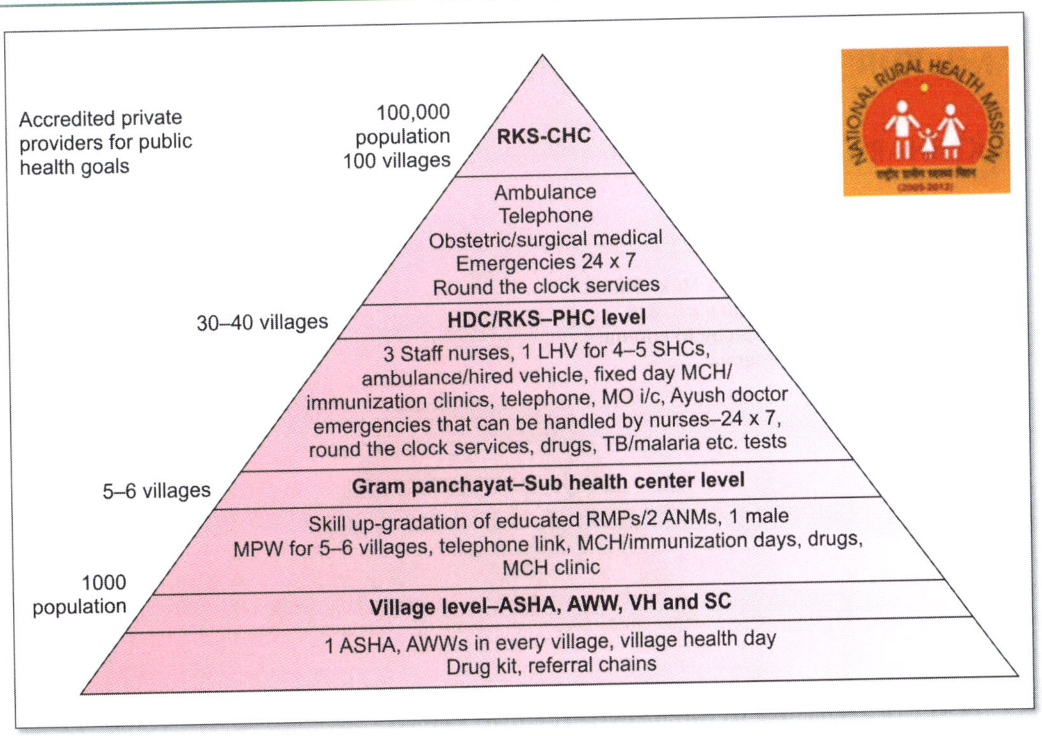

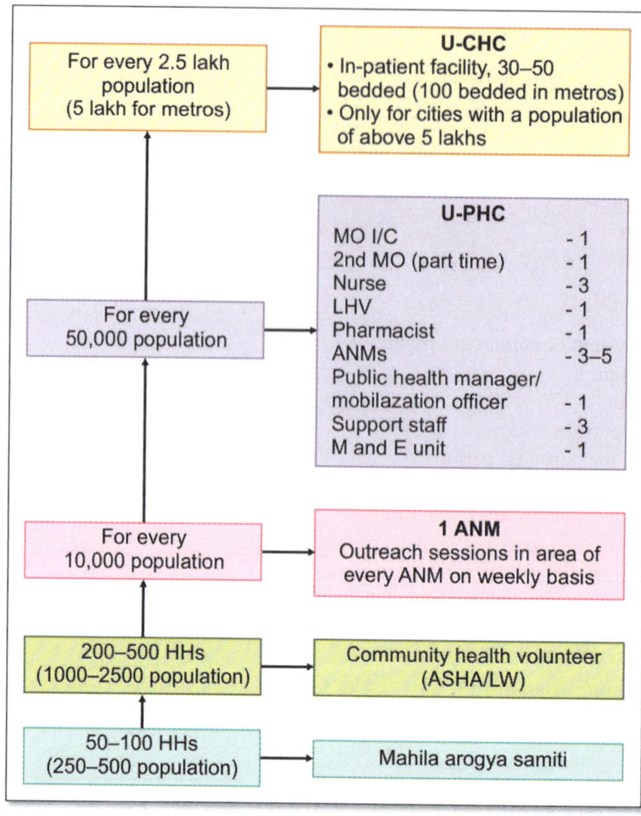

ANNEXURE 15: 2018–19 UPDATE NEW INITIATIVES BY MoHFW

ANEMIA MUKT BHARAT

Targets

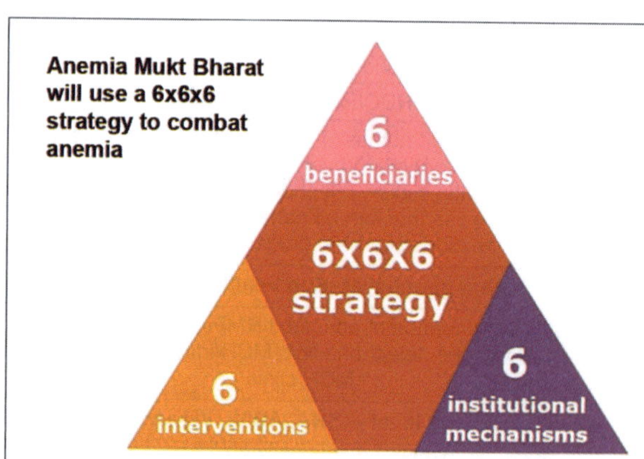

Prophylactic Iron and Folic Acid Supplementation (2018 - Guidelines)

Eligible beneficiary	Age group	Dosing schedule	Dose	Iron + Folic acid composition
Children	6-59 months	Biweekly	1 ml IFA syrup from 50 ml auto-dispenser bottle	20 mg elemental iron + 100 mcg folic acid

Contd...

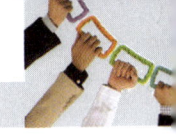

Eligible beneficiary	Age group	Dosing schedule	Dose	Iron + Folic acid composition
Children	5-9 years	Weekly	1 IFA tablet - sugar coated pink color	45 mg elemental iron + 400 mcg folic acid
Adolescent boys	10-19 years – school going	Weekly	1 IFA tablet – sugar coated blue color	60 mg elemental iron + 500 mcg folic acid
Adolescent girls	10-19 years – school going and out of school	Weekly	1 IFA tablet – sugar coated blue color	60 mg elemental iron + 500 mcg folic acid
Women of reproductive age group	Under mission parivar vikas	Weekly	1 IFA tablet – sugar coated red color	60 mg elemental iron + 500 mcg folic acid
Pregnant females and lactating mothers	Pregnant + lactating (0-6 months)	Daily starting from 4th month throughout pregnancy and for 180 days postpartum	1 IFA tablet – sugar coated red color	60 mg elemental iron + 500 mcg folic acid

Deworming Dose and Regime (2018 - Guidelines)

National deworming day program: Biannual deworming is done on 10th February and 10th August every year

Age category	Age	Dose and regime
Children	12-24 months	½ tablet (200 mg) biannual dose
Children	24 – 59 months	1 tablet – 400 mg Biannual dose
Children	5-9 years	
School going adolescent boys and girls	10-19 years	
Out of school adolescent girls	10 – 19 years	
Reproductive age group females	20-49 years	
Pregnant and lactating females	Lactating female 0-6 months	1 tablet 400 mg, Single dose in 2nd trimester

AYUSHMAN BHARAT

Elements are:

- Comprehensive primary health care by Health and wellness centers
- PM JAY - Prime Minister Jan Arogya Yojana – providing health protection cover to poor and vulnerable families
  - PM JAY (Pradhan Mantri Jan Arogya Yojana) benefits:
    - Financial health protection to 10.74 crore poor, deprived rural families and identified occupational categories of urban workers' families as per the latest Socio-Economic Caste Census (SECC) data
    - Approx. 50 crore beneficiaries
    - Benefit cover of ₹500,000 per family per year (on a family floater basis)
    - For any primary, secondary tertiary level care for any disease and 1350 medical packages including surgery, medical and day care treatments, cost of medicines and diagnostics

PM SURAKSHIT MATRITVA SAHYOG YOJNA

Objectives of the Program

- Ensure at least one antenatal check-up for all pregnant women in their second or third trimester by a physician/specialist
- Free ANC on 9th of every month in the empanelled health facility
- Improve the quality of care during antenatal visits. This includes ensuring provision of the following services:
  - All applicable diagnostic services
  - Screening for the applicable clinical conditions
  - Appropriate management of any existing clinical condition such as Anemia, Pregnancy induced hypertension, Gestational Diabetes etc.
  - Appropriate counseling services and proper documentation of services rendered
  - Additional service opportunity to pregnant women who have missed antenatal visits
  - Identification and line-listing of high risk pregnancies based on obstetric/medical history and existing clinical conditions.
  - Appropriate birth planning and complication readiness for each pregnant woman especially those identified with any risk factor or comorbid condition.

- Special emphasis on early diagnosis, adequate and appropriate management of women with malnutrition.
- Special focus on adolescent and early pregnancies as these pregnancies need extra and specialized care

ANNEXURE 16: 2018–19 UPDATE POPULATION NORMS

Health personnel	Population norms
Doctor	1 per 3500
Nurse	1 per 5000
Health worker (Male or female)	1 per 5000 (Plains) or 3000 (Hills)
Health assistant (Male or female)	1 per 30000 (Plains) or 20000 (Hills)
Pharmacist	1 per 10000
Lab technician	1 per 10000
USHA (Urban worker)	1 per 2500
ASHA (23 days annual training)	1 per 1000
Trained dai	1 per 1000
Village health guide	1 per 1000
Anganwadi worker (4 months training)	1 per 400–800 (Plains) or 300–800 (Hills)

HEALTH CARE SYSTEM

		Subcenter	PHC	CHC
Level of care		Primary	Primary	Secondary
Population	Plains	5,000	30,000	1,20,000
	Hilly and Tribal areas	3,000	20,000	80,000
Staff		3–4 staff	13–14 (basic) (Desirable 18–21)	Basic - 45–46 Desirable 50–52
Maintenance		Central government	State government	State government
Radial distance covered		2.6	6.6	15.6

ANNEXURE 17: 2018–19 UPDATE TRIBAL HEALTH IN INDIA

Scheduled tribe are described under the article 366 (25) of the Indian Constitution

DEMOGRAPHIC PROFILE

- Highest number of tribal population –
- Madhya Pradesh > Maharashtra > Odisha > Rajasthan
  - Overall highest concentration is in north eastern states
  - 90% tribal population resides in rural areas
- Basic demographic indicators

Indicator	Value	Remarks
Sex ratio	990	-
TFR	2.48	Higher than national average 2.2
Literacy rate (2011)	59%	Lower than national average of 74%
Life expectancy	63.9 years	Lower than national average of 67.5 years
Institutional deliveries	68%	Lower than national average of 78.9%
Infant mortality rate	44.4	Lower than national average of 34
Under five mortality rate	57.1	Lower than national average of 39
Neonatal mortality rate	31.3	Lower than national average of 23.2
Fully immunized	55.8%	Lower than national average of 62%
Underweight for age	45.3%	Lower than national average of 35.7%

Contd...

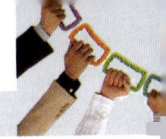

MORBIDITY PROFILE IN TRIBAL POPULATION

Tuberculosis

- **Prevalence rate:** 703 per Lac population - Very high than country profile of 256 cases per lac population for prevalence of tuberculosis
- **Strategies:**
  - Enhance and strengthen Early Diagnosis and prompt treatment
  - Improve standard of care
  - Launch of 'MTDV' – Mobile TB Diab = gnostic Vans with X-ray and sputum testing facility

Leprosy

- 18.9% of all Leprosy cases are from the ST's
- **Strategy:**
  - Improvement in budget allocation, IEC and involvement of NGO's

Malaria and Vector Borne Diseases

- ST's constitute
- 30% of all malaria cases in India
  - 60% of all falciparum cases in India
  - 50% of deaths due to malaria in India
- Vector borne disease is a high priority public health problem in tribal population
- **Strategy:** Improve budget, 100% central assistance

Other Public Health Problems in Tribal Population

- Hypertension – 25% prevalence in tribal population
- Blindness
- Genetic diseases as thalassemia, sickle cell disease
- Tobacco use (72% prevalence of tobacco use)
- Animal bites, accidents and violence

Health Care Services in Tribal Population

- To improve manpower, health care facility in tribal areas norms:
- Subcenter per 3000 population
- PHC's per 20,000 population

ANNEXURE 18: NATIONAL HEALTH POLICY (2017)—TARGETS

KA elimination	2017
Lymphatic filariasis	2017
Leprosy elimination	2018
IMR < 28	2019
MMR to <100	2020
HIV '90-90-90'	2020
Safe water and sanitation	2020
Reduce occupational injury by 50%	2020
Establish Health surveillance	2020
DALY regular tracking trend by	2022
Life expectancy at birth from 67.5 to 70 Years	2025
Reduction in TFR by	2025
Reduce under-5 mortality to 23	2025
NNMR <16 and SBR <10	2025

Contd...

TB cure rate >85%, case detection >70%	2025
Blindness prevalence <0.25/1000	2025
Premature mortality from CVD, cancer, diabetes by 25%	2025
Increase utilization of health services by 50%	2025
ANC coverage >90%	2025
Skilled attendance at birth >90%	2025
Fully immunized >90%	2025
Family planning >90%	2025
HTN and diabetes-controlled status >80%	2025
Reduction in Tobacco use <30%	2025
Stunting reduction <40%	2025
Health expenditure to 2.5% of GDP	2025
All IPHS standard to be implemented	2025

ANNEXURE 19: SUSTAINABLE DEVELOPMENT GOALS

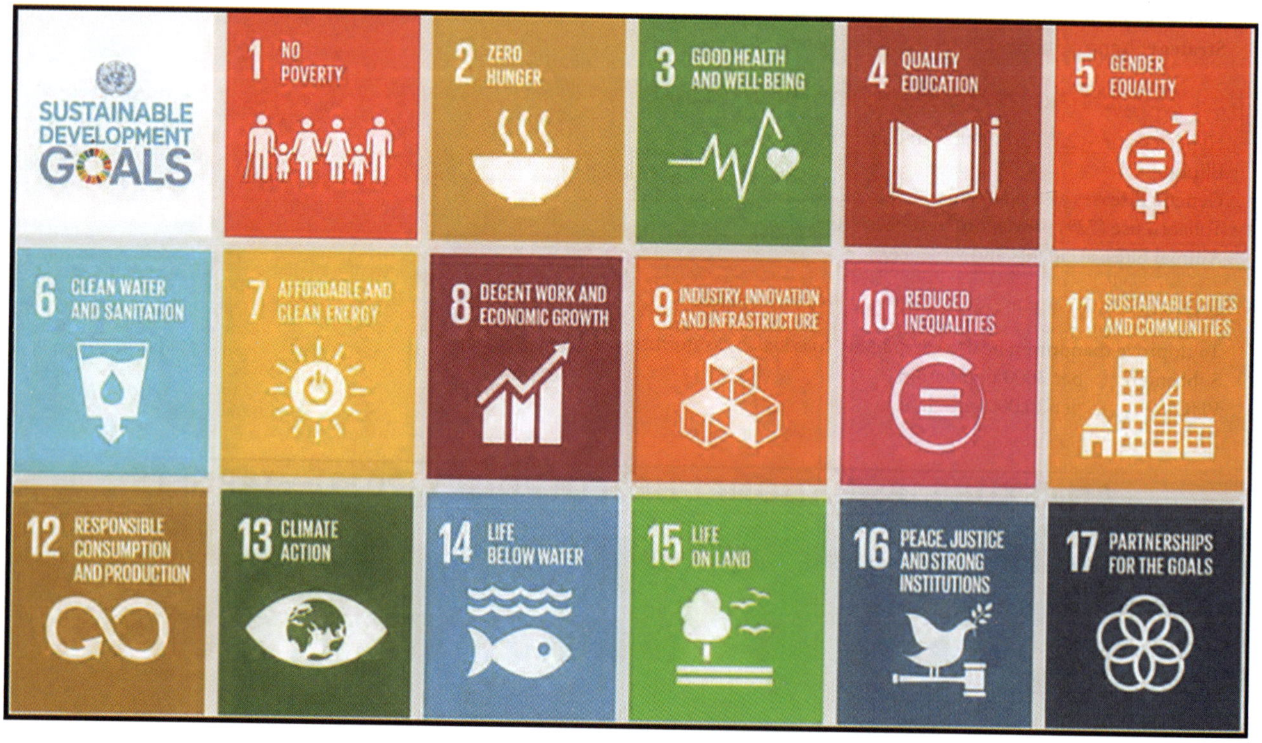
SUSTAINABLE DEVELOPMENT GOALS
1 NO POVERTY
2 ZERO HUNGER
3 GOOD HEALTH AND WELL-BEING
4 QUALITY EDUCATION
5 GENDER EQUALITY
6 CLEAN WATER AND SANITATION
7 AFFORDABLE AND CLEAN ENERGY
8 DECENT WORK AND ECONOMIC GROWTH
9 INDUSTRY, INNOVATION AND INFRASTRUCTURE
10 REDUCED INEQUALITIES
11 SUSTAINABLE CITIES AND COMMUNITIES
12 RESPONSIBLE CONSUMPTION AND PRODUCTION
13 CLIMATE ACTION
14 LIFE BELOW WATER
15 LIFE ON LAND
16 PEACE, JUSTICE AND STRONG INSTITUTIONS
17 PARTNERSHIPS FOR THE GOALS

GOAL #3

The specific target are as below:

Goal	Target
3.1	By 2030, reduce global MMR <70
3.2	By 2030, reduce ▪ Neonatal mortality rate <12 per 1000 Live births ▪ Under five mortality rate <25 per 1000 Live births
3.3	By 2030, end epidemics of AIDS, TB, Malaria and neglected tropical disease
3.4	By 2030, reduce by 1/3rd premature deaths from non-communicable diseases

Contd...

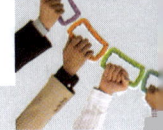

Goal	Target
3.5	Prevention and treatment of substance abuse
3.6	By 2020, halve the number of global deaths and injuries from road traffic accidents
3.7	By 2030, ensure universal access to RTI/STI services, family planning services
3.8	Universal health coverage, access to vaccines, essential medicines and all
3.9	By 2030, reduce deaths from chemicals, air and water pollution and contamination
3a	Strengthen tobacco control implementation
3b	Support research and development of vaccines and new treatment
3c	Increase health financing and recruitment development
3d	Enhance capacity of all countries for early warning, risk reduction and management of national and global health risks

SUSTAINABLE DEVELOPMENT GOALS - "SURVIVE – THRIVE & TRANSFORM HEALTH"

Important Points to Remember

- Reduce global maternal mortality to less than 70 per 100,000 live births
- Reduce newborn mortality to at least as low as 12 per 1,000 live births in every country
- Reduce under-five mortality to at least as low as 25 per 1,000 live births in every country
- End epidemics of HIV, tuberculosis, malaria, neglected tropical diseases and other communicable diseases
- Reduce by one-third premature mortality from non-communicable diseases and promote mental health and well-being

SDG Targets on Infectious Diseases

Specific Plan—Main Targets 2030	
Ending the epidemic of AIDS	Reduce the annual number newly infected with HIV by 90% and the annual number of people dying from AIDS-related causes by 80% (compared with 2010)
Ending the epidemic of TB	▪ 90% reduction in TB deaths ▪ 80% reduction in TB incidence rate (to less than 20 per 100,000 population) ▪ Zero TB-affected families facing catastrophic costs due to TB
Ending the epidemic of malaria	▪ 90% reduction in global malaria mortality rate ▪ 90% reduction in global malaria case incidence ▪ Malaria eliminated from at least 35 countries ▪ Re-establishment of malaria prevented in all countries identified as malaria-free
Ending the epidemic of NTDs	90% reduction in the number of people requiring interventions against NTDs
Control hepatitis	95% decline in new cases of chronic HBV infection between 2010 and 2030; 80% reduction in new cases of chronic HCV infection over the same period; 65% reduction in HBV-and HCV-related deaths
Combat waterborne diseases	▪ No one practices open defecation (by 2025) ▪ Everyone uses a basic drinking-water supply and handwashing facilities at home ▪ Everyone uses adequate sanitation when at home (by 2040) ▪ All drinking-water supply, sanitation and hygiene services are delivered in progressively affordable, accountable and financially and environmentally sustainable manner

12 Points High Focus Areas by WHO-2019

- Accessible, approachable, affordable – Universal health coverage
- Measles outbreak to be controlled
- Zero polio transmission and health for all
- Ebola case management and drug trials
- Road safety and RTA prevention
- Neonatal care and essential services
- Climatic change – air safety
- Prevent hearing loss
- Global influenza strategy
- Accelerate – End TB - strategy
- Human genome editing program
- Food safety

ANNEXURE 20: MCH INDICATORS

ANC in WRA (Women of reproductive age) = 84%
ANC in 1st TM (Trimester) 59%
Neonatal tetanus immunization 89%
Institutional delivery 79%

MMR (Maternal mortality ratio) 130
MM Rate (Maternal mortality rate) 8.8
Lifetime risk 0.3%

Indicators	India	India Stats (NFHS 4 – 2015-2016)
Maternal Mortality Ratio (MMR)	167/100000 MDG Target –109/Lakh, SDG Target (2030)- <70/Lakh Highest MMR[Q] –Assam (300) >UP and Uttarakhand (285) Lowest MMR – Kerala (61) Target -100 (by 2017–12th Five year plan)	130/lac LB
Maternal mortality rate@		8.8
Adult life time risk of maternal death#	0.4%	0.3%
TT coverage in pregnancy	89 %	89%
ANC coverage (4 ANC Visits)	51% (Rural -45, Urban -66)	59%
Institutional deliveries	78.9% (Rural- 75, Urban -88.7)	79%
Delivery by trained personnel	81.4% (Rural-78, Urban -90)	89% rural, 75% rural
Postnatal checkup (Within 2 days of delivery)	62.4 % (Rural-58.5, Urban -71.7)	81.4%
Crude birth rate	India -20.4 (Rural -22.7, Urban -17.4)	India -20.4 (Rural -22.7, Urban -17.4)
Total fertility rate	2.2, Target -2.1 (by 2017-12th Five year plan) Highest –UP -3.2	2.2, Target -2.1 (by 2017-12th Five year plan)
Couple protection rate	53.5, Target -65 (by 2017-12th Five year plan)	53.5, Target -65 (by 2017-12th Five year plan)

@Maternal mortality rate = number of maternal deaths among females age group 15–49 years (per lakh)
#The life time risk is defined as the probability that at least one women of reproductive age(15-49) will die due to child birth or puerperium assuming that chance of death is uniformly distributed across the entire reproductive span. The formula is:

$$\text{Lifetime risk} = 1 - \left(1 - \frac{\textit{maternal mortality rate}}{100{,}000}\right)$$

ANNEXURE 21: INDICATORS OF HEALTH CARE SERVICES

INDICATORS

Global health indicator	Life expectancy
Socio-economic development	Life expectancy
Health care delivery indicators	▪ Doctor population ratio ▪ Doctor nurse ratio ▪ Population bed ratio ▪ Population per subcenter ▪ Population per trained birth attendant

Contd...

Utilization indicators	▪ Proportion of children Fully immunized ▪ Proportion of ANC in pregnant females ▪ Couple protection rate ▪ Bed occupancy rates ▪ Average length of stay ▪ Bed turnover ratio
Socio-economic indicators	▪ Annual growth rate ▪ Per capita GNP ▪ Unemployment rate ▪ Dependency ratio ▪ Literacy rates ▪ Family size ▪ Per capita calorie available
Health policy indicators	▪ Proportion of GNP spent on health ▪ Proportion of budget for primary health care
Quality of life indicator	Physical quality of life index
Basic needs indicator (indicator for the International labor organization - ILO)	▪ Calorie consumption ▪ Access to water ▪ Life expectancy ▪ Deaths due to disease ▪ Illiteracy ▪ Doctor/nurse per population ▪ Rooms per person ▪ GNP per capita
Disability person type indicator	▪ Limitation of mobility indicator ▪ Limitation to perform activity of daily life
Disability event type indicator	▪ Work loss days ▪ DALY (disability adjusted life years)
Morbidity indicators	▪ Incidence and prevalence ▪ Notification rates ▪ Hospital admission, OPD rates
Mortality indicators	▪ Crude death rate ▪ Case fatality rates ▪ Proportional mortality rates

MCH INDICATORS

Overall development of country (WHO)	IMR
Overall social development of country (UN or UNICEF)	Under five mortality rate
Quality of delivery service	MMR
International comparisons of health care services	Perinatal mortality rate

ANNEXURE 22: MCH—CHILD DEVELOPMENT

ICDS

Nutrition supplement guidelines

Age	Calorie	Proteins (g)	Financial (per child/day)
Child 6–72 months	500 calories	12–15 g	₹6
Pregnant and nursing mothers	600 calories	18–20 g	₹7
Severe malnourished 7–72 months	800 calories	20–25 g	₹9

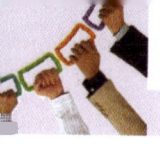

RIGHTS OF CHILD

Article 24—employment of children below <14 years of age
Article 39—prevent abuse of children of tender age
Article 45—free compulsory education for all children age <14 years

COMPOSITION OF BREAST MILK

Type	Time	Appearance	Composition	Function
Colostrum	First 3-4 days after birth	Yellowish and thick	▪ More antibodies and WBC ▪ Anti-infective agents (lactoferrin, lysozyme, lactoperoxidase, complements, proline-rich polypeptides) ▪ Rich in vitamins A, D, E & K ▪ Less fats ▪ More proteins and IG (IgA, IgM, IgG) ▪ Rich in growth factors– EGF, FGF	Protection against infection has a mild laxative effect helps to pass early stools
Transitional milk	4 days to 10-14 days	Thinner, lighter in color	More fat, sugar, calories & vitamins Less IG & proteins	Supplies adequate calories needed by the baby
Mature milk	2 weeks after the baby is delivered	Thinner	More fat, protein, water, lactose, energy (71 cal/100 mL)	Supplies all the nutrients needed for normal growth
Preterm milk	When a preterm baby is delivered		More calories, fat, proteins, sodium, IG, lactoferrin, Zn, macrophages Less lactose, calcium, phosphorus	Supplies more energy which is needed for rapid growth
Foremilk	At the start of feed	Watery	Rich in proteins, sugar, vitamins, minerals and water	Satisfies baby's thirst
Hind milk	At the end of feed	Thick	Richer in fat content	Provides energy, satisfies baby's hunger and nutritional demands

ANNEXURE 23: BIOMEDICAL WASTE 2016 GUIDELINES

Categories	Waste types	Includes	Treatment and disposal
Yellow	Human anatomical waste	Human tissues, organs, body parts, fetus	Incineration Plasma Pyrolysis Deep burial Or Autoclave/microwave
	Animal waste	Animal tissues, body parts, organs, carcasses, fluids, blood	
	Soiled waste	Items contaminated with blood, and fluids, including cotton, dressing, soiled plaster casts, linen, beddings	
	Expired or Discarded medicines and Cytotoxic drugs	Outdated contaminated and discarded medicine	Return to Manufacturer Incineration Encapsulation
	Chemicals	Chemical used in disinfection (insecticides) or in production of biologicals	
	Chemical Liquid waste	Waste from lab and washing, cleaning, housekeeping and disinfecting activities	Resource recovery followed by pretreatment and discharge into drains
	Discarded linen, mattresses, beddings contaminated with blood or body fluid		Nonchlorinated chemical disinfection followed by Incineration or Plasma
	Microbiology and Biotechnology waste	Lab waste, live vaccine, toxins	Incineration Pre-treat to sterilize with nonchlorinated chemicals on-site as per NACO or WHO

Contd...

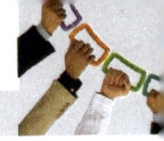

Categories	Waste types	Includes	Treatment and disposal
Red	Contaminated Waste (Recyclable)	Tubing, Bottles, IV tubes and sets, Catheters, Urine bags, Syringes (without needles and fixed needle syringes) and vacutainers with needle cut and gloves	Autoclaving Micro-waving/ Hydroclaving followed by shredding or mutilation and waste
White	Waste sharps	Needles, syringes, blades, scalpels, glass	Autoclaving or Dry Heat Sterilization followed by shredding or mutilation or encapsulation in metal container or cement concrete
Blue	Glassware Metallic Body Implants	Broken or discarded and	Glassware Metallic Body Implants

PSM ANNEXURES AND LAST MINUTE REVISION

ANNEXURE 24: FORMULAS IN COMMUNITY MEDICINE

1. Expected number of live births = $\dfrac{\text{Birth rate (per 1000 population)} \times \text{population}}{1000}$
2. Number of pregnancies (expected) = $\dfrac{\text{Birth rate (per 1000 population)} \times \text{population}}{1000}$ + pregnancy waste factor (10% of expected live births)
3. Vaccine requirement (expected) = Expected live births × number of doses per child × vaccine multiplicative factor
4. Child death rate = $\dfrac{\text{Number of deaths of children age 1-4 years}}{\text{Total number of children aged 1-4 years in the middle of the year}} \times 1000$
5. Child mortality rate = $\dfrac{\text{Number of deaths of children less than 5 years}}{\text{Total number of live births in the same year}} \times 1000$
6. Child mortality rate = $\dfrac{\text{1000-under five mortality rate}}{10}$
7. Maternal mortality ratio = $\dfrac{\text{Number of deaths of mothers due to pregnancy or related causes}}{\text{Total number of live births in the same year}} \times 100{,}000$
8. Maternal mortality rate = $\dfrac{\text{Number of deaths of mothers due to pregnancy or related causes}}{\text{Total number of women age 15-49 years}} \times 100{,}000$
9. Lifetime maternal mortality risk = $\dfrac{1-(\text{1-maternal mortality rate})}{100{,}000}$
10. Case fatality rate = $\dfrac{\text{Number of deaths due to a particular disease}}{\text{Total number of cases of the same disease}} \times 100$
11. Proportional mortality rate = $\dfrac{\text{Number of deaths due to a particular disease}}{\text{Total deaths in a year}} \times 100$
12. Cause specific death rate = $\dfrac{\text{Number of deaths due to a particular disease}}{\text{Mid-year population}} \times 1000$
13. Attack rates = $\dfrac{\text{Total number of cases in an area during a specified period}}{\text{Total population at the start of period}} \times 100$
14. Secondary attack rate = $\dfrac{\text{Total number of cases arising from the primary case within an incubation period}}{\text{Total number of susceptible contacts}} \times 100$
15. Digestibility coefficient = $\dfrac{\text{Amount of amino acid absorbed from the food}}{\text{Amount of protein ingested}}$
16. Biological value = $\dfrac{\text{Amount of nitrogen retained for body mass}}{\text{Amount of amino acid absorbed from the food}}$

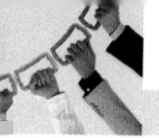

17. Net protein utilization = Digestibility coefficient × Biological value = $\frac{\text{Amount of nitrogen retained for body mass}}{\text{Amount of protein ingested}}$

18. Annual growth rate = $\frac{\text{Crude birth rate - Crude death rate}}{10}$

19. Crude birth rate (CBR) = $\frac{\textit{Number of live births during the year}}{\textit{Mid-year population}} \times 1000$

20. Crude death rate (CDR) = $\frac{\textit{Number of deaths during the year}}{\textit{Mid-year population}} \times 1000$

21. Standardized mortality ratio = $\frac{\textit{Observed deaths}}{\textit{Expected deaths}} \times 1000$

22. General fertility rate (GFR) = $\frac{\textit{Number of live births in a year}}{\textit{Mid-year female population in age group 15-49 years}} \times 1000$

23. General marital fertility rate (GMFR) = $\frac{\textit{Number of live births in a year}}{\textit{Mid-year married female population in age group 15-49 years}} \times 1000$

24. Age specific fertility rate (ASFR) = $\frac{\textit{Number of live births in a particular age-group}}{\textit{Mid-year female population of the same age group}} \times 1000$

25. Age specific marital fertility rate (ASMFR) = $\frac{\textit{Number of live births in a particular age-group}}{\textit{Mid-year married female population of the same age group}} \times 1000$

26. Total fertility rate (TFR) = $\frac{5 \times \Sigma_{19-49}^{15-49} ASFR}{1000}$

27. Total marital fertility rate (TMFR) = $\frac{5 \times \Sigma_{15-19}^{45-49} ASMFR}{1000}$

28. Gross reproduction rate (GRR) = $\frac{5 \times \Sigma_{15-19}^{45-49} \textit{ASFR for female live births}}{1000}$

29. Infant mortality rate (IMR) = $\frac{\textit{Number of infant deaths during the year}}{\textit{Number of live births during the same year}} \times 100$

30. Neonatal mortality rate (NnMR) = $\frac{\textit{Number of infant deaths age<29 days during the year}}{\textit{Number of live births during the same year}} \times 100$

31. Early neonatal mortality rate (E-NnMR) = $\frac{\textit{Number of infant deaths age<7 days during the year}}{\textit{Number of live births during the same year}} \times 1000$

32. Late neonatal mortality rate (L-NnMR) = $\frac{\textit{Number of infant deaths age 7 days to < 29 days during the year}}{\textit{Number of live births during the same year}} \times 1000$

33. Post neonatal mortality rate (P-NnMR) = $\frac{\textit{Number of infant deaths age 29 days to <1 year during the year}}{\textit{Number of live births during the same year}} \times 1000$

34. Perinatal mortality rate (PnMR) = $\frac{\textit{Number of still births and infant deaths of<7 days during the year}}{\textit{Number of still births and live births during the same year}} \times 1000$

35. Still birth rate(SBR) = $\frac{\textit{Number of still births during the year}}{\textit{Number of still briths and live births during the same year}} \times 1000$

36. Pearls index = $\frac{\textit{Total accidental pregnancies}}{\textit{Total women months of exposure}} \times 100 \times 12$ (months in a year)

37. Relative risk (Risk Ratio) = $\frac{\textit{Incidence exposed}}{\textit{Incidence in exposed}}$

38. Attributable risk proportion = $\frac{\textit{Incidence exposed – incidence in nonexposed}}{\textit{Incidence in exposed}}$

39. Population attributable risk = $\frac{\textit{Incidence in total group – incidence in nonexposed}}{\textit{Incidence in total group}}$

40. Sensitivity = $\frac{\textit{True positive}}{\textit{True positive + False negative}} \times 100$

41. Specificity = $\frac{\textit{True negative}}{\textit{True negative + False positive}} \times 100$

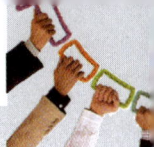

42. False negative error rate = $\frac{\textit{False negative}}{\textit{True positive + False negative}} \times 100$

43. False positive error rate = $\frac{\textit{False positive}}{\textit{True negative + False positive}} \times 100$

44. Positive predictive value = $\frac{\textit{True positive}}{\textit{True positive + False positive}} \times 100$

45. Negative predictive value = $\frac{\textit{True negative}}{\textit{True negative + False negative}} \times 100$

46. Positive predictive value (Bayes formula) = $\frac{\text{Sensitivity} \times \text{Prevalence}}{(\text{Sensitivity} \times \text{Prevalence}) + ((1 - \text{specificity}) \times (1 - \text{prevalence}))} \times 100$

47. Negative predictive value (Bayes formula) = $\frac{\text{Specificity} \times \text{(1-Prevalence)}}{(\text{Specificity} \times (1 - \text{Prevalence}) + ((1 - \text{sensitivity}) \times \text{prevalence}))} \times 100$

48. Youden's Index = (sensitivity + specificity) - 1

49. Accuracy of a screening test = $\frac{\textit{True positive + True negative}}{\textit{True positive + true negative + false positive + false negative}} \times 100$

50. Likelihood ratio for positive test = $\frac{\textit{Sensitivity}}{\textit{1 - specificity}} \times 100$

51. Relative risk reduction (RRR) = $\frac{\textit{Event rate in exposed group - Event rate in Control (Nonexposed) group}}{\text{Event rate in control (nonexposed) } \textit{group}} \times 100$

52. Absolute risk reduction (ARR) = Event rate in experimental (exposed) group – Event rate in control (nonexposed) group

53. Number needed to treat (NNT) = $\frac{1}{\text{ARR}} = \frac{1}{\text{Experimental event rate - Control Event Rate}} \times 100$

54. Regression variable (y) = a + bx + e,
Where a = regression constant or the intercept at 'y'
b = slope of curve, x is the independent variable, e = error

55. Median
In case of odd number of observations
Median
= $[n + 1/2]^{th}$ observation
In case of even number of observations
Median
= $[(n/2) + (n/2+1)]/2]^{th}$ observation

56. Mode
Mode = Mean – 3 (Mean –Median) or 2 Median – 2 Mean

57. Mean (sample: X) = $\Sigma\frac{x}{n}$

58. Mean deviation (MD) = $\frac{\Sigma(x - \bar{x})}{n}$

59. Standard deviation (SD) (Sample size >30) = $\sqrt{\frac{[\Sigma(x - \bar{x})^2]}{n}}$

60. Standard deviation (SD) (Small sample – Sample size < 30) = $\sqrt{\frac{[\Sigma(x - \bar{x})^2]}{n - 1}}$

61. Variance = SD^2

62. Coefficient of variance (CV) = $\left[\frac{SD}{\bar{x}}\right] \times 100$

63. Standard normal deviate or Z score = $(x - \bar{x})/\sigma$, (σ standard deviation)
$= \frac{\textit{Observed value-expected value}}{\textit{Standard deviation}}$

64. Standard error of mean (SEM) = $\frac{SD}{\sqrt{n}}$

65. Standard error of proportion (SEP) = $\sqrt{\frac{pq}{n}}$
Where
p = prevalence
q = 100 – prevalence

66. Standard error of difference between 2 means (SEDM) = $\sqrt{\frac{(SD_1)^2}{n} + \frac{(SD_2)^2}{n} + \ldots}$

67. Degree of Freedom (dF) (for qualitative data) = (c – 1) (r – 1); c = Number of columns; n = Number of rows

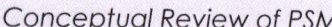

68. Degree of Freedom (dF) (for quantitative data) = n – 1, where n = number of observations or sample size
69. Coefficient of determination (CD) = r^2, where r = coefficient of correlation
70. Power of a test = 1 – β where β is type II error
71. Sample size in quantitative studies $4pq/L^2$, where p = prevalence, q = 1 – p, and L = absolute error
72. Accuracy = (Sensitivity × Prevalence) + (specificity) (1 – prevalence)
73. Pretest odds = Pretest probability/[1 – pretest probability]
74. Post-test probability = Post-test odds/[Post-test odds + 1]
75. Post-test odds = Pretest odds × LR (LR = Likelihood ratio)

ANNEXURE 25: EVOLUTION IN MEDICINE AND WHO'S WHO

Atreya	First Indian Physician and teacher
Charaka	Father of Indian medicine For his book – 'Charaka Samhita'
Susruta	Father of Indian surgery For his book – Susruta Samhita
Laws of Manu	Code on personal hygiene
Horus	Egyptian God of health
Hygiea	Goddess of health
Panacea	Goddess of medicine
Dhanvantri	Hindu God of medicine
John Snow	Father of epidemiology
Cholera	Father of public health
Fracastorius	Founder of epidemiology
Hippocrates	Father of medicine
David Lawrence Sackett	Father of evidence-based medicine
Gordon Guyatt	Founder of evidence-based medicine
Pattenkofer	Multifactorial causation of disease
McMahon	Web of causation of disease
Edward Jenner	(Coined the term) Vaccination
Louis Pasteur	Germ theory of disease
James Lind	Study on vitamin C and scurvy
Doll and hill	Study on smoking and lung cancer
Framingham study	Study on cardiovascular risks and morbidity profile
Multi centric growth reference study	To assess growth pattern in children across different countries (Brazil, Ghana, India, Norway, Oman and the USA)
Accord trial	Assessment of cardiovascular risks and diabetes

Table 10: Nobel Prize Winners

Nobel Laureates	Year	Discovery
Yoshinori Ohsumi	2016	Mechanism of Autophagy
William C. Campbell and Satoshi Ōmura	2015	Discovery of a novel therapy against infections caused by roundworm parasites
John O'Keefe, May-Britt Moser and Edvard I. Moser	2014	Discovery of cells that constitute a positioning system in the brain
Rothman, Schekman and Südhof	2013	Discovery of machinery regulating vesicle transmission in cells
Sir John B. Gurdon and Shinya Yamanaka	2012	Mature cells can be reprogrammed to become pluripotent

Contd...

Nobel Laureates	Year	Discovery
Beutler and Hoffmann Ralph M. Steinman	2011	Discovery on activation of innate immunity Discovery of dendritic cell and its role in adaptive immunity
Robert G. Edwards	2010	In vitro fertilization
Murray and E. Donnall Thomas	1990	Organ and cell transplantation
Robert Koch	1905	Investigations and discoveries in relation to tuberculosis
Ronald Ross	1902	Life cycle of plasmodium
Beadle and Tatum Joshua Lederberg	1958	Genes act by regulating definite chemical events Genetic recombination and organization of genetic material of bacteria
Frederick Sanger	1958 and 1980	Structure of proteins (Insulin) and base sequence of nucleic acids
Paul Muller	1948	DDT as a contact poison against arthropods
Alexander Fleming	1945	Discovery of penicillin
I.P. Pavlov	1904	Physiology of digestion
Ilya Ilyich Mechnikov and Paul Ehrlich	1908	Work on Immunity
Kary Mullis	1944	PCR method

ANNEXURE 26: INFECTIOUS DISEASE EPIDEMIOLOGY—REMEMBER POINTS

DAY DISEASES

First disease	Rubeola/Measles/Hard measles/14-day measles
Second disease	Scarlet Fever (due to streptococcus pyogenes)
Third disease	Rubella/German measles/3-day measles
Fourth disease	Filatow-Dukes' Disease/Staphylococcal Scalded Skin Syndrome/Ritter's disease
Fifth disease	Erythema infectiosum (due to Erythrovirus (Parvovirus) B19)
Sixth disease	Exanthem subitum/Roseola infantum (due to Human Herpes Virus 6/7)

TRENDS IN INFECTIONS

Seasonal trends are seen in-
Measles, rubella, varicella, cerebral meningitis, Gastroenteritis etc.
Cyclic trends are seen in-
Measles- every 2-3 years, Rubella, Influenza pandemic
Secular trends are seen in-
Diphtheria, Diabetes mellitus, polio, Tuberculosis, Typhoid, Lung Cancer

TYPES OF CARRIERS OF INFECTIONS

Carrier by type	Incubatory carrier	Shed infectious agent in incubation period of disease	Measles, Mumps, Polio, Pertussis, Influenza, Diphtheria and Hepatitis B
	Healthy carrier	Continue to shed the infectious agent without suffering from overt disease	Polio, Cholera, Meningococcal meningitis, Salmonellosis and Diphtheria
	Convalescent carrier	Continue to shed the infectious agent during period of convalescence	Typhoid fever, Dysentery (bacillary and amebic), Cholera, Diphtheria and Pertussis

Contd...

Carrier by duration	Temporary carrier	Shed infectious agent for short periods	Incubatory/Convalescent or healthy
	Chronic carrier	Excrete infectious agent (intermittently or continuously) for indefinite period	Reintroduce disease into areas free of infection (e.g. Malaria)
Carriers by portal of exit	Urinary carriers, intestinal carriers, respiratory carriers		

PERIODS OF ISOLATION

Periods of Isolation Recommended

Disease	Duration of isolation
Chickenpox	Until all lesions crusted; usually about 6 days after onset of rash
Measles	From the onset of catarrhal stage through 3rd day of rash
German measles	None, except that women in the first trimester or sexually active, non immure women in child-bearing years not using contraceptive measures should not be exposed
Cholera, Diphtheria	3 days after tetracyclines started, until 48 hours of antibiotics (or negative cultures after treatment)
Shigellosis Salmonellosis	Until 3 consecutive negative stool cultures
Hepatitis A	3 weeks
Influenza	3 days after onset
Polio	2 weeks adult, 6 weeks paediatric
Tuberculosis (sputum +)	Until 3 weeks of effective chemotherapy
Herpes zoster	6 days after onset of rash
Mumps	Until swelling subsides
Pertussis	4 weeks or until paroxysms cease
Meningococcal meningitis Streptococcal pharyngitis	Until the first 6 hours of effective antibiotic therapy are completed

CHEMOPROPHYLAXIS

Chemoprophylaxis is protection from or prevention of disease.

- Causal prophylaxis → Prevention of infection by early elimination of invading causal agent.
- Clinical prophylaxis → Prevention of clinical symptoms (not necessarily elimination of infection)

Table 11: Chemoprophylaxis of various diseases

Disease	Chemoprophylaxis
▪ Influenza	▪ Oseltamivir for contacts with chronic disease
▪ Meningococcal meningitis	▪ Ciprofloxacin and Minocycline or Rifampicin (House-hold and close community contact) + Immunization (A and C)
▪ Cholera	▪ Tetracycline or Furazolidone (House-hold contacts)
▪ Bacterial conjunctivitis	▪ Erythromycin ophthalmic ointment
▪ Diphtheria	▪ Erythromycin and 1st dose of vaccine
▪ Pneumonic plague	▪ Tetracycline for contacts
▪ Malaria	▪ Short term (<6 weeks)- Doxycycline/Chloroquine/Mefloquine ▪ Long term - Proguanil/Mefloquine (if tolerated)
▪ Tuberculosis	▪ Isoniazid (10 mg/kg x 6 months)

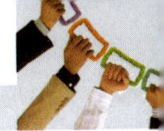

ANNEXURE 27: LIST OF DISEASES UNDER ESI, IDSP, NOTIFIABLE DISEASES

LIST OF DISEASES UNDER ESI

- **Infectious diseases**
  - Tuberculosis
  - Leprosy
  - Chronic Empyema
  - AIDS
- **Neoplasms**
  - Malignant diseases
- **Endocrine, nutritional and metabolic disorders**
  - Diabetes Mellitus-with proliferative retinopathy/diabetic foot/nephropathy.
- **Disorders of nervous system**
  - Monoplegia
  - Hemiplegia
  - Paraplegia
  - Hemiparesis
  - Intracranial Space Occupying Lesion
  - Spinal Cord Compression
  - Parkinson's disease
  - Myasthenia Gravis/Neuromuscular Dystrophies
- **Diseases of eye**
  - Immature Cataract with vision 6/60 or less
  - Detachment of Retina
  - Glaucoma
- **Diseases of cardiovascular system**
  - **Coronary artery disease:**
    - Unstable Angina
    - Myocardial infraction with ejection less than 45%
  - Congestive heart failure- Left, Right
  - Cardiac valvular diseases with failure/complications
  - Cardiomyopathies
  - Heart disease with surgical intervention along with complications
- **Chest diseases**
  - Bronchiectasis
  - Interstitial lung disease
  - Chronic obstructive lung diseases (COPD) with congestive heart failure (Cor Pulmonale)
- **Diseases of the digestive system**
  - Cirrhosis of liver with ascites/chronic active hepatitis
- **Orthopaedic diseases**
  - Dislocation of vertebra/prolapse of intervertebral disc
  - Non-union or delayed union of fracture
  - Post-traumatic surgical amputation of lower extremity
  - Compound fracture with chronic osteomyelitis
- **Psychoses**
  - Sub-group under this head are listed for clarification
    - Schizophrenia
    - Endogenous depression
    - Manic depressive psychosis (MDP)
    - Dementia
- **Others**
  - More than 20% burns with infection/complication
  - Chronic renal failure
  - Reynaud's disease/Burger's disease.

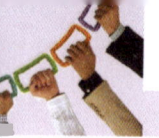

LIST OF DISEASES UNDER IDSP

Syndromic Case Surveillance

It has six syndromes—cough, fever, acute flaccid paralysis (AFP), diarrhea, jaundice, unusual death

Probable Case Surveillance

- Acute diarrheal disease (including acute gastroenteritis)
- Bacillary dysentery
- Viral hepatitis
- Enteric fever
- Malaria
- Dengue/dengue hemorrhagic fever/dengue shock syndrome (DHF/DSS)
- Chikungunya
- Acute Encephalitis syndrome
- Meningitis
- Measles
- Diphtheria
- Pertussis
- Chicken pox
- Fever of unknown origin (PUO)
- Acute respiratory infection (ARI)/Influenza like Illness (ILI)
- Pneumonia
- Leptospirosis
- Acute flaccid paralysis<15 years of age
- Dog bite
- Snake bite
- Any other state specific disease (Specify)
- Unusual syndromes not captured above (Specify clinical diagnosis)

Laboratory Case Surveillance

- Dengue/DHF/DSS
- Chikungunya
- Japanese encephalitis (JE)
- Meningococcal meningitis
- Typhoid fever
- Diphtheria
- Cholera
- Shigella dysentery
- Viral hepatitis A
- Viral hepatitis E
- Leptospirosis
- Malaria
    - Plasmodium vivax (PV)
    - Plasmodium falciparum (PF)

LIST OF DISEASES NOTIFIABLE UNDER INTERNATIONAL HEALTH REGULATIONS

[Q]*Notifiable cases under International Health Regulations—*

- Cholera
- Plague
- Yellow fever
- Small pox
- Relapsing fever
- Salmonellosis
- Polio
- Influenza
- SARS
- Malaria
- Rabies
- Louse borne typhus fever

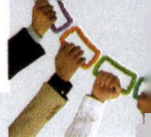

ANNEXURE 28: INCUBATION PERIOD OF DISEASES

Skin Infections/Rashes		
Disease	**Incubation period**	**Period of communicability**
Chickenpox	10–21	2 days before rash until all sores have crusts (6–7 days)
Fifth disease (Erythema infectiosum)	4–14	7 days before rash until rash begins
Hand, foot, and mouth disease	3–6	Onset of mouth ulcers until fever gone
Impetigo (strep or staph)	2–5	Onset of sores until 24 hours on antibiotic
Lice	7	Onset of itch until 1 treatment
Measles	8–12	4 days before rash until 4 days after rash appears
Roseola	9–10	Onset of fever until rash gone (2 days)
Rubella (German measles)	14–21	7 days before rash until 5 days after rash appears
Scabies	30–45	Onset of rash until 1 treatment
Scarlet fever	3–6	Onset of fever or rash until 24 hours on antibiotic
Shingles (contagious for chicken pox)	14–16	Onset of rash until all sores have crusts (7 days) (Note: No need to isolate if sores can be kept covered.)
Warts	30–180	Minimally contagious
Respiratory Infections:		
Bronchiolitis	4–6	Onset of cough until 7 days
Croup/Coryza	2–5	Onset of cough until fever gone
Diphtheria	2–5	Onset of sore throat until 4 days on antibiotic
Influenza	1–2	Onset of symptoms until fever gone
Sore throat, strep	2–5	Onset of sore throat until 24 hours on antibiotic
Sore throat, viral	2–5	Onset of sore throat until fever gone
Tuberculosis	6–24 months	Until 2 weeks on drugs (Note: Most childhood TB is not contagious.)
Whooping cough	7–10	Onset of runny nose until 5 days on antibiotic
Intestinal Infections:		
Diarrhea, bacterial	1–5	Variable – depends on organism
Diarrhea, giardia	7–28	Variable – depends on organism
Diarrhea, traveller's	1–6	Variable – depends on organism
Diarrhea, viral (Rotavirus)	1–3	Variable – depends on organism
Hepatitis A	14–50	2 weeks before jaundice begins until jaundice resolved (7 days)
Pinworms	21–28	Minimally contagious, staying home is unnecessary
Vomiting, viral	2–5	Variable – depends on etiology
Other Infections:		
Infectious mononucleosis	30–50	Onset of fever until fever gone (7 days)
Meningitis, bacterial	2–10	7 days before symptoms until 24 hours on IV antibiotics in hospital
Meningitis, viral	3–6	Onset of symptoms and for 1–2 weeks
Mumps	12–25	5 days before swelling until swelling gone (7 days)
Conjunctivitis	1–5	Mild infection, staying home is unnecessary
Conjunctivitis with suppuration	2–7	Onset of pus until 1 day on antibiotic eye drops

ANNEXURE 29: VACCINE STRAINS AND IMMUNIZATION

MALARIA VACCINE - MOSQUIRIX

Mosquirix - RTS,S is the first, and to date the only, vaccine that has demonstrated it can significantly reduce malaria in children. In clinical trials, the vaccine was found to prevent approximately 4 in 10 malaria cases, including 3 in 10 cases of life-threatening severe malaria

Details for RTS,S Vaccine (Mosquirix ™)

- RTS, S is a scientific name given to this malaria vaccine candidate and represents its composition.
- The 'R' stands for the central repeat region of Plasmodium (P.) falciparum 'circumsporozoite protein (CSP);
- The 'T' for the T-cell epitopes of the CSP;
- The 'S' for hepatitis B surface antigen (HBsAg).
- These are combined in a single fusion protein ('RTS') and co-expressed in yeast cells with free HBsAg.
- The 'RTS' fusion protein and free 'S' protein spontaneously assemble in 'RTS,S' particles.
- The vaccine is administered via intramuscular injection (preferably to the deltoid region), over 3 dosing periods, each 1 month apart, which is consistent with administration of other WHO EPI vaccines. The product is stable for 3 years when stored at temperatures between 2 and 8°C, but must be used within 6 hours of reconstitution
- Financial partner: GSK, Bill and Melinda Gates foundation, World Bank

STRAINS OF VACCINE

BCG	Danish 1331
OPV	Sabin
IPV	Salk
Measles	▪ Edmonston Zagreb ▪ Schwartz strain
Mumps	Jeryll lynn
Rubella	RA 27/3
Chicken pox	OKA
Influenza/Flu vaccine	Quadrivalent vaccine ▪ An A/Michigan/45/2015 (H1N1)pdm09-like virus; ▪ A/Switzerland/8060/2017 (H3N2)-like virus ▪ B/Colorado/06/2017-like virus (B/Victoria/2/87 lineage) ▪ B/Phuket/3073/2013-like virus (B/Yamagata/16/88 lineage).
Meningitis	A, C, W135, Y strain
JE vaccine	▪ SA 14-14-2 (live vaccine) ▪ Nakayama strain (killed vaccine)
Malaria vaccine	Mosquirix (RTS,S/AS01 strain) (WHO approval for community use in Africa)
Dengue	CYD/TDV vaccine
Leprosy vaccine	▪ MIP - Mycobacterium indicus pranii vaccine (under trial) ▪ BCG vaccine (partial protection)
HIV vaccine	▪ rAAV – recombinant adeno associated viral vaccine ▪ AIDSVAX
Typhoid vaccine	▪ Typhoral 21 a (live vaccine) ▪ Vi polysaccharide vaccine
Cholera	▪ Dukoral (WC-rBS - whole cell recombinant beta subunit) ▪ Sanchol ▪ Euvichol
Pneumococcal	▪ Pneumococcal conjugate vaccine – PCV 23
Yellow fever vaccine	17 D vaccine

Active and Passive Immunization

Both active and passive vaccination can be given to-

- Diphtheria
- Hepatitis B
- Rabies
- Tetanus

Heat and Freeze Sensitivity of Vaccine

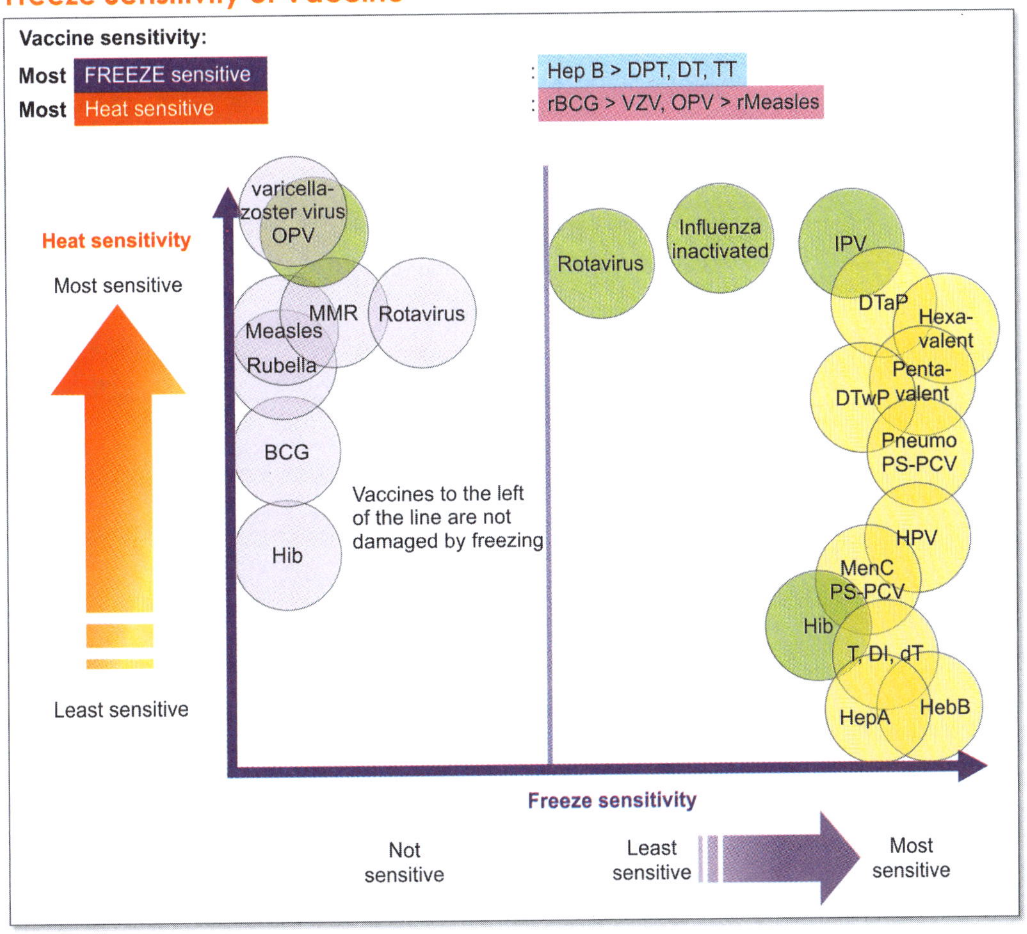

ANNEXURE 30: DAYS OF PUBLIC HEALTH IMPORTANCE

30th January	Anti-leprosy day
2nd Wednesday of March	No smoking day
8th March	International Women's day
15th March	World disabled day
24th March	World TB day (WHO Official)
7th April	World health day (WHO Official)
25th April	World malaria day (WHO Official)
8th May	World red cross day
31st May	No tobacco day (WHO Official)

Contd...

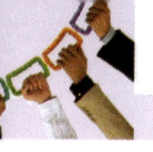

5th June	World environment day
14th June	World blood donor day (WHO Official)
26th June	International day against drug abuse & illicit trafficking
1st July	Doctors day
1st July (30th June)	Mid-year population counting day
11th July	World population day
28th July	World hepatitis day (WHO Official)
8th September	World literacy day
28 September	World rabies day
29th September	World heart day
1st October	International day for geriatric population
1st October	National voluntary blood donation day
2nd Wednesday of October	World disaster reduction day
9th October	World sight day
10th October	World mental health day
10th October	World blindness day
24th October	UN day
24th October	World Polio Day
29th October	World stroke day
10th November	Universal immunization day
1st December	World AIDS day (WHO Official)
3rd December	International day of disabled persons
10th December	Human rights day
Last week April	World Immunization week (WHO Official)
1-7 August	World breastfeeding week
12-18 November	World antibiotic awareness week (WHO Official)
10th February and 10th August	Handwashing days
1-7 September	National nutrition week
October	World cancer awareness month

"ZERO MALARIA STARTS WITH ME"

WORLD MALARIA DAY—25th April 2019

World TB Day - It's Time
World Leprosy day - ending discrimination, stigma and prejudice
World Health day - universal health coverage - everyone, everywhere
World rabies day - share the message save a life
Anti tobacco day - tobacco and lung health

ANNEXURE 31: ENVIRONMENT AND INSTRUMENTS OF PUBLIC HEALTH IMPORTANCE

DIFFERENCE BETWEEN RAPID AND SLOW SAND FILTER

Features	Rapid sand filter	Slow sand filter
Space	Occupies very little space	Occupies large area
Rate of filtration	200 m.g.a.d	2-3 m.g.a.d
Effective size of sand	0.4–0.7 mm	0.2 –0.3 mm
Preliminary treatment	Coagulation sedimentation	Plain sedimentation
Washing	Back washing	By scraping sand bed
Mechanism of action	Essentially physical	Physical & mechanical
Loss of head allowed	6–8 feet	4 feet
Removal of turbidity	Good	Good
Removal of color	Good	Fair
Removal of bacteria	98–99%	99.9 – 99.99%
Suitability	For big cities	For small towns

INSTRUMENTS OF PUBLIC HEALTH IMPORTANCE

Instruments	Public Health Importance
Ice lined refrigerator	Cold chain temperature maintenance
Dial thermometer	Cold chain temperature monitoring
Horrock's apparatus	Chlorine demand estimation in water
Chlorinator, chloronome	Mixing/regulating the dose of chlorine in water
Chloroscope	Measuring level of residual chlorine in drinking water
Winchester Quart bottle	Assess physical & chemical quality of drinking water
Kata thermometer	Assess cooling power of air and air velocity
Anemometer/venturimeter	Assess air/wind velocity
Hygrometer, sling psychrometer & Assman psychrometer	Assess air humidity
Mercurial barometer, aneroid barometer	Atmospheric pressure
Wind vane	Assess air/wind direction
Salter's scale	Field instrument for low birth weight
Infantometer	Length of infants
Stadiometer	Weight of adults
Shakir's tape	Mid-arm circumference
Sound level meter	Measure intensity of sound
Band frequency analyser	Characteristic of sound
Audiometer	Assess hearing ability
Lactometer	To check for milk quality
Hydrometer	Check for solid soil particles in water
	Uses
	Maintains cold chain
	Cold chain temperature monitoring
	Measures birthweight
	Mid-arm circumference measurement
	Measures length of infant
Barometer (Aneroid/Mercury)	Atmospheric pressure

Contd...

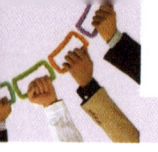

Assman psychrometer	Air humidity
	Air humidity
Dry bulb/Wet bulb/Six's maximum minimum, silvered thermometer	Air temperature
Globe thermometer	Radiant heat
Campbell-Stokes sunshine recorder	Number of hours of sunshine in the day
	Air/wind velocity
	Assess cooling power of air and air velocity
	Air/wind direction
	Assess physical and chemical quality of drinking water
	Measures level of residual chlorine in water
Colorimeter	Determine Color of water (prescribed upper limit 15 TCU, optimum-5 TCU)
Jackson candle turbidimeter	Determines turbidity of water (prescribed upper limit 5 unit)
	Estimation of chlorine demand in water
	Mixes chlorine in water
	Hearing ability assessment
Octave band frequency analyzer	Indicates whether intensity of sound is high or low pitched
	Intensity of sound in Decibel
Pattern Kopler test	Measures CO_2 content of air
Symons rain gauze	Measures precipitation (rain, snow, hail, dew and frost)
Pocket dosimeter	Cumulative radiation exposure to an individual
Stevenson screen	Measures air temperature

ANNEXURE 32: DISINFECTION PROCEDURES

Materials	Methods of sterilisation & disinfection
Faeces, urine, vomitus	Bleaching powder, cresols, formalin, burning, autoclaving, boiling
Sputum	Burning (most effective) 5% cresol for 1 hr
Serum, body fluids, bacterial vaccines	Water bath, vaccine bath
Glassware – syringes, petri dishes, test tubes, flasks, surgical instruments	Hot air oven
Cystoscope, Endoscope	Glutaraldehyde for 20 mins (preferred) (or ethylene dioxide)
Rubber, plastic & polythene tubes, disposable syringes	Glutaraldehyde for 20 mins (preferred) (or ethylene dioxide)
Dressing, aprons, gloves	Autoclaving
Sharp instruments	5% cresol
Suture materials without catgut	Autoclaving
Catgut	Ionizing radiation
Rubber or plastic disposable goods, disposable syringes, bone and tissue grafts, adhesive dressing	Ionizing radiation
OT sterilisation	Formaldehyde gas
Wards, laboratory, OT floor space	Formaldehyde gas, cresol
Skin	Tincture iodine, spirit (70 % alcohol), Savlon
Culture media	Autoclaving
Culture media with egg, serum or sugar	Tyndallisation

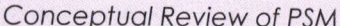

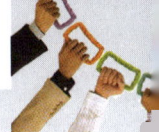

ANNEXURE 33: GRADING AND CUT OFF CRITERIA

CUT OFF CRITERIA FOR URINARY IODINE EXCRETION RATE

Median urinary iodine (μg/L) in School-age children (6 year or older)	Iodine intake	Iodine status
<20	Insufficient	Severe iodine deficiency
20–49	Insufficient	Moderate iodine deficiency
50–99	Insufficient	Mild iodine deficiency
100–199	Adequate	Adequate iodine nutrition
200–299	Above requirements	May pose a slight risk of more than adequate iodine intake in these populations
≥300	Excessive	Risk of adverse health consequences (Iodine–induced hyperthyroidism, autoimmune thyroid disease

GRADING CRITERIA FOR AFB IN SPUTUM

Table 12: Grading of AFB Smears

Examination	Result	Grading	No. of fields to be examined
More than 10 AFB per oil immersion field	Positive	3+	20
1–10 AFB per oil immersion	Positive	2+	50
10–99 AFB per 100 oil immersion fields	Positive	1+	100
1–9 AFB per 100 oil immersion fields	Scanty	Record exact number seen	200
No AFB per 100 oil immersion fields	Negative	–	100

INTELLECTUAL DISABILITY SEVERITY GRADING

Table 13: Classifications of intellectual disability severity

Severity Category	Approximate Percent distribution of cases by severity	DSM-IV Criteria (severity levels were based only on IQ categories)	DSM-5 Criteria (severity classified on the basis of daily skills)	AAIDD Criteria (severity classified on the basis of intensity of support needed)
Mild	85%	Approximate IQ range 50–69	Can live independently with minimum levels of support	Intermittent support needed during transitions or periods of uncertainty
Moderate	10%	Approximate IQ range 36–46	Independent living may be achieved with moderate levels of support, such as those available in group homes	Limited support needed in daily situations
Severe	3.5%	Approximate IQ range 20–35	Requires daily assistance with self-care activities and safety supervision	Extensive support needed for daily activities
Profound	1.5%	IQ<20	Requires 24-hour care	Pervasive support needed for every aspect of daily routines

AAIDD: American Association on Intellectual and Developmental Disabilities

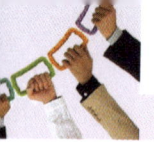

ANNEXURE 34: HEALTH COMMUNICATION

Socratic approach – 2 way communication
Didactic approach – 1 way communication

GROUP APPROACHES

Approaches to Health education	Components of each group	Salient features
Demonstrations	Groups of audience with 1 demonstrator	Carefully planned presentation to show how to perform a skill or a step by step procedure. The demonstration is done in front of an audience who are the learners. It is high impact on the audience.
Group discussion	Group size 6–10 members including 1 group leader and 1 recorder	Group of people discussing over a common point. The group leader manages the events, thoughts and promotes each member participation. It is effective tool for health awareness, attitude change.
Panel discussion	Comprises a chairman or moderator, 4– 6 expert speakers	▪ 4–6 persons who are qualified to talk about the topic sit and discuss a given problem/topic in front of a target group or audience ▪ Extremely effective method of education ▪ Passive audience
Symposium	Presenters and small group of audience	▪ Series of speeches/lectures on a selected subject ▪ Each person presents an aspect briefly ▪ Audience may raise questions in the end ▪ Chairman makes a comprehensive summary at the end of symposium ▪ Good tool for integrated teaching
Workshop	Series of meetings usually >4, Total workshop may be divided into smaller groups	▪ Emphasis is on individual work within the group to impart training ▪ It is focused on hands-on-training for the participants
Role playing	Demonstrator audience not >25	▪ Situation is dramatized by a talent group ▪ Usually used for creating awareness for social problems, of disease with social stigma
Conferences & seminars		It is a series of educative sessions by experts from the field. The conference must have a theme and the speakers share experiences, prospective strategies around the theme
Delphi approach		▪ It is a special way for having an organized communicating between groups comprising of experts from various fields ▪ This technique is implied at administrative levels or higher levels for providing a solution to a complex task involving many fronts and fields of expertise

ANNEXURE 35: NUTRITION REQUIREMENTS—RECOMMENDED DIETARY ALLOWANCE

Table 14: Recommended daily allowances for Indians —2010

Group [Male = 60 kg, Female = 55 kg]	Net Energy (Kcal/day)	Protein (g/day)	Visible Fat (g/day)	Calcium (mg/day)	Iron (mg/day)	Vitamin A (Retinol) mcg/day	Ascorbic Acid (mg/day)	Folate (mcg/day)	Iodine (mcg/day)
Sedentary worker male	2,320	60	25	600	17	600	40	200	150 mcg
Moderate worker male	2,730		30						
Heavy worker male	3,490		40						
Sedentary worker female	1,900	55	20	600	21	600	40	200	150 mcg
Moderate worker female	2,230		25						

Contd...

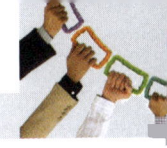

Group [Male = 60 kg, Female = 55 kg]	Net Energy (Kcal/day)	Protein (g/day)	Visible Fat (g/day)	Calcium (mg/day)	Iron (mg/day)	Vitamin A (Retinol) mcg/day	Ascorbic Acid (mg/day)	Folate (mcg/day)	Iodine (mcg/day)
Heavy worker female	2,850		30						
Pregnant women	+350	78	30	1200	35	800	60	500	250 mcg
Lactating women 0–6 months	+600	74	30	1200	21	950	80	300	290 mcg
Lactating women 6–12 months	+520	68							
Infant [0–6 months]	92 Kcal/kg/day	1.16 g/kg/day	–	500	46 mcg/kg/day	350	25	25	
Infant [6–12 months]	80 Kcal/kg/day	1.69 g/kg/day	19		05				

ANNEXURE 36: ONCOGENIC INFECTIONS

Organism	Neoplasm
Human papilloma virus (Papovaviridae)	SCC of cervix, vulva, penis Oropharyngeal carcinoma
HSV type 2	Cervical carcinoma
Hepatitis B virus (Hepadnaviridae)	Hepatocellular carcinoma
Hepatitis C virus (Flaviviridae)	Hepatocellular carcinoma Lymphoplasmacytic lymphoma
HTLV-I (Retroviridae)	Adult T-cell leukemia/lymphoma
HTLV-II (Retroviridae)	T-cell variant of hairy cell laukemia
HTLV-III (Retroviridae)	AIDS related malignancies Non Hodgkins Lymphoma Kaposi sarcoma SCC of urogenital tract Diffuse large B-cell lymphoma Burkitt's lymphoma
Epstein barr virus (Herpesviridae)	Mixed cellularity hodgkin's Nasopharyngeal carcinoma (anaphastic), African Burkitt's lymphoma
	Post organ transplant lymphoma Primary CNS diffuse large B-cell lymphoma, Extranodal NK/T cell lymphoma (nasal type)
H. pylori	Gastric malt lymphoma Gastric cancer
Human herpes virus 8	Primary effusion lymphoma Multicentric castleman's disease
Schistosoma haematobium	Bladder cancer (squamous cell)
Clonorchis	Cholangiocarcinoma
Opisthorchis	Cholangiocarcinoma

ANNEXURE 37: VITAMINS AND DEFICIENCY DISORDERS

Water soluble vitamin	Functions	Deficiency syndromes
Vitamin A	A component of visual pigment Maintenance of specialized epithelia Maintenance of resistance to infection	Xerophthalmia, Increased chance of Infections (especially measles)

Contd...

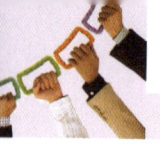

Water soluble vitamin	Functions	Deficiency syndromes
Vitamin B1 (thiamine)	As pyrophosphate, is coenzyme in decarboxylation reactions	Dry and wet beriberi, Wernicke syndrome, Korsakoff syndrome
Vitamin B2 (riboflavin)	Converted to coenzymes flavin mononucleotide and flavin adenine dinucleotide, cofactors for many enzymes in intermediary metabolism	Ariboflavinosis, cheilosis, stomatitis, seborrheic dermatitis
Vitamin B3 Niacin	Incorporated into nicotinamide adenine dinucleotide and NAD phosphate, involved in a variety of redox reactions	Pellagra
Pantothenic acid	Incorporated in coenzyme A	Burning foot syndrome
Vitamin B6 (Pyridoxine)	Derivatives serve as coenzymes intermediary reactions	Cheilosis, glossitis, dermatitis, peripheral neuropathy
Vitamin B7 Biotin	Cofactor in carboxylation reactions	Dermatitis
Folate	Essential for transfer and use of 1-carbon units in DNA synthesis	Megaloblastic anemia, neural tube defects
Vitamin B12	Required for normal folate metabolism and DNA synthesis, maintenance of myelinisation of spinal cord tracts	Megaloblastic pernicious anemia
Vitamin C	Serves in many oxidation reduction reactions and hydroxylation of collagen	Scurvy
Vitamin D	Facilitates intestinal absorption of calcium and phosphorus and mineralization of bones	Rickets in children osteomalacia in adults
Vitamin E	Major antioxidant; scavenges free radicals	Spinocerebellar degeneration, Peripheral neuropathy, Testicular atrophy sterilization
Vitamin K	Co factor in hepatic carboxylation of procoagulants–factors II, VII, IX and X and protein C and protein S	Coagulopathy

ANNEXURE 38: ZOONOSES AND VECTOR BORNE DISEASES

WATER BORNE DISEASES CLASSIFICATION

Water borne diseases	Occur due to drinking contaminated water, transmitted by faeco-oral route	Typhoid, cholera, Dysentery, Viral Hepatitis A
Water washed diseases	Infections of outer body surface which occur due to inadequate use of water or improper hygiene	Scabies, trachoma, typhus, bacillary dysentery, amoebic dysentery
Water-based diseases	Infections transmitted through an aquatic invertebrate animal	Schistosomiasis, Dracunculiasis
Water breeding diseases	Infections spread by insects that depend on water	Malaria, filariasis, dengue, yellow fever, Onchocerciasis

Terms	Definition	Examples
Anthropozoonoses	Infections transmitted from animals to man	Rabies, Plague, Anthrax, Hydatidosis, Trichinosis
Zooanthroponoses	Infections transmitted from man to animals	Human TB in cattle
Amphixenosis	Infection transmitted in either direction between animals and humans	Trypanosoma cruzi, schistosoma japonicum
Direct zoonoses	Infections transmitted from infected to susceptible vertebrate host by direct contact/fomite/vector	Rabies, Brucellosis, Trichinosis
Cyclozoonoses	Involves more than one species for disease transmission	Taeniasis, echinococcosis

Contd...

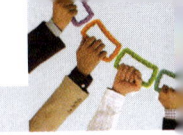

Terms	Definition	Examples
Meta zoonoses	Infections transmitted biologically through invertebrate vectors	Plague, schistosomiasis
Saprozoonoses	Involves non animal developmental site or reservoir for disease transmission	Mycoses, Larva migrans
Epizootic	Outbreak of disease in animal population	Anthrax, influenza, rabies, brucellosis, rift valley fever, Q fever, Japanese encephalitis
Enzootic	Endemic of disease occurring in animals	Anthrax, Brucellosis, Rabies, Bovine TB, Endemic typhus, Tick typhus
Epornithic	Outbreak of disease in bird population	Japanese encephalitis

VECTOR AND DISEASE

Vector	Disease
Anopheles mosquito	▪ Malaria ▪ Filaria (not in India)
Culex mosquito	▪ Bancroftian filariasis ▪ Japanese encephalitis ▪ West Nile fever ▪ Viral arthritis (Epidemic/polyarthritis)
Aedes mosquito	▪ Yellow fever (not in India) ▪ Dengue ▪ Dengue hemorrhagic fever ▪ Chikungunya fever ▪ Rift valley fever ▪ Filaria (not in India)
Mansonoides mosquito	▪ Malayan (Brugian) filariasis ▪ Chikungunya fever
Housefly	Typhoid and paratyphoid fever, diarrhea, dysentery, cholera, gastroenteritis, amoebiasis, helminthic infestations, poliomyelitis, conjunctivitis, trachoma, anthrax, yaws, etc.
Sandfly	Kala-azar, oriental sore, sandfly fever, oroya fever
Tsetse fly	Sleeping sickness
Louse	Epidemic typhus, relapsing fever, trench fever, pediculosis
Rat flea	Bubonic plague, endemic typhus, chiggerosis, hymenolepis diminuta
Blackfly	Onchocerciasis
Reduviid bug	Chagas disease
Hard tick	Tick typhus, viral encephalitis, viral fevers, viral haemorrhagic fever, (e.g., kyasanur forest disease), tularemia, tick paralysis, human babesiosis
Soft tick	Q fever, relapsing fever
Trombiculid mite	Scrub typhus, Rickettsial-pox
Itch-mite	Scabies
Cyclops	Guinea-worm disease, fish tapeworm (D. latus)
Cockroaches	Enteric pathogens

ANNEXURE 39: COMMON NAMES OF ILLICIT DRUGS

- **Marijuana (smoked, swallowed):** Blunt, dope, ganja, grass, herb, joint, bud, Mary Jane, pot, reefer, green, trees, smoke, skunk, weed
- **Hashish (smoked, swallowed):** Boom, gangster, hash, hash oil, hemp
- **Heroin (injected, smoked, snorted):** Diacetylmorphine: smack, horse, brown sugar, dope, junk, skag, skunk, white horse, China white; cheese

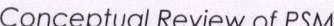

- **OPIUM (smoked, swallowed):** Laudanum, paregoric: big O, black stuff, block, gum, hop
- **Cocaine (snorted, smoked, injected):** Cocaine hydrochloride: blow, bump, C, candy, Charlie, coke, crack, flake, rock, snow
- **Amphetamine (swallow, snorted, smoked, injected):** Biphetamine, Dexedrine: bennies, black beauties, crosses, hearts, LA turnaround, speed, truck drivers
- **Methamphetamine (swallowed, snorted, smoked, injected):** Desoxyn: meth, ice, crank, chalk, crystal, fire, glass, go fast, speed
- **Mdma (methylenedioxymethamphetamine):** Ecstasy, Adam, clarity, Eve, lovers' speed, Molly
- **LSD:** Lysergic acid diethylamide: acid, blotter, cubes, microdot, yellow sunshine, blue heaven
- **Psilocybin:** Magic mushrooms, purple passion, shrooms, little smoke
- **Anabolic steroid:** Anadrol, Oxandrin, Durabolin, Depo-Testosterone, Equipoise: roids, juice, gym candy, pumpers
- **Inhalants:** Solvents (paint thinners, gasoline, glues); gases (butane, propane, aerosol propellants, nitrous oxide); nitrites (isoamyl, isobutyl, cyclohexyl): laughing gas, poppers, snappers, whippets

ANNEXURE 40: INSTITUTES OF PUBLIC HEALTH

Institutes	Location
Central Labor Institute	Mumbai
Regional Labor Institutes	Kanpur, Kolkata and Chennai
Central Mining and Research Station, CSIR	Dhanbad
Industrial Toxicology Research Center	Lucknow
National Institute of Occupational Health	Ahmedabad
National Environmental Engineering Research Institute	Nagpur

Other Institutes	Location
National Institute of Nutrition	Hyderabad
Central Leprosy Teaching and Research Institute	Chengalpattu
Central Family Planning Institute	New Delhi
International Institute for Population Studies	Mumbai
Indian Council of Medical Research	New Delhi
Blood Group Reference Center	Mumbai
All India Institute of Hygiene and Public Health	Kolkata
All India Institute of Mental Health	Bengaluru
National Tuberculosis Institute	Bengaluru
National Center for Diseases Control (Formerly National Institute of Communicable Diseases)	New Delhi
Central Research Institute	Kasauli
National Institute of Health and Family Welfare	New Delhi
Haffkine Institute	Mumbai
National Institute of TB and Respiratory Diseases (Formerly LRS Institute of TB and Allied Diseases)	New Delhi
National Institute of Virology	Pune
National JALMA Institute for Leprosy	Agra
National Institute for Research in Tuberculosis	Chennai
National Institute of Mental Health and Neurosciences (NIMHANS)	Bengaluru
Vector Control Research Center	Puducherry
Central Drug Research Institute	Lucknow

Section

A

Medical Research

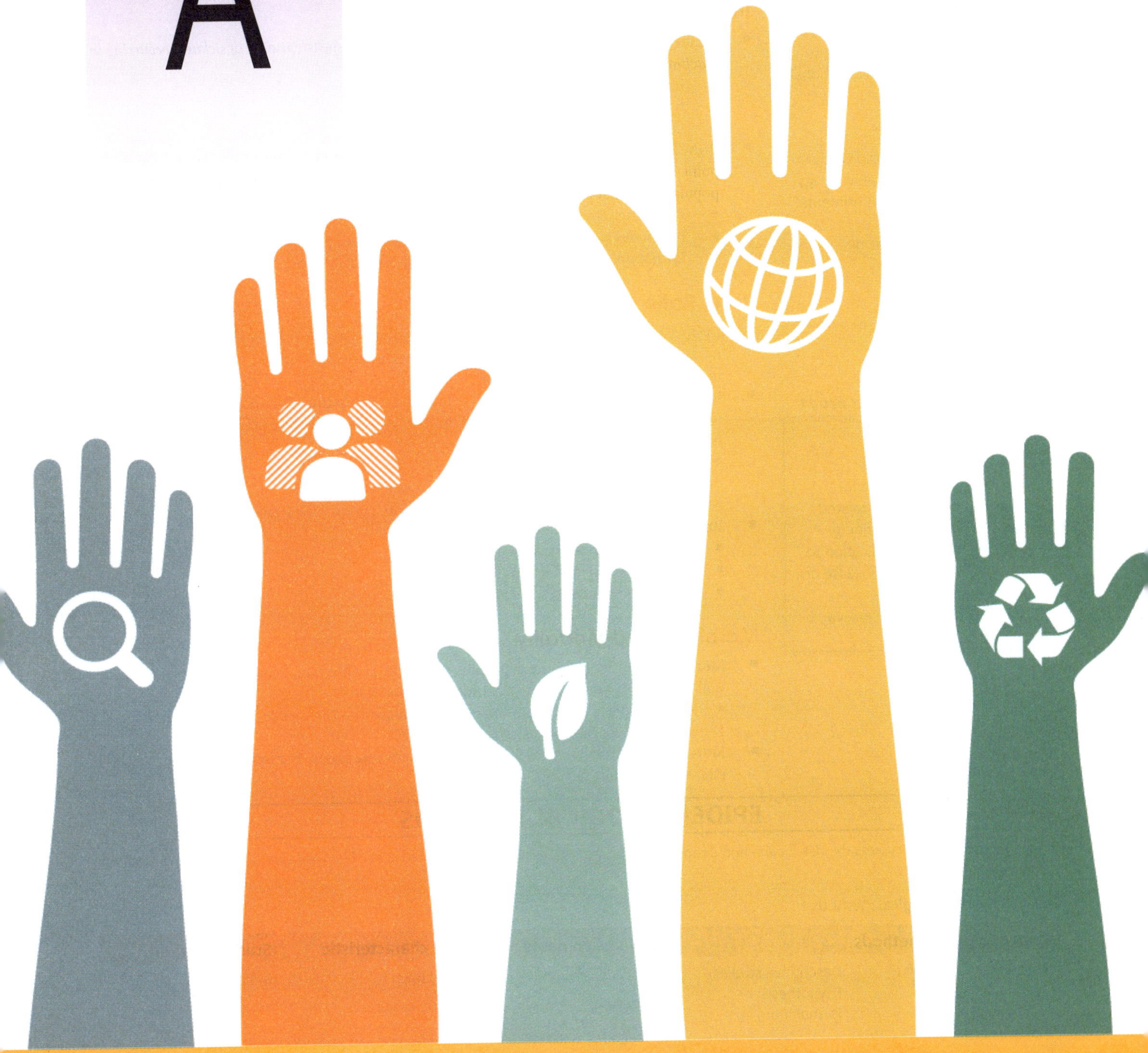

Basic Principles of Epidemiology

Chapter Outline

Must Remember

Epidemiology

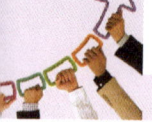

- Epidemiology is study of frequency, distribution and determinants of health related states or events in a defined population and its application to control or prevent the disease or health related events.

(Definition of epidemiology given by John Murray Last, 1988)

BASIC EPIDEMIOLOGICAL TOOLS

Incidence-Prevalence

- **Incidence**[Q] is "*number of new cases of a disease or new spells/episodes of sickness occurring in a defined population during a specified time period*".
  - Incidence is a rate
  - It not affected by the duration of the disease.
  - Disease rate is an incidence rate that measures occurrence of disease in a population.
- **Prevalence** is total number of all individuals who have an attribute or disease at a particular point of time – **(Point prevalence)** or in a particular period (**Period prevalence)** in the population at that point in time or midway through the period.
  - Prevalence is a proportion
  - It includes all current cases (old and new) in a given population.
  - ***Limitation:*** It is not ideal for studying disease etiology or causation.

Rate, Ratio and Proportion

- **Ratio:** The numerator is not a part of the denominator. It is relationship in size between 2 random variables. Numerator and denominator may involve an interval of time or may be instantaneous in time
- **Rate: The numerator is part of the bigger denominator.** It is occurrence of an event (disease/death) or change in the pattern of an event in a defined population in a specified time period
  - Example:
    - **Incidence rate:** Number of new cases in a given time
    - **Attack rate:** It is the number of cases in a given time frame
- **Proportion:** Numerator is a part of the denominator.
  - It is expressed as a percentage.
  - Time interval is not required
  - Example: Prevalence, case fatality rate.

Morbidity and Mortality

- **Morbidity** is defined as "any departure, subjective or objective, from a state of physiological well-being". It approximates to sickness or disease state
  - Three aspects are commonly studied frequency (incidence and prevalence rates), duration (disability rate) and severity (CFR).
- **Mortality:** Refers to death as an event in a given time frame. For example, Infant mortality rate, maternal mortality ratio.

EPIDEMIOLOGICAL METHODS

It is a formal method to assess the risk factors and define causation for a disease or health related state. The various epidemiological methods are given as in Table 1.

Table 1: Epidemiological methods

Epidemiological methods		Study design name	Study characteristic	Study based on
Observational studies	Descriptive studies (Hypothesis formulation)	Case study	Single subject	Individual
		Case series, case reports	Multiple cases	Individual
	Analytical studies (Hypothesis testing)	Cross sectional	Survey, sample of population	Individual
		Case control	Sample of cases and control	Individual
		Cohort study	A group of individuals with common characteristic	Individual
		Ecological study	A defined population	Population groups

Contd...

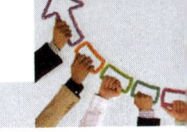

Epidemiological methods	Study design name	Study characteristic	Study based on
Experimental studies	Pre-post study design		Patients
	Randomized control trial		Patients
	Field trial		Healthy people
	Community trial		Community or group of individuals
Evidence based medicine	Systematic reviews		Research studies
	Meta-analysis		Research studies

Hence, we can discuss three gross epidemiological methods
- Observational study designs
- Experimental study designs
- Evidence-based medicine

OBSERVATIONAL STUDY DESIGNS

Case Study

Usually conducted for an atypical case. It involves in depth understanding of disease determinants in that particular single case. It is a type of descriptive study.

Case Series

Done as descriptive study of understanding the determinants of disease and disease in terms of time, place or person.

These types of studies help in formulating the hypothesis.

Cross-sectional Study

Cross-sectional/Prevalence study—is a single examination of a cross-section of population at one point in time
- Unit of study is the individual
- More useful for chronic diseases
- It does not involve a follow up, hence is also known cross-sectional study or snapshot of the population
- May not be a good measure to assess risk factors for diseases which are acute in nature or fatal
- This study helps us in estimating the total number of present cases (or the prevalence of the disease)
- The study includes survey of the population, or sample of the total population.

Case Control Study

It is the 1st technical approach towards testing a causal hypothesis. It has 3 distinct features:
- Both exposure and outcome (disease) have occurred before the start of the study
- Study proceeds backwards from **effect to cause**
- The study starts with selection of study population including people with disease or without disease.
- It is a type of analytical study.

Cohort Study

- Cohort is a group of individuals with common characteristic
- It is a type of analytical study.
- Cohorts are identified prior to appearance of the disease under investigation
- The cohort group should be essentially free from disease at the time of start of the study and then the study groups are observed over a period of time to determine the frequency of disease among them
- The study proceeds forward from **cause to effect**.

Must Remember

Expected errors in cohort study:
- May have a misclassification error
- Berksonian bias
- Recall bias

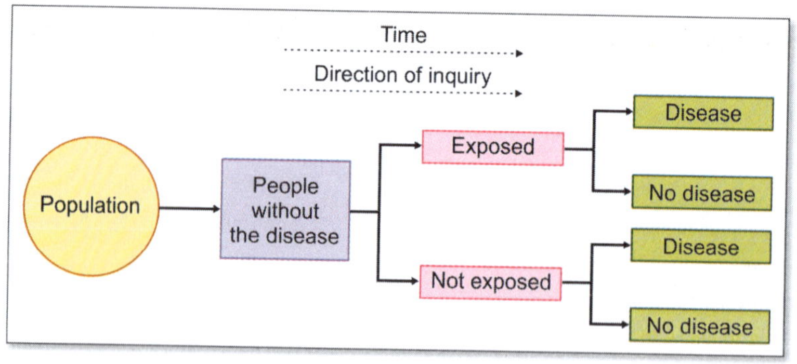

Fig. 1: Cohort study

Other Types of Cohort Study

Nested Case-control Study

- Cut down cost of cohort study.
- Cases and controls are chosen from a defined cohort (Where information on exposure/risk factor being studied is available)
- Additional information on cases and controls, selected for the study is collected and analysed.
- **Advantage:** Economical, Temporal association is maintained, recall bias is eliminated, useful when measurement of exposure is expensive

Open or Dynamic or Concurrent Cohort

Involves a selection of dynamic cohort group. The challenge is to avoid or at least to minimize the selection bias to as low as possible and yet to maintain the openness of cohort group to provide the results with the best possible time effect or adjusting for the trends of disease over time

Closed or Fixed or Nonconcurrent Cohort

It involves selection of a cohort group which is fixed and does not change over time. Usually this method of cohort selection may be deployed for measurement of disease that do not change over time (or over years) and which are not grossly affected by change in lifestyle or habits of the humans over time.

Prospective or Retrospective Cohort

- **Prospective cohort:** The cohort is chosen and follow-up is done with time. (Refer to Figs 2 and 3)
- **Retrospective cohort:** Sometimes, data from past medical records or any record may be taken and observation of the event (disease) is done in the present time (which may have already occurred). (Figs 4 and 5)

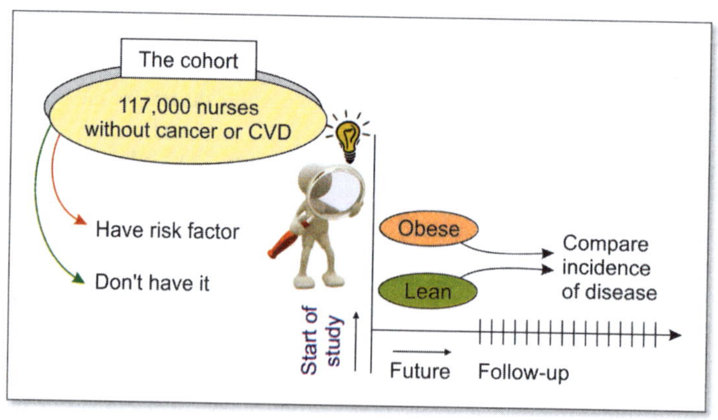

Fig. 2: Prospective cohort

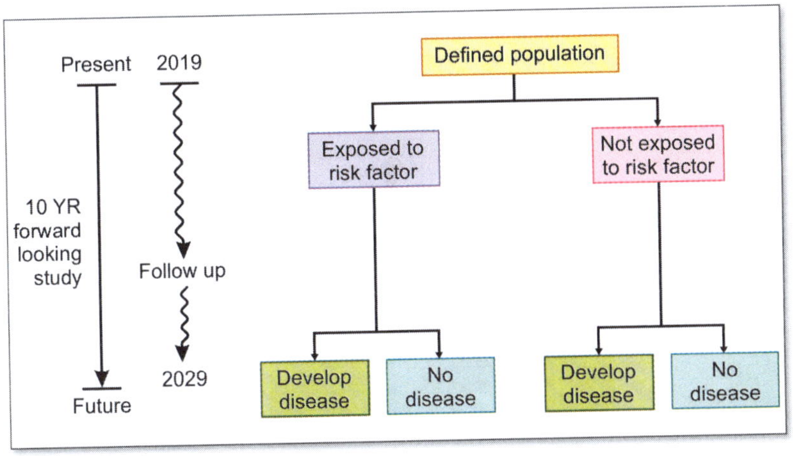

Fig. 3: Prospective cohort

- **Problems in retrospective cohort design**
  - The data collected may not be valid or it may be difficult to trace the individuals starting from back date.
  - The cohort may also have changed the life style or risk exposure quantification should always be done to ensure no classification errors.

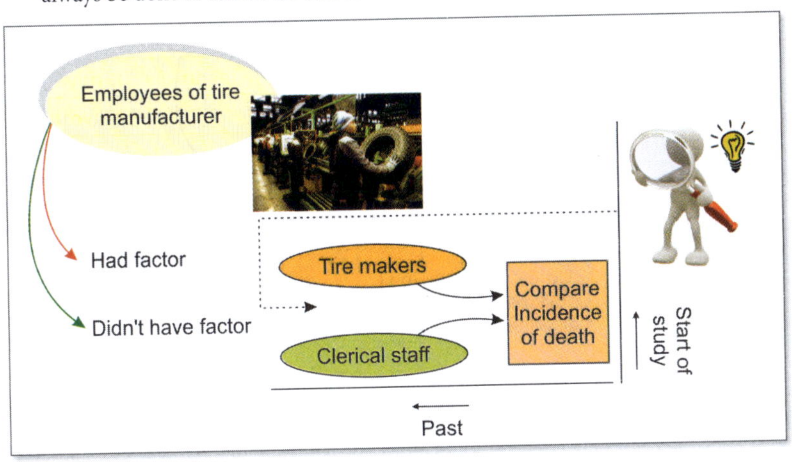

Fig. 4: Retrospective cohort

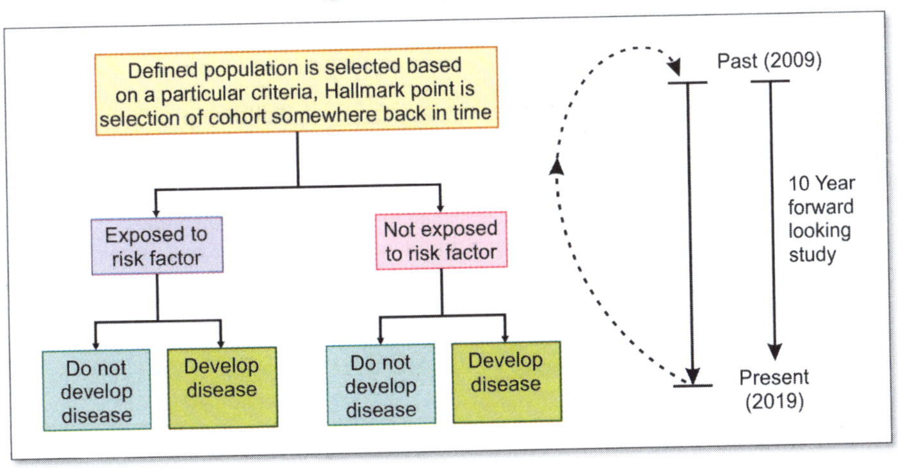

Fig. 5: Retrospective cohort

Must Remember

Disadvantages of cohort design:
- Long, time taking, expensive studies
- Follow up is essential
- Expected errors:
  - May have a misclassification error
  - Selection bias
  - Attrition bias

Mixed Cohort (Ambispective) Cohort

It involves both retrospective and prospective cohort. (Fig. 6)

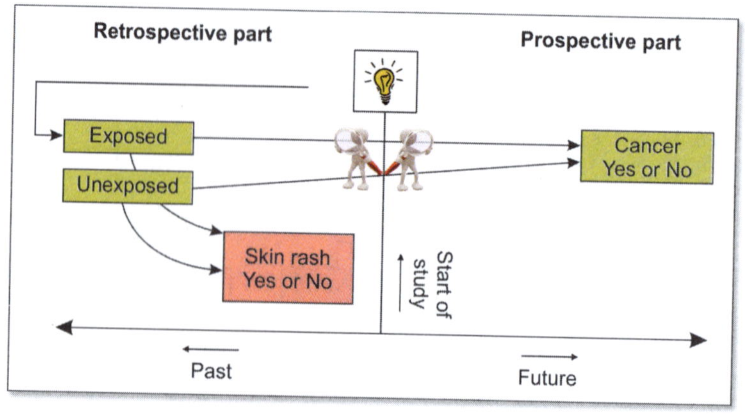

Fig. 6: Mixed cohort

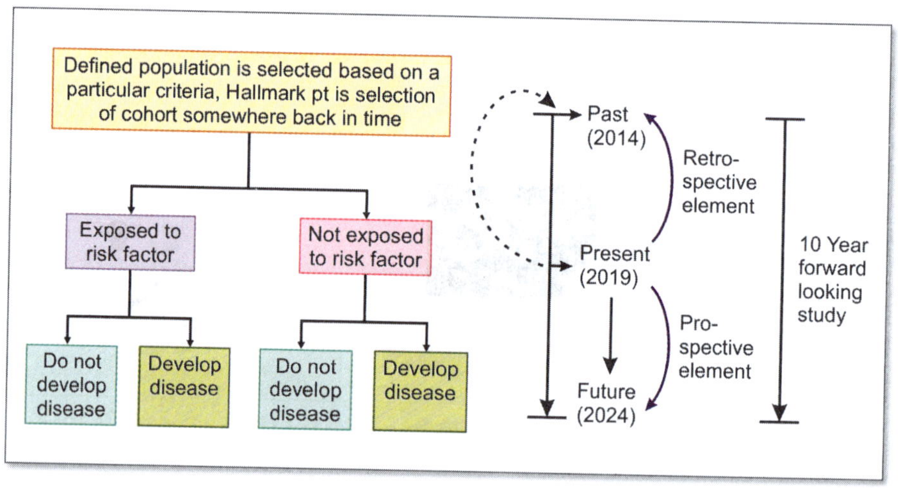

Fig. 7: Ambispective (Mixed) cohort

Good to Remember

Table 2: Summary of prospective, retrospective and ambispective cohort

	Baseline	Follow-up
Prospective cohort	Assessed at the time of start of study	In future date
Retrospective cohort	Assessed at some time in past using historical data or cohorts	In present date (the outcome has already occurred)
Ambispective cohort	Assessed at some time in past using historical data or cohorts	In future date (note that the outcome may have occurred in some, but final assessment is done in a future date)

Good to Remember

Table 3: Summary of case control/cohort studies

Case control study	Cohort study
*Commences from "**effect to cause**". Exposure and Outcome have occurred before start of Investigation*	*Commences from "**cause to effect**". Cohorts are identified prior to appearance of the disease (or outcome) under investigation*
We look for if the suspected cause occurs more often in those with the disease than among those without the disease	We look for if the disease occurs more frequently in those exposed, than in those not exposed
No Attrition	Attrition is a major problem
Quick results and relatively easy to carry out	Takes a long time
Involves fewer subjects	Involves large number of subjects
Suited for study of rare diseases	Suited for study of rare exposure
Cheaper	Costly
No follow up is needed	Follow up is an integral part
Odds ratio is obtained	Incidence rate, RR and AR, PAR are obtained
We get information on several etiological agent or risk factors	We get information on more than one disease outcome from single etiological agent
1st approach to testing a causal hypothesis	Used to test precisely formulated hypothesis
Recall bias, Selection bias is an issue	No recall bias

Must Remember

Table 4: Application of different observational study designs

Objective	Ecological	Cross-sectional	Case-control	Cohort
Unit of study	Population	Individual	Individual	Individuals
Helps to determine	Correlation of variables at large population levels	▪ Association of various risk factors ▪ Determine prevalence of disease	▪ Association of various risk factors ▪ Determine Odds ratio	▪ Association of risk factors ▪ Assessment of causation ▪ Proves temporality ▪ Determine the Risk ratio ▪ Attributable and population attributable risks ▪ Determine the incidence of disease
Investigation of rare disease	++++	–	++++	–
Investigation of rare cause	++	–	–	++++
Testing multiple effects of cause	+	++	–	++++
Study of multiple exposures and determinants	++	++	+++	+++
Measurements of time relationship	++	–	+	++++
Direct measurement of incidence	–	–	+	++++
Investigation of long latent period	–	–	+++	–

High Yield Points

Study of choice:
- **Rare disease:** Case control study
- **Rare risk factor:** Cohort study
- **Rare (expensive) investigation:** Nested case control study

High Yield Points

- However, the ecological studies are basically useful in 'co-relating' events rather than describing the events in terms of causation
- The ecological fallacy is a type of confounding specific to ecological studies. It occurs when relationships which exist for groups are assumed to also be true for individuals

Good to Remember

The ecological studies would best suit in case of:
- The purpose of the study is to monitor population health so that public health strategies may be developed and directed;
- The purpose of the study is to make large-scale comparisons, e.g., comparisons between countries
- Helps in migration, occupation, social class studies
- The purpose of the study is to study the relationship between population-level exposure to risk factors and disease, or in order to look at the contextual effect of risk factors on the population
- Measurements at individual level are not available, e.g. confidentiality might require that individuals are anonymized by aggregation of data to small area level; or
- The disease under investigation is rare, requiring aggregation of data for any analysis to be carried out.

Correlational/Ecological Studies

- Use population as unit of analysis. (Population can be of countries, States – usually to compare genotypic distinct population)
- Use database from entire population to compare frequency of a particular disease/attribute

Advantages

- Helps in evaluating the disease exposure relationship
- Usually based on records from the whole population

Must Remember

Table 5: Advantages and disadvantages of various observational designs

	Ecological	Cross-sectional	Case-control	Cohort
Probability of:				
Selection bias	NA	Medium	High	Low
Recall bias	NA	High	High	Low
Loss to follow-up	NA	NA	Low	High
Confounding	High	Medium	Medium	Medium
Time required	Low	Medium	Medium	High
Cost	Low	Medium	Medium	High

INTERPRETATION OF OBSERVATIONAL STUDIES

Strength of Association in Case Control Studies

Odds Ratio (Cross Product Ratio)

- It is a measure of the strength of the association between exposure and outcome obtained in a case control study
- It is the ratio of the odds of exposure among the cases to the odds of exposure among the controls

Table 6: Odds ratio

	Diseased	Nondiseased
Exposed	a	b
Nonexposed	c	d

Then the odds ratio is computed by taking the ratio, of odds, where the odds in each group is computed as follows:

$$OR = (a/b)/(c/d)$$
$$= ad/bc$$

Strength of Association in Cohort Study

Relative Risk or Risk Ratio

- It reflects how many times exposure to a risk factor increases the risk of contracting the disease.
- **Formula:** $\frac{\text{Incidence in exposed}}{\text{Incidence in nonexposed}}$

Risk Difference (Attributable Risk)

- The risk difference focuses on absolute effect of the risk factor, or the excess risk of disease in those who have the factor compared with those who don't

- It provides a measure of the public health impact of the risk factor, and focuses on the number of cases that could potentially be prevented by eliminating the risk factor
- **Formula:** $\frac{\text{Incidence in exposed}}{\text{Incidence in nonexposed}}$

Attributable Risk Proportion or Percentage

- It is the proportion of disease in the exposed group that could be prevented by eliminating the risk factor
- It indicates the amount of disease that might be eliminated if the exposure being studied is controlled or eliminated.
- Expressed as a **percentage**, it is the extent to which the disease being studied can be attributed to the exposure.

Formula # 1 : $\frac{\text{Incidence in exposed} - \text{Incidence in nonexposed}}{\text{Incidence in exposed}} \times 100$

Formula # 2 : $\frac{RR - 1}{RR} \times 100$

Population Attributable Risk Proportion

- It indicates the proportion of disease in the population attributable to the exposure and that can be eliminated if the exposure is avoided completely

Formula # 1 : $\frac{\text{Incidence in exposed} - \text{Incidence in nonexposed}}{\text{Incidence in exposed}} \times 100$

Formula # 2 : $\frac{Ppop^{*}\ (RR - 1)}{Ppop^{*}\ (RR - 1) + 1} \times \mathbf{100}$

Where:

- *Ppop* = Proportion of exposed subjects in total population
- RR = Risk ratio
- P(exp) = Proportion of cases that have exposure

Interpretation of "Significant" Odds Ratio/Risk Ratio

Interpreting the 'real' association for factors under study by odds ratio and statistical methods

- **Example:** Researcher conducts a case control study to evaluate the risk factors for low birth weight in 200 females attending the ANC clinic and admitted under labor room in department of gynecology. The outcome was 100 females with low birth weight babies and another 100 females with normal (or above median) birth weight babies. The females were then asked questions based on the factors influencing pregnancy and its outcomes. The results obtained from the study as are given Table 7.

Table 7: Results obtained from the study example stated above

S. no	Variable	OR	95% CI
1.	Low Fat intake	0.4	0.01 – 1.09
2.	Low Carbohydrate intake	4.7	0.8 – 9.5
3.	High protein Intake	0.5	0.01 – 0.95
4.	Alcohol	5.6	1.2 – 9.5
5.	Number of hours of watching TV	1.3	0.95 – 2.1
6.	Number of hours of Physical exercise	0.7	0.62 – 0.73
7.	Stress levels	2.1	1.5 – 3.8
8.	Smoking	5.01	4.85 – 6.3

Analysis of the results obtained:

So, if we now plot the odds ratio obtained from the study on a distribution curve and along-side the 95% confidence intervals range, we depict the results as follows:

3 High Yield Points

Odds ratio (OR) interpretation

- OR < 1 → negative association (The factor under stay is protective factor)
- OR = 1 → no association
- OR > 1 → positive association (The factor under stay is risk factor)

Relative risk (RR) interpretation

- RR < 1 → negative association (The factor under stay is protective factor)
- RR = 1 → no association
- RR > 1 → positive association (The factor under stay is risk factor)

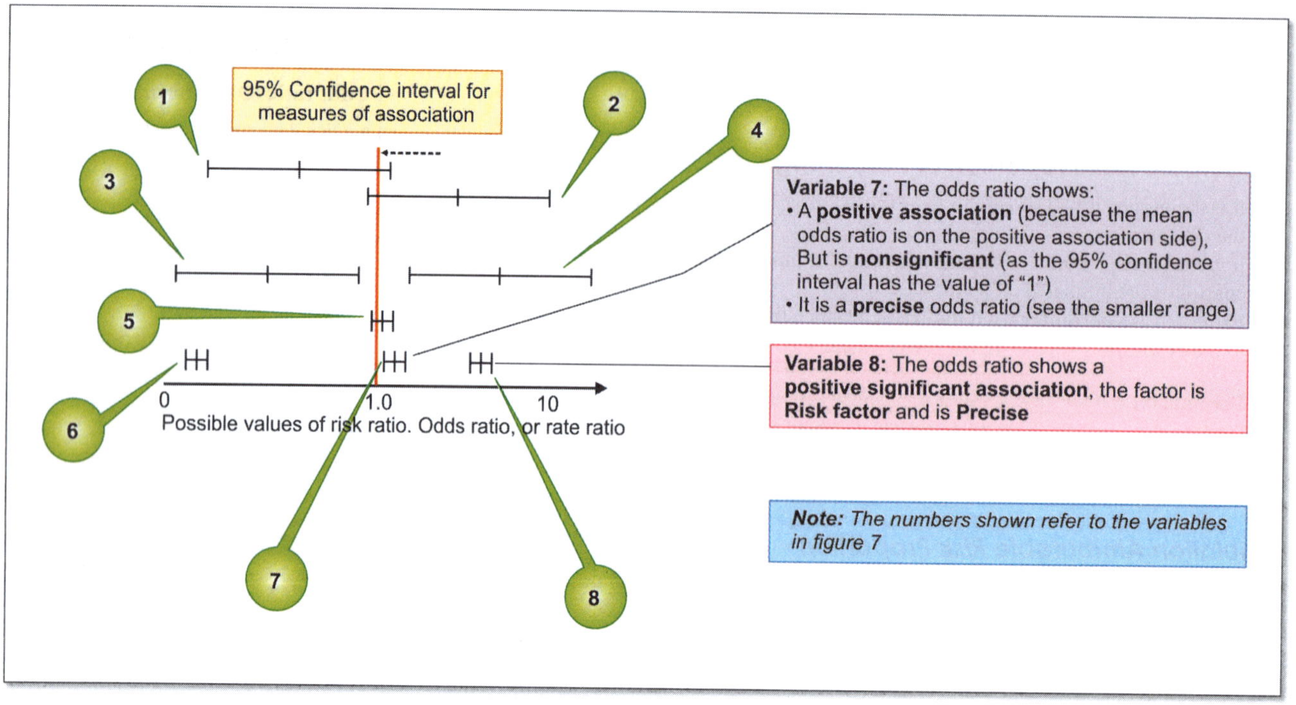
95% Confidence interval for measures of association
1
2
3
4
5
6
7
8
0
1.0
10
Possible values of risk ratio. Odds ratio, or rate ratio
Variable 7: The odds ratio shows:
• A **positive association** (because the mean odds ratio is on the positive association side), But is **nonsignificant** (as the 95% confidence interval has the value of "1")
• It is a **precise** odds ratio (see the smaller range)
Variable 8: The odds ratio shows a **positive significant association**, the factor is **Risk factor** and is **Precise**
Note: *The numbers shown refer to the variables in figure 7*

Now let's analyze the Odds ratio of different variables and comment on each of them.

Table 8: Interpretation summary from example in Table 7

Variable	OR	95% CI	Our Comments
Low Fat intake	– 0.4	0.01 – 1.09	A non-significant, but negative association and is non precise
Low Carbohydrate intake	4.7	0.8 – 9.5	A non-significant, but positive association and is non precise
High protein Intake	– 0.5	0.01 – 0.95	A significant, negative association and is non precise
Alcohol	5.6	1.2 – 9.5	A significant, positive association and is non precise
Number of hours of watching TV	1.3	0.95 – 2.1	A non-significant, positive association and is precise
Number of hours of Physical exercise	– 0.7	0.62 – 0.73	A significant, negative association and is precise
Stress levels	2.1	1.5 – 3.8	A significant, positive association and is precise
Smoking	5.01	4.85 – 6.3	A highly significant, positive association and is precise

Good to Remember

Trick

- Positive or negative association may be commented by – the absolute Odds ratio mean value
- Significant, non-significant may be commented by – inclusion of the value "1" in the 95% confidence interval range
- Precise, non-precise may be commented by – the range of the 95% confidence interval

EXPERIMENTAL STUDY DESIGNS

In an experimental study, the investigator determines through a controlled process the exposure for each individual (clinical trial) or community (community trial), and then tracks the individuals or communities over time to detect the effects of the exposure.

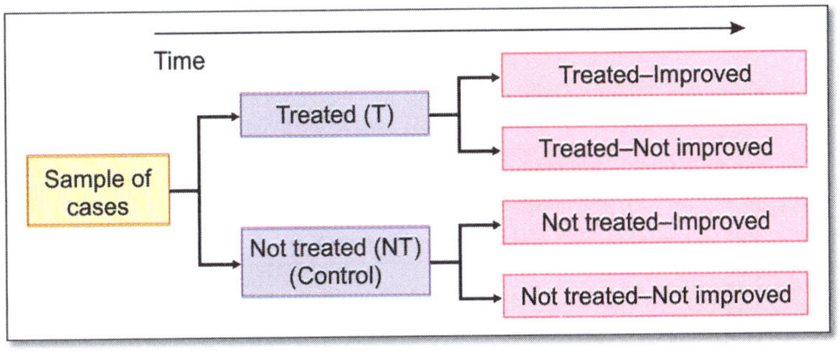

Fig. 8: Experimental study design

Example 1: In a clinical trial of a new vaccine, the investigator may randomly assign some of the participants to receive the new vaccine, while others receive a placebo shot. The investigator then tracks all participants, observes who gets the disease that the new vaccine is intended to prevent, and compares the two groups (new vaccine vs. placebo) to see whether the vaccine group has a lower rate of disease.
Example 2: Similarly, in a trial to prevent onset of diabetes among high-risk individuals, investigators randomly assigned enrollees to one of three groups—placebo, an antidiabetic drug, or lifestyle intervention. At the end of the follow-up period, investigators found the lowest incidence of diabetes in the lifestyle intervention group, the next lowest in the antidiabetic drug group, and the highest in the placebo group.

Randomized Clinical Trial (RCT)

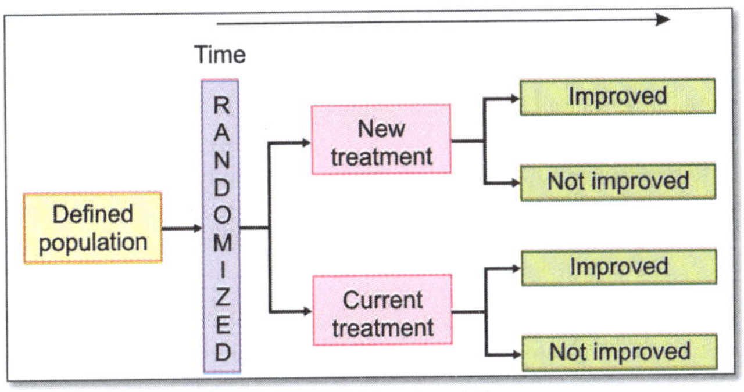

Fig. 9: Randomized trial design

Randomization: Randomization refers to the practice of using chance methods (random number tables, flipping a coin, etc.) to assign subjects to treatments. Using this method the selected subjects maybe randomly allocated to different study groups, where the chance is known and always equal. This type of statistical approach towards allocating subjects may provide a strong platform for the research study and negate selection (or allocation) bias in the study design.

Crossover Study Design

In crossover designs, each study participant receives all treatments that are being investigated, but at different times. The order in which a study participant receives the treatments maybe randomized. For example, patient A is randomized to receive Treatment #1 for a period of time. After completing Treatment #1, the patient then "crosses over" and receives Treatment #2. Usually between treatments is a period of time called a washout when no treatment is delivered. (Fig. 10)

In some crossover designs, particularly ones with more than two treatments, patients may not receive all treatments under investigation (partial crossover or incomplete block), but would receive more than one.

Advantages

- The patient serves as his or her own control – reducing inter-subject variability
- Even smaller sample sizes may be evaluated with reasonable accuracy and precision and detecting small effect size.

5 Good to Remember

Advantages of RCT

- Helpful in assessing the value of new therapies to combat acute diseases in developing countries
- Can evaluate a single variable in a precisely defined patient group
- Prospective design
- Eliminates bias by comparing two otherwise identical groups
- Allows for meta-analysis

Disadvantages of RCT

- Ethical issues – regarding the control group or the non-interventional group
- Expensive and time consuming
- Not always properly conducted – too few subjects, too short a time period
- Influence of sponsorship, need to show a positive effect of the intervention
- Not proper randomization or proper blinding

4 High Yield Points

Randomization:
- It is done at the time of allocation to groups
- It removes selection bias
- It is known and equal chance of selection

Example:

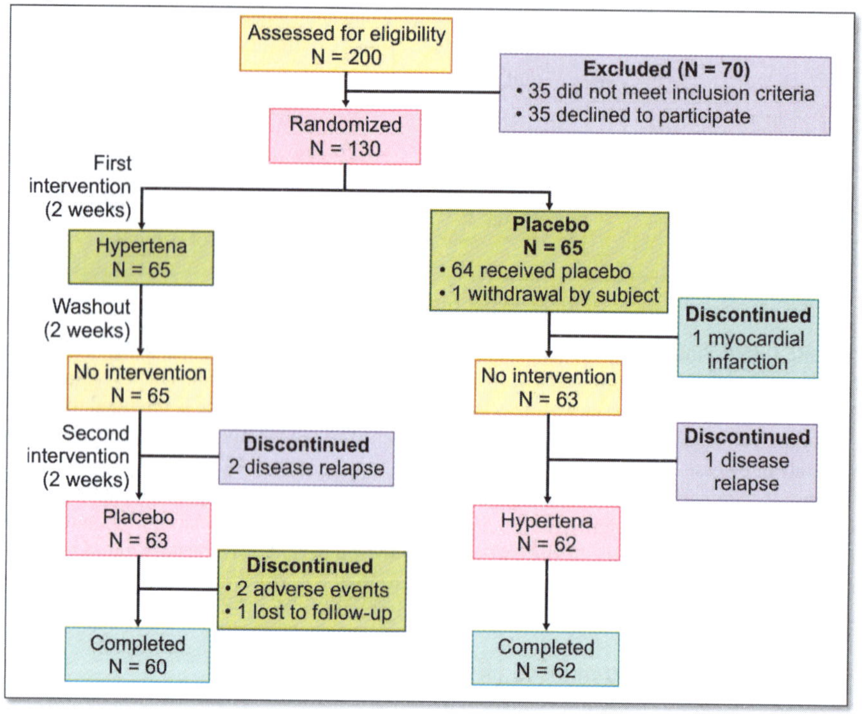

Fig. 10: Example of crossover study design

Community Trial

A community intervention study targets the whole community and not individuals. High-risk lifestyles and behaviors are influenced more by community norms than by individual preferences. Interventions are tested in the actual natural conditions of the community, and cheaper

Advantage

The community trial can evaluate a public health intervention in natural field circumstances.

Example: Community Intervention Trial for Smoking Cessation (COMMIT): Cohort results from a four-year community intervention.

Field Trial

Involve people who are disease-free but presumed to be at risk. Thus the data collection for the field trial is usually from the field in the general population. The field trial is usually deployed to measure the effect of interventions which tend to reduce exposure or the risk factor rather than measuring the outcomes or health related effects.

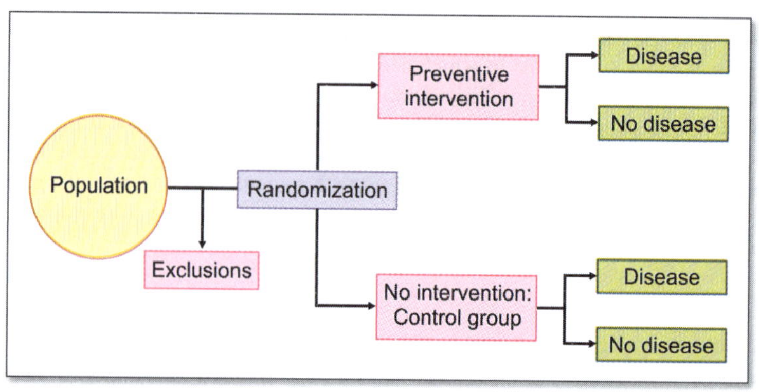

Fig. 11: Data collection for field trial

5 High Yield Points

Limitations of community trial
- Random allocation of the communities maybe difficult
- Other supporting studies maybe required to evaluate the final outcome assessment

Clinical Trials for Testing of New Drugs or Interventions

- **Phase I trial:** Initial studies to determine the metabolism and pharmacologic actions of drugs in humans, the side effects associated with increasing doses, and to gain early evidence of effectiveness; may include healthy participants and/or patients.
- **Phase II trial:** Controlled clinical studies conducted to evaluate the effectiveness of the drug for a particular indication or indications in patients with the disease or condition under study and to determine the common short-term side effects and risks. The new treatment might be tested in a somewhat larger group (80-200) to get more information about effectiveness and potential side effects at different dosages.
- **Phase III trial:** Expanded controlled and uncontrolled trials after preliminary evidence suggesting effectiveness of the drug has been obtained, and are intended to gather additional information to evaluate the overall benefit-risk relationship of the drug and provide adequate basis for physician labeling." These are typically conducted in larger groups (200-40,000) to formally test effectiveness and establish the frequency and severity of side effects compared to no treatment, or, compared to currently used treatments ("usual care")
- **Phase IV** refers to postmarketing "surveillance" to collect information regarding risks, benefits, and optimal use. This phase can be particularly important for identifying rare, but potentially devastating side effects.

6 High Yield Points

Field trial, in contrast to clinical trial, involve people who are healthy but presumed to be at risk; data collection takes place "in the field," usually among non-institutionalized people in the general population

Interpretation of Experimental Designs

- **As treated analysis (per-protocol analysis)** – does not preserve randomization
- **Intention to treat analysis** - randomization is accounted. This method of analysis also accounts for the drop-outs, crossovers and loss to follow up cases while the study process.

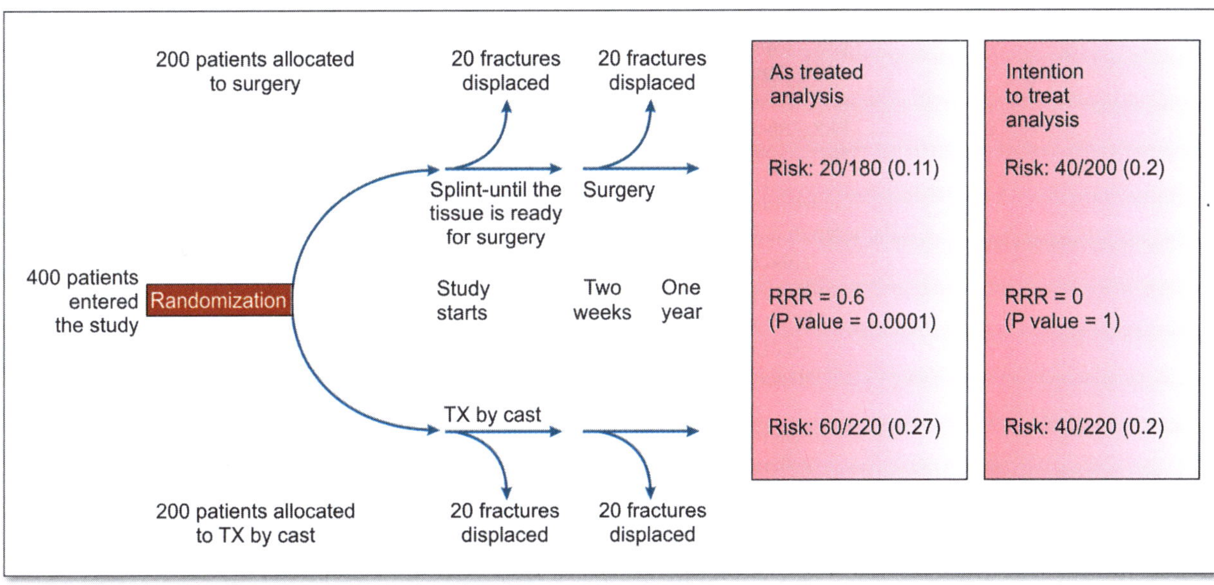

Fig. 12: The importance of the intention-to-treat principle is demonstrated by this example. In this trial, 400 patients were equally randomized either to the surgical arm or to the nonsurgical arm and each of the interventions had a similar effect. The surgery requires a two-week preparation period in which the patients are treated with a splint, and during this period 10% of the fractures in each group displaced; 10% of the fractures in each group also displaced in the following year. Performance of an "as-treated analysis" will lead to the conclusion that the surgical treatment is superior to the nonsurgical therapy, with a relative risk reduction (RRR) of 0.6 (p = 0.0001). An intention-to-treat analysis will not lead to this erroneous conclusion.

Source: Adapted, with modifications, from: Montori VM, Guyatt GH. Intention-to-treat principle. CMAJ. 2001;165:1339–41.

Number Need to Treat (NNT)

Concept: NNT offers a measurement of the impact of a medicine or therapy by estimating the number of patients that need to be treated in order to have an impact on one person. The concept is statistical, but implicative, for we know that not everyone is helped by a medicine or intervention — some are benefitted, some are harmed, and some are unaffected. The NNT tells us how many of each is expected to happen.

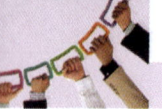

Example:

Researchers are evaluating a drug "G" for efficacy in preventing the long-term complications for Coronary artery disease in diabetic patients. The pharmaceutical company claims that drug "G" is more effective in preventing myocardial infarction in Diabetics compared to conventional OHA being used. The 5-year RCT results are shown below:

Example #1

	Number of patients on drug G	**Number of patients on control drug**	**Total**
	Experimental group (E)	Control group (C)	
Event (E) (MI happened)	10 (EE)	25 (CE)	35
Non Event (N) (no MI happened)	990 (EN)	975(CN)	1965
Total	1000 (ET)	1000 (CT)	2000

Abbreviations used:

EE – Number of events in experimental group
EN – Number of "No-event" in experimental group
ET – Total in experimental group
CE - Number of events in control group
CN – Number of "No-event" in control group
CT – Total in control group
EER – Experimental group event rate
CER – Control group event rate
ARR - Absolute risk reduction
RRR – Relative risk reduction
NNT – Number needed to treat

Can we find out – how many patients be treated with drug "G" to prevent one case of Myocardial infarction..?

This concept is given by NNT – which is the number of patients to be treated with drug "G" in order to prevent a negative outcome (i.e. MI)

Event rate in Experimental group (EER) = EE/ET
Event rate in control group (CER) = CE/CT
Hence, Absolute risk reduction (ARR) = Event rate in control group (CER) – Event rate in experimental group (EER)
Relative risk reduction (RRR) = (CER-EER)/CER
Risk ratio = EER/CER (ratio of the risks in each group)
ODDS ratio = (EE/EN) ÷ (CE/CN) (cross product ratio)
Number needed to treat = 1/ARR = 1 ÷ (CER-EER)

Hence in the example #1, we can assess:
EER = 10/1000
CER = 25/1000
So ARR = CER-EER = (10/1000) – (25/1000) = 15/1000 = 0.015
So, NNT = 1/ARR = 1 ÷ (15/1000) = 1000/15 = 66.66 ÷ 67
So, we need to treat 67 individuals with drug "G" to prevent MI in one person.
Remember: The lower the NNT, the more is the effectivity of the drug

Validity of Study

Validity is an expression of the degree to which a test is capable of measuring what it is intended to measure.

- **Internal validity** is the degree to which the results of an observation are correct for the particular group of people being studied
- **External validity** or generalizability is the extent to which the results of a study apply to people not in it (or, for example, to laboratories not involved in it). Internal validity is necessary for, but does not guarantee, external validity, and is easier to achieve

EVIDENCE-BASED MEDICINE

Systematic Reviews

- Systematic reviews are types of literature reviews that collect and critically analyze multiple research studies or papers
  - The systematic reviews may use methods of collective analyzing the multiple researches which may answer a research question or assess the effect of intervention(s) using methods that are selected before one or more research questions are formulated
  - It is a structured methodology to analyze and finalize the effect

Meta-analysis

- This approach is the aggregation of information leading to a higher statistical power and more robust point estimate from multiple studies, thus eliminating smaller errors arising from any individual studies.
- However, in performing a meta-analysis, an investigator must make choices which can affect the results, including deciding how to search for studies, selecting studies based on a set of objective criteria, dealing with incomplete data, analyzing the data, and accounting for or choosing not to account for publication bias.
- **Quorom** is the acronym used for the Quality of Reporting of Meta-analyses standards developed by QUOROM group
- **Prisma (Preferred Reporting Items for Systematic Reviews and Meta-analyses):** These are predefined set of items to assess systematic reviews and meta-analysis to assess the final effect of the intervention
- **Chochrane:** As its core is the collection of Cochrane Reviews, a database of systematic reviews and meta-analyses which summarize and interpret the results of medical research.

Forest Plot

It is a graphical display of estimated results from a number of scientific studies addressing the same question, along with the overall results.

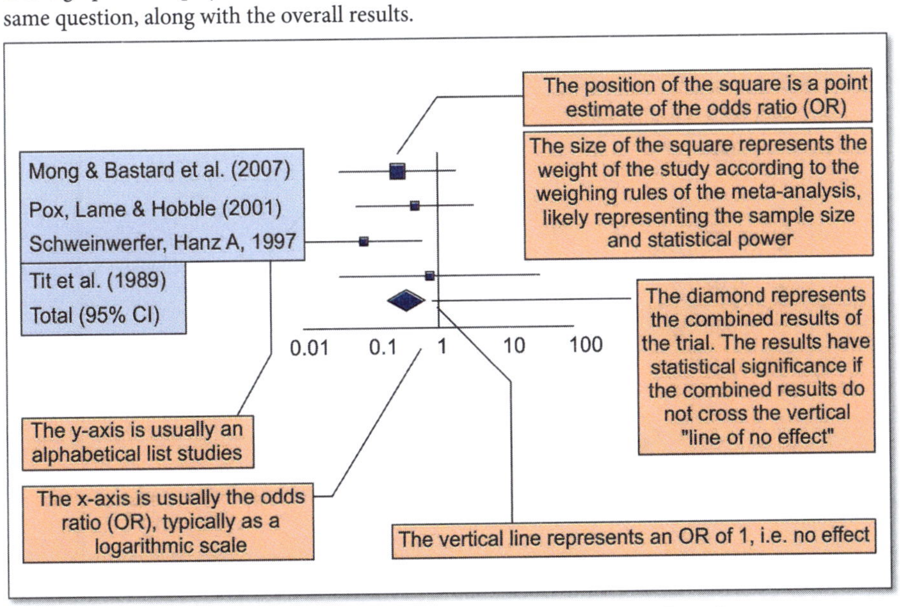

Fig. 13: Forest plot by graphical display of estimated results

Issues in Meta-analysis

Publication Bias (File Drawer Effect)

A *funnel plot* is a graph designed to check for the existence of publication bias; funnel plots are commonly used in systematic reviews and meta-analyses.

Good to Remember

- Father of evidence-based medicine—David Sackett
- Founder of evidence-based medicine—Gordon Guyatt

Must Remember

Why do we get a publication bias..?

- Trials could not be included in the meta-analysis because they were not published owing to non-significant treatment effects
- Trials reporting significant treatment effects were cited more often in publications, increasing the likelihood of being identified and included in the meta-analysis
- Trials were not included because they were published in inaccessible languages
- Inclusion of a trial because of.. (any other reason, not cited..!)

In the absence of publication bias, it assumes that studies with high precision will be plotted near the average, and studies with low precision will be spread evenly on both sides of the average, creating a roughly funnel-shaped distribution. **Deviation from this shape can indicate publication bias (or a file drawer effect)**

- **A funnel plot without a file drawer problem:** Almost equal distribution of the studies is seen below

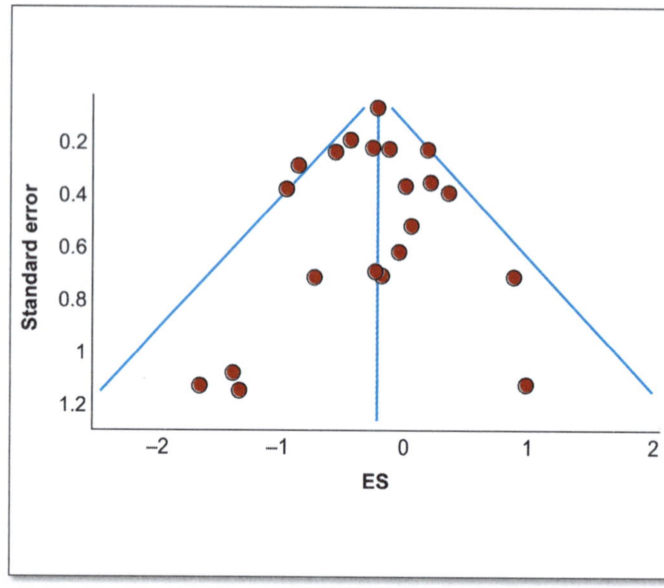

Fig. 14: Funnel plot without a file drawer problem

- **A funnel plot with a file drawer problem:** As seen in the funnel graph, most studies are placed in the left side of the funnel, depicting a bias towards publication of the negative result studies.

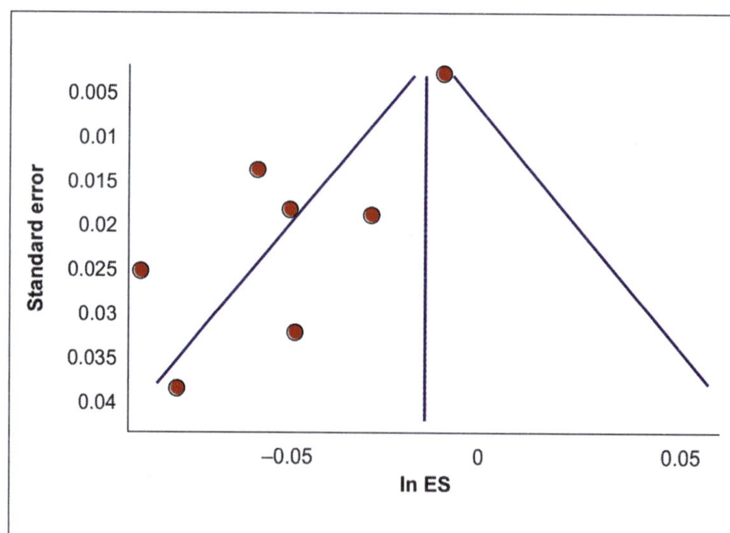

Fig. 15: Funnel plot with a file drawer problem

ERRORS IN EPIDEMIOLOGY

- **Random error:** May be due to a sampling error, individual biological variation or measurement error.
- **Systematic error** is known as Bias.

Bias

Table 9: Classification of bias

Common types of systematic errors in statistical studies	
Selection biases	*Inappropriate selection or poor retention of study subjects* ▪ **Ascertainment (sampling) bias:** Study population differs from target population due to nonrandom selection methods ▪ **Nonresponse bias:** High nonresponse rate to surveys/questionnaires can cause errors if nonresponders differ in some way from responders ▪ **Berkson bias:** Disease studied using only hospital-based patients may lead to results not applicable to target population ▪ **Prevalence (Neyman) bias:** Exposures that happen long before disease assessment can cause study to miss diseased patients that die early or recover ▪ **Attrition bias:** Significant loss of study participants may cause bias if those lost to follow-up differ significantly from remaining subjects
Observational biases	*Inaccurate measurement or classification of disease, exposure, or other variable* ▪ **Recall bias:** Common in retrospective studies, subject with negative outcomes are more likely to report certain exposures than control subjects ▪ **Observer bias:** Observers misclassify data due to individual differences in interpretation or preconceived expectations regarding study ▪ **Reporting bias:** Subject over or under-report exposure history due to perceived social stigmatization ▪ **Surveillance (detection) bias:** Risk factor itself causes increased monitoring in exposed group relative to unexposed group, which increases probability of identifying a disease

How to Decrease Bias from a Study Design?

- **Randomization:** Helps in reducing the chance of selection bias
- Blinding

Must Remember

Hawthorne effect: Change in attitude while under observation. It is an effect observed in follow up, long-term studies

Blinding

It is a formal method for decreasing the chance of systematic errors in the study design. Blinding is a fundamental tool to reduce bias in conducting clinical trials, whether it is blinding of patients, of physicians, or of the investigators who assign participants to each condition. Thus, blinding may be:

- **Single blind**
  - Where only the subject (or patient) is blind. It is the most basic type of blinding (Fig. 16).

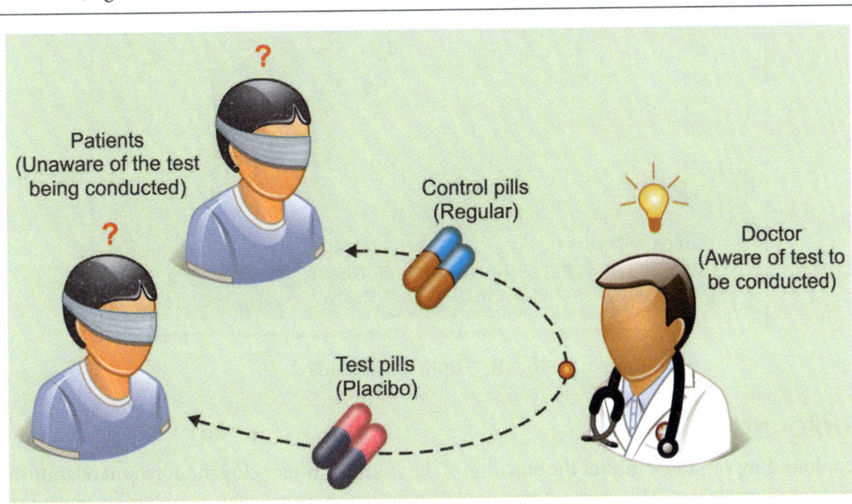

Fig. 16: Single blind clinical trial

- **Double blind**
  - Where both subject and the experimenter or the observer is blind (Fig. 17).
  - Random assignment of test subjects to the experimental and control groups is a critical part of any double-blind research design. It helps control for the placebo effect, observer bias, experimenter's bias
  - It is the main core of the RCT designs and is most commonly used in research methods.

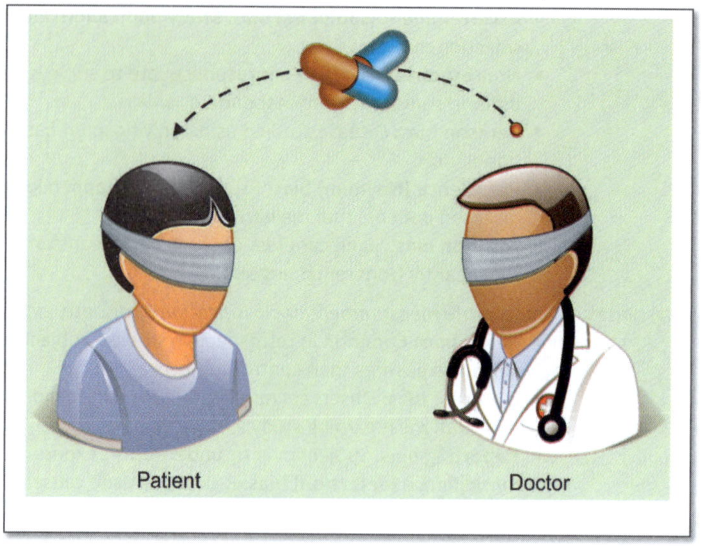

Fig. 17: Double blind clinical trial

- **Triple blind**
  - Where the subject, observer and the analyzer (the person who may conduct randomization or allocation of subjects or the statistician) are blind (Fig. 18)
  - It is the most robust of all, giving higher power and validity to the study design, though most difficult and may require advance version of planning and research methodology.
    * When an outcome such as death is the measure in the study, usually blinding is not required or done

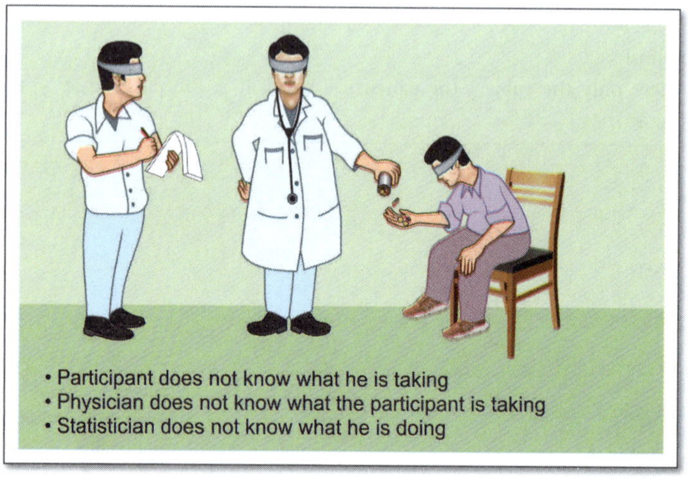

• Participant does not know what he is taking
• Physician does not know what the participant is taking
• Statistician does not know what he is doing

Fig. 18: Triple blind study

Confounding

A confounding variable can alter the outcome of the study by influencing the apparent relationship between two variables. The confounder can either mask the relationship—making it appear as if there is no relationship, when really, there is, or the confounder can make it seem that there is a relationship when in fact there is no relation.

Positive confounding is when the observed association is biased away from the null. In other words, it overestimates the effect.

Negative confounding is when the observed association is biased toward the null. In other words, it underestimates the effect.

Example: Age is a confounding factor because it is associated with the exposure (meaning that older people are more likely to be inactive), and it is also associated with the outcome (because older people are at greater risk of developing heart disease).

Example 1:

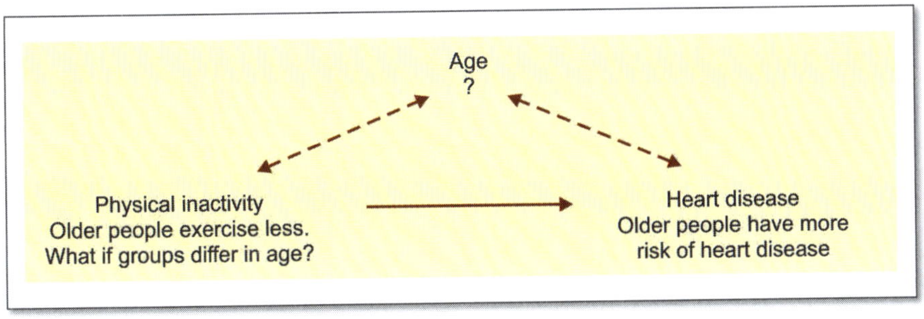

Fig. 19: Age confounding factor

Example 2:

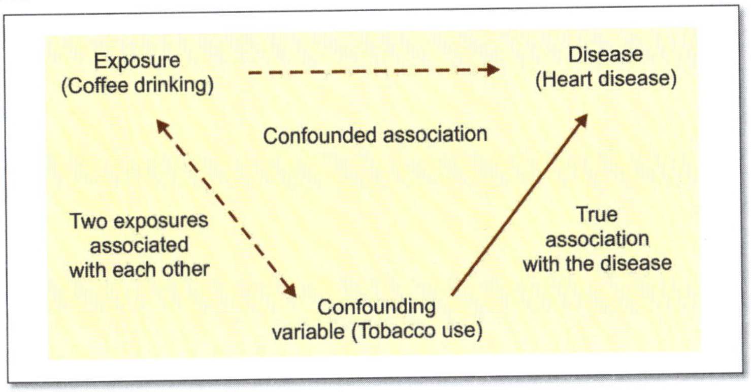

Fig. 20: Disease confounding factor

How to reduce confounding effect:

- **Matching** – in case the confounding variable is known
- **Randomization** – is the ideal way to control confounders, especially in experimental study designs
- **Standardization** – maybe adopted to control for age as confounding variable
- **Stratification**—usually is an easy approach for control of confounders, especially in the analysis phase rather than designing phase. It may not control for all confounders and is of limited use in larger study designs and higher statistical analysis with multiple variables.
- **Regression**—is the most robust measure while analysis of the study.

Effect Modification

Effect modification results when an external variable positively or negatively impacts the effect of an existing risk factor on the disease of interest.

If the variable is a confounder, there will be no significant difference in risk between the stratified groups as the confounding effects are now removed. However, if the variable is instead an effect modifier, there will be a significant difference between the 2 groups.

7 Good to Remember

When an outcome such as death is the measure in the study, usually blinding is not required or done

8 Good to Remember

Features of confounders:

- Associated with risk factor
- Associated with dependent or the outcome variable
- The confounder will lead to the disease both directly and indirectly under the effect of the confounder

7 High Yield Points

Confounding may lead to:

- Increase variance
- Useless results
- Bias
- Absurd correlation (which might show an effect which was not there or show blunted effect of an existing association)

8 Must Remember

Burden of genetic diseases in a community is determined by gene pool, breeding pattern and migration.

8 High Yield Points

Effect modification can be distinguished from confounding by performing a stratified analysis centering on the variable of interest.

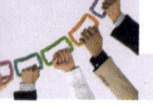

Multiple Choice Questions

1. In comparison to a placebo, the number of adverse outcomes with a drug was seen. What is the relative risk reduction for the drug? *(AIIMS Nov 2017)*

	Total patients	Adverse outcome
Placebo	1000	50
Drug	1000	10

a. 0.05 b. 0.01
c. 0.4 d. 0.8

2. A radiotherapist prescribes a new drug combination of chemotherapy and immunotherapy for metastatic melanoma. It prolongs the survival but does not cure cancer. Which of the following is true in this situation? *(AIIMS May 2017)*

a. Incidence reduces and prevalence increases
b. Incidence remains the same and prevalence increases
c. Incidence reduces and prevalence remains the same
d. Incidence increases and prevalence reduces

3. The following are the disease frequencies in a population. Based on the number of cases which of the following is the correct match *(AIIMS May 2017)*
Disease 1: Number of cases last week 42 this week 43
Disease 2: Number of cases last week 2 and present week 42
Disease 3: Number of cases last week 6 and present week 1

a. Endemic, epidemic, sporadic
b. Endemic, sporadic, epidemic
c. Sporadic, endemic, epidemic
d. Pandemic, endemic, sporadic

4. Ratio of incidence of a disease among the exposed to the incidence among nonexposed is: *(Recent Question 2018)*

a. Odds ratio b. Relative risk
c. Absolute risk d. Attributable risk

5. Unit of ecological study is: *(Recent Question 2018)*

a. Population b. Individual
c. Healthy people d. Patient

6. Incidence of a disease is 4 per 1000/year in a population. Calculate the period prevalence in two years? *(AIIMS May 2017)*

a. 8/1000 b. 4/1000
c. 2/1000 d. 6/1000

7. Framingham heart study is: *(Recent Question 2017)*

a. Cohort
b. Case control
c. Interventional
d. Cross-sectional

8. From 1970-1995, 500 people were monitored. Exposed to smoking 400, nonexposed 100. Out of 400 exposed 50 developed the lung cancer and out of 100 nonexposed 5 developed the lung cancer. Calculate relative risk:

a. 1.2 b. 2.5
c. 12.5 d. 1.5

9. Calculate odds ratio from the given table:

	Disease	Nondiseased
Exposed	33	53
Nonexposed	2	27
	35	82

a. 32 b. 8.4
c. 88.4 d. 11.4

10. When some people develop a disease after exposure from a primary case, it is known as: *(Recent Question 2017)*

a. Incidence b. Prevalence
c. Lead time d. Secondary attack rate

11. Relative risk calculation is done for:

a. Cohort study b. Case control study
c. Cross sectional study d. Ecological study

12. Framingham heart study comes under:

a. Cohort b. Case control
c. Cross sectional study d. Ecological study

13. Hospital patient admission rate differs in different hospitals with different disease. This causes which type of bias:

a. Subject bias b. Investigator bias
c. Berksonian bias d. Analyzer bias

14. Lung cancer patients : 300 smokers and 300 nonsmokers, 10 year history taken. What can be calculated?

a. Prevalence b. Incidence
c. RR d. Odds ratio

15. In situation of an epidemic, what is the medical officer's first role/first to do: *(Recent Question 2017)*

a. Do diagnosis and submit
b. Find out at risk population
c. Find out about number of cases
d. Confirm epidemic whether it exists in real

16. Which of the following is not a utilization rate:

a. Population bed ratio
b. Average length of stay
c. Bed turnover ratio
d. Bed occupancy rate

17. Which is correct about Prevalence(P), incidence(I) and duration(D):

a. $I = P \times D$ b. $P = I \times D$
c. $D = P \times I$ d. All are correct

18. Because of cross-sectional study: *(Recent Question 2016)*

a. We can measure prevalence
b. We can measure incidence
c. We can measure both
d. Best for justification of causation

19. Odds ratio is related to:

a. Relative risk b. Incidence
c. Prevalence d. Attributable risk

20. The preferred epidemiological study for rare diseases is:

a. Cohort study b. Case control study
c. Cross-sectional study d. Case study

Ans.

1.	d
2.	b
3.	a
4.	b
5.	a
6.	a
7.	a
8.	b
9.	b
10.	d
11.	a
12.	a
13.	c
14.	d
15.	d
16.	a
17.	b
18.	a
19.	a
20.	b

Most Recent Questions of 2019-18 are given at the end of MCQs

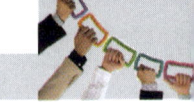

21. **Framingham coronary heart disease study is the example of:** *(Recent Question 2016)*
 a. Cohort study b. Prospective
 c. Retrospective d. Descriptive
22. **Natural history of disease is determine by:**
 a. Case control study b. Cohort study
 c. RCT d. Ecological studies
23. **When we are investigating the relationship between steroid contraceptive and breast cancer, if the women taking these contraceptives are younger than those in the comparison group, they would be at a lower risk of breast cancer since this disease becomes common with increasing age. The age factor in this case is called:** *(Recent Question 2016)*
 a. Selection bias b. Berksonian bias
 c. Confounding factor d. Interviewer bias
24. **Confounding factor:**
 a. It is evenly distributed in case and control
 b. Associated with both exposure and outcome
 c. Not associated with exposure
 d. It is not a risk factor of disease
25. **Lung cancer develops in 30% of patients cigarette smokers. This indicates:** *(Recent Question 2016)*
 a. Relative risk b. Attributable risk
 c. Incidence d. Population attributable risk
26. **Attributable risk is:**
 a. Incidence among exposed/Incidence among non-exposed
 b. (Incidence among exposed – Incidence among non-exposed)/Incidence among exposed
 c. (Incidence among exposed – Incidence among non exposed)/Incidence among non-exposed
 d. Incidence among non-exposed /Incidence among exposed
27. **Calculation of RR:**
 a. Incidence of disease among exposed/incidence of disease among unexposed
 b. Incidence of disease among exposed/incidence of disease among total population
 c. Cross product ratio
 d. It is never more than 1

INCIDENCE

28. **In epidemiology, disease frequency is measured by :**
 a. Incidence and prevalence b. Incidence only
 c. Prevalence only d. Attack rate
29. **Population at risk is used as denominator in calculation of:**
 a. Mortality rate b. Incidence
 c. Prevalence d. Relative risk
30. **When a new treatment is developed that delays deaths but does not produce recovery from a chronic disease, which of the following will occur:**
 a. Prevalence of the disease will decrease
 b. Incidence of the disease will increase
 c. Prevalence of the disease will increase
 d. Incidence and prevalence of the disease will decrease
31. **Incidence rate is calculated from**
 a. Case-control
 b. Prospective trial
 c. Retrospective trial
 d. RCT
32. **An expert in the field of public health is required to estimate the magnitude of health problem. Which rate would be calculate for this?**
 a. Incidence b. Prevalence
 c. Cause specific mortality d. Proportionate mortality rate
33. **A study was conducted to estimate the Annual parasitic incidence for malaria. All persons in the village were examined for smear examination. The results are as mentioned below**

	Number of persons	Number of new cases in two years
Persons in household with known cases of malaria	500	10
Households without any known case of malaria	5000	50

What is the incidence per 1000-person years for households with malaria cases
 a. 0.1 b. 0.01
 c. 1 d. 10

For Q 34–36

Data from an investigation of an epidemic of German measles in a remote village are given in the table below:

Age group (years)	Number in population	Number Ill (symptomatic)	Number not Ill but with antibody rise (asymptomatic	Number Unifected	Percent infected
0–19	204	110	74	20	90
10–19	129	70	46	13	90
20–39	161	88	57	16	90
40–59	78	42	28	8	90
60+	42	2	2	38	10
Total	614	312	207	95	

34. **Which expression represents the calculation to determine the incidence of illness for all age groups (as a percentage)?**
 a. 95/519 × 100 = 18.3 per 100 population
 b. 207/614 × 100 = 33.7 per 100 population
 c. 207/519 × 100 = 39.9 per 100 population
 d. 312/614 × 100 = 50.8 per 100 population
35. **Which of the following calculation represents the percentage of infection that is subclinical?**
 a. 95/519 × 100 = 18.3% b. 207/614 × 100 = 33.7%
 c. 207/519 × 100 = 39.9% d. 312/614 × 100 = 50.8%
36. **Based on the age-specific infection rates, when did German measles previously occur in this village in relation to the current epidemic?**
 a. 1 to 9 years ago b. 10 to 19 years ago
 c. 20 to 39 years ago d. 60 years ago

Ans.

21. a	22. b
23. c	24. b
25. b	26. b
27. a	28. a
29. b	30. c
31. b	32. b
33. d	34. d
35. c	36. d

Most Recent Questions of 2019-18 are given at the end of MCQs

37. **A village with 2000 population was surveyed for one year and 10 were found to be disease. Assuming that the disease lasts for 2 years, annual prevalence is:**
    a. 10/4000 per 1000 population
    b. 20/2000 per 1000 population
    c. 10%
    d. 0.5%
38. **Total number of cases in given population at a given time is:**
    a. Incidence b. Prevalence
    c. Attack rate d. Odds ratio
39. **After the volunteers for a study have been questioned about use of smokeless tobacco and examined for lesions of the mouth, the data on the 400 individuals are tabulated as follows:**

Age group	Males		Females	
	Using smokeless tobacco	Oral lesions	Using smokeless tobacco	Oral lesions
15–19 years	30	12	30	1
20–24 years	50	36	50	13
25–29 years	50	32	50	8
30–34 years	50	23	50	8
> 35 years	20	6	20	2

In this study, which measure of disease occurrence can be calculated?
    a. Incidence rate b. Cumulative incidence rate
    c. Odds ratio d. Prevalence
40. **Prevalence of disease in a community can be found out by**
    a. Case-control study b. Cohort study
    c. Cross-sectional study d. Analytical study
41. **What is not true about cross-sectional study?**
    a. Estimate for prevalence for disease
    b. Confirms the etiology of disease
    c. Evaluate the disease pattern in the community
    d. Evaluate the association of risk factors
42. **Prevalence of a disease:**
    a. Can only be determined by a cohort study
    b. Is the number of new case in a defined population
    c. Describe the balance between incidence, mortality and recovery
    d. Is the best measure of disease frequency in etiological studies
43. **For calculation of incidence denominator is taken as:**
    a. Mid-year population *(Recent Question 2012)*
    b. Population at risk
    c. Total number of cases
    d. Total number of deaths
44. **In a town of population 5000, 500 are myopic on January 1, 2011. Number of new myopia cases is 90 till December 31, 2011. Calculate the incidence of myopia per thousand population in year 2011.** *(AIIMS Nov 2012)*
    a. 0.018 b. 0.02
    c. 0.05 d. 20
45. **All about incidence are false except:**
    a. Not affected by duration *(Recent Question 2012)*
    b. More than prevalence
    c. Measures old and new cases
    d. Used for chronic conditions
46. **Incidence of a disease in a population of 30,000 with 300 new cases is:**
    a. 0.1 per 1000 b. 10 per 1000
    c. 100 per 1000 d. 1 per 1000
47. **Which of the following studies can find out the incidence of disease?** *(Recent Question 2015)*
    a. Cohort study
    b. Case control study
    c. Cross-sectional study
    d. RCT
48. **All the following are true regarding incidence rate except:** *(Recent Question 2015)*
    a. Number of new cases in a specified population in a specific period of time
    b. Secondary attack rate is a special incidence rate
    c. Use is generally restricted to acute conditions
    d. Useful to find the magnitude of the disease problem in the community
49. **Which of the following is used as an indicator of efficacy of hospital services and health programs:** *(Recent Question 2015)*
    a. Prevalence b. Incidence
    c. Case fatality rate d. Secondary attack rate
50. **All statements are true about the incidence of disease except:**
    a. Incidence rate falls if a new drug is effective in reducing deaths from the disease
    b. Incidence measures absolute risk of developing disease
    c. Incidence falls if a prevention program is effective
    d. Incidence is probability that a healthy individual will develop the disease during a specified period.
51. **Incidence is best studied by:** *(AIIMS May 10, Nov 08)*
    a. Retrospective studies
    b. Prospective studies
    c. Cross sectional
    d. Case control
52. **From 1st January to 30th June 2019, 22 new cases of TB were reported per 1,65,000 population. But during this period 120 suspected cases of TB were registered. What will be incidence rate for TB in the population?**
    a. 133 per 10,00,000 population
    b. 270 per 10,00,000 population
    c. 75 per 10,00,000 population
    d. 90 per 10,00,000 population

PREVALENCE

53. **A new intervention can decrease the mortality of disease but not cure it, which of the following is true?**
    a. Incidence will decrease *(AIIMS Nov 2015)*
    b. Prevalence will increase
    c. Incidence will increase
    d. No change
54. **If a disease has three times more incidence in females as compared to males and same prevalence in both males and females, true statement will be:**
    a. It is highly fatal in females
    b. More survival in females
    c. Better prognosis in males
    d. Less fatal in females

Ans.
37. d 38. b 39. d 40. c 41. b 42. c 43. b 44. d 45. a 46. b 47. a 48. d 49. b 50. a 51. b 52. a 53. b 54. a

Most Recent Questions of 2019-18 are given at the end of MCQs

55. **True regarding prevalence is:** *(JIPMER 2015)*
 a. Cannot be used to determine the health needs of a community
 b. Independent of incidence
 c. Independent of duration
 d. Measures all cases

56. **When the term "Prevalence rate" is used without any qualification, it is taken to mean as?**
 a. Period prevalence rate
 b. Annual prevalence rate
 c. Point prevalence rate
 d. Mean duration prevalence rate

57. **In population of 5000, number of new cases of TB is 500; old cases in the same population are 150. What is the prevalence of TB:** *(Recent Question 2014)*
 a. 9% b. 12%
 c. 13% d. 18%

58. **Prevalence is a:** *(Recent Question 2013)*
 a. Rate b. Ratio
 c. Proportion d. Mean

59. **A district has total population 10 lacs, with under 16 population being 30%. The prevalence of blindness is 0.8/1000 among under 16 population. Calculate total number of blind among under 16 population in the district:** *(AIIMS Nov 2012)*
 a. 240 b. 2400
 c. 24000 d. 240000

MORATLITY AND MORBIDITY RATES

60. **Age adjusted death rate is calculated for all except?** *(AIIMS Nov 2015)*
 a. To allow communities with different age structures to be compared
 b. To allow comparison of both sex
 c. To allow comparison of different age in relation to injuries or accidents
 d. To allow comparison of cancer prevalence in different strata

61. **Age specific death rate can be used for all of the following except:**
 a. Compare different causes within the same population
 b. Compare injuries/accidents between different sexes
 c. Compare injuries/accidents between different age groups
 d. Identify specific age groups at risk for preventive action

62. **Proportional mortality rate is:** *(New Question 2012)*
 a. Rate b. Ratio
 c. Proportion d. None

63. **In proportional mortality rate for a specific disease, denominator is:**
 a. Mid-year population during that year
 b. Population at risk in a specific area
 c. Total death in that year
 d. Attributable death of a particular disease

64. **Direct standardization is used to compare the mortality rates between two countries because of difference in:**
 a. Cause of death
 b. Numerator
 c. Age distribution
 d. Denominators

DESCRIPTIVE EPIDEMIOLOGY

65. **Spot maps for diseases are used in epidemiology to depict**
 a. Local distributions b. Rural urban variations
 c. International variations d. National variations

66. **Hypothesis is not tested by**
 a. Descriptive studies b. Analytical studies
 c. Case control studies d. Cohort studies

67. **Discovery of cholera by John Snow was a ……**
 a. Cohort study b. Cross sectional study
 c. Natural experiment study
 d. Clinical trial

ANALYTICAL EPIDEMIOLOGY

68. **Which is not an analytical study**
 a. Case control b. Cohort study
 c. RCT d. Cross-sectional

69. **Cross-sectional study is:**
 a. Longitudinal study b. Prospective study
 c. Retrospective study d. Prevalence study

70. **A person found correlation between fatty food intake and a disease due to obesity. He did this by collecting data from the food manufacturers and hospital respectively. Such a study is:** *(AIIMS May 2012)*
 a. Ecological study
 b. Cross-sectional disease
 c. Psychological study
 d. Experimental study

71. **Which of the following epidemiological method is a observational study** *(Recent Question 2015)*
 a. Randomized control trials
 b. Field trials
 c. Ecological study
 d. Community intervention study

72. **A study was done in 3 states to see the mean blood pressure in each community. Health workers were assigned and they visited each house in the three communities. Mean blood pressure is each community was found and compared. What type of study design is represented here?**
 a. Cohort study b. Cross Sectional study
 c. Case control study d. Field trial

73. **In a study conducted on typhoid carrier in three villages with three different water sources. Investigations were done and the carrier status were calculated and compared. The type of study is:**
 a. Field trial b. Cross sectional study
 c. Cohort study d. Case-control study

74. **Follow up is not required in which of the following study:** *(PGI Pattern)*
 a. Prospective study b. Retrospective study
 c. Cross-sectional study d. Longitudinal study
 e. Cohort study

75. **Least time consuming study design to ascertain association between lung cancer and smoking?**
 a. Cohort
 b. Case control
 c. Cross sectional
 d. RCT

Ans.

55. d	56. c
57. c	58. c
59. a	60. b
61. b	62. c
63. c	64. c
65. a	66. a
67. c	68. c
69. d	70. a
71. c	72. b
73. b	74. b
75. c	

CASE CONTROL STUDY

76. Which type of study design would you use to test a hypothesis in limited recourses and time?
a. Cohort study b. Case control study
c. RCT d. Field trial

77. In a study of the cause of lung cancer patients who had the disease were matched with control by age, sex, place and social class. The frequency of cigarette smoking was then compared on the two groups of with and without lung cancer. What type of study was this?
a. Prospective cohort study b. Case control study
c. Retrospective cohort study
d. Case series study

78. The most feasible design to assess the relationship between "breast cancer" and risk factor as "OCP use" can be established by
a. Cohort study b. Case control study
c. Randomized trial d. Non-randomized trial

79. A research organization wishes to estimate the risk of bronchial cancer in people who smoke bidi "unfiltered, hand rolled – herbal cigarettes". 200 bronchogenic cancer patients and 400 Ca pancreas patients were enrolled for the study to assess the risk of bidi smoking and lung cancer. The results reported 81% of lung cancer patients were bidi smokers, while 17% of pancreatic cancer patients were bidi smokers. This is an example of:
a. Cross sectional study b. Case series
c. Case control study d. Cohort study

80. "Risk ratio" may be a proxy indicator for:
a. Number needed to harm
b. Attributable risk
c. Population attributable risk
d. Odds ratio

81. Not an advantage of case control studies:
a. Cost effective and inexpensive
b. Odds ratio can be calculated
c. Relative risk can be calculated
d. Useful in rare diseases

82. Study of a person who has already contracted the disease is known as:
a. Cohort study b. Case control study
c. Control cohort study d. None of the above

83. Which of the following is the most useful study design in a hospital setting?
a. Cohort b. Case control
c. Cross sectional d. Longitudinal

84. All of the following are true about case control study except
a. Long duration
b. Inexpensive
c. Odds ratio can be derived
d. Recall bias may be present

85. Odds ratio, is calculated from:
a. Cohort study b. Cross sectional study
c. Case control study d. Randomized controlled trial

86. Study of a person who has already contracted the disease is called:
a. Case control b. Cohort
c. Control cohort d. None of the above

87. The following statement is wrong regarding case control study
a. It is useful for rare disease
b. Early to do the study
c. Incidence can be calculated
d. It is a retrospective study

88. Which one of the following statement regarding case control studies is correct?
a. Used for rare disease
b. Incidence rate can be calculated
c. Treatment can be formulated
d. Takes long time for the results

89. A total of 500 patients with thyroid cancer are identified and surveyed by patient interviews with reference to past exposure to radiation. The study design most appropriately illustrates
a. Case series report b. Case-control study
c. Case report d. Clinical trial

90. Case reference study is the other name for: ***(Recent Question 2015)***
a. Case control study b. Cohort study
c. Prospective study d. Ecological study

91. All the following are advantages of case control studies except: ***(Recent Question 2015)***
a. Rapid studies
b. Study of several different etiological factors
c. No attrition problems
d. Can distinguish causes and associated factors

92. Which of the following rate can be obtained from case control studies: ***(Recent Question 2015)***
a. Odds ratio
b. Relative risk
c. Attributable risk
d. Population attributable risk

93. True about case control study is:*(Recent Question 2014, 12)*
a. Not possible for rare disease
b. Odds ratio cannot be calculated
c. Attributable risk cannot be calculated
d. Bias is not seen

94. Regarding case control study true is: ***(JIPMER 2014)***
a. Useful for rare diseases
b. Incidence can be calculated
c. Takes longer time
d. Relative risk can be calculated

95. A study on association between smoking and lung cancer to be done in a relatively quick time. Which of the study design is preferred:
a. Case control
b. Cohort study
c. Randomized controlled study
d. Cross sectional study

96. Features of case control study is/are: ***(PGI May 2013)***
a. Useful for study of rare diseases
b. Large sample size required
c. Association measure by relative risk
d. Study multiple potential risk factors of a disease
e. Higher accuracy rate

Ans.

76. b
77. b
78. b
79. c
80. d
81. c
82. b
83. b
84. a
85. c
86. a
87. c
88. a
89. a
90. a
91. d
92. a
93. c
94. a
95. a
96. a, d

97. **Which one of the following statement regarding case control studies is correct:** *(Recent Question 2012)*
   a. Used for rare diseases
   b. Incidence rate can be calculated
   c. Treatment can be formulated
   d. Takes long time for the result

98. **All of the following are advantages of case control studies except:** *(Recent Question 2013)*
   a. Useful in rare diseases
   b. Relative risk can be calculated
   c. Odds ratio can be calculated
   d. Cost effective and inexpensive

99. **Confounding can be eliminated by all except:** *(AIIMS May 2012)*
   a. Matching b. Blinding
   c. Randomization d. Multivariate analysis

100. **A study revealed lesser incidence of carcinoma colon in pure vegetarians than nonvegetarians by which it was concluded that beta-carotene is protective against cancer. This may not be true because the vegetarian subject may be consuming high fiber diet which is protective against cancer. This is an example of:** *(AIIMS May 2012, 10)*
   a. Multifactorial causation
   b. Causal association
   c. Confounding factor
   d. Common association

101. **Confounding can be removed by:**
   a. Assign confounders equally to both cases and controls
   b. Stratification
   c. Matching
   d. All of the above

102. **In a study done to establish smoking as a risk factor for a disease, out of 50 cases, 30 were smokers, while there were 10 smokers out of another 50 healthy control. The Odds ratio is:**
   a. 3 b. 6
   c. 5 d. 10

COHORT STUDY

103. **The association between low birth weight and maternal smoking during pregnancy can be studied by obtaining smoking histories from women at the time of the prenatal visit and then subsequently correlating birth weight with smoking histories. What type of study is this?**
   a. Clinical trial
   b. Cross-sectional
   c. Cohort (Prospective)
   d. Case-control (retrospective)

104. **Community physician take action based on:**
   a. Population attributable risk
   b. Relative risk
   c. Attributable risk
   d. Odds ratio

105. **Relative risk is measured by:**
   a. Incidence among non-exposed/incidence among exposed
   b. Incidence among exposed/incidence among non-exposed
   c. Incidence among non-exposed/total incidence
   d. Incidence among exposed/total incidence

106. **The ratio between incidences among exposed and non-exposed persons is called**
   a. Attributable risk
   b. Positive predictive value
   c. Relative risk
   d. Odds ratio

107. **The best indicator to determine maximum benefit to the community through preventive intervention strategies is**
   a. Relative risk
   b. Attributable risk
   c. Absolute risk
   d. Odds ratio

108. **The results in a nonrandomized study to find role of cigarette smoking in causation of Ca Gall Bladder is shown below. Calculate the Attributable risk is**

	GB cancer	Total
Smokers	20	2000
Nonsmokers	40	4000

   a. 0%
   b. 20%
   c. 10%
   d. 50%

109. **True about cohort studies is:**
   a. Proceeds from cause to effect
   b. Cohorts are identified prior to the appearance of disease under investigation
   c. Study groups are observed over a period of time to determine the frequency of disease among them
   d. All of the above

110. **Which of the following statements is not correct?**
   a. A cohort study is more expensive in comparison with case—control study.
   b. A cohort study starts with people exposed to risk factor or suspected cause while case—control study starts with disease.
   c. A long follow-up period is often needed with delayed results in a cohort study yields relatively quick results.
   d. A cohort study is more appropriate when the disease or exposure under investigation is rare in comparison with case— control study.

111. **The ratio between the incidence of disease among exposed and nonexposed is called**
   a. Causal risk b. Relative risk
   c. Attributable risk d. Odds ratio

112. **All of the following are true about cohort studies except**
   a. Costly b. Useful for rare disease
   c. Prospective d. Necessary for incidence

113. **True statements concerning cohort studies include all the following except:**
   a. Cohort studies are longitudinal in design
   b. Subjects are selected on the basis of characteristics present before the onset of the condition being studied
   c. Subjects are observed over time to determine the frequency of occurrence of the condition under study
   d. Cohort studies are necessary to estimate the prevalence of disease

Ans.

97. a
98. b
99. b
100. c
101. d
102. b
103. c
104. a
105. b
106. c
107. b
108. a
109. d
110. d
111. b
112. b
113. d

Most Recent Questions of 2019-18 are given at the end of MCQs

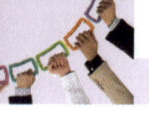

114. Incidence is calculated from
a. Prospective cohort study
b. Retrospective cohort study
c. Cross-sectional study
d. Case-control study

115. Most appropriate method to know about contribution of risk factor to disease
a. Relative risk
b. Attributable risk
c. Absolute risk
d. Odd's ratio

116. If relative risk is one, the type of association between Disease and Agent is
a. Strong association   b. Casual association
c. No association   d. Negative association

117. Which of the following study design, give you the incidence
a. Case control study   b. Cohort study
c. RCT   d. Descriptive cross sectional

118. Cohort study is which type of study:
a. Prospective   b. Retrospective
c. Ambispective   d. All

119. Framingham Heart Study is an example of:
a. Cohort study
b. Case-control study
c. Cross-sectional study
d. RCT

120. All of the following are true about Cohort study except:
a. Expensive
b. Chronic disease can be studied
c. Incidence rate can be calculated
d. Starts with the disease

121. In studying the association between disease and exposure factor, a study design which allows the study of multiple outcomes for a given exposure is:
a. Cohort study   b. Ecological study
c. Cross sectional study   d. Case-control study

122. True about cohort study are all except:
a. Long follow up required
b. Large number of subjects required
c. Less expensive
d. Not done for rare diseases

123. The following are true regarding cohort studies except ***(Recent Question 2015)***
a. Dose-response ratio can be calculated
b. Incidence can be calculated
c. Suitable to study rare diseases
d. Yields information about more than one disease outcome

124. About 1200 adults were randomly selected for a prospective study of the effect of a new drug x. The drug will be given for 5 years and its association with cataract is studied. What type of study is this? ***(JIPMER 2015)***
a. Case control study   b. Cohort study
c. Randomized clinical trial   d. Cross sectional study

125. Which of the following is true about cohort study:
a. Disease to risk factor study ***(Recent Question 2014)***
b. Effect to cause study
c. Not associated with attributable risk
d. Associated with antecedent causation

126. 20 pregnant women were asked about the history of smoking when they came for regular antenatal visit and then followed up to see how many of them had low birth weight babies. What is the type of study?
a. Case control ***(Recent Question 2014)***
b. Prospective cohort
c. Cross sectional
d. Ecological

127. Natural history of a disease is best studied with:
a. Longitudinal studies
b. Cross-sectional studies
c. Trials
d. None

128. Natural history of disease is best studied by:
a. Cross-sectional study
b. Cohort
c. Case control study
d. Any of the above

129. Which of the following is correct with respect to a planned prospective cohort study for *H. pylori* and IBD in gastroenterology ward
a. Enroll all patients in whom endoscopy is done
b. Enroll all patient taking proton pump inhibitor
c. Exclude patient diagnosed with inflammatory bowel disease
d. Exclude patient positive for urea breath test for *H. pylori*

130. Cause to effect progression is seen in all except
a. Case control study
b. Ecological study
c. Cohort study
d. Randomized control trail

BIAS

131. 'Systematic error in the determination of the association between the exposure and disease, is termed as:
a. Chance   b. Probability
c. Bias   d. Confounding

132. Berksonian bias refer to the bias arising from :
a. Different rate of admission to the hospital
b. The cases not being representative of the general population
c. Presence of confounding bias
d. Improper selection of case

133. Recall information bias is unlikely to affect cohort studies because
a. Data collection is prospective
b. Large number of subjects is usually included
c. Exposure is usually determined prior to disease occurrence
d. Actual relative risk can be determined

134. Recall bias mostly associated with which study design:
a. Case control study   b. Cohort
c. RCT   d. Field trial

135. Which of the following is true regarding Berkesonian bias:
a. Systematic differences in characteristic between cases and control
b. Cases and controls are asked questions about their past history
c. Error in sampling
d. Different rates of admission in hospital

Ans.
114. a
115. a
116. c
117. b
118. d
119. a
120. d
121. a
122. c
123. c
124. b
125. d
126. b
127. a
128. b
129. c
130. a
131. c
132. a
133. c
134. a
135. d

Most Recent Questions of 2019-18 are given at the end of MCQs

136. Double blind study means:
a. Observer is blind about the study
b. Person or groups being observed are blind about the study
c. Both observer and observed group is blind
d. Interpreters and analyzer are blind about study

137. The purpose of double blind study is to:
a. Avoid subject bias
b. Avoid observer bias and sampling variation
c. Reduce the effect of sampling variation
d. Avoid subject bias and sampling variation

138. The purpose of a double-blind study is to
a. Reduce the effects of sampling variation
b. Avoid observer and subject bias
c. Avoid observer bias and sampling variation
d. Avoid subject bias and sampling variation

139. Double blind studies are done while conducting
a. Case-control studies b. Cohort studies
c. Experimental studies d. Meta. analysis

140. Randomization is useful to eliminate:
a. Observer bias b. Selection bias
c. Patient bias d. Sampling bias

141. Randomization is useful to eliminate:
a. Observer bias b. Selection bias
c. Patient bias d. Sampling bias

142. In case control study confounding can be prevented by
a. Randomization b. Matching
c. Double blinding d. Triple blinding

143. Confounding bias can be eliminated by all Except:
a. Matching b. Blinding
c. Randomization d. Multivariate analysis

144. Matching reduces which bias in case control study:
a. Selection bias b. Response bias
c. Confounding factor d. Berkesonian bias

145. Matching is done in case control study to eliminate:
a. Confounding factor b. Bias
c. Sampling error d. Relative risk

146. The use of matching as a technique to control for confounding is most appropriate for which type of study design?
a. A large-scale cohort study
b. A case-control study with a small number of cases
c. A clinical trial with a factorial design
d. A cross-sectional study with multiple variables

147. Which one of the following is true regarding confounding factor except
a. It is associated with exposure under investigation
b. It is distributed equally in study and control groups
c. It is associated both with exposure and disease
d. It is related to matching in case control study

148. Randomization is useful to eliminate:
a. Observer bias
b. Selection bias
c. Subject bias
d. Sampling bias

149. A statistical procedure by which the study participants are allocated into "study" and "control" groups is called:
a. Stratified sampling b. Randomization
c. Blinding d. Comparative study

150. Selection bias can be eliminated by:
a. Removing confounding effect *(Recent Question 2015)*
b. Matching
c. Blinding
d. Selection of a representative study group of cases and control from the population

151. When we are investigating the relationship between steroid contraceptive and breast cancer, if the women taking these contraceptives are younger than those in the comparison group, they would be at a lower risk of breast cancer since this disease becomes common with increasing age. The age factor in this case is called: *(Recent Question 2015)*
a. Confounding factor b. Selection bias
c. Interviewer bias d. Berksonian bias

152. Confounding factor can be eliminated by all except:
a. Blinding *(Recent Question 2015)*
b. Randomization
c. Matching
d. Standardization

153. A researcher wishes to compare blood lipid profile of smokers and nonsmokers. But is concerned that the Smokers might differ from Nonsmokers in their diet, exercise, etc. This is an example of: *(AIIMS May 2015)*
a. Recall bias b. Information bias
c. Hawthorne bias d. Selection bias

154. A study done to establish relationship between Smoking and Lung cancer found that association was more in people who exercised less and less in people who exercise more. Here exercise is a: *(AIIMS May 2015)*
a. Selection Bias b. Effect modifier
c. Confounding factor d. Collinear factor

155. Berksonian bias is a type of:
a. Selection bias b. Interviewer bias
c. Information bias d. Recall bias

156. Hospital patient admission rate differs in different hospitals with different disease. This causes which type of bias:
a. Subject bias b. Investigator bias
c. Berksonian bias d. Analyzer bias

157. Selection bias occurs during:
a. Treatment b. Analysis
c. Recruitment d. Observation

158. Berksonian bias is due to:
a. Presence of confounding factors in both cases and control
b. Questioning the case more thoroughly as compared to controls
c. Different rates of admission to hospital due to different disease
d. Better recall by the cases as compared to controls

159. Selection bias can be eliminated by:
a. Randomization b. Single blinding
c. Double blinding d. Matching

160. Bias can be eliminated by all except:
a. Matching b. Blinding
c. Randomization d. Multivariate analysis

161. Hawthorne effect is seen in:
a. Case control study b. Cohort study
c. Cross sectional study d. Retrospective Cohort study

Ans.
136. c
137. b
138. b
139. c
140. b
141. b
142. b
143. b
144. c
145. a
146. b
147. b
148. b
149. b
150. d
151. a
152. a
153. d
154. b
155. a
156. c
157. c
158. c
159. a
160. d
161. b

Most Recent Questions of 2019-18 are given at the end of MCQs

RR/AR/PAR OR MEASURES OF EFFECT

162. The difference in incidence rates of disease (or deaths) between an exposed group and nonexposed group is known as:
a. Relative risk
b. Attributable risk
c. Population attributable risk
d. Odds ratio

163. In a population of 9000, 2100 were alcoholic, 70 of the alcoholics developed cirrhosis and 23 nonalcoholic developed cirrhosis. What is the attributable risk ?
a. 40% b. 60%
c. 70% d. 90%

164. The formula for relative risk is: *(New Question 2015)*
a. $(I_{exposed} - I_{nonexposed})/ I_{exposed} \times 100$
b. $(I_{total} - I_{nonexposed})/ I_{total} \times 100$
c. $I_{exposed}/ I_{nonexposed}$
d. $(I_{total} - I_{exposed})/ I_{total}$

165. If the relative risk is 1, then which of the following statement is true:
a. There is a positive association between the cause and effect
b. If the cause is there, then it will decrease the occurrence of the effect
c. Cannot be commented upon because of inadequate data
d. There is no increase in risk because the effect occurs in both groups

166. Definition of population attributable risk: *(AIIMS Nov 2014)*
a. Risk of disease among exposed as compared to nonexposed
b. Difference in risk of exposed and nonexposed groups
c. Estimate of amount disease that can be reduced if risk factor is modified/eliminated
d. Extent to which disease can be attributed to risk factor under study

167. In a cohort study to ascertain association between a risk factor and disease, the risk ratio was 1. What does this signify?
a. No association between risk factor and disease
b. Positive association between risk factor and disease
c. Negative association between risk factor and disease
d. Data is insufficient to comment

168. Attributable risk is defined as:
a. Incidence among exposed divided by incidence among nonexposed
b. Incidence among exposed minus incidence among nonexposed/incidence exposed
c. Incidence among nonexposed minus incidence among exposed/incidence exposed
d. Incidence among nonexposed divided by incidence among exposed

169. Strength of association between a putative risk factor and a disease is measured by: *(AIIMS Nov 2016)*
a. Attributable risk b. Absolute risk
c. Relative risk d. Magnitude of p-value

170. Relative risk is calculated in *(Recent Question 2013)*
a. Cross sectional study b. Cohort study
c. Case control study d. None

171. Relative risk calculation is done from
a. Cohort study b. Case control study
c. Cross sectional study d. Ecological study

172. Attributable risk means *(Recent Question 2012)*
a. Fatality of a disease
b. Disease risk ratio between exposed and non-exposed
c. Risk difference between exposed and non-exposed
d. Communicability of a disease

EXPERIMENTAL EPIDEMIOLOGY

173. Double blinding means:
a. Blinding subject only
b. Blinding both interviewer and subject
c. Blinding patient
d. Blinding interviewer and analyzer

174. Full form of CONSORT is:
a. Common standard for reporting trial
b. Consolidated standard for reporting trial
c. Critical standards for reviewing trials
d. None of the above

175. All of the following are true regarding Meta-analysis except:
a. It is a statistical technique that combines result from several independent studies on a specific topic
b. It is not meant to identify risk factors
c. It seeks to increase statistical power by increasing the sample size
d. Validity does not depend on quality of systemic review

176. Which of the following is not a feature of Systematic Review? *(Recent Question 2015)*
a. Meta-analysis always done
b. Search for literature is compulsory using explicit search strategy
c. Criterion based critical appraisal of findings of the included studies
d. Research question always focused

177. Best study design for exposure and outcome association is?
a. RCT b. Cohort
c. Ecological d. Cross-sectional

178. The best evidence for making a clinical decision is obtained through which type of study? *(Recent Question 2015)*
a. Cohort b. Case-control
c. RCT d. Ecological study

179. Which of these is not true about randomization in a clinical trial?
a. Reduces confounding
b. Decreases selection bias
c. Ensure comparability of two groups
d. Increases external validity of the trial

180. Maximum Rate of Drug failure is seen in which phase of Clinical trial:
a. 1 b. 2
c. 3 d. 4

181. In clinical trials one can take care of the effects of un-known confounders by:
a. Matching cases and controls
b Randomization of study subjects
c. Proper selection of cases and controls
d. Properly measuring exposure and outcome

Ans.
162. b
163. d
164. c
165. d
166. c
167. a
168. b
169. c
170. b
171. a
172. c
173. b
174. b
175. d
176. a
177. a
178. c
179. d
180. b
181. b

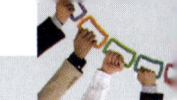

182. **True regarding double blinding placebo controlled clinical trial is:** *(Recent Question 2013)*
   a. Some patients are not treated
   b. The clinician does not know which treatment is given to the patient
   c. 50% of the patients do not know what drug they receive
   d. Everybody receives both the drug
183. **Evidence-based medicine is:**
   a. Clinical trials to prove adverse effects of drug
   b. Clinical trials to prove safety of drug
   c. Use of various research findings for taking decision about best patient care
   d. All the above
184. **Maximum tolerated dose of a new drug is evaluated in which phase of clinical trial:** *(Recent Question 2013)*
   a. 1   b. 2
   c. 3   d. 4

ASSOCIATION AND CAUSATION

185. **Which criteria is not included in causal relationship?**
   a. Temporal   b. Coherence
   c. Sensitivity   d. Specificity
186. **A study shows maternal mortality is higher in institutional deliveries than in home deliveries. This is an example of**
   a. Spurious association   b. Temporal association
   c. Indirect association   d. Multifactorial causation
187. **The strength of association between putative risk factor and a disease is measured by:**
   a. Attributable risk   b. Relative risk/odds ratio
   c. Magnitude of p value   d. Absolute risk
188. **Suspected cause preceding the observed effect is an example of:** *(Recent Question 2013)*
   a. Coherence
   b. Temporality
   c. Biological plausibility
   d. Specificity
189. **Study of time, place, person is known as:**
   a. Randomized controlled trial
   b. Descriptive epidemiology
   c. Analytical epidemiology
   d. Experimental epidemiology
190. **Study of time, place and person distribution of health related event is known as:**
   a. Descriptive epidemiology
   b. Experimental epidemiology
   c. Analytical epidemiology
   d. Clinical epidemiology
191. **All of the following statements concerning meta analysis are true except:**
   a. A study in which the units of analysis are populations or groups, rather than individuals
   b. Used to enhance the statistical power of research findings where number in studies available are too small
   c. Is applied by pooling results of small, randomized, controlled trials when no single trial has large enough numbers to reach a statistical significance
   d. It combines results from different studies to obtain a numerical estimate of overall effect
192. **All the following statements concerning meta-analysis are true EXCEPT.**
   a. It is a study in which the units of analysis are populations or groups of people, rather than individuals.
   b. It is used to enhance the statistical power of research findings where number in available studies are too small
   c. It is applied by pooling results of small, randomized, controlled trials when no single trial has large enough numbers to reach statistical significance
   d. It combines results from different studies to obtain a numerical estimate of an overall effect.

RCT

193. **Experimental epidemiology deals with:**
   a. Epidemics
   b. Intervention
   c. Screening of disease
   d. Early diagnose
194. **A major issue in conducting randomized control trial (RCT) is**
   a. Information bias
   b. Lead time bias
   c. Berksonian bias
   d. Ethics
195. **A new drug is to be evaluated for its therapeutic effect. The best study design will be**
   a. Cross-sectional survey
   b. Case-control design
   c. Natural experiment
   d. Randomized controlled trial
196. **A randomized, double-blinded trial finds that oral corticosteroids are superior to placebo in hastening the resolution of otitis media with effusion. Possible reasons why this study might have given a falsely positive result include**
   a. The sample size may have been too small
   b. The apparent effect might be a result of chance
   c. Non-stringent inclusion criteria may have led to inclusion of some subjects in the study who did not really have otitis media with effusion
   d. Any of above could be the possibility
197. **Crossover study is done when:**
   a. Control and case are the same
   b. Case and control are different
   c. Control is same and case is different
   d. Case is the same and control is different
198. **The most important part of a control trial is:**
   a. Selection of study group
   b. Selection of control group
   c. Randomization
   d. Analysis
199. **A total of 100 newly diagnosed patients with thyroid cancer are allocated to treatment with either surgical alone or surgical + radiation treatment. What is the study design?**
   a. Case series report
   b. Case control study
   c. Cross over trial design
   d. Randomized intervention clinical trial

Ans.

182. b
183. c
184. a
185. c
186. a
187. b
188. b
189. b
190. a
191. a
192. a
193. b
194. d
195. d
196. b
197. a
198. c
199. d

Most Recent Questions of 2019-18 are given at the end of MCQs

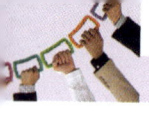

200. A recent multi-centric RCT study demonstrates the efficacy of new drug for lowering of cholesterol levels. As a public health consultant, which of the following would be disadvantage of making treatment guidelines based on large RCTs?
a. Cannot compare the standard drug and new drug in terms of efficacy
b. Cannot replicate the results from RCTs to the real world
c. The effect observed in the RCT may be biased of higher alpha errors
d. Cannot compare for the difference in cost of treatments with new or standard drugs

201. Community intervention study:
a. Cross sectional study b. Cohort study
c. Fields trial d. Co relational study

202. A public health physician wants to study the load of hypertension in community to design a health program for prevention of hypertension. Which is the most useful design for this case?
a. Cross sectional b. Case control series
c. Cohort d. RCT designs

203. Using cross sectional disease , we can determine the:
a. Temporal association between exposure and exposure and outcome
b. Odds ratio
c. Burden of disease in population
d. Incidence of the disease

204. Hypothesis are derived from:
a. Non-randomized clinical trials
b. Randomized clinical trials
c. Cohort study
d. Case series study

205. Longitudinal studies:
a. Are economical b. Are efficient
c. Single outcome
d. For identifying risk factors of disease

206. Association is best implicated by:
a. Case control study b. Prospective study
c. Cross sectional study d. Experimental epidemiology

207. Group of people worked at uranium mines for 5 years. Among them few developed cancer due to uranium exposure. Which type of association would it be?
a. Biological plausibility b. Coherence of association
c. Temporal association d. Spurious association

208. All of the following are true regarding RCT except
a. Double binding is done to remove investigator bias
b. Drop outs are excluded from the study
c. Randomizations is the heart of a control trial
d. 1st step in RCT is drawing up a protocol

209. A new drug was developed as thrombolytic therapy for acute MI. The large RCT showed a 30% decline in the mortality, within 3 weeks of MI due to MI or its complications compared to a standard drug ($p<0.01$ at 95% CI). Which of the following is our first concern as critical review of research
a. Was the trial blinded?
b. What happened to surviving patients in the next year?
c. What was the power of the study?
d. What percentage of patients in each group actually had a myocardial infarction?

210. In the context of epidemiology, the following are important criteria for making causal inferences except
a. Strength of association b. Consistency of association
c. Coherence of association d. Predictive value

211. Consider the following criteria of association:
1. Temporal association 2. Biological plausibility
3. Sensitivity of association 4. Specificity of association
The criteria which are necessary to show cause and effect between agent and disease would include:
a. 1 and 3 b. 2, 3, and 4
c. 1, 2, and 4 d. 1 and 2

212. The occurrence of two variable more often than would be expected by chance is called:
a. Correlation b. Confounder
c. Bias d. Association

213. Study unit of ecological study is:
a. Individual b. Society
c. Population d. Community

214. Incidence of disease is 4 per 1000 per year. The disease has duration of 2 years in the population. Calculate the 2 year prevalence rate of the disease
a. 4/1000
b. 2/1000
c. 6/1000
d. 8/1000

215. Risk among exposed by risk among non-exposed is defined to be?
a. Odds ratio
b. Attributable risk
c. Relative risk
d. None of the above

216. Which of the following studies is used to estimate the prevalence of risk factor or behavior?
a. Cross-sectional studies
b. Randomized controlled trials
c. Cohort studies
d. Quasi designs

Ans.
200. d
201. c
202. a
203. c
204. d
205. d
206. d
207. c
208. b
209. b
210. d
211. c
212. d
213. c
214. d
215. c
216. a

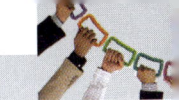

Most Recent Questions (2019–2018)

217. Incidence is defined as: *(PGI Nov 2018)*
a. Number of new cases in an area
b. Number of new cases and old cases in a time period from an area
c. Incidence depends on the duration
d. Incidence depends on morbidity
e. Incidence is a proportion

218. True regarding Odd-ratio: *(PGI May 2018)*
a. Calculated in case-control study
b. Calculated in cohort study
c. Closely related to relative risk
d. It is a cross-product ratio calculated by 2 × 2 table
e. Measure the strength of the association between risk factor and outcome

219. A randomized clinical trial was conducted to evaluate a novel drug vs placebo. Which of the following statistical results will give a positive information about the usefulness of the novel drug *(JIPMER Nov 2018)*
a. Odds ratio 4.7 ; with 95% CI 0.1 – 9.6
b. Odds ratio 0.5 ; with 95% CI 0.4 - 0.6
c. Odds ratio 1.7 ; with 95% CI 0.02 – 1
d. Odds ratio 2.7 ; with 95% CI 1.0 – 9.6

220. Study design of choice for testing circadian variation of fat content in expressed breast milk of mothers of preterm infant: *(AIIMS May 2019)*
a. Case control
b. Prospective cohort
c. Ecological Study
d. Cross sectional

221. Confounding is removed by all except *(AIIMS May 2019)*
a. Matching
b. Randomization
c. Restriction
d. Blinding

222. Cross product ratio is calculated in which study: *(Recent Question 2019)*
a. Case control study
b. Cohort study
c. Cross sectional study
d. Ecological study

223. Confounding factor is defined as: *(Recent Question 2019)*
a. Factor associated with both the exposure and the disease & is distributed unequally in study and control groups
b. Factor associated with exposure only & is distributed unequally in study and control groups.
c. Factor associated with both the exposure and the disease & is distributed equally in study and control groups
d. Factor associated with the disease & is distributed equally in study and control groups

Ans.
217. a, c
218. a, c, d, e
219. b
220. b
221. d
222. a
223. a

Answers with Explanations

1. Ans. (d) 0.8

Step 1: Lets reframe the table as per our understanding

	Experimental (Drug) group (E)	Control (Placebo) group (C)	Total
Adverse outcome (E)	10 (EE)	50 (CE)	
No adverse outcome (N)	(EN)	(CN)	
	1000	1000	

Step 2: Lets complete the table and find the missing values

	Experimental (Drug) group (E)	Control (Placebo) group (C)	Total
Adverse outcome (E)	10 (EE)	50 (CE)	60
No adverse outcome (N)	990 (EN)	950 (CN)	1940
	1000 (ET)	1000 (CT)	

Step 3:
EE = experimental group events
EN = experimental group no event
ET – experimental group total
CE = control group event
CN = control group no event
CT = control group total
EER = experimental group event rate
CER = control group event rate
ARR = absolute risk reduction
RRR = relative risk reduction
NNT = number needed to treat
Now we also know that,
EER = EE/ET = (10/1000)
CER = CE/CT = (50/1000)
ARR = CER – EER = (50/1000) – (10/1000) = 40/1000 = 0.04
RRR = (CER-EER) / CER = 0.04/0.05 = 0.8
NNT = 1/ARR = 1/0.04 = 25

2. Ans. (b) Incidence remains the same and prevalence increases

Ref: Park 24th edition, Pg. 66

Since the drug is prolonging survival and does not cure it; eventually the disease prevalence rate would increase as more people would be recorded as living with this disease. However, logically the number of cases of cancer per year would remain same. Hence we can comment, the drug will increase prevalence but the incidence is unaltered.

3. Ans. (a) Endemic, epidemic, sporadic

Ref: Park 24th edition, Pg. 98

4. Ans. (b) Relative risk

5. Ans. (a) Population

6. Ans. (a) 8/1000

Its simple, incidence is number of cases in a particular time. So as per the MCQ, the incidence is 4/1000 in year or 4 cases will be observed in a year. Hence in two years, 8 (4 + 4) cases will be observed in a 1000 population.

7. Ans. (a) Cohort

Ref: K. Park 24th ed. p 389-90

8. Ans. (b) 2.5

Ref: K. Park, 24th ed. p 94

	Lung cancer	No lung cancer	
Exposed	50	350	400
Nonexposed	5	95	100
			500

Risk in exposed = 50/400 = 0.125
Risk in nonexposed = 5/100 = 0.05
Relative risk = Risk in exposed/Risk in nonexposed
= 0.125/0.05 = 2.5

9. Ans. (b) 8.4

Ref: K. Park, 24th ed. p 78

	Diseased	Nondiseased
Exposed	33	53
Nonexposed	2	27
	35	82

Odds ratio = (a/c)/(b/d)
= a*d/b*c (cross product ratio)
= 33*27 / 53*2
= 8.4

10. Ans. (d) Secondary attack rate

Ref: K. Park, 24th ed. p 105

11. Ans. (a) Cohort study

Ref: K. Park, 24th ed. p 83

12. Ans. (a) Cohort

Ref: K. Park, 24th ed. p 85

13. Ans. (c) Berksonian bias

Ref: K. Park, 24th ed. p 78

14. Ans. (d) Odds ratio

Ref: K. Park, 24th ed. p 79

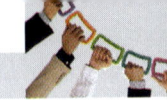

15. Ans. (d) Confirm epidemic whether it exists...

Ref: K. Park, 24th ed. p 141

16. Ans. (a) Population bed ratio

Ref: K. Park, 24th ed p 26

17. Ans. (b) P = I × D

Ref: K. Park, 24th ed. p 66

18. Ans. (a) We can measure prevalence

Ref: K. Park, 24th ed. p 74

19. Ans. (a) Relative risk

Ref: K. Park, 24th ed. p 80

20. Ans. (b) Case control study

Ref: K. Park, 24th ed. p 79

21. Ans. (a) Cohort study

Ref: K. Park, 23rd ed. p 371

22. Ans. (b) Cohort study

Ref: K. Park, 24th ed. p 39

Since cohort studies start from the risk factor and follow up is done to observe the occurrence of disease, hence there are a few direct advantages from a cohort study:

- We can estimate the natural course of disease
- We can estimate the temporal relationship of probable causative factor and disease
- We can estimate the incidence, risk ratios, attributable risk proportion

23. Ans. (c) Confounding factor

Ref: K. Park, 24th ed. p 77

Confounding factor:

- Is present in both the groups to be assessed (but in un-equal proportions)
- It is associated with both disease and the risk factor

24. Ans. (b) Associated with both exposure and outcome

Ref: K. Park, 23rd ed. p 72

25. Ans. (b) Attributable risk

Ref: K. Park, 24th ed. p 83

26. Ans. (b) (Incidence among exposed – Incidence among nonexposed)/Incidence among exposed

Ref: K. Park, 24th ed. p 83

27. Ans. (a) Incidence of disease among exposed /incidence of disease among unexposed

Ref: K. Park, 24th ed. p 83

INCIDENCE

28. Ans. (a) Incidence and prevalence

Inherent in the definition of epidemiology is measurement of frequency of the disease in terms of rates, ratio and proportions. Example include: incidence rate, prevalence rates, death rates. Given this MCQ – the option of attack rates is also a suitable option to be marked, but as we have a single option correct, we should go along with option A – both incidence and prevalence.

Note: Attack rates are also special incidence rates. They do not consider time as a variable and are used for short duration (usually communicable) diseases.

29. Ans. (b) Incidence

30. Ans. (c) Prevalence of the disease will increase

Note: Factors increasing the prevalence of disease are, long duration of disease, decrease the cure rate of disease, decrease the death rate due to the disease and decreasing the incidence of disease

31. Ans. (b) Prospective trial

(Also known as cohort studies or follow up study designs)

32. Ans. (b) Prevalence

Prevalence is best established by cross-sectional study

33. Ans. (d) 10

The number of persons under survey for 2 years for household with malaria are 500.

$$Incidence = \frac{\text{(number of new cases)}}{\text{(Total population at risk or surveyed)}}$$

$$Incidence = \frac{10}{500 \times 2 \text{ years}} = 10 \text{ cases per 1000 person years}$$

(In people living in household with previous cases of malaria)

34. Ans. (d) 312/614 x 100 = 50.8 per 100 population

The incidence of illness (as a percentage) is the

$$Incidence = \frac{\text{(number of cases who have symptomatic illness}}{\text{(Total population at risk or surveyed)}}$$

$$Incidence = \frac{312}{614} \times 100$$

35. Ans. (c) 207/519 × 100 = 39.9%

Percentage of subclinical infections

$$= \frac{\text{(Number of subclinical cases)}}{\text{[Total number of infected individuals (clincal+subclinical)]}}$$

$$\text{Percentage of subclinical infections} = \frac{207}{519} \times 100 = 39.9\%$$

36. Ans. (d) 60 years ago

From the data in the table, it is observed that the age group 0-59 years shows a uniform percentage of infection as 90%. While in age group > 60 years, it is only 10%.

The low attack rate in this age group may be explainable on basis of development of immunity in this age group probably due to a mass prior exposure at least 60 years prior to the survey.

37. Ans. (d) 0.5%

Prevalence: It is the total number of cases present (both old and new) in an area in a population

In the MCQ, the total cases found in the survey = 10

Population under survey = 2000

$$Prevalence = \frac{\text{Total cases}}{\text{Population under survey}} \times 100 = 0.5\%$$

[Note: controversial point: For technical and practical reasons, the prevalence is expressed as a percentage (proportion) and incidence is expressed as rate per 1000 population per unit time]

38. Ans. (b) Prevalence

39. Ans. (d) Prevalence

Cross-sectional studies allow one to estimate the prevalence (the number of existing cases at one point in time divided by the population at risk) but not incidence (number of new cases occurring over a period of time divided by the population at risk and the period of time at risk).

The prevalence of oral lesions in male is higher than in females.

The other options in the MCQ as incidence rates can be calculated in follow up studies and not a cross sectional study as is in the MCQ.

Similarly, Odds ratios are calculated in case control studies.

Cross sectional studies help estimate the risk factors and asses the prevalence of a disease.

40. Ans. (c) Cross-sectional study

Cross-sectional studies, known as "prevalence study:' is the simplest form of an observational study. It is based on a single examination of a cross-section of population at one point in time and more useful for chronic disease.

41. Ans. (b) Confirms the etiology of disease

The etiology of the disease cannot be estimated by a cross sectional study.

The causation of disease (or etiology) may be best measured by cohort (follow up) studies.

Cross-sectional study – salient features:

- Estimate for the prevalence of the disease
- Evaluation for the risk factors for the disease
- Asses the epidemiological determinants as pattern of disease – host factors, age groups and other related variables maybe assessed.

42. Ans. (c) Describe the balance between incidence, mortality and recovery

43. Ans. (b) Population at risk

Ref: K. Park, 24th ed p65

Incidence is "*Number of new cases of a disease or new spells/ episodes of sickness occurring in a defined population during a specified period of time*".

$$\text{Incidence rate} = \frac{\text{Number of new cases of specific disease during a given time period}}{\text{Population at risk during that period}}$$

44. Ans. (d) 20

Ref: K. Park, 24th ed p65

$$\text{Incidence rate} = \frac{90}{4500} \times 1000 = 20 \text{ per } 1000$$

45. Ans. (a) Not affected by duration

Ref: K. Park, 24th ed. p 66

46. Ans. (b) 10 per 1000

Ref: K. Park, 24th ed. p 105

New cases = 300

Population = 30,000

Incidence = 300/30,000 = 10 per thousand

47. Ans. (a) Cohort study

Ref: K. Park, 24th ed. p 83

Incidence is concerned with the occurrence of new cases of a disease among susceptible in a population over a period of time. Hence, it is best studied by prospective studies – E.g. Cohort Study

48. Ans. (d) Useful to find the magnitude of the disease problem in the community

Ref: K. Park, 24th ed. p 65

Incidence[Q] Its **use is more often** restricted to acute conditions

- To take action to control disease
- To study etiology, pathogenesis, distribution of disease, efficacy of preventive and therapeutic measures
- To formulate and test etiological hypotheses.

Also Know......................

- **Prevalence** gives an estimate of magnitude of health/ disease problem in the community and helps identify high-risk population.

49. Ans. (b) Incidence

Ref: K. Park, 24th ed. p 66

50. Ans. (a) Incidence rate falls if a new drug...

Ref: K. Park, 24th ed. p 65

Incidence[Q] is absolute risk of developing disease

Prevalence = Incidence × Duration

If a new drug is effective in reducing deaths from the disease but does not cure the disease, it will result in increase in the duration of disease and prevalence; however the incidence will remain the same

Effective prevention program is essential for reducing incidence

51. Ans. (b) Prospective studies

Ref: K. Park, 24th ed. p 84

52. Ans. (a) 133 per 10,00,000 population

Ref: K. Park, 24th ed. p 65

Here, Number of new cases of TB during a given time period (1st Jan 2019 to 30th June 2019)= 22

Population at risk= 165000

So, Incidence rate = (22/165000) × 10, 00,000 = 133 per 10,00,000 population

Also Know........................

- An increase in new cases denotes increase in Incidence. Suspect cases are not considered

PREVALENCE

53. Ans. (b) Prevalence will increase

Ref: K. Park, 24th ed. p 66

Prevalence = Incidence × Duration

Here, the intervention decreases the mortality but does not cure the disease; hence it will result in increase in the duration of disease and consequently increase in Prevalence

Also Know........................

Factors leading to rise in prevalence

- Immigration (moving in) of diseased people
- Emmigration (moving out) of healthy people
- Low cure rates (Death is averted)
- Low fatality and chronic diseases (long duration)
- Prevention program- Decrease in occurrence of new cases

54. Ans. (a) It is highly fatal in females

Ref: K. Park, 24th ed. p 66

Prevalence is same in male and female and Incidence(Females) = 3 × Incidence (Male)

Hence, Incidence (Female) × Duration (Female) = Incidence (Male) × Duration (Male) or

3 × Incidence (Male) × Duration (Female) = Incidence (Male) × Duration (Male)

Duration (Female)= 1/3 Duration (Male)

That implies, disease has high fatality or better cure in females

55. Ans. (d) Measures all cases

Ref: K. Park, 24th ed. p 66

Prevalence measures all current cases (old and new) in a given population

Uses of Prevalence

- Estimate magnitude of health/disease problem in the community and identify potential high-risk populations.
- Administrative and planning purposes, e.g., hospital beds, manpower needs, rehabilitation facilities, etc.

56. Ans. (c) Point prevalence rate

Ref: K. Park, 24th ed. p 66

57. Ans. (c) 13%

Ref: K. Park, 24th ed. p 66

$$\text{Prevalence} = \frac{\text{All current cases (Old + New) at any given point or period of time}}{\text{Estimated population at that point or period of time}} \times 100$$

$$= \frac{650}{5000} \times 100 = 13\%$$

58. Ans. (c) Proportion

Ref: K. Park,-59, 23rd ed. p 61 Epidemiology, Leon Gordis, 4th ed.p-43

Prevalence is the number of all cases (old + new) of a disease or health condition in a defined geographic area at a given point or period of time amongst the population of the defined geographic area at that point or period of time.

Or

The proportion of the population affected by the disease at any point or period of time.

- Since, Numerator is a part of the denominator, hence it is a proportion

Also Know........................

- Prevalence is measured by cross sectional study[Q].

59. Ans. (a) 240

Ref: K. Park, 24th ed. p 66

Total population = 10,00,000, Under 16 population = 30% of 10 lacks = 30/100* 10,00000 = 3,00,000

The Prevalence of blindness in Under 16 population = 0.8/1000

So, Number of blind in Under 16 population = 0.8/1000*300000 = 240

MORATLITY AND MORBIDITY RATES

60. Ans. (b) To allow comparison of both sex

Ref: K. Park, 24th ed. p 63

"Age adjusted death rate" removes confounding effect of different age structures in population and helps compare mortality. Adjustment can be made for age, sex, race, parity, etc.

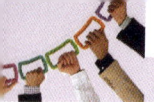

61. Ans. (b) Compare injuries/accidents between different sexes

Ref: K Park 24th ed. p 62

Advantages of Specific Death Rate

- Helps identify groups "at risk" for preventive action
- Compare different causes within the same population
- Compare injuries/accidents/death between different sub groups of the population

62. Ans. (c) Proportion

Ref: K. Park, 24th ed. p 63

Proportional mortality rate is number of deaths due to a particular cause (or in a specific group) per 1000 total deaths.
- It reflects the relative importance of a specific disease or disease group.

Also Know......................

- It is a measure of burden of disease

63. Ans. (c) Total death in that year

Ref: K Park 24th ed. p 63

64. Ans. (c) Age distribution

Ref: K. Park, 24th ed. p 63

- Age adjustment or standardization removes the confounding effect of different age structures
- Standardization can be done in 2 ways – direct and indirect

Direct Standardization

- Age specific rate death rate of the population whose crude death rate is to be adjusted/standardized is applied to the standard population (Composition -numbers in each age and sex group is known).
- Feasible only if the actual age specific rates of the population are available.

Indirect Standardization or SMR

- It is ratio of the total number of death in the study group to number of expected death in the study group, had it experienced the death rates of a standard population.

$$SMR = \frac{\text{Observed death}}{\text{Expected death}} \times 100$$

SMR > 100 → Study group has higher mortality risk than that of the standard population.

SMR < 100 → Study group has lower mortality risk than the standard population.

- **Advantage:** Permits adjustment for age and other factors where age specific rates are not available.

Also Know......................

- Survival analysis, Life table, Regression and Multivariate analysis are other methods of indirect standardization

DESCRIPTIVE EPIDEMIOLOGY

65. Ans. (a) Local distributions

Ref: K Park, 24th ed. p 72

Spot maps display geographical locations of cases and rates (area with high/low frequency)
- **Spot map** were used by John Snow to display occurrence of cholera relative to the famous pump in Broad street
- Clustering of cases on a spot map suggest a common infection source or risk factor shared by all the cases.
- It helps localizing the source of infection

Rate Maps

- Geographical areas are shaded as per the differences in values (prevalence, incidence or mortality)
- Areas with the highest rates are shaded with darkest shades or brightest colors

66. Ans. (a) Description studies

Ref: K. Park, 24th ed. p 71

Descriptive studies *contribute to research by –*
- *Describing variations in disease occurrence by time, place and person*
- *Provide clue to disease etiology and help in the formulation of etiological hypothesis.*
- *Provide data on magnitude of disease, types of disease problems in the community, morbidity/mortality rates and ratios*
- *Provide background data for planning, organizing and evaluating preventive and curative services*
- **Descriptive studies** *are the 1st phase of an epidemiological investigation*

67. Ans. (c) Natural experiment study

Ref: K. Park, 24th ed. p 91

Natural experiment study: Natural circumstances mimic an experiment.

Examples: Migrant study, Natural calamities (i.e. Famine, Earthquake), Accidents, Atomic bombing

ANALYTICAL EPIDEMIOLOGY

68. Ans. (c) RCT

Ref: K. Park, 24th ed. p 67

69. Ans. (d) Prevalence study

Ref: K. Park, 24th ed. p 74

Cross-sectional Study or Prevalence Study

- Unit of study is the individual
- It is based on a single examination of a cross-section of population at one point in time. There is no follow up
- More useful for chronic diseases.
- Informs about distribution of disease in a population.
- Yields no information on incidence, natural history of disease, time sequence or etiology

Longitudinal study involves repeated observations in the same population, over a period of time by follow-up examination.

- **Advantage:** Yields natural history of disease, Incidence rate and helps identify risk factors of disease.[Q]
- **Disadvantage:** Difficult to organize and Time/Resource consuming

70. Ans. (a) Ecological study

Ref: K. Park, 24th ed. p 67

Ecological study or "*Correlational study*".

- Unit of study is population or group of people.
- It provides an indirect evidence or clue, which can be further elaborated

Example: Increase in sale of antiarrhythmic drug and an increase in deaths due to asthma.

71. Ans. (c) Ecological study

Ref: K. Park, 23rd ed. p 62

72. Ans. (b) Cross-sectional study

Ref: K. Park, 24th ed. p 74

73. Ans. (b) Cross-sectional study

Ref: K. Park, 24th ed. p 74

74. Ans. (b) Retrospective study; (c) Cross-sectional study

Ref: K. Park, 24th ed. p 74, 81

75. Ans. (c) Cross-sectional

Ref: K. Park, 24th ed. p 74

Cross-sectional/Prevalence study involves no follow up, hence is Least time consuming

CASE CONTROL STUDY

76. Ans. (b) Case control study

77. Ans. (b) Case control study

78. Ans. (b) Case control study

79. Ans. (c) Case control study

80. Ans. (d) Odds ratio

Odds ratio is closely related to relative risk. The derivation of odds ratio is based on three assumptions:

- The disease being investigated must be relatively rare.
- The cases must be representative of those with the disease.
- The control must be representative of those without the disease.

81. Ans. (c) Relative risk can be calculated

Advantages of case control studies:

- Relatively easy to carry out and inexpensive
- Requires comparatively few subjects.
- Particularly suitable to investigate *rare* diseases or diseases about which little is known.
- Several different etiological factors may be assessed at a single time
- Risk factors can be identified and rational prevention and control programs can be established
- *Odds ratio (OR)* can be derived from a case control study. Odds ratio is a measure of the strength of the *association* between risk factor and outcome.
- Ethical issues and problems related to loss to follow up (attrition) is less

Disadvantages:

- Temporality (causation factor assessment) may not be established
- May have a recall bias

82. Ans. (b) Case control

Case control study is also known as retrospective studies. This method has three distinct features.

- Both exposure and outcome (disease) have occurred before the start of the study.
- The study proceeds backwards from effect to cause.
- It uses a control or comparison group to support or refute an inference.

83. Ans. (b) Case control

In hospital settings, the case control studies maybe easy to conduct as the cases are already there in the hospital as patients. The controls can either be selected from the healthy accompanying individuals or from other non-related departments.

Extra edge: Sometimes the cases maybe almost equal to the controls (in selected diseases) from the case control study done in a single hospital, which maybe catering to a specific type of disease. This may lead to a special bias known as Berksonian bias.

84. Ans. (a) Long duration

Case control or retrospective study

- Case control study is relatively inexpensive.
- Is suited for rare diseases
- It gives only odds ratio
- Incidence, prevalence and attributable risk can not be calculated
- For incidence, cohort study, and for prevalence, cross-sectional study is required.

85. Ans. (c) Case control study

- Odds ratio is calculated from *case control study*. It is a measure of the *strength of the association* between the risk factor and outcome.
- Relative risk can be calculated only from a *cohort study*.

86. Ans. (a) Case control

Cross-sectional studies

- Observational study or *prevalence* study

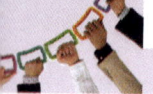

- Useful for *chronic* disease when interest is distribution of disease
- Less expensive/less time required in establishing relationship.

Longitudinal studies

- Useful to study the *natural history* of disease and its *future* outcome.
- Identifies the *risk factors* of disease
- Finds out the incidence of disease but *more expensive and more time consuming.*

87. Ans. (c) Incidence can be calculated

Case control studies, often called 'retrospective studies' are a common first approach to test a hypothesis.

Case-control study or retrospective study has 3 features:

- Both exposure and outcome have occurred before the start of study.
- The study proceeds backwards from effect to cause, (so called retrospective study)
- It uses a control group to come to inference.
- Matching of cases and controls to eliminate confounding factors is done in this study.
- Odds ratio can be calculated but not incidence

88. Ans. (a) Used rare disease

Advantages of case control studies:

- Easy and Rapid.
- Inexpensive
- Requires few subjects
- Used for Rare diseases
- No risk to subjects
- Different etiological factors can be studied.
- Risk factors can be identified.
- No attrition problems ethical problems

Disadvantages of case - control studies

- Bias problems (memory or recall bias)
- Difficulties in selection.
- Incidence can't be measured
- Not suited for evaluation of therapy.
- No difference between causes and associated factors.

89. Ans. (a) Case series report

It cannot be considered as a case control study, as 500 cases of thyroid cancer patients are assessed for the radiation exposure. There is no control group for comparison of the results.

90. Ans. (a) Case control study

Ref: K. Park, 24th ed. p 67

91. Ans. (d) Can distinguish causes and associated factors

Ref: K. Park, 24th ed. p 79

Advantages of Case Control Study

- It is rapid and inexpensive (compared with cohort studies)
- It requires fewer subjects and is relatively easy to do
- It is suitable to investigate rare diseases or diseases about which little is known.
- There is no risk to subjects and no attrition problem.
- Allows the study of several different etiological factors
- Multiple risk factors can be identified. (Prevention and Control program can be framed)
- Minimal ethical problems
- It yields exposure rate among cases and controls, Odds ratio and Risk ratio

Disadvantages of Case Control Study

- Limited to one outcome variable
- Potential bias from selection of cases and controls, measuring exposure (Relies on recall or past records, accuracy of which is uncertain and also difficult to validate; sometimes impossible)
- Does not establish sequence of events
- Potential survivor bias
- Does not yield absolute risk (Incidence cannot be measured)
- Does not distinguish between cause and associated factors
- Not suited for evaluation of therapy or prophylaxis of disease

92. Ans. (a) Odds ratio

Ref: K. Park, 24th ed. p 78

93. Ans. (c) Attributable risk cannot be calculated

Ref: K. Park, 24th ed. p 79

Case control study is the 1st approach towards testing a causal hypothesis. It has 3 distinct features:

- Both exposure and outcome (disease) have occurred before the start of the study
- Study proceeds backwards from **effect to cause.**
- A control group is used to support or refute an inference.

Also Know........................

- Cohort study yields Attributable risk, incidence risk and Relative risk (AIR)

94. Ans. (a) Useful for rare disease

Ref: K. Park, 24th ed. p 79

95. Ans. (a) Case control

Ref: K. Park, 24th ed. p 79

Case control study commences from "effect to cause". Exposure and Outcome have occurred before start of investigation hence it yields quick results.

Cohort study and RCT involve follow up of the exposed population for a long period of time until outcome start to appear.

Cross-sectional study tells us about the frequency and distribution of disease/risk factors/health-related event in a defined population at a particular point/period in time

96. Ans. (a) Useful for study of rare disease; (d) Study multiple potential risk factors of a disease

Ref: K. Park, 24th ed. p 79

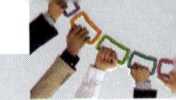

97. Ans. (a) Used for rare disease

Ref: K. Park, 24th ed. p 79

98. Ans. (b) Relative risk can be calculated

Ref: K. Park, 24th ed. p 79

99. Ans. (b) Blinding

Ref: K. Park, 24th ed. p 88

Also Know.......................

- **Blinding** technique eliminates **Bias** (systematic error in the determination of the association between exposure and disease)

100. Ans. (c) Confounding factor

Ref: K. Park, 24th ed. p 77

Confounding factor is one that is:
- Associated with both exposure and disease
- Distributed unequally in study and control groups.
- Itself, independently a "risk factor" for the disease

101. Ans. (d) All of the above

Ref: K. Park, 24th ed. p 77

102. Ans. (b) 6

Ref: K. Park, 24th ed. p 78

Here, on making a 2 × 2 contingency table, we get

Suspected or risk factors	Cases (Disease present)	Control (Disease absent)
Smokers	*30 (a)*	*10 (b)*
Non smokers	*20 (c)*	*40 (d)*
Total	*50*	*50*

$$\text{Odds ratio} = \frac{a \times d}{b \times c} = \frac{30 \times 40}{20 \times 10} = 6$$

COHORT STUDY

103. Ans. (c) Cohort (Prospective)

This is a typical example of a prospective cohort study as the study subjects are categorized as smokers or non-smokers in the prenatal period. The outcome of pregnancy is followed up and groups are compared.

104. Ans. (a) Population attributable risk

105. Ans. (b) Incidence among exposed/incidence among non exposed

Relative risk is the ratio of the incidence of the disease or death among exposed and the incidence among non-exposed. It is direct measure of the strength of the association/between suspected cause and effect. It is calculated by:

$$\text{Relative risk} = \frac{\text{Incidence of disease (or death) among exposed}}{\text{Incidence of disease (or death) among non exposed}}$$

106. Ans. (c) Relative risk

107. Ans. (b) Attributable risk

108. Ans. (a) 0%

Attributable risk indicates association between risk factor and disease. Attributable risk is often expressed as a percent. It is expressed as

Attributable risk

$$= \frac{\text{Incidence in exposed} - \text{incidence in nonexposed}}{\text{Incidence in exposed}} \times 100$$

Here,

Incidence in exposed = 20/2000 = 0.01

Incidence in non-exposed = 40/4000 = 0.01

$$\text{so, } \textit{attributable risk} = \frac{0}{0.01} \times 100 = 0$$

109. Ans. (d) All of the above

Cohort study is a type of analytical study which is usually done to obtain additional evidence to refute or support the existence of an association between suspected cause and disease. Cohort is defined as a group of people who share common characteristic or experience within a defined time period. The features of cohort studies are as under:
- Cohorts are identified prior to the appearance of disease under investigation.
- Study groups are observed over a period of time to determine the frequency of disease among them.
- Proceeds from cause to effect.

110. Ans. (d) A cohort study is more appropriate when the disease or exposure under investigation is rare in comparison with case— control study

111. Ans. (b) Relative risk

112. Ans. (b) Useful for rare diseases

Cohort study: Proceeds from "cause to effect".
- Starts with people exposed to risk factor or suspected cause
- Tests whether disease occurs more frequently in those exposed, than in those not similarly exposed.
- Reserved for testing of precisely formulated hypothesis.
- Involves larger number of subjects.
- Long follow-up period often needed, involving delayed results; Inappropriate when the disease or exposure under investigation is rare.

113. Ans. (d) Cohort studies are necessary to estimate the prevalence of disease

- In cohort studies, a group of subjects is defined on the basis of certain baseline characteristics and followed over time for the development of the disease (or other outcome) under study.

- Incidence, relative risk, attributable is calculated from cohort studies
- If a suitable cohort can be identified from past records, a retrospective cohort study is possible.
- Prevalence can be estimated from cross-sectional studies and cohort studies are not required for prevalence estimation

114. Ans. (a) Prospective cohort study

115. Ans. (a) Relative risk

Relative risk (RR) is the ratio of the incidence of the disease (or death) among exposed and the incidence among nonexposed.

- Some authors use the term "risk ratio" to refer to relative risk

116. Ans. (c) No association

117. Ans. (b) Cohort study

118. Ans. (d) All

Ref: K. Park, 24th ed. p 81

Types of Cohort Study

- **Prospective/concurrent:** Exposure status is ascertained at beginning of study and the cohort is followed up into future.
- **Retrospective/historical:** Exposure is ascertained from past records and outcome is ascertained at the beginning of study
- **Combined retrospective and prospective:** Exposure is ascertained from past records and follow-up and measurement of outcome continue into the future

119. Ans. (a) Cohort study

Ref: K. Park, 24th ed. p 85

Framingham Heart Study (A Cohort Study)

- It started in 1948 in Framingham (Massachusetts). A sample of 5,127 men and women, 30-62 years of age and free of cardiovascular disease at start of study were enrolled.
- Many "exposures" were defined, including smoking, obesity, elevated blood pressure, elevated cholesterol levels, low levels of physical activity, and other factors.
- The population was observed over time to determine which individuals developed or already had the "exposure(s)" of interest and, later on to determine which ones developed the cardiovascular outcome(s) of interest.
- New coronary events were identified by examining the study population every 2 years and by daily surveillance of hospitalizations at the only hospital in Framingham.

120. Ans. (d) Starts with the disease

Ref: K. Park, 24th ed. p 84

Advantages of Cohort Study

- Multiple health effects (outcome) related to single exposure can be studied
- Temporal association (Exposure must precede outcome) is established
- Yields RR, AR, PAR and Incidence
- Minimal potential for selection bias–At time of measurement of exposure outcomes are not known
- Dose-response ratios can also be calculated
- Effect of rare exposure can be studied

Disadvantages of Cohort Study

- Long follow up (Problem may have no relevance by time study is complete)
- Involves a very large number of subjects
- Expensive
- Restricted to study of limited number of exposures measured at start of study.
- Administrative problems - loss of experienced staff, loss of funding and extensive record keeping
- Attrition (loss to follow up) - migration, loss of interest in study or refusal to provide required information
- Selection of comparison groups is a limiting factor
- There may be changes in the standard methods or diagnostic criteria of disease over prolonged follow-up.
- Study itself may alter people's behavior.
- Ethical problems

Indication for Cohort Study

- Good evidence of an association between exposure and disease
- Exposure is rare
- Attrition of study population can be minimized (cohort is stable, cooperative and accessible)
- Ample funds are available
- Interval between exposure and development of disease is short
- Reliable past records/other data sources (retrospective study)

121. Ans. (a) Cohort study

Ref: K. Park, 24th ed. p 84

122. Ans. (c) Less expensive

Ref: K. Park, 24th ed. p 80

123. Ans. (c) Suitable to study rare diseases

Ref: K. Park, 24th ed. p 80

Suitable study design for rare diseases is cross sectional study and rare exposure is Cohort study

124. Ans. (b) Cohort study

Ref: K. Park, 24th ed. p 84

The study proceeds from cause to effect in a cohort of 1200 adults – Hence a Cohort Study

125. Ans. (d) Associated with antecedent causation

Ref: K. Park, 24th ed. p 84

Cohort Study

- *Commences from "**cause to effect**". Cohorts are identified prior to appearance of disease (or Outcome) being studied*
- *It tests whether disease occurs more frequently in those exposed, than in those not similarly exposed*
- *Starts in present and continues into future.*

- *Used to test precisely formulated hypothesis (with sufficient evidence)*

126. Ans. (b) Prospective cohort

Ref: K. Park, 24th ed. p 81

*The study commenced from "**Cause**" i.e. exposure to smoking towards "**Effect**" i.e. incidence of low birth weight.*
Repeated follow up were done
Hence, it is a prospective cohort study

127. Ans. (a) Longitudinal studies

Ref: K. Park, 24th ed. p 75

***Longitudinal study** involves repeated observations in the same **population**, over a period of time by means of follow-up examination.*
- *Advantage: Used to study natural history of disease, Incidence rate and Identifying risk factors of disease.*[Q]
- *Disadvantage: Difficult to organize and time consuming*

128. Ans. (b) Cohort

Ref: K. Park, 24th ed. p 39

Natural history of disease[Q] is the progression of a disease over time from the prepathogenesis phase (earliest phase) to its termination as recovery, disability or death *in absence of any treatment or prevention*
- Natural history of diseases can be best studied using a cohort study[Q].

129. Ans. (c) Exclude patient diagnosed with inflammatory bowel disease

Ref: K. Park, 24th ed. p 81

Cohort study - Cohorts are identified prior to appearance of disease (or Outcome) being studied

130. Ans. (a) Case control study

Ref: K. Park, 24th ed. p 76

BIAS

131. Ans. (c) Bias

132. Ans. (a) Different rate of admission to the hospital

133. Ans. (c) Exposure is usually determined prior to disease occurrence

134. Ans. (a) Case control study

135. Ans. (d) Different rates of admission in hospital

Berksonian bias is a special example of bias. It is named after Dr. Joseph Berkson, who recognized this problem. The bias arises because of the different rates of admission to hospitals for people with different diseases (hospital cases and controls).

136. Ans. (c) Both observer and observed group is blind

Single blind trial	The participant is not aware whether he belongs to the study group or control groups
Double blind trial	Neither the doctor nor the participant is aware of the group allocation and the treatment received.
Triple blind trial	The subject, investigator and the person analyzing the data are all 'blind'

137. Ans. (b) Avoid observer bias and sampling variation

138. Ans. (b) Avoid observer and subject bias

Blinding: In order to reduce bias, "blinding" is adopted, which will ensure that the outcome is assessed objectively. Blinding is done in three ways.
- Single blind trial: Participant is not aware whether he belongs to the study or control group.
- Double blind trial: Neither the doctor nor the participant is aware of the group allocation and the treatment received. Most frequently used method.
- Triple blind trial: The participant, the investigator, and the person analyzing the data are all "blind'

139. Ans. (c) Experimental studies

Double blinding is a procedure usually adopted in interventional studies where different interventions (treatment) are given to different groups. To decrease the effect of an unintentional subject bias while receiving two different treatments for same disease, blinding is done. The best answer here would be option C, experimental study designs

Note: Blinding is done to remove subject and observer bias. It may be done in selected case control studies or cohort studies also.

In the above MCQ, the single best answer is interventional studies

140. Ans. (b) Selection bias

Randomization is a statistical procedure by which the participants are allocated into different groups. It allows comparability and eliminate **subject bias**. The observer or investigator does not determine the group for allocation of study participants, rather it is based on robust randomization methods for a **known and equal chance of allocation** into the groups

141. Ans. (b) Selection bias

142. Ans. (b) Matching

Blinding is a procedure to eliminate subject or observer bias

143. Ans. (b) Blinding

144. Ans. (c) Confounding factor

Matching is defined as the process by which controls are selected in such a way that they are similar to cases with regard to certain relevant selected variables, which are known to influence the outcome of disease and which, if not adequately matched for comparability, could distort or confound the results.

A confounding factor is defined as one, which is, associated both with exposure and disease, and is distributed unequally in study and control groups.

145. Ans. (a) Confounding factor

A confounding factor is the one which is associated both with exposure and disease, and is distributed unequally in study and control groups e.g., smoking is a confounding factor while studying etiological role of alcohol in esophageal cancer because smoking is associated with alcoholism and is also an independent risk factor for esophageal cancer. Thus, the role of alcohol consumption in causing esophageal cancer can be determined only if influence of smoking is neutralized by having matched controls in the study.

146. Ans. (b) A case-control study with a small number of cases

Matching is a technique used in the design of the study to control for <u>confounding</u>. Subjects enrolled in a study are matched for age, gender, smoking, or any variable that is not being analyzed.

In case control studies, it is very important to match the cases and control to eliminate the chances of confounding.

Confounders are variable which are associated with both disease and risk factor and if unequally distributed may affect the outcome of the research. Hence, it is important to match the cases and control for the probable confounding variables in the study.

Now these confounding variables can only be matched if the study sample size is somewhat smaller and manageable.

On the other hand, Randomization is used in clinical trials to control <u>confounding</u>

Matching is not done in descriptive studies or the cross-sectional studies.

147. (b) It is distributed equally in study and control groups

"Confounding factor" is associated both with exposure and disease, and is distributed unequally in study and control groups.

Confounding factors have the following characteristics:

- Associated with both disease and the risk factor
- Distributed unequally among the two groups
- It itself is a risk factor for causing the disease

148. Ans. (b) Selection bias

Randomization is a statistical procedure by which the participants are allocated into groups. The investigator does not have control over allocation to either the treatment group or the placebo group. This specifically removes 'selection bias'.

149. Ans. (b) Randomization

150. Ans. (d) Selection of a representative study...

Ref: K. Park, 24th ed. p 78

Selection bias occurs when cases and controls in a study are not representative of cases and controls in population.

- *It can be best* eliminated by prevention (i.e. Selection of a representative study group)

Also Know........................

Recall bias -Bias resulting from differential ability of study subjects to recall previous exposure. (People with disease recall past events in more detail than those without disease) occurs in retrospective study[Q] (Case control study)
Lead time bias is apparent increase in survival of patients whose disease is detected by screening.

Also Know........................

Interviewers bias – Interviewer questions 'cases' in more detail compared to 'controls' regarding history of exposure to suspect casual factor.
Interviewer knows the hypothesis and also who the cases are. It can be eliminated by equal interview time for both cases and controls.[Q] and by double blinding.[Q]

151. Ans. (a) Confounding factor

Ref: K. Park, 24th ed. p 77

Confounding factor is one that is:

- Associated with both exposure and disease
- Distributed unequally in study and control groups.
- It is itself, independently a "risk factor" for the disease

152. Ans. (a) Blinding

Ref: K. Park, 24th ed. p 77

Confounding factor can be eliminated by:

- **Matching** (Group or By pairs)- Controls and Cases are similar with regard to certain selected variables (e.g. age), known to influence outcome of disease.
- **Stratification:** Confounders are equally distributed amongst case and control group
- **Randomization:** It is a statistical procedure for allocation of participants to "study" and "control" groups, to receive or not to receive a preventive or therapeutic intervention. It eliminates "bias" and allows for comparability.
- **Multivariate analysis** is used to estimate the strength of the associations while controlling for several confounding variables simultaneously. (Basic epidemiology, 2nd ed., Bonita and Beagle hole p-57)

153. Ans. (d) Selection bias

Ref: K. Park, 24th ed. p 78

154. Ans. (b) Effect modifier

Ref: Encyclopedia of Epidemiologic Methods, Mitchell H Gail, Jacques Benichou. P-336

Effect modifier is a variable that differentially (positively and negatively) modifies the observed effect of a risk factor on disease status.

- The magnitude of the effect of an exposure on the outcome

will vary according to the presence of a third factor (Effect Modifier)

- Different groups have different risk estimates when effect modification is present
- For effect modification true relation must be there between outcome (disease) and independent variable (risk factor) E.g. Malnutrition increases the impact of an exposure (i.e. high bilirubin) on an outcome (i.e. brain damage).

Effect Modifier Needs to be Studied to

- Define high-risk subgroups for preventive actions,
- Increase precision of effect estimation by taking into account groups that may be affected differently,
- Increase the ability to compare across studies that have different proportions of effect-modifying groups, and
- Aid in developing a causal hypotheses for the disease

155. Ans. (a) Selection bias

Ref: K. Park, 24th ed. p 78

Berksonian Bias

- *Occurs in studies on hospitalized patients*
- *Results due to different rates of admission to hospitals for people having different diseases*
- *Cases' (i.e. those who have a risk factor or disease) are more frequently admitted to a hospital in comparison to either 'cases' (without the risk factor or disease) and 'control'.*
- *Avoided by choosing controls from a population of healthy subjects or from a variety of disease condition*

156. Ans. (c) Berksonian Bias

Ref: K. Park, 24th ed. p 78

Selection bias occurs during recruitment when cases and controls are selected in such a way that they are not representative of cases and controls in population.

- *It can be best* eliminated by prevention (i.e. Selection of a representative study group)

157. Ans. (c) Recruitment

Ref: K. Park, 24th ed. p 78

158. Ans. (c) Different rates of admission to hospital due to different disease

Ref: K. Park, 24th ed. p 78

159. Ans. (a) Randomization

Ref: K. Park, 24th ed. p 87

Randomization ensures that researcher has no control on allocation of participants to either study or control group, thus eliminates "selection bias"

160. Ans. (d) Multivariate analysis

Ref: K. Park, 24th ed. p 87

Also Know........................

- Bias refers to any systematic error in determination of association between exposure and disease.

Bias arises due to noncomparability between study and control groups. It leads to false conclusions (increase or decrease in Relative Risk)

Techniques to Eliminate Bias

- **Matching:**
  - Matching is ideal for removing confounding bias
  - Types of matching→ Group matching, Pair matching.
- **Blinding** eliminates
  - Observer bias (i.e. Investigator measuring a outcome may be influenced if he knows beforehand the particular procedure or therapy to which the patient has been subjected)
  - Bias in evaluation (Investigator may subconsciously give a favorable report to outcome of the trial).
- **Randomization**
  - It ensures that every individual has an equal chance of being allocated into either group
  - Multivariate analysis may be used for treatment for unknown confounders.

161. Ans. (b) Cohort study

Ref: Internet- Wikipedia

Hawthorne effect: *Study subjects improve or modify an aspect of their behavior being measured simply in response to the fact that they are being studied and not in response to any particular experimental manipulation.*

RR/AR/PAR OR MEASURES OF EFFECT

162. Ans. (b) Attributable risk

Ref: K. Park, 24th ed. p 83

Attributable risk (Risk difference)

- *It is the difference in incidence rate of disease between those exposed and those not exposed to a risk factor.*
- *It indicates the amount of disease that might be eliminated if the exposure being studied is controlled or eliminated.*
- *It is expressed as a percentage, it is the extent to which the disease being studied can be attributed to the exposure.*

163. Ans. (d) 90%

Ref: K. Park, 24th ed. p 83

Attributable risk (Risk difference)

$$= \frac{\text{(Incidence of disease among exposed} - \text{Incidence of disease among nonexposed)}}{\text{Incidence of disease among exposed}} \times 100$$

From the MCQ, we know that:

Exposed population (alcoholics) = 2100
Non-exposed = 9000-2100 = 6900
Incidence among exposed = 70/2100
Incidence among non-exposed = 23/6900
= ((70/2100) – (23/6900))/(70/2100)
= ((1/30 – (1/300))/(1/30)
= (0.03 – 0.003)/0.03
= 0.027/0.03 = 0.9 × 100 = 90%

164. Ans. (c) $I_{exposed}/I_{nonexposed}$

Ref: K. Park, 24th ed. p 83

Relative risk or Risk ratio =

$$\frac{\text{Incidence of disease (or Outcome) among exposed}}{\text{Incidence of disease (or Outcome) among nonexposed}}$$

- It shows how many times exposure to a cause/factor being studied increases the risk of an outcome.
- It is an indicator of strength of association between exposure and outcome

165. Ans. (d) There is no increase in risk...

Ref: K. Park, 24th ed. p 83

Relative Risk (RR)

- RR = 1 indicates no association
- RR > 1 indicates "positive" association (E.g. RR = 3 means a 3 times higher incidence of disease in exposed group compared to unexposed.)
- RR < 1 indicates "Negative" association (E.g. RR = 0.5 means a 50% reduction in incidence of disease in exposed group compared to unexposed.)

166. Ans. (c) Estimate of amount disease...

Ref: K. Park, 24th ed. p 83

***Population Attributable risk** = Incidence of disease in population – Incidence of disease in people not exposed to suspected factor*

- *It is a measure of the excess incidence of disease in population attributable to the exposure*

Population Attributable Risk Proportion

$$= \frac{\text{Population Attributable Risk}}{\text{Incidence of disease in population}} \times 100$$

- *It indicates the proportion of disease in the population attributable to the exposure and that can be eliminated if the exposure is avoided completely*

167. Ans. (a) No association between risk factor...

Ref: K. Park, 24th ed. p 83

168. Ans. (b) Incidence among exposed minus incidence among nonexposed/incidence exposed

Remember:

Relative risk = Incidence exposed/Incidence nonexposed

Attributable risk = Incidence exposed – Incidence nonexposed

Attributable risk proportion =

$$\frac{\text{Incidence exposed} - \text{Incidence nonexposed}}{\text{Incidence exposed}} \times 1000$$

Note: Usually, until specified, the term "attributable risk" may denote AR proportion and is expressed in percentages.

169. Ans. (c) Relative risk

Ref: K. Park, 24th ed. p 94

Measures of Strength of Association

- Odds ratio
- Relative risk
- Dose-response/Duration response relationship

170. Ans. (b) Cohort study

Ref: K. Park, 24th ed. p 83

Also Know........................

- ***Case control study yields*** → Exposure rate among cases and controls and Odds ratio.
- ***Cohort study yields*** → Relative Risk, Attributable Risk, Population Attributable Risk and Incidence

171. Ans. (a) Cohort study

Ref: K. Park, 24th ed. p 83

172. Ans. (c) Risk difference between exposed...

Ref: K. Park, 24th ed. p 83

Attributable Risk (AR) or **"Risk Difference"** is *the difference in incidence rate of disease (or outcome) between those exposed and those not exposed to a risk factor.*

EXPERIMENTAL EPIDEMIOLOGY

173. Ans. (b) Blinding both interviewer and subject

Ref: K. Park, 24th ed. p 88

174. Ans. (b) Consolidated standard for reporting trial

Ref: BMJ 2010;340:c332Enhancing the Quality and Transparency Of health Research. http://www.equator-network.org/reporting-guidelines

Reporting Guidelines for Different Study Design

Randomized Control Trials	CONSORT	Consolidated Standards of Reporting Trials
Observational studies	STROBE	STrengthening the Reporting of OBservational studies in Epidemiology
Systematic reviews	PRISMA	Preferred Reporting Items for Systematic Reviews and Meta.Analyses
Case reports	CARE	CAse. REport
Qualitative research	SRQR	Standards for Reporting Qualitative Research
Diagnostic/ prognostic studies	STARD	Standards for Reporting of Diagnostic Accuracy
Quality improvement studies	SQUIRE	Standards for Quality Improvement Reporting Excellence

Contd...

Economic evaluations	CHEERS	Consolidated Health Economic Evaluation Reporting Standards
Study protocols	SPIRIT	(Standard Protocol Items: Recommendations for Interventional Trials

175. Ans. (d) Validity does not depend on quality of systemic review

Ref: Basic epidemiology, 2nd ed. Bonita and Beagle hole p-81

Meta-analysis is statistical synthesis of data from separate but similar (comparable) studies (particularly RCT), leading to a quantifiable summary of the pooled results.

- No new data is collected; it combines the results of several trials.
- It is a retrospective research, subject to the methodological deficiencies of each included study.
- Steps in meta-analysis include:
  - Formulating the problem and study design
  - Identifying relevant studies
  - Excluding poorly conducted studies or those with major methodological flaws
  - Measuring, combining and interpreting the results.
- It allows comparisons to be made between studies even if they used different measures of outcome.
- Advantage –No ethical issues, low cost

Purpose of Meta-analysis

- To summarize a large and complex body of literature on a topic
- To resolve conflicting reports in the literature
- To clarify or quantify the strengths and weaknesses of studies on a topic
- To document the need for a major clinical trial
- To avoid the time and expense of conducting a clinical trial
- To make comparisons of interventions more objective and accurate
- To identify areas in which insufficient research has been performed or additional research may not be necessary
- To increase statistical power by combining many smaller studies
- To improve the precision of an estimated treatment effect
- To detect smaller treatment effects than have been reported
- To investigate variations in treatment effects through subgroup (or stratified) analysis
- To improve the generalizability of known treatment effects.

176. Ans. (a) Meta-analysis is always done

Ref: Cochrane Handbook for Systematic Reviews of Interventions Version 5.1.0 (updated March 2011

A systematic review attempts to collate all empirical evidence that fits pre-specified eligibility criteria in order to answer a specific research question.

The key characteristics of a systematic review are:

- A clearly stated set of objectives with predefined eligibility criteria for studies
- An explicit reproducible methodology to minimize bias
- A systematic search to identify all studies that would meet the eligibility criteria
- Assessment or Critical appraisal of the validity of the findings of the included studies
- Systematic presentation and synthesis of the characteristics and findings of the included studies.
- Many systematic reviews contain meta-analyses (But not always)

177. Ans. (a) RCT

Ref: Basic epidemiology, 2nd ed. Bonita and Beagle hole p-95

Relative ability to "prove" causation in different types of study:

Study design	Ability to "prove" causation
Meta-analysis and Systematic Review	*Strongest*
RCT	*Strong (Gold Standard)*
Cohort	*Moderate*
Case control	*Moderate*
Cross sectional	*Weak*
Ecological/ Case Series or Report	*Weak*

178. Ans. (c) RCT

Ref: Basic epidemiology, 2nd ed. Bonita and Beaglehole p-95

179. Ans. (d) Increases external validity of the trial

Ref: K. Park, 24th ed. p 87

Randomization Ensures

- Investigator has no control over allocation of participants to study or control group thus eliminates "selection bias"
- Comparability of two groups for demographic, behavioral, genetic characteristics etc. except for exposure status.
- Equal distribution of known covariates (like **Matching)** and unknown covariates or confounders (not possible by **Matching)**
- Randomization increases internal validity of a trial.

External validity or Generalizability is concerned with the clinical usefulness of the results.

Also Know.......................

- *If the internal validity is rotten, there can be no meaningful external validity.*

180. Ans. (b) 2

Ref: Targeted Regulatory Writing Techniques: Clinical Documents for Drugs and biologics. Linda Fossati Wood, MaryAnn Foote

Maximum Rate of Drug failure is seen in phase 2 of Clinical trial- Reasons being

- Poor risk: benefit ratio (risk of using drug outweigh benefit)
- Poor study design
- Wrong endpoint
- Lack of statistical power

181. Ans. (b) Randomization of study subjects

Ref: K. Park, 24th ed. p 87

182. Ans. (b) The clinician does not know which treatment is given to the patient

Ref: K. Park, 24th ed. p 88

Blinding is a technique to ensure that the outcome is assessed objectively. It takes care of subject variation, observer bias and evaluation bias.

- *Single blind: The participant is not aware whether he belongs to study group or control group*
- *Double blind trial: Neither investigator nor participant is aware of group allocation and treatment received*
- *Triple blind trial: The participant, investigator and the person analyzing the data are all "blind".*

Also Know......................

- Most ideal blinding technique is Triple blinding and **most frequently used** method is Double blinding.

183. Ans. (c) Use of various research findings for...

Ref: Izet Masic, Milan Miokovic et al, Evidence Based Medicine - New Approaches and Challenges, Acta Inform Med. 2008; 16(4): 219–225.

Evidence-based medicine refers to putting evidence into practice.

- EBM integrates clinical experience and patient values with the best available research information

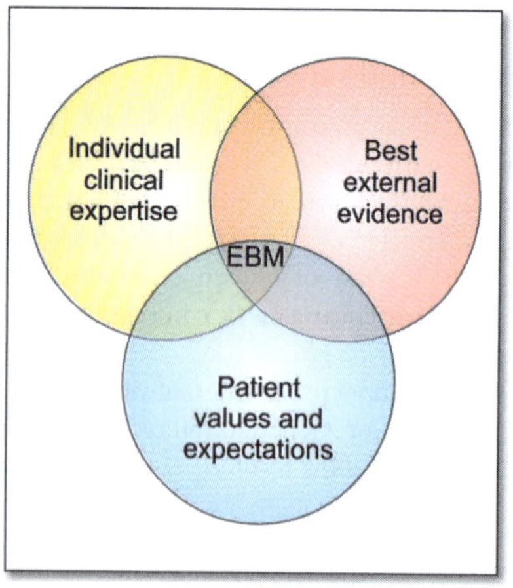

184. Ans. (a) 1

Ref: Targeted Regulatory Writing Techniques: Clinical Documents for Drugs and biologics. Linda Fossati Wood, Mary Ann Foote

Phase I

- Done on a small number of patients or healthy volunteers (i.e. 20 to 80)
- **Objective:** To find out Maximally Tolerated Dose (MTD), enlist toxic and pharmacological effects of the drug.

ASSOCIATION AND CAUSATION

185. Ans. (c) Sensitivity

Ref: K. Park, 24th ed. p 49; 24th ed. p 94

Criteria for Judging Causality (Hill Criteria)

- *Temporal association – (Exposure to a cause must precede the onset of a disease, to allow for induction and latency)*
- *Strength of association –(Relative risk, Dose-response, Duration -response relationship)*
- *Specificity of the association – a "one-to-one" relationship between cause and effect.*
- *Consistency–Results are replicated when studied in different settings and using different methods.*
- *Biological plausibility – Association agrees with current understanding of response of cells, tissues, organs, etc. Lack of biological mechanism does not rule out possibility of a cause and effect relationship.*
- *Coherence of association – coherence with known facts thought to be relevant.*

Also Know......................

- Specificity of the association is most difficult criteria to establish in chronic and also in acute diseases and conditions.
- Specificity supports causal interpretation but lack of specificity does not negate it.

186. Ans. (a) Spurious association

Ref: K. Park, 24th ed. p 92

Spurious association means that the observed association between outcome and suspected factor is not real.

- Selection bias is a very important cause leading to a spurious association

187. Ans. (b) Relative risk/odds ratio

Ref: K. Park, 24th ed. p 95

- Measures of strength of association—Odds ratio, Relative risk, Dose-response, Duration-response relationship

188. Ans. (b) Temporality

Ref: K. Park, 24th ed. p 95

189. Ans. (b) Descriptive epidemiology

Procedure in descriptive studies

- Defining the population to be studied.
- Defining the disease under study.
- Describing the disease by time, place and person
- Measurement of disease
- Comparing with known indices
- Formulation of etiological hypothesis

190. Ans. (a) Descriptive epidemiology

191. Ans. (a) Study in which the units of analysis are populations or groups, rather than individuals

Meta-analysis combines result from different studies and through statistical methods, calculates an overall estimate of the effect.

Ecological studies use data based on groups of people rather than individuals. Associations observed on an aggregate mat not represent associations on an individual level. (ecological bias or ecological fallacy)

192. Ans. (a) It is a study in which the units of analysis are populations or groups of people, rather than individuals

Meta analyses combine results from several studies and, through statistical methods, calculate an overall estimate of effect Ecological studies use data based on groups of people rather than individuals. Associations observed on an aggregate level may not represent associations on an individual level (ecological bias or ecological fallacy).

RCT

193. Ans. (b) Intervention

194. Ans. (d) Ethics

Information bias: May be in studies involving subjective retrieval of information. Can be found as recall bias in case control studies

Lead time bias: Is a bias arising in case a screening test is able to diagnose a disease condition early in the natural course of disease, but there is no significant change in mortality pattern or there is no alteration in the prognosis of the disease. This would lead to a virtual higher survival rates and lower mortality rates

Berksonian bias: Is a typical bias associated with a hospital-based case control study, where the cases would be similar to the control, if selected from the same hospital. It is due to differential hospital admission rates.

195. Ans. (d) Randomized controlled trial

Explanation:

For new program or new therapies, the randomized controlled trial is the best method of evaluation.

196. Ans. (b) The apparent effect might be a result of chance

As a general rule, the false negative errors maybe associated more with placebo, double blinded RCT designs.

If sample size is small – more chance to have a 'null' effect or Falsely negative result

If inclusion criteria would have been problem, it would have had affected both the groups, as randomization is done after selection of the study participants for allocation into the two groups

Chance error is false positive errors

197. Ans. (a) Control and case are the same

Crossover Study

- Used where patient serves as his own control.

The advantage of cross over design is: better analysis, no need of intricate randomization procedures.

A few disadvantages are:

- If the drug of interest cures the disease
- If the drug is effective only during a certain stage of the disease
- If the disease changes radically during the period of time required for the study
- The disease is acute or fatal
- The drug is having a long half life
- Chances of subject bias is very high especially if double blinding is not done

198. Ans. (c) Randomization

Randomization is the "heart" of a control trial. It will give greatest confidence that the groups are comparable so that like can be compared with like.

199. Ans. (d) Randomized intervention clinical trial

200. Ans. (d) Cannot compare for the difference in cost of treatments with new or standard drugs

In RCT or any clinical trials, the efficacy of the drug or intervention is definitely determined. But the major area of concern before such is drug is approved for public policy, is cost of treatment. Cost benefit or cost effective analysis help in determining the costs and assessment from public health point.

201. Ans. (c) Fields trial

202. Ans. (a) Cross sectional

To estimate the load of disease – we need to find the prevalence, which is given by the cross-sectional studies

203. Ans. (c) Burden of disease in population

Burden of disease means to find prevalence of disease in population

204. Ans. (d) Case series study

Hypothesis formulation is usually done at the level of descriptive studies, which may also sometimes include the cross sectional studies.

Hypothesis testing is usually done by the analytical studies. These studies help us assess for the presumptive hypothesis and try to prove the existence of such causality in nature.

Experimental studies are of course, without doubt, the best studies to ascertain the effect of drugs or preventive measures as vaccines or any preventive health strategy in a community level setting.

205. Ans. (d) For identifying risk factors of disease

In longitudinal studies, observations are repeated in the same population over a prolonged period of time by means of follow-up examinations. Longitudinal studies are useful:

- To study the natural history of disease and its future outcome
- For identifying risk factors of disease
- For finding out incidence rate or rate of occurrence of new cases of disease in the community.

206. Ans. (d) Experimental epidemiology

Criteria for judging causality

- Temporal association

- Strength of association
- Specificity of the association
- Consistency of the association
- Biological plausibility
- Coherence of the association

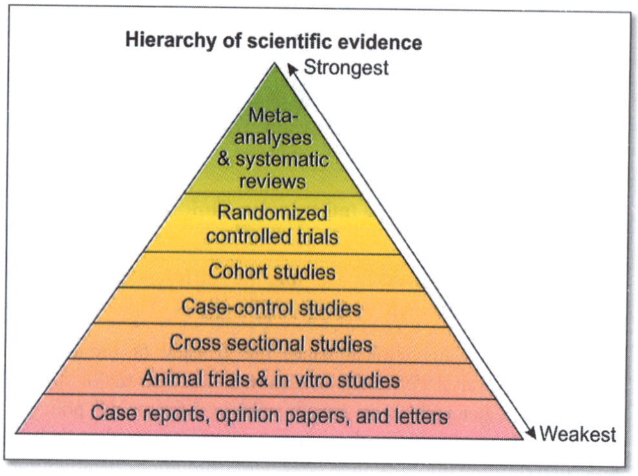

207. Ans. (c) Temporal association

The stress of the MCQ statement is for uranium workers working in a mine and later they developed the disease of interest. The MCQ is pointing towards the spatial distribution of events in 'Time dimension" i.e. the risk factor happened "BEFORE" the disease. Hence the answer – temporality.

Note: Temporality means: Distribution of events in "Dimension of Time"

208. Ans. (b) Drop outs are excluded from the study

Basic steps in conducting a RCT include the following:

- Drawing up a protocol
- Selecting reference and experimental populations
- Randomization
- Manipulation or intervention
- Follow-up
- Assessment of outcome
  - Randomization is the "heart" of a control trial. It controls for confounding bias
  - Follow-up: This implies examination of the experimental and control group subjects at defined intervals of time, in a standard manner, with equal intensity, under the same given circumstances, in the same time frame till final assessment of outcome.
  - Attrition: Loss to follow up during the course of the clinical trial
  - Double blind trial: The trial is so planned that neither the doctor nor the participant is aware of the group allocation and the treatment received.

209. Ans. (b) What happened to surviving patients in the next year?

Option discussion:

- Blinding: Usually not of major concern in large RCT's and moreover, when mortality is the end point.
- Power is not relevant with p-value 0.01 at 95% confidence interval
- In the RCT design the total MI cases must have been taken and then randomized to the interventional group or the control group and further compared. So obviously, the number of MI cases would have been predetermined in both the groups with a reasonable statistical base.

In RCT's involving use of drugs for acute and fatal conditions as acute MI, the final outcome to be assessed should have been 'all-cause mortality" rather than mortality due to "MI or its complications". Also another point of concern is the increase in longevity, does it delay death in such cases or there is just over 3 week postponement.

Though all the options in the MCQ should be looked upon for a clear and concise critical review of research, but the single best suitable option seems to be is Option B.

210. Ans. (d) Predictive value

Bradford Hill and others have pointed out that the likelihood of a causal relationship is increased by the presence of the following criteria:

- Temporal association
- Strength of association
- Specificity of association
- Consistency of association
- Biological plausibility
- Coherence of the association.

211. Ans. (c) 1, 2, and 4

212. Ans. (d) Association

213. Ans. (c) Population

The ecological study determines and compares a variable from one geographical area to another. The unit of study is the whole population rather than an individual.

Cohort Studies	A cohort (group) of individuals with exposure to a chemical and a cohort without exposure are followed over time to compare disease occurrence
Case Control Studies	Individuals with a disease (*e.g., cancer*) are compared with similar individuals without the disease to determine if there is an association of the disease with prior exposure to an agent
Cross-Sectional Studies	The prevalence of a disease or clinical parameter among one or more exposed groups is studies. For example, the prevalence of respiratory conditions among furniture makers
Ecological Studies	The incidence of a disease in one geographical area is compared to that of another area. For example, cancer mortality in areas with hazardous waste sites as compared to areas without waste sites

Study design	Strengths	Weaknesses
Ecological	Very inexpensive Fast Easy to assign exposure levels	Inaccuracy of data Inability to control for confounders Difficulty identifying or quantifying denominator No demonstrated temporality
Case-crossover	Reduces some-types of bias Good for acute health outcomes with a defined exposure Cases act as their own control	Selection of comparison time point difficult Challenging to execute Prone to recall bias No demonstrated temporality
Cross-sectional	Inexpensive Timely Individualized data Ability to control for multiple confounders Can assess multiple outcomes	No temporality Not good for rare diseases Poor for disease of short duration No demonstrated temporality
Case-control	Inexpensive Timely Individualized data Ability to control for multiple confounders Good for rare diseases Can assess multiple exposures	Cannot calculate prevalence Can only assess one outcome Poor selection of controls can introduce bias May be difficult to identify enough cases Prone to recall bias No demonstrated temporality
Retrospective and prospective cohort	Temporality demonstrated individualized data Ability to control for multiple confounders Can assess multiple exposures Can assess multiple outcomes	Expensive Time intensive Not good for rare disease

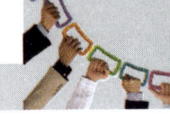

214. Ans. (d) 8/1000

Prevalence of disease may be calculated as:

Prevalence = incidence × duration

= 4/1000 × 2 years = 8/1000 population

215. Ans. (c) Relative risk

$$\text{Relative risk} = \frac{\textit{incidence (or risk) among exposed group}}{\textit{incidence (or risk) among the nonexposed group}}$$

216. Ans. (a) Cross-sectional Studies

Recall:

Cross-sectional studies:

- Also gives us the prevalence
- Survey is conducted
- Is known as snapshot of the population

Cohort study

- Incidence may be found
- Follow up is done, prospective study
- Risk ratio, attributable risks are estimated

Quasi designs; nonrandomized, partial designs

217. Ans. (a) Number of new cases in an area; (c) Incidence depends on the duration

Option	T/F	Comment
Number of new cases in an area	T	Yes, correct. Incidence is number of new cases in an area in a defined time period
Number of new cases and old cases in a time period from an area	F	No, Prevalence is the number of old and new cases

Contd...

Option	T/F	Comment
Incidence depends on the duration	T	Yes correct
Incidence depends on morbidity	F	No, morbidity is sickness or illness due to a disease
Incidence is a proportion	F	No, Incidence is a special rate. It is always expressed as per unit time.

218. Ans. (a) Calculated in case-control study; (c) Closely related to relative risk; (d) It is a cross-product ratio calculated by 2 × 2 table; (e) Measure the strength of the association between risk factor and outcome

Option	T/F	Remarks
Calculated in case-control study	T	Yes, correct. It is calculated in case control studies
Calculated in cohort study	F	No, it is calculated in case control only
Closely related to relative risk	T	Yes, correct. In fact, OR is an approximation of Relative risks for rare diseases
It is a cross-product ratio calculated by 2 × 2 table	T	Yes, correct.
Measure the strength of the association between risk factor and outcome	T	Yes correct. if the OR < 1 – implies – negative association or a protective factor OR = 1 – implies – no association OR > 1 – implies – positive association or a risk factor

219. Ans. (b) Odds ratio 0.5 ; with 95% CI 0.4 - 0.6

As we see in this data, there are two general rules for assessment:
Rule 1. The more extreme is the value of the ODDS ratio the more significant (stronger) is the association of data to be evaluated.
Rule 2. It is always required to see for the 95% confidence interval as well. Within the range of 95% confidence interval if the Odds Ratio value '1' lies in between the range, the Odds ratio is 'not significant' hence we discard the rule #1

Odds ratio 4.7 with 95% CI 0.1–9.6	High Odds ratio, but is NON Significant as the 95% CI contains the value 1 in between
Odds ratio 0.5 with 95% CI 0.4–0.6	This is Negative Association and the 95% Confidence interval is also < 1. so we interpret this as 'significant Negative association'
Odds ratio 0.7 with 95% CI 0.02–1	Negative association, but is NON Significant as the 95% CI contains the value 1 in between
Odds ratio 2.7 with 95% CI 1.0–9.6	Positive association, but is NON Significant as the 95% CI contains the value 1 in between

The clinical implication of the study result is that there is a protective effect of the new drug and it has a significant negative association, with Odds ratio 0.5 with 95% CI 0.4-0.6

220. Ans. (b) Prospective cohort

This is a typical study to ascertain the fat content in breast milk for a sample of females who have delivered in a specified time. A sample cohort of females maybe selected for the study and evaluation for fat content is done at regular follow ups.

221. Ans. (d) Blinding

Known Confounders are Removed by Matching

Confounding can be controlled by:

- Matching – is done at designing stage – especially for case control studies
- Restriction – involves restricting participation in the study to individuals who are similar in relation to the confounder. For example, a study restricted to non-smokers only will eliminate any confounding effect of smoking.
- Randomization using random allocation – usually used in clinical trials
- Stratification – analyze the association of exposure and outcome within a stratum of the confounding variable.
- Standardization – control for effects of age and gender
- Multivariate regression

Blinding is adopted to control Bias

222. Ans. (a) Case control study

Ref: Park 25th Ed. Pg 81

For case control studies – odds ratio is calculated for cohort studies – relative risk, attributable risk, population attributable risks are calculated

223. Ans. (a) Factor associated with both the exposure and the disease & is distributed unequally in study and control groups

Ref: Park 25th Ed. Pg 80

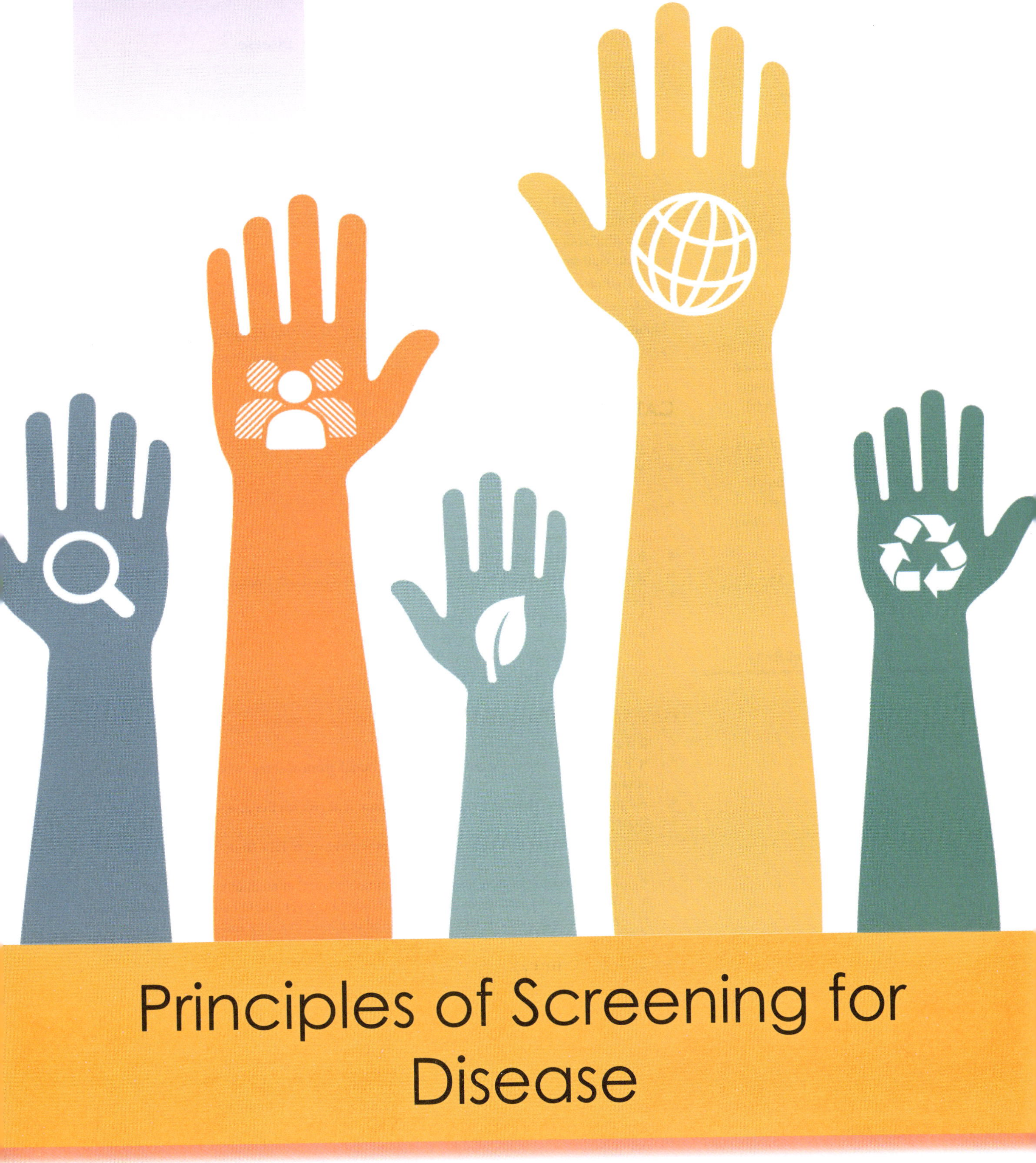

Principles of Screening for Disease

Chapter Outline

- Introduction
- Categories of Screening
  - Prescriptive Screening
  - Presumptive (Prospective, Predictive Screening)
- Types of Screening Methods
  - Mass Screening
  - High-risk Screening
  - Multiphasic Screening
- Usefulness of Screening
- Concept of Screening
  - Events in Course of Disease and Screening Time
  - Lead Time Bias
- Assessment of a Screening Test
  - Properties of a Screening Test
  - Predictive Value of a Screening Test
  - Points to Remember
  - Likelihood Ratio
    - Concept of Likelihood Ratio
    - Application of Likelihood Ratio (Pre- and Post-test Probability of the Test)
  - Point to Remember
  - Combination Array of Tests
    - Remember
- Statistical Interpretation of Screening Tests Receiver-Operator Characteristic Curves (ROC)
  - Interpreting the ROC
  - Interpretation–Validity, Accuracy, Precision
    - Validity
    - Accuracy
    - Precision (or Reliability)

INTRODUCTION

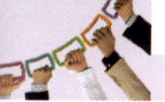

Screening denotes the search for unrecognized disease or defect in apparently (or outwardly) healthy persons by the application of rapid diagnostic tests, examinations or procedures.

Table 1: Examples of screening for disease

Screening Tests	Diseases
Blood cholesterol	Cardiovascular disease
Fecal occult blood	Colorectal cancer
Breast Self-Examination and Mammography	Breast cancer
Prostate Specific Antigen	Prostate cancer
Papanicolaou Test (Pap smear), Visual Inspection with 5% Acetic acid	Cervical cancer
Glucose Tolerance Test	Diabetes mellitus
Guthrie Test (Heel prick blood in a newborn 7–10 days post birth) Tandem Mass Spectrometry (New method replaces Guthrie test)	Phenylketonuria
TSH, T_4 (Umbilical cord blood)	Neonatal hypothyroidism
ELISA and RAPID	HIV
Bimanual Oral Inspection	Oral cancer
Alpha Fetoprotein (AFP)	Developmental anomaly in fetus

CATEGORIES OF SCREENING

- Prescriptive screening
- Presumptive screening

Prescriptive Screening

- It is a usually a secondary type of prevention
- It is done to find the disease in early phase in an individual
- It is used for prevention of complications or sequel or death from a disease
- Examples:
  - Mammography for breast cancer
  - PAP smear for cancer cervix
  - Blood glucose testing for diabetes
  - Visual acuity for refractive errors

Presumptive (Prospective, Predictive Screening)

- It is a usually a primary type of prevention
- It is done to prevent (or protect) an individual from disease, when he/she is at risk of obtaining the disease
- For prevention of disease, assuming the person is at risk for the disease
- Examples:
  - HIV screening for blood donation – for prevention of HIV transmission to the recipient of blood donation
  - HIV screening in ANC cases for prevention of mother to child transmission
  - Tracking of hypertension in young children for prevention of cardiovascular morbidity
  - Health check for persons to be employed in a food industry and so on...

TYPES OF SCREENING METHODS

Mass Screening

When all members of a population are screened for disease it is called mass screening. This is very costly and the yield of cases is usually too small to warrant such a screening procedure.

High-risk Screening

High-risk screening or selective screening refers to the situation where tests are offered only to those individuals who are at high risk of developing a specific disease. This makes the screening process more focused and reduces the overall costs.

Multiphasic Screening

Multiphasic screening is done in phases:

- **Example:** For assessment of tuberculosis, The Mantoux test can be done first, following by CXR and further followed by sputum testing in all those who are tested as Mantoux positive and CXR positive
- **Example:** For assessment of COPD in community, questionnaire-based interview method may be adopted first to screen individuals with possibility of and obstructive airway disease, further PFT (pulmonary functions tests may be done in screened positive patients from the initial phase screening level

High Yield Points

A good screening tool is:

- Acceptable
- Affordable
- Good validity

USEFULNESS OF SCREENING

Screening is most useful for:

- Disease with higher number of subclinical or undiagnosed cases
- Disease with long latent period
- Disease which has a good screening test (or tool)
- The screening test should be
  - Easy to carry out
  - Able to find (or diagnose) disease in a relatively early stage of the course of disease
  - Affordable and cost effective
  - Acceptable by the general community
- The disease should have an appropriate treatment or good quality management, so that if diagnosed early should be treatable and have good prognosis

CONCEPT OF SCREENING

Events in Course of Disease and Screening Time

- This is the natural course of the disease

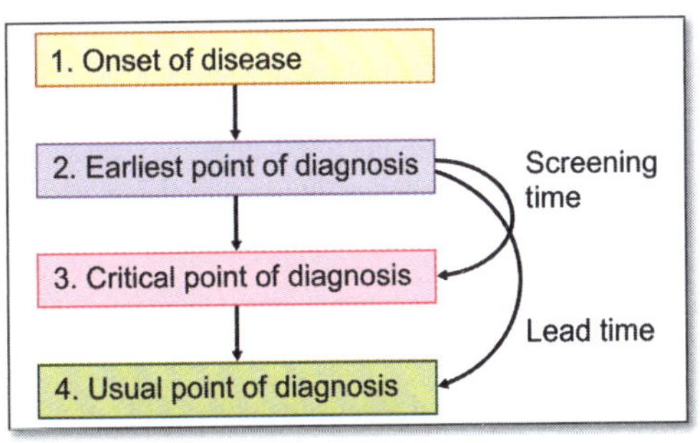

Fig. 1: Concept of screening

- The individual with the disease will usually present to the physician at point #4, – i.e. the usual point of diagnosis and not at the point of start or the onset of the disease (i.e. point # 1 or 2)
- A screening test would be most useful at the point of the onset of the pathogenesis phase, rather than at the point of the start of the disease

So,

- The time difference between the earliest possible point of diagnosis and the critical point of diagnosis is known as – **Screening time**
- The time difference between the earliest possible point of diagnosis and the usual point of diagnosis is known as the – **Lead time**

Thus we understand that for some diseases the screening test may be applied early in the natural course of the disease. It is of utmost importance that while in the process of detecting the pathology early, the medical science should also take the responsibility of treating the disease in better way so as to provide early relief and escape from the sequel of the disease.

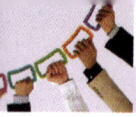

Must Remember

Lead time bias:

Sometimes, the disease, if detected early, but does not alter the natural course of disease or no additional life span has been gained – rather the patient may even be subject to added anxiety as the patient must live for longer with knowledge of the disease, may distort the results and appear to decrease the mortality rates or increase the survival rates. This error is known as lead time bias. The lead time bias may affect the five year survival analysis.

Lead Time Bias

As seen previously, the screening test help us identify the disease EARLY in the natural course of disease, so that the treatment is initiated early and hence prolong the survival. This obvious jump in time – from point of usual diagnosis to the first possible point of diagnosis is known as LEAD time.

A systematic error (bias) in Lead time is : when erroneously, the treatment for a disease is not available or there is no change in the prognosis of disease, then a mere early diagnosis of disease would imply an **apparent increase in survival** due to detecting a health condition such as cancer at an early stage, when there is no actual effect **on survival, just a longer period with the diagnosis**.

ASSESSMENT OF A SCREENING TEST

	Disease +	Healthy (nondiseased)
Test +	True positive (TP)	False positive (FP)
Test –	False negative (FN)	True negative (TN)

Now let's see the different parts of the table:

- True positive (TP) -The population who was **diseased** and was **tested positive** by the screening test
- True Negative (TN) -The population who was **healthy** and was **tested negative** by the screening test
- False Negative (FN) -The population who was **diseased** and was wrongly identified as **test negative** by the screening test
- False Positive (TP) -The population who was **healthy** and was wrongly identified as **test positive** by the screening test

Properties of a Screening Test

Sensitivity: The term was introduced by 'Yerushalmy' in 1940

It is the ability of a test to correctly identify those having the disease, and expressed as the percentage of diseased persons, showing the test result positive.

Formula:

$$Sensitivity = \frac{TP}{TP + FN} \times 100 = \frac{True\ positive}{Total\ diseased} \times 100$$

Meaning: If the sensitivity of a screening test is 95% it means that 95% of the diseased persons are correctly identified as 'True positives' and remaining 10 percent of diseased persons are wrongly identified as not having the disease, because the test is negative (Falsely negative).

Specificity: It is the ability of the test to correctly identify those 'not having' the disease. It is expressed as the percentage of test negative persons out of total healthy (non-diseased) individuals

Formula:

$$Specificity = \frac{TN}{TN + FP} \times 100 = \frac{True\ negatives}{Total\ healthy} \times 100$$

Meaning: If the specificity of a test is 80%, it means that 80% of the non-diseased will be correctly 'ruled-out' for the diseased and will be 'true negatives'

False Negative Error Rate (FNER): These are the percentage of diseased persons who are wrongly identified as not having the disease, because the test result is negative.

$$FNER = \frac{FN}{TP + FN} \times 100 = \frac{False\ negatives}{Total\ diseased} \times 100$$

False Positive Error Rate (FPER): These are the percentage of healthy persons who may be wrongly identified as having the disease, because the test result is positive.

$$FPER \frac{FN}{TP + FN} \times 100 = \frac{False\ positive}{Total\ healthy} \times 100$$

Predictive Value of a Screening Test

Positive Predictive Value (PPV): This is indicator for usability of the screening test in a population. It is the probability (expressed as percentage) of an individual to actually have the disease in case the person is tested positive.

$$PPV = \frac{TP}{TP + FN} \times 100 = \frac{True\ positive}{Total\ test\ positives} \times 100$$

Meaning:

If the PPV for a screening test is 95%, it means that if the test is positive for a case, there is 95% chance for the person to actually have a disease

Negative Predictive Value: It is the probability (expressed as percentage) of an individual being actually free from disease given that the test report is negative for the case

$$NPV = \frac{TN}{TP + FN} \times 100 = \frac{True\ negatives}{Total\ test\ negatives} \times 100$$

Note:

The predictive values for a test are related to the utility of the screening test for diagnosing a condition in general community. It relates to the 'YIELD' of a screening test

The predictive values (both positive predictive and negative predictive value) can also be determined by:

- Sensitivity
- Specificity
- Prevalence of the disease

This may be given by the Bayes probability theorem as follows:

$$PPV = \frac{\text{Sensitivity} \times \text{Prevalence}}{(\text{Sensitivity} \times \text{Prevalence}) + (1-\text{specificity}) \times (1-\text{prevlence})} \times 100$$

$$NPV = \frac{\text{Specificity} \times (1-\text{Prevalence})}{(\text{Specificity} \times 1-\text{Prevalence}) + (1-\text{sensitivity}) \times \text{prevalence}} \times 100$$

The positive predictive value is directly proportional to the prevalence of the disease in the community and is also maximally affected by the same.

If the prevalence of a certain disease is higher in the population, the PPV is a reliable indicator for diagnosing the disease, whereas, if the disease is rare in community (low prevalence), the PPV will be low due to higher false positivity rate.

Table Summary:

Sensitivity	=	TP/D+		NPV	=	TN/T–
FNER	=	FN/D+		FNER	=	False negative error rate
Specificity	=	TN/D–		FPER	=	False positive error rate
FPER	=	FP/D–		PPV	=	Positive predictive value
PPV	=	TP/T+		NPV	=	Negative predictive value

10 Must Remember

- Sensitivity – probability of being tested positive in diseased individuals
- Specificity – probability of being tested negative in healthy individuals
- Positive predictive value – probability of being diseased, if the test result is positive
- Negative predictive value – probability of being healthy, if the test result is negative

11 Must Remember

Predictive value of a positive test

$$PPV = \frac{\textit{Sensitivity} \times \textit{Prevalence}}{(\textit{Sensitivity} \times \text{Prevalence}) + (1\text{-}\textit{specificty}) \times (1\text{-}\textit{prevalence})} \times 100$$

Predictive value of a negative test

$$= \frac{\text{Specificity} \times (1\text{-Prevalence})}{(\textit{Specificity} \times 1\text{-Prevalence}) + (1\text{-}\textit{sensitivity} \times \textit{prevalence})} \times 100$$

Points to Remember

- False-positive error is more serious compared to false-negative error
- False-positive test corresponds to the type 1 error or alpha error
- False-negative test corresponds to the type 2 error or Beta error
- For screening tests, sensitivity of the test is important
- For diagnostic tests, specificity of the test is essential
- Higher false positive is due to:
  - Low specificity
  - Low prevalence
  - High sensitivity

Likelihood Ratio

Concept of Likelihood Ratio

Likelihood ratios (LR) in medical testing are used to interpret diagnostic tests. Basically, the LR tells you how likely a patient has a disease or condition. The higher the ratio, the more likely

10 High Yield Points

How does prevalence influence the PPV or NPV

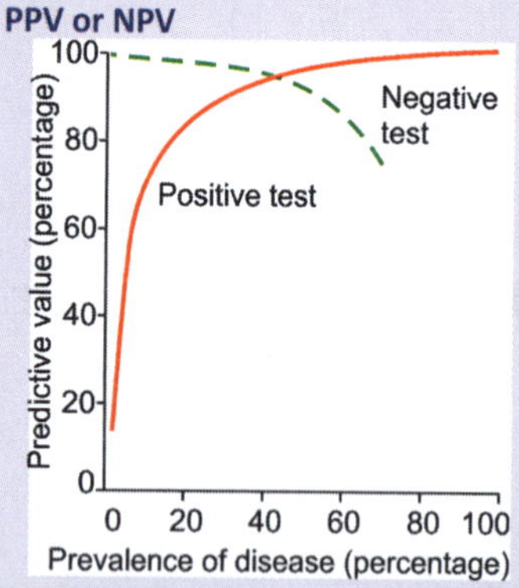

9 Good to Remember

Likelihood Ratio

For a positive test: $\frac{\text{Sensitivity}}{\text{1–specificity}}$

For a negative test: $\frac{\text{1–Sensitivity}}{\text{specificity}}$

they have the disease or condition. Conversely, a low ratio means that they very likely do not. Therefore, these ratios can help a physician to rule in or rule out a disease

As the results of tests can be either positive or negative, so there are two ratios:

- **Positive LR:** This tells you how much to increase the probability of having a disease, given a positive test result. The ratio is: Probability a person with the condition **tests positive** (a true positive)/probability a person without the condition tests positive (a false positive).
- **Negative LR:** This tells you how much to decrease the probability of having a disease, given a negative test result. The ratio is—Probability of a person with the condition tests negative (a false negative) /probability of a person without the condition tests negative (a true negative).

Sensitivity and specificity are an alternative way to define the likelihood ratio:

- **Positive LR** = sensitivity/(100–specificity).
- **Negative LR** = (100–sensitivity)/specificity.

The Likelihood ratio (LR) is the likelihood that a given test result would be expected in a patient with a specific disease as compared to the likelihood that that same result would be expected in a patient without the disease. The LR is used to assess the usefulness of a test for a particular condition. An example is discussed below:

Example:

A patient age 55 years, with chronic cough has a peak expiratory flow rate (PEFR) of 180 L/min. The review of literature reports that 90% of patients diagnosed as COPD were having PEFR < 200 l/min, while 10% of non-COPD cases also had a PEFR of <200 L/min. so, we can conclude that if the PEFR is <200 L/min, there is 9 times more chance of person to suffer from COPD than from other causes of chronic cough. This concept is known as 'likelihood ratio'

Application of Likelihood Ratio (Pre- and Post-test Probability of the Test)

Let us assume that using spirometry for diagnosis of chronic bronchitis yield the following results:

- Prevalence of 30% in community
- Sensitivity of the test = 95%
- Specificity = 90%

Step 1. Find the likelihood ratio for positive test

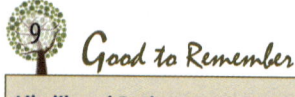

Likelihood ratio for a positive test =

$$LR+=\frac{\textit{Sensitivity}}{(1\text{-specificity})}=\frac{100}{(100-90)}=\frac{95}{10}=9.5$$

Step 2. Find the pre-test odds

Chances of person to have chronic bronchitis before the test = Pre-test probability = prevalence of disease = 30%

Pre-test odds (The odds of a person to have disease) = p / (1–p)

$$=\frac{100}{(100-30)}=\frac{30}{70}=0.43$$

Step 3. Find the post-test odds

The post-test odds (the odds of a person to have disease with a positive test)

$$\text{ODDS}_{\text{post-test}}=\text{Odds}_{\text{pre-test}}\times \text{LR}$$
$$=0.43\times 9.5=4.07$$

Hence,

$$\text{Post-test probability}=\text{ODDS}_{\text{post-test}}/(\text{ODDS}_{\text{post-test}}+1)$$
$$=\frac{4.07}{(4.04+1)}=\frac{4.07}{5.07}=0.803$$

This may also be expressed as positive predictive value: 0.803 * 100 = 80.3%

The positive predictive value corresponds to the post test probability of 80.3%, which implies that 80.3% of all the spirometry positive cases will presumably have chronic bronchitis in reality.

Note: The PPV may also be directly calculated from the probability Bayes theorem as follows,

$$PPV=\frac{\text{Sensitivity}\times\text{Prevalence}}{(\text{Sensitivity}\times\text{Prevalence})+(1-\text{specificity})\times(1-\text{prevlence})}\times 100$$

$$PPV=\frac{95\times 30}{(95\times 30)+(1-90)\times(1-30)}\times 100=80.3\%$$

Point to Remember

Pretest probability of the test is corresponding to the prevalence of the disease, whereas

Post-test probability of a positive test is corresponding to the positive predictive value of the test

Combination Array of Tests

The screening tests may be combined into an array of tests which may be further of two types:

Sequential tests are applied for a disease condition (part A of image below). This type of testing method is known as 'Test in series'

Simultaneous testing for a condition using a combination of tests (part B of image below), the result is usually interpreted as any test positive, the disease condition is diagnosed, and the treatment may be started. This type of testing method is known as 'Tests in parallel'

Features of combining the tests:

- If multiple tests are applied in series, the specificity of the complete testing panel increases (and sensitivity decreases)
- If multiple tests are applied in parallel mode, the sensitivity of the testing panel increases (and specificity decreases)

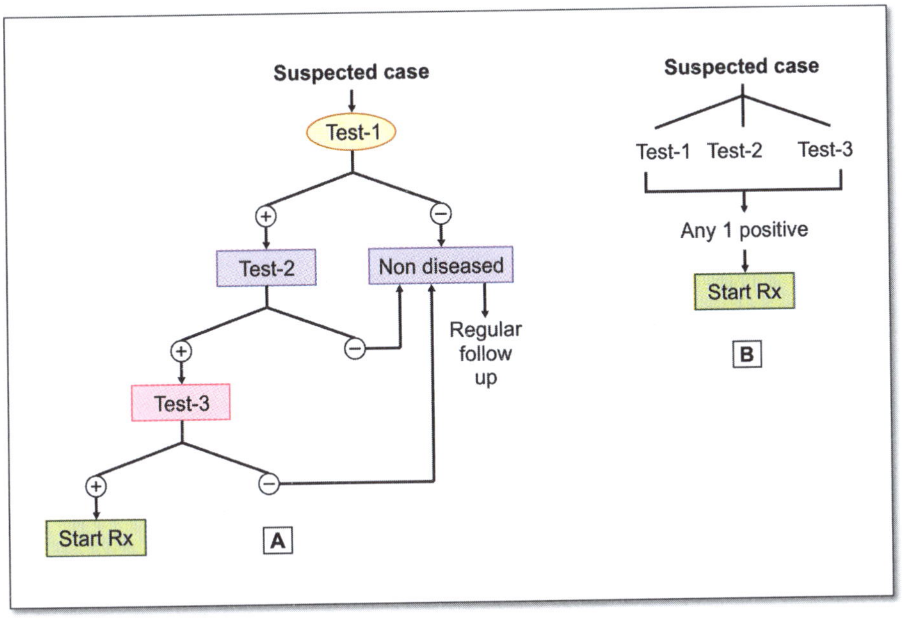

Remember

Screening Test	Net sensitivity	Net specificity	Net PPV	Net NPV
Series	Decrease	Increase	Increase	Decrease
Parallel	Increase	Decrease	Decrease	Increase

STATISTICAL INTERPRETATION OF SCREENING TESTS RECEIVER-OPERATOR CHARACTERISTIC CURVES (ROC)

Receiver operating characteristic (ROC) curve is the plot that depicts the trade-off between the sensitivity and (1-specificity) across a series of cut-off points when the diagnostic test is continuous or on ordinal scale (minimum 5 categories). This is an effective method for assessing the performance of a diagnostic test.

It is drawn between sensitivity and 1-specificity for a test (Fig. 2).

11 High Yield Points

Area under the ROC curve is considered as an effective measure of inherent validity of a diagnostic test.

12 **Must Remember**

Post-test odds = Pretest odds × Likelihood ratio

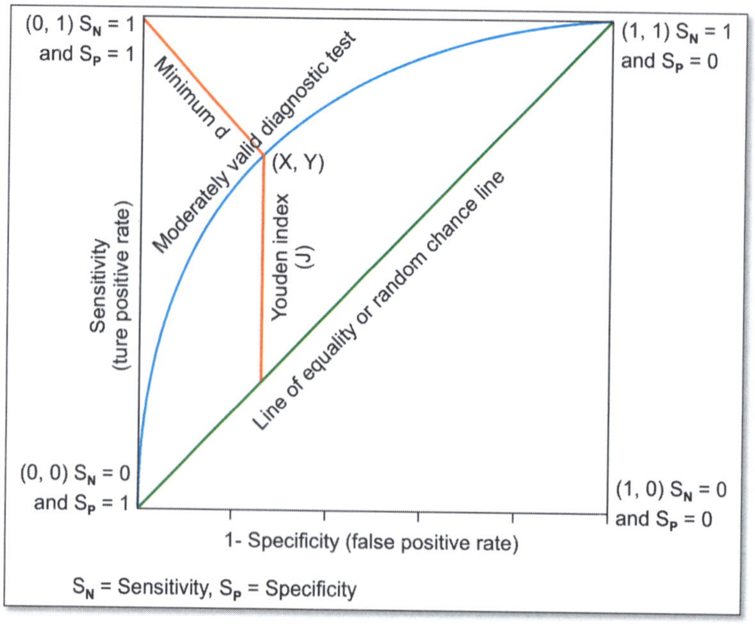

Fig. 2: Receiver-operator characteristic curves

13 **Must Remember**

Features of the ROC:

- ROC is independent of the prevalence of the disease (as it is based on sensitivity and specificity of the disease)
- Two or more diagnostic tests can be visually compared on ROC

Interpreting the ROC

If we look at the graph in figure 3, ROC is drawn between sensitivity and 1-specificity.
For a good test:

- The sensitivity should be high – i.e. the result point should be higher up in the graph
- The 1-specificity (false positive rate) should be lowest as possible – i.e. the result point should be most toward left in the graph

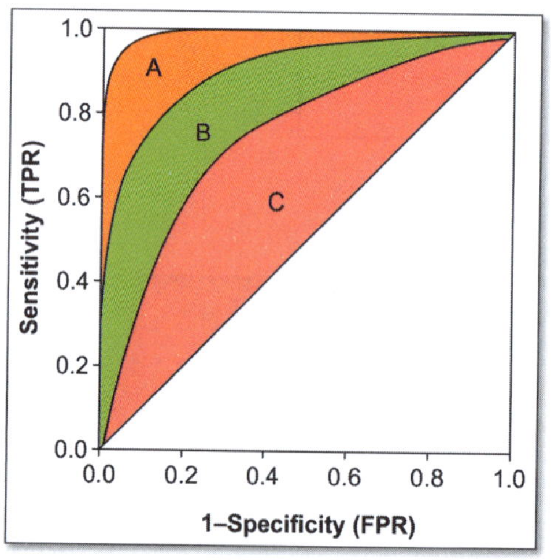

Fig. 3: ROC between sensitivity and 1–Specificity

12 **High Yield Points**

Youden Index

- Youden's Index (delta p') = (sensitivity + specificity) – 1
- It is a way of summarizing the performance of a diagnostic test.
- Its value ranges from 0 to 1, and has a zero value when a diagnostic test gives the same proportion of positive results for groups with and without the disease, i.e. the test is useless. A value of 1 indicates that there are no false positives or false negatives, i.e. the test is perfect.
- Usually not used as single index, but in combination with assessment of precision of the test

Thus the best test would be the curve which has the maximum area under the curve (Fig. 3).

Also in the Figure 2, we can see the Youden's index. It is a measure for the usefulness of the test and also to find the optimum cut off for the investigation.

The Youden's Index is the index for 'area under curve'. The higher the Youden's index, the better the test is for a particular condition. Youden's Index is given by formula: (sensitivity + specificity) – 1. The value ranges from 0 to 1

0 = not useful test, 1 = highly useful test

As we can see here, the best investigation is curve 'A', which has maximum sensitivity and lowest false positive (or 1-specificity).

Hence, we can grossly say that the best investigation is one which has the curve, which is most upwards and left on ROC (at intercept 0, 1).

The use of ROC are:

- Finding optimal cut-off point to least misclassify diseased or non-diseased subjects
- Evaluating the discriminatory ability of a test to correctly pick diseased and non-diseased subjects
- Comparing the efficacy of two or more tests for assessing the same disease
- Comparing two or more observers measuring the same test (interobserver variability).

Interpretation–Validity, Accuracy, Precision

Validity

- It refers to the diagnostic or criterion validity. It measures the extent to which the results obtained from a screening test are within a desired range for a disease condition
- The validity of the results of the screening test are measured and expressed in terms of
    - Sensitivity
    - Specificity

Measures of the Diagnostic Validity:

- Construct validity – refers to the basic foundation for the research principle. It accounts for the hypothesis and method to tests for the hypothesis
- Content Validity: the extent to which 'all components' of a variable are taken into consideration
- Criterion validity: it is the extent to which the results from the investigation are related to the outcome. Example – to what degree does S. Ferritin studies predict the anemic status of a person or obesity for CAD in a patient.
    - Concurrent validity – when the result of investigation and outcome are measured at same time
    - Predictive validity – when the results may be valid to predict an outcome.
    - Eg:
        - Obesity has high predictive validity for coronary artery disease
        - S. Ferritin levels have a reasonable concurrent validity for anemia as outcome
- Discriminant validity: the extent to which the investigation may be able to differentiate from other diseases of similar group

Note: Validity is a term used in Statistics. It may be applicable in different types as:

For study Designs and research methods:

- Internal validity: when the results obtained from the study are applicable to the same population with a high degree of authenticity or causal relationship.
    - It is determined by research methodology and robust design of the study
    - It is also affected by confounding and bias in the study
- External validity: when the results obtained are applicable to other populations or different places. It relates to concern that – if the results can be generalized to larger populations?
    - It is largely determined by the sample size of the study
- Ecological validity: when the results obtained from the experimental research study are applicable to the real world

Accuracy

- It is the degree of closeness of a measured/calculated quantity to its actual value.
    - **Tests for accuracy:** Mean chart, Levy Jennings [LJ] chart, Shewhart control chart
    - The accuracy of an investigation/test may also be measured by:

$$\textit{Accuracy of a screening test} = \frac{\textit{true positive} + \textit{true negative}}{\textit{true positive} + \textit{true negative} + \textit{false positive} + \textit{false negative}}$$

Precision (or Reliability)

- Also known as repeatability or reliability or precision or reproducibility
- It means the test must give consistent results when repeated more than once on the same individual or material, under similar conditions
- Repeatability depends on - Observer variation (intra observer and interobserver), biological variation and Technical Errors relating instrument/methods

10 **Good to Remember**

The test which is most towards the 0,1 value (up and left corner) on the graph is the best curve

13 *High Yield Points*

R Charts (Range charts)

- Tells about the stability of the test results (or repeatability)

14 *High Yield Points*

LJ Charts

These are used for quality control testing in laboratories. These charts are graphical presentation for the closeness to the mean value (hence may be a measure for both validity, variability (precision) and closeness to the central (mean) value.

11 *Good to Remember*

Efficacy/Efficiency/Effectivity

- **Efficacy:** It is measure of outcome in terms of effect produced at a particular input level. It pertains to vaccine, drugs or any intervention (Roughly corresponding to the potency or dose of the drug)
- **Efficiency:** It is a measured in controlled conditions to know the effect of the agent or intervention, i.e. Does intervention "work" under ideal, "laboratory" conditions?
- **Effectiveness:** It is the measure of accuracy or success of a diagnostic or therapeutic technique, when carried out in an average clinical environment, i.e. if we administer the agent in a "real-life" situation, is it effective?

Tests for precision - Range (R) chart, LJ charts

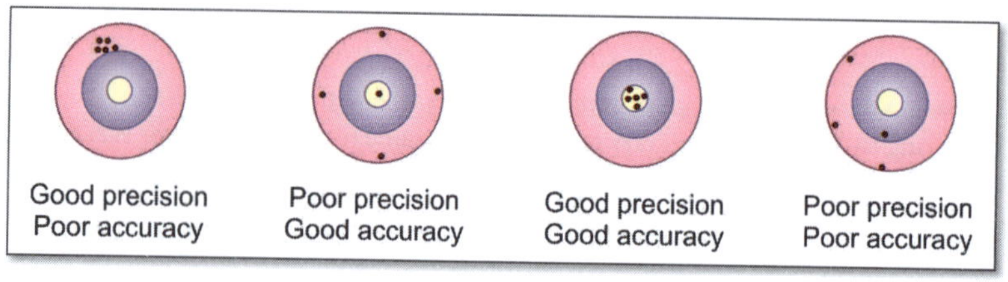

Fig. 4: Tests for precision - Range chart, LJ charts

Example 1: R chart for complete blood count over the days of hospitalization

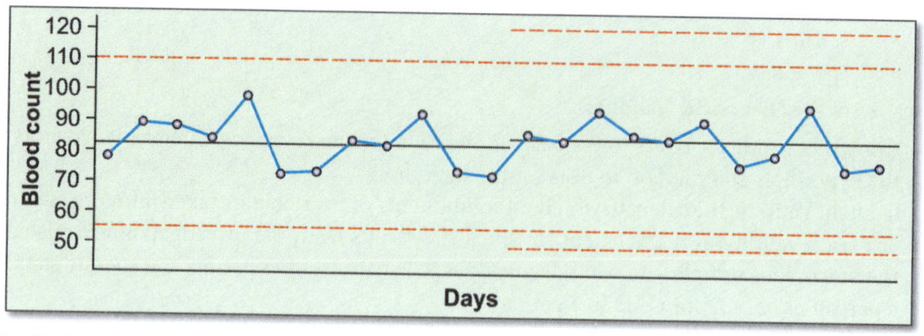

Fig. 5: Mean ($\bar{x}$) and range chart of complete blood count over the days of hospitalization

Example 2: Range chart of potassium levels in hospitalized patient

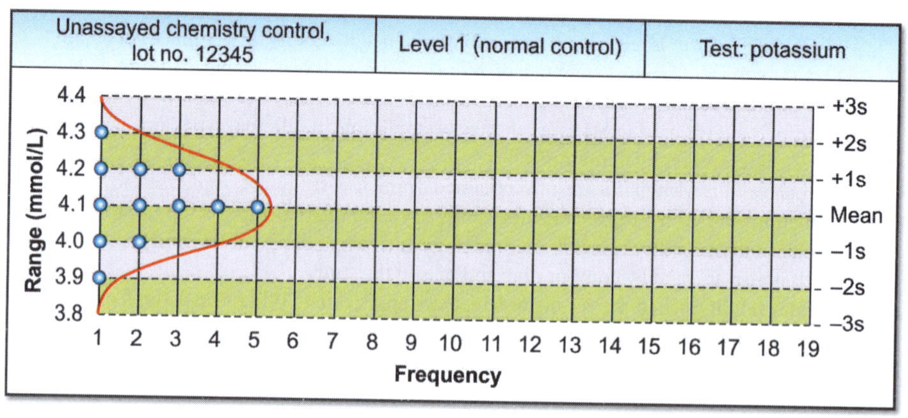

Fig. 6: Range chart

Example 3: LJ chart of blood sugar levels

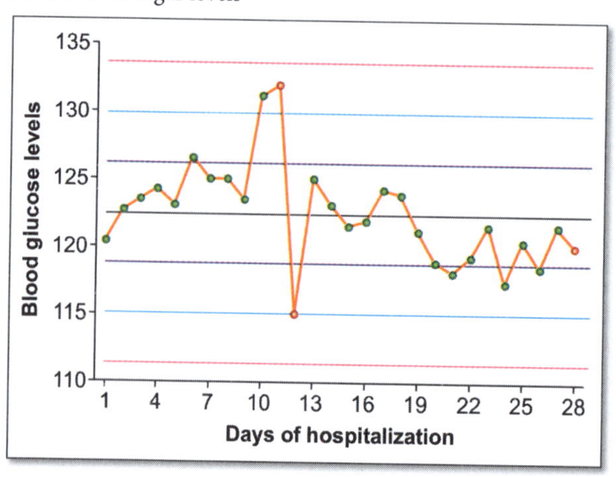

Fig. 7: Levey-jennings chart of blood sugar levels with mean 122 mg/dL, SD = 9.65, CV% = 3.83

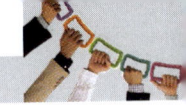

15 High Yield Points

Yield of Test: The number of cases detected

- It can be estimated from the positive predictive value.
- Sensitivity and specificity are characteristics of the test and are only influenced by the test characteristics and the criterion of positivity that is selected.
- The positive predictive value of a test, or the yield, is very dependent on the prevalence of the disease in the population being tested. The higher the prevalence of disease is in the population being screened, the higher the positive predictive values (and the yield).
- The primary means of increasing the yield of a screening program is to target the test to groups of people who are at higher risk of developing the disease

Multiple Choice Questions

1. **The sensitivity of a diagnostic test is very high. What does it signify.** *(AIIMS Nov 2017)*
   a. If it is positive, the patient has the disease
   b. If it is negative, the patient does not have the disease
   c. If the disease is rare, and the test comes positive, patient is likely to have the disease
   d. If the disease is prevalent in the population, a patient is likely to have the test positive.
2. **A diabetes screening trial on 1000 random individuals, 100 patients were found to be diabetic using a gold standard investigation, out of which 90 were tested positive using a new screening method. Calculate the sensitivity of the new investigation?** *(Recent Question 2018)*
   a. 90 /1000 b. 9 /1000
   c. 90 /100 d. 90 /900
3. **A new test in red line has been designed to diagnose a disease condition. The test is being applied to both normal and diseased population. The graph of which is given below. Which of the following is correct regarding the new test** *(AIIMS May 2017)*

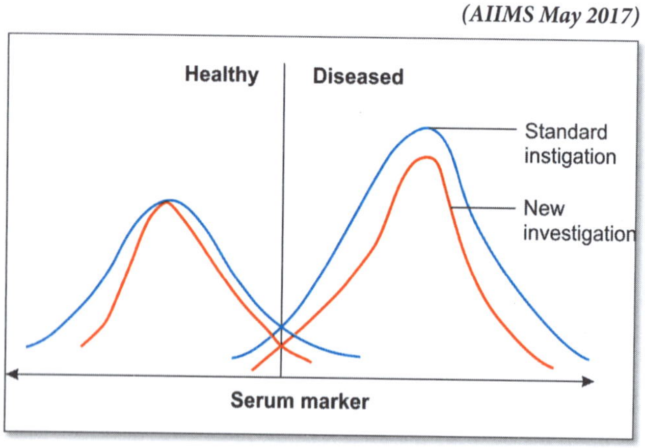

   a. High sensitivity and high specificity
   b. High sensitivity and low specificity
   c. Low sensitivity and low specificity
   d. Low sensitivity and high specificity
4. **A pharmaceutical company introduced a new pregnancy kit. It shows out of 100 pregnant women, 99 were positive and out of 100 nonpregnant women, 90 negative. Sensitivity is:** *(Recent Question 2017)*
   a. 95% b. 97%
   c. 98% d. 99%
5. **Sensitivity formula is:**
   a. TP/TP + FP × 100 b. TN/TN + FN × 100
   c. TP/TP + FN × 100 d. TN/FP + TN × 100
6. **All the following are true regarding screening with reference to periodic health examination, except:**
   a. Requires little physician-time
   b. Capable of wide application
   c. Relatively inexpensive
   d. The physician is required to administer the test
7. **Time lag between first possible detection and usual time of diagnosis is:** *(Recent Question 2017)*
   a. Screening time b. Lead time
   c. Serial interval d. Generation time
8. **True positives are defined as:**
   a. Patient tested positive without having disease
   b. Patient tested positive and having disease
   c. Patient tested negative without having disease
   d. Patient tested negative but having disease
9. **The ability of a test to correctly diagnose the percentage of sick people who are having the condition is called?**
   a. Sensitivity b. Specificity
   c. Positive predictive value d. Negative predictive value
10. **A new screening test was designed for a disease. In a population of 10,000, thousand persons were selected for the study. The Gold standard test showed 100 persons as test positive and diagnosed as diseased, while a new investigation showed 180 individuals as tested positive. Out of total tested positive, 81 individuals were those who were also diagnosed as diseased using the gold standard test. The sensitivity of the new test would be:**
    a. 45% b. 65%
    c. 81% d. 35%

SCREENING

11. **A screening test (when compared to diagnostic test) is characterized by which of the following:**
    1. Done on healthy individuals *(Recent Question 2017)*
    2. Done on unhealthy people
    3. More accurate 4. Less accurate
    5. Less expensive 6. More expensive
    7. Not a basis for treatment
    8. Used as a base for treatment

    Select the correct answer using the code given below
    a. 2, 4, 5 and 8 b. 1, 3, 5 and 8
    c. 2, 3, 6 and 7 d. 1, 4, 5 and 7
12. **Which of the following type of screening is most productive?**
    a. Mass screening b. High risk screening
    c. Monophasic screening d. Multiphasic screening
13. **Use of clinical or laboratory tests to detect disease in individuals seeking health care for other reasons is called:**
    a. Screening b. Case finding
    c. Diagnosis d. Monitoring
14. **VDRL test to detect syphilis in pregnant women is an example of:** *(Recent Question 2016)*
    a. Mass screening b. Case finding
    c. Diagnostic test d. Surveillance
15. **A disease must fulfill all of the following criteria for screening, except:**
    a. The disease should be an important health problem
    b. The natural history of the diseases should be adequately understood
    c. Facilities for the confirmation of the diagnosis are not available
    d. There is an effective treatment

Ans.

1.	d
2.	c
3.	a
4.	d
5.	c
6.	d
7.	b
8.	b
9.	a
10.	c
11.	d
12.	b
13.	b
14.	b
15.	c

Most Recent Questions of 2019-18 are given at the end of MCQs

16. A disease considered for screening should fulfil which of the following criteria: *(Recent Question 2016)*
a. Prevalence should be <3/1000
b. High case fatality rate
c. Should have an effective treatment
d. There could be minor gaps in natural history of disease

17. When people are primarily screened for their own benefit it is called:
a. Prescriptive screening b. Prospective screening
c. Multiphasic screening d. High risk screening

18. Screening of cervical cancer in lower socioeconomic groups is an example of:
a. Mass screening b. High-risk screening
c. Multiphasic screening d. Prospective screening

19. Screening is done because of all except:
a. To test for infection or disease in a population or in individuals who are not seeking health care
b. Presumptive identification of unrecognized disease
c. Search for unrecognized diseases or defect by means of rapidly applied test, examinations or other procedures in apparently healthy individuals
d. Use of clinical or laboratory tests to detect disease in individual seeking health care for other reasons

20. Best time to screen is breast self-examination (BSE) is:
a. 1 week before menstruation
b. 1 week after menstruation
c. During ovulation
d. 2–3 days post – ovulation

21. Criteria for a disease fit for screening include:
a. It should be an important public health problem
b. Facilities should be available for confirmation
c. There should be sufficiently long time available
d. All of the above

22. Example of multiphasic screening is:
a. Chest X-ray for TB on large population
b. Annual health check up
c. Pap smear in old females
d. Mammography in all young females

23. Benefit of screening is: *(Recent Question 2016)*
a. Prevention of disease/cancer
b. Early treatment of disease
c. Provide rehabilitation
d. Diagnosing all the missing cases

24. In case of PAP smear being a screening test for carcinoma cervix which of the following statement it is not true: *(Recent Question 2016)*
a. Visual inspection of cervix is good enough in patient >65 years old and regular PAP screening is not needed
b. In case of HPV testing negative the test can be repeated once in 5 years
c. If PAP smear did not show any abnormality the test can be repeated in 3 years
d. The screening can be intense between 25 and 40 years as it the most needed time

25. In which of the following disease, screening procedure increases the overall survival maximum?
a. Childhood leukemia b. Lung cancer
c. Colon cancer d. Ovarian cancer

26. Screening is not useful for which of the following cancer
a. Carcinoma colon b. Breast carcinoma
c. Prostate carcinoma d. Testicular carcinoma

27. Screening test for breast and genital tract malignancy is all except: *(Recent Question 2016)*
a. CA- 125 b. Mammography
c. Endometrial aspiration d. Pap smear

28. Which of the following is not useful as a screening method?
a. Pap smear for cervical cancer
b. CA – 125 for ovarian cancer
c. Endometrial washing for endometrial cancer
d. USG in endometrial cancer

29. In the following natural history of disease. Which is B-X duration:

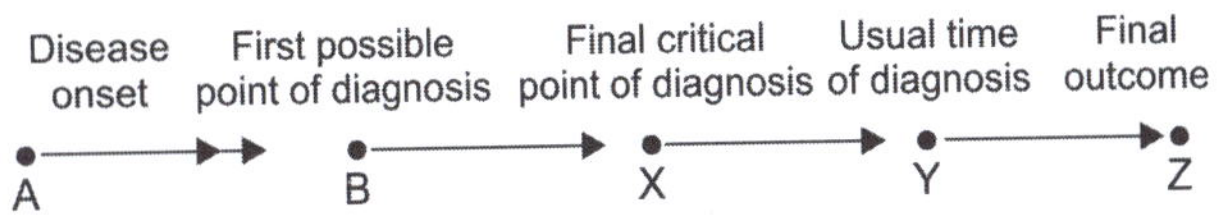

a. Lead time b. Lag time
c. Screening time d. None

30. In following figure, which point is usual time of diagnosis:

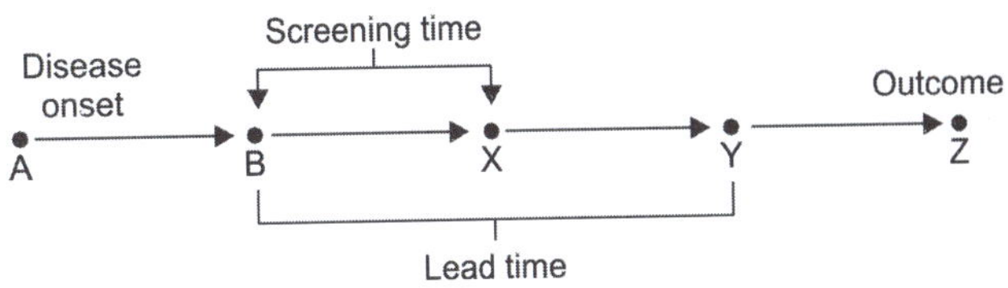

a. A b. B
c. X d. Y

31. Time between first possible point of diagnosis to final critical point of disease is: *(Recent Question 2015)*
a. Lag time b. Lead time
c. Screening time d. Log time

32. Lead time is defined is as:
a. Time between diagnosis and treatment
b. Time between points where the diagnosis is made by screening test to usual diagnosis.
c. Time between disease onset and outcome
d. Time between usual time of diagnosis and outcome

33. 'Lead time' refers to the time between:
a. Disease onset and first critical diagnosis
b. Disease onset and first possible point of detection.
c. First possible point of detection and first critical diagnosis.
d. First point of detection and usual time of diagnosis.

34. Most specific screening test for vitamin D deficiency is:
a. 7- dehydrocholesterol b. 1, 5 dihydroxy Vitamin D
c. 25 hydroxy Vitamin D d. Serum calcium levels

35. Screening is recommended for a condition when:
a. Low case fatality rate
b. Diagnostic tools not available
c. No effective treatment available
d. Early diagnosis can change disease course because of effective treatment

36. Screening of diseases is which type of prevention? *(Recent Question 2016)*
a. Primordial b. Primary
c. Secondary d. Tertiary

Ans.

16. c
17. a
18. b
19. a
20. b
21. d
22. b
23. b
24. a
25. c
26. d
27. a
28. b
29. c
30. d
31. c
32. b
33. d
34. c
35. d
36. c

Most Recent Questions of 2019-18 are given at the end of MCQs

37. **Most reliable test for screening diabetes mellitus is:**
    a. GTT b. Glycosylated haemoglobin
    c. Fasting blood sugar d. Urine for sugar
38. **Blood screening is not done for:** ***(Recent Question 2015)***
    a. HIV b. HBV
    c. EBV d. HCV
39. **Screening of cervical cancer at PHC level is done by:**
    a. History of clinical examination
    b. Colposcopy
    c. Visual Inspection with acetic acid
    d. PAP smear
40. **Screening strategy for prevention of blindness from diabetic retinopathy according to the NPCB involves:**
    a. Opportunistic screening
    b. High-risk screening
    c. Mass screening
    d. Screening by primary care physician

PRECISION/RELIABILITY

41. **If one person examines a blood-smear and finds malaria parasite while a second person examines the same slide and finds it normal, this is called:** ***(Recent Question 2015)***
    a. Intraobserver variation
    b. Interobserver variation
    c. Biological variation
    d. Errors relating to technical methods
42. **The following variation in a test can be reduced by repeat measurements over time:**
    a. Intraobserver variation b. Interobserver variation
    c. Biological variation d. Technical faults

VALIDITY

43. **The ability of a screening test to distinguish those who have disease from those who don't have is called:**
    a. Validity b. Reliability
    c. Precision d. Acceptability
44. **Which of the following is NOT a component of validity of a screening test?** ***(Recent Question 2014)***
    a. Sensitivity b. Specificity
    c. Precision d. Predictive value

PREDICTIVE VALUE OF A POSITIVE/NEGATIVE TEST

45. **Denominator of negative predictive value is:**
    a. TP + FP b. TP + FN
    c. TN + FN d. TN + FP
46. **CA 125 marker levels for screening of ovarian cancer was measured. 60 out of 100 patients with positive test results had Ca Ovary and 20 out of 100 tested negative had Ca Ovary confirmed by histopathology. Calculate the positive predictive value:**
    a. 60% b. 80%
    c. 75% d. 90%
47. **NPV is given by the formula:** ***(Recent Question 2014)***
    a. True positives/(True positives + False positives) × 100
    b. True negatives/(False negatives + True negatives) × 100
    c. True positives/(True positives + False negatives) × 100
    d. True negatives/(False positives + True negatives) × 100
48. **The performance of a screening test is measured by:**
    a. Sensitivity b. Specificity
    c. Predictive value d. Reliability
49. **If the prevalence of a disease in a locality increases, the positive predictive value of a screening test for the disease will:** ***(Recent Question 2014)***
    a. Increase b. Decrease
    c. Remain the same d. None
50. **Positive predictive value is a function of sensitivity, specificity and.....**
    a. Incidence
    b. Prevalence
    c. Negative predictive value
    d. Accuracy
51. **Numerator in calculating positive predictive value:**
    a. True positive b. False positive
    c. True negative d. False negative
52. **True statement about Positive Predictive Value is:**
    a. It increases with prevalence
    b. It decreases with prevalence
    c. No relation with prevalence
    d. Doubles with decrease in prevalence
53. **If the prevalence of a disease in a population increases, the predictive value of a positive tests:**
    a. Increases
    b. Decreases
    c. Remains constant
    d. Becomes compromised
54. **If prevalence is increased, which of the following will be seen:** ***(Recent Question 2014)***
    a. Sensitivity increase
    b. Specificity decrease
    c. Increase positive predictive value
    d. Decrease positive predictive value
55. **In a population of 10000 people, the prevalence of a disease is 20%. The sensitivity of a screening test is 95% and specificity is 80%. The positive predictive value of the test will be:** ***(Recent Question 2013)***
    a. 54.3% b. 45.7%
    c. 15.3% d. 98.5%
56. **A diagnostic test for a particular disease has a sensitivity of 0.90 and a specificity of 0.60. A single test is applied to each subject in the population in which the diseased population is 20%. Probability of a person, negative to this test, has no disease is**
    a. 80% b. 70%
    c. 95% d. 72%
57. **The diagnostic power of a test is reflected by:**
    a. Sensitivity
    b. Specificity
    c. Predictive value
    d. Population attributable risk

SENSITIVITY AND SPECIFICITY

58. **Sensitivity formula is**
    a. TP/TP+FP × 100 b. TN/TN+FN × 100
    c. TP/TP+FN × 100 d. TN/FP+TN × 100

Ans.

37.	a
38.	c
39.	d
40.	b
41.	b
42.	c
43.	a
44.	c
45.	c
46.	a
47.	b
48.	c
49.	a
50.	b
51.	a
52.	a
53.	a
54.	c
55.	a
56.	c
57.	c
58.	c

59. **(A/[A + C]) × 100 will be the formula for:**

Test result	Persons with disease	Persons without disease	Total
Positive	A	B	A+B
Negative	C	D	C+D

a. Specificity b. Sensitivity
c. PPV d. NPV

60. **Denominator in sensitivity is:**
a. Total number of healthy people
b. Total number of diseased people
c. Total number of people showing positive results
d. Total number of people showing negative results

61. **Numerator in case of sensitivity is:**
a. True positives b. True Negatives
c. False Positive d. False Negative

62. **A pharmaceutical company introduced a new pregnancy kit. It shows out of 100 pregnant women, 99 were positive and out of 100 non pregnant women, 90 negative. Sensitivity is:** *(Recent Question 2013)*
a. 95 b. 97
c. 98 d. 99

63. **More false positive cases in a screening test is due to:**
a. Low prevalence b. High specificity
c. High PPV d. Low sensitivity

64. **Numerator in case of sensitivity is:**
a. False positives b. False negatives
c. True negatives d. True positives

65. **Sensitivity measures:** *(Recent Question 2013)*
a. True positive b. False positive
c. True negative d. False negative

66. **Which of the following is included in the formula for calculating sensitivity of a screening test?**
a. True positive b. True negative
c. Total negative d. False positive

67. **If the cut-off point of a screening test is lowered then:**
a. Sensitivity ↑, Specificity ↓
b. Sensitivity ↑, Specificity ↑
c. Sensitivity ↓, Specificity ↓
d. Sensitivity ↓, Specificity ↑

68. **During a screening 5000 persons were screened for a disease. Among the 500 diseased, 350 reported True positive and out of 4500 healthy, 3000 reported True negative. Which of the following is correct about this screening test?**
a. Sensitivity 70% b. Specificity 70%
c. Sensitivity 80% d. Specificity 80%

69. **Recently a latex agglutination test was approved for detection of meningitis, calculate the sensitivity and specificity based on the given findings?**

	Test (+)	Test (–)
Diseased	27	3
Non diseased	5	95

a. 90% sensitivity and 95% specificity
b. 90% sensitivity and 90% specificity
c. 95% sensitivity and 95% specificity
d. 95% sensitivity and 90% specificity

70. **If a test is 90% specific, then:** *(Recent Question 2014)*
a. 90% of disease persons will be true positive
b. 10% of diseased person will be false negative
c. 90% of non-diseased persons will be true negative
d. 10% of non-diseased persons will be false negative

71. **A test has sensitivity of 90% and specificity 95%. True statement:**
a. The test is likely to be useful for general screening
b. Sensitivity = True positive/(True positive + False negative)
c. Sensitivity indicates the test is negative when disease is present
d. 10% positive tests are false positive

72. **Number of false positive in a screening test will be high because of:** *(Recent Question 2014)*
a. High specificity b. Low sensitivity
c. High prevalence d. Low prevalence

73. **The following results of a screening test will burden diagnostic facilities and bring discredit to screening program:**
a. True negatives b. True positive
c. False negatives d. False positives

74. **A city has a population of 10,000 with 500 diabetic patients. A new diagnostic test gives true positive result in 350 patients and false positive result in 1900 patients. Which of the following is/are true regarding the test?**
a. Prevalence is 5% b. Sensitivity is 70%
c. Specificity is 80% d. Sensitivity is 80%
e. Specificity is 70%

75. **Validity includes:** *(Recent Question 2016)*
a. Sensitivity and specificity
b. Precision
c. Acceptability
d. None

76. **Which of the following is/are true about a screening test?**
a. Sensitivity is 1 – false positive rate
b. Specificity is 1 – false negative rate
c. Posttest possibility is pre test probability multiplied by prevalence
d. Predictive value does not depend on prevalence
e. None of the above

77. **Most important factor for a test to be a good screening test is:** *(Recent Question 2015)*
a. Specificity b. Sensitivity
c. Reliability d. Predictive value

78. **Most number of false positives by a screening test is because:**
a. High specificity b. High sensitivity
c. High prevalence d. Low sensitivity

79. **All of the following characteristics are of importance in a screening test, except:**
a. Low sensitivity b. High safety margin
c. High sensitivity d. High specificity

80. **A new test for diabetes was carried out of the 80 people who were tested positive (+ve), it was found that actually 40 had diabetes and out of 9920 people who were tested negative (–ve) only 9840 did not have the disease actually. The sensitivity of this new test is:** *(Recent Question 2015)*
a. 33% b. 50%
c. 65% d. 99%

Ans.

59. b
60. b
61. a
62. d
63. a
64. d
65. a
66. a
67. a
68. a
69. a
70. c
71. b
72. d
73. d
74. a, b,
75. a
76. e
77. b
78. b
79. d
80. a

81. A screening test was used for assessment of Hypertension among middle aged population in a district. In the urban area the prevalence of depression was known to be 25% and in the rural area it was 2.5%. Which of the following comments regarding the screening test is true?

a. Sensitivity of the test in urban area would be 10 times that of in rural area
b. Specificity of the test in urban area would be 10 times that of in the rural area
c. Specificity of the test in the urban area would be 1/10th of that in the rural area sensitivity will be the same in two areas
d. The predicative values of the test would vary between rural and urban areas

82. In a study to evaluate the use of creatine kinase (CK) as a diagnostic test for acute myocardial infarction (AMI), 360 consecutive patients were admitted to CCU with suspected AMI. A CK level of 180 IU was selected as normal. Among 360 patients 220 had AMI out of which 180 were positive for CK. Out of 140 who did not have AMI, 50 were positive for CK. What is probability that a patient who has not suffered AMI will have a negative CK?

(Recent Question 2016)

a. 50% b. 60%
c. 70% d. 80%

83. A test which produces similar results when repeated, but values obtained are not close to actual. The test will be termed as:

a. Precise but inaccurate b. Precise and accurate
c. Imprecise and accurate d. Imprecise and inaccurate

84. Study the following table carefully and Calculate the sensitivity of diagnostic test.

	Disease	Healthy
Test +	40	225
Test –	10	225

a. 45%
b. 20%
c. 80%
d. 50%

85. While comparing two diagnostic tests, computerized tomography (CT) and radionuclide (RN) scanning to detect brain tumor it was seen that, at 90% sensitivity the CT scan gives 5% false-positives and the RN scan gives 50% false-positives. It can be said that:

a. The ROC curve for CT scan will be on the right of the ROC for the RN scan
b. The ROC curve for RN scan will to the right of the ROC for the CT scan
c. For a lower false-positive rate, RN scan will have a higher sensitivity
d. For a given false-positive rate CT scan will have a lower positive predictive value

86. If a test has cut off value at point Z, it will have:

a. High PPV
b. Low PPV
c. Low Sensitivity
d. High Specificity

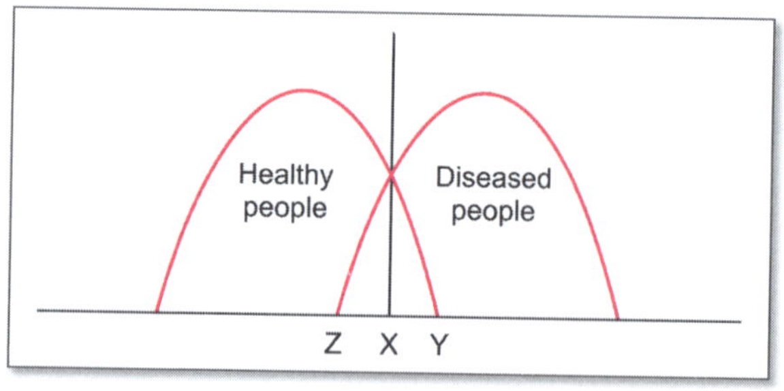

87. A screening test was applied to a population of 1000 individuals, out of which 95 were tested positive from a new investigation. On comparing with the gold standard, 100 individuals were found to be diseased out of which 90 were tested positive from the new investigation. What is the sensitivity of the new investigation?

a. 90/1000
b. 95/1000
c. 90/100
d. 95/100

88. A doctor uses a highly sensitive test on a patient and the result is positive. What does this mean?

a. If it is a rare disease, this can be considered positive
b. Highly unlikely that patient has the disease
c. If the prevalence is high, then the patient has the disease
d. Both A and C

89. A gynecologic oncology research institute isolates a potential tumor marker for endometrial cancer. A large multicenter study is then performed to evaluate serum levels of the tumor marker in women with and without endometrial cancer. The following curves are generated using the results of the study.
Clinical researchers decide to use the tumor antigen to develop a confirmatory test for patients with suspected endometrial cancer. During preliminary design of the test, the cutoff point for positive/negative results is set at point A.

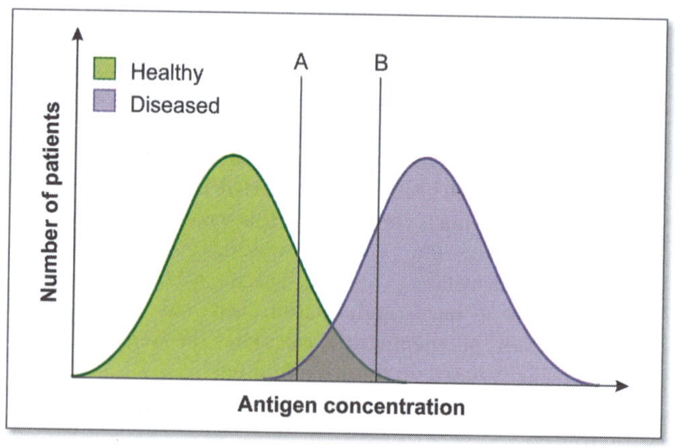

If the cutoff point is moved from A to B, the specificity of the test will change in which of the following ways?

a. Cannot be determined
b. Decreased
c. Increased
d. Unchanged

Ans.

81. d
82. c
83. a
84. c
85. b
86. b
87. c
88. c
89. c

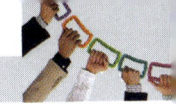

Most Recent Questions (2019–2018)

90. Pick the right answer when 2 screening tests are done in series: *(AIIMS Nov 2018)*
- a. Increased sensitivity and decreased specificity
- b. Increased specificity and decreased sensitivity
- c. Increased sensitivity and increased specificity
- d. Decreased sensitivity and decreased specificity

91. Screening test over confirmatory test, which of the following is/are correct statements *(PGI Nov 2018)*
- a. Higher Sensitivity
- b. Higher Specificity
- c. Higher Negative predictive value
- d. Lower Positive predictive value
- e. Lower False negative rates

92. Screening tests should be: *(PGI May 2018)*
- a. More specific
- b. Expensive
- c. Low sensitivity
- d. Easy to perform
- e. Difficult to perform

93. Probability of a person with positive test result having the disease is given by: *(Recent Question 2019)*
- a. Sensitivity
- b. Specificity
- c. Positive predictive value
- d. Negative predictive value

Ans.

90. b
91. a, e
92. a, d
93. c

Answers with Explanations

1. Ans. (d) If the disease is prevalent in the population, a patient is likely to have the test positive

	Diseased	Healthy	
Test positive	A	B	A+B
Test negative	C	D	C+D
	A+C	B+D	A+B+C+D

Sensitivity – A/A + C
PPV – A/A + B
Specificity – D/B + D
NPV – D/C + D
Sensitivity: probability of having test positive in people with disease
PPV – probability of being diseased if the test is positive
Specificity – probability of having test negative in people who are healthy
NPV – probability of being healthy if the test is negative
Hence, if the Sensitivity is high, it means higher chance of having test positive in a person who is diseased.
Option A, might also look to be the answer, but it is the probability of having disease in person who is 'tested positive' this is given by the positive predictive value

2. Ans. (c) 90 /100

	Diabetes	Healthy	
Test +	90		
Test -	10		
	100	900	1000

Sensitivity = 90/100 = 90%

3. Ans. (a) High sensitivity and high specificity

Ref: Park 23rd edition, Pg. 141

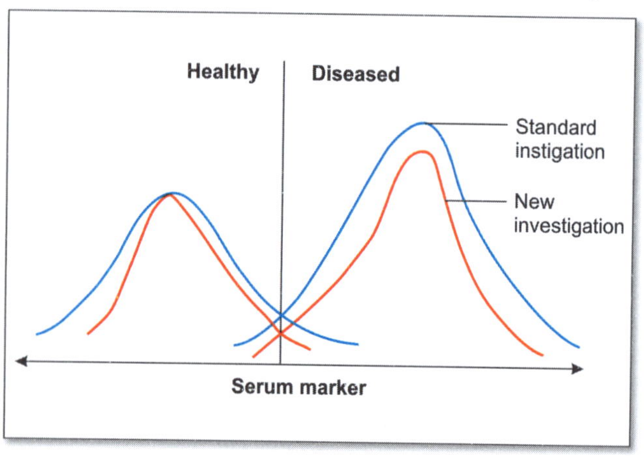

As we see in the image, the area under curve for diseased individuals who may be falsely classified as healthy (because of the cut-off) are called as false negatives and on the other side of cutoff point are the falsely positives.

Hence, if we look at the diagram, we find that the false negatives and false positive are lesser for the red color line (or the new test) compared to the blue color line (or the standard investigation). This implies that the new investigation has a higher sensitivity (low false negatives) and higher false positive (lower false positives) compared to the standard investigation.

4. Ans. (d) 99%

Ref: K. Park, 24th ed. p 149

	Pregnant	Nonpregnant
Kit +ve	99 (TP)	10 (FP)
Kit –ve	1 (FN)	90 (TN)
	100	100

TP = 99
TN = 90
FP = 10
FN = 1
So,
Sensitivity is: TP/(TP + FN)
= 99/100 * 100 = 99%

5. Ans. (c) TP/TP + FN × 100

Ref: K. Park, 24th ed. p 149

6. Ans. (d) The physician is required to administer the test

Ref: K. Park, 24th ed. p 145

7. Ans. (b) Lead time

Ref: K. Park, 24th ed. p 146

8. Ans. (b) Patient tested positive having disease

Ref: K. Park, 24th ed. p 149

9. Ans. (a) Sensitivity

Ref: K. Park, 24th ed. p 149

10. Ans. (c) 80%

Ref: K. Park, 24th ed. p 149

	Dis +	Dis –	
Test +ve	81 (TP)	99 (FP)	180
Test –ve	19 (FN)	801 (TN)	
	100	900	1000

Information provided in MCQ
Values deduced from the information provided
Hence,
Sensitivity = TP/TP + FN
= 81/81+19
= 81/100 *100
= 81%

SCREENING

11. Ans. (d) 1, 4, 5 and 7

Ref: K. Park, 24th ed. p 145

Screening test	Diagnostic test
▪ Done on apparently healthy *persons*[Q]	▪ Done on those with indications or sickness
▪ Applied to groups	▪ Applied to individual patients, all possible diseases are considered
▪ Test results are arbitrary and final	▪ Diagnosis is not final (can be modified with new evidence).
▪ Based on one criterion or cut-off point.	▪ Based on evaluation of a number of symptoms, signs and laboratory findings
▪ Less accurate	▪ More accurate
▪ *Less expensive*[Q]	▪ More expensive
▪ Not a basis for treatment	▪ Used as a basis for treatment
▪ Initiative comes from the investigator	▪ Initiative comes from a patient with a complaint
▪ Test must be – Reliable, Valid, Efficient, Practical and give good yield	▪ The test must be –Reliable, Valid and Efficient

12. Ans. (b) High risk screening

Ref: K. Park, 24th ed. p 147

- ***High risk or selective screening*** is screening applied selectively to high risk groups. E.g. Screening for cancer cervix in the lower social groups. *It is effective and economical*[Q]. (Most productive)

13. Ans. (b) Case finding

Ref: K. Park, 24th ed. p 146

Opportunistic screening or Case finding is use of clinical and/or laboratory tests *to detect disease in individuals seeking health care for other reason*[Q]; E.g. - VDRL to detect syphilis in pregnant women consulting doctor for some other purpose.

14. Ans. (b) Case finding

Ref: K. Park, 24th ed. p 146

15. Ans. (c) Facilities for the confirmation of the diagnosis are not available

Ref: K. Park, 24th ed. p 147

Refer to WHO criteria for Screening in theory section

16. Ans. (c) Should have an effective treatment

Ref: K. Park, 24th ed. p 147

17. Ans. (a) Prescriptive screening

Ref: K. Park, 24th ed. p 146

Uses of Screening

- Prescriptive screening or case detection
- Prospective screening or control of disease
- Research
- As an educational opportunity

18. Ans. (b) High-risk screening

Ref: K. Park, 24thed p-147

Women in the lower socioeconomic groups are at high risk of developing cancer cervix.
Hence, screening for cancer cervix in the lower socioeconomic groups constitutes S***elective or High risk screening***

Also Know.......................

- High risk screening is effective and economical

19. Ans. (a) To test for infection or disease in a population or in individuals who are not seeking health care

Ref: K. Park, 24th ed. p 145

20. Ans. (b) 1 week after menstruation

Ref: How to Perform a Breast Self-Examination. John Hopkins. http://www.hopkinsmedicine.org/healthlibrary/printv.aspx?d=85,P00135

A breast self-exam is a check-up a woman does at home to look for changes or problems in the breast tissue.
- Women can practice BSE at about 20 years of age and continue lifelong, even during pregnancy and after menopause.
- Breast self-examination can be performed every month.
- Best time for self-breast exam is
  - About 3–5 days after start of period
  - Post menopause- a certain day—such as the first day of each month

21. Ans. (d) All of the above

Ref: K. Park, 24th ed. p 147

22. Ans. (b) Annual health check up

Ref: K. Park, 24th ed. p 147

Multiphasic screening is application of two or more screening tests in combination to a large number of people at one time.
- Annual Health Checkup may involves application of 2 or more tests in combination

23. Ans. (b) Early treatment of disease

Ref: K. Park, 24th ed. p 146

Also Know......................

Screening comes under secondary level of prevention and the mode of intervention is early diagnosis and treatment

24. Ans. (a) Visual inspection of cervix is good enough in patient >65 years old and regular PAP screening is not needed

Ref: K. Park, 24th ed. p 147, 407

- Screening is most productive when applied to high risk groups. Incidence of cervical cancer increases sharply from 25–40 years of age and then levels off and declines.
- Hence, intense screening is advisable in the age group 25 -40 years age group.

Screening of Cervical Cancer

Also Know......................

Present strategy is Visual Inspection after application of freshly prepared 5% Acetic acid solution with/without magnification (VIA or VIAM)

- Well-defined opaque acetowhite lesions close to squamocolumnar junction or well-defined circumorificial acetowhite lesion or dense acetowhite ulceroproliferative growth on cervix constitute a positive test

FOGSI – 2017-2018 Update on Ca cervix screening guidelines:

	Good resource setting	Limited resource setting
Modality	HPV testing ▪ Primary HPV testing ▪ Co-testing (HPV & Cytology) Cytology Colposcopy and biopsy VIA	VIA Colposcopy ± Biopsy
Target Age Group (years)	25–65	30–65 (In postmenopausal women, screening with VIA may not be as effective)
Age to start (years)	Cytology at 25 Primary HPV Testing/ Co-testing at 30 years	30 years
Frequency	Primary HPV Testing or Co-testing - every 5 years Cytology – every 3 years	Every 5 years (at least 1-3 times in a lifetime)
Age to stop	▪ 65 years with consistent negative results in last 15 years ▪ Women with no prior screening should undergo tests once at 65 years and, if negative, they should exit screening.	
Follow-up method after treatment; interval	HPV testing (preferred) or Cytology 12 months	VIA (12 monthly)
Screening in hysterectomized women	▪ Following hysterectomy in which cervix was removed for benign causes : no need for screening, unless there is history of previous cervical intraepithelial neoplasia ▪ Absence of cervix must be confirmed by clinical records or examination ▪ If indications for hysterectomy unclear, screening may be performed at clinician's discretion	
F/up with CIN in hysterectomy HPE report	Need to be screened with HPV at 6 months and 18 months	

Contd...

25. Ans. (c) Colon cancer

Ref: CMDT 2014, page-1571

Cancers for which Screening can lead to an improvement in outcome include:

- Cancers of the breast
- Cancer cervix
- Cancer colon
- Cancer prostate
- Cancer oral cavity
- Cancer skin.

Also Know......................

Screening is not useful if

- Method of early detection does not exist (e.g. Cancer of the Pancreas)
- No apparent localized stage (e.g., Leukemia)
- Distant metastases occur early, even from a small primary tumor (e.g., Lung or Ovarian cancer)

Effective Screening requires a test that will[Q]

- Specifically detect early cancers or premalignancies,
- Be cost effective
- Result in improved therapeutic outcomes.

26. Ans. (d) Testicular carcinoma

Ref: CMDT 2014, page-1571

27. Ans. (a) CA-125

Ref:Multiplesources, http://www.uptodate.com/contents/ovarian-cancer-screening-beyond-the-basics?source)

CA 125 tumor marker is a protein that is higher than normal in approximately 80% of women with ovarian cancer.

High CA 125 level is also found in :
- Endometriosis
- Uterine fibroids
- Liver disease (cirrhosis)
- Pelvic infections
- Other cancers, including endometrial, breast, lung, and pancreatic cancer.
- 1% healthy women (Levels change during the menstrual cycle)

As a result, CA 125 is not recommended as a stand-alone screening test for ovarian cancer.

28. Ans. (b) CA-125 for ovarian cancer

Ref: Multiple sources, http://www.uptodate.com/contents/ ovarian-cancer-screening-beyond-the-basics?source)

29. Ans. (c) Screening time

Ref: K. Park, 24th ed. p 146

- Screening time is the time lag between the 1st possible point of diagnosis and Final critical point of diagnosis.
- ***Lead time*** is the advantage gained by screening[Q]. *It is the period between diagnosis by early detection and usual time of diagnosis.*[Q]

30. Ans. (d) Y

Ref: K. Park, 24th ed. p 146

Refer to theory section

31. Ans. (c) Screening time

Ref: K. Park, 24th ed. p 146

32. Ans. (b) Time between point where the diagnosis is made by screening test to usual diagnosis

Ref: K. Park, 24th ed. p 146

- The time difference between the earliest possible point of diagnosis and the critical point of diagnosis is known as – **Screening time**
- The time difference between the earliest possible point of diagnosis and the usual point of diagnosis is known as the– **Lead time**

33. Ans. (d) First point of detection and usual time of diagnosis

Ref: K. Park, 24th ed. p 146

34. Ans. (c) 25 hydroxy Vitamin D

Ref: Clinical Laboratory Medicine by McClatchey, 2/e p446

Vitamin status	Best screening test
Vitamin D	Serum 25 Hydroxy Vitamin D3 level by RIA, Nephelometry, or HPLC
Vitamin E	Ratio of alpha-tocopherol to total plasma lipid
Vitamin K	Prothromin time
Vitamin B1(thiamine)	Erythrocyte or whole blood transketolase activity.
Vitamin B2(Riboflavin)	RBC Glutathione Reductase Activity (Before and After addition of FAD)
Niacin	Urine metabolites, N1- methylnicotinamide and its pyridoxine.
Vitamin B6 (Pyridoxine)	Enzyme assay, Radioimmunoassay or HPLC methods.
Vitamin C (Ascorbic-acid)	Measured by colorimetric, flurometric and HPLC method

Contd...

35. Ans. (d) Early diagnosis can change disease course because of effective treatment

Ref: K. Park, 23rd ed. p 137

36. Ans. (c) Secondary

Ref: K. Park, 24th ed. p 46

"***Screening***" is a secondary level of prevention.
- It seeks to diagnose diseases early among apparently healthy/ asymptomatic individuals to improve outcome.

37. Ans. (a) GTT

Ref: K. Park, 24th ed. p 413

Epidemiological screening of Diabetic mellitus –Glucose Tolerance Test (2-hour value after 75 g oral glucose) alone or with FBS is considered most reliable

Also Know......................

- Standard oral GTT is the cornerstone of diagnosis of diabetes.

38. Ans. (c) EBV

Ref: Standards For Blood Banks and Blood Transfusion Services, National AIDS Control Organisation Ministry of Health and Family Welfare, Government of India, 2007, p-33

Mandatory Screening of Blood Samples for Infectious disease at Blood Bank is done for

- Syphilis - by VDRL/RPR Method/TPHA.
- Viral Hepatitis A, Hepatitis B (HBsAg) and Hepatitis C (anti HCV) by ELISA/Rapid test
- HIV 1and 2 antibodies using ELISA/Rapid
- Malarial parasites using a validated and sensitive antigen test

39. Ans. (c) Visual inspection with acetic acid

Ref: K. Park, 24th ed. p 405

At PHC level- Screening for cancer cervix is done using PAP smear [Lab, Equipment and Trained personnel are available]
- *Visual inspection with 5% acetic acid (VIA), VIA with magnification (VIAM) and visual inspection post application of Lugol's iodine (VILI) are alternative screening tests.*

- *Sensitivity is similar to cytology based screening.*
- *It is easy to carry out and appropriate for peripheral health workers.*

40. Ans. (b) High Risk Screening

Ref: K. Park, 24th ed. p 414

Screening Strategy for prevention of blindness from diabetic retinopathy as per NPCB is

- *High Risk Strategy* [For NIDDM][Q]- Screening is applied selectively to high -risk target population groups.
- *There is no special high risk strategy for IDDM.*

PRECISION/RELIABILITY

41. Ans. (b) Interobserver variation

Ref: K. Park, 24th ed. p 148

Observer Variation

- Intraobserver (or within observer)-Variation between repeated observations by the same observer on the same subject or material at the same time.
  - Minimized by taking average of several replicate measurements at the same time.
- Interobserver or between observer–
  - Variation between different observers on the same subject or material.
  - Minimized by (a) standardization of procedures (b) intensive training of all observers (c) making use of two or more observers for independent assessment, etc.

42. Ans. (c) Biological variation

Ref: K. Park, 24th ed. p 148

Biological (or Subject) Variation

- It is associated with physiological variables e.g. BP, blood sugar, serum cholesterol, etc.
- It occurs due to (a) Changes in the parameters observed, (b) Variations in the way patients perceive their symptoms and answer, (c) Regression to the mean.
- Biological variation is tested by repeat measurements over time.

VALIDITY

43. Ans. (a) Validity

Ref: K. Park, 24th ed. p 148

Validity (Accuracy) is the degree of closeness of a measured/ calculated quantity to its actual value.

- *It has 2 components - Sensitivity and Specificity*[Q].

44. Ans. (c) Precision

Ref: K. Park, 24th ed. p 148

Sensitivity, Specificity and Predictive accuracy are *inherent properties of a screening test*

Types of Validity

Criterion-related validity (predictive validity)	It is consistency of test results with those of a Reference criterion standard (Gold Standard)
Construct validity	Consistency of test results with other tests that measure similar characteristics. It may or may not be quantifiable, depending on the parameters used in its assessment
Content validity	Inclusion of questions representative of the qualities of the test attempts to measure
Face validity	Appearance that a test is adequate for its intended purpose. It encompasses factors like readability and unambiguity of test questions and the overall appearance of the examination.
Internal validity	It measures if the test could have led to an erroneous conclusion. Errors of chance, Bias, Confounding
External validity or Generalizability	It is concerned with the clinical usefulness of the results or broader application

Criterion validity (*predictive validity) is the best measure of validity*

PREDICTIVE VALUE OF A POSITIVE/NEGATIVE TEST

45. Ans. (c) TN + FN

Ref: K. Park, 24th ed. p 150

$$\text{Negative predictive value} = \frac{\text{True negative [TN]}}{\text{True negative [TN] + False negative [FN]}} \times 100$$

- ***Negative* Predictive value [NPV]** is the probability that a patient with a negative test result truly does not have the disease or Ability of a test to identify all those who do not have the disease from all those who tested negative

Also Know......................

- NPV is inversely proportional to prevalence of disease in population

46. Ans. (a) 60%

Ref: K. Park, 24th ed. p 150

As per the MCQ:

- Total test positive patients = 100
- Ca ovary confirmed out of test positive = 60
- Total test negative patients = 100
- Ca ovary confirmed out of test negative cases = 20

So, now if e construct the 2 × 2 table:

	Dis +	Dis –	Total
Test +	60		100
Test –	20		100
Total			200

PPV = 60/100 = 60%
NPV = 80/100 = 80%

47. Ans. (b) True negatives/(False negatives + True negatives) × 100

Ref: K. Park, 24th ed. p 149

48. Ans. (c) Predictive value

Ref: K. Park, 24th ed. p 150

***"Predictive value"** of a screening test reflects the diagnostic power of the test.*[Q]

49. Ans. (a) Increase

Ref: K. Park, 24th ed. p 150

Positive Predictive Value** [PPV] **is the probability that a patient with a positive test result has in actual the disease or Ability of a test to identify all those who have the disease from all those who tested positive.

Also Know.......................

- PPV is same as Post-test probability of a disease in a population. It is directly proportional to prevalence of disease.

50. Ans. (b) Prevalence

Ref: K. Park, 24th ed. p 150

Predictive accuracy depends upon *sensitivity, specificity and disease prevalence*

51. Ans. (a) True Positive

Ref: K. Park, 24th ed. p 149

52. Ans. (a) It increases with prevalence

Ref: K. Park, 24th ed. p 150

As prevalence increases, accuracy of "Predictive value" of a positive screening test increases

53. Ans. (a) Increases

Ref: K. Park, 24th ed. p 150

54. Ans. (c) Increase positive predictive value

Ref: K. Park, 24th ed. p 150

55. Ans. (a) 54.3%

Ref: K. Park, 24th ed. p 149

Population = 10000 and Prevalence of a disease = 20%.
Number of diseased = 20/100 × 10,000 = 2000
Sensitivity of screening test = 95%, So TP = 95/100 × 2000 = 1900

Specificity of screening test = 80%, So TN = 80/100 × 8000 = 6400

Diseased		Not diseased	Total
Positive	1900 [TP]	X = 1600 (8000-6400) FP	3500
Negative	Y = 100 (2000-1900) FN	6400 [TN]	6500
Total	2000	8000	10000

$$\text{Positive predictive value} = \frac{\text{True positive [TP]}}{\text{(True positive [TP] + False positive[FP])}}$$

$$= \frac{1900}{3500} \times 100 = 54.3\%$$

56. Ans. (c) 95%

Ref: K. Park, 24th ed. p 149-50

We know that predictive values can be calculated from the Bayes formula, as follows:

$$\text{PPV} = \frac{\text{Sensitivity} \times \text{Prevalence}}{\text{Sensitivity} \times \text{Prevalence} + (1 - \text{Specificity}) \times (1 - \text{Prevalence})}$$

$$\text{NPV} = \frac{\text{Specificity} \times (1 - \text{Prevalence})}{(1 - \text{Sensitivity}) \times \text{Prevalence} + \text{Specificity} \times (1 - \text{Prevalence})}$$

However, another approach to this problem may be as follows:

Given in the MCQ

- Sensitivity – 0.9
- Specificity – 0.6
- Prevalence – 20%
- **Calculate – NPV?**

	Disease +	Healthy
Test +	True positive (TP)	False positive (FP)
Test –	False negative (FN)	True negative (TN)

Step – 1 – use prevalence for D+ (assuming the total population to be 100)
So, D+ –20
Hence, The D– will be 80 (100–20)

	Disease +	Healthy	Total
Test +	True positive (TP)	False positive (FP)	
Test –	False negative (FN)	True negative (TN)	
Total =	20	80	100

Step 2
Use sensitivity to calculate true positive
Sensitivity (Sn) = TP/D+
∴ TP = Sn * D+
⇒ TP = 0.9 * 20 = 18
Hence, FN = (D+) – TP
⇒ **FN = 20 – 18 = 2**

	Disease +	Healthy	Total
Test +	18	False positive (FP)	
Test –	2	True negative (TN)	
Total =	20	80	100

Step 3
Use specificity to calculate true negative
Specificity (Sp) = TN/D–
∴ TN = Sp * D-
⇒ TN = 0.6 * 80 = 48
Hence, FP = (D–) – TN
⇒ **FP = 80 – 48 = 32**

	Disease +	Healthy	Total
Test +	18	32	
Test –	2	48	
Total =	20	80	100

Hence,
NPV = TN / T+
= 48/50 = 96%

57. Ans. (c) Predictive value

Ref: K. Park, 24th ed. p 150

SENSITIVITY AND SPECIFICITY

58. Ans (c) TP/TP+FN x 100

Ref: K. Park, 24th ed. p 149

Sensitivity: Probability of having test positive in people who are diseased

	Disease +	Healthy
Test +	True positive (TP)	False positive (FP)
Test –	False negative (FN)	True negative (TN)

Sensitivity = TP / D+

59. Ans. (b) Sensitivity

Ref: K. Park, 24th ed. p 149

Test result	Persons with disease	Persons without disease	Total
Positive	A (TP)	B (FP)	A+B
Negative	C (FN)	D (TN)	C+D

(A/A + C) × 100 = TP/TP + FN × 100 = Sensitivity

60. Ans. (b) Total number of diseased people

Ref: K. Park, 24th ed. p 149

$$\text{Sensitivity} = \frac{\text{True positive [TP]}}{\text{True positive [TP] + False negative [FN]}} \times 100$$

Denominator = TP (Have the disease and are tested positive) + FN (Have the disease but tested negative)= Total diseased cases

61. Ans. (a) True Positive

Ref: K. Park, 24th ed. p 149

If Sensitivity increases → TP increases and FN decreases.[Q]

62. Ans. (d) 99

Ref: K. Park, 24th ed. p 149

99 pregnant women could be identified by the test out of 100 pregnant women , So sensitivity is 99%
90 non pregnant women could be identified by the test out of 100 non pregnant women , So specificity is 90%

Also Know........................

- *If Sensitivity increases → TP increases and FN decreases.*[Q]
- *If Specificity increases → TN increases and FP decreases.*[Q]

63. Ans. (a) Low Prevalence

Ref: K. Park, 24th ed. p 150

False-positive means the patients who does not have the disease, is told to be having the disease
High false positive results is seen when
- Test has low specificity [or high sensitivity][Q]
- Low prevalence even with high specificity[Q]

64. Ans. (d) True positives

Ref: K. Park, 24th ed. p 149

65. Ans. (a) True positives

Ref: K. Park, 24th ed. p 149

66. Ans. (a) True positive

Ref: K. Park, 24th ed. p 149

67. Ans. (a) Sensitivity ↑, Specificity ↓

Ref: K. Park, 24th ed. p 151

If the cut-off of a screening test is lowered → Sensitivity ↑, Specificity ↓
If the cut-off of a screening test is raised → Sensitivity ↓, Specificity ↑

Factors that Decide the cut off are

- Disease prevalence- If prevalence is high, cut off is set at a lower level
- Disease-If the disease is lethal and early detection improves prognosis, cut off is set at a lower level

68. Ans. (a) Sensitivity 70%

Ref: K. Park, 24th ed. p 149

Test Result	Diseased	Non Diseased	Total
Positive	350 [TP]	1500 [FP]	1850
Negative	150 [FN]	3000 [TN]	3150
Total	500	4500	5000

$$\text{Sensitivity} = \frac{[TP]}{[TP]+FP]} \times 100 = \frac{350}{500} \times 100 = 70\%$$

$$\text{Specificity} = \frac{[TP]}{[TN]+[FP]} \times 100 = \frac{3000}{4500} \times 100 = 66.7\%$$

69. Ans. (a) 90% Sensitivity and 95% Specificity

Ref: K. Park, 24th ed. p 149

Sensitivity is given by the formula:

$$Senstivity = \frac{True\ positive}{Total\ diseased} \times 100$$

In the MCQ, the 2 × 2 Table is reconstructed as below:

	Total diseased	Total healthy
Test +	27 (TP)	5 (FP)
Test –	3 (FN)	95 (TN)

Hence,

$$Sensitivity = \frac{27}{30} \times 100 = 90\%$$

$$Specificity = \frac{True\ negative}{Total\ healthy} \times 100 = \frac{95}{100} \times 100 = 95\%$$

70. Ans. (c) 90% of non-diseased persons will be true negative

Ref: K. Park, 24th ed. p 149

Sensitivity – "Rule OUT" a disease if the test is "Negative"
Specificity = "Rule IN" a disease, if the test is positive

71. Ans. (b) Sensitivity = True positive/(True positive + False negative)

Ref: K. Park, 24th ed. p 149

72. Ans. (d) Low prevalence

Ref: K. Park, 24th edp-149-51

Remember:

The false positive will be high in case of:

- Low specificity
- Low prevalence
- High sensitivity

73. Ans. (d) False positive

Ref: K. Park, 24th ed. p 150

74. Ans. (a) Prevalence is 5%; (b) Sensitivity is 70%; (c) Specificity is 80%

Ref: K. Park, 24th ed. p 149

	Disease +	Healthy	Total
Test +	$350^{\$}$	$1900^{\$}$	
Test –	150	7600	
Total =	$500^{\$}$	9500	$10{,}000^{\$}$

\$ = Information provided in MCQ
Prevalence = D+ / total population
= 500/10,000 *100 = 5%

$$Sensitivity = \frac{True\ positive}{Total\ diseased} \times 100 = \frac{350}{500} \times 100 = 70\%$$

$$Specificity = \frac{True\ negative}{Total\ healthy} \times 100 = \frac{7600}{9500} \times 100 = 80\%$$

75. Ans. (a) Sensitivity and specificity

Ref: K. Park, 24th ed. p 149-50

76. Ans. (e) None of the above

Ref: K. Park, 23rd ed. p 139-140) NMS Preventive medicine and public health, 2nd edition, p-75, 24th ed. p 149-50

A few formulae to remember:

- $Sensitivity = \frac{True\ positive}{Total\ diseased} \times 100$
- $Specificity = \frac{True\ negative}{Total\ healthy} \times 100$
- $PPV = \frac{TP}{TP + FP} \times 100 = \frac{True\ positive}{Total\ test\ positives} \times 100$
- $NPV = \frac{TN}{TN + FN} \times 100 = \frac{True\ negatives}{Total\ test\ negatives} \times 100$
- *False positive rate = 1 – Specificity or Specificity = 1 – False positive rate*
- *False negativity rate = 1 – Sensitivity or Sensitivity = 1 – False Negative rate*
- *Positive LR = sensitivity/(100 – specificity).*
- *Negative LR = (100 – sensitivity)/specificity.*
- Pre-test odds = p / (1 – p)
- Post-test probability = $ODDS_{post\text{-}test}/(ODDS_{post\text{-}test} + 1)$
- $ODDS_{post\text{-}test} = Odds_{pre\text{-}test} \times LR$

77. Ans. (b) Sensitivity

Ref: K. Park, 24th ed. p 149

78. Ans. (b) High sensitivity

Ref: K. Park, 24th ed. p 149-50 Sensitivity and specificity are inversely related[Q]

79. Ans. (d) High specificity

For a screening test to have a better utility, it is necessary that it should be highly sensitive to be able to detect maximum individuals with disease. This obviously does come at an expense of higher false positive tests, but at large, high sensitivity is the main parameter for the initial screening tests.

Also Know....................

- For screening tests, usually a low cut off is selected, whereas
- For diagnostic tests, usually a higher cut-off is selected to ensure minimum false positives for a common disease

80. Ans. (a) 33%

Ref: K. Park, 24th ed. p 149

	Disease +	Healthy	Total
Test +	$40^{\$}$	40	$80^{\$}$
Test –	80	$9840^{\$}$	$9920^{\$}$
Total =	120	9880	

$ = Information provided in MCQ

Sensitivity = TP/TP + TN

= 40/120 × 100 = 33%

81. Ans: (d) The predicative values of the test would vary between rural and urban areas

	Diseased (D+)	Healthy (D-)	
Test +	True positive (TP)	False positive (FP)	PPV = TP/ TP + FP
Test –	False negative (FN)	True negative (TN)	NPV = TN/ TN + FN
	Sensitivity = TP/ TP + FN	Specificity = TN/ TN + FP	

Hence if we look and analyze the table more closely, it may be observed that the sensitivity and the specificity is essentially a function of the test – i.e. the proportion of test positive in diseased (sensitivity) and test negative in the healthy (specificity). The sensitivity and specificity of the test is a feature of the test and would not vary among the populations with change in the prevalence

Whereas, the predictive value (positive) is probability (or chance) of having disease in people who are tested positive, would obviously be more affected by the prevalence of the disease, than anything else. And the same would also be true for the negative predictive value of the test.

Hence, we can conclude: If the prevalence varies in two populations, the most affected will be the predictive values and not the sensitivity and specificity of the test.

82. Ans. (c) 70%

As per the MCQ, 360 patients were admitted to the CCU with "suspected – MI" out of which

- Total population under study 360
- Number of diseased: 220 (cases who had AMI)
- Number of nondiseased: 140 (who did not have AMI)
- True positive cases = 180 (positive for CK and had AMI)
- False positive cases = 50 (who did NOT have AMI and were positive for CK)

We need to find the "Negative predictive value"

	Diseased	Non Diseased
Positive	TP (180)$	FP (50)$
Negative	FN (40)	TN (90)
Total	220$	140$

$ = information provided in the MCQ

- **Prevalence** = Total number of cases/Mid-year population = 220/360 × 100 = 61%
- **Negative predictive value** = TN/TN + FN × 100 = 90/ (40+90) × 100 = 69.2%

83. Ans. (a) Precise but inaccurate

The test is said to be giving similar results every time. This means that the test has high precision.

However, the test results are noted to be away from the actual value, hence, we may term the test as precise but inaccurate

84. Ans. (c) 80%

Sensitivity of the test is calculated by: TP / TP+FN

	Disease	Healthy
Test +	TP	FP
Test –	FN	TN

Hence,

Sensitivity = TP / TP+FN

= 40 / (40+10) = 40/50 = 80%

85. Ans. (b) The ROC curve for RN scan will to the right of the ROC for the CT scan

The ROC curves are drawn between – Sensitivity and 1-specificty

Recall that:

- Sensitivity corresponds to the true positive
- Specificity corresponds to the true negative
- False positive error corresponds to 1 – specificity
- False negative error corresponds to 1 – sensitivity

Now, as per the MCQ:

At a set sensitivity (of 90%), the CT has lower False positive errors (5%) compared to Radio-Nucleotide scanning (50%). Hence in the ROC curve, at the same sensitivity, the curve for CT will lie more towards left side (lower false positive error) compared to Radio-nucleotide scan.

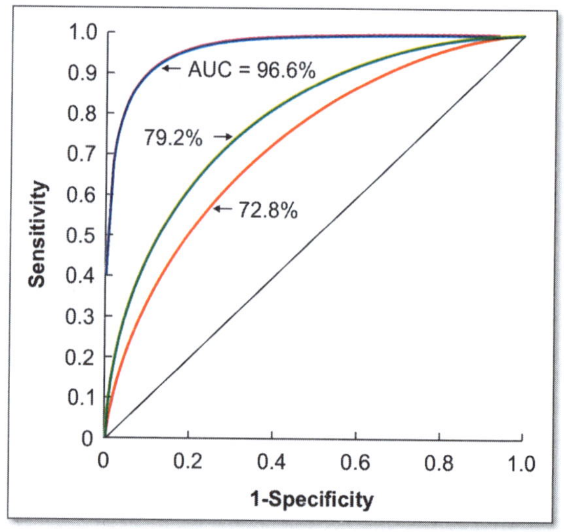

86. Ans. (b) Low PPV

Ref: K. Park, 24th ed p-151

- If a test has cut off value at point Z, it will have-High Sensitivity, High False Positive and Low PPV
- If a test has cut off value at point Y, it will have-High Specificity
- Cut off point is decided on basis of disease prevalence (high prevalence, low cut off), fatality or prognosis of disease

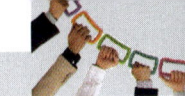

87. Ans. (c) 90/100

As the MCQ reads, 90 were tested positive out of 100 diseased individuals, the sensitivity will be given by 90/100
The calculation is as follows:

	Dis +	Dis -	Total
Test +	90		95
Test -			
Total	100	900	1000

88. Ans. (c) If the prevalence is high, then the patient has the disease

It's a slightly tricky MCQ -
Sensitivity: The probability of person to be tested positive if he was diseased.
Positive predictive value: The probability of person to be diseased if the test result is positive

So, for an investigation, with positive test on a highly sensitive test…means, the true positive are more.

Now, the MCQ is asking for chance of having disease with a positive result from a highly sensitive test - in other words, the MCQ is asking for the positive predicative value.

We should also know that, in case of more common disease prevalence, the true positive is more and higher positive predicative value.

So, if the prevalence is higher and the test result is positive, there is higher chance that the person actually has the disease

89. Ans. (c) Increased

High Specificity
If the Cut of is at Point A: there is lesser False negative, but higher False positives

Now, if the cut-off is moved to point B, there are lesser false positive and higher False negatives.

Hence at Point B, there is lesser False positives, or higher Specificity.

90. Ans. (b) Increased specificity and decreased sensitivity

When screening tests are combined, the combined sensitivity and specificity of the whole array of test will change.

- If the tests are combined in series – the specificity increases, and the sensitivity decreases
- If the tests are combined in parallel – the sensitivity increases, and the specificity decreases

91. Ans. (a) Higher Sensitivity, (e) Lower False negative rates

Option	T/F	Comment
Higher Sensitivity	T	Yes correct
Higher Specificity	F	Not technically correct, as higher specificity we would like to mark for a confirmatory or diagnostic test and not a screening test, as in this MCQ
Higher Negative predictive value	F	No not correct, as predictive values are properties of an investigation which further depend on sensitivity, specificity, and prevalence. The predicative values are dependent on these inputs and not vice versa
Lower Positive predictive value	F	No, not correct
Lower False negative rates	T	Yes, a lower 'false negative' rates implies a higher sensitivity

92. Ans. (a) More specific, (d) Easy to perform

Discussion

Option	T/F	Remarks
More specific	T	Yes correct, it should have high sensitivity and a reasonably high specificity as well
Expensive	F	No, it should not be expensive. a good screening test is affordable, acceptable by society and with good validity (in terms of high sensitivity and validity)
Low sensitivity	F	No, it should not be expensive. a good screening test is affordable, acceptable by society and with good validity (in terms of high sensitivity and validity)
Easy to perform	T	Yes, correct
Difficult to perform	F	No, not correct

93. Ans. (c) Positive predictive value

Ref: Park 25th Ed. Pg 152

NOTES

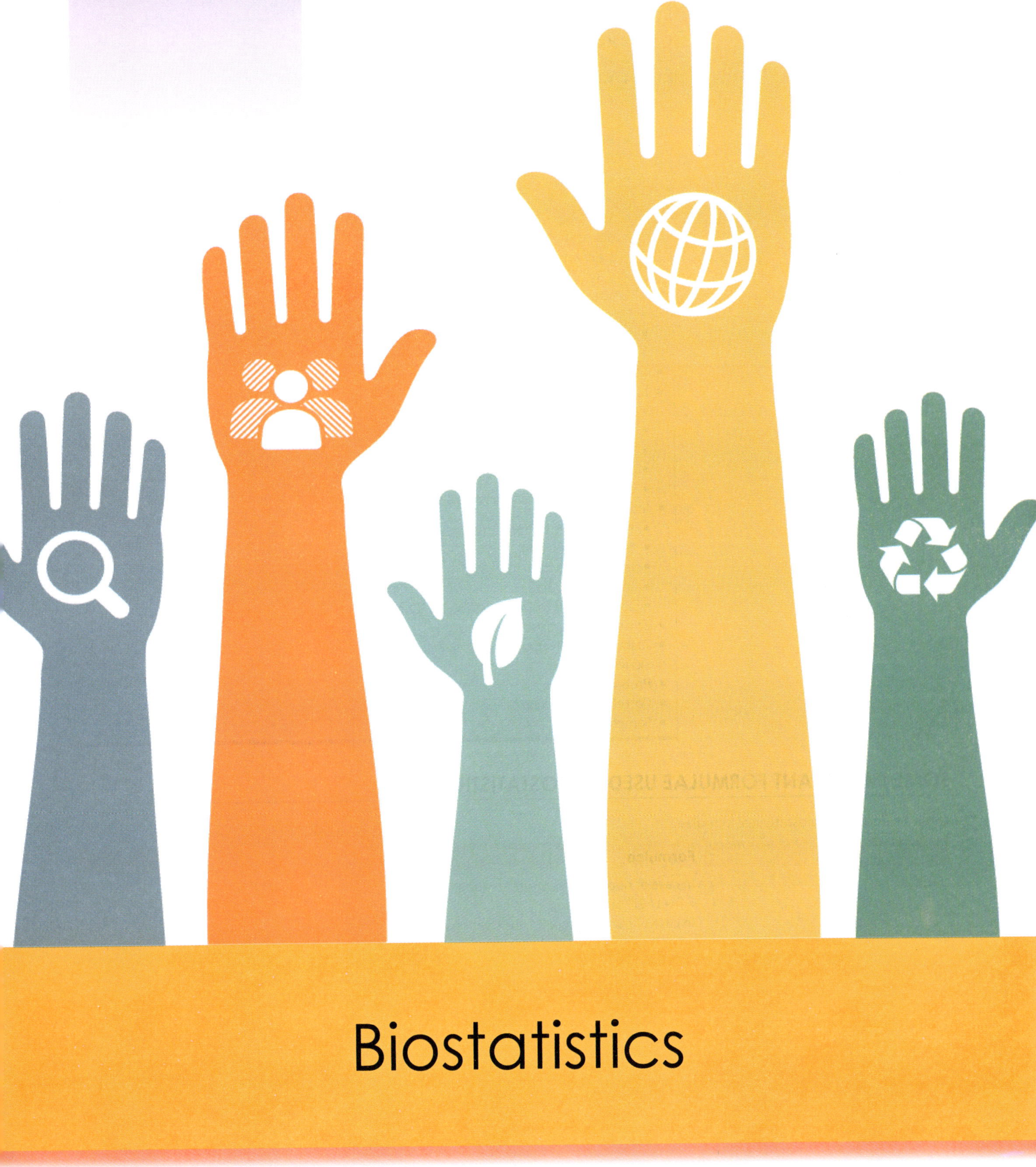

Biostatistics

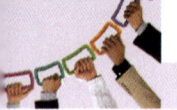

Chapter Outline

SOME IMPORTANT FORMULAE USED IN BIOSTATISTICS

Table 1: Important biostatistical formulae

	Formulae
Median	In case of odd number of observations Median = $[n+1/2]^{th}$ observation In case of even number of observations Median = $[(n/2) + (n/2+1)]/2]^{th}$ observation
Mode	Mode = Mean – 3(Mean –Median)
Mean (sample: X)	$= \Sigma\frac{x}{n}$
Mean deviation (MD)	$= \frac{\Sigma(x-\bar{x})}{n}$

Contd...

	Formulae
Standard deviation (SD) (Sample size ≤ 30)	$= \sqrt{\frac{[\Sigma(x-\bar{x})^2]}{n-1}}$
Coefficient of variance (CV)	$= \left[\frac{SD}{\bar{x}}\right] \times 100$
Standard normal deviate or Z score	$= (x-\bar{x})/\sigma$ where, σ is the standard deviation
Standard error of mean (SEM)	$= \frac{SD}{\sqrt{n}}$
Standard error of proportion (SEP)	$= \sqrt{\frac{pq}{n}}$
Standard error of difference between 2 mean (SEDM)	$= \sqrt{\frac{(SD_1)^2}{n} + \frac{(SD_2)^2}{n} + \ldots}$
In chi square test, Degree of Freedom (dF)	= (c – 1) (r – 1); c = Number of columns; n = Number of rows
Coefficient of determination (CD)	$= r^2$, where r = coefficient of correlation
Power of a test	$= 1 - \beta$ where β is type II error
Sample size in quantitative studies	$4pq/L^2$, where p= prevalence, q = 1-p, and L = absolute error
Accuracy	= (Sensitivity x Prevalence) + (specificity) (1-prevalence)
Pretest odds	= Pretest probability/[1 – pretest probability]
Post-test probability	= Posttest odds / [Posttest odds + 1]
Post-test odds	= pretest odds × LR (LR = Likelihood ratio)
Number needed to treat	= 1 / (Experimental event rate – Control event rate)
Absolute risk reduction = Event rate in exposed - Event rate in control group	
Relative risk reduction = $\frac{\text{(Event rate in exposed - Event rate in control group)}}{\text{Event rate in control group}}$	

DATA

Types of Data

Data: Is a set of values to obtaining useful information. The data may further be composed of

- Constants (which do not change)
- Variables (values which change)

The numeric (metric) variables may be of various types as:

- Discrete variable – where the values are based on a count from "whole values". A value of fraction between one value and next closest value cannot be taken. Example – number of children, type of disease, grade of disease, blood group
- Continuous variable – where any value may be taken in -between the set of real numbers. Example: height, weight, time, temperature.

Table 2: Basic differences between types of data

	Quantitative data	Qualitative data
Data type	Measurable data Usually continuous	Countable data Usually discrete
Mathematical tool used	Mean, median and mode	Percentages, ratios, proportions
Examples	Height, weight, Blood pressure, age, pulse rate	▪ Types of diseases – colon cancer and breast cancer ▪ Gender: Male or female ▪ Height categories – tall or short ▪ Grade of disease – mild, moderate or severe ▪ Age categories: Young, adult or old

Scale of Data

Nominal data: Categorical variable for data which does not have any order
Ordinal Scale: Categorical variable with an inherent order property.
Interval scale: Where the interval between the values is meaningful. There is usually no absolute zero in this data scale.
Ratio scale: It has all the properties of an interval variable, and also has a clear definition of zero point. Variables like height, weight, clearance of drug are ratio variables. There is a true Zero point beyond which there are no values.

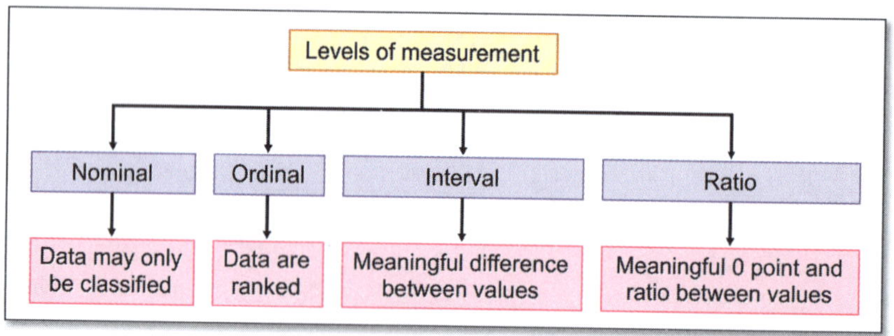

Fig. 1: Levels of measurement

Table 3: Examples of various scales

	Nominal Scale	Ordinal Scale	Interval Scale	Ratio Scale
Characteristic	Categorical data and NO specific order	Categorical data WITH an inherent order	Metric data WITHOUT an absolute zero and NO start point	Metric data WITH an absolute zero
			The interval between the values is of value	The ratios of the values may be calculated
Examples	Type of disease Religion Dichotomous data	Grade, stage of disease Severity of disease	Degree Celsius Degree Fahrenheit	Hb, weight, LDL, HDL, S. Creatinine Temperature in kelvin units

Other 'Qualitative' Scales of Data

- **Summative scale - LIKERT Scale**
  - It converts individual qualitative ordinal ratings to a quantity
  - It is based on an "agree-disagree" continuum
  - Example:

    I am happy with the medical services in the hospital.
    Strongly agree – agree – okay – disagree – strongly disagree

- **Cumulative (or summative) scale – GUTTMAN Scale**
  - It is measured in a binary (yes/no) answers and ascertain the 'opinion' of respondents.
  - Feature: The options of a questionnaire "follow a hierarchy" – that a yes to any item implies yes to all the preceding (or subsequent) items
  - Example

    The following question shows attitude towards depression

Please answer YES or NO to the following questions:	[YES]	[NO]
Depression affects many people	[ ]	[ ]
Depressed people should seek medical help	[ ]	[ ]
Medication can help with depression	[ ]	[ ]
All depressed people can be helped with the right medication	[ ]	[ ]

Data Presentation

Table 4: Quantitative and qualitative variables of data presentation

Quantitative Variables	Qualitative Variables
▪ Column charts - Histogram ▪ Frequency polygon / curve ▪ Ogive ▪ Line diagram ▪ Scatter plot ▪ Box and whisker plot	▪ Column charts - Bar chart ▪ Pie chart ▪ Pictogram ▪ Spot maps ▪ Venn diagrams

Histogram

- It is a pictorial diagram of frequency distribution used for continuous and ordered data[Q] (Fig. 2)

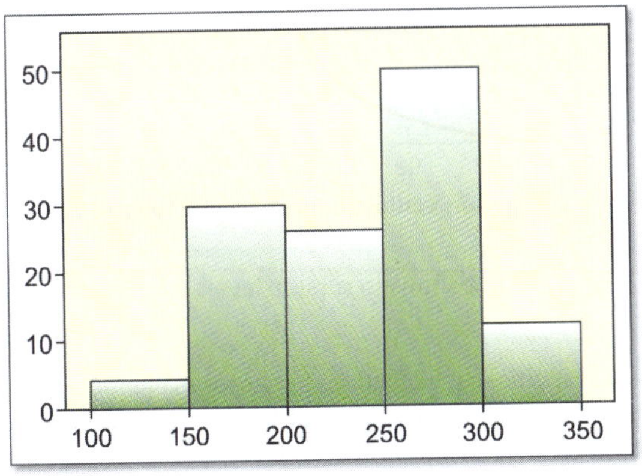

Fig. 2: Histogram

- It has a series of blocks adjacent to each other with no intervening space and area of each block is proportional to the frequency[Q]
- Class intervals are given along the horizontal axis and frequencies along the vertical axis
- Histogram is the most commonly used method of presentation of grouped frequency distribution of continuous and discontinuous data.

Frequency Polygon

It is an area diagram which is formed by joining the mid-points of the histogram blocks.[Q] It has the same area as the histogram, if the width of all class intervals are the same.

Frequency Curve

If number of observations is very large and group interval is reduced and frequency polygon loses its angulations resulting in a smooth curve known as Frequency curve (Fig. 3)

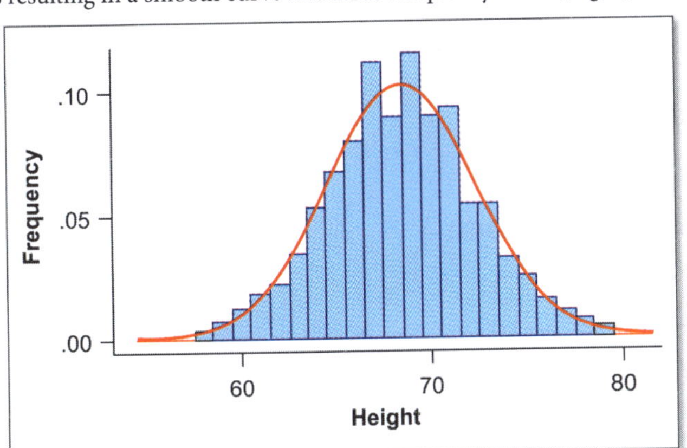

Fig. 3: Frequency curve for height in a population

Cumulative Frequency Curve or Ogive

- It is a graph, showing cumulative frequency distribution of quantitative data
- Curve is plotted by taking the variable on X-axis and cumulative frequency on Y-axis.
- Median can be calculated from Ogive[Q]

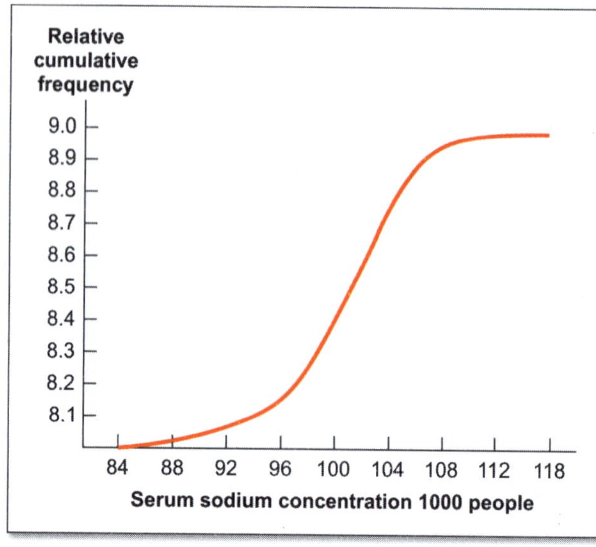

Fig. 4: Ogive showing sodium levels in a population

Bar Diagram

Bar diagram compares magnitude of frequencies in categories of mutually exclusive discrete data. (Length of the bar is proportional to the magnitude to be represented).

- **Simple bar chart:** Vertical or horizontal bars, separated by space for neatness and clear presentation.
- **Multiple bar chart or compound bar chart:** Two or more bars can be grouped together
- **Component bar chart:** Bars may be divided into two or more parts. Each part represents a certain item and is proportional to the magnitude of that particular item.

Pie Charts

- Areas of segments of a circle (depends upon the angle at center) are compared
- It usually represents the sectoral presentation of the data in a circle with percentages (and not in absolute numbers).[Q]

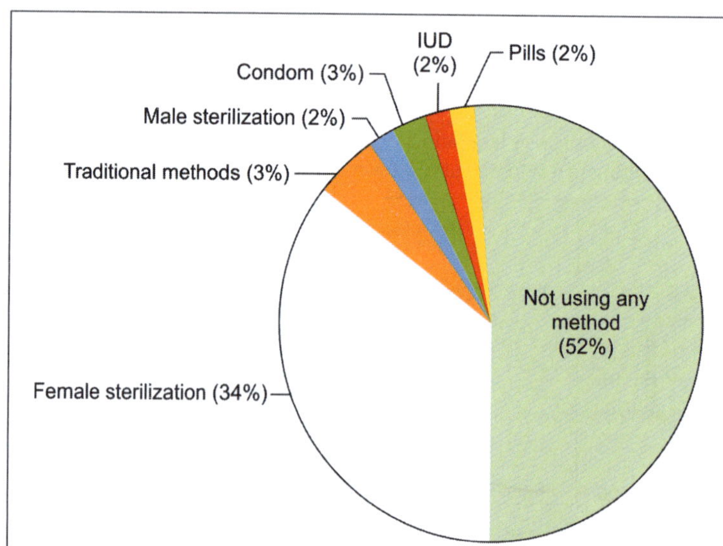

Fig. 5: Pie chart showing use of methods of contraception by community

Pictogram (a form of Bar Chart)

- For general population purpose presentation of statistical values or data. It may provide a meaningful interpretation to the observer (who may not have a technical background)
- Small pictures or symbols are used to present data.
- Fractions of picture can be used to represent numbers smaller than the value of a whole symbol.

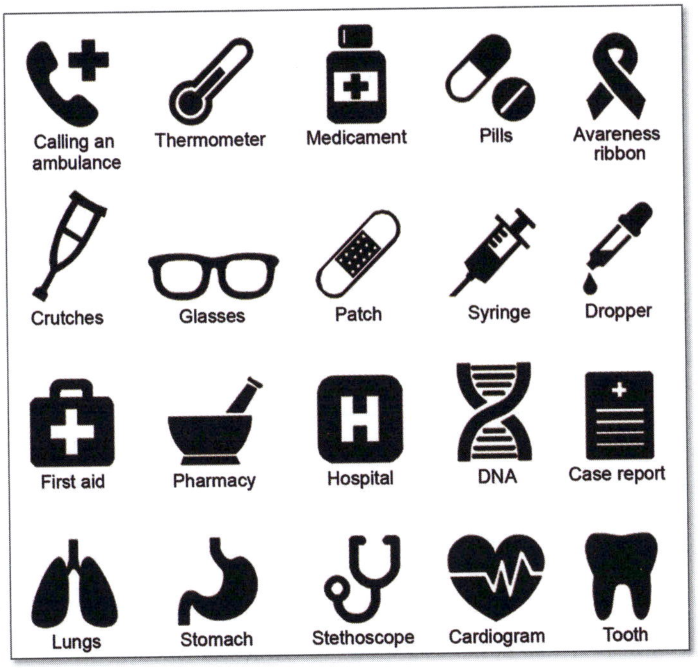

The use of symbols or pictures instead of written data may help in better, easier and faster communication and interpretation of data.

Example: Use of symbols for patient education is better than simple writing and may help patients understand better.

Line Diagram

- Also known as line charts, run diagrams
- A line chart is often used to visualize a trend in data over intervals of time – a time series – thus the line is often drawn chronologically (Fig. 6)

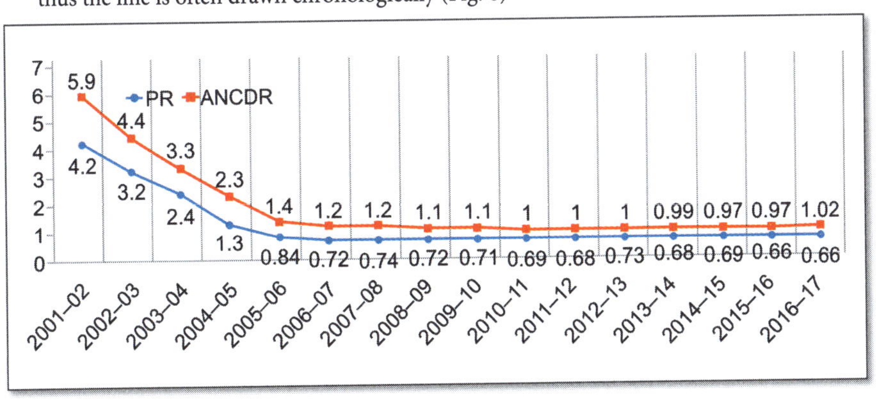

Fig. 6: Line chart for leprosy cases

Scatter Diagram or Correlation Diagram

- A typical type of presentation with the following features:
  - Drawn between two variables
  - Shows the correlation between variables

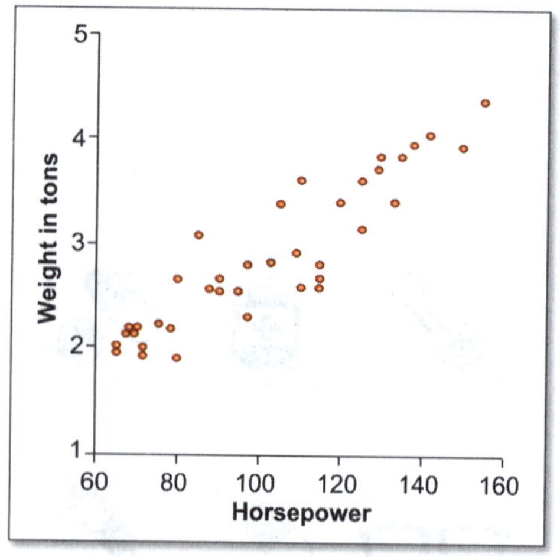

Fig. 7: Scatter diagram showing correlation between the variable

Spot Map

Spot maps and rate maps display geographical locations of cases or rates

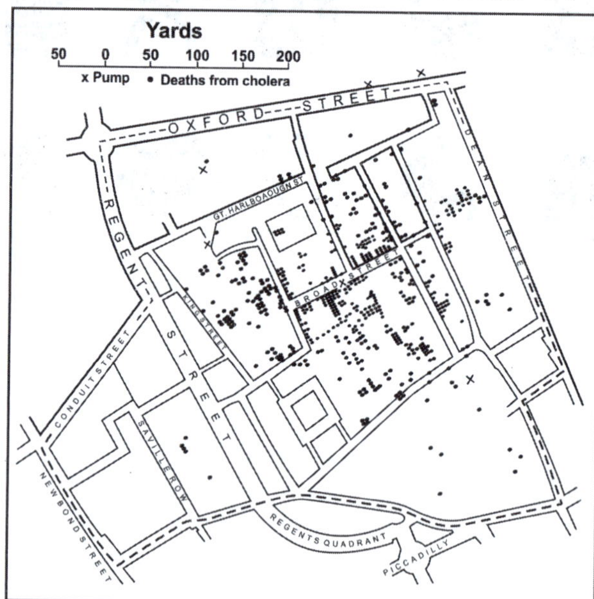

Fig. 8: Spot map for the deaths from cholera in Central London (1854), by Dr John Snow

Box and Whisker

- A unique presentation of quantitative data using the quartiles Q (measure of location) as units for display

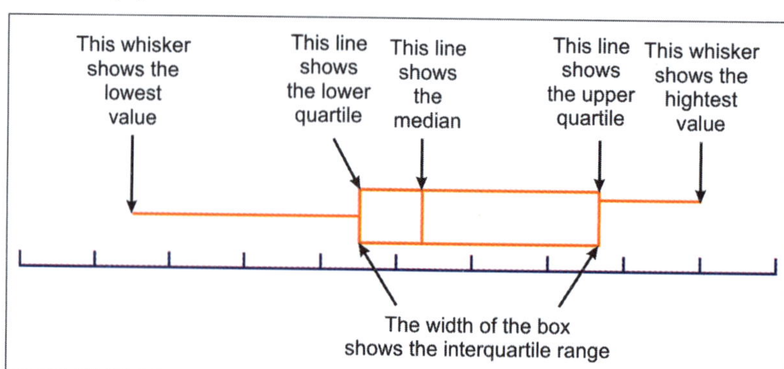

Fig. 9: Box and whisker presentation of data

High Yield Points

Box and whisker plots-

- Tell about the data distribution, the spatial spread and skewness of the data
- It is useful in interpreting large data and in higher statistical interpretation and presentations as forest plots

- It is helpful in general assessment for the trend of the data in respect to higher of lower values. Each of the quartile is composed of 25% of the data which further show whether more values are toward the lower extreme or the higher extreme.

Stem and Leaf Design

6	8
7	58
8	536687755
9	84031839776171319996
10	71015462796276457785
11	1466070
12	238
13	6
14	1

Fig. 10: Stem and leaf design of representing data

A good way to display the discrete data though may occasionally be used as well for a continuous scale. Basic design of the SAL (stem and leaf) design is to have display of data showing the trend of data spread with respect to the variable.

Venn Diagrams

The characteristics are represented by circles and the diagram represents logical overlaps.

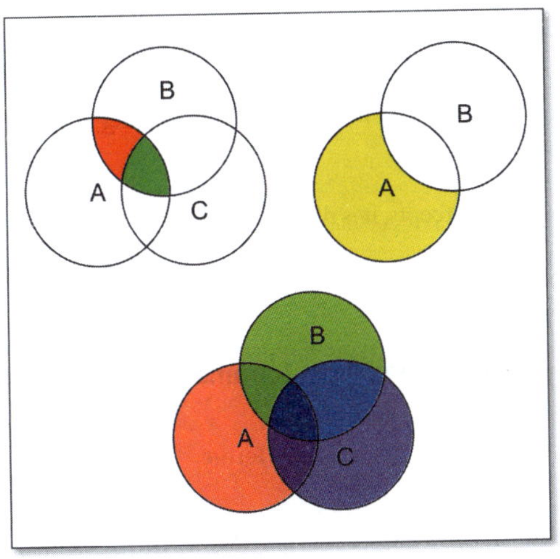

Fig. 11: Venn diagrams

> 17 *High Yield Points*
>
> - **Advantage:** Easy to calculate and understand
> - Mean is most influenced by abnormal or extreme values in the distribution.[Q]

MEASURES OF CENTRAL TENDENCY

Mean (X, μ)

- It is widely used and is the most useful of statistical averages
- Calculation: Individual observations are added together and divided by number of observations

Types of Mean

- **Arithmetic mean** is the sum of all values of a set of observations divided by number of observations
- **Geometric mean** is the Nth root of the product of N observations. It is used for exponential data sets or data with very extreme values

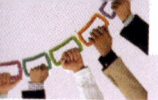

- **Harmonic mean** is the reciprocal of arithmetic mean or the reciprocal of individual observations
- **Weighted mean:** Mean of individual classes are multiplied by total number of individuals in that class and sum of all such products is divided by total number of individuals in all classes.

Median

- Data is arranged in ascending or descending order of magnitude and the value of the **middle observation** is located, known as median
- In case of even number of items or values, average of the two middle values is taken[Q]

Mode

- It is the **most frequently occurring value** in a series of value or observation
- It is the only average that can be applied to qualitative data[Q]
- There can be more than one mode for a series of data and even no mode in a series of data
- Used primarily for bimodal distribution.
- Mode may be calculated as: mode = 3 median – 2 mean

Features

- Most commonly used measure for central tendency — Mean
- Most affected by extreme values (or outliers) in data — Mean
- Data with outliers, the preferred measure for central tendency — Median
- Most robust measure for central tendency — Mode
- Histogram may help estimate all the measures of central tendency – mean, median and mode

MEASURES OF LOCATION

Measure for location: To find the 'location' of a single value in a set of numbers constituting the Data Set, The data may be divided into 'EQUAL' parts using intercepts, so as to simplify the process of locating a value in the data.
Example:
If the data is divided using 2 intercepts, it is divided into 3 equal parts, each part named as "Tertile" – Tertile 1, tertile 2 and tertile 3

So, if we divide the data into a number of equal parts using intercepts, the part (or portion) size would vary as shown below:

Number of intercepts	Data divided into	Name	Median location
2	Three sections	Tertile	Between (Tertile) T1 and T2
3	Four sections	Quartile	At (quartile) Q2
4	Five sections	Quintile (pentile)	Between (Pentile) P2 and P3
7	Eight sections	Octile	At (octile) O4
9	Ten sections	Decile	At (decile) D5
99	Hundred sections	Percentile	At (centile) C50

Uses
Widely used measures of location are – quartiles and percentiles.
Percentiles are used for

- Display of marks scored by students in relation to the maximum marks obtained in a particular exam – percentile rank
- Assessment of growth pattern in children – growth charts
- As a measure of comparison of metric variables in a population

MEASURES OF DISPERSION

Range

- It is the simplest measure of dispersion
- It is the difference between highest and lowest figures in a given sample
- In grouped data, range is the difference between mid-points of the extreme categories

Mean Deviation

- It is the average of the deviations from the arithmetic mean
  Mean deviation = $\Sigma(x - \bar{x}) / n$

Variance

The variance (σ^2) is a measure of how far each value in the data set is from the mean.
It is derived as:

- Subtract the mean from each value in the data. This gives you a measure of the distance of each value from the mean.
- Square each of these distances (so that they are all positive values), and add all of the squares together.
- Divide the sum of the squares by the number of values in the data set.
- Formula:
  Variance (v) = $\Sigma(x - \bar{x}) / n$ where,
  $\bar{x}$ = sample mean
  x = observed value
  n = sample size

Standard Deviation

It is denoted by the Greek letter sigma (σ) [for population] or by initials SD [for a sample]
SD gives us an idea of 'spread' of dispersion

$$\text{Standard deviation} = \sqrt{\text{Variance}}$$

$$SD = \sqrt{\frac{\sum(x - \bar{x})^2}{n}}$$

Where,
$\bar{x}$ = sample mean
x = observed value
n = sample size

Standard deviation is given by the formula - Root Mean Square Deviation (root of mean of squared deviations)

It is the best measure for dispersion

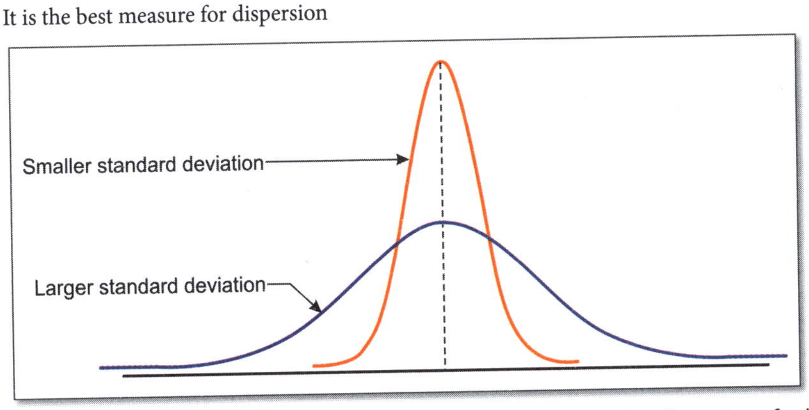

Fig. 12: Interpreting standard deviation (SD): Larger the SD, greater the dispersion of values

18 High Yield Points

Median - Advantage:
- It is least influenced by abnormal or extreme values in the distribution
- Used for numeric data that is skewed and for ordinal data.

14 Must Remember

Mode = Mean – 3 (Mean – Median)

12 Good to Remember

Note: "σ" is symbol for Standard Deviation

15 Must Remember

$$\text{Variance} = \frac{\sum(x - \bar{x})^2}{n - 1}$$

19 High Yield Points

(Remember: **RMSD** - **R**oot of **M**ean of **S**quared **D**eviations)

16 Must Remember

Note: For small samples the SD is calculated as:

$$SD = \sqrt{\frac{\sum(x - \bar{x})^2}{n - 1}}$$

20 High Yield Points

It is the best and most frequently used measure of deviation.[Q]

Application of Standard Deviations

- Estimation of the sample size [Sample Size $\propto \frac{1}{SD}]^{Q}$
- Estimation of range of variation or deviation of observations about mean
- Summarizes the variation of a large distribution in one figure and defines normal limits of variation
- Used to calculate relative deviate or Z score Q (refer topic: Normal distribution curve)
- Estimate the
  - Coefficient of variation (discussed below)
  - Standard errors (discussed below)

Coefficient of Variation (CV):

- It is the ratio between the standard deviation and the mean
- Formula: Coefficient of variation (CV) = SD/mean × 100
- Interpretation: The higher the coefficient of variation, the greater the level of dispersion around the mean and conversely – the lower the coefficient of variation, the more precise the data
- Use: It is frequently used to compare and evaluate relative risks.

Standard Error

Standard error: is the variation in the sample means from the actual population mean.

- Standard error is a measure of the 'chance variation' by taking different samples from a population
- It is inversely proportional to the sample size of the population. The larger the sample size from a population, the smaller will be the chance variation (or the standard error)
- Uses:
  - For estimating the confidence intervals
  - For estimating the degree of chance variation from different sample study

Measures of Standard Error

The Standard error may be calculated in different terms as:

- Standard error of mean:
  - May be calculated for quantitative data, with measure of central tendency as 'mean'
  - The variation in the sample 'mean' from the population mean
  - Formula: *Standard error for means (SEM)* = $\frac{SD}{\sqrt{n}}$ × 100, where n = sample size
- Standard error of proportions
  - Maybe calculated for qualitative data, with measure for central tendency as proportions
  - Is the measure for variation in the sample proportions
  - Formula: *Standard error of proportions (SEP)* = $\sqrt{\frac{PQ}{n}}$ × 100, where
    P = Prevalence as proportion
    Q = 100 – Prevalence
    n = sample size

INFERENTIAL STATISTICS

Normal Distribution Curve (NDC)

If we take a large population and check for any variable as BP, height, weight, serum cholesterol, the distribution would be something like as shown in the figure below:

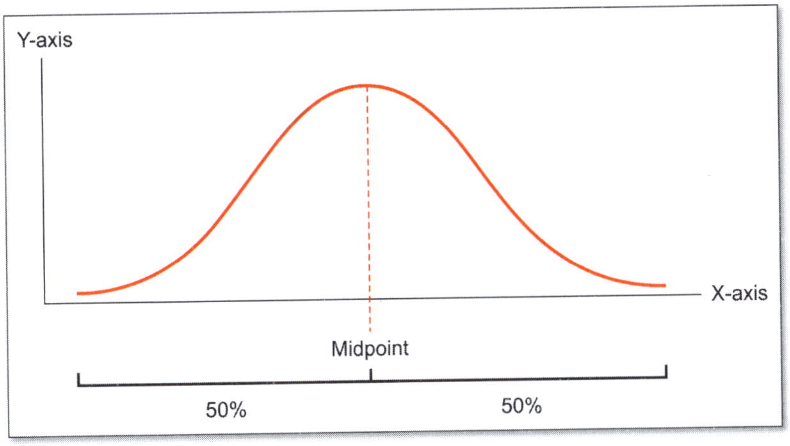

Fig. 13: Normal distribution curve

- This is known as a normal distribution curve, also known as Gaussian distribution curve

Features of the normal distribution curve:

- It is a bell shaped, bilaterally symmetrical curve
- The mean = median = mode, they all coincide
- The ends never touch the baseline
- The area under curve = 1
- The variance = 1, The SD = 1

Whenever, the data collected is from a large homogenous population or whenever the data is normally distributed (i.e. shows a normal distribution curve pattern), it will always also have the following characteristics:

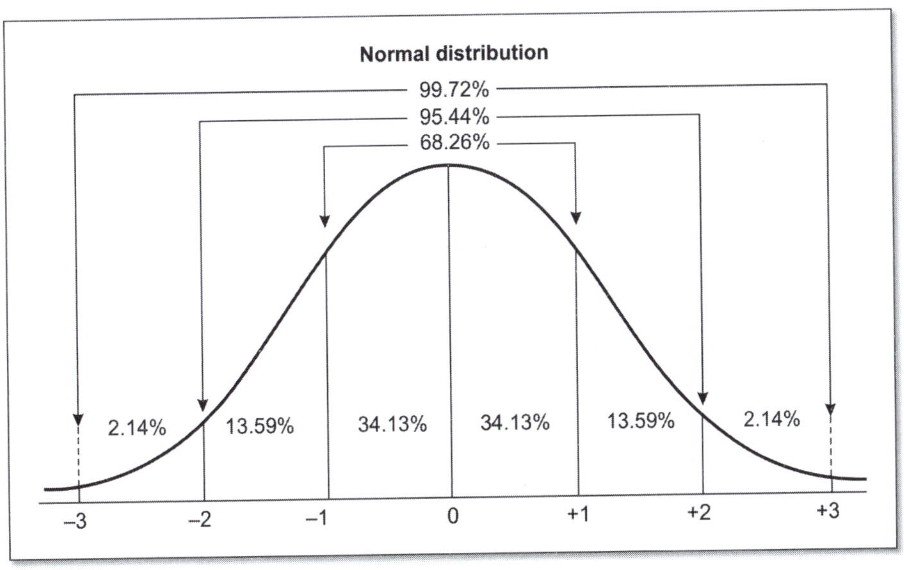

Fig. 14: Characteristic or normal distribution

Thus in a normal distribution curve:

- Within ± 1 SD comprises of 68.23% (~68%) of the total observations
- Within ± 2 SD comprises of 95.45% (~95%) of the total observations
- Within ± 3 SD comprises of 99.7% (~99%) of the total observations

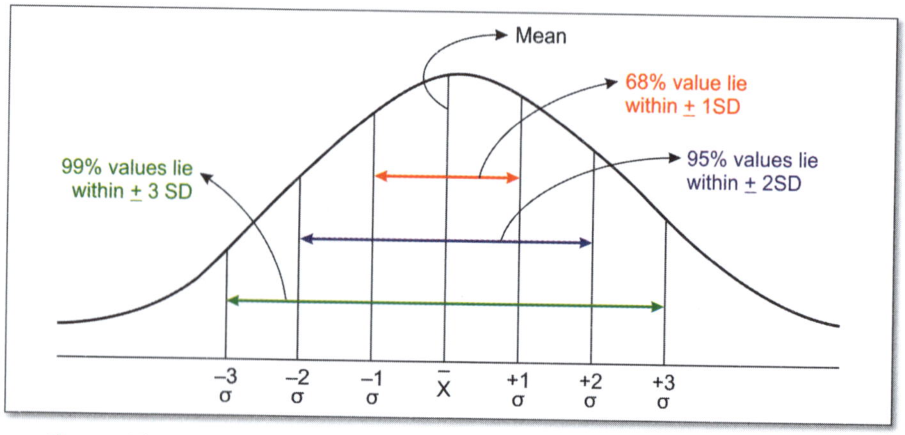

Fig. 15: The normal distribution curve, where x̄ is mean and σ is standard deviation

Z Score (Standard Deviate)

- In a Normal distribution curve, we may calculate the Z-Scores
- The Z-scores tell about the location of the value in terms of Standard deviations away from the mean (hence Z-scores is also known as ***standard deviate***)
- Formula: It is denoted by 'Z' and is given as:

$$Z\ score = \sqrt{\frac{\text{Observed value Expected value}}{\text{Standard deviation}}}$$

Inference

- In a normal distribution curve (NDC), the observations within 95% of population zone is considered as normal
- Hence, In a NDC, the observations lying within ± 1.96 SD ~ 2 SD is the normal zone

21 *High Yield Points*

Concept of normal zones in a normal distribution curve (NDC)

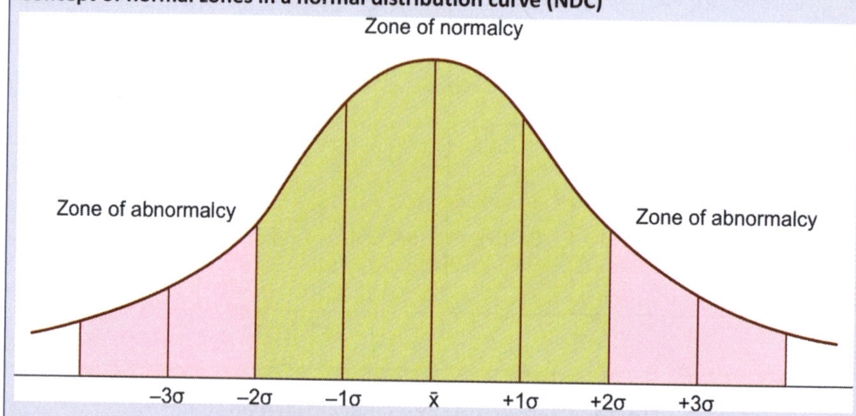

Fig. 16: Zone of normalcy in normal distribution curve

Standard Errors (SE)

- When a number of random samples (with different sample means) are drawn from a population
- Frequency distribution of all sample means drawn from the same population shows normal distribution about the population mean (μ)
- Variation of sample mean is measured in terms of SE (i.e. Standard deviations of sample mean from population mean)

So, the normal distribution can be drawn for the deviations of sample means (in terms of standard errors) from the population mean, using confidence intervals.

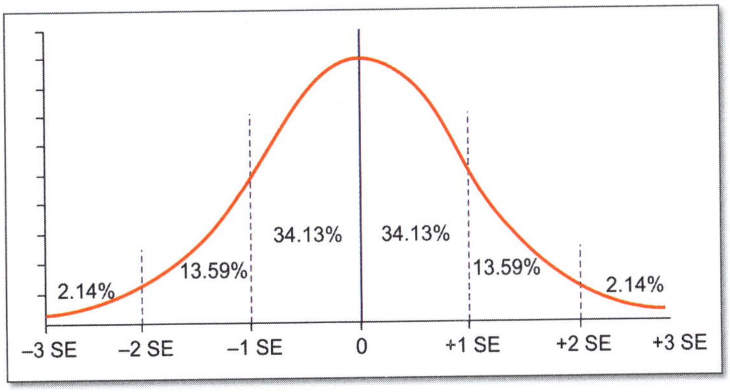

Fig. 17: The standard errors on a normal distribution curve

where, now the population mean is at point 0 in the NDC, and the range of 68%, 95% and 99% are the confidence limits, lying within

± 1 SE = 68.26% confidence limits
± 2 SE = 95.44% confidence limits
± 3 SE = 99.73% confidence limits

22 High Yield Points

The Confidence limits

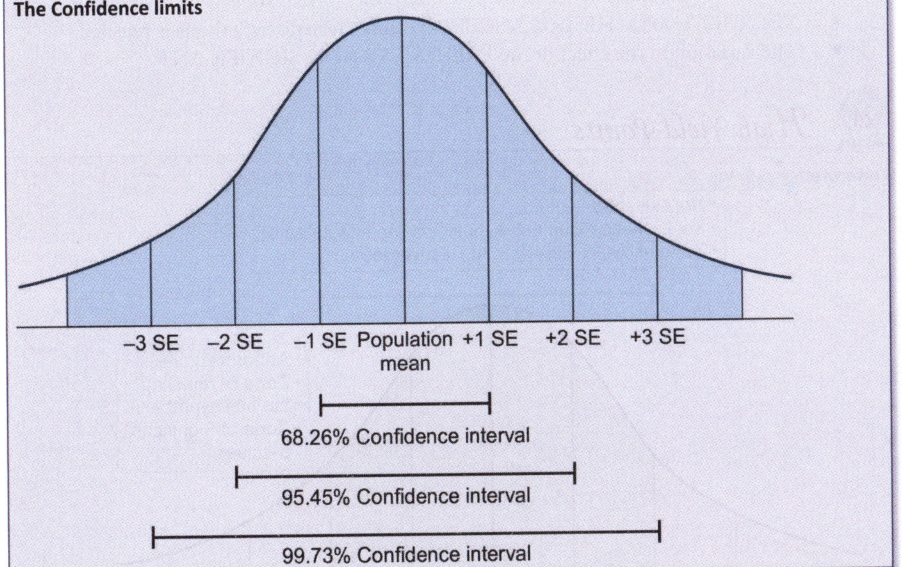

Fig. 18: Confidence limits in terms of SE

23 High Yield Points

Hence if we reconsider the image 14 and 16 and 19 we may understand that:

- p-values <0.05 lie in the abnormal zone and the null hypothesis is rejected (and the alternate hypothesis is accepted or the effect is found in the study)
- p-values >0.05 lie within the normal zone and the null hypothesis is accepted (and the alternate hypothesis is rejected or no effect is found in the study).

Calculating Confidence Intervals from Standard Error

The standard error is the measure of chance variation and the confidence limits of the standard errors may be calculated as:

- Finding the confidence limits for parametric (quantitative) data
  Formula: Confidence limits = sample mean ± (Z * SEM)
- Finding the confidence limits for non-parametric (qualitative) data expressed as proportions
  Formula: Confidence limits = sample prevalence (as proportions) ± (Z * SEP)

Where, Z = standard deviate, SEM = standard error for means, SEP = standard error for proportions

17 Must Remember

X = (mean or prevalence) ± Z(SE)
This formula may be used to estimate the:

- Confidence limits
- Percentiles

Use the

- SEM for data with mean or metric data or quantitative data
- SEP for data with percentages or prevalence or proportions or qualitative data

p-Values and the Normal Distribution Curve

- p-values are the probability values
- p-values tell about the probability of rejecting (or accepting) the null hypothesis
- p-Values range from 1 to 0 (1 is the maximum probability, 0 is the minimum probability)
- p-value = 0.05 correspond to the ±2 SE or the 95.44% confidence limits

A few definitions:

Null hypothesis(H_0):

- Is the initial speculated hypothesis
- The objective of the study is – find out if this observation is just by chance or is it a real variation
- This hypothesis is 'nullified' and hence is termed as 'null hypothesis'

Alternate hypothesis (H_1):

- Is the research hypothesis or the maintained hypothesis

Example:

We wish to establish the association of selenium intake and risk of CAD

Research hypothesis (alternate hypothesis): selenium intake protects from CAD

Null hypothesis: selenium intake has no effect on CAD

Interpretation of p-value

- If the p-value from the study is <0.05 (less than 0.05), it implies that:
  - The observed results of the study lie OUTSIDE the normal zone
  - The NULL HYPOTHESIS IS REJECTED, and alternate hypothesis is accepted.
  - The variation in the effect or the VALUES ARE SIGNIFICANT

Conversely,

- If the p-value from the study is > 0.05 (higher than 0.05), it implies that:
  - The observed results of the study lie INSIDE the normal zone
  - The NULL HYPOTHESIS IS ACCEPTED, and alternate hypothesis is rejected.
  - The variation in the effect or the VALUES ARE NON-SIGNIFICANT

24 *High Yield Points*

Interpreting p-Value

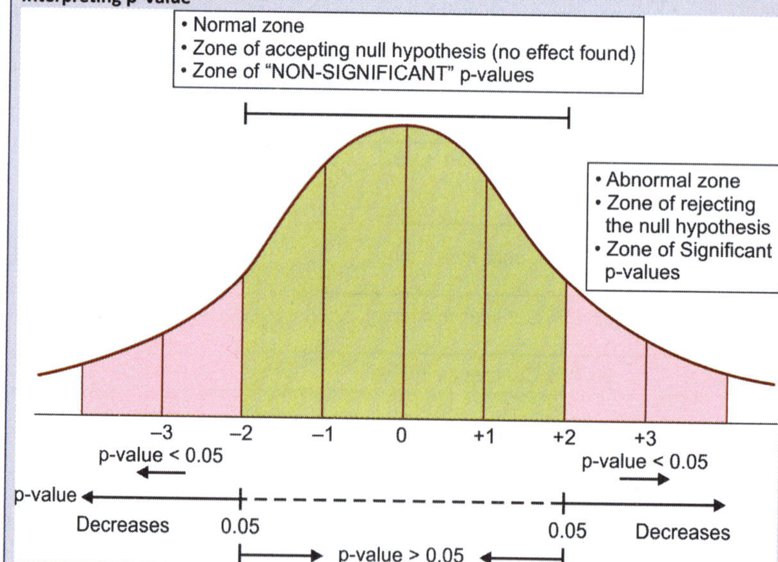

Fig. 19: Interpreting p-value in normal distribution curve

Computing Percentiles from the Normal Distribution Curve

Sometimes, the research may require estimating the population below a certain cutoff expressed in percentiles. The Standard normal distribution curve maybe used to estimate for the percentiles.

Example:

The mean BMI for adults in a population was found to be 30 and standard deviation of 5.

So, what is the 90th percentile for the BMI in the population?

We already know that the median is the 50th percentile, the first quartile is the 25th percentile, and the third quartile is the 75th percentile

The 90th percentile is the BMI that holds 90% of the BMIs below it and 10% above it, as illustrated in the figure below.

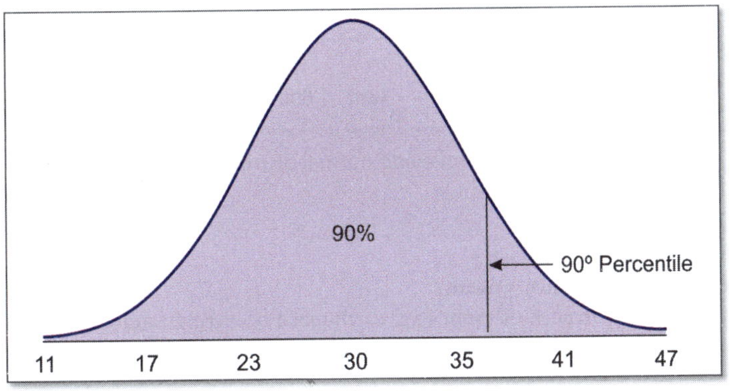

Standard distribution of male BMI showing the 90th percentile somewhere to the right of the mean of 30.

So, we find the 'Z' value which corresponds to the value of 0.90 in the "standard normal distribution table". We find that the Z-value at 0.90 is 1.28, hence now the 90th percentile is calculated as:

$x = \mu + Z\sigma$

X = variable

μ = mean

σ = standard deviation

$x = 30 + 1.28\,(5) = 36.4$

Thus, we can say that 90 percent of the population is having BMI below 36.4 and 10% have BMI higher than 36.4

The commonly used percentiles and Z-score from the Standard distribution table is given below:

Percentile	Z
1st	−2.326
2.5th	−1.960
5th	−1.645
10th	−1.282
25th	−0.675
50th	0
75th	0.675
90th	1.282
95th	1.645
97.5th	1.960
99th	2.326

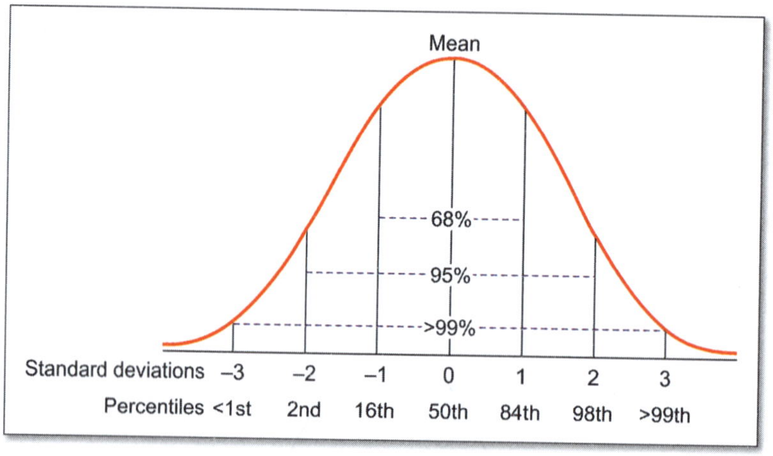

Fig. 20: Percentile and normal distribution curve

Other Distributions

Poisson distribution (variance = mean)

- Probability of occurrence of event (e.g. earthquake occurring randomly) in a given time period is indefinitely small and 'n' the number of observations is very large.

Binomial Distribution

- Distribution of outcome from a series of data characterized by 2 mutually exclusive [Dichotomous] categories.
- Population under observation can be divided into 2 groups, one with a certain characteristic and other without it.
- Uniform distribution or rectangular distribution
- A distribution in which all events occur with equal frequency. It does not occur very often.

Log Normal Distribution

It is a skewed distribution when graphed using a arithmetic scale but a normal distribution when graphed using a logarithmic scale

ERRORS IN BIOSTATISTICS

There may be two types of errors in biostats

- Type 1 error (corresponds to False positive error or Alpha error)
- Type 2 error (corresponds to False negative error or Beta error)

Type 1 Error

- False interpretation of an event or false observation, which in reality DOES NOT EXIST
- The NULL hypothesis was TRUE and the Study REJECTS it erroneously
- "REJECT a TRUE null hypothesis" – "False positive error"
- It depends on the significance level set for the study
- The probability of making type I error is known as α
- Example:
  - The investigation concludes that the patient has disease, but in reality, the patient DOES NOT have disease
  - The study reports that the drug is useful for a particular disease, which in reality was NOT USEFUL
  - A study shows that the medical treatment is cure for disease, which in reality DOES NOT cure the disease

Alpha Value

- It is the probability of making a type 1 error in the study
- A study sets a significance level (p-value) of 0.05, which corresponds to alpha value of 5%.
- This means that if the results are significant, there is 5% chance that the results obtained are not the true variation and are because of chance
- An α of 0.05 indicates that the researcher is willing to accept a 5% chance that the study is wrong when we reject the null hypothesis. To lower this risk, the research must use a lower value for α

Type II Error

- When a study fails to find an effect, which was present in reality.
- The NULL hypothesis was FALSE, and the Study ACCEPTS it erroneously
- "ACCEPT a FALSE null hypothesis" - "False Negative Error"
- It depends on the power of the study and the sample size of the study
- The probability of making type II error is known as β
- Example:
  - The study fails to find an effect which in reality did exist
  - The study reports that the drug is not useful for a particular disease, which in reality was USEFUL
  - An investigation declared the person as disease free, while in reality was diseased

Example:

A study is conducted to find the effectivity and use of a novel monoclonal antibody (drug x) for Bronchial Asthma Cure. A randomized control trial was conducted using the drug 'x' and the drug 'e'

Null hypothesis (H_0) – the new drug is same as the existing drug

Alternate hypothesis (H_1) – The new drug is BETTER than the existing drug

The study was done and the results obtained were that the drug 'x' is superior than Drug 'e' with p-value of 0.02. Hence, we REJECT our null hypothesis.

Now in reality the null hypothesis could have been true to false, so there are multiple options as shown below

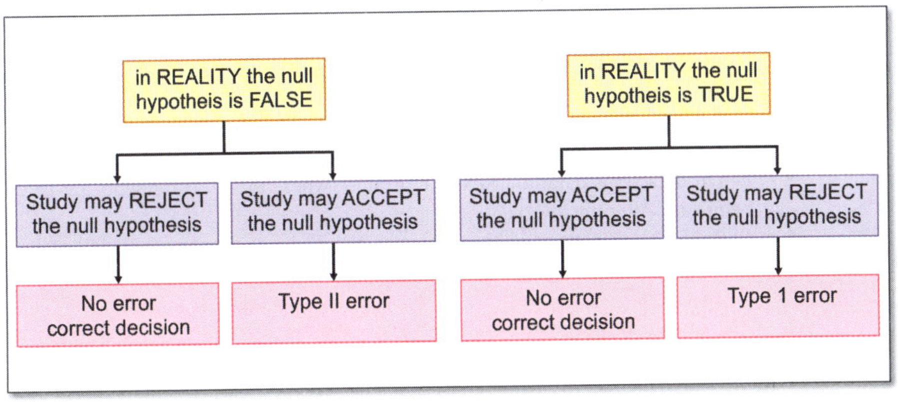

We can also depict this information in a 2 × 2 table as below:

		Truth in the population	
		Null hypothesis is FALSE	**Null hypothesis is TRUE**
Study results	Effect Found (Null hypothesis rejected)	Correct decision	Type I error (probability = α)
	No effect found (Null hypothesis Accepted)	TYPE II error (probability = β)	Correct decision

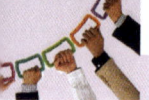

TESTS FOR SIGNIFICANCE

- The Test of significance is a mathematical procedure for comparison of data for a variation between two or more groups or two or more recordings in a single group
- The tests for significance may be parametric tests (for quantitative data) or nonparametric tests (for Qualitative data):

Table 5: Parametric and nonparametric test for qualitative data

Testing groups – situation	Parametric test	Nonparametric test
Testing association between two qualitative variables		Chi square test
Comparison of two **independent groups**	t-test for independent samples	Wilcoxon rank sum test
Comparison of data between **paired observations** (usually single group – before and after)	t-test for paired observation	Wilcoxon rank sign test
Comparison of several groups **(three or more groups)**	ANOVA	Kruskal-Wallis test
Assessment of relationship between two variables	Pearson correlation for linear relation	Spearman rank correlation

Table 6: Tests used in various number of groups

Between one group	Paired t-test	McNemar's test
Between two groups	Unpaired t-test	Chi square test
Between 3 or more groups	ANOVA	Kruskal-Wallis test

Brief explanation for various tests of significance (ToS):

Parametric tests:

- t- test – is a universal test for significance for quantitative parametric data with mean as measure of central tendency
  - Paired t-test
    - Comparing the means in a 'paired' data set
    - Paired data set is data in a **SINGLE** group – where the measurements are taken before and after the intervention
    - Example: Mean Hemoglobin levels were compared in a group of 10 individuals before and after giving 1 month of IFA supplements.
  - Unpaired t-test
    - Also known as independent sample t-test
    - Comparing the means in an un-paired data set
    - Un-paired data set means – TWO groups. Where the measurements were taken in independent groups
    - Example: Mean Hemoglobin levels were compared for 20 individuals. 10 persons were selected for giving the new IFA tablets, while another 10 persons were given a standard therapy in terms of only folic acid supplements
- Z-test: is a universal test for significance for large sample (sample size > 30)
- ANOVA -is the Test of significance (ToS) for three or more data groups with quantitative data
  - Example: Mean Hemoglobin levels were compared in three different villages. The first group of individuals from village 1 was given nutrition supplements, second sample from village 2 was given the new formulation IFA tablet, and the third sample from village 3 was given the standard folic acid tablet. The change in the HB levels was noted and statistically compared for assessment of effect of the interventions using the ANOVA test for significance.
- Chi square test

Concept of Chi Square Test

Chi square test is measure for the test of significance for nonparametric data set.
Remember: The chi square (is based on the frequencies and not the parameter of the values
Note: Expected values (E) are calculated by:

$$E = \sqrt{\frac{Row\ total \times Column\ total}{Total\ population}}$$

and,
chi square (χ^2) is

$$(\chi^2) = \sqrt{\frac{(\text{Observed}-\text{expected})^2}{\text{expected value}}}$$

the degree of freedom (dF) in chi square table is calculated as
dF = (row – 1) x (column – 1)

Note that:

Degree of freedom is :

- In chi square test, DF = (c – 1) (r – 1); c = Number of columns; n = Number of rows
- In unpaired ' t' test, DF = n1+ n2 – 2, where n1 and n2 are number of observation in each series
- In paired 't' test, DF = n – 1
- In testing the significance of correlation, DF = n – 2, n is the number of paired measurements

Other Tests of Significance

- Wilcoxon rank test – for ordinal data
  - Single group or grouped data – Wilcoxan rank SIGN test
  - Multiple groups or ungrouped data – Wilcoxan rank SUM test
- For small sample size
  - Value in a cell (in nonparametric tests) is less than 5 – Fischer exact test
  - Very small sample (parametric test) – Yates correction
- F-test (variance test): For comparison of multiple groups
- **Dixon Q Test:** For data with outliers
- **Kappa stats:** To check for the level of agreement between two or more independent groups
- **Cronbach alpha score:** For assessment of the internal consistency of the questionnaire

The Cronbach alpha score ranges from 0-1. score greater than 0.7 is considered very good and acceptable.

- Cohen's kappa statistics (k) is done to check for the inter rater agreement between various groups. It is given by the formula

$$\kappa \equiv \frac{P_o - P_e}{1 - P_e}$$

Where,
p_o is the observed probability of agreement between the observers.
p_e is the expected or hypothetical probability of chance agreement

- **Kolmogorov-Smirnov test:** To check for normalcy of data
- **Bland Altman analysis:** For evaluation of gold standard (or a standardized) test with a new investigation
- ANOVA (<u>AN</u>alysis <u>O</u>f <u>VA</u>riance) describes effect of one independent qualitative variable on a dependent quantitative variable.

SKEW

- Skew means a deviation from the normal shape and structure
- In some cases, the data is not showing a normal distribution, in the sense, that it does not have the mean coinciding with the median and the mode.

25 *High Yield Points*

Remember: Chi square value at probability value 0.95 (95% confidence) at dF 1 is 3.84

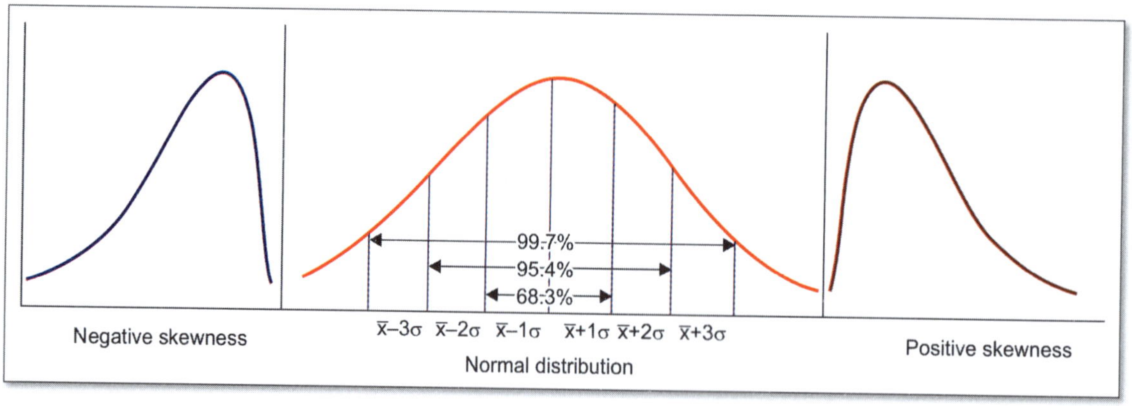

Fig. 21: Skew diagram

26 High Yield Points

Remember:

In the Right skew:
Mean > Median > Mode
In the Left Skew
Mode > Median > Mean

Right Skew

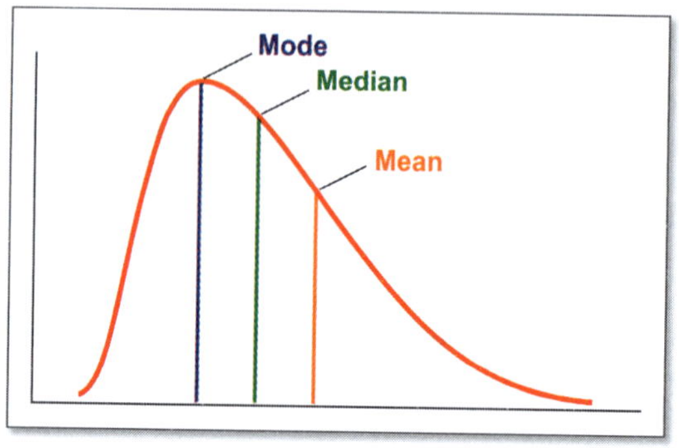

Fig. 22: Right skew

- Right skew (positive skew)
- Tail toward the right
- Large number of low scores and small number of high values.
- In right skew mean has the highest value
- The mean is the maximum value
- Mean is greater than median, which is greater than mode in Right skew

Left Skew

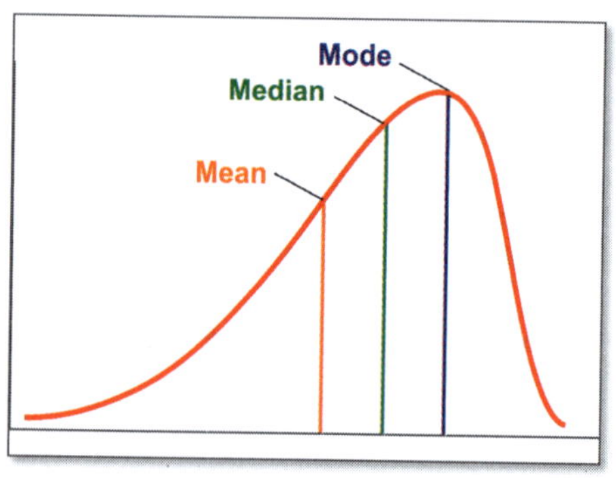

Fig. 23: Left skew

- Left skew (Negative skew)
- Tail toward the left
- Large number of high scores and small number of low values
- In left skew mode has the highest value
- The mode is greater than median is greater than mean in a left skew

PROBABILITY

Probability, as we know, is the chance of an event to happen. Or the chance of an outcome to occur. Odds on the other hand is the chance of event to 'not' occur. It is given by the formula p/(1–p)

Let's take an example:

In a region the blood group was distributed among individuals as follows:

- Blood group A – 30% (or probability of 0.3)
- Blood group B – 40 % (or probability of 0.4)
- Blood group AB – 10% (or probability of 0.1)
- Blood group O – 20% (or probability of 0.2)

  Also, the Tuberculosis prevalence - 2% (or probability of 0.02)

  So, the chance to find a random person with blood group B is 40%.

Rule of multiplication

1. What is the chance to find two individuals and both of them to be blood group B.

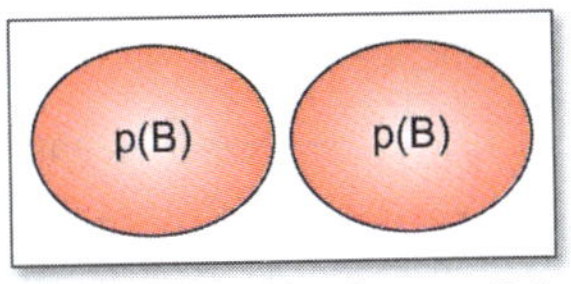

Probability of finding 2 persons and both with blood group B is

Answer is: p(B) × p(B)

= 0.4 × 0.4 = 0.16 (or 16% chance)

Rule of Addition

2. What is the chance to find two people, with Blood group A or B

Now, in this case, the variables (Blood group) as we know are mutually exclusive (that is there is not a chance that both can occur in the same individual). So,

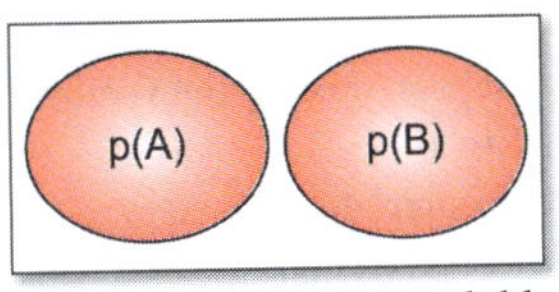

Probability of finding 2 persons with blood group A or with blood group B is

Ans is: p(A) + p(B)

= 0.3 + 0.4 = 0.7 (or 70% chance)

3. What is the chance to find two people, with TB and Blood group A.

So, in this case the variables are not mutually exclusive, i.e. both can occur in an individual. And we use the **rule of multiplication**

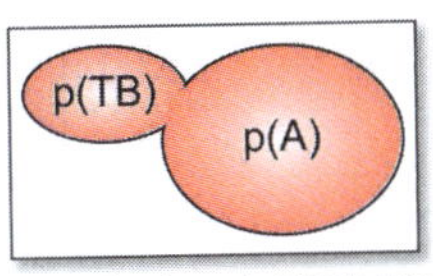

Hence the probability of finding an individual with TB 'AND' blood group A is

= P(TB) × p(A)

= 0.02 × 0.3 = 0.06 (or 6% chance)

4. What is the chance to find two people, with TB "OR" Blood group A.

So, in this case the variables are not mutually exclusive, i.e. both can occur in an individual and hence, we use the **Rule of addition**

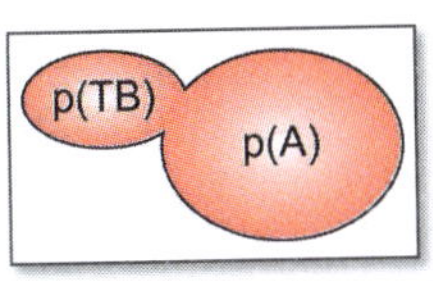

Hence the probability of finding an individual with Tuberculosis 'OR' blood group A is

= P(TB) + p(A)

= 0.02 + 0.3 = 0.32 (or 32% chance)

Hint for MCQ Exams:

- Rule of multiplication: For **combined occurrence** of two or more independent events.
  - The Boolean operator used is: [Both] , [AND]. The statement will say probability of event 'A' **and** event 'B'
- Rule of addition: For mutually exclusive events or when 'Either or Any' of event is desired
  - The Boolean operator used is: [OR], [EITHER], [ANY]. The statement will say probability of event 'A' **or** event 'B'
- Odds is given by formula = p/(1-p), where p = probability

27 *High Yield Points*

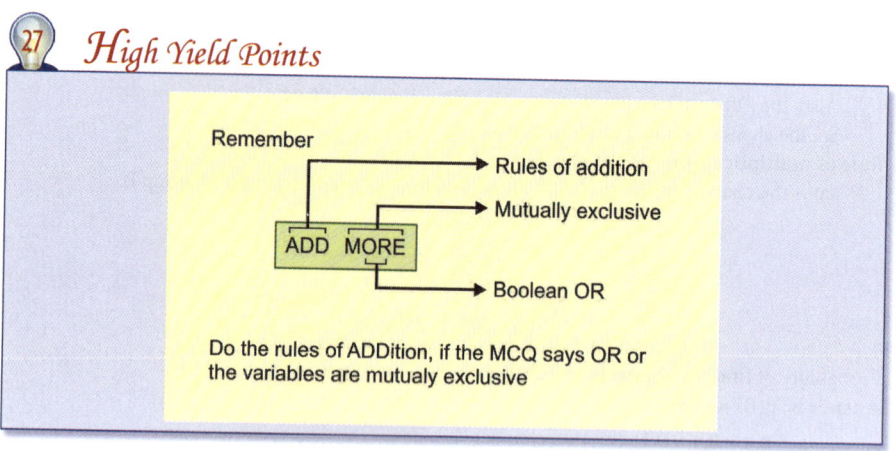

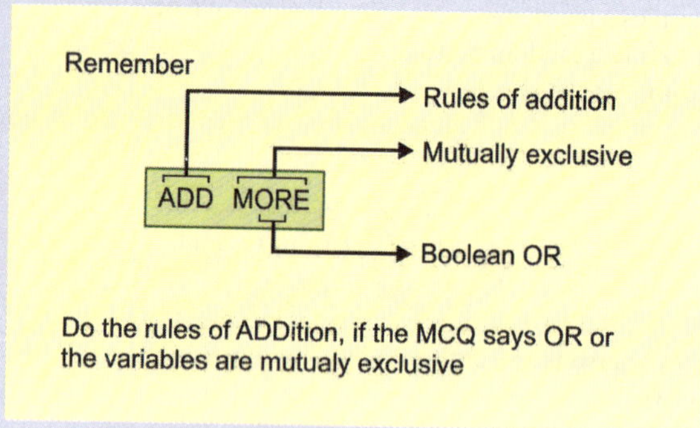

Remember
Rules of addition
Mutually exclusive
ADD MORE
Boolean OR
Do the rules of ADDition, if the MCQ says OR or the variables are mutualy exclusive

CORRELATION AND REGRESSION

Correlation Analysis

In technical terms is the statistical association between two variables. It tells about the strength and direction of association

- The linear correlation is often represented by the symbol 'r', known as Pearson correlation
  The value of 'r' ranges from –1 to + 1
  'r' value = –1 is perfect negative correlation
  'r' value = + 1 is perfect positive correlation

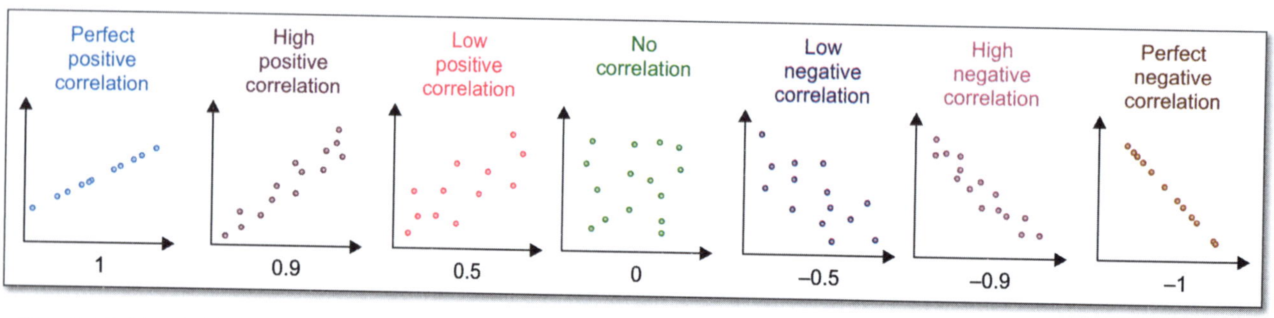

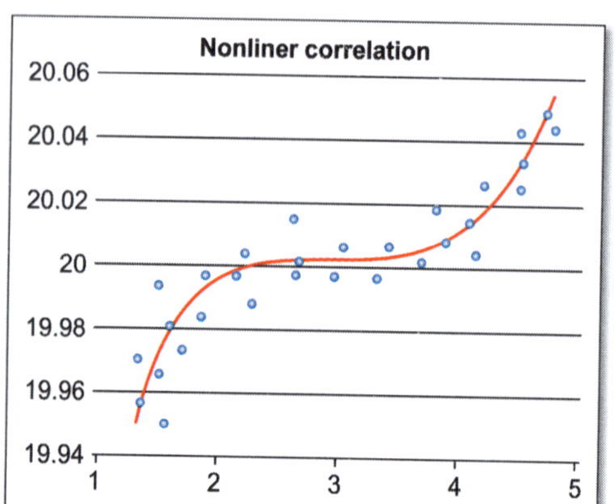

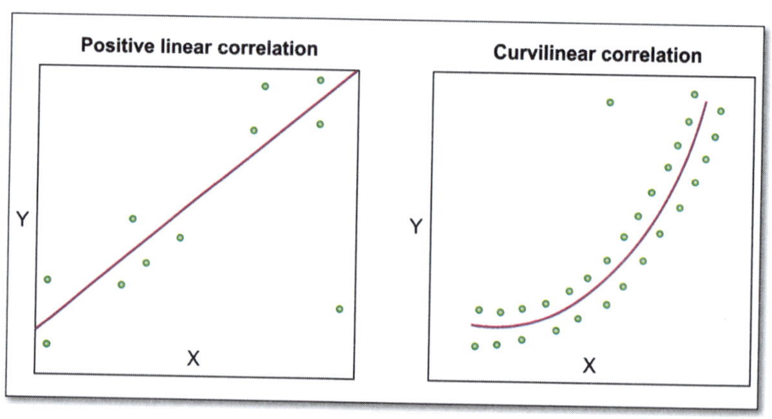

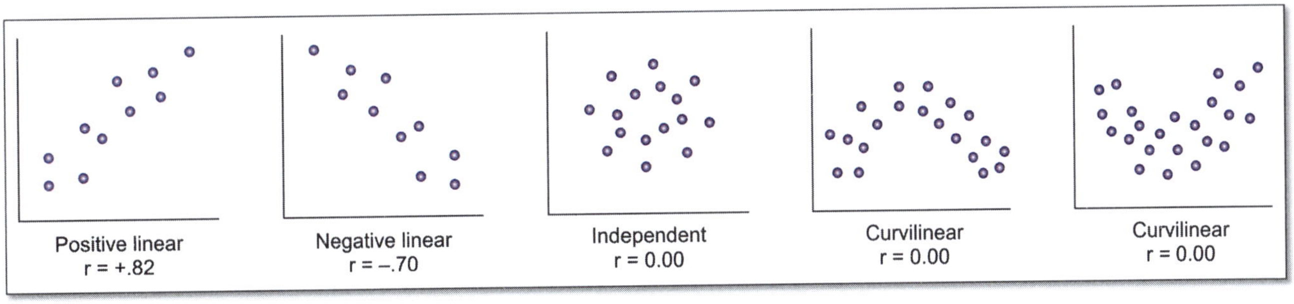

Fig. 24: Statistical correlation

- **Coefficient of determination** is given by the formula r^2. The square of the coefficient (or r^2) is equal to the percent of the variation in one variable that is related to the variation in the other. If the r = 0.5, means 26% of variation in the outcome variable (or dependent) is due to a unit change in the input (or independent) variable.

Regression Analysis

- Regression analysis is a mathematical model to describe the effect of ≥ 1 independent variable on a dependent variable
- Linear regression describes effect of one independent variable on a dependent variable.
- Multiple linear regression describes effect of two or more independent variable on a dependent variable.
- Nonlinear regression involves more complex mathematical forms, including logarithmic functions.
- Logistic regression describes effect of multiple independent (Qualitative, Quantitative or Mixed) variable on dichotomous qualitative variable.
- Regression coefficient is average change in dependent variable for each unit of independent variable.

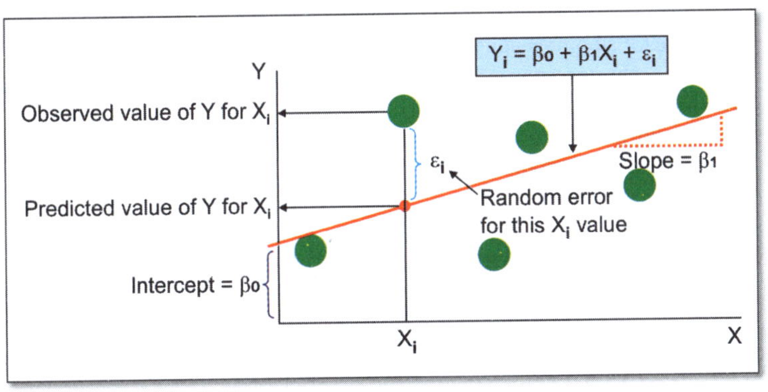

Fig. 25: Regression analysis

SAMPLING

The formula for sample size calculation is:

$$\text{Sample size} = \frac{4PQ}{L \times L}$$

P = prevalence

Q = 100 – prevalence

L = allowable error

(remember – allowable error is the absolute number expressed as percentage of the population mean or expected true value)

Nonrandom or nonprobability sampling:

- Convenient sampling –
  - The sample is selected with convenience without any set selection criteria

28 High Yield Points

Regression equation:

y = a + bx + e

where,

y = dependent variable;

a = regression constant

= intercept of slope on Y

b = slope coefficient; (slope of the curve)

x = independent variable;

e = error

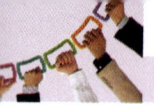

- It is easy to carry out
- Example: 10 patients were selected from the surgery ward for study on patient satisfaction in a hospital

- Purposive sampling
  - With any secondary intention for data advantage
- Quota sampling
  - Predetermined group of sampling. The data is segmented into arbitrary groups, and the population is selected based on convenience or purpose.
- Snowball sampling
  - Is a special technique of sampling, where a small group of population is selected and then the selected subjects would recruit more subjects for the study.
  - Used for "hidden" diseases, or difficult to access population – as drug abusers, commercial sex workers, rare risk factors, or special featured groups

Random sampling or Probability sampling methods:

- Simple random sampling
  - Merits are: Each and every individual has an equal chance of being selected in the sample hence the sample is assured of being representative.
  - Sample selection can be done by different methods like using lottery method or random number table method
  - It does not have observer bias or selection bias.
- Systematic sampling
  - Based on sampling fraction technique. After enumerating the units, they are selected at a predetermined interval
  - It is Simple and convenient method of sampling, needs less time and work, easy administration in the field, but is inferior compared to the simple random sampling.
- Stratified random sampling
  - It gives different population subgroups an equal chance of being selected
  - This ensures that a prespecified number of individuals is given adequate representation hence reduces bias and none is over or under reported
  - It is best done if the population is nonhomogeneous.
- Cluster sampling
  - Best done for a homogenous population
  - To increase the operational feasibility, in the first step, "groups" rather than individuals, are selected and in the final stage, all the individuals in the identified cluster or randomly selected individuals from group are examined
  - Usually used for evaluation of programs or schemes
  - May be associated with a bias due to intercluster variation in the groups.

Population Proportionate to Size Sampling

When samples from different sized subgroups are used and sampling is taken with the same probability, the chances of selecting a member from a large group are less than selecting a member from a smaller group. For example:

- If one sample city has 20,000 individuals, the probability of a member being selected would be 1/20,000 or .005%.
- If another sample had 10,000 members, the chance of a member being selected would be 1/10,000 or .01%.

Image-Based Questions

1. The statistical diagram shown in figure is referred to as:

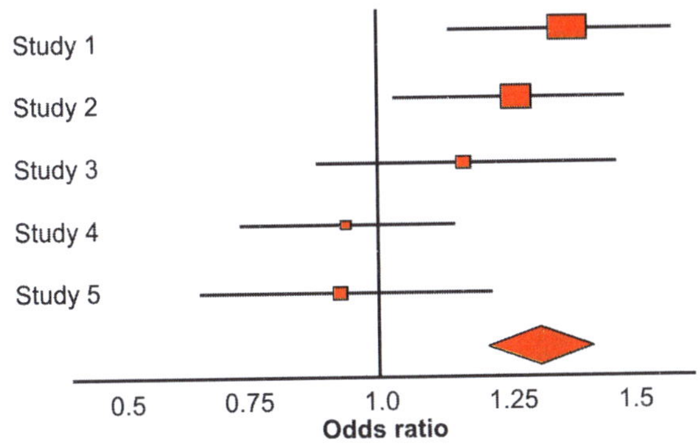

a. Funnel plot
b. Forest plot
c. Stem and Leaf plot
d. Box and Whisker plot

2. The statistical diagram shown in figure is referred to as:

82	0 2
83	0 2 4
84	0 2 8 9
85	0 0 4 4 5 6 7 9
86	0 0 0 0 2 2 4 5 6 8 9
87	0 0 2 7 8 9
88	0 0 2 4 6 7
89	0 2 6
90	0 0 0 0 3 3 7 8

a. Funnel plot
b. Forest plot
c. Stem and Leaf plot
d. Box and Whisker plot

3. The statistical diagram shown in figure is referred to as:

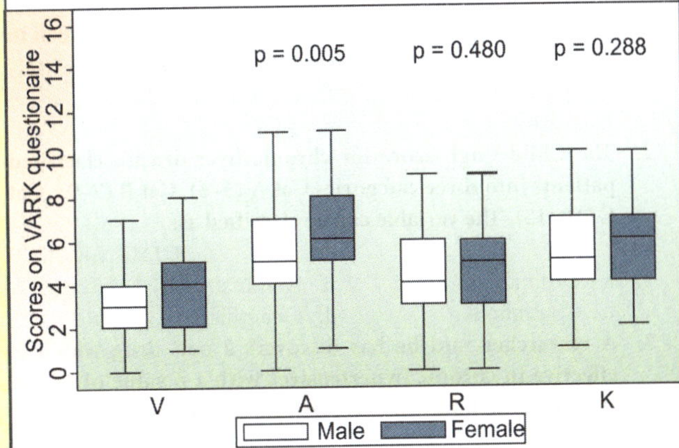

a. Funnel plot
b. Forest plot
c. Stem and Leaf plot
d. Box and Whisker plot

4. Identify the diagram shown in figure:

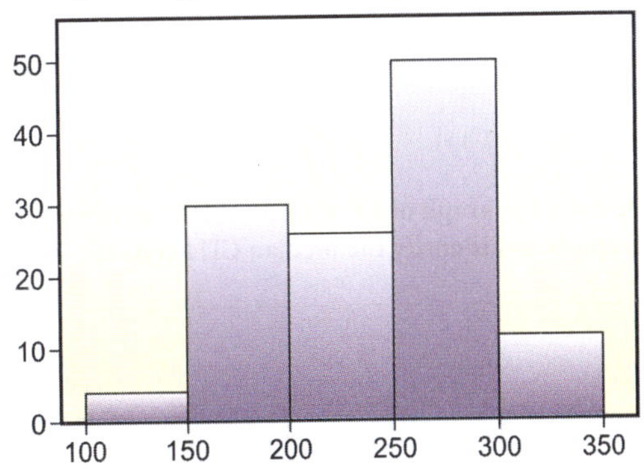

a. Simple bar chart
b. Frequency Diagram
c. Component bar chart
d. Histogram

Answers of Image-Based Questions

1. **Ans. (b)** **Forest plot**
2. **Ans. (c)** **Stem and Leaf plot**
3. **Ans. (d)** **Box and Whisker plot**
4. **Ans. (d)** **Histogram**

Multiple Choice Questions

1. When comparing the relationship between two variables, a significant correlation was found between them (P < 0.5), though none existed in reality. What type of error is seen in this study? ***(AIIMS Nov 2017)***

a. α-1 b. α error
c. β error d. 1-β

2. The Child Pugh score for chronic liver disease classified patients into three categories Cat A (5–6), Cat B (7–9), Cat C (10–15). The variable can be classified as: ***(AIIMS Nov 2017)***

a. Ordinal b. Nominal
c. Continuous d. Quantitative

3. A researcher said he has discovers a new drug which is effective in chronic hypertensives with a p value of <0.10. Which of the following is true regarding the same ***(AIIMS May 2017)***

a. The test is 90% reproducible
b. 90% of test results could have occurred by chance
c. Not more than 10% of the people benefitted by the drug could be due to chance
d. 90% of patients will be benefitted by giving the drug

4. A study was conducted with the objective to compare the incidence of postpartum depression in mother as compared to the sex of the child. For assessment Edinburg Depression scaled score (EDSS) was used. The study was divided into mothers with male baby as one group to be compared with mothers with female baby. Which of the following statistical test will be used to determine the association? ***(AIIMS May 2017)***

a. Student's t test b. Chi-square test
c. ANOVA d. Paired t Test

5. Below is the graph of CD4 count in HIV patients. From the graph below identify the median CD4 count. ***(AIIMS May 2017)***

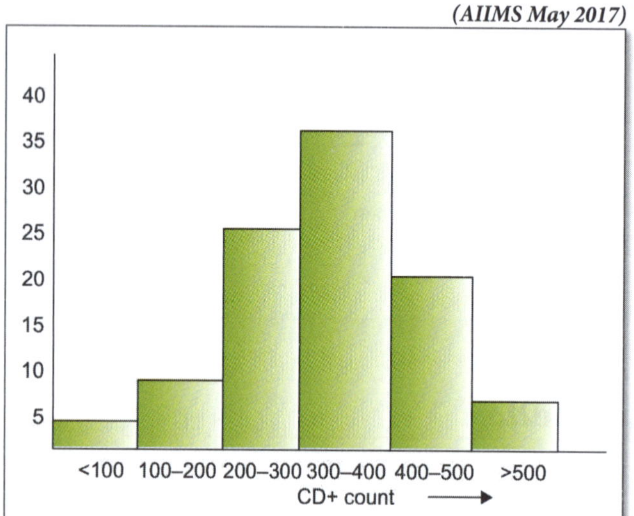

a. 350 b. Above 350
c. Below 350 d. Between 300–400

6. After applying a statistical test, an investigator gets the P value as 0.4. This means: ***(AIIMS May 2017)***

a. The probability of finding a significant difference is 0.4
b. The probability of declaring a significant difference, when there is truly no difference, is 0.4
c. The difference is not significant 60 times and significant 40 times
d. The power of the test used is 60%

7. All of the following are Non-parametric test, except: ***(Recent Question 2018)***

a. Chi square test b. Z test
c. Wilcoxon Rank sum test d. Kruskal-Wallis 'H' test

8. In a normal distribution curve, the area between three standard deviation on either side of the mean is equal to:

a. 68% b. 75%
c. 99% d. 100%

9. Systemic Random sampling: ***(Recent Question 2017)***

a. Random numbers are use
b. Picking every 5th or 10th unit at regular interval
c. Numbers of possible sample is not reduced significantly
d. None

10. A study was done to compare Haemoglobin levels in two different villages. IFA tablets was given to village A and nutritional modifications was given to village B. The change in haemoglobin levels was assessed in each group. the test of significance to be used is:

a. Chi square test
b. t-test
c. ANOVA test
d. Kruskal wallis test

TABULATION, CHART AND DIAGRAM

11. The data description shown below is referred to as:

5	3				
6	8	9	5		
7	9	2	0	2	
8	4	7	9	5	3
9	0	4			

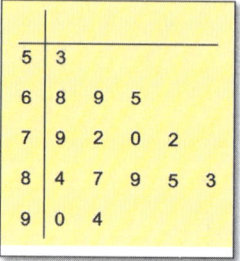

a. Stem and leaf diagram b. Box whisker plot
c. For rest plot d. Funnel plot

12. The following diagram is used to show the trend of events with passage of time: ***(Recent Question 2017)***

a. Histogram b. Frequency polygon
c. Line diagram d. Pictogram

13. A popular method of presenting data to the man in the street and those who cannot understand orthodox charts is:

a. Histogram b. Frequency polygon
c. Line diagram d. Pictogram

Ans.

1. b
2. a
3. c
4. b
5. d
6. b
7. b
8. c
9. b
10. b
11. a
12. c
13. d

Most Recent Questions of 2019-18 are given at the end of MCQs

14. The Statistical diagram shown below is referred to as:

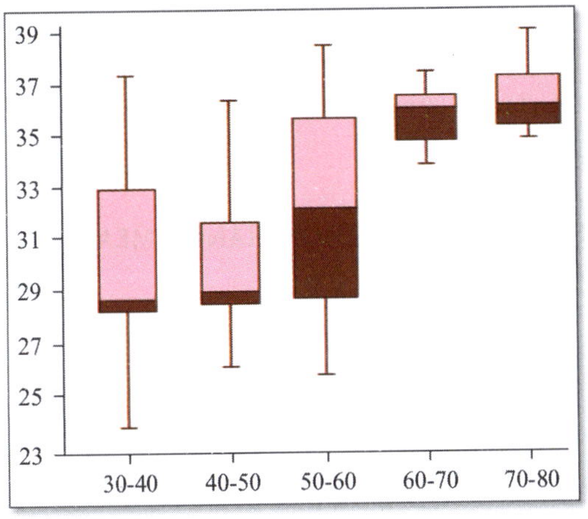

a. Funnel plot b. Forest plot
c. Stem and Leaf plot d. Box and Whisker plot

15. Which of the following diagram/chart is used to present qualitative data?
a. Line diagram b. Scat diagram
c. Pie chart d. Histogram

16. Which of the following diagram is used to find out the relationship between two variables?
a. Pictogram b. Bar diagram
c. Histogram d. Scatter diagram

17. Histogram is used as method of graphical presentation for:
a. Qualitative data
b. Quantitative and continuous data
c. Quantitative and discrete type
d. Nominal data

18. A popular method of presenting data to the man in the street and those who cannot understand orthodox charts is:
a. Histogram b. Frequency polygon
c. Line diagram d. Pictogram

19. Blood pressure was measured for 200 persons. The first quartile BP was 94 mm Hg and third quartile BP was 110 mm Hg. How many persons will have a BP between 3rd and 4th quartile? *(Recent Question 2017)*
a. 100 b. 50
c. 25 d. 150

20. A doctor takes history from a diabetic patient and makes a chart to know about joint involvement. Which chart would he prefer? *(Recent Question 2017)*
a. Pie chart
b. Venn diagram
c. Histogram
d. Tree diagram

21. All of the following are continuous variable, except:
a. Weight in kg
b. Blood group (A, B, AB, O)
c. Age in years and months
d. Height in cm

22. Scatter diagram is used for: *(Recent Question 2016)*
a. Two plot cumulative frequency
b. Relationship between two variables
c. Trend of event with passage of time
d. Symbol used to present data

23. Which of the following is/are true about use of Bar diagram? *(PGI Pattern)*
a. Comparison of 2 categorical data which are not-additive
b. Comparison of 2 categorical data which are proportional percentage contribution of categories
c. Pie chart is used for comparison of 2 categorical data which are proportional percentage contribution of categories
d. Comparison of magnitude of different frequencies in discrete data
e. Comparison of continuous data

24. Ogive is: *(Recent Question 2016)*
a. Bar chart
b. Histogram
c. Cumulative frequency curve
d. Frequency polygon

25. Correlation between two variables is plotted in:
a. Pie chart b. Histogram
c. Frequency polygon d. Scatter diagram

26. Scatter diagram is used for: *(Recent Question 2016)*
a. Two plot cumulative frequency
b. Relationship between two variables
c. Trend of event with passage of time
d. Symbol used to present data

27. Test used to compare two qualitative data is:
a. Paired T-test b. Unpaired T-test
c. Chi-square test d. AVOVA

28. Trends can be represented by: *(Recent Question 2016)*
a. Scatter diagram b. Bar diagram
c. Line diagram d. Pie chart

29. Best way to plot the change of incidence of disease over time is:
a. Histogram b. Line chart
c. Scatter diagram d. Ogive

30. Best method to show trend of events with passage of time is:
a. Line diagram b. Bar diagram
c. Histogram d. Pie chart

31. Graph to correlate two quantitative data is: *(Recent Question 2015)*
a. Histogram
b. Scatter diagram
c. Line diagram
d. Frequency curve

32. The best graphic representation of frequency distribution of data gathered of a continuous variable is:
a. Simple bar b. Histogram
c. Line diagram d. Multiple bar

TYPES OF SCALES

33. Nominal data example is:
a. Types of hospitals
b. Severity of pain
c. Height
d. Grades of obesity

34. Old men with BP 210/110 mm Hg are classified as severe hypertension. This type of data is: *(Recent Question 2015)*
a. Categorical
b. Numerical
c. Quantitative
d. Continuous

Ans.

14. d
15. c
16. d
17. b
18. d
19. b
20. d
21. b
22. b
23. a, c, d
24. c
25. d
26. b
27. c
28. c
29. b
30. a
31. b
32. b
33. a
34. a

35. An old man with hypertension and BP 210/110 mm Hg is classified into severe hypertension. Scale used is:
a. Nominal b. Ordinal
c. Interval d. Ratio

36. All of the following are example of nominal scale, except: ***(Recent Question 2015)***
a. Race b. Sex
c. Body weight d. Socio economic status

37. When the number of observation is 25, the number of class interval must be:
a. 25 b. 15
c. 10 d. 5

38. In a study following interpretation are obtained: Satisfied, Very satisfied, Dissatisfied. Which type of scale is this?
a. Nominal b. Ordinal
c. Interval d. Ratio

39. Likert scale is: ***(Recent Question 2015)***
a. Ordinal scale b. Normal scale
c. Variance scale d. Categorical scale

MEASURES OF CENTRAL TENDENCY (MEAN/MEDIAN/MODE)

40. True regarding the following observation 1, 2, 2, 4, 6 is
a. Mean = 3 b. Median = 3
c. Mode = 3 d. Standard deviation = 1

41. Mean diastolic BP in 125 females aged be 18-60, was found to be 70 mm Hg with SD of 10 mm Hg. What will be the 5th percentile value? ***(Recent Question 2015)***
a. 67.5 b. 50.4
c. 89.6 d. 40

42. In a distribution, the one which is present in greatest frequency is called:
a. Mean b. Median
c. Mode d. Standard deviation

43. In a positively skewed distribution:
a. Mean< Median
b. Mean< Mode
c. Median > Mode
d. Longer tail towards lower values of the variable

44. True regarding the distribution of weights of a group of students: 70, 70, 70, 75, 79, 83, 84, 85 is:
a. Median 77 b. Mode 70
c. Range 8 d. Mean 77
e. Normal distribution

45. In a survey of Sleep apnea scores among 10 persons, highest recoded value was 58 , but was wrongly recorded as 85. The effect on final results will be: ***(Recent Question 2014)***
a. Mean will remain same and Median will be Increased
b. Mean will be Increased, Median will remain same
c. Both Mean and Median will be Increased
d. Mean will be Increased and Median decreased

46. Smoking history of a smoker for last 6 years is as follows. 1st year - 5 cigarettes per day. In subsequent 3 years half pack, 1 pack in the 5th year and 2 pack per day in the last year. True statement for Mean, median and mode of number of sticks are: ***(Recent Question 2014)***
a. 16, 10, 15 b. 16, 10, 10
c. 10, 10, 16 d. 16, 10, 5

47. Which of the following measures of central tendency can have more than one value?
a. Median b. Mode
c. Mean d. None

48. Most frequently occurring value in a group of data:
a. Mean b. Mode
c. Median d. Standard deviation

MEASURES OF DISPERSION (RANGE, MEAN DEVIATION AND SD)

49. Following are measures of dispersion, except:
a. Range
b. Mean or average deviation
c. Standard deviation
d. Correlation and regression

50. 1.95 Standard Deviation (SD) includes what percentage of values or sample in a distribution
a. 99% b. 95%
c. 68% d. 50%

51. In a normal distribution curve, the area between three standard deviation on either side of the mean is equal to:
a. 99% b. 95%
c. 75% d. 68%

52. Variance is equal to the square of:
a. 'P' value b. Mean deviation
c. Standard deviation d. Standard error of mean

53. Measuring variation between two different units is done through: ***(Recent Question 2014)***
a. Variance b. Coefficient of variation
c. Standard deviation d. Range

54. True statements regarding Standard Deviation is/are:
a. 1 SD covers 95% values in a distribution
b. It indicates the distribution of variables
c. It is the most commonly used method of dispersion
d. Applicable only for normal distributions
e. It is a better indicator of variance than range

55. In a group of pregnant females mean hemoglobin level was 10.6 g/dL with Standard deviation of 2gm/dL, 5% pregnant females in this group will have their hemoglobin level below:
a. 8.6 g/dL b. 7.31 g/dL
c. 6.6 g/dL d. 5.0 g/dL

56. Formula for Standard Deviation [SD], in case where sample size is < 30 is:
a. $\sqrt{[\Sigma(x-\bar{x})^2]\rho}$ b. $\sqrt{[\Sigma(x-\bar{x})^2]/\eta\text{-}1}$
c. $\sqrt{[\Sigma(x-\bar{x})^2]/\eta}$ d. $\sqrt{[\Sigma(x-\bar{x})^2]/\rho-1}$

57. If the birth weight of each of the 10 babies born in an hospital in a day is found to be 2.8 kg, then the standard deviation of this sample will be: ***(Recent Question 2013)***
a. 2.8 b. 0
c. 1 d. 0.28

58. Most common deviation used in social medicine is:
a. Mean
b. Range
c. Variance d. Standard deviation

Ans.
35. b
36. c
37. d
38. b
39. a
40. a
41. b
42. c
43. c
44. a,b,d
45. b
46. b
47. b
48. b
49. d
50. b
51. a
52. c
53. b
54. b,c,e
55. b
56. b
57. b
58. d

59. **Dispersion of data is measured by:**
   a. Coefficient of correlation
   b. Range
   c. Standard deviation
   d. Coefficient of variation
   e. Normal distribution curve

60. **Measures of dispersion all, except:** *(Recent Question 2013)*
   a. Range
   b. Mean or average deviation
   c. Standard deviation
   d. Correlation and regression

NORMAL DISTRIBUTION

61. **The following box plot shows the distribution of three sets of data around the mean. What is the correct sequence of inference from this box plot?** *(Recent Question 2013)*

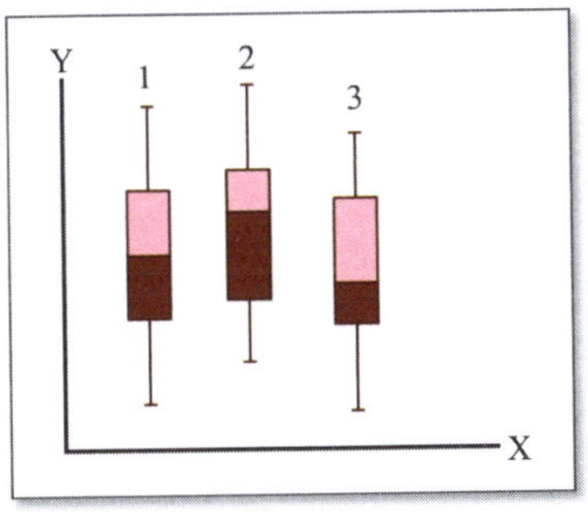

   a. 1-Normal distribution, 2- Positive skewed, 3-Negative skewed
   b. 1-Normal Distribution, 2- Negative skewed, 3- Positive skewed
   c. 1- Negative skewed, 2- Positive skewed, 3- Normal distribution
   d. 1- Positive skewed, 2- Normal distribution, 3-Negative skewed

62. **If the mean, median and mode are 10, 16 and 22 respectively, the distribution is:** *(Recent Question 2013)*
   a. Positively skewed b. Negatively skewed
   c. Symmetric d. Normal

63. **True statement about standard normal curve is**
   a. Equal distribution on either side of the curve
   b. The total area under the curve is 2
   c. Its mean is 1
   d. Standard deviation is 0

64. **Not true regarding standard normal curve:**
   a. Mean < median
   b. The total area under the curve is 1
   c. Its mean is zero
   d. Standard deviation is 1 (s)

65. **In standard normal curve, mean is:**
   a. Equal to standard deviation
   b. Zero
   c. <1
   d. 1

66. **Z score criteria applicable to a:** *(Recent Question 2014)*
   a. Normal distribution b. Chi-square test
   c. Paired t test d. Skewed deviation

67. **Continuous distribution is shown by**
   a. Weibull curve b. Normal distribution
   c. Poisson distribution d. Binomial distribution

68. **What will be the 95% confidence interval in a study estimated prevalence of 10% and 100 being their sample size?**
   a. 4–16
   b. 2–18
   c. Inadequate information to calculate 95% CI
   d. 7–13

69. **An obstetrician used APGAR score to assess health of 30 newborn infants. The result showed most of them with score >7. Then the:** *(Recent Question 2014)*
   a. Data is symmetrical
   b. Data is negatively skewed
   c. Data is positively skewed
   d. Data is symmetrically skewed

70. **In a center the number of nodes dissected during 20 modified radical mastectomy were plotted in the form of a cure and there are three marking on the below curve. Based on the distribution type of curve which of the following is correct:**

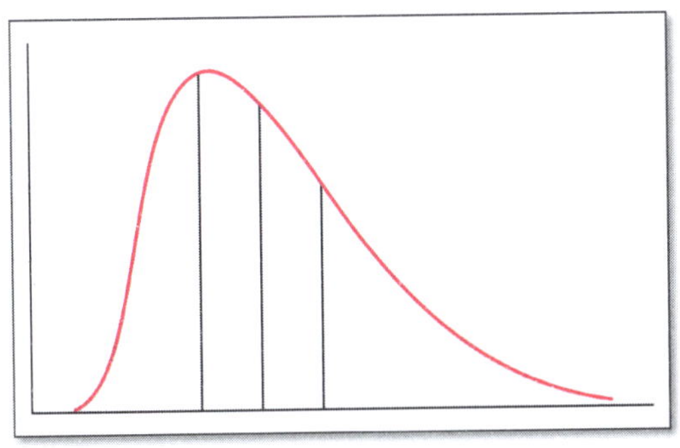

   a. Mean > median > mode
   b. Mode > median > mean
   c. Median > mode > mean
   d. Mode > mean > median

71. **There is a population of 2000 people with mean hemoglobin being 13.5 g% having a normal distribution. What proportion of population constitutes proportion more than 13.5 g%?**
   a. 0.25 b. 0.50
   c. 1 d. 0.34

72. **In a population of 100, the prevalence of candida was found to be 80%. What is the 95% confidence interval for the study conducted.** *(Recent Question 2015)*
   a. 78–82% b. 76–84%
   c. 72–88% d. 74–86%

73. **For a negatively skewed data mean will be:**
   a. Less than median b. More than median
   c. Equal to median d. One

74. **In the left skewed curve, true statement is:**
   a. Mean = median b. Mean < Mode
   c. Mean > mode d. Mean = mode

75. **How much population falls between median and median plus one standard deviation in a normal distribution:**
   a. 0.34 b. 0.68
   c. 0.17 d. 0.47

Ans.

59.	b, c, d, e
60.	d
61.	b
62.	b
63.	a
64.	a
65.	b
66.	a
67.	b
68.	a
69.	b
70.	a
71.	b
72.	c
73.	a
74.	b
75.	a

Most Recent Questions of 2019-18 are given at the end of MCQs

76. Pearson's skewness coefficient is: *(Recent Question 2015)*
a. (3 × [Mean – Median])/SD
b. (3 × [Median – Mean])/SD
c. SD/[Mean – Median]
d. SD/[Median – Mean]

77. Z score is for which type of distribution:
a. Binominal
b. Normal distribution curve
c. 't' test
d. Chi square test

78. Which of the following statements about confidence limits/interval is true?
a. Smaller the confidence level larger will be the confidence interval
b. Less variable the data, wider will be the confidence interval
c. Sample size does not affect the confidence interval
d. 95% confidence interval will cover 2 standard errors around the mean

SAMPLING

79. A researcher selects all possible samples from a population and plots their means on a line graph. What is this distribution referred to as: *(Recent Question 2015)*
a. Sample distribution
b. Sampling distribution
c. Population distribution
d. Parametric distribution

80. In a study with prevalence of 10%. Calculate the sample size for across sectional study if relative precision 20%, alpha error-5% and power of the study 80%:
a. 3600
b. 400
c. 900
d. 600

81. Cluster sampling is done for collecting data on:
a. Drug users
b. Nonhomologous groups
c. Immunization coverage
d. Contraceptive use

82. True statement regarding systematic sampling is:
a. Every unit has an unequal chance of being selected
b. Sampling Interval depends on total number of samples
c. Sampling is done is stages
d. Small homogenous populations give best results

83. If subjects are assigned according to the potential factor that will influence the outcome of the study, then the sampling is: *(Recent Question 2015)*
a. Systemic random sampling
b. Stratified random sampling
c. Simple random sampling
d. Clustered random sampling

84. In an epidemiological study, every 10th person was selected from the population. This is an example of:
a. Cluster random sampling
b. Simple random sampling
c. Stratified random sampling
d. Systematic random sampling

85. 50% population having disease with the estimated prevalence to be 45-55% with 95% of probability of identifying them minimum sample size required is:
a. 100
b. 200
c. 300
d. 400

86. Simple random sampling is ideal for:
a. Vaccinated people
b. Heterogeneous population
c. Homogeneous population
d. All of the above

87. Stratified sampling is ideal for:
a. Hetrogeneous data
b. Homogeneous data
c. Both
d. None

88. Children surveyed in cluster sampling for coverage of national immunization programme in:
a. 30 cluster of 5 children
b. 20 cluster of 5 children
c. 30 cluster of 10 children
d. 30 cluster of 7 children

89. In a study first school are sampled, then sections and finally student, this type of sampling is known as:
a. Stratified sampling
b. Simple random sampling
c. Cluster sampling
d. Multistage sampling

90. All of the following comes under random sampling method, except:
a. Quota sampling
b. Simple random sampling
c. Stratified sampling
d. Cluster sampling

91. A village was divided into 5 sub groups, for a survey. The sample was drawn by selecting people randomly from these subgroups. What type of sampling was done?
a. Simple random sampling
b. Stratified random sampling
c. Cluster sampling
d. Systematic random sampling

92. Which sampling method is used in assessing immunization status of children under an immunization programme?
a. Quota sampling
b. Multistage sampling
c. Stratified sampling
d. Cluster sampling

TEST OF SIGNIFICANCE

93. Which of the following is used to compare two independent means? *(Recent Question 2014)*
a. Chi-square test
b. Student's test
c. McNemar's Chi-square test
d. Paired test

94. Criteria for applying t-test is: *(Recent Question 2014)*
a. Non-Random samples
b. Qualitative data
c. Variable asymmetrically distributed
d. Sample size <30

95. P value is significant when it is less than:
a. 1
b. 0.5
c. 0.1
d. 0.05

96. Degree of freedom for a contingency table with 3 rows and 6 columns is: *(Recent Question 2014)*
a. 2
b. 3
c. 10
d. 18

97. Not true regarding Chi-square test:
a. To find the significance of difference between two proportions
b. To find any association between two attributes occurring together
c. To test the goodness of fit
d. Chi-square curve is negatively skewed

Ans.

76. a
77. b
78. d
79. b
80. c
81. c
82. b
83. b
84. d
85. d
86. c
87. a
88. d
89. d
90. a
91. b
92. d
93. b
94. d
95. d
96. c
97. d

Most Recent Questions of 2019-18 are given at the end of MCQs

98. All of the following are tests of significance, except:
a. t test
b. Z test
c. Standard Deviation
d. Chi-square test

99. Type I statistical error is said to have occurred if:
a. Null hypothesis is true and is accepted
b. Null hypothesis is false but is accepted
c. Null hypothesis is true but is rejected
d. Null hypothesis is false and is rejected

100. If we say that there is no significant association between two variable and if truly an association exists. Then it is called as: ***(Recent Question 2014)***
a. Type I error
b. Type II error
c. Systematic error
d. Random error

101. True statement regarding significance testing is:
a. Type 1 error is to reject alternate hypothesis when is should be accepted
b. Type 2 error is to accept alternate hypothesis when it should be rejected
c. Probability associated with type 1 error is significant
d. The significant level is always set to 5%

102. In a study, two groups of newborns were assessed (based on low or normal birth weight) for the intake of nutritional supplement (yes or no) by mother. Suggest an appropriate test of significance: ***(Recent Question 2013)***
a. Paired t test
b. Chi-square test
c. Unpaired t test
d. Fischer's exact test

103. Power of study can be increased by:
a. Increasing a error
b. Decreasing b error
c. Decreasing a error
d. Increasing b error

104. Type 1 sampling error is classified as:
a. Alpha error
b. Beta error
c. Gamma error
d. Delta error

105. The intraocular pressure (IOP) was measured in a population of 400 people above the age of 65. The mean IOP was 25 and standard deviation was 10. What is the range that would contain the IOP of 95% of the population:
a. 23–27 b. 21–29
c. 24–26 d. 22–28

106. In a population of 100000, hemoglobin of 100 women is estimated with standard deviation of 2 g%. What is the standard error: ***(Recent Question 2013)***
a. 1 b. 0.1
c. 2 d. 0.2

107. When we say "the difference is significant" it means that:
a. It is likely by chance and $p > 0.05$
b. It is unlikely by chance and $p < 0.05$
c. It is unlikely by chance and $p > 0.05$
d. It is likely by chance and $p < 0.05$

108. Rejecting a null hypothesis when it is true is called as:
a. Type 1 error
b. Type 2 error
c. Type 3 error
d. Type 4 error

109. Q – test is used to detect:
a. Outliers
b. Interquartile range
c. Difference of means
d. Difference of proportions

110. Test used to compare two proportions is/are:
a. Paired T test
b. Unpaired T test
c. ANOVA
d. Fischer's exact test
e. Chi square test

111. Appropriate statistical method to compare two means is:
a. Chi square test b. Students T test
c. Odd ratio d. Correlation coefficient

112. Chi square test 5 rows/4 columns, degree of freedom is:
a. 9 b. 12
c. 16 d. 20

113. Degree of freedom of contingency table with 3 rows and 6 columns is: ***(Recent Question 2013)***
a. 2 b. 3
c. 10 d. 18

114. ANOVA is used
a. To compare means in two groups
b. To compare means in three or more groups
c. To compare means in one group before and after intervention
d. To find correlation

115. Not required for Chi square test: ***(Recent Question 2013)***
a. Null hypothesis
b. Degree of freedom
c. Means in different groups
d. Proportion in different groups

116. Chi square test is for:
a. Standard error of mean
b. Standard error of proportion
c. Difference between population means
d. Difference between population proportion

117. Degree of freedom for 2 × 2 contingency table is:
a. 1 b. 0
c. 2 d. 4

118. Test used to compare Kaplan – Meier survival curve is:
a. ANOVA
b. Bland Altman analysis
c. Chi square test
d. Cox proportional hazard test

119. An investigator finds out that 5 independent factors influence the occurrence of a disease. Comparison of multiple factors responsible for a disease can be assessed by: ***(Recent Question 2014)***
a. Multiple linear regression
b. ANOVA
c. Kruskal-Wallis one way analysis of variance by ranks
d. Multiple logistic regression

Ans.

98. c
99. c
100. b
101. c
102. b
103. b
104. a
105. c
106. d
107. b
108. a
109. a
110. d, e
111. b
112. b
113. c
114. b
115. c
116. b
117. a
118. d
119. d

Most Recent Questions of 2019-18 are given at the end of MCQs

CORRELATION AND REGRESSION

120. The following scatter plot of 4 different samples shows the correlation between weight and height in the samples. What will be the approximate net correlation coefficient as from the image given below. What will be the net correlation coefficient?

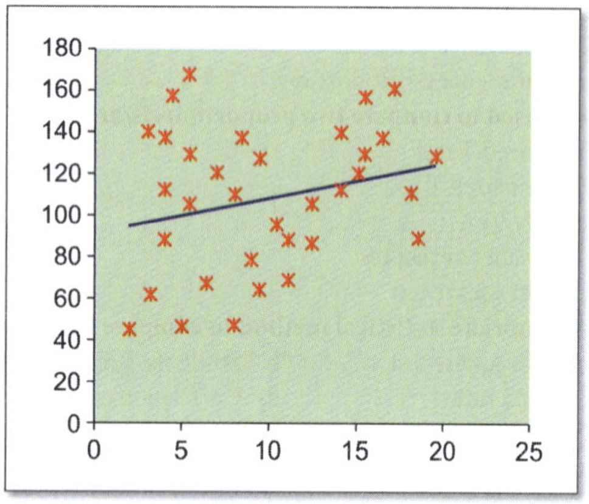

a. + 1 b. + 0.25
c. – 1.5 d. + 1.5

121. Correlation coefficient lies between:

a. –1 to +1
b. –1 to 0
c. 0 to 1
d. 1 to 100

122. Pearson coefficient is used for: ***(Recent Question 2015)***

a. Differences in proportion
b. Comparison of more than 2 means
c. Comparison for variance
d. Correlation

123. In an agreement between SpO_2 of two groups with and without micropore in a pediatric population the values spotted is as below. Which of the following is true?

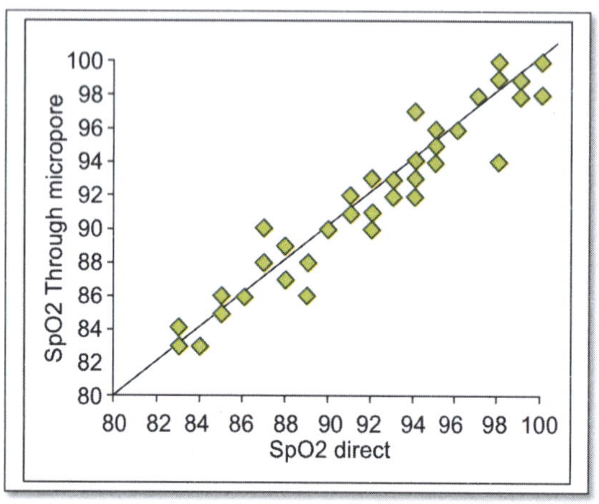

a. There is no agreement between the two groups
b. The two groups have a constant relation with a variation of 3%
c. The is no association between the two groups
d. The curve shows a regression line means correlation

124. Which of the following is correct regarding the below pic?

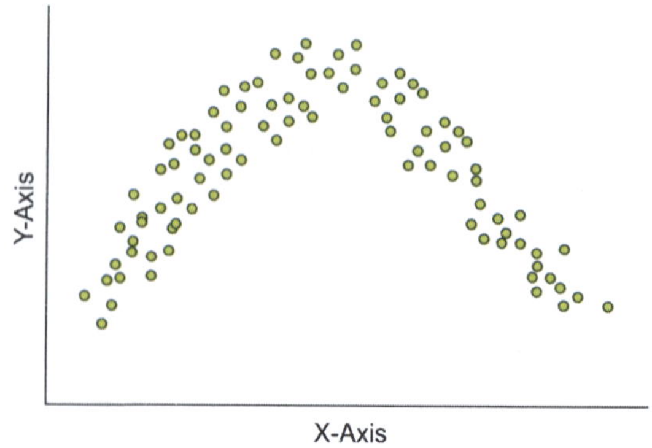

a. Nonlinear relationship b. Linear relationship
c. Nothing can be inferred d. Positive co-relation found

125. Change in the frequency of one variable can be estimated from the change in other variable by:

a. Regression b. Correlation
c. Bar diagram d. Scatter Diagram

126. Pearson or spearman coefficient is used for evaluation of:

a. Differences in proportion
b. Comparison of more man 2 means
c. Comparison of variance
d. Correlation

127. Correlation in height and weight are measured by:

a. Coefficient of variation b. Range of variation
c. Correlation coefficient d. None

128. Mosquito density decreases as height increases in:

a. Positive correlation b. Negative correlation
c. Bi directional d. Zero correlation

129. Strong correlation is signified by an correlation coefficient of: ***(Recent Question 2013)***

a. Zero b. 1
c. Less than 1 d. More than 1

130. Threshold of measurable data can be determined by:

a. ROC curve b. Frequency polygon
c. Histogram d. Scatter diagram

131. All of the following are true regarding the Ratio except

a. Numerator is component of denominator
b. Numerator is not a component of denominator
c. Numerator and denominator are related values
d. It is expressed as variable a:b

132. The diagram that indicates the frequency represented by an area in columns corresponding to quantitative data is called as

a. Bar diagram b. Pie diagram
c. Histogram d. Pictogram

133. Which one of the following represent frequency of quantitative data?

a. Histogram b. Line diagram
c. Simple bar chart d. Component bar chart

134. Dispersion of data is measured by

a. Mean b. Mode
c. Median d. Standard Deviation

135. Most commonly used measure of dispersion is

a. Mean b. SD
c. Mean deviation d. Mode

Ans.

120. b
121. a
122. d
123. d
124. a
125. a
126. d
127. c
128. b
129. b
130. a
131. a
132. c
133. a
134. d
135. b

136. Standard deviation represents
a. Distribution b. Dispersion
c. Correlation d. Comparison

137. Confidence limit is calculated by using
a. Mean and standard error
b. Mean and standard deviation
c. Median and standard deviation
d. Median

138. Variability from mean is measured by
a. SD b. Variance
c. Mean d. Mode

139. Root mean square deviation is derived from
a. SD b. Mean derivative
c. Mode d. Median

140. Test of association between two variables is done by
a. Chi square b. Correlation
c. Regression d. Anova - test

141. If the size of the random sample is increased, we would expect *[PGI Pattern]*
a. The mean to decrease
b. The standard error of the mean to decrease
c. The standard deviation to decrease
d. The sample variance to increase
e. The coefficient of variation will increase

142. Most important test of significance to find the strength of association between two non-parametric data sets is
a. Standard error of difference of mean
b. Regression coefficient test
c. Student's test
d. χ^2 test (Chi-square test)

143. A coefficient of correlation value of r = +0.8 indicates
a. Strong positive relationship between two variables
b. A strong negative relationship between two variables
c. An insignificant association between two variables
d. One variable is the cause of the other variable

144. What is the method of sampling in which the units are picked up at regular intervals from the universe?
a. Simple random sampling
b. Systematic random sampling
c. Stratified random sampling
d. Snowball sampling

145. Which of the following results gives the reader the most information concerning statistical significance, sample size, and strength of association?
a. A relative risk of 2.5 with a 95 percent confidence interval of 2.0 to 3.1
b. A p value of 0.4 and a relative risk of 0.6
c. A relative risk of 5.0 with a 95 percent confidence interval of 0.1 to 9.8
d. A p value of <0.05 and a relative risk of 2.5

146. All the following statements concerning statistical inference are true EXCEPT:
a. A test of statistical significance does not prove causality
b. A statistically significant test assesses the probability of a "chance" occurrence
c. A statistically significant test supports the null hypothesis
d. A confidence interval does not address whether an association is due to bias.

147. Assuming that Visual inspection for Ca cervix has a sensitivity of 90 percent and a specificity of 98 percent, and that consecutive tests are independent, what is the probability that a woman with cervical cancer will have a negative screening VIA (visual inspection with acetic acid) for two consecutive years?
a. 1/10 b. 2/10
c. 4/10 d. 1/100

148. The probability of being born with condition A is 0.10 and the probability of being born with condition B is 0.50. If condition A and B are independent, what is probability of being born with either condition A or condition B but not both?
a. 0.05 b. 0.40
c. 0.50 d. 0.55

149. Which statement is true concerning measures of central tendency ?
a. If more outlying observations are smaller than the rest of the values , the data are skewed to the right
b. If more outlying observation is larger than the rest of the values, the median will be smaller than the mean
c. If the data are skewed to the left , the means is larger than the median
d. The median is more sensitive than the means to extreme observation

150. Weight in kg is:
a. Normal variable b. Discrete variable
c. Confounding variable d. Continuous variable

151. In a standard normal curve, mean ± 2 standard deviation covers:
a. 60% b. 65%
c. 99% d. 95%

152. Which of the following measures the central tendency of frequency distribution:
a. Mean deviation b. Standard deviation
c. Median d. Range

153. Coefficient of correlation is calculated to find:
a. Value of other variable if the value of one variable is known
b. Whether there is significant association between two variables
c. Difference between two proportions
d. Standard deviation

154. True about 'standard deviation' is:
a. Measures the spread of dispersion
b. Defined as root means square deviation
c. Measures the dispersion of values about the mean
d. All of the above

155. True about a negatively skewed data:
a. Mode is Less than median
b. Mode is More than median
c. Mode is equal to median
d. No correlation

156. Which is the best distribution to study the daily admission of head injury patients in a trauma care center?
a. Poisson distribution
b. Nominal distribution
c. Binomial distribution
d. Uniform distribution

Ans.
136. b
137. b
138. a
139. a
140. b
141. b, c
142. d
143. a
144. b
145. a
146. c
147. d
148. d
149. b
150. d
151. d
152. c
153. b
154. d
155. b
156. a

157. Not a marker of association
a. P value b. Odds ratio
c. Correlation coefficient d. Alpha value

158. In a particular trial, the association of lung cancer with smoking is found to be 40% in one sample and 60% in another sample. What is the best to compare the results?
a. ANOVA b. Fischer test
c. Chi Square test d. Paired T test

159. All of the following about standard error (SE) are true except?
a. Standard error for difference in means is calculated for parametric data
b. As the sample size increase standard error increases
c. It is a measure of the extent to which the sample means deviate from the true population mean
d. SE is inversely related to the square root of the sample size

160. The correlation coefficient between two variables x and y of -0.99 shows:
a. No association b. Weak association
c. Strong association d. None of the above

161. To measure the disease probability, Bayes' theorem uses all parameters except one:
a. Pretest probability of disease
b. Test sensitivity
c. Test specificity
d. Predictive value of the test

162. A study to compare the hemoglobin level was conducted on alcoholics before and after consumption. The statistical method used to find significance is
a. Chi square test b. Unpaired t test
c. Paired T test d. Mann Whitney test

163. Pearson's skewness coefficient is?
a. Mean–mode/SD
b. Mode–mean/SD
c. SD/mean–mode
d. SD/median–mode

164. The mean blood pressure of a group of people is 105. The standard deviation was 10. 95% of the population will lie within how much range:
a. 95-115
b. 85-125
c. 75-135
d. 104-106

165. If the systolic blood pressure in a population has a mean of 130 mm Hg and a median of 140 mm Hg. The distribution is said to be:
a. Symmetrical
b. Positively skewed
c. Negatively skewed
d. Either positively or, negatively skewed depending on the standard deviation

166. Which of the following statements is correct with regard to Confidence limits?
a. Smaller the confidence level, the wider the interval.
b. The lesser variable our data, the wider is the confidence interval
c. The width of the confidence interval is independent of sample size
d. Confidence interval for 95% 'is wider than 70%

167. In a study, the remission rate of the new drug was found to be equal to the remission rate of a drug already in use with a p value 0.04. Which of the following is true?
a. Insufficient data to compare the two drugs
b. Both drugs are effective
c. Both drugs are ineffective
d. Power of study is 60%

168. A clinical trail was conducted with 15225 hypertensive patients allotted in the intervention group (New drug) and control group (Old drug) respectively Results of the research study are given in the following table•
Calculate the absolute risk reduction (ARR) and relative risk reduction (RRR):

	Control group (old drug)	Intervention Group (new drug)
Developed HT complications	1800	1620
Did not develop HT complications	13425	13605
Total subjects	15225	15225

a. ARR = 10% and RRR = 0.9
b. ARR = 1% and RRR = 0.9
c. ARR = 1% and RRR = 9.9
d. ARR = 10% and RRR = 9.9

169. Chronic liver disease is classified into Child—Pugh class A to C, employing the added score from above. Class A: 5-6, B: 7-9, C: 10-15. This is ....scale:
a. Ordinal
b. Nominal
c. Qualitative
d. Continuous

170. In a statistical study for calculating the effect of drug on patient's sugar level, the test showed significant difference, whereas in reality there was no difference. This is due to:
a. Beta error
b. Gamma error
c. Alpha error
d. Power of the test

171. A group of investigators conduct a study to evaluate the association of serum homocysteine levels and myocardial infarction. The study concludes that high levels of homocysteine is associated with MI with a risk ratio of 1.05 and a p value of 0.01. which of the following statement is true for the study:
a. There is an excess of 5% chance that high homocysteine may cause MI
b. There is 1% chance that there is no association
c. There is 95% chance that the Confidence interval includes RR of 1
d. There is 95% chance that there is no correlation

172. Calculate the 95% confidence interval for a study to estimate the Anemia prevalence showing result as 10% in a sample size of 100 individuals.
a. 4–16
b. 2–18
c. 7–13
d. Inadequate information to calculate 95% CI

Ans.
157. d
158. c
159. a
160. c
161. d
162. c
163. a
164. b
165. c
166. d
167. b
168. c
169. a
170. c
171. b
172. a

Most Recent Questions of 2019-18 are given at the end of MCQs

173. The estimated prevalence for Diabetes mellitus in a population is 10%. The researcher wishes to find the prevalence of DM in a community with 95% confidence limits and within a range of 8-12%

a. 200
b. 300
c. 400
d. 900

174. Which is true regarding the Kolmograph Smirnov test

a. Used to find the spearman correlation between two variables
b. It is used to assess for equality of distribution of non-parametric data
c. It is to determine agreement between qualitative parameters
d. To find the significance between two ordinal grouped data set

175. Unlinked testing is done for

a. Finding missing cases
b. Commercial sex workers
c. ANC
d. Blood donations

176. While testing the health hazards on a group of people after giving a new drug and/or placebo. The following results were obtained. Based on these results what is the absolute risk reduction and relative risk reduction in %?

	Total subjects	Complications
New drug	1000	100
Placebo	2000	400

a. 10% and 50%
b. 0.1% and 0.9%
c. 1% and 50%
d. 0.1% and 9%

177. A new drug treatment is shown to reduce the incidence of a complication of a disease by 50%. If the usual incidence of this complication were 1% per year, how many patients with this disease would have to be treated with this medication for 1 year to prevent one occurrence of this complication?

a. 20
b. 50
c. 100
d. 200

Most Recent Questions (2019–2018)

178. In a clinical trial, blood pressure was measured between 2 independent groups following treatment, which of the following test will be suitable as at test of significance? ***(AIIMS Nov 2018)***

a. Paired t-test
b. Unpaired t-test
c. ANOVA
d. Chi-square

179. In a clinical trial, blood pressure was measured between in a group of patients before and after treatment, which of the following test will be suitable as at test of significance? ***(AIIMS Nov 2018)***

a. Paired t-test
b. Mann Whitney U test
c. Student test
d. ANOVA

180. Which of the following true regarding the following image: ***(AIIMS Nov 2018)***

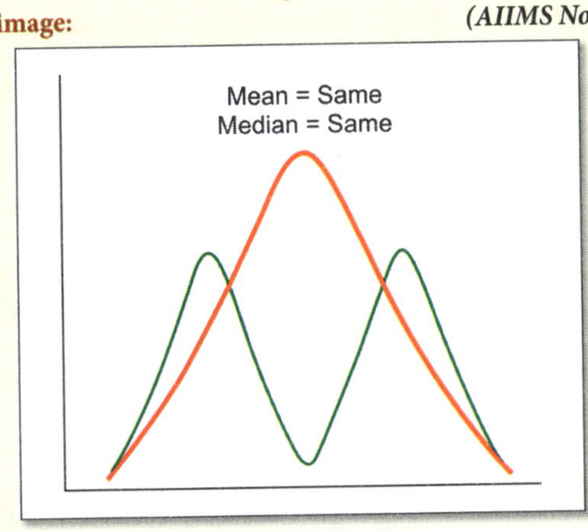

a. Mean = Median = Mode
b. Mean = Median, not equal to Mode
c. Mean = Mode, not equal to Median
d. Mean, Median and Mode are not equal

181. All of the following related with the following image is right; except: ***(AIIMS Nov 2018)***

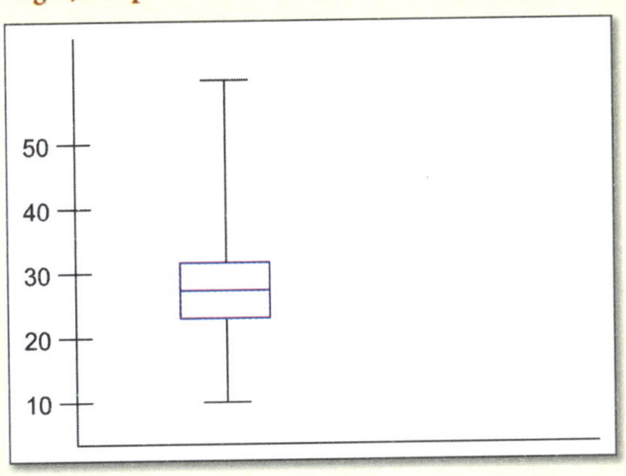

a. Negatively skewed
b. Positively skewed
c. 75% values are above 25 mg
d. Median is 50 mg

Ans.

173. d
174. b
175. d
176. a
177. d
178. b
179. a
180. b
181. b

182. Order of least margin of error in the graph given below is? ***(AIIMS May 2018)***

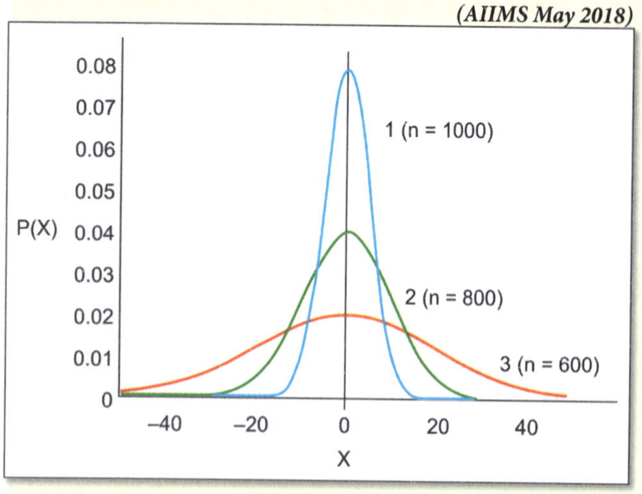

a. 3>2>1 b. 3>1>2
c. 1>2>3 d. 1=2=3

183. All of the following can be analyzed with chi square test except? ***(AIIMS May 2018)***

a. Sex and stage of cancer
b. Heart rate/min and Age
c. Benign or malignant, and type of surgery
d. Age group and cancer state

184. Weight of a group of students is measured in pounds. Thereafter they are given diet and supplements for a year and the weight is recorded again. The test best used is- ***(JIPMER Nov 2018)***

a. Paired t test b. Unpaired t test
c. Mc Nemar d. None of these

185. In a study with a new treatment, there were reported 36 deaths/ treatment failures out of sample of 120. With a new treatment, 26 treatment failures were reported from a sample size of 130. How many patients should be treated to avert 1 death? ***(AIIMS May 2019)***

a. 100 b. 10
c. 250 d. 160

186. A study was done to assess the risk factors for Breast cancer in 100 females from urban cities. A statistical graph and analysis is shown below. ***(AIIMS May 2019)***

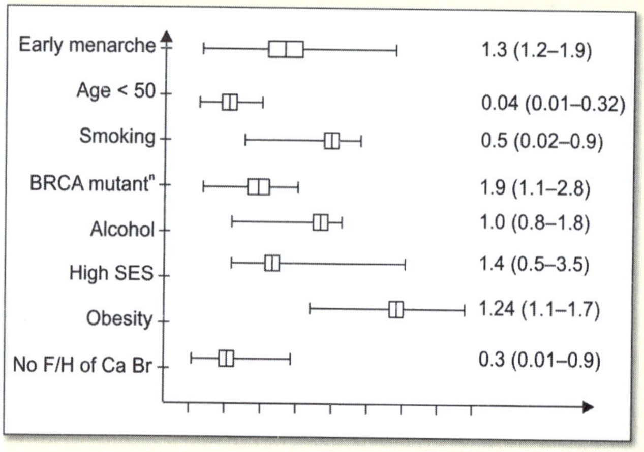

How many risk factors may be ascertained from the statistical analysis of the research

a. 3 b. 4
c. 5 d. 6

187. Look at the image below find the correct corresponding option ***(AIIMS May 2019)***

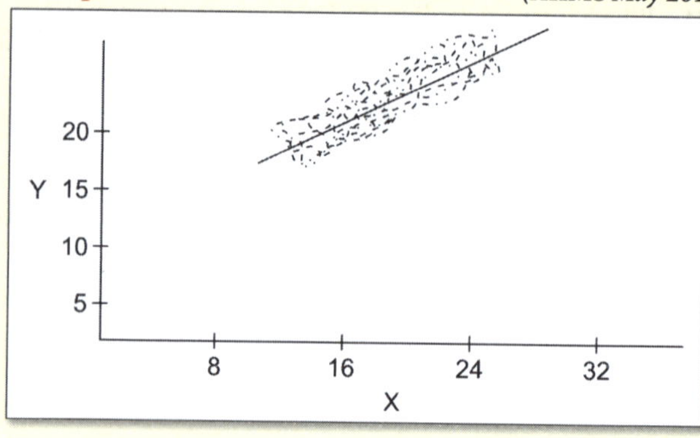

a. y = 10 + x b. x = 10 + y
c. y = 11 + 2x d. x = 11 + 2y

188. The bone mineral density along with gestational age is plotted from two different researches. Which of the following is true for the relation between BMD and gestational age ***(AIIMS May 2019)***

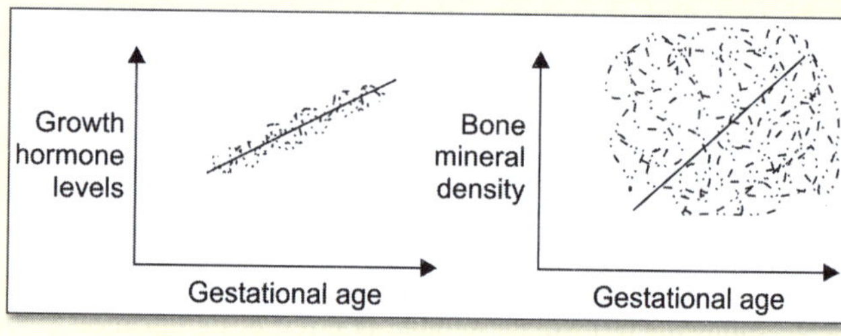

a. Strength of relation is same in A and B
b. Strength of relation is more in A than in B
c. Strength of relation is more in B than in A
d. Variation in variables is more with A than with B

189. A study was conducted to assess the effect of an intervention for certain disease. The p-values for two similar researches A and B with 95% confidence limits, was found to be 0.02 and 0.001 respectively using test 'x' and 'y' with a control group. Based on preliminary analysis, the results may be interpreted as: ***(AIIMS May 2019)***

a. Study A is more precise than Study B and the population size in study A is higher than Study B
b. Study B is more precise than Study A and the population size in study B is higher than study B
c. Both study A and B show a significant variation and both interventions have similar statistical significance
d. Both 'x' and 'y' show a significant variation, but study-B is more significant than Study-A
e. Data is not sufficient to compare the investigations

Which of the following options are correct?

a. If a, b, c are correct
b. If a and c are correct
c. If b and d are correct
d. If all four (a, b, c, & d) are correct

Ans.

182. a
183. b
184. a
185. b
186. a
187. c
188. b
189. c

190. A study was conducted on two different sample. The sample A had the mean value 110 ± 11 while the sample B had mean value of 18 ± 3. which of the following statement is correct: ***(AIIMS May 2019)***

a. Sample A more than Sample B
b. Sample B more than Sample A
c. Variation in sample B is approximately 4 times that in sample A
d. It cannot be ascertained from information provided

191. Seasonal variation of a disease studied in children in a group in June to July and in august to September in another group of similar characteristics from the same area. The test of significance used to compare the data is: ***(AIIMS May 2019)***

a. Chi square b. Paired t
c. Wilcoxan rank test d. ANOVA

192. Best chart to represent incidence of disease over a period of time: ***(Recent Question 2019)***

a. Histogram b. Bar chart
c. Scatter plot d. Line diagram

193. Test of significance used for 2 or more groups using qualitative data (proportions): ***(Recent Question 2019)***

a. ANOVA
b. Chi-square test
c. Fischer's test
d. Paired T test

194. Identify the graph

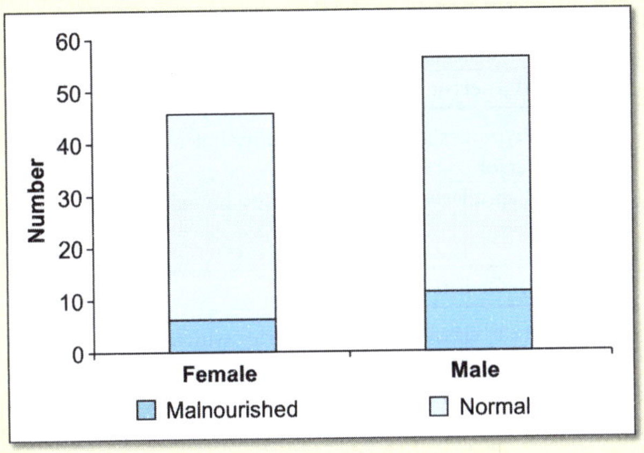

a. Histogram b. Simple bar chart
c. Multiple bar chart d. Component bar chart

195. Test of significance used for 2 independent means is: ***(Recent Question 2019)***

a. Paired t test b. Unpaired t test
c. ANOVA d. Chi-square test

196. In a normal curve what is the area that comes under 1 standard deviation: ***(Recent Question 2019)***

a. 50% b. 68%
c. 95% d. 100%

Ans.

190. b
191. a
192. d
193. b
194. d
195. b
196. b

Answers with Explanations

1. Ans. (b) α error

If null hypothesis was true in reality but rejected in research –alpha error

If null hypothesis was false in reality but accepted in research – beta error

2. Ans. (a) Ordinal

The data is classified into categories which have an inherent order, hence this would be an ordinal data

3. Ans. (c) Not more than 10% of the people benefitted by the drug could be due to chance

Ref. Oxford Handbook of Medical Statistics, Pg. 248

Comment: Since the p-value is 0.1, i.e. the probability of having the observed result by chance is 10% or in other words, not more than 10% of the people benefitted by the drug could be due to chance.

4. Ans. (b) Chi-square test

Ref. Oxford Textbook of Medical Statistics, Pg. i, ii, 252 Park 23rd edition, pg. 852

5. Ans. (d) Between 300–400

Ref: Oxford Handbook of Medical Statistics, p 182

As we can see from the graph:

CD4 count	Number of observations	Cumulative frequency
<100	5	5
100–200	10	15
200–300	25	50
300–400	35	85
400–500	20	105
>500	8	113

Thus among 113 individual observations, the median would lie at 56th–57th individual observation—which is lying in column (in chart) number 4, i.e. between 300-400 CD4.

6. Ans. (b) The probability of declaring a significant difference, when there is truly no difference, is 0.4

7. Ans. (b) Z test

8. Ans. (c) 99%

Ref: K. Park, 24th ed. p 886

9. Ans. (b) Picking every 5th or 10th unit at regular interval

Ref: K. Park, 24th ed. p 887

10. Ans. (b) t-test

Ref: K. Park, 24th ed. p 889; Oxford Textbook of Medical Statistics, P i, ii, 252 Park

TABULATION, CHART AND DIAGRAM

11. Ans. (a) Stem and leaf diagram

Ref: Dr. Avijit Hazra : Biostatistics. Part 1 – Descriptive Statistics. RGUHS J Pharm Sci | Vol 3 | Issue 3 | Jul–Sep, 2013

Stem-and-Leaf Plot

- It was introduced by John Wilder Tukey.
- It combines the features of a diagram and a table.
- It depicts frequency distribution as well as individual data values for numerical data.
- Data is examined to determine the last significant digit (leaf) and this is 'attached' to the previous digits (stem item).
- Stem items are arranged in ascending or descending order vertically. A vertical line is drawn to separate stem from leaf.
- Figures to the left of the vertical line comprise the stem, while those to the right comprise the leaf.
- The number of digits in the leaf equals the number of observations in the data set.
- Drawback–It becomes cumber-some with large data sets.

12. Ans. (c) Line diagram

Ref: K. Park, 24th ed. p 883

Line Diagram

- Line diagrams are used to show the trend of events with the passage of time. The variable is represented on the X-axis and frequencies of observations are represented on Y-axis.

13. Ans. (d) Pictogram

Ref: K. Park, 23nd ed. p 846; 24th ed. p 883

Pictogram (A form of Bar Chart)

- Method of presenting data to "man on street"
- Small pictures or symbols are used to present data.
- Fractions of picture can be used to represent numbers smaller than the value of a whole symbol.

14. Ans. (d) Box and Whisker plot

Ref: Dr Avijit Hazra: Biostatistics. Part 1 – Descriptive Statistics. RGUHS J Pharm Sci | Vol 3 | Issue 3 | Jul–Sep, 2013

Box-and-Whiskers Plot (or Box Plot)

- It was introduced by Turkey in 1970.
- It is a graphical representation of numerical data based on five-figure summary – minimum, 25th percentile, median (50th percentile), 75th percentile and maximum values.
- A rectangle is drawn extending from the lower quartile to the upper quartile, with the median dividing this 'box' but not necessarily equally.

- Lines ('whiskers') are drawn from the ends of the box to the extreme values.
- Outliers may be indicated beyond the extreme values by dots or asterisks
- Whiskers have lengths not exceeding 1.5 times the interquartile range.
- The whole plot may be aligned vertically or horizontally.
- Ideal for summarizing large samples and are being increasingly used.
- Multiple box plots, arranged side by side, allow ready comparison of data sets.

15. Ans. (c) Pie chart

Ref: K. Park, 24th ed. p 883

Refer to theory

16. Ans. (d) Scatter diagram

Ref: K. Park, 24th ed. p 884

Scatter Diagram or Correlation Diagram

- It is a graphical presentation of correlation between two different quantitative variables.
- One variable is represented on X axis and other on Y axis.
- Perpendiculars drawn from the axis readings meet to give a scatter point. (There are as many points as there are individuals in the observation). When all the points are plotted, it forms a scatter plot.
  - *Direction of scatter helps to determine the presence or absence of association.*[Q]
  - *If scatter takes the direction midway between the 2 axis, it signifies +ve association [correlation]*[Q]
  - *If it takes a direction at right angle to midway scatter, it signifies –ve association[correlation]*[Q]
  - *A haphazard scatter represents neither positive nor negative association.*

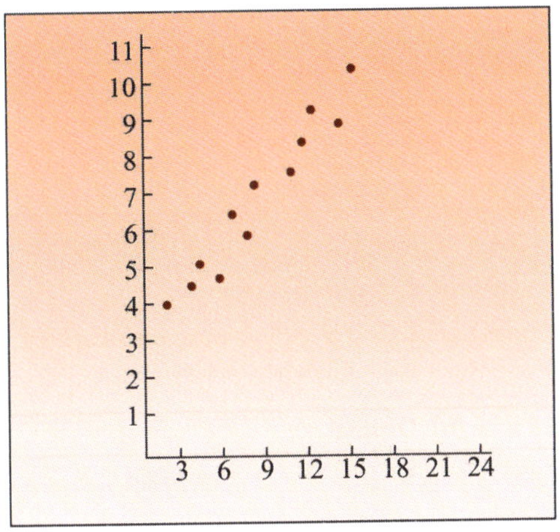

Positive association

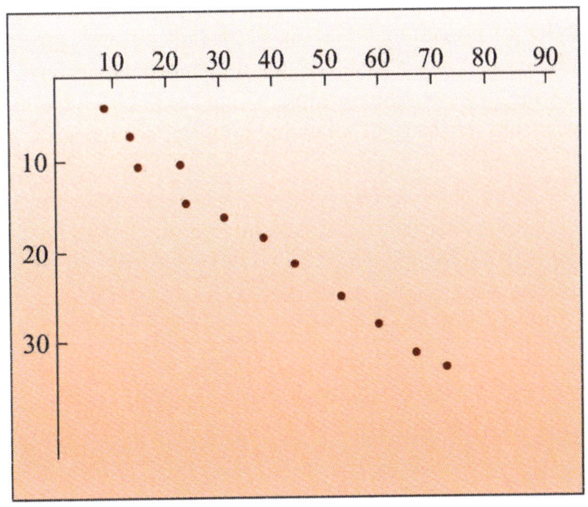

Negative association

17. Ans. (b) Quantitative and continuous data

Ref: NMS Preventive medicine and public health, 2nd ed. p-48

Qualitative data	Quantitative data
Also called discrete or finite data.[Q] People with a characteristic [Yes/Having or No/not having] are counted.	*Also called infinite or continuous data.*[Q]Eg. BP, Weight → can have a range of values.
Expressed in → *Rate, Ratio or Proportion*	Expressed in → *Mean, SD, Correlation*
Represented as Bar diagram, Pie diagram, Pictogram, Spot map	Represented as Histogram, Frequency polygon, Frequency curve, Ogive, Scatter diagram.
Measured on a nominal scale	Measured on a ordinal or metric scale

18. Ans. (d) Pictogram

Ref: K. Park, 24th ed. p 883

19. Ans. (b) 50

Ref: Community medicine Recent advances, Suryakanta,3rd ed. p-665-66

Quartile** divides the total frequencies in equal parts in order of magnitude. **A** **quartiles divides the total frequencies into 4 equal parts, each part having 25% of total observation

Here, 1st quartile BP = 94 mm Hg and 3rd quartile BP = 110 mm Hg and N = 200

Number of patient in the sample expected to have a BP between 3rd and 4th Quartile = 25 % of observations = 50

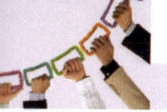

Also Know

Common Quartiles

- *Median* → divides the total frequencies into 2 equal parts, each part having 50 % of total observations
- *Quartiles* → divide the total frequencies into 4 equal parts, each part having 25% of total observation.
- *Quintiles* → divide the total frequencies into 5 equal parts, each part having 20% of total observation.
- *Deciles* → divide the total frequencies into 10 equal parts, each part having 10% of total observation.
- *Centile or percentile* → Divides total frequencies into 100 equal parts, each part having 1% of total observation.

20. Ans. (d) Tree diagram

Ref: Introductory Probability and Statistics. Kozak, R.A., Staudhammer, C.L., Watts, S.B. p-39

Dendrogram or Tree Diagram

- It is a systemic procedure for listing all possible outcomes in a sample space or an event. It is a two-dimensional diagram representing a tree of relationships.
- It moves from left to right following a logical sequence of time
- It can be more complicated with increasing outcomes. In some situations it can have different number of choices for each successive step

21. Ans. (b) Blood group (A, B, AB, O)

Ref: NMS Preventive medicine and public health, 2nd ed. p-48

Continuous

- Continuous → data for which unlimited number of possible values exist.
- Continuous variables accept decimal numeric values e.g. height, weight, BMI, Hemoglobin level etc.

22. Ans. (b) Relationship between two variables

Ref: K. Park, 24th ed p-884

23. Ans. (a) Comparison of 2 categorical data ..., (c) Pie chart is used for comparison of 2...(d) Comparison of magnitude of different ...

24. Ans. (c) Cumulative frequency curve

Ref: KK Sharma, Arun Kumar, Statistics in Management Studies, p-79

Refer to theory

25. Ans. (d) Scatter diagram

Ref: K. Park, 24th ed p-884

26. Ans. (b) Relationship between two variables

Ref: K. Park, 24th ed p-884

27. Ans. (c) Chi-square test

28. Ans. (c) Line diagram

Ref: K. Park, 24th ed. p 883

29. Ans. (b) Line chart

Ref: K. Park, 24th ed. p 883

30. Ans. (a) Line diagram

Ref: K. Park, 24th ed. p 883

31. Ans. (b) Scatter diagram

Ref: K. Park, 24th ed. p 884

32. Ans. (b) Histogram

Ref: NMS Preventive medicine and public health, 2nd ed. p-48

TYPES OF SCALES

33. Ans. (a) Type of Hospitals

Ref: K. Park, 23nd ed. p 845, NMS Preventive medicine and public health, 2nd ed. p-48-49; 24th ed. p 882

34. Ans. (a) Categorical

Ref: High yield biostatistics, 1st ed.p-5

Ordinal/Categorical Data

- Data can be placed in a meaningful order e.g. 1st, 2nd and 3rd or mild, moderate or severe.

35. Ans. (b) Ordinal

Ref: High yield biostatistics, 1st ed. p-5

36. Ans. (c) Body weight

Ref: High yield biostatistics, 1st ed. p-5

Nominal Scale

- Data is divided into qualitative categories or group (e.g. Male or Female, Urban/Semi urban/ Rural)
- There is no order or ratio.
- Dichotomous scale → Nominal data can be put into only two possible categories or group.

37. Ans. (d) 5

Ref: Introduction To Statistics, P.K.Giri and J.Bannerjee, 6th ed. p-103

Class Intervals (Grouped Frequencies)

- Must be exhaustive-must include the entire range of the data.
- Must be mutually exclusive

Number of Class Intervals: No hard and fast rule exists. As a working rule

- 15–20 class intervals are considered ideal for a total frequency of >1000
- 10–15 class intervals are considered ideal for a total frequency of around 1000

- 7–8 class intervals are considered ideal for a total frequency 200

Here, since number of observations is just 25, five to seven intervals are usually sufficient to give a graphical portrayal of the data.

38. Ans. (b) Ordinal

Ref: High yield biostatistics, 1st ed. p-5

39. Ans. (a) Ordinal

Ref: High yield biostatistics, 1st ed. p-5

MEASURES OF CENTRAL TENDENCY (MEAN/MEDIAN/MODE)

40. Ans. (a) Mean = 3

Ref: K. Park, 24th ed. p 884

41. Ans. (b) 50.4

Ref: http://sphweb.bumc.bu.edu/otlt/MPH-Modules/BS/BS704_Probability/BS704_Probability10.html

In a normal data distribution, mean represents the 50th percentile. So, in the above question 70 mm Hg is the 50th percentile. The nth percentile is given by the following formula: nth percentile = mean + SD x Z, where Z is the quantile function on standard normal distribution.

Z values for commonly used percentiles	
1st	–2.326
5th	–1.645
10th	–1.282
25th	–0.675
50th	0
75th	0.675
90th	1.282
95th	1.645
99th	2.326

In the above question, n = 5, hence, 5th percentile = 70 + 10* (–1.645) = 53.55

42. Ans. (c) Mode

Ref: K. Park, 24th ed. p 884

Mode is the most frequently occurring value in a series of value or observation.

43. Ans. (c) Median > Mode

Ref: Community medicine Recent advances, Suryakanta, 3rd ed. p-671-72

Skewed or Asymmetrical Distribution

Skewness	Interpretation
Positive (Mean > Median> Mode) Q	*Skewness is to the right* (Tail is towards right) → Large number of low scores and small number of high scores.
Negative (Mean < Median<Mode) Q	*Skewness is to the left* (Tail is towards left) → Large number of high scores, small number of low scores)

44. Ans. (a) Median 77 (b) Mode 70 (d) Mean 77

Ref: K. Park, 24th ed. p 884

45. Ans. (b) Mean will be Increased, Median will...

Ref: K. Park, 24th ed. p 884

- Mean is the sum of individual observations divided by number of observations and is *influenced by extreme values*

Here, 85 in place of 58 results in an increased sum of individual observations, hence mean will be increased

- Median is the value of the middle observation, hence will remain unchanged as number of observations is still same.

46. Ans. (b) 16, 10, 10

Ref: K. Park, 24th ed. p 884

Assuming, 1 pack has 20 cigarettes. The distribution of smoking habits over a period of 6 years is as follows

Year	1st	2nd	3rd	4th	5th	6th
No. of Cigarettes	5	10	10	10	20	40

Mean = 95/6 = 15.8, Median = 10, Mode = 10

47. Ans. (b) Mode

Ref: K. Park, 24th ed p-884

48. Ans. (b) Mode

Ref: K. Park, 24th ed. p 884

MEASURES OF DISPERSION (RANGE, MEAN DEVIATION AND SD)

49. Ans. (d) Correlation and regression

Ref: K. Park, 24th ed. p 889

50. Ans. (b) 95%

Ref: K. Park, 24th ed. p 886

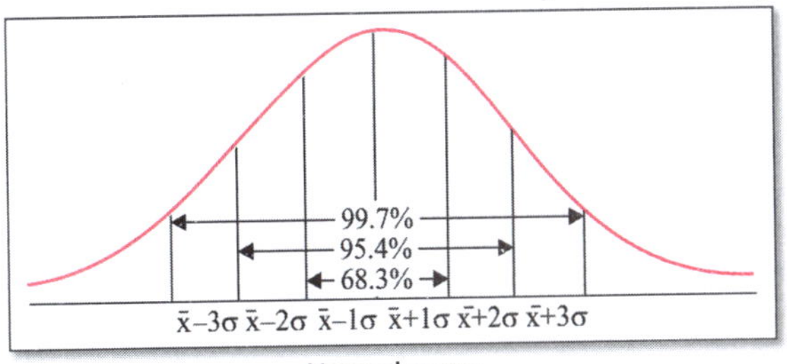

Normal curve

"Confidence limits"

- Area between *1SD on either side of mean includes approximately 68 %* of values in distribution[Q]
- Area between *2SD on either side of the mean will cover approximately 95 % of the values.* [Q]
- Area between *3SD on either side of the mean will cover approximately 99.7 % of the values.*[Q]

51. Ans. (a) 99%

Ref: K. Park, 24th ed. p 886

52. Ans. (c) Standard deviation

Ref: S Lal, Textbook of Community Medicine, 4th ed. p-367

Variance is a measurement of the spread between individual values in a data set.

- Variance of zero indicates that all values are identical.
- Variance is always non-negative.
- Square root of variance is standard deviation.

Variance = $\Sigma(x-\bar{x})^2 / n$

53. Ans. (b) Coefficient of variation

Ref: S Lal, Textbook of Community Medicine, 4th ed. p-368

Coefficient of variance [CV] is *Standard deviation expressed as "percentage of mean".*[Q]

- It is a ratio, has no units of measurement[Q]
  - CV= [SD/Mean] × 100

54. Ans. (b) It indicates the... (c) It is the most commonly ... (e) It is a better indicator...

Ref: K. Park, 24th ed. p 885

Standard Deviation *is the best and most frequently used measure of deviation.*[Q]

It is defined as "Root - Means Square - Deviation."

- SD gives us an idea of *'spread' of dispersion* → Larger the SD, greater the dispersion of values about mean
- *1 SD covers approximately 68 %* of values in distribution[Q] *on either side of mean*

55. Ans. (b) 7.31 g/dL

Ref: K. Park, 24th ed p886

2 SD covers approximately 95% of the values in a distribution *on either side of the mean. Hence 95% of* pregnant females will have their mean hemoglobin level between 6.6 g/dL and 14.6 g/ dL.

1SD covers approximately 68 % of the values in a distribution *on either side of the mean. Hence 68% of* pregnant females will have their mean hemoglobin level between 8.6gm/ dL and 12..6 g/ dL.

- 2.5% of pregnant females will have their mean hemoglobin level below 6.6 g/dL and 16% will have their mean hemoglobin level below 8.6 g/L.

Hence, the Answer is 7.3 (most likely)

56. Ans. (b) $\sqrt{[\Sigma(x-\bar{x})^2]/ \eta\text{–}1}$

Ref: K. Park, 24th ed p-885

57. Ans. (b) 0

Ref: K. Park, 24th ed. p 885

Here, deviation from mean =0 (Since birth weight of each of the 10 babies born is 2.8 kg, Mean = 2.8)

Hence, SD = 0

58. Ans. (d) Standard deviation

Ref: K. Park, 24th ed. p 885

59. Ans. (b) Range, (c) Standard, deviation, (d) Coefficient of variation, (e) Normal distribution curve

Ref: K. Park, 24th ed. p 885

60. Ans. (d) Correlation and regression

Ref: K. Park, 24th ed p 885

NORMAL DISTRIBUTION

61. Ans. (b) 1-Normal distribution, 2-Negative skewed, 3-Positive skewed

Ref: Community medicine Recent advances, Suryakanta, 3rd ed. p 671-72

	Skewness	Interpretation
No skewness or Normal distribution Equal number of low and high scores Box -1 (median divides the 'box' into equal halves)	Positive (Mean > Median> Mode)[Q] or Right sided (Tail is towards right) Large number of low scores and small number of high scores	Negative (Mean < Median < Mode) [Q] or Left sided (Tail is towards left) Large number of high scores, small number of low scores)

62. Ans. (b) Negatively skewed

Ref: Community medicine Recent advances, Suryakanta, 3rd ed. p-671-72

Here, Mean < Median < Mode, hence it is a Negatively skewed distribution.

63. Ans. (a) Equal distribution on either side...

Ref: K. Park, 24th ed. p 886

Refer to theory

64. Ans. (a) Mean < median

Ref: K. Park, 24th ed. p 886

65. Ans. (b) Zero

Ref: K. Park, 24th ed. p 886

66. Ans. (a) Normal distribution

Ref: K. Park, 24th ed. p 885

Relative deviate or Standard normal variate or *Z score* is the measure of distance of a value (x) from the mean ($\bar{x}$) of a normal distribution curve in units of SD.

$$Z = (x-\bar{x}) / \sigma$$

67. Ans. (b) Normal distribution

Ref: Handbook for Clinical Research: Design, Statistics, and Implementation. P-88

Major Types Data Distribution

- Discrete data - Binomial distribution, Poisson distribution, Geometric distribution, Hypergeometric distribution
- Continuous data -Normal, Exponential, Uniform, Weibull

Also Know........................

- Weibull distribution is a continuous probability distribution to represent decreasing failure rate, constant failure rate or increasing failure rate.

68. Ans. (a) 4–16

Ref: Ray M. Merrill, Thomas C. Timmreck, Introduction to Epidemiology, 4th edition, p-92

Sample estimate is a point estimate of population rate.
The confidence Interval tells us the precision of an estimated sample rate (e.g. Prevalence =10%). It is the range of values in which the population rate is likely to fall.
Formula to calculate the confidence interval is:
CI = mean (or prevalence) ± Z * SE
Where, Z = standard deviate multiplier. The values for 'Z' are as follows:
68% confidence interval = 1
95% confidence interval = 1.96 ~ 2
99% confidence interval = 2.58
The standard error (SE) is calculated for the mean or the proportions as follows:

$$\text{SE for Mean} = \frac{SD}{\sqrt{n}}$$

$$\text{SE for Proportions} = \sqrt{\frac{PQ}{n}}$$

Where, P = Prevalence; Q = 100 – Prevalence
So, in this MCQ

$$CI = 10 \pm 2 \times \sqrt{\frac{10 \times 90}{100}}$$

$$= 10 \pm 2 \times 3$$
$$= 10 \pm 6$$
$$= 4 - 16$$

69. Ans. (b) Data is negatively skewed

Ref: The Apgar Score Pediatrics Volume 136, number 4, October 2015

APGAR Score is a scoring system devised by Dr Virginia Apgar for rapid assessment of clinical status of the newborn infant at 1 minute of age and need for prompt intervention to establish breathing

- Apgar score comprises 5 components: (1) color; (2) heart rate; (3) reflexes; (4) muscle tone; and (5) respiration.
- Each of these components is given a score of 0, 1, or 2.
- Neonatal Encephalopathy and Neurologic Outcome report defines a 5-minute Apgar score of 7 to 10 as reassuring, a score of 4 to 6 as moderately abnormal, and a score of 0 to 3 as low in the term infant and late-preterm infant

70. Ans. (a) Mean > median > mode

Ref: Community medicine Recent advances, Suryakanta, 3rd ed. p-671-72

71. Ans. (b) 0.50

Ref: K. Park, 24th ed. p 886

In a normal distribution, Mean divides the area under the curve into 2 equal halves.

- 50% of values lie above and 50% of values lie below mean (mode or median)

72. Ans. (c) 72–88%

The confidence Interval tells us the precision of an estimated sample rate. Formula to calculate the confidence interval is:
CI = mean (or prevalence) ± Z * SE
Where, Z = standard deviate multiplier. The values for 'Z' are as follows:
68% confidence interval = 1
95% confidence interval = 1.96 ~ 2
99% confidence interval = 2.58
The standard error (SE) is calculated for the mean or the proportions as follows:

$$\text{SE for Mean} = \frac{SD}{\sqrt{n}}$$

$$\text{SE for Proportions} = \sqrt{\frac{PQ}{n}}$$

Where, P = Prevalence ; Q = 100 – Prevalence
So, in this MCQ

$$CI = 80 \pm 2 \times \sqrt{\frac{80 \times 20}{100}}$$

$$= 80 \pm 2 \times 4$$
$$= 80 \pm 8$$
$$= 72 - 88$$

73. Ans. (a) Less than median

Ref: Community medicine Recent advances, Suryakanta, 3rd ed. p-671-72

74. Ans. (b) Mean < Mode

Ref: Community medicine Recent advances, Suryakanta, 3rd ed. p-671-72

75. Ans. (a) 0.34

Ref: K. Park, 24th ed. p 886

76. Ans. (a) (3 × [Mean–Median])/SD

Ref: Schaums's outlines of Theory and problems of statistics, 4th ed. p-125

Skewness is the degree of asymmetry, or departure from symmetry, of a distribution.

- Pearson's first coefficients of skewness

$$= \frac{\text{Mean} - \text{Mode}}{\text{SD}}$$

- Pearson's second coefficients of skewness

$$= \frac{3(\text{Mean} - \text{Median})}{\text{SD}}$$

- Quartile coefficient of skewness

$$= \frac{(Q_3 - Q_2) - (Q_2 - Q_1)}{Q_2 - Q_1}$$

Kurtosis is the degree of peakedness of a distribution relative to a normal distribution.

- A distribution having a relatively high peak is called **leptokurtic**, flat-topped peak is called **platykurtic**., not very peaked or very flat-topped, is called **mesokurtic**.

Also Know........................

- Moment coefficient of kurtosis [b2] is measure of kurtosis → It is Positive for a leptokurtic, Negative for a platykurtic, Zero for normal distribution.

77. Ans. (b) Normal distribution curve

Ref: K. Park, 24th ed 886

78. Ans. (d) 95% confidence interval will cover 2 standard errors around the mean

Ref: K. Park, 24th ed. p 886-87

Standard Error is the variation of sample means about population mean

SE for Proportions = $\sqrt{\frac{PQ}{n}}$

Distribution of sample means follows normal distribution, where the 95% of sample means lie within 2 SE on either side of the true or population mean.

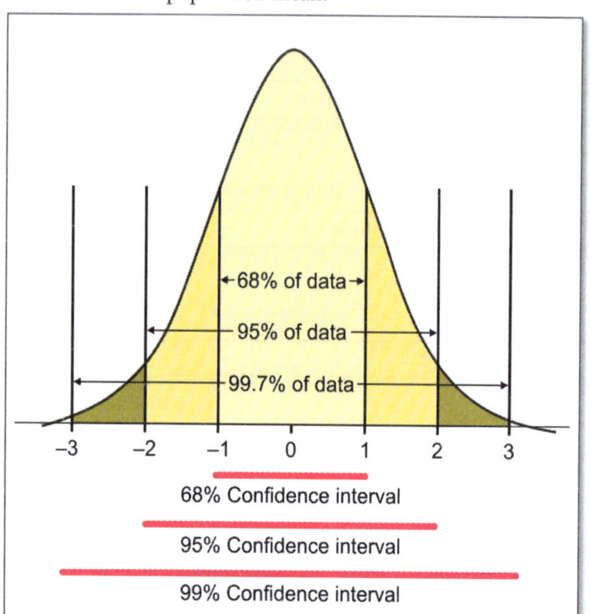

SAMPLING

79. Ans. (b) Sampling distribution

Ref: David C. Le Blanc. Statistics: Concepts and Applications for Science, Volume 2, p 118

Population distribution is the probability distribution for individual values of a variable X obtained if the entire population were measured.

Sampling distribution – It is the probability distribution for values of sample mean X of all possible samples drawn from a population to arrive at population mean (μ)

- Central Limit Theorem – If the sample size is sufficiently large, shape of sampling distribution of mean X will be normal irrespective of shape of population distribution.
- How far population distribution is from normal will determine the sample size. More skewed the population distribution, larger the sample size needed for Sampling distribution to be normal

80. Ans. (c) 900

Ref: Community medicine Recent advances, Suryakanta, 3rd ed. p-675

Minimum sample size for prevalence (cross-sectional studies) at 95% confidence interval is calculated using the formula:

Sample size = 4pq/L2

Where, p = prevalence; q = 1–p; L = Permissible error in estimation of prevalence

Given :- value of ($z_{\alpha=0.95}$) = 1.96≈2

Prevalence(P) = 10%, Q = 1–P

Relative Precision(l) = 20% of the prevalence i.e = 20 * 10/100 = 2

So n = $(1.96)^2$ * 10*90/$(2)^2$ = 4*900/4 = 900

81. Ans. (c) Immunization coverage

Ref: S. Lal, Text book of community medicine,4th ed. p- 370

Cluster Sampling

- It involves 2 stages
  - 1st stage → we select clusters
  - 2nd stage → we select households within the cluster [by simple random sampling].
- Sampling frame is a list of clusters with size of population.
- To ensure that everyone has the same chance of getting selected to sample
  - We select different number of households per cluster according to its population size [difficult to maintain quality control]

OR

  - Use PPS (Probability proportional to size) method → a constant number of households per cluster are selected
- *Advantage* → Easy, Rapid, Simple and Cheaper[Q]
- *Disadvantage* → High sampling error.
- *Use* → To evaluate **immunization coverage,** Diarrheal disease survey, Leprosy elimination monitoring Survey.

82. Ans. (b) Sampling interval depends on total...

Ref: K. Park, 24th ed. p 887

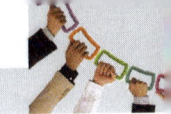

Systematic Random Sampling

- If the sample to be drawn is "n" and total population is "N". Then sampling interval 'r" = N/n
- A unit is selected at random and other units are selected by adding "r" to previous selected number (every r^{th} unit at regular intervals is picked)
- Each unit in sampling frame has equal chance of being selected, but number of possible samples is greatly reduced.
- Preferred when population is large, scattered and not homogenous

Also Know.......................

- Advantage - No sampling frame is required.

83. Ans. (b) Stratified random sampling

Ref: K. Park, 24th ed. p 887

Stratified Random Sample

- Population is divided into homogenous sub groups [strata] based on the characteristic being studied
- Simple random sampling is done from each strata.
- *Precision of the estimate of the characteristic being studied is increased.*
- Sample is drawn in a way that *each portion of sample represents a corresponding part of universe.*
- *It is ideal if the population is heterogenous* with respect to the characteristic under study or when the *characteristic is influenced by different sections of the population*, viz. Religion [Hindus, Muslims], age-groups etc.

Population → Stratification for homogenous Subgroups → Random selection for sample from these subgroups

84. Ans. (d) Systematic random sampling

Ref: K. Park, 24 th ed p 887

85. Ans. (d) 400

Ref: Community medicine Recent advances, Suryakanta, 3rd ed. p-675

The Sample Size Determinants

- Precision (d) → Amount of sampling error [Absolute or relative] that can be tolerated.
- Level of significance [commonly set at 5% (p = 0.05)]
- Prevalence (p) [for qualitative characteristic]
- Standard deviation (SD) [for quantitative characteristics]

The formula for Sample size for quantitative characteristics at 95% Confidence Interval is = $\frac{(1.96)^2 \times SD^2}{L^2}$

Sample size for qualitative characteristics at 95% CI = $\frac{(1.96)^2 \times P \times Q}{L^2}$

Where, SD = Standard Deviation; P = Prevalence; Q = 100 – Prevalence; L = Allowable error

So, in this MCQ

Prevalence (P) = 50%

Q = 50

L = 45-55% = ± 5%

Sample size = $\frac{(1.96)^2 \times P \times Q}{L^2}$ (and we can assume 1.96 to be approximate for ~ 2)

$= \frac{2 \times 2 \times 50 \times 50}{5^2} = 400$

86. Ans. (c) Homogeneous population

Ref: K. Park, 24th ed 887

87. Ans. (a) Hetrogeneous data

Ref: K. Park, 24th ed. p 887

88. Ans. (d) 30 cluster of 7 children

Ref: S. Lal, Text book of community medicine,4th ed. p- 370

In coverage evaluation survey of immunization, WH0 30 Cluster Sampling is used

- *7 children, 12-23 months of age are chosen from each of the 30 clusters by moving in one direction till the desired number of children are complete*
- Total respondents = 210

89. Ans. (d) Multistage sampling

Ref: Suryakanta, Community Medicine Recent Advances, 3rd ed. p-674

Multistage Sampling

- Sampling is done in stages, using random techniques.
- Useful when large population (country/state) is to be studied with limited resources.
- The sample size is reduced progressively in stages, till a representative sample is obtained to cut down cost
- E.g. Hook worm survey in district- 10% Talukas are chosen, followed by 10% villages and then everyone in the 10th house has his/her stool examined

Advantage: Flexibility in sampling, Saves cost and time

Disadvantage: Sampling error is increased, Sampling units are of unequal size at different stages

Multiphase Sampling

- Basic information is collected on a larger sample size followed by successive collection of more specific information for successive sub-samples out of the earlier sample. E.g. TB Prevalence survey
- When not enough funding is available
- Cost of collection varies from one phase to another

90. Ans. (a) Quota sampling

Ref: K. Park, 23nd ed. p 850, Community Medicine Recent Advances, Suryakanta, 3rd ed. p-672-73

Sampling Methods	
Random/probability/ non purposive	**Nonrandom/non probability/purposive**
Simple random sampling	Convenience sampling
Systematic random sampling	Quota sampling

Contd...

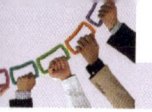

Sampling Methods	
Random/probability/ non purposive	**Nonrandom/non probability/purposive**
Stratified random sampling	Snow ball sampling
Multistage random sampling	Clinical trial sampling
Cluster sampling	

Quota sampling: It is like stratified sampling, but instead of sampling randomly the participants to come from each stratum, the survey samplers themselves choose the people subjectively from each stratum until sufficient people have been chosen.

Convenience sampling: Sampling units which are accessible easily and conveniently are selected. Easy to use, but may add strong biases. It can give accurate results when the population is homogeneous.

Snow ball sampling: Referral from initial known subjects is used to reach additional subjects. It is costly and time consuming.

It does not provide a representative sample. It is used when subjects are rare or variable is associated with some stigma/ taboo. E.g. Survey of RTI/STI in sex workers

91. Ans. (b) Stratified random sampling

Ref: K. Park, 23nd ed. p 850, Community Medicine Recent Advances, Suryakanta, 3rd ed. p 67-743; 24th ed. p 887

92. Ans. (d) Cluster sampling

Ref: S. Lal, Text book of community medicine, 4th ed. p 370

Also Know......................

- Simple random sampling is the "GOLD STANDARD" sampling method.

TEST OF SIGNIFICANCE

93. Ans. (b) Student's test

Ref: Methods in biostatistics by Mahajan, 7th ed. p 127

Student 't' test [Devised by William Sealy Gosset]

Based on "t" distribution [a continuous, symmetrical, bell shaped, unimodal distribution of infinite range. It is similar in shape to normal distribution, but more spread out].

Application

- To find the significance of difference between two means.
- To evaluate the null hypothesis for continuous (quantitative) variables (e.g. height, weight).
- **Student t test for single small sample** → compares a single sample mean with population mean.
- Student t test for independent samples (**Unpaired t test**) → compares mean of 2 small samples [< 30 size].
- Student t test for paired samples (**Paired t test**) → compares mean of 2 small paired samples [< 30 size].

94. Ans. (d) Sample size <30

Ref: Methods in biostatistics by Mahajan, 7th ed. p-127

Student 't' test comparing means of two samples assumes:

- Each of the two populations compared follow a normal distribution.
- Two populations being compared have the same variance.
- The rule of sample size <30 is not absolute. T-test may be applied to larger populations if variance is unknown. Numerically, when n >30, t and z statistic are close, or in other words, t distribution is close to normal distribution.

However, in the above alternatives, sample size<30 would be the closest match.

95. Ans. (d) 0.05

Ref: S Lal, Textbook of community medicine,4th ed. p-376

*If the calculated **p value** is less than predetermined alpha value [taken as 0.05 or 5%], the relationship/association is inferred as statistically significant and null hypothesis is rejected.*

96. Ans. (c) 10

Ref: K. Park, 24th ed p-889

Degree of freedom (d.f) = (r – 1) × (c – 1), r represents rows and c as columns

Hence d.f = (3 – 1) × (6 – 1) = 10

97. Ans. (d) Chi-square curve is negatively skewed

Ref: K. Park, 23nd ed.p-852 , Community Medicine Recent Advances, Suryakanta, 3rd ed. p-684-85; 24th ed. p 889

Chi- square test (χ^2) was developed by Karl Pearson

- It is a non parametric test, *used for qualitative data (e.g. proportions)*
- ***Applications***
  - To test for any *significant difference between two proportions.* Q
  - *Used as a test of goodness of fit* (determines whether observed frequency distribution differs from theoretical distribution [i.e. normal, binomial or Poisson) by chance or the sample is drawn from a different population)
  - *To test if any association between two events or discrete attributes is real or by chance*
  - To test the strength of the association between exposure and disease in a cohort study, an unmatched case-control study, or a cross-sectional study
- ***Advantage***: It can also be used when more than two groups are to be compared.

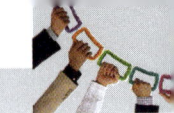

Also Know.......................

- **McNemar's** test is used to test the strength of the association between exposure and disease in a matched case control study.
- **Characteristic of chi**-square curve: The mean of a Chi Square distribution is its degrees of freedom. Chi Square distributions are positively skewed, with the degree of skew decreasing with increasing degrees of freedom. As the degrees of freedom increases, the Chi Square distribution approaches a normal distribution.

98. Ans. (c) Standard Deviation

Ref: K. Park, 24th ed. p 887

***Standard Deviation** is the best and most frequently used measure of deviation* or dispersion[Q]

- Larger the SD, greater the dispersion of values about mean

Tests of Significance – Refer to Annexure -18.2

99. Ans. (c) Null hypothesis is true but is rejected

Ref: S Lal, Textbook of community medicine,4th ed. p-377

Null hypothesis assumes that there is no significant difference between 2 samples, whatever difference occurs is by chance.

Null hypothesis	Accepted	Rejected
True	Correct conclusion	Type I (α) error
False	Type II (β) error	Correct conclusion

Type I Error or α Error

- *Rejecting a null hypothesis when actually it is true*[Q] (a statistically significant difference is found between two groups when actually there is no difference).
- If null hypothesis is false there can be no type I error.
- Probability of a type I error is equal to alpha.
- Multiple comparisons and repeated testing for significance increase likelihood of type I error

Also Know.......................

- Type I error is important in *sample size determination and* statistical testing for significance.

Type II Error or β Error

- *Acceptance of a null hypothesis as true when actually it is false.*[Q]
- The study fails to find a statistically significant difference when actually there is a difference.
- If null hypothesis is true there can be no type II error.
- Probability of a type II error is equal to beta.
- *It is inversely related to type I error.*

Also Know.......................

- Type II error or b error is used to determine the power of study = 1 – β

100. Ans. (b) Type II error

Ref: S Lal, Textbook of community medicine,4th ed. p-377

101. Ans. (c) Probability associated with type 1...

Ref: S Lal, Textbook of community medicine,4th ed. p-377

102. Ans. (b) Chi-square test

Ref: K. Park, 24 nd ed. p-889

Here, the birth weight of two group of new born children (Low or Normal) is to be assessed based on receipt or nonreceipt of food supplement in mothers (Received –Yes/No)

Hence the most appropriate statistical test is Chi-square test

103. Ans. (b) Decreasing b error

104. Ans. (a) Alpha error

Ref: S Lal, Textbook of community medicine,4th ed. p-377

105. Ans. (c) 24–26

Ref: K. Park, 24th ed p-886-87

Standard error of mean = SE = S/ η = 10/ √400= 0.5

- Frequency distribution of all sample means drawn from the same population shows normal distribution about the population mean (m).
- Variation of sample mean is measured in terms of SE (i.e. SD of sample mean from population mean)

95 % of sample means lie within limits of 2 SE on either side of the true or population mean

Range of IOP, that would contain 95% of population = Mean ±2 SE = 25 ±2X 0.5 = 24 to 26

106. Ans. (d) 0.2

Ref: K. Park, 24th ed. p 886-87

The standard error (SE) is calculated for the mean or the proportions as follows:

$$\text{SE for Mean} = \frac{SD}{\sqrt{n}}$$

$$= \frac{2}{\sqrt{100}} = 2/10 = 0.2$$

107. Ans. (b) It is unlikely by chance and p < 0.05

Ref: S Lal, Textbook of community medicine,4th ed. p-376

108. Ans. (a) Type 1 error

Ref: S Lal, Textbook of community medicine,4th ed. p-377

109. Ans. (a) Outliers

Ref: Steven Walfish, Pharmaceutical Technology, Nov 2, 2006. A Review of Statistical Outlier Methods

Methods for Detecting Outliers

- Plotting data using histograms, scatter plots, or a box plot.

- Extreme studentized deviate test for a normally distributed sample with more than 10 observations.
- Dixon test based on ordered statistics (based on the ratio of the ranges) is ideal
  - For small samples
  - If data is not normally distributed

110. Ans. (d) Fischer's exact test, (e) Chi square test

Ref: K. Park, 23rd ed. p 852, Field Epidemiology, Michael B. Gregg, 3rd ed; 24th ed. p 889

Also Know......................

- Fisher's exact is used when both dependent and independent variable are nominal. It is considered "Gold Standard" for a 2 × 2 table and is preferred over Chi square test when the expected numbers in the 2 × 2 table are small.
- ANOVA is parametric equivalent of the Kruskal-Wallis test.

111. Ans. (b) Student T test

Ref: Methods in biostatistics by Mahajan, 7th ed. p-127

112. Ans. (b) 12

Ref: K. Park, 24th ed. p 889

113. Ans. (c) 10

Ref: K. Park, 24th ed. p 889

114. Ans. (b) To compare means in three or more...

Ref: S Lal, Textbook of community medicine, 1st ed. p-379

ANOVA is used to compare the mean values of a quantitative (continuous) variables and when comparison involves more than two comparison groups.

- E.g. Comparison of BP levels in 4 different groups, with study participants in each group having only one of four different antihypertensive medications.
- Null hypothesis for the ANOVA test is that all of the group means are equal to each other in the population.

Also Know......................

- ANOVA- Dependent variable is Quantitative, whereas independent variable is Qualitative
- ANCOVA- Dependent variable is Quantitative, whereas independent variable is Qualitative or Quantitative
- MANOVA- Both Dependent variable and independent variable are Qualitative

115. Ans. (c) Means in different groups

Ref: K. Park, 23nd ed.p-852 , Community Medicine Recent Advances, Suryakanta, 3rd ed. p-684-85

116. Ans. (b) Standard error of proportion

Ref: K. Park, 24th ed. p 889

117. Ans. (a) 1

Ref: K. Park, 24th ed. p 889

118. Ans. (d) Cox proportional hazards test

Ref: Viv Bewick, Liz Cheek, Jonathan Ball, Statistics review 12: Survival analysis. Crit Care. 2004; 8(5): 389–394.

Comparison of Kaplan – Meier survival curve is done using

Log Rank Test

- Test the null hypothesis "No difference exists between the population survival curves (i.e. the probability of an event occurring at any time point is the same for each population).
- Limitation-It does not allow other explanatory variables to be taken into account.

Cox's Proportional Hazards Model

- Similar to a multiple regression model -Enables difference between survival times of groups of patients to be tested while allowing for other factors.
- 'Hazard' is the probability of dying given the patients have survived up to a given point in time or risk of death at that moment. It is the dependent variable.
- Hazard ratio is independent of time- If risk of death at a particular point in time in one group is, 3 times that in the other group, then at any other time it will still be 3 times that in the other group

119. Ans. (d) Multiple logistic regression

Ref: NMS Preventive Medicine and public health. 2nd ed. p 70- 71, Epidemiology and biostatistics, Bryan Kestanbaum, p 182, Encyclopedia of statistics.

Regression analysis is the mathematical model to describe the effect that one or more independent variables have on a dependent/outcome variable

Linear regression → describes the effect of one independent variable on a dependent variable. y= a + bx ['x' is independent and 'y' is dependent variable, b = regression coefficient, 'a' is y axis intercept (y for x = 0)]

Multiple linear regression→describes effect of two or more independent variable on a dependent variable.

y = a + b 1x 1 + b 2x 2 + b nx n. [Here each dependent variable has its own regression coefficient]

Nonlinear → involves more complex mathematical forms, including logarithmic functions.

Multiple Logistic Regression

- Applied when out come variable is measured on a dichotomous scale and independent variables [≥2] are measured either on numerical continuous or numerical discrete or categorical dichotomous scale.
- *It is used to adjust statistically the estimated effects of each variable in the model for differences in the distributions of and associations among the other independent variables.*

Here, dependent variable is occurrence of a disease – Yes or No [**dichomatous**] and there are 5 independent factors that influence the occurrence of disease and we want to compare the effect of independent factors on disease occurrence.

So, while calculating the effect of a single factor we need to neutralize the confounding effect of other 4 independent factors. This can be done using **Multiple logistic regression**

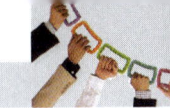

CORRELATION AND REGRESSION

120. Ans. (b) **+0.25**

As seen in the MCQ image the slope of the regression line approximate towards the correlation coefficient value of +0.25. Further clarity on approximate correlation coefficient may be understood from the graphs given below.

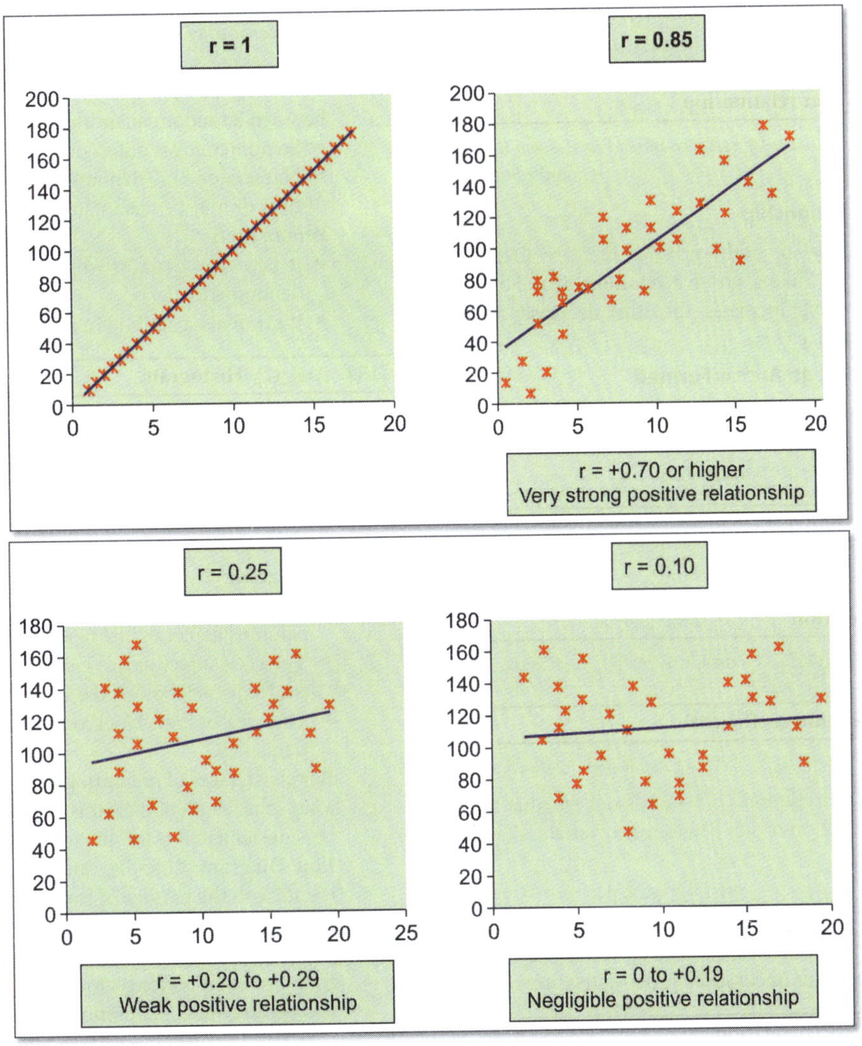

Note: Averaging correlation coefficient: We can calculate an average correlation coefficient but NOT by simply calculating the mean of the coefficients. Firstly, must transform each correlation coefficient using Fisher's Z, calculate the mean of the z values, then back-transform to the correlation coefficient.

121. Ans. (a) **–1 to +1**

Ref: k Park, 24th ed. p 889-90

Correlation coefficient ["r"] lies between - 1.0 and + 1.0.

- "r" near +1 → signals a strong positive association. [If one variable increases the other also increases]
- "r" near - 1 → signals a strong negative association [when one variable increases the other decreases.]
- r = 0 → signals no association

122. Ans. (d) **Correlation**

Ref: Piyush Gupta, Textbook of Community Medicine, Pp-658

Types of Correlation Coefficients

- **Pearson product-moment correlation coefficient:** It measures the strength and direction of linear relationship between two ungrouped normally distributed variables.
- **Intraclass correlation:** It describes how strongly units in the same group resemble each other.
- **Rank correlation:** It describes relationships between rankings of different variables or different rankings of the same variable
- **Spearman's rank correlation coefficient:** It measures how well the relationship between two variables can be described by a function. It is used for grouped data, not normally distributed

- **Kendall tau rank correlation coefficient:** It is a measure of the portion of ranks that match between two data sets

123. Ans. (d) The curve shows a regression line means correlation

Ref: k Park, 24th ed p-889-90

In the above figure increase in SpO_2 values of the two different groups show a positive correlation. (If one variable increases the other also increases) signaling a positive association

124. Ans. (a) Nonlinear relationship

Ref: Allen Rubin, Statistics for Evidence-Based Practice and Evaluation, 3rd edition , p-207

Curvilinear Relationship

Values (Frequency) of both variables increase together up to a certain point (like a positive **relationship**) and then as value of one variable increases, the other decreases (negative **relationship**) or vice versa.

On a Scatterplot, an Arch is Formed

Example- Strength and age: When we are younger, we are weaker; when we are older, we are stronger; but when we become very old, we are weaker again

125. Ans (a) Regression

Ref: K. Park, 24th ed p-889

126. Ans. (d) Correlation

Ref: Community medicine Recent advances, AH Suryakanta, 3rd ed. p

127. Ans. (c) Correlation coefficient

Ref: K. Park, 24th ed. p 889-90

Co-efficient of Correlation ("r")→finds out whether there is significant association or not between two variables (x and y) in 'n' individuals.

$$r = \frac{S(x-\bar{x})(y-\bar{y})}{\sqrt{\Sigma(x-\bar{x})^2\,\Sigma(y-\bar{y})^2}}$$

Correlation does not necessarily prove causation.

128. Ans. (b) Negative correlation

Ref: K. Park, 24th ed. p 889-90

129. Ans. (b) 1

Ref: K. Park, 24th ed. p 889-90

130. Ans. (a) ROC Curve

Ref: Leon and Gordis, Epidemiology 4thedition, p-92-96

ROC (Receiver Operating Characteristic) **allows optimal specification of test sensitivity and specificity.**

- ***A ROC curve plots test sensitivity on Y-axis vs. 1 – specificity on X-axis.***[Q]
- When a ROC has been established for a test, any one of several sensitivity and specificity combinations may be evaluated for suitability in test application and contrasted with potential alternate tests.
- Perfect ROC has 100% sensitivity and specificity

131. (a) Numerator is component of denominator

Ratio: It is a direct number expressing the quantity in relation to another quantity or it may express a relation in size between two random quantities

- The numerator is not a component of the denominator.
- The numerator and denominator may involve an interval of time or may be instantaneous in time.
- It is expressed in the form of a:b or a/b

Rates: It is a measure of disease frequency. It expresses relation between 2 random quantities.

- So numerator is not a component of denominator.
- Numerator and denominator may involve an interval of time or may be instantaneous in time.

Proportion:

- It is a type of ratio which always includes numerator in denominator.
- It expresses a relation in magnitude of a part of the whole.

132. Ans. (c) Histogram

The diagram that indicates the frequency represented by an area corresponding to number of continuous type is called histogram

133. Ans. (a) Histogram

Histogram:

- It is a pictorial diagram of frequency distribution with columns depicting the magnitude of data set
- The class intervals are given along the horizontal axis and the frequencies along the vertical axis.
- The area of each block or rectangle is proportional to the frequency.

Bar charts: way of presenting a set of numbers by the length of a bar - the length of the bar is proportional to the magnitude to be represented. It is for qualitative data

Line Diagram: Line diagrams are used to show the trend of events with the passage of time.

Pie charts: Instead of comparing the length or a bar, the areas of segments of a circle are compared. The degree in the circle are representation for sectoral data presentation.

Pictogram: Small pictures or symbols are used to represent the data.

134. Ans. (d) Standard Deviation

Significance of standard deviation - that it is an abstract number; that it gives us an idea of the spread' of the dispersion; that the larger the standard deviation, the greater the dispersion of values about the mean.

135. Ans. (b) SD

SD is the most frequently used measure of deviation.
S.D (Root means-square-deviation) denoted by sigma (σ)

136. Ans. (b) Dispersion

Standard deviation is a measure of dispersion

137. Ans. (b) Mean and standard deviation

Confidence limits:

In a normal curve:

- The area between one standard deviation on either side of the mean ($x \pm 1\sigma$) will include approximately 68 percent of the values in the distribution.
- The area between two standard deviations on either side of the mean ($x \pm 2\sigma$) will cover most of the values (95%).
- The area between ($x \pm 3\sigma$) will include 99.7 percent of the values.
- These limits on either side of the mean are called as "Confidence limits".

138. Ans. (a) SD

139. Ans. (a) SD

In simple terms, standard deviation is defined as "Root - Means - Square - Deviation."

It is the variation or dispersion of the values from the mean

140. Ans. (b) Correlation

Correlation: It is a statistical measure to assess the degree and direction of association between two variables as weight and height, age and FEV, triglyceride levels and hypertension and so on.

- We construct a scatter plot between the two variables
- Calculate the coefficient of correlation (r), which ranges from –1 to +1
- If
  - $r = 0$, means no correlation
  - $r < 0$, means negative correlation - one value increase and the other decrease
  - $r > 0$, means positive correlation – an increase in one value will increase the other value also

Regression: If wish to know in an individual case the value of one variable, knowing the value of the other, we calculate what is known as the regression coefficient of one measurement to the other.

141. Ans. (b) The standard error of the mean to decrease; (c) The standard deviation to decrease

If the sample size (denoted by symbol n) is increased, then the standard deviation and its other derivation will be affected.

- Mean is given by the formula
  - Mean = $\frac{\Sigma x}{n}$
  - So, as sample size will increase, the sum of observation will also increase, hence the net effect on mean may remain unchanged.
  - The change in the mean cannot be calculated in terms of increase or decrease, but the probability of the mean to be closer to true (or actual) mean will increase. In other words, the variability of data will decrease
- Standard deviation is given by the formula:
  - SD = $\sqrt{\frac{(x-\bar{x})^2}{n-1}}$
  - Hence, we see SD $\propto \frac{1}{\sqrt{n}}$
  - So, as sample size will increase the SD will decrease
- Standard error of mean is given by the formula
  - SEM = $\frac{SD}{\sqrt{n}}$
  - Hence, we see SEM
  - So, as sample size will increase the SEM will decrease
- Variance is given by the formula
  - V = SD^2
  - And SD $\propto \frac{1}{\sqrt{n}}$
  - So, as sample size will increase the SD will decrease and Variance will also decrease
- Coefficient of variation is given by the formula
  - CoV = $\frac{SD}{Mean}$
  - And SD $\propto \frac{1}{\sqrt{n}}$
  - So, as sample size will increase the SD will decrease and the coefficient of variation will also decrease

Please note:

- The Standard error of means vary directly with the standard deviations.
- Greater the SD, greater will be the SE as will happen in small samples.
- Sampling error or chance variation has to be minimized by reducing the SD which can be done only by taking a large sample

142. Ans. (d) χ^2 test (Chi-square test)

Chi-square test is applied to find association between two events occurring together when there are more than two classes or more than two samples.

- It is used for non-parametric data or qualitative data
- Appropriate when both predictor and outcome variables are dichotomous
- Example: Comparison of prevalence of hypertension in town A and town B, or prevalence of low birth weight babies in two groups of data sets and so on …

143. Ans. (a) Strong positive relationship between two variables

Coefficient of correlation is a measure of extent or degree of relationship between two variables (x or y) represented by symbol

Types of correlation:

- Perfect negative correlation—if r is +1, it indicates strong positive association.
- Perfect negative correlation— If the value of 'r' is –1 indicates strong negative association.
- No correlation—if r = 0, it indicates no association between x and y, e.g., height and pulse rate.

144. Ans. (b) Systematic random sampling

145. Ans. (a) A relative risk of 2.5 with a 95 percent confidence interval of 2.0 to 3.1

The 95% confidence interval is a measure for the range within which the values will lie in 95% of the time.

If the confidence interval contains a value of '1' for relative risk, that means 95% of times there will not be a significant association (as we can see in the option C of the MCQ)

Option B and option D are not the correct answer, as they simply give us the p-values and the relative risk.

Option C gives the confidence interval, but the confidence interval range (0.1–9.8) contains the value '1' and hence is 'not' a significant result.

146. Ans. (c) A statistically significant test supports the null hypothesis

Null hypothesis: there is no difference of effect between the groups or data sets.

A p-value < 0.05 – rejects the null hypothesis and accepts the alternate hypothesis, i.e. the effect IS FOUND

A p-value > 0.05 – accepts the null hypothesis and rejects the alternate hypothesis, i.e. the effect IS NOT FOUND. Thus a statistically significant test supports the alternate hypothesis and rejects the null hypothesis.

A statistically significant test does not prove causality or determine the errors in a study.

147. Ans. (d) 1/100

The probability of having a negative result in female with cervical cancer = false negative error rate.

FNER = 100 – sensitivity% = 100 – 90 = 10% i.e. probability of 0.1

The multiplicative rule applies to independent events. The probability to have:

FNER for two years = p[A] * p[B] = 0.1*0.1 = 0.01 = 1/100

Note: The *higher the sensitivity, the lower the probability of false negative tests as they are repeated.*

148. Ans. (d) 0.55

For two events or conditions, the probability that either will occur is the sum of their probabilities, minus the probability that both will occur. This is illustrated in the following figure:

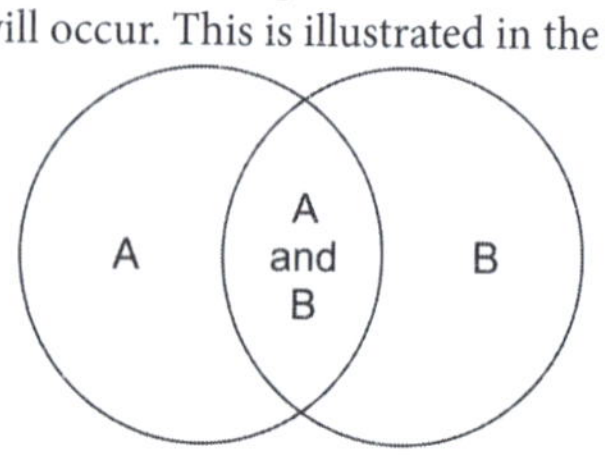

Probability of condition A = p[A] = 0.1
Probability of condition B = p[B] = 0.5
So,

- Probability of having condition [A] OR condition [B]
  Using the 'rule of addition'
  p[A] or p[B] = p[A] + p[B] = 0.1+0.5 = 0.6
- Probability of having condition [A] AND condition [B]
  Using the 'rule of multiplication'
  Both p[A] and p[B] = p[A] * p[B] = 0.1 * 0.5 = 0.05
- Probability of having condition [A] or condition [B], but NOT both
  p[A] or p[B] but not both = {p[A] + p[B]} – {p[A]*p[B]} = (0.1+0.5) – (0.1*0.5) = 0.6-0.05 = 0.55

149. Ans. (b) If more outlying observation is larger than the rest of the values, the median will be smaller than the mean

When more outlying values are larger than the rest of the values, the data are said to be skewed to the *right*, and the median is *smaller* than the mean.

If more outlying values are smaller than the rest, the data are said to be skewed to the *left*, and the median is larger than the mean.

These distributions can be illustrated as follows:

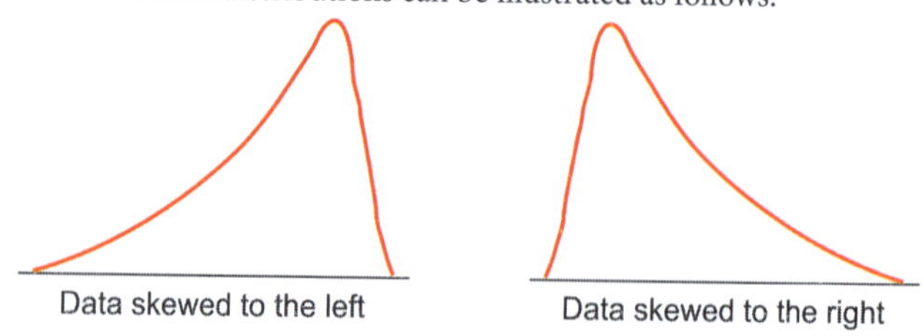

The median is more robust than the mean because it is less sensitive to extreme observations and is a more appropriate measure of central tendency when extreme values are part of the data set.

150. Ans. (d) Continuous variable

Continuous variable: where the values on scale have infinite value and any value is possible for a variable. Example: weight in Kgs, gms, miligrams and so on..

Discrete variable: which can take only certain values. Example: number of people with pancreatic cancer, number of anemic population, blood groups, color of hair and so on…

151. Ans. (d) 95%

- In a standard normal curve:
  - Mean ± 1 standard deviation covers 68.3 % of values,
  - Mean + 2 standard deviations cover 95.4 % of values,
  - Mean ±3 standard deviations cover 99.7% of values in the distribution.

152. Ans. (c) Median

- **Measures of central tendency of frequency distribution are**
  - Mean
  - Median
  - Mode
- **Measures of variation or dispersion of frequency distribution are**
  - Range
  - Mean deviation
  - Standard deviation

153. Ans. (b) Whether there is significant association between two variables

- Coefficient of correlation is calculated to establish or rule out the presence of *significant association* between two variables.
- The correlation coefficient has a value between *–1.0 and +1.0.*

154. Ans. (d) All of the above

Standard deviation is also called root mean square deviation. It measures dispersion of values about the mean

155. Ans. (b) Mode is More than median

Skew to the LEFT

- If more outlying values are smaller than the rest, data are said to be skewed to left
- Data have longer tail among lower values
- Mode > Median > mean. The mode is the maximum value in measure of central tendency

Skewed to Right (Positively skewed)

- If more outlying values are larger than the rest, data are said to be skewed to right
- Data have longer tail among higher values
- Mode < Median < mean. The mean is the highest value

156. 4. Ans. (a) Poisson distribution

Poisson Distribution

In probability theory and statistics, the Poisson distribution is a discrete probability distribution that expresses the probability of a number of events occurring in a fixed period of time if these events occur with a known average rate and independently of the time since the last event. The Poisson distribution can also be used for the number of events in other specified intervals such as distance, area or volume.

- The number of cars that pass through a certain point on a road (sufficiently distant from traffic lights) during a given period of time.
- The number of spelling mistakes one makes while typing a single page.
- The number of phone calls at a call center per minute.
- The number of times a web server is accessed per minute.
- The number of road kill (animals killed) found per unit length of road.
- The number of mutations in a given stretch of DNA after a certain amount of radiation.
- The number of unstable nuclei that decayed within a given period of time in a piece of radioactive substance. The radioactivity of the substance will weaken with time, so the total time interval used in the model should be significantly less than the mean lifetime of the substance.

157. Ans. (d) Alpha value

p value, OR and correlation Coefficient are all markers of association except the value of alpha which is a test criterion or level for deciding whether to accept or reject a null hypothesis, also known as type I error. According to convention, if P is less than or equal to 0.05, it is regarded as statistically significant.

The smaller the P value, the greater the statistical significance or probability that the association is not due to chance alone.

However, the statistical association (p value) does not imply causation.

Odds Ratio is a measure of the strength of association between the risk factor and outcome.

A correlation coefficient simply expresses the strength and direction of association or relationship between two quantitative variables, signified by 'r'. Values of r varies from −1 to +1; the strength of the relationship is indicated by the size of the coefficient, whereas its direction is indicated by the sign.

158. Ans. (c) Chi Square test

Since proportion between 2 groups is to be compared, Chi Square test would be used.

159. Ans. (a) Standard error for difference in means is calculated for parametric data

SE is inversely related to the square root of the sample size hence as the sample increases the SE decreases and not increases. The other statements regarding SE are true.

160. Ans. (c) Strong association

The correlation coefficient is the quantitative measure for the degree, and direction of association between two quantitative variables.

The value for correlation coefficient (r) is interpreted as:

- r = 0 — no correlation
- r = +1 — perfect positive correlation
- r = −1 — perfect negative correlation
- the plus (+) or minus (−) sign indicate the direction of correlation
- the value of 'r' lies between
  - 0 and 0.3 – weak correlation
  - 0.3 and 0.7 – moderate correlation
  - 0.7 and 1 – strong correlation

161. Ans. (d) Predictive value of-the-test

Bayes theorem is a simple mathematical way to calculate the post-test probability (Positive predictive value) of disease from three parameters:

- The pretest probability of disease
- Sensitivity of the test
- Specificity of the test

162. Ans. (c) Paired T test

This is a study to assess the hemoglobin levels (quantitative, parametric data) in a group of individuals 'before and after' consumption of alcohol.

So, it is a single group and data is parametric. The test of significance to be used is a 'paired t-test'

The tests of significance used are:

- Parametric tests
  - Paired t-test – for single group – before and after comparisons
  - Unpaired t-test – for two independent groups
  - ANOVA test – to compare 3 or more than 3 groups
  - Z- test – is used for large sample data
- Nonparametric tests
  - McNemar's test is a statistical test used on paired nominal data. It is applied to 2 × 2 contingency tables with a dichotomous trait, with matched pairs of subjects
  - Wilcoxan matched pairs – to compare the medians in a paired data. It can also be used for ordinal data in a single group
  - Spearman test – for correlations
  - Chi square test – used for comparison of percentages in 2 or more groups

163. Ans. (a) Mean–mode/SD

Normal distribution is a bell-shaped distribution of data where the mean, median and mode all coincide.

Skewness – is abnormal distribution of data – either to the right or to the left

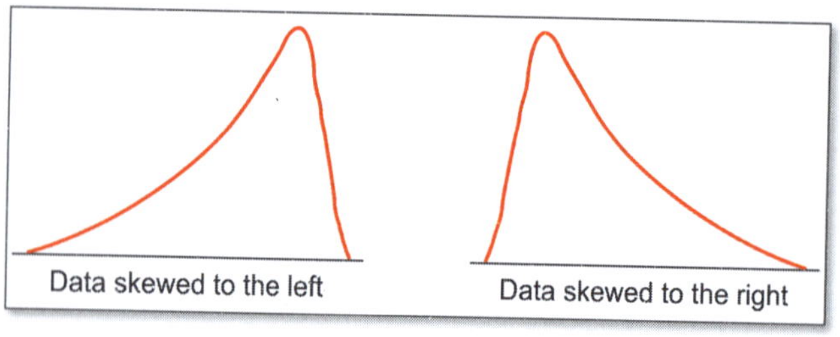

The degree of skewness is calculated by the pearson's skewness coefficient (Sk)

$$Sk = \frac{mean-mode}{SD}$$

It may also be calculated as:

$$Sk = \frac{3\ (mean-median)}{SD}$$

If the mode is not available or is not affirmative for the representation of the central tendency

Interpretation:

Sk indicates the difference in distribution of the sample data from the normal distribution data.

- A value of zero means no skewness at all.
- A large negative value means the distribution is negatively skewed.
- A large positive value means the distribution is positively skewed.

164. Ans. (b) 85-125

95% confidence interval includes values within 2 standard deviations of the mean (+/–2 SD). Since the SD is 10, twice of the SD would be 2X 10 = 20. Hence, $\mu \pm 2SD = 105 \pm 20 = 85–125$

165. Ans. (c) Negatively skewed

Negatively skewed distribution

- Skewed to the left
- Have relatively large number of high scores and small number of low scores
- Mean < median < mode
- The mode is the highest value

Positively skewed distribution

- Skewed to the right
- Have relatively large number of low scores and small number of very high scores
- Mean> median> mode
- The mean is the highest value

166. Ans. (d) Confidence interval for 95% is wider than 70%

The interpretation is as follows:

- The larger the sample size
- Smaller is the tendency for dispersion of the values
- Smaller is the variation in the data sets
- Smaller is the variation in the confidence levels

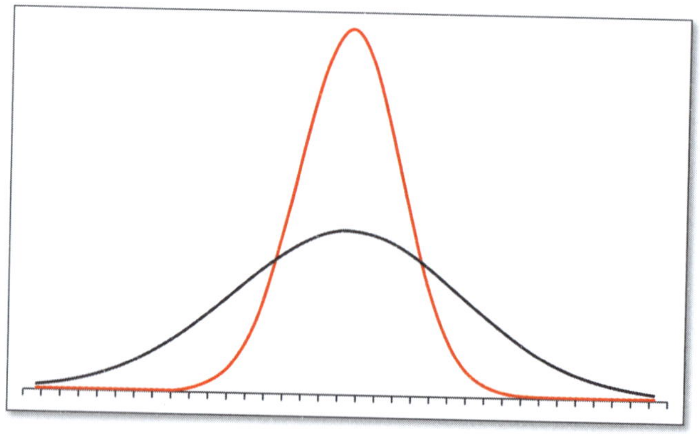

As seen in the image:

The study with 'red' color line, the sample size is more and the variations in the sample is lesser and smaller confidence intervals

The study with 'black' color line, the sample size is lesser and the variations in the sample is greater and larger or wider confidence intervals

167. Ans. (b) Both drugs are effective

In this MCQ, the new developed drug is as effective as the currently used standard drug. The p-value is found to be 0.04, which is lesser than the cut-off points of p-value 0.05 with 95% confidence interval

Remember:

95% confidence interval corresponds to 0.05 p-value.

P value < 0.05 are interpreted as SIGNIFICANT p-values and the null hypothesis is rejected (while the alternate hypothesis is accepted)

168. Ans. (c) ARR = 1% and RRR = 9.9

This is an experimental study design. and we can assess for the relative risk reduction, absolute risk reduction, and the number need to treat

The relative risk reduction is different from the relative risk (or the risk ratio)

The relative Risk reduction is given by the formula:

The event rate in exposed group (EER – Experimental group Event Rate) = $\frac{1620}{15225}$ = 10.64%

The event rate in Control group (CER – control group Event Rate) = $\frac{1800}{15225}$ = 11.82%

The Absolute risk reduction is = Event rate in experimental (exposed) group - Event rate in control (non-exposed) group

ARR = 10.64 – 11.82 = (-) 1.18% absolute reduction

$$RRR = \frac{\textit{event rate in exposed group-Event rate in Control (Non Exposed) group}}{\text{Event rate in control (non exposed) } \textit{group}} \times 100$$

$$RRR = \frac{10.64\text{-}11.82}{11.82} = \frac{(-)1.18}{11.82}\ (-)\ 9.9\%\ \text{relative reduction}$$

169. Ans. (a) Ordinal

This is a direct example of categorical data. Also, there's an inherent order in the data and the grading for liver disease severity is done, based on Child Pugh classification.
This type of data is known as ordinal data

170. Ans. (c) Alpha error

- Alpha error
  - When the research finds a significant difference, which in reality does not exist
  - The null hypothesis is rejected which was actually true
- Beta Error
  - When the research study could not (or does not) find a difference, while in reality the difference exists
  - The null hypothesis was accepted which was actually false.

171. Ans. b. There is 1% chance that there is no association

Recall that, the p-value of 0.01 corresponds to alpha level of 1%, or 0.1 probability of observing an effect just by chance. Hence option B is correct

172. Ans. (a) 4–16

Sample estimate is a point estimate of population rate.

The confidence Interval tells us the precision of an estimated sample rate (e.g. Prevalence =10%). It is the range of values in which the population rate is likely to fall. Formula to calculate the confidence interval is:

CI = mean (or prevalence) ± Z * SE

Where, Z = standard deviate multiplier. The values for 'Z' are as follows

68% confidence interval = 1

95% confidence interval = 1.96 ~ 2

99% confidence interval = 2.58

The standard error (SE) is calculated for the mean or the proportions as follows:

$$\text{SE for Mean} = \frac{SD}{\sqrt{n}}$$

$$\text{SE for Proportions} = \sqrt{\frac{PQ}{n}}$$

Where, P = Prevalence; Q = 100 – Prevalence

So, in this MCQ

$$CI = 10 \pm 2 * \sqrt{\frac{10*90}{100}}$$
$$= 10 \pm 2 * 3$$
$$= 10 \pm 6$$
$$= 4 - 16$$

173. Ans. (d) 900

The sample Size Determinants

- Precision (d) → Amount of sampling error [Absolute or relative] that can be tolerated.
- Level of significance [commonly set at 5% (p = 0.05)]
- Prevalence (p) [for qualitative characteristic]
- Standard deviation (SD) [for quantitative characteristics]

The formula for Sample size for

Quantitative characteristics at 95% Confidence Interval is $= \frac{(1.96)^2 \times SD^2}{L^2}$

Sample size for qualitative characteristics at 95% CI $= \frac{(1.96)^2 \times P \times Q}{L^2}$

Where, SD = standard deviation; P = Prevalence ; Q = 100 – Prevalence ; L = allowable error

So, in this MCQ

Prevalence (P) = 10%

Q = 90

L = 8-12% = ± 2% (absolute allowable error)

Sample size $= \frac{(1.96)^2 \times P \times Q}{L^2}$ (and we can assume 1.96 to be approximate for ~ 2)

$$= \frac{2 \times 2 \times 10 \times 90}{2^2} = 900$$

174. Ans. (b) It is used to assess for equality of distribution of non-parametric data

Nonparametric **test** of the equality of continuous, one-dimensional probability distributions that can be used to compare a sample with a reference probability distribution (one-sample K–S **test**), or to compare two samples (two-sample K–S **test**).

175. Ans. (d) Blood donations

Note:

HIV screening in apparently healthy individuals is a presumptive screening for HIV.

HIV testing in ANC females is called as "Opt Out Testing"

HIV testing in blood donations is "Unlinked anonymous testing"

176. Ans. (a) 10% and 50%

	Event (complications)	No event (No complications)	Total
Experimental group	100	900	1000
Control (Placebo) group	400	1600	2000
	500	2500	3000

Control group Event Rate (CER) = 400/2000 = 0.2

Experimental group Event rate (EER) = 100/1000 = 0.1

Absolute risk reduction (ARR) =

= CER – EER

= 0.2-0.1 = 0.1 = 10%

Relative Risk reduction (RRR) =

= (CER-EER)/CER

= (0.2-0.1) / 0.2

= 0.5 = 50%

177. Ans. (d) 200

Number Needed to Treat (NNT): Is the minimum number of patients to be treated with the drug to observe a positive effect in a person and to prevent a bad outcome as death or complication.

NNT = 1/ARR

CER = 1%

EER = event rate reduction of 50%, i.e. = 0.5%

So, ARR = CER – EER

ARR = 1 – 0.5 = 0.5% = 0.005
NNT = 1/ARR = 1/0.005 = 200

178. Ans. (b) Unpaired t-test

For parametric data (or quantitative variable) – paired t test, unpaired t-test or Z test is used

For non-parametric data (or qualitative variable) – Chi square tests, wilcoxan rank test, kruskal wallis tests are used

In the MCQ, the blood pressures (which is a quantitative variable or parametric data) are to be compared between two groups, so the direct answer would be unpaired t-test

179. Ans. (a) Paired t-test

For parametric data (or quantitative variable) – paired t test, unpaired t-test or Z test is used

For non-parametric data (or qualitative variable) – Chi square tests, wilcoxan rank test, kruskal wallis tests are used

In the MCQ, the blood pressures (which is a quantitative variable or parametric data) are to be compared in a single group as before intervention and after intervention, so the direct answer is 'paired t-test' will be used

180. Ans. (b) Mean = Median, not equal to Mode

We can see from the image, there are two curves – red color and a green color curve

- The red color curve probably shows a normal distribution with the maximum values are towards the center, so we can say the mean ~ median ~ mode.
- The green color curve shows a bimodal distribution (with two peaks). the average would be towards the center, but definitely the modes are different

So, we may answer as:

Mean = median for both curves. While the mode is different for red and green color curves

181. Ans. (b) Positive skew or Right skew.

As we see in the MCQ image, most of the values are lying towards the lower side, with a few outlier values more than the 30 point mark.

So, if we just take the box and whisker pictographically as presented below:

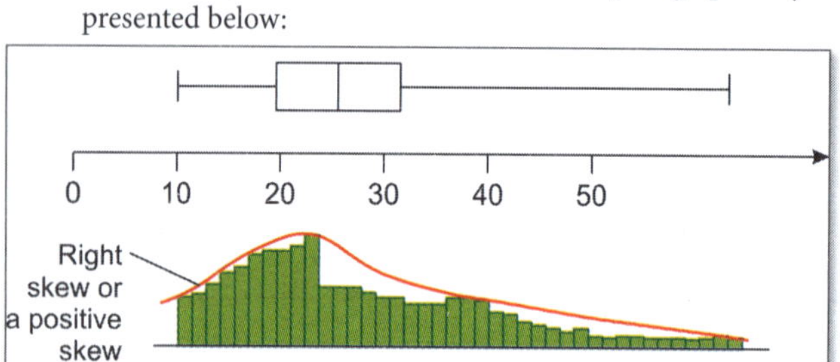

We see that most of the values are towards the left side with a few outliers towards the right side. Hence this forms a RIGHT SKEW also known as POSITIVE SKEW

182. Ans. (a) 3>2>1

Ref: Biostatistics Principles and Practice by B. Antonisamy and Mcg raw hill publication, Pg.44-45 Park 25th edition, Pg 913

Note that:

- The margin of error is inversely proportional to sample size (SE $\alpha \frac{1}{n}$).
- The larger the sample, the smaller is the error and the closer the values are to the actual or the true value

Hence if we see the graph, we see that curve 3 is with least sample size and the values are more spread out away from the central value, while the curve 1 has highest sample and the values are more concentrated near the central value.

Hence the answer should be margin of error is least for 1 and highest for curve #3

183. Ans. (b) Heart rate/min and Age

Ref: Biostatistics Principles and Practice by B Antonisamy, Mcg raw hill publication, pg. 117 Park 25th edition 915

The data given in the options are:

Option	Category of data	Test of significance
▪ Sex and stage of cancer	Nominal data, non-parametric data	Chi square test
▪ Heart rate/min and Age	Ratio scale, quantitative data	t – test
▪ Benign or malignant, and type of surgery	Nominal data, qualitative data, non-parametric data	Chi square test
▪ Age group and cancer state	Categorical data, non-parametric data	Chi square test

Testing groups – situation	Parametric test	Non parametric test
Testing association between two qualitative variables		Chi square test
Comparison of two **independent groups**	t-test for independent samples	Wilcoxon rank sum test (Ordinal data)
Comparison of data between **paired observations** (usually single group – before and after)	t-test for paired observation	Wilcoxon rank sign test (Ordinal data)
Comparison of several groups **(three or more groups)**	ANOVA	Kruskal wallis test (independent groups, nominal data)
Assessment of relationship between two variables	Pearson correlation for linear relation	Spearman rank correlation

184. Ans. (a) Paired t test

The weight of students is measured in pounds (quantitative variable, parametric data) and pre-post testing was done. This is clear example of a 'paired t-test'

Refer to theory section for more details

185. Ans. (b) 10

In this MCQ we need to calculate the 'Number NEED to TREAT'

Solution

- The MCQ provides us with following information: The failure rates in
  - New treatment group (experimental group) – 26 out of 130
  - Previous treatment group (control group) – 36 out of 120

Step 1: Make a BOX

	Treatment failure – event	No treatment failure	Total
Experimental group	26		130
Control group	36		120
			250 samples

so, we make a complete box as

	Treatment failure – event	No treatment failure	Total
Experimental group	26	130-26 = 104	130
Control group	36	120-36 = 84	120

Step 2: Calculate the Risk of event in EACH group

- Event rate in experimental group (EER) = 26/130 = 0.2
- Event rate in control group (CER) = 36/120 = 0.3

Step 3: Calculate the Risk reduction and Number need to Treat

- Absolute Risk reduction = CER – EER = 0.3 – 0.2 = 0.1
- Number needed to Treat = 1/ARR = 1 / 0.1 = 10

So, we need to treat atleast 10 persons to decrease the treatment failure rate by 1.

186. Ans. (a) 3

Ref: Biostats Simplified for PGME, Pg 53

As we can see in the image, the risk factors under consideration are:

Variables – potential associated factors	Risk assessment – Odds ratio	95% confidence interval range
Early menarche	1.3	1.2 – 1.9
Age < 50 years	0.04	0.01 – 0.32
Smoking history	0.5	0.02 – 0.9
BRCA mutation	1.9	1.1 – 2.8
Alcohol	1	0.8 – 1.8
High SES	1.4	0.5 – 3.5
Obesity	1.24	1.1 – 1.7
No family history of breast cancer	0.3	0.01 – 0.9

Contd...

General rules to interpret the Odds / Risk ratio with 95% confidence intervals on multiple regression analysis:

- Look at the confidence interval range –
  - If the range starts or ends with '1', it is a non-significant odds ratio
  - If the 95% confidence Interval range has the value '1' within the range – interpret as a non- significant odds ratio
  - For a significant odds ratio, the 95% confidence interval should not have value '1' within it
- Look at the risk assessment measure (i.e. Odds ratio or risk ratio)
  - If the risk assessment = 1 interpret as non-significant association
  - If the risk assessment measure > 1 interpret as positive and significant association. The factor is risk factor
  - If the risk assessment measure < 1 interpret as positive and significant association. the factor is risk factor

Variables – potential associated factors	Risk assessment – Odds ratio	95% confidence interval range	Comment
Early menarche	1.3	1.2 – 1.9	Positive and significant association - risk factor
Age < 50 years	0.04	0.01 – 0.32	Negative and significant association – protective factor
Smoking history	0.5	0.02 – 0.9	Negative and significant association – protective factor
BRCA mutation	1.9	1.1 – 2.8	Positive and significant association -risk factor
Alcohol	1	0.8 – 1.8	Positive, but non-significant association
High SES	1.4	0.5 – 3.5	Positive, but non-significant association
Obesity	1.24	1.1 – 1.7	Positive and significant risk factor
No family history of breast cancer	0.3	0.01 – 0.9	Negative and significant association – protective factor

187. Ans. (c) y = 11 + 2x

Ref: Biostats Simplified for PGME, Pg 97

Solution: We know that:
Regression means to predict a value based on another variable.
The regression equation is expressed as:
Regression equation:
$y = a + bx + e$
where,
y = dependent variable;
a = regression constant = intercept of slope on Y
b = slope coefficient; (slope of the curve)
x = independent variable;
e = error
The intercept on y we can estimate is somewhere around 10 or 11, with the slope of the line, given as 2 so the best suited option is – option C

188. Ans. (b) Strength of relation is more in A than in B

Ref: Biostats Simplified for PGME, Pg 96

Scatter Plot A

- The values are more concentrated towards the median vector or the correlation coefficient curve.
- This shows a positive correlation

Scatter Plot B

- The values are more dispersed around the median vector or the correlation coefficient curve
- This shows a very less correlation (or no correlation)

Note:

- Correlation coefficients are used to measure the strength of the relationship between two variables. The more closer and concentrated the values are on scatter, the more stronger is the relation between two variables (and Vice versa)
- Pearson correlation is the one most commonly used in statistics. This measures the strength and direction of a linear relationship between two variables.
- Values always range between -1 (strong negative relationship) and +1 (strong positive relationship).
- Values at or close to zero imply weak or no relationship.
- Correlation coefficient values less than +0.6 or greater than -0.6 are not considered significant.

189. Ans. (c) B & D are correct

Ref: Biostats Simplified for PGME, 73

Must Remember Point

95% confidence level corresponds to

- Z score ± 1.96 SE
- p value 0.05
- Alpha error 5%

General Guiding Principles

Observation from study	Interpretation	Comment
In both the interventions, the p value is less than 0.05	Both the interventions are considered as significant	Null hypothesis is rejected
The p-value with 'x' = 0.02 And with 'y' = 0.001	The lower the p-value → the higher is significance and stronger is the effect and lesser the alpha errors	The significance for 'y' is more than 'x' and hence 'y' intervention has a stronger statistical effect on the disease

So, we may Conclude that

- The study B (p-value 0.001) has a higher significance and shows a stronger effect of the intervention 'y' compared to the control group
- The intervention 'x' in the study A is also significantly better than the control group intervention (P-value 0.02).
- The study A shows a higher significance and a stronger effect compared to the study B
- The study with lower p-values, will be more significant and correspond to lower error and higher sample size

190. Ans. (b) Sample B more than Sample A

Ref: Biostats Simplified for PGME, Pg 34

The dispersion of data is measured using:

- Coefficient of variation (CV) is a measure of relative variability of data set. We can directly compare the variability in two different populations using the CV

$$CV = \frac{SD}{mean}$$

Sample A

Mean = 110
Standard deviation = 11

$$\text{Coefficient of variation} = \frac{SD}{mean} \times 100 = \frac{11}{110} \times 100 = 16\%$$

Sample B

Mean = 18
Standard deviation = 3

$$\text{Coefficient of variation} = \frac{SD}{mean} \times 100 = \frac{3}{18} \times 100 = 16\%$$

So, we may interpret this as: Sample B has higher variability compared to sample A

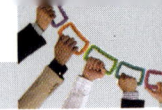

Note:

The standard error (SE) is a measure of variation for random variables, providing a measurement for the spread. The smaller the spread, the more accurate the dataset. It is calculated for a data set with SD's, sample size and confidence limits. It is given by the formula:

$$\text{SE (mean)} = \frac{\text{SD}}{\sqrt{n}}$$

191. Ans. (a) Chi Square test

Ref: Biostats Simplified for PGME, Pg 75-80

The chi square test is to compare the non-parametric data like prevalence of disease or number of cases in an area in two independent sample groups.

Other Tests of Significance in the MCQ

- Paired t-test – used for quantitative data
- Wilcoxan rank test – for ordinal data
- ANOVA – Analysis of variance is a test for parametric data (quantitative variables) for comparing three or more groups.

192. Ans. (d) Line diagram

Ref: Mukhmohit's Biostats simplified for PGMEE, Pg 9

Presentation of Data

- Quantitative data – histogram, frequency polygons
- Correlation between two variables – scatter plot
- Trend of events over time – line chart
- Qualitative data – bar charts, Pie charts

193. Ans. (b) Chi-square test

Ref: Park 25th Ed. Pg 915

Chi square is a method for testing the significance of difference between two proportions. It can be used for two or more than two groups.

194. Ans. (d) Component bar chart

Ref: Mukhmohit's Biostats simplified for PGMEE, Pg 11

195. Ans. (b) Unpaired t test

Ref: Mukhmohit's Biostats simplified for PGMEE, Pg 78

196. Ans. (b) 68%

Ref: Mukhmohit's Biostats simplified for PGMEE, Pg 64, Park 25th Ed. Pg 912

Remember - within

± 1 SD	68% of values lie
± 2 SD	95% of the values lie
± 3 SD	99% of the values lie

NOTES

Section

B

Preventive Medicine

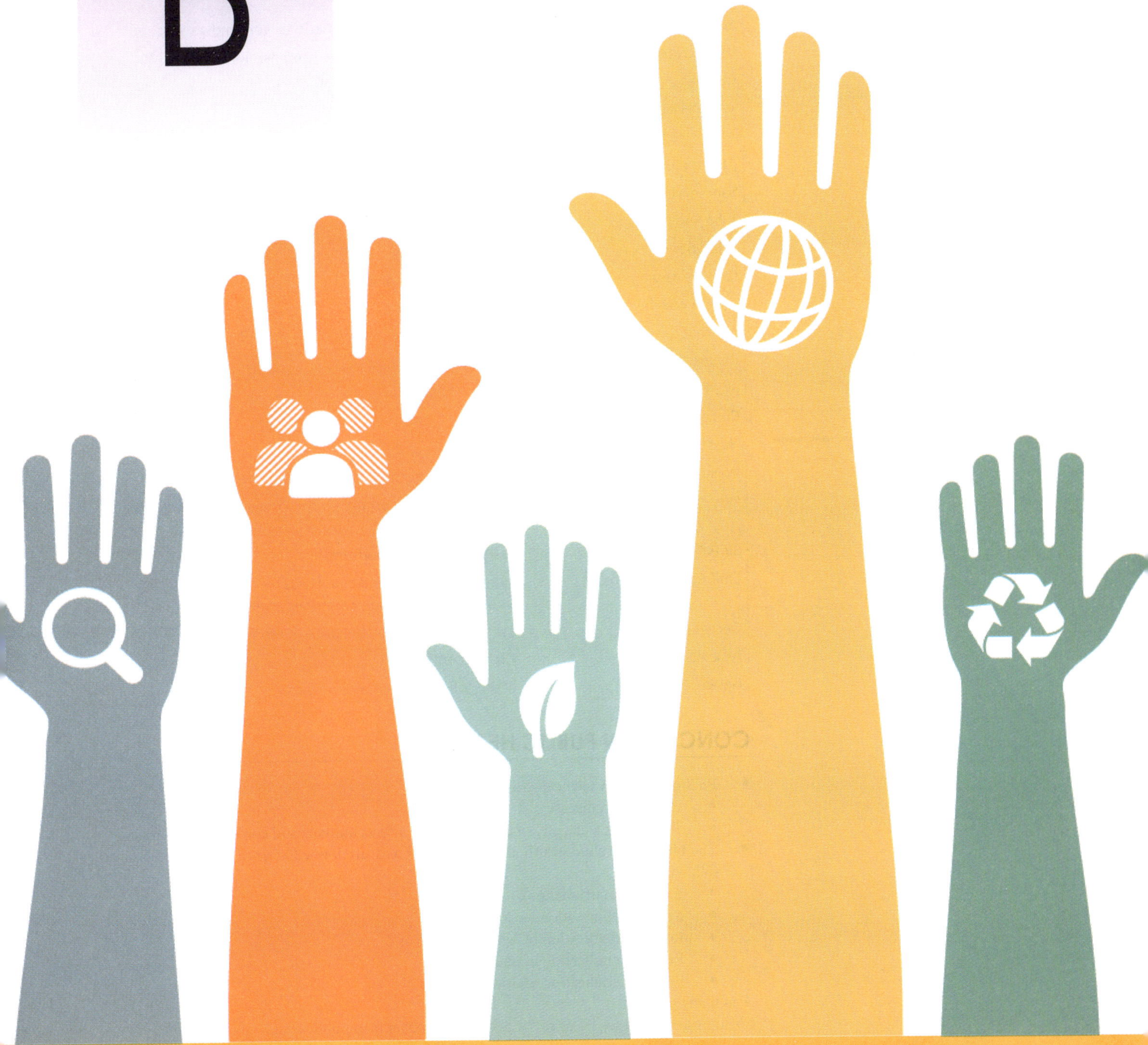

Evolution and Concepts in Community Medicine

Chapter Outline

TITLES IN PUBLIC HEALTH

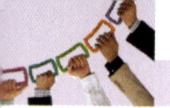

Scientists	Titles
Dhanvantari	Hindu God of Medicine[Q]
Sushruta	Father of Plastic and Cosmetic Surgery/Indian Surgery[Q]
Hippocrates (Greek Medicine)	Father of Medicine[Q], 1st true epidemiologist[Q]
Charaka	Father of Indian Medicine[Q]
Joseph Lister	Father of Antisepsis[Q]
Ambroise Pare	Father of Modern Surgery
Atreya (800 BC)	First great Indian physician and teacher
Samuel Hanemann	Father of Homeopathy[Q]
John Snow	Father of Epidemiology
Aristotle	Father of Biology
Louis Pasteur	Father of Bacteriology
Gregor Mendel	Father of Genetics
Andreas Vesalius	Father of Modern Anatomy, 1st man of modern science
Claude Bernard	Father of Physiology
Sigmund Freud	Father of Psychoanalysis
Cholera	Father of Public Health[Q]
Hospitals	Ivory towers of disease
William Farr	Father of modern epidemiological surveillance
Langmuir	Founder of 20th century epidemiological and public health surveillance
Sir Patrick Manson	Father of tropical medicine
Emil Adolf von Behring	1st nobel prize in medicine (1901)—Worked on serum therapy and developed diphtheria vaccine
Gerty Cori	1st woman to win Nobel prize in Medicine (1947)
Aesculapius	His staff entwined by a snake is the symbol of medicine
Galen	Father of experimental physiology

CONCEPTS IN PUBLIC HEALTH

- Public health is a science which deals with
  - Uprooting a disease
  - To conquer a disease, so that it no more affects humans and community at large.
- The efforts of public health as an organized and disciplined science are evident from the following facts:
  - Eradication of smallpox
  - Regional elimination for measles
  - Regional eradication of "wild" polio virus
  - Regional eradication of malaria
  - Regional eradication of dracunculiasis

And many others…

So, to understand this, let us revise a few basic concepts in public health.

NATURAL HISTORY OF DISEASE

- **Natural History of Disease**[Q] is the progression of a disease over time from the prepathogenesis phase (earliest phase) to its termination as recovery, disability or death *in absence of any treatment or prevention.*
- Natural history of diseases can be best studied using a cohort study[Q]

Table 1: Prepathogenesis and pathogenesis phases of disease

Prepathogenesis phase (Man in the middle of disease)	Pathogenesis phase
▪ Interaction occurs between agent, host and environment ▪ *Disease agent has not entered man* (It is the period before onset of disease in man) ▪ All of us are in the prepathogenesis phase of many communicable and non-communicable diseases ▪ Possible level of prevention is primary	▪ *Disease agent enters man and* multiplies, resulting in disease progression ▪ Infection may be clinical or subclinical; typical or atypical or host may become a carrier (e.g. Diphtheria, Polio, etc.) ▪ Final outcome is recovery or *disability or death* ▪ Possible level of prevention is secondary and tertiary[Q]

THEORIES OF DISEASE CAUSATION

- ***Germ Theory of Disease***[Q] states 1:1 relationship between causal agent and disease. *It was given by Louis Pasteur*[Q].

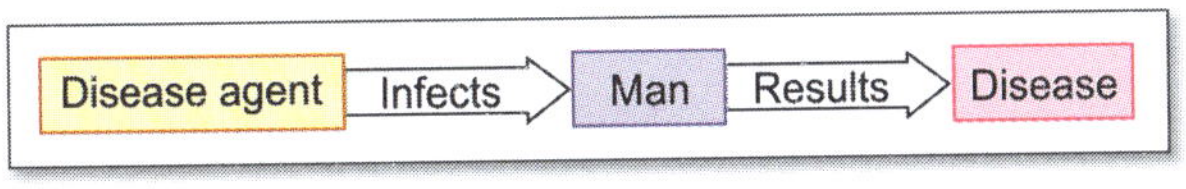

- ***Epidemiological triad***[Q]: Disease results from disturbance in equilibrium between agent, host and environmental factors
- ***Multifactorial causation***[Q]**:** Proposed by Pettenkofer of Munich[Q] Disease results from interaction of multiple factors
- ***Theory of "Web of Causation":*** Proposed by McMahon and Pugh[Q] to explain causation of noncommunicable disease. *It states that* multiple factors interact like "web of a spider" with each factor having its own relative importance and modify the effect of each other
  - To prevent a disease, a few *"weak links"* in the interlacing webs need to be identified and acted upon
- Theory of "Necessary" and "Sufficient" cause proposed by Rothman
  - ***Necessary cause:*** Its presence is essential for disease to occur. But it may or may not be able to cause the disease by itself alone
  - ***Sufficient cause:*** Its presence will always result in disease.
  - Necessary cause may by itself be a sufficient cause, e.g. HIV for AIDS
  - Necessary cause by itself may not be a sufficient cause, e.g. *M. tuberculosis* for TB disease
  - In most noncommunicable diseases an optimum mix of multiple factors (No single necessary cause) is needed to produce the "sufficient cause"
- ***Miasma theory:*** Proposed by *William Furr*. It states that human diseases were due to bad clouds
- **Iceberg phenomenon**[Q]**:**
  - *Disease in a community is comparable to an iceberg*
  - ***Water line*** *represents the demarcation between apparent and inapparent disease.*
  - **Screening** *applies to submerged portion*, whereas **diagnosis** *applies to tip of the iceberg.*

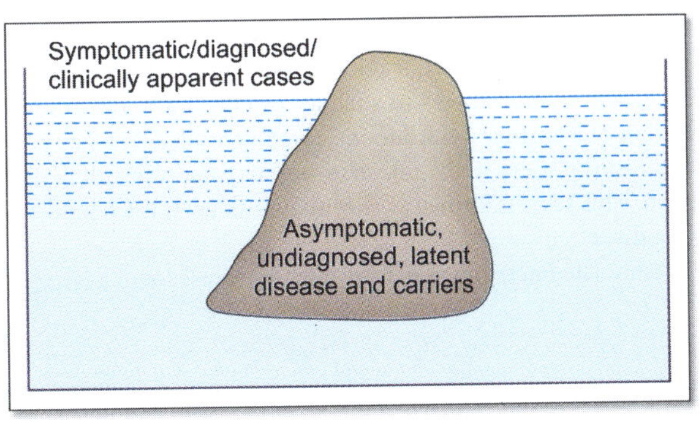

Fig. 1: Iceberg phenomenon

29 **High Yield Points**

- **Risk factor** is an attribute/ exposure significantly associated with development of disease or a determinant that if modified by intervention reduces the possible of occurrence of the disease.
- **Spectrum of disease**[Q] is graphic representation of variation in disease manifestation (sub-clinical infection at one end and fatal illness at other, with mild /moderate/severe illness in between).
- WHO has defined health but not disease.

- *Iceberg phenomenon is seen mostly in diseases with subclinical infections*[Q] e.g. Rubella, mumps, polio, diphtheria, JE, hepatitis A and B and Influenza.
- It is of *no use* in disease like measles, tetanus, rabies, chicken pox, etc. which have no subclinical infection.
- The larger the submerged portion, larger is the utility of the screening tool in the community.

EPIDEMIOLOGICAL TRIANGLE

- The triad consists of an external **agent**, a **host** and an **environment** in which host and agent are brought together, causing the disease to occur in the host.
- A **vector**, an organism which transmits infection by conveying the pathogen from one host to another without causing disease itself, may be part of the infectious process.
- The transmission occurs when the agent leaves its **reservoir** or **host** through a **portal of exit**, is conveyed by a **mode of transmission** to enter through an appropriate **portal of entry** to infect a **susceptible host**.
- Transmission may be **direct** (direct contact host-to-host, droplet spread from one host to another) or **indirect** (the transfer of an infectious agent from a reservoir to a susceptible host by suspended air particles, inanimate objects (vehicles or fomites) or animate intermediaries (vectors).

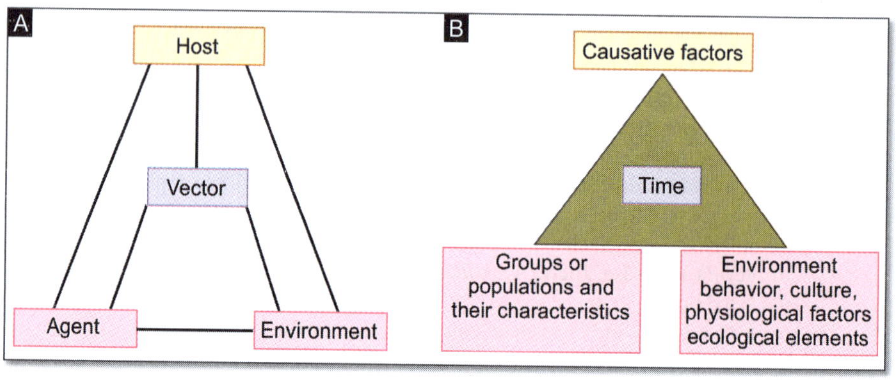

Figs 2A and B: (A) Epidemiological triangle; (B) Modern epidemiological triangle—advanced model of the triangle of epidemiology

HOW TO CONTROL A DISEASE? CONCEPT OF CONTROL

Control

As the public enforcement acts upon a disease, the disease frequency obviously tends to decline. The stage where the disease is no more a public health problem is known as "Control phase". E.g. Hepatitis, malaria, tuberculosis, blindness, obesity.

Elimination

As the further actions and interventions of public health would happen, the disease frequency drops (control phase) and then it lowers to such an extent, that there are no new cases found because of interruption of transmission from one case to another. The key point is the agent (or the pathogen or organism) present in the universe, but may not transmit because of interruption of transmission chain. This stage is known as elimination stage. It is a temporary stage just before extermination of the disease.

Elimination is complete *interruption of transmission* of disease in a large geographic region.

Eradication

Just as we achieve an elimination phase, i.e. organism exists but may not transmit to the host or carrier. Henceforth, obviously, after some time the organism also shall cease to exist (as it may find any host to invade and multiply). This stage is known as eradication stage. It is usually a permanent stage meaning—termination of pathogen or the causative microorganism.

Also Know......................

- *Elimination is an intermediate goal between control and eradication.*[Q] Regional elimination is precursor to eradication.
- *Disease eliminated from India are:*
  - *Leprosy (2005,<1/10000),*
  - *Yaws (2016),*
  - *Maternal and Neonatal Tetanus (2015, <1/1000 live birth).*
- *Those targeted for elimination are:*
  - *Kala-azar,*
  - *Lymphatic filariasis*
  - *Tuberculosis*

- It is an "**all or none phenomenon**"[Q]. Once eradicated, the disease no longer occurs in the population
- Only disease globally eradicated till date is **smallpox**[Q]
- Diseases with potential for global eradication are [Q]**polio, measles and, Dracunculosis** (eradicated from India).

CONCEPT OF PREVENTION

- Primordial prevention – prevention of the occurrence of risk factors
- Primary prevention – prevention of the occurrence of disease
- Secondary prevention – prevention of the occurrence of complications from disease
- Tertiary prevention – Prevention of the occurrence of disability or fatality due to a complication from the disease
- Quaternary prevention – Quaternary prevention is the set of health activities to mitigate or avoid the consequences of unnecessary or excessive intervention of the health system.

13 Good to Remember

Quaternary prevention: It is a new term denoting—actions taken to identify patients at risk of over-treatment, to protect them from new medical procedures and ethically acceptable alternatives to be advised

Table 2: Levels of preventions and modes of interventions

Levels of preventions	Modes of interventions	Examples
Primordial	Individual and mass education	Discourage adoption of high-risk behavior in a population where it does not exist. E.g. Smoking, drinking in societies where it is not prevalent yet.
Primary	Health promotion	▪ Health education ▪ Environment modification, e.g. Provision of safe water, sanitary latrines, control of insects and rodents, etc. ▪ Lifestyle and behavioral changes, e.g Exercise and meditation ▪ Improvement in overall socioeconomic status of the population ▪ Promotion of breastfeeding ▪ Promotion of small family norms ▪ Marriage counseling
	Specific protection	▪ Immunization ▪ Chemoprophylaxis ▪ Nutrition supplement, e.g. IFA, Vitamin A, Iodine ▪ Protection against occupational hazards, accident, carcinogen, etc. ▪ Avoidance of allergens ▪ Control of consumer product quality and safety of food and drug ▪ Control of air pollution, noise control, chlorination of water ▪ Use of helmets and seat belts to protect against head injuries ▪ Use of mosquito net ▪ Personal hygiene and environmental sanitation ▪ Contraception
Secondary	Early diagnosis	Screening (Pap smear, self-breast examination, mammography) active case search, medical examination of school children, infants and young children, industrial workers
	Treatment	▪ DOTS ▪ MDT for leprosy ▪ Dental filling and tooth extraction

Contd...

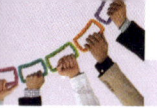

Levels of preventions	Modes of interventions	Examples
Tertiary	Disability limitation	▪ Resting affected limbs in neutral position to prevent stress on paralyzed muscle ▪ Plaster cast to a patient with Colles' fracture ▪ Rest, morphine, oxygen and streptokinase to a patient of Acute MI
	Rehabilitation	▪ School for blind ▪ Reconstructive surgery ▪ Arranging for schooling of child suffering from PRPP ▪ Provision of hearing aids, artificial limb, and calipers ▪ Restoration of capacity to earn a livelihood (Vocational) ▪ Restoration of family and social relation (Social) ▪ Restoration of personal dignity and confidence (Psychological).

MONITORING AND SURVEILLANCE

Monitoring[Q]

It is performance and analysis of *routine measurements to detect any change in environment or health status of a population*, e.g. Monitoring of air pollution, water quality, growth and nutritional status, etc.

(Note: in monitoring we keep on checking the data to help us plan for future inputs and outcomes – may be related to evaluation of program)

Surveillance[Q]

It is continuous scrutiny of factors that determine occurrence and distribution of disease and other conditions of ill health. It is a continuous supervision of activities which help in close watch and ability to complete the desired results in the session.

Types

- **Passive:** Patient comes to doctor with complain of cough >2 weeks. (RNTCP).
- **Active:** Data is collected actively by health system, e.g. Health worker actively searches for leprosy cases (NLEP), collects blood slides every fortnightly for malaria (NVBDCP).
- **Sentinel:** Detects missing cases and supplements notified cases. E.g. HIV sentinel surveillance

30 High Yield Points

Active surveillance yields true morbidity

INDICATORS OF HEALTH

Human Development Index (HDI)

- It is an index *of quality of life*[Q].
- It combines three dimensions–
  - *Longevity (life expectancy at birth)*[Q]
  - *Knowledge (Mean years of schooling and expected years of schooling)*[Q]
  - *Income (GNI per capita in purchasing power parity in US dollars)*[Q]
- *Each dimension has maximum and minimum values. For each dimension of* HDI, individual indices are computed by using formula:

$$\textbf{Dimension Index} = \frac{\textit{Actual value} - \textit{Minimum value}}{\textit{Maximum value} - \textit{Minimum value}}$$

- *HDI values range between 0 and 1*[Q] and is the geometric mean of three-dimension indices [$HDI = I_{Life\ 1/3} \times I_{Education\ 1/3} \times I_{Income\ 1/3}$].
- HDI is indicator of achievements in basic human capabilities of a country (i.e. Long life, education and decent standard of living).

18 Must Remember

Diseases under WHO International Surveillance are: Rabies, Malaria, Polio, Salmonellosis, Louse born typhus fever, Influenza human and Relapsing fever. [**Mnemonic →** RMPSLIR]

Inequality-adjusted Human Development Index

The difference between the inequality-adjusted human development index (IHDI) and HDI is the human development cost of inequality, also termed – the loss to human development due to inequality. The IHDI allows a direct link to inequalities in dimensions, it can inform policies toward inequality reduction, and leads to better understanding of inequalities across population and their contribution to the overall human development cost.

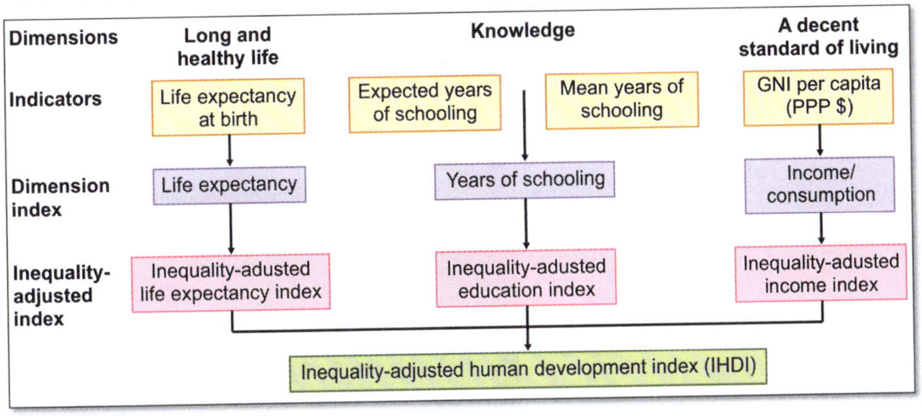

Fig. 3: Inequality-adjusted human development index (IHDI)

Physical Quality of Life Index (PQLI)

- Combines three indicators:
  - *Infant mortality*[Q],
  - *Life expectancy at age 1 year*[Q] *and*
  - *Literacy.*[Q]
- Performance of individual countries is measured on a scale of 0 to 100. [0 = worst and 100 = Best]
- PQLI (0–100) is the average of the 3 indicators with equal weightage to each of them.
- *Per capita GNP is not taken into consideration* (does not measure economic growth).[Q]
- It measures results of social, economic and political policies and seeks to complement GNP.
- Ultimate objective is to attain a PQLI of 100 **(India, PQLI is 65)**.

Human Poverty Index (HPI)

- Introduced in 1978. Measures average deprivation in basic dimensions of human development.
- ***HPI 1*** is used for developing countries (India = 28%). It measures
  - Vulnerability to death at a relatively early age *(Probability at birth of not surviving to the age of 40 year).* **(P_1)**
  - Exclusion from reading and communication *(Adult literacy rate).* **(P_2)**
  - Lack of access to decent standard of living/economic provisioning. **(P_3)** (It is the unweighted *average of two indicators.)*
    - Percentage of population not using an improved water source.
    - Percentage of children underweight for age.

$$HPI_1 = \left[\frac{1}{2}(p_1^{\alpha} + p_2^{\alpha} + p_3^{\alpha})\right]^{\frac{1}{\alpha}}, \text{ where Alpha} = 3.$$

- **HPI 2** – Used for developed countries. It measures:
  - P_1 is vulnerability to death at a relatively early age *(Probability at birth of not surviving to age of 60 years).*
  - P_2 is exclusion from reading and communication [*% of adults (Age 16-65)* lacking functional literacy skills].
  - P_3 is lack of access to decent standard of living/economic provisioning *(% of population living below poverty line).*
  - P_4 is social exclusion [Rate of long-term unemployment (*12 months or more*)]

$$HPI_2 = \left[\frac{1}{4}(p_1^{\alpha} + p_2^{\alpha} + p_3^{\alpha})\right]^{\frac{1}{\alpha}}, \text{ where alpha} = 3$$

31 High Yield Points

As per 2015 ratings—India falls in the medium HDI category, with an HDI of 0.624[Rank 131][Q]
- Norway, Australia and Switzerland have highest HDI values.
- D.R. of Congo, Niger have lowest HDI values.

14 Good to Remember

HDI measures the standard of living

32 High Yield Points

PQLI measures the quality of life

15 Good to Remember

PQLI is applicable for international and national comparison.

Multidimensional Poverty Index (MPI)

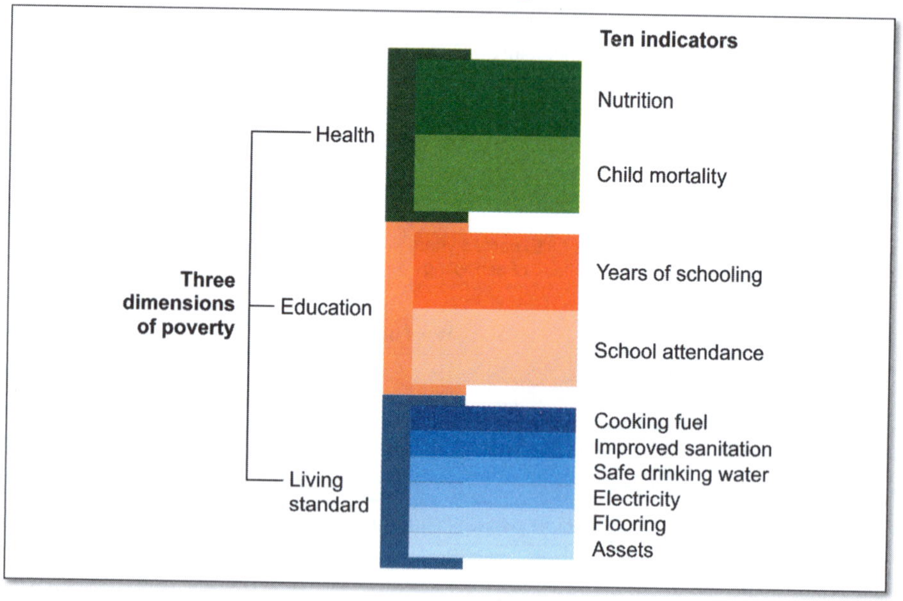

Fig. 4: Indicators of multidimensional poverty index

16 Good to Remember

The MPI assesses poverty at the individual level. If someone is deprived in a third or more of ten (weighted) indicators (Fig. 4), the global index identifies them as "MPI poor" and the extent – or intensity – of their poverty is measured by the number of deprivations they are experiencing.

Gender-related Development Index (GDI)

- Highlights the achievements in basic human development adjusted for gender inequalities.
- It has three components:
  - Long and healthy life *(Male and Female life expectancy at birth)*
  - Knowledge *(Male adult literacy rate + Male Gross Enrolment Ratio and Female adult literacy rate + Female GER)*
  - Decent standard of living *(Male and Female estimated earned income).*

Gender Empowerment Measure (GEM)

- Measures gender inequalities in economic and political opportunities.
- It measures three components:
  - Political participation and decision making *(Female and male share of parliamentary seats)*
  - Economic participation and decision making *(Female and male share of positions as Legislators, senior official/managers and female and male share of professional and technical positions)*
  - Power over economic resources (*Female and male estimated earned income).*

WHO–HEALTH FOR ALL INDICATORS

- **Health policy indicators:** Political commitment, resource allocation, equity of distribution of health services, community involvement, organizational framework and managerial process.
- ***Social and economic indicators:*** GDP or GNP, housing, income, food availability.
- ***Indicators for the provision of health care:*** Availability, accessibility, utilization and quality of care.
- **Standard of living** has been defined by WHO as "Income and occupation, standards of housing, sanitation, nutrition, level of provision of health, educational, recreational and other services (used individually as measures of socioeconomic status) may collectively be used as an index of Standard of living".
- Inequalities in standards of living are due to difference in per capita GNP of people in different countries.
- **Level of living** (Used in United Nations documents) has 9 components: health, food consumption, education, occupation and working condition, housing, social security, clothing, recreation and leisure and human rights.

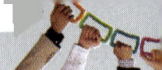

INTERNATIONAL CLASSIFICATION OF DISEASE – 11TH REVISION (2018)

ICD Classification

Reference classifications by WHO are:

- International classification of diseases (ICD)
- International classification of functioning disability and health (ICF)
  - Body Functions and Structures
  - Environmental and personal factors
- Internal classification of health interventions (ICHI)
  - Classification of interventions covering acute care, primary care, rehabilitation, assistance with functioning, prevention, public health, and ancillary services

ICD defines the universe of diseases, disorders, injuries and other related health conditions, listed in a comprehensive, hierarchical fashion that allows for:

- Easy storage, retrieval and analysis of health information for evidenced-based decision-making;
- Sharing and comparing health information between hospitals, regions, settings and countries; and
- Data comparisons in the same location across different time periods.

ICD 11 Characteristics

- The classification has integrated digital and electronic health record system
- It has three volumes
  - Volume 1 Tabular list
  - Volume 2 Reference list
  - Volume 3 Alphabetical list
- 26 chapters are defined, which are alphanumeric with 'Arabic' system of numbering

Table 3: Difference between ICD 10 and ICD 11 revision

ICD 10	ICD 11
Chapter in roman numerical	Chapter number is Arabic
3-character categories and further 10 sub-categories	4-character category and 2 sub-categories
First character is not corresponding to chapter	First character of the code always relates to the chapter
21 Chapters	26 Chapters
	New chapters: ▪ Sleep wake disorders ▪ Immune system disorders (separate chapter) ▪ Codes for special purposes ▪ Traditional medicine conditions
	Terminal letter 'Y' is reserved for the residual category 'other specified' and the terminal letter 'Z' is reserved for the residual category 'unspecified'
	All ICD-11 categories have a short and a long description
	All ICD-11 categories include separate information on anatomy, etiology and other aspects that can be accessed for search purposes, or when browsing in the tabular list

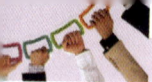

Chapter List under ICD 11

ICD-11 Mortality and Morbidity Statistics

- Certain infectious or parasitic diseases
- Neoplasms
- Diseases of the blood or blood-forming organs
- Diseases of the immune system
- Endocrine, nutritional or metabolic diseases
- Mental, behavioural or neurodevelopmental disorders
- Sleep-wake disorders
- Diseases of the nervous system
- Diseases of the visual system
- Diseases of the ear or mastoid process
- Diseases of the circulatory system
- Diseases of the respiratory system
- Diseases of the digestive system
- Diseases of the skin
- Diseases of the musculoskeletal system or connective tissue
- Diseases of the genitourinary system
- Conditions related to sexual health
- Pregnancy, childbirth or the puerperium
- Certain conditions originating in the perinatal period
- Developmental anomalies
- Symptoms, signs or clinical findings, not elsewhere classified
- Injury, poisoning or certain other consequences of external causes
- External causes of morbidity or mortality
- Factors influencing health status or contact with health services
- Codes for special purposes
- Traditional medicine conditions—Module I
- V supplementary section of functioning assessment
- X extension codes

DISABILITY AND IT'S MEASURES

Impairment

- Impairment is any loss or abnormality of psychological, physiological or anatomical structure or function.
- It may be visible or invisible, temporary or permanent, progressive or regressive.
- An impairment may lead to secondary impairment, e.g. Leprosy leading to damaged nerves (*primary impairment*) in turn may lead to plantar ulcers (*secondary impairment*)

Disability

Disability is restriction or lack of ability to perform any activity in a manner or within a range considered normal for a human being for his age, sex, etc. due to impairment.

Handicap

- **Handicap** is a disadvantage to an individual, because of an impairment/disability that limits him to perform a role expected of him and considered normal (with respect to age, sex, social and cultural factors) for that individual.
- It has 7 major categories: Blindness, hearing disability, orthopedic handicap (Most common), multiple disabilities, mental retardation, speech disability and others.

> 33 *High Yield Points*
>
> **Anatomical impairment**
>
> **Dysfunction**—inability to do activity
> **Disability**—inability to do activity
> **Handicap**—social disadvantage for getting work or job

Disability Indicators

Health-Adjusted Life Expectancy

- It is the number of years a newborn is expected to live in full health, based on current morbidity and mortality.
- This term HALE was previously known as DALE.

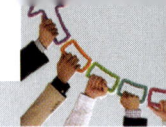

Disability-Adjusted Life Year

- It is the number of years lost in the healthy life of an individual due to disability
- One DALY is "one lost year of healthy life". It is a measure of the burden of disease in a defined population and the effectiveness of the interventions.

Sullivan's Index

- This is computed by subtracting the duration of bed disability (during life) from the expectation of life at birth
- This is a better indicator for disability due to disease
- For example, if the expectation of life is 62.6 years for an Indian and the disability days is 7.6 years, the Sullivan's index is 62.6–7.6 = 55 years.

Indian Disability and Assessment Scale

- A scale for measuring and quantifying disability in mental disorders
- The Persons with Disability Act 1995 includes mental illness as disability. The persons with mental illness are eligible to avail all the benefits under the persons with Disability Act 1995. The disabled people need disability certificate showing more than 40% disability from the competent authority to avail the benefits.

Diagnostic Categories

Patients with only following diagnosis as per ICD or DSM criteria are eligible for disability benefits:

- Schizophrenia
- Bipolar disorder
- Dementia
- Obsessive compulsive disorder

Duration of Illness

The total duration of illness should be at least 2 years.

Scores for Each Item

0 – No disability
1 – Mild disability
2 – Moderate disability
3 – Serve disability
4 – Profound disability
Total Score (range 0-20)

Score of

0	No disability = 0% disability
1-7	Mild disability = <40% disability
8-13	Moderate disability
14-19	Severe disability
20	Profound disability

19 Must Remember

The disability act covers seven disabilities:

- Blind
- Low vision
- Deaf and dumb
- Leprosy cured
- Mentally retarded
- Orthopedic handicap
- Mental illness

Right to Disability Act 2016

- Bill for the rights of persons with disabilities was passed by Indian Parliament on December 28, 2016
- The types of disabilities have been increased from existing 7 to 21 and the Central Government will have the power to add more types of disabilities. The 21 disabilities included are given below:
    1. Blindness
    2. Low-vision
    3. Leprosy cured persons
    4. Hearing impairment (deaf and hard of hearing)
    5. Locomotor disability
    6. Dwarfism

7. Intellectual disability
8. Mental illness
9. Autism spectrum disorder
10. Cerebral palsy
11. Muscular dystrophy
12. Chronic neurological conditions
13. Specific learning disabilities
14. Multiple sclerosis
15. Speech and language disability
16. Thalassemia
17. Hemophilia
18. Sickle cell disease
19. Multiple disabilities including deaf/blindness
20. Acid attack victim
21. Parkinson's disease

- Speech and language disability and specific learning disability have been added for the first time.
- Acid attack victims have been included
- Dwarfism, muscular dystrophy has been indicated as separate class of specified disability
- Three blood disorders have been included as new categories of disability these are thalassemia, hemophilia and sickle cell disease

Must Remember

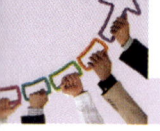

- Speech and language disability and specific learning disability have been added for the first time.
- Acid attack victims have been included.
- Dwarfism, muscular dystrophy have been indicated as separate class of specified disability.
- The New categories of disabilities also included three blood disorders *Thalassemia, Hemophilia and Sickle-cell disease.*

Disability-related Schemes Launched by GOI

1. **Sahyogi:** Revamped scheme for caregivers to persons with disability
2. **Samarth:** Early intervention for special education and vocational training
3. **Niramaya:** Health insurance scheme for any person below the poverty line with the four disabilities under the National Trust
4. **ADIP Scheme:** Scheme of assistance to disabled persons for purchase/fitting of aids/ appliances
5. Accessible India campaign under ministry of social justice and empowerment (Fig. 5)
6. Right to Disability Act 2016 (see text above)

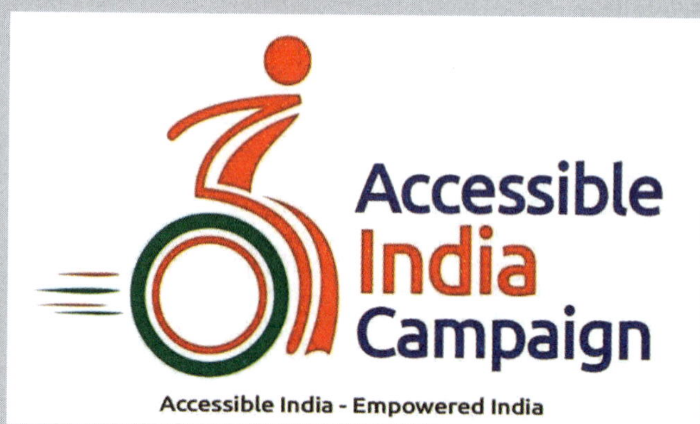

Fig. 5: Accessible India campaign

Image-Based Questions

1. Identify the scientist shown in the figure:

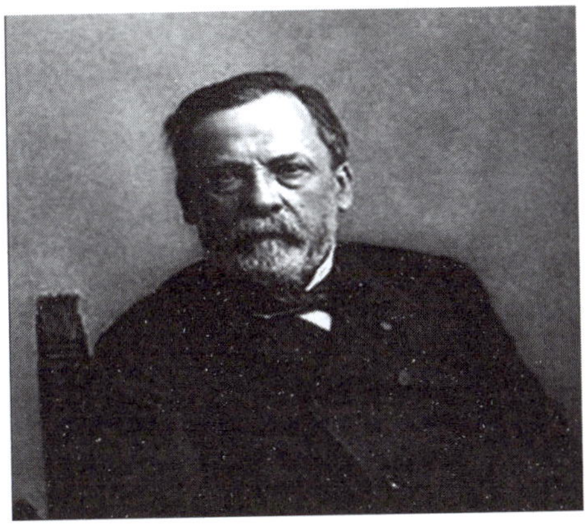

a. Edward Jenner
b. Ronald Ross
c. Robert Koch
d. Louis Pasteur

2. The scientist in figure is given the title:

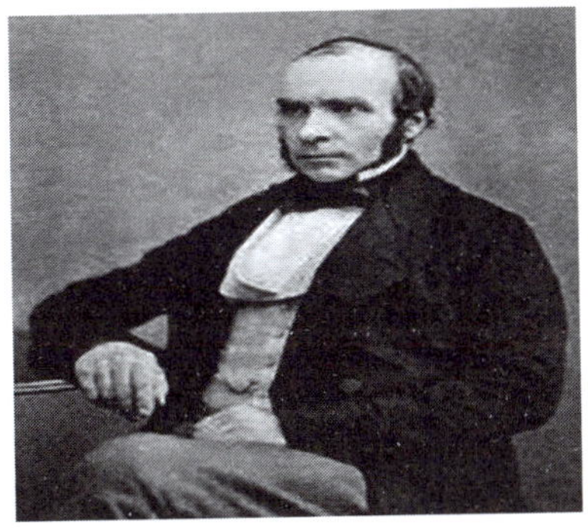

a. Father of Public Health
b. Father of Epidemiology
c. Father of Modern medicine
d. Father of Tropical Medicine

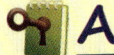

Answers of Image-Based Questions

1. **Ans. (d)** **Louis Pasteur**

2. **Ans. (b)** **Father of Epidemiology**

Multiple Choice Questions

1. **Which point in the below natural history of disease marks the onset of symptoms?** *(AIIMS May 2017)*

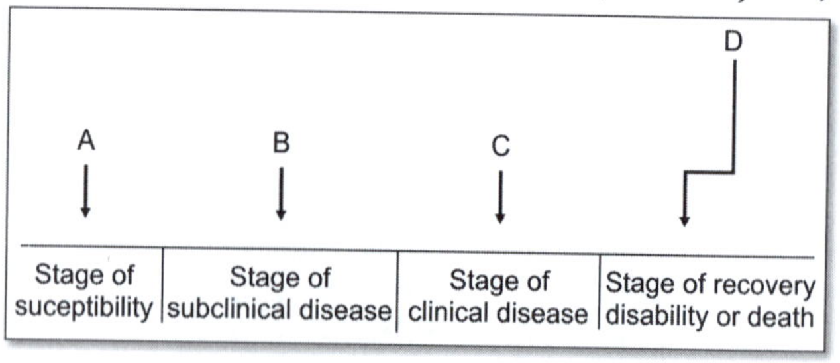

   a. A b. B
   c. C d. D
2. **True about Human development index (HDI):** *(PGI May 2017)*
   a. Adult literacy rate range from 0 to 100
   b. HDI score range is 0-10
   c. Life expectancy at birth range from 25 years to 85 years
   d. GDP per capita range from 25$ to 50000$
   e. HDI score range is 0-1
3. **True about PQLI:**
   a. Literacy rate, birth rate, life expectancy at birth
   b. Life expectancy at 1 year, IMR, literacy rate
   c. Life expectancy at birth, income, literacy rate
   d. Soon to be replaced by GNP
4. **Fetal cardiac monitoring is a type of:** *(Recent Question 2017)*
   a. Primary prevention
   b. Secondary prevention
   c. Tertiary prevention
   d. Primordial prevention
5. **True about Sentinel surveillance:** *(Recent Question 2017)*
   a. Includes notifiable cases
   b. Done through evaluation of sub center reports
   c. Done by anganwadi worker
   d. Increase reporting bias
6. **Who is regarded as Father of modern surgery:**
   a. Orfila
   b. Ambroise Pare
   c. Sushrutha
   d. Hippocrates
7. **The value of Human Developmental Index in India is:** *(Recent Question 2013, 2015)*
   a. 0.500 b. 0.62
   c. 0.505 d. 0.540
8. **Sullivian index:**
   a. Measures life expectancy adjusted without disability or free of disability
   b. Measures disability
   c. Measures life expectancy
   d. Measures life years adjusted with disability
9. **All of the following indicators are included in physical quality of life index (PQLI), except:** *(Recent Question 2016)*
   a. Literacy rate
   b. Infant mortality rate.
   c. Life expectancy at age one
   d. Per capita income
10. **Which of the following measures the deprivations in basic dimensions of human development?** *(Recent Question 2016)*
   a. Human development index
   b. Physical quality of life index
   c. Gender related development index
   d. Human poverty index
11. **The highest point in spectrum of health is:** *(Recent Question 2015)*
   a. Positive health
   b. Better health
   c. Death
   d. Freedom from sickness
12. **Disease control is aimed at all the following, except:**
   a. Reducing the financial burden to the community
   b. Reducing the incidence of disease
   c. Reducing the duration of disease
   d. Interruption of transmission of disease
13. **The prevention of emergence or development of risk factors in countries or population groups in which they have not yet appeared is called:** *(Recent Question 2015)*
   a. Tertiary prevention
   b. Primary prevention
   c. Secondary prevention
   d. Primordial prevention
14. **Which of the following is primordial prevention?**
   a. Screening b. Chemoprophylaxis
   c. Quitting smoking d. Vaccination
15. **Food fortification is an example of:** *(Recent Question 2014)*
   a. Health promotion
   b. Early diagnosis and treatment
   c. Disability limitation
   d. Specific protection
16. **Hand washing to prevent nosocomial infection is an example of:** *(Recent Question 2013)*
   a. Tertiary prevention
   b. Primary prevention
   c. Secondary prevention
   d. Primordial prevention
17. **In 1980, ICIDH (International Classification of Impairment, Disability and Handicap) was published by the WHO as a manual of classification relating to the consequences of disease. In an accident, a person lost his leg. According to ICIDH this is an example for:**
   a. Disability b. Impairment
   c. Handicap d. Disease

Ans.

1. c
2. a, e
3. b
4. b
5. a
6. b
7. b
8. a
9. d
10. d
11. a
12. d
13. d
14. c
15. d
16. b
17. b

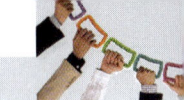

DISCOVERIES AND CONTRIBUTIONS

18. Pioneer in the concept of specific protection by immunization was: *(JIPMER 2015)*
a. Edward Jenner b. Robert Koch
c. Chinese d. James Lind

19. James lind is known for: *(Recent Question 2013, 2012)*
a. Germ theory of disease
b. Multifactorial causation of disease
c. Prevention of scurvy by citrus fruits
d. Web of causation

BOOKS AND TITLES

20. First true epidemiologist:
a. Aristotle b. Hippocrates
c. John Snow d. James Lind

21. Who is regarded as Father of modern surgery? *(Recent Question 2015)*
a. Sushrutha
b. Ambroise Pare
c. Hippocrates
d. Orfila

22. Father of Evidence Based Medicine is: *(AIIMS May 2014)*
a. Sackett b. Da Vinci
c. Hippocrates d. Tolstoy

23. Father of Indian medicine: *(Recent Question 2015)*
a. Charaka b. Sushrutha
c. Samuel Hahnemann d. Pampana

PRIMITIVE MEDICINE

24. Which system of medicine is said to be the world's first organized body of medical knowledge?
a. Indian b. Chinese
c. Egyptian d. Roman

25. World's first organized body of medical knowledge was:
a. Greek b Mesopotanian
c. Chinese d. Egyptian

26. Principle of Chinese medicine is: *(New Question 2013)*
a. Yang b. YIn
c. Both d. None

REVIVAL OF MEDICINE

27. Theory of web causation was given by: *(Recent Question 2013)*
a. Mc Mohan and Pugh
b. Pettenkofer
c. John Snow
d. Louis Pasteur

HUMAN DEVELOPMENT INDEX

28. Human Development Index includes which of the following: *(AIIMS May 2015)*
a. Infant mortality rate
b. Life expectancy at birth
c. Life expectancy at 1 yeard. Adult literacy rate

29. Human development index includes?
a. Knowledge b. Infant mortality
c. Disability rate d. Urbanization rate

30. Human Development Index *(HDI)* does not include:
a. Mean Years of schooling b. Life expectancy at age 1
c. Real GDP per capita d. Adult literacy rate

31. In construction of Education Index in HDI which is true: *(AIIMS May 2014)*
a. 2/3 adult literacy considered
b. 1/3 gross enrolment considered
c. Gross enrolment of secondary education is considered and not primary education
d. Minimum and maximum values are used based on global data

32. Which of the following is not a component of human development index? *(JIPMER 2015)*
a. Life expectancy at 1 year
b. Knowledge
c. Per capita income
d. Life expectancy at birth

33. According to classification by Human development index, India belongs to:
a. High HDI
b. Medium HDI
c. Low HDI
d. Very Low HDI

34. Human development index measures:
a. Deprivation in basic dimensions of human development
b. Achievement in basic dimensions of human development
c. Quality of life
d. Level of living

35. Age limit for HDI in India is: *(Recent Question 2013)*
a. 25 to 85 yrs b. 25 to 50 yrs
c. 15 to 45 yrs d. 50 to 75 yrs

36. Refering to HDI, India ranks at:
a. 43 b. 62
c. 133 d. 545

37. About HDI, all are true, except:
a. Life expectancy at birth
b. GDP
c. Life expectancy at 1 year
d. Education

38. HDI includes: *(PGI Nov 2010)*
a. Infant mortality rate
b. Life expectancy at birth
c. Life expectancy at 1 year
d. Longetivity
e. GDP

HUMAN POVERTY INDEX

39. The following is not true about components of HPI-I
a. Probability at birth of not surviving to age 60
b. Adult literacy rate
c. % of population not using an improved water source
d. % of children underweight for age

40. Not included in the human poverty index is: *(AIIMS May 2013)*
a. % of population not surviving up to 40 yrs of age
b. Undernutrition for age
c. Occupation
d. % population not using safe water source

41. Poverty index does not include:
a. Long life
b. Knowledge
c. Standard of living
d. Income

Ans.

18.	a
19.	c
20.	b
21.	b
22.	a
23.	a
24.	b
25.	c
26.	c
27.	a
28.	b
29.	a
30.	b
31.	d
32.	a
33.	b
34.	b
35.	a
36.	c
37.	c
38.	b, d
39.	a
40.	c
41.	d

PHYSICAL QUALITY LIFE INDEX (PQLI)

42. True regarding PQLI are all, except: ***(Recent Question 2015)***
a. 0 – 100
b. Kerala state has low per capita income but high PQLI
c. It measures economic growth
d. Includes infant mortality, life expectancy at age one and literacy

43. Physical quality of life index in a composite based on the following, except: ***(Recent Question 2013)***
a. Infant mortality rate
b. Literacy rate
c. Maternal mortality ratio
d. Life expectancy at age one

44. PQLI is: ***(Recent Question 2013)***
a. Disability indicator
b. Quality of life indicator
c. Standard of living indicator
d. Level of living indicator

45. True about PQLI:
a. Literacy rate, birth rate, life expectancy at birth
b. Life expectancy at 1 year, IMR, literacy rate
c. Life expectancy at birth, income, literacy rate
d. Soon to be replaced by GNP

46. All of the following indicators are included in physical quality of life index (PQLI), except:
a. Infant mortality rate
b. Life expectancy at age one
c. Literacy rate
d. Per capita income

47. The value of PQLI value lies between: ***(Recent Question 2014, 15)***
a. 0 and 1 b. 0 and 10
c. 0 and 100 d. 1 and 10

48. Human living standards can be compared in different countries by: ***(Recent Question 2013)***
a. HDI b. PQLI
c. HPI d. DALY

NATURAL HISTORY OF DISEASE/THEORIES OF DISEASE CAUSATION

49. Natural history of disease is best studied by:
a. Cross sectional study b. RCT
c. Case-control study d. Cohort study

50. Basis of Biomedical concept of health is:
a. Absence of pain
b. Social and psychological factors
c. Equilibrium between man and environment
d. Germ theory of disease

51. Epidemiological triad constitutes:
a. Agent, Host and Environmental factors
b. Endemic, Epidemic and Outbreak
c. Time place and person distribution
d. Incidence, Prevelence and disease load

52. The highest point in spectrum of health is: ***(New Question 2015)***
a. Positive health
b. Better health
c. Freedom from sickness
d. Death

53. In today's world all are true about Positive health, except:
a. It is dependent on social, economic and cultural factors
b. It means peace of body and mind
c. It is like a mirage because of changing environment
d. It is change in behavior with respect to change in future

54. A subjective state of a person who feels aware of not being well is ***(Recent Question 2015)***
a. Disease b. Illness
c. Sickness d. Negative health

55. Epidemiological triad comprise of all, expect: ***(Recent Question 2014)***
a. Host b. Environmental factor
c. Agent d. Investigator

56. Optimum unit of preventive, curative and promotive health care is:
a. Appropriateness b. Availability
c. Adequacy d. Comprehensiveness

57. In the concept of Advanced Epidemiological triad , agent is replaced by:
a. Causative factors b. Determinant
c. Bacteria and Virus d. Risk factor

58. "Web of causation of disease", which statement is most appropriate?
a. Mostly applicable for common disease
b. Requires complete understanding of all factors associated with causation of disease
c. Epidermiological ratio
d. Helps to suggest ways to interrupt the risk of transmission

59. BEINGS model of disease causation does not include: ***(Recent Question 2013)***
a. Spiritual factors b. Social factors
c. Religious factors d. Social factors

60. Transition from increased prevalence of infectious pandemic disease to manmade disease is known as: ***(AIIMS Nov 2012)***
a. Paradoxical transition
b. Reversal of transition
c. Epidemiological transition
d. Demographic transition

DISEASE ERADICATION/CONTROL/ ELIMINATION

61. Disease control is aimed at all the following, except: ***(Recent Question 2015)***
a. Reducing the incidence of disease
b. Reducing the duration of disease
c. Reducing the financial burden to the community
d. Interruption of transmission of disease

62. Consider the following statements: ***(AIIMS Nov 2014)***
The term disease control describes ongoing operations aimed at reducing the
1. Incidence of disease
2. Financial burden to the community
3. Effects of infection including both physical and psychological complications
4. Duration of diseases and its transmission

About the above statement true is:
a. 1, 2 and 3 are correct
b. 1, 3 and 4 are correct
c. 1, 2 and 4 are correct
d. 1, 2, 3 and 4 are correct

Ans.

42. c
43. c
44. b
45. b
46. d
47. c
48. a
49. d
50. a
51. a
52. a
53. d
54. b
55. d
56. d
57. a
58. d
59. c
60. c
61. d
62. d

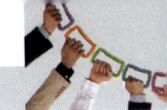

63. **Disease control implies all, except:**
   a. Effects of infection including its complications
   b. Financial Burden to the community
   c. Duration of disease and risk of transmission
   d. Virulence

64. **Disease elimination is helped by:**
   a. Herd immunity b. Isolation
   c. Quarantine d. None

65. **Zero incidence is:** *(Recent Question 2013)*
   a. Elimination of disease b. Eradication of disease
   c. Elimination of infection
   d. Eradication of infection

66. **All of the following are eradicable disease, except:**
   a. Tuberculosis b. Guineaworm
   c. Poliomyelitis d. Measles

67. **The disease which are likely to be eradicated in within foreseeable future are all, except:** *(Recent Question 2015)*
   a. Polio b. Measles
   c. Yellow fever d. Dracunculiasis

MONITORING AND SURVEILLANCE

68. **Analysis of routine measurement aimed at detecting changes in environment is:** *(Recent Question 2013)*
   a. Monitoring b. Surveillance
   c. Isolation d. Evaluation

69. **A method of identifying the missing cases and thereby supplementing the notified cases is called:** *(Recent Question 2015)*
   a. Monitoring
   b. Sentinel surveillance
   c. Sample registration system
   d. Census

70. **Actual target of surveillance is:** *(Recent Question 2015)*
   a. Disease prevention b. Health planning
   c. Disease monitoring d. Disease eradication

71. **Sentinel surveillance is for:** *(Recent Question 2013)*
   a. Border districts
   b. For malaria surveillance
   c. Effective sanitary surveillance
   d. Supplementary to routine surveillance

72. **Morbidity in a community is best estimated by:**
   a. Sentinel surveillance
   b. Passive surveillance
   c. Active surveillance
   d. Monitoring

73. **Missing cases are detected by:**
   a. Active surveillance b. Passive surveillance
   c. Sentinel surveillance d. Monitoring

ICEBERG PHENOMENON

74. **Iceberg phenomenon is not shown by:** *(Recent Question 2015)*
   a. Rabies b. Tuberculosis
   c. Hypertension d. Ancylostomiasis

75. **Iceberg phenomonon is shown by:**
   a. Rabies b. Measles
   c. Tetanus d. Influenza

76. **Iceberg phenomenon is not shown by the following disease:** *(Recent Question 2015)*
   a. Polio b. Diphtheria
   c. Typhoid d. Measles

77. **The floating tip of the iceberg represents cases:**
   a. Clinical b. Latent
   c. Presymptomatic d. Inapparent

INDICATORS OF HEALTH

78. **The condition of life resulting from the combination of the effects of the complete range of factors such as those determining health, happiness, education, social and intellectual attainments, freedom of action, justice and freedom of expression is defined as:** *(Recent Question 2015)*
   a. Quality of life b. Standard of living
   c. Level of living d. Positive health

79. **Burden of disease is given by:** *(Recent Question 2013)*
   a. Incidence b. Crude death rate
   c. Cause specific death rate d. Proportional mortality rate

80. **Indicator for health status of community is:**
   a. IMR b. MMR
   c. Bed occupancy ratio d. DALY

81. **Which of the following is not a utilisation rate:**
   a. Population bed ratio b. Bed occupancy rate
   c. Bed turnover ratio d. Average length of stay

82. **Not a utilisation rate:**
   a. Population per PHC b. Bed occupancy rate
   c. % of infants fully immunized
   d. Proportion of people using various methods of family planning

DISABILITY RATES

83. **The following indicator is not an event type indicator of disability:**
   a. Number of days of restricted activity
   b. Bed disability days
   c. Limitation to perform the basic activities of daily living
   d. School loss days

84. **A measure of overall disease burden, expressed as a number of years lost due to ill-health, disability or early death:**
   a. Health adjusted life expectancy
   b. Quality adjusted life years
   c. Disability free life expectancy
   d. Disability adjusted life years

85. **One DALY is:**
   a. One lost year of healthy life
   b. One year spent in poor health
   c. One year of life lived in perfect health
   d. One year lost to disability

86. **The 'overall burden of diseases' is best detected by:**
   a. Sullivan's index
   b. Quality adjusted life years (QALY)
   c. Human developmental index
   d. Disability adjusted life years (DALY)

87. **DALE has been replaced by:** *(Recent Question 2013)*
   a. DALY b. QALY
   c. HALE d. DFLE

Ans.

63. d
64. a
65. b
66. a
67. c
68. a
69. b
70. b
71. d
72. c
73. c
74. a
75. d
76. d
77. a
78. a
79. a
80. a
81. a
82. a
83. c
84. d
85. a
86. d
87. c

88. Which of the following is true about DALYs?
a. Life is adjusted for disease
b. Premature death is adjusted for disability
c. Life expectancy free of disability
d. Years lost to premature death and years lived with disability adjusted for severity of disability

89. One DAILY signifies: *(Recent Question 2013)*
a. 1 year of disease free life
b. 1 lost year of healthy life
c. 1 month of bed ridden life
d. None of theses

90. Sullivan index is:
a. Measures disability
b. Measures life years adjusted with disability
c. Measures life expectancy adjusted without disability or free of disability
d. Measures life of expectancy

PRIMORDIAL PREVENTION

91. The prevention of emergence or development of risk factors in countries or population groups in which they have not yet appeared is called: *(Recent Question 2015)*
a. Primordial prevention b. Primary prevention
c. Secondary prevention d. Tertiary prevention

92. The key action areas identified in the Ottawa Charter of health promotion are all of the following, except:
a. Build a healthy public policy
b. Create a social security system
c. Reorientation of health services
d. Strengthening community action for health

93. Examples of primordial prevention are?
1. Health Education
2. Treatment of hypertension
3. Screening for cervical cancer
4. Changing lifestyles to prevent stress

Choose the correct combination
a. 2 and 4 b. 2 and 3
c. 1 and 3 d. 1 and 4

94. Which level of prevention is applicable in a population without any risk factor? *(Recent Question 2014)*
a. Primordial prevention
b. Primary prevention
c. Secondary prevention
d. Tertiary prevention

95. Childhood obesity prevention is a type of: *(JIPMER 2014)*
a. Primordial prevention
b. Primary prevention
c. Secondary prevention
d. Tertiary prevention

96. CAD primordial prevention is by:
a. Life style changes b. Coronary bypass
c. Treatment of CAD d. None

97. Which of the following is health promotion, i.e. First level of prevention? *(Recent Question 2013)*
a. PAP smear
b. Use of helmet
c. Root canal treatment
d. Encouraging physical activity

98. Food fortification is an example of:
a. Health promotion
b. Prevention of food adulteration
c. Early diagnosis and treatment
d. Disability limitation

99. Special protection includes: *(PGI Pattern Question)*
a. Personality development
b. Immunization against specific disease
c. Specific nutritional diet
d. Protection from occupational hazard
e. Environmental modification

100. Primary prevention includes all of the following, except? *(PGI Nov 2010)*
a. Helmets b. Contraception
c. Pap smear d. Vaccines

101. An example of primary prevention is?
a. Measles vaccination
b. Smoking cessation after a heart attack
c. Self-breast examination for lumps
d. Cervical cytology screening

102. Use of seat-belt while driving car is an example of:
a. Health promotion
b. Specific protection
c. Early diagnosis and treatment
d. Disability limitation

103. Hand washing to prevent nosocomial infection is an example of: *(Recent Question 2013)*
a. Primordial prevention b. Primary prevention
c. Secondary prevention d. Tertiary prevention

104. Improving the standard of living is an example of
a. Primordial prevention
b. Primary prevention
c. Secondary prevention
d. Tertiary prevention

105. Not a method of primary prevention:
a. Salt reduction b. Weight reduction
c. Exercise promotion d. Early diagnosis

106. Desks provided with table top to prevent neck problem is an example of: *(Recent Question 2013)*
a. Primordial prevention b. Primary prevention
c. Secondary prevention d. Disability limitation

107. Immunization is: *(Recent Question 2013)*
a. Primary prevention b. Econdary prevention
c. Tertiary prevention d. Disability limitation

108. Primary prevention includes: *(PGI Pattern Question)*
a. Marriage counseling
b. Health education
c. Pap smear
d. Self-breast examination
e. Health promotion

SECONDARY PREVENTION

109. An action which halts the progress of a disease at its incipient stage and prevents complications is called: *(Recent Question 2015)*
a. Primordial prevention b. Primary prevention
c. Secondary prevention d. Tertiary prevention

Ans.
88. d
89. b
90. c
91. a
92. b
93. d
94. a
95. a
96. a
97. d
98. a
99. b, c, d
100. c
101. a
102. b
103. b
104. b
105. d
106. b
107. a
108. a, b, e
109. c

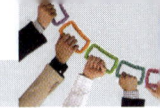

110. **True regarding secondary prevention:**
a. Reduction of risk factors
b. Reduction of incidence
c. Reduction of prevalence
d. Reduction of complication

111. **Secondary prevention of carcinoma cervix includes?**
a. PAP smear b. Circumcision
c. Family planning d. Personal hygiene

112. **Fetal cardiac monitoring is a type of:**
a. Primary prevention b. Secondary prevention
c. Tertiary prevention d. Primordial prevention

113. **Monitoring of blood pressure which type of prevention, except:** *(New Question 2014)*
a. Primordial b. Primary
c. Secondary d. Tertiary

114. **Patient is on psychotherapy, what is the level of prevention:** *(Recent Question 2014)*
a. Primordial b. Primary
c. Secondary d. Tertiary

115. **Screening of the disease is which type of prevention:** *(Recent Question 2013)*
a. Primordial prevention
b. Primary prevention
c. Secondary prevention
d. Tertiary prevention

116. **School health checkup comes under ....Level of prevention:** *(Recent Question 2013)*
a. Primordial prevention
b. Primary prevention
c. Secondary prevention
d. Tertiary prevention

117. **Target group in secondary prevention:** *(Recent Question 2013)*
a. Healthy individuals b. Patients
c. Animals d. Children

TERTIARY PREVENTION

118. **Any restriction or lack of ability to perform an activity within the range that is considered normal for a human being is called:** *(Recent Question 2015)*
a. Disease b. Impairment
c. Disability d. Handicap

119. **In 1980, ICIDH (International Classification of Impairment, Disability and Handicap) was published by the WHO as a manual of classification relating to the consequences of disease. In an accident, a person lost his leg. According to ICIDH this is an example for:** *(Recent Question 2015)*
a. Disease b. Impairment
c. Disability d. Handicap

120. **Abnormality in impairment is** *(Recent Question 2015)*
a. Physiological b. Psychological
c. Anatomical d. Any of the above

121. **Components of IDEAS are all except All India**
a. Self-care b. Rehabilitation
c. Communication d. Work

122. **Which of the following is the most logical sequence:** *(Recent Question 2013)*
a. Impairment – Disease – Disability – Handicap
b. Disease –Impairment – Disability – Handicap
c. Disease –Impairment – Handicap – Disability
d. Disease– Handicap –Impairment – Disability

123. **Disability limitation is which mode of intervention for:** *(AIIMS May 2008)(New Question 2013)*
a. Primordial prevention b. Primary prevention
c. Secondary prevention d. Tertiary prevention

124. **Any loss or abnormality of psychological, physiological or anatomical structure or function is:** *(AIIMS Nov 2006)*
a. Impairment b. Disability
c. Handicap d. Disease

MISCELLANEOUS

125. **For optimum utilization of health services in a hospital, Red turnover interval should always be:**
a. Slightly positive b. Largely negative
c. Slightly negative d. Largely negative

INFECTIOUS DISEASE EPIDEMIOLOGY

126. **The performance and analysis of routine measurements aimed at detecting changes in the environment or in the health status of the population is called:**
a. Evaluation
b. Surveillance
c. Situational analysis
d. Monitoring

127. **Continuous scrutiny of the factors that determine the occurrence and distribution of disease and others conditions of ill-health is known as surveillance. The National Health Program of India collects data for morbidity and mortality mainly by which type of surveillance?**
a. Active surveillance
b. Passive surveillance
c. Sentinel surveillance
d. None of these

MODERN MEDICINE AND MEDICAL REVOLUTION

128. **Which events occurred before 1900 AD:** *(PGI Nov 2010)*
a. Establishment of seat of social medicine at Oxford
b. Epidemiological work on cholera by John Snow
c. Work on scurvy by James Lind
d. Use of BCG vaccine
e. Chadwick work on cholera in London

129. **Evidence-based medicine refers to:**
a. Clinical trials to prove adverse effects of drugs
b. Clinical trials to prove safety of drugs
c. Use of various research finding for taking decisions about best patients care
d. All of the above

Ans.

110. c
111. a
112. b
113. c
114. c
115. c
116. c
117. b
118. c
119. b
120. d
121. b
122. b
123. d
124. a
125. a
126. d
127. b
128. b, c, e
129. c

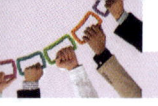

Answers with Explanations

1. Ans. (c) C

Ref: Park 24th edition, p. 40

2. Ans. (a, e) Adult literacy rate range from 0 to 100; (e) HDI score range is 0-1

3. Ans. (b) Life expectancy at 1 year, IMR, literacy rate

Ref: K. Park, 24th ed. p 17

4. Ans. (b) Secondary prevention

Ref: K. Park, 24th ed. p 46

5. Ans. (a) Includes notifiable cases

Ref: K. Park, 24th ed. p 45

6. Ans. (b) Ambroise Pare

Ref: K. Park, 24th ed. p 5; 23rd ed p 5, Refer to Annexure 1.2-for important Titles and Honours

7. Ans. (b) 0.62

Ref: K. Park, 24th ed. p 18; 23rd ed. p 18; UNDP, HDI values 2013 http://hdr.undp.org

8. Ans. (a) Measures life expectancy adjusted without disability or free of disability

Ref: K. Park, 21st ed. p 25

9. Ans. (d) Per capita income

Ref: K. Park, 24th ed. p 17

10. Ans. (d) Human poverty index

Ref: K. Park, 24th ed. p 17

11. Ans. (a) Positive health

Ref: K. Park, 24th ed. p 16,18

12. Ans. (d) Interruption of transmission of disease

Ref: K. Park, 24th ed. p 44

13. Ans. (d) Primordial prevention

Ref: K. Park, 24th ed. p 45

14. Ans. (c) Quitting smoking

Ref: K. Park, 24th ed. p 45

15. Ans. (d) Specific protection

Ref: K. Park, 24th ed. p 47

16. Ans. (b) Primary prevention

Ref: K. Park, 24th ed. p 45

17. Ans. (b) Impairment

Ref: K. Park, 24th ed. p 48

DISCOVERIES AND CONTRIBUTIONS

18. Ans. (a) Edward Jenner

Ref: K. Park, 24th ed. p 6

19. Ans. (c) Prevention of scurvy by citrus fruits

Ref: K. Park, 24th ed. p 6

James Lind was a naval surgeon who advocated intake of fresh fruit and vegetables for prevention of scurvy

BOOKS AND TITLES

20. Ans. (b) Hippocrates

Ref: K. Park, 24th ed. p 3

21. Ans. (b) Ambroise Pare

Ref: K. Park, 24 th p 5 Refer to Annexure 2 Titles in Public Health

22. Ans. (a) Sackett

Ref: Richard Smith, Evidence Based Medicine- an oral history, BMJ 2014; 348

Evidence-Based Medicine is conscientious, explicit and judicious use of currently available best scientific evidence in decision making for providing clinical care to individual patients.
"**Evidence-Based Medicine**" term was coined by Gordon Guyatt.
"**Father of Evidence-Based Medicine**" is David Sackett.

23. Ans. (a) Charaka

Ref: K. Park, 24th p 2, Textbook of Community Medicine, B Rao Thirunavalli, 3rd ed. p 2

Indian sages associated with Ayurveda are

- Atreya (800 BC—Taught Medicine)
- Sushrutha (500 BC—Father of Indian Surgery)
- Charaka (200 BC—Father of Indian Medicine)

PRIMITIVE MEDICINE

24. Ans. (b) Chinese

Ref: K. Park, 24th ed. p 2

25. Ans. (c) Chinese

Ref: K. Park, 24th ed. p 2

26. Ans. (c) Both

Ref: K. Park, 24th ed. p 2

REVIVAL OF MEDICINE

27. Ans. (a) Mc Mohan and Pugh

Ref: K. Park, 24th p-39

Theories of Disease Causation

- Tridosha theory—Ayurveda
- Theory of four humors—Greek medicine
- Theory of contagion—Fracastoro (Italian physician).
- Theory of Spontaneous Generation—Aristotle
- Miasma theory [disease attributed to noxious air and vapors]—William Furr.
- Germ theory of disease—Louis Pasteur
- Multifactorial causation of disease– Pattenkofer

HUMAN DEVELOPMENT INDEX

28. Ans. (b) Life expectancy at birth

Ref: K. Park, 24th ed. p 17-18

Also Know........................

HDI [Human Development Index] is an index *of quality of life*[Q]. It combines 3 dimensions

- *Longevity (life expectancy at birth)*[Q]
- *Knowledge (Mean years of schooling and Expected years of schooling)*[Q]
- *Income (Per capita GNI in purchasing power parity US dollar)*[Q]

29. Ans. (a) Knowledge

Ref: K. Park, 24th ed. p 24

30. Ans. (b) Life expectancy at age 1

Ref: K. Park, 24th ed p-17

31. Ans. (d) Minimum and maximum values are ...

Ref: K. Park, 24th ed. p 17

Each component of HDI has maximum and minimum values,

$$\text{Dimension Index} = \frac{\textit{Actual value} - \textit{Minimum value}}{\textit{Maximum value} - \textit{Minimum value}}$$

Also Know........................

Education Index-

- Dimension index is calculated for mean year of schooling (Average number of years of education received by people ≥25 year age) and expected year of schooling (i.e. Years of schooling a child can expect to receive as per current age specific enrolment rates).
- A geometric mean of resultant indices is calculated.
- Formula for dimension index is reapplied to geometric mean so calculated using minimum value 0 and maximum valve 0.978. [Combined Education Index].

32. Ans. (a) Life expectancy at 1 year

Ref: K. Park, 24th ed. p 17-18

33. Ans. (b) Medium HDI

Ref: K. Park, 24th ed. p 18

***As per 2015 ratings**-India falls in the medium HDI category, with an HDI of 0.609 [Rank 130]*[Q]

34. Ans. (b) Achievement in basic dimensions of human development

Ref: K. Park, 24th ed. p 17-18

HDI is indicator of achievements in basic human capabilities of a country (i.e. Long life, Education and Decent standard of living)

Human Poverty Index (HPI) (1978), measures average deprivation in basic dimensions of human development

35. Ans. (a) 25 to 85 yrs

Ref: K. Park, 24th ed. p 17-18

36. Ans. (c) 133

Ref: K. Park, 23rd ed. p 17-18. UNDP, HDI values 2013 http://24th ed p-18 hdr.undp.org/

Also Know........................

HDI is indicator of achievements in basic human capabilities of a country (i.e. Long life, Education and Decent standard of living).

***2015**–India falls in the medium HDI category, with an HDI of 0.609 [Rank 130]*[Q]

- HDI → ≥ 0.9 = Very High, 0.8-0.899 = High (Developed countries), 0.5-0.799 = Medium (Developing country) and < 0.5 = Low (underdeveloped country).

37. Ans. (c) Life expectancy at 1 year

Ref: K. Park, 24th ed. p 17-18

38. Ans. (b, d) (b) Life expectancy at birth (d) Longetivity

Ref: K. Park, 24th ed. p 17-18

HUMAN POVERTY INDEX

39. Ans. (a) Probability at birth of not surviving...

Ref: K. Park, 21rd ed. p-16

HPI 1 is used for developing countries [India = 28%]. It measures

- P_1 is vulnerability to death at a relatively early age *[Probability at birth of not surviving to the age of 40 year]*.
- P_2 is exclusion from reading & communication *[Adult literacy rate]*
- P_3 is lack of access to decent standard of living/economic provisioning. [It is unweighted *average of 2 indicators*].

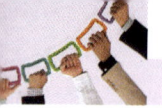

- Percentage of population not using an improved water source
- Percentage of children underweight for age.

HPI 1 = $[1/3 (P_1^{alpha} + P_2^{alpha} + P_3^{alpha}.]^{1/alpha}$, where Alpha = 3.

HPI 2 – Used for developed countries

40. Ans. (c) Occupation

Ref: K. Park, 21st ed. p 16

41. Ans. (d) Income

Ref: K. Park, 21st ed. p 16

PQLI [PHYSICAL QUALITY LIFE INDEX]

42. Ans. (c) It measures economic growth

Ref: K. Park, 24th ed. p 17

	PQLI	HDI
Dimensions	▪ *Infant mortality* ▪ *Life expectancy at age 1 year* ▪ *Literacy.*[Q]	▪ Life expectancy at birth ▪ Mean years of schooling and Expected years of schooling ▪ GNI per capita in purchasing power parity in US$
Range	**0–100.** Ultimate objective is to attain a PQLI of 100	0–1
Calculation	Arithmetic mean of the 3 dimensions	Geometric mean of three dimension indices
Current value	65	0.609

PQLI does not measure economic growth (GNI is not considered). It measures results of social, economic & political policies.

- It intends to complement, not replace GNP
- Applicable for international and national comparison.

43. Ans. (c) Maternal Mortality Ratio

Ref: K. Park, 24th ed. p 17

Maternal Mortality Ratio is Health status indicator not a component of PQLI.

Health Status Indicators

- Infant mortality rate,
- Child mortality rate (1–4 years),
- Life expectancy at birth,
- Maternal mortality ratio,
- Disease specific mortality & morbidity (incidence/prevalence/disability),
- % low birth weight,
- Nutritional status.

44. Ans. (b) Quality of life indicator

Ref: K. Park, 24th ed. p 17-18

Quality of life –

- *It is the "subjective" component of wellbeing.*
- *It has been defined by WHO as: "the condition of life resulting from the combination of the effects of the complete range of factors such as those determining health, happiness (including comfort in the physical environment and a satisfying occupation), education, social and intellectual attainments, freedom of action, justice and freedom of expression".*

Also Know......................

- Concept of "level of living" is a objective evaluation of wellbeing

Quality of Life Indicators

- *PQLI*
- *HDI*

45. Ans. (b) Life expectancy at 1 year, IMR, literacy rate

Ref: Life expectancy at 1 year, IMR, literacy rate Park 23rd ed. p 17; 24th ed. p 17

46. Ans. (d) Per capita income

Ref: K. Park, 24th ed. p 17

47. Ans. (c) 0 and 100

Ref: K. Park, 24th ed. p 17

48. Ans. (a) HDI

Ref: K. Park, 24th ed. p 17

NATURAL HISTORY OF DISEASE/THEORIES OF DISEASE CAUSATION

49. Ans. (d) Cohort study

Ref: K. Park, 24th ed. p 39

Natural History of Disease[Q] is the progression of a disease over time from the prepathogenesis phase (earliest phase) to its termination as recovery, disability or death *in absence of any treatment or prevention.*

- *Natural history of diseases can be best studied using a cohort study*[Q].

50. Ans. (a) Absence of pain

According to the biomedical model, health constitutes the freedom from disease, pain, or defect, making the normal human condition "healthy." It focuses on purely biological factors and excludes psychological, environmental, and social influences.

51. Ans. (a) Agent, Host and Environment factors

Ref: K. Park, 24th ed. p 37

Epidemiological triad

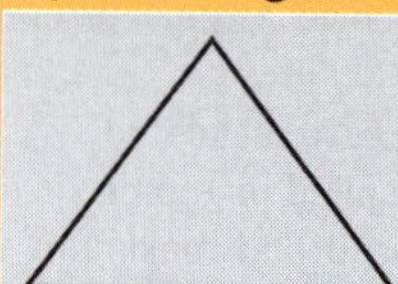

Disease results from disturbance in the fine equilibrium between Agent, Host and Environmental factors.

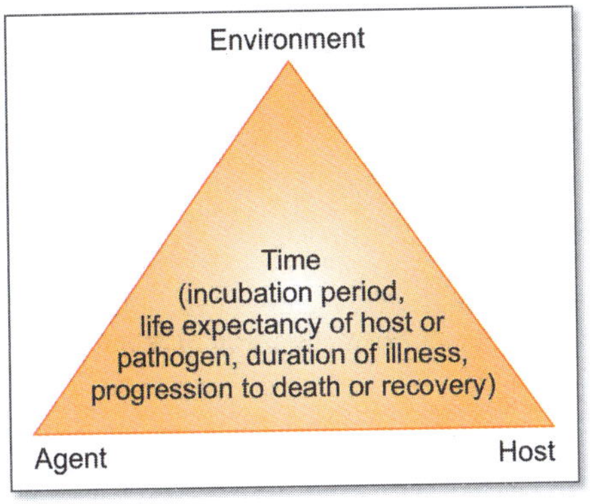

Triangle of Epidemiology

- It is based on the communicable disease model.
- It shows the interaction between agent, host, environment and time.
- Time here is concerned with the incubation period, life expectancy of host or pathogen, duration of the illness, progression to death or recovery useful in investigation of disease and epidemics

52. Ans. (a) Positive health

Ref: K. Park, 24th ed. p 16,18

Positive Health

- Positive health means "perfect functioning" of the body and mind.
- It is highest point of health-disease spectrum.

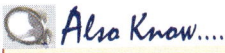

Also Know........................

- The lowest point in health-disease spectrum is Death.

Spectrum of health

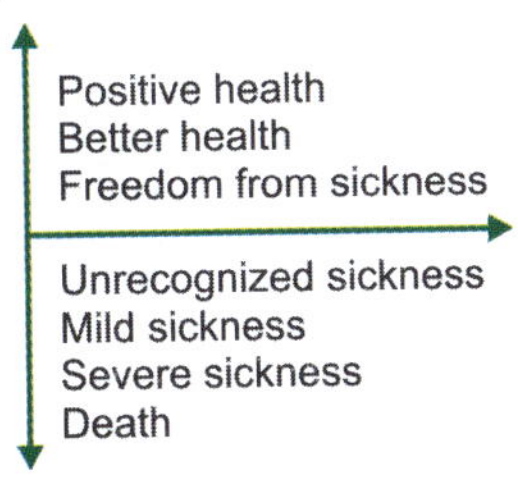

53. Ans. (d) It is change in behavior with respect...

Ref: K. Park, 24th ed p-16

Positive Health

- It depends on medical, economic, cultural and social factors in the community
- It is the ability to change continually, in the face of changing conditions of life

54. Ans. (b) Illness

Ref: K. Park, 24th ed. p 37

Illness is a subjective state of the person who feels aware of not being well.

Sickness is a state of social dysfunction i.e. A role that an individual assumes when ill.

55. Ans. (d) Investigator

Ref: K. Park, 24th ed. p 37

56. Ans (d) Comprehensiveness

Ref: Textbook of PSM, Mahajan and Gupta, 4th ed p- 635

Comprehensive Health Care – includes promotive, protective, curative and rehabilitative health care.

57. Ans. (a) Causative factors

Ref: K. Park 24th ed p- 38

Advanced Epidemiological Triad

Agent: Replaced by causative factor [Multiple cause of a disease, disability, injury and death]
Host: Replaced by Groups or population
Environment: Replaced by Environment behavior, culture, physiological factors, ecological factors

It seeks to identify multiple factors of disease and to prioritize them for modification or amelioration to prevent or control disease

58. Ans. (d) Helps to suggest ways to interrupt...

Ref: K. Park, 24th ed. p 39

Theory of "Web of Causation" was proposed by *McMahon and Pugh.*

- It was formulated to explain causation of *non-communicable diseases.*
- Multiple factors interact with each other similar to web of a spider and modify the effect of each other.
- Each factor has its own relative importance.

To prevent a disease, we need to identify and act on the "*weakest links*" in the inter-lacing webs.

59. Ans. (c) Religious factors

Ref: Textbook of Community Medicine, Rajvir Bhalawar, p-19

"BEINGS" model of disease causation is a new concept according to which human disease and their consequences are a result of complex interplay of nine different factors –

- **B** → *Biological factors and Behavioral factors [lifestyles]*
- **E** → *Environmental factors* [Physical, Chemical and Biological]
- **I** → *Immunological factors*
- **N** → *Nutritional factors*
- **G** → *Genetic factors*
- **S** → *Social factors, Spiritual factors and Services factors* [Related to health care services].

Also Know........................

Epidemiological Wheel Theory

- Human disease is compared to a *wheel*, with a *central hub representing genetic factors* and peripheral portion representing the environmental factors.
- Peripheral portion has spokes that divide it into sub components (social, biological and physical).
- Relative sizes of each components is in proportion to its contribution to the disease and vary in every disease.

60. Ans. (c) Epidermiological transition

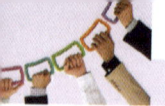

Ref: Robert E. McKeown, The Epidemiologic Transition: Changing Patterns of Mortality and Population Dynamics. Am J Lifestyle Med 2009 Jul 1; 3 1 Suppl: 19S–26S.

"Epidemiologic Transition" refers to changes in

- Population growth trajectories and composition (age distribution).
- Pattern of mortality that includes increase in life expectancy and reordering of relative importance of different cause of death.

Also Know......................

- R. Omran formulated the theory of epidemiologic transition.

DISEASE ERADICATION/CONTROL/ ELIMINATION

61. Ans. (d) Interruption of transmission of disease

Ref: K. Park, 24th ed. p 44

Disease control means reducing the disease transmission to a level where it is no more a public health problem.

- Disease agent persists in the community at very low levels.
- A state of equilibrium is established between disease agent, host and environment. E.g. Malaria control

Disease control involves ongoing activities that seek to reduce:[Q]

- Incidence of disease
- Duration of disease and risk of transmission
- Effects of infection (physical and psychosocial complications)
- Financial burden to the community.

Also Know......................

- Control activities focus on *primary prevention or secondary prevention*.
- Interruption of disease transmission is called Elimination

62. Ans. (d) 1, 2, 3 and 4 are correct

Ref: K. Park, 24th ed. p 44

63. Ans. (d) Virulence

Ref: K. Park, 24th ed. p 44

64. Ans. (a) Herd immunity

Ref: K. Park, 24th ed. p 44, 107

Herd immunity provides an immunological barrier (resistance. To spread of disease in human population.

- It offers group protection much more than that offered by immunization of individuals
- Elements contributing to herd immunity are
  - Occurrence of clinical and subclinical infection
  - Immunization
  - Herd structure (never constant)
- If herd immunity is high, an epidemic is unlikely to occur.
- High levels of herd immunity, resulting in reduced number of susceptible persons may lead (not necessarily) to elimination of disease. E.g. Diphtheria and Poliomyelitis.

Also Know......................

- Herd immunity does not protect an individual in case of Tetanus.
- Herd immunity is determined by serological surveys (serological epidemiology).
- Herd structure (host species, presence/distribution of alternative animal hosts, vectors, environment & social factors) determines immunity status of herd.

65. Ans. (b) Eradication of disease

Ref: K. Park, 24th ed. p 44

Eradication means termination of all transmission of infection by extermination of infectious agent (tear out by roots[Q])

- It is a '*all or none phenomenon*'[Q] (i.e. once eradicated disease will no longer occur in the population)
- It refers to cessation of infection and disease worldwide

66. Ans. (a) Tuberculosis

Ref: K. Park, 24th ed. p 44

67. Ans. (c) Yellow fever

Ref: K. Park, 24th ed. p 44

Eradication

- *Candidate diseases for global eradication are*[Q]– Polio, Measles, Guinea worm (eradicated from India).
- *Candidate diseases for elimination are*[Q] –Neonatal Tetanus, Kala-azar, Lymphatic filariasis.

Also Know......................

- One disease eradicated till date is **Smallpox**.

MONITORING AND SURVEILLANCE

68. Ans. (a) Monitoring

Ref: K. Park, 24th ed. p 44

Monitoring is performance and analysis of routine measurements to detect changes in environment or health status of population.

Monitoring	Surveillance
Part of a broader concept covered by surveillance	Broader concept
One time activity	Continuous process
No, inbuilt action component	It is data collection for action.
No feedback present	Feedback present
Requires careful planning and use of standardized procedures/methods of data collection.	Requires professional analysis & sophisticated judgement of data

69. Ans. (b) Sentinel surveillance

Ref: K. Park, 24th ed. p 45

Surveillance *is continuous scrutiny of factors that determine occurrence & distribution of disease/other condition of ill health.*

- **Sentinel surveillance** seeks to identify missed cases [not identified by routine notification] and supplement notified cases. E.g. *sentinel surveillance*
  - A small number of health units (Sentinel sites) are selected to report cases of disease or death.
  - Data collected is extrapolated to entire population to estimate disease prevalence in the total population.
  - *Advantage:* Reporting biases are minimized, feedback of information to providers is simplified.

Also Know........................

Other Types of Surveillance

- *Passive*– Data reports itself to health system. E.g. Patient comes to doctor with cough > 2 week. (RNTCP).
- *Active*- Data is collected actively by health system E.g. HW actively searches for Leprosy cases (NLEP), collects blood slides every fortnightly for malaria (NVBDCP). It yields true morbidity.

70. Ans. (b) Health planning

Ref: K. Park, 24th ed. p 45

Objectives of Surveillance

- To provide information about new and changing trends in health status of a population, e.g., morbidity, mortality, nutritional status, environmental hazards, health practices etc.
- To provide feedback for policy modification and to redefine objectives
- To provide timely warning of public health disasters.

71. Ans. (d) Supplementary to routine surveillance

Ref: K. Park, 24th ed. p 45

72. Ans. (c) Active Surveillance

Ref: S Lal, Textbook of community medicine, 4th edition, p- 311

73. Ans. (c) Sentinel surveillance

Ref: K. Park, 24th ed. p 45

ICEBERG PHENOMENON

74. Ans. (a) Rabies

Ref: K. Park, 24th ed. p 44, 294

Iceberg phenomenon is seen mostly in diseases with subclinical infections e.g. Rubella, Mumps, Polio, Diphtheria, JE, Hepatitis A and B, Influenza.

- Tuberculosis, hypertension and Ancylostomiasis are diseases with subclinical infections hence show the Iceberg phenomenon.
- Iceberg phenomenon is not seen in diseases with no subclinical infection. e.g. Measles, Tetanus, Rabies, chicken pox etc.

75. Ans. (d) Influenza

Ref: K. Park, 24th ed. p 44, 294

76. Ans. (d) Measles

Ref: K. Park, 24th ed. p 44

77. Ans. (a) Clinical

Ref: K. Park, 24th ed. p 44

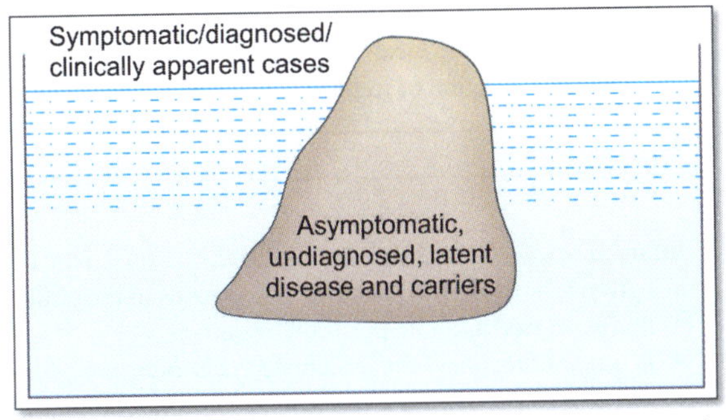

Iceberg phenomenon states that disease in a community is comparable to an iceberg.

- **Tip of iceberg (above waterline)** represents apparent (Symptomatic/Diagnosed/Clinically apparent) disease i.e. what the physician/clinician sees.
- **Submerged portion (below waterline)** represents inapparent disease (Asymptomatic, Undiagnosed, Latent disease and carriers). It is of concern for epidemiologist.
- ***Water line*** *represents the demarcation between apparent and inapparent disease.*

Also Know........................

- **Screening** *applies to submerged portion* and **diagnosis** *applies to tip of ice berg.*

INDICATORS OF HEALTH

78. Ans. (a) Quality of life

Ref: K. Park, 24th ed. p 16-17

Quality of Life

- It is a subjective component of wellbeing evaluated by assessing a person's subjective feeling of happiness and unhappiness.

Level of living and Standard of living are Objective component of wellbeing

Also Know........................

WHO QOL is an instrument to measure Quality of Life.

- WHO QOL (100 Items) has four items for each of 24 facets of quality of life and 4 items relating to the overall quality of life and general health facet.
- WHO QOL BREF has 26 Items that cover 4 domains of life.
  - Physical health
  - Psychological health
  - Social relationships
  - Environment.

79. Ans. (a) Incidence

Ref: K. Park, 24th ed. p 25

Burden of disease in a community (e.g. Mental illness, Rheumatoid arthritis etc. is expressed by **Morbidity indicators** –

- Incidence, Prevalence, Notification rates, Attendance rates at OPD, Admission/Readmission/Discharge rates, Duration of hospital stay, Sickness Spells or Absence from work/school.
- *It supplement mortality data to give a complete picture of health status of a population.*
- Drawback- Subclinical or Inapparent conditions [i.e. Submerged portion of iceberg of disease] are overlooked

80. Ans. (a) IMR

Ref: K. Park, 24th ed. p 24

Infant mortality rate is the ratio of deaths under 1 year of age in a given year to the total number of live births in the same year

- It is expressed as a rate per 1000 live births.
- *It is one of the most universally accepted indicator of health status of entire population and of socioeconomic conditions under which they live*[Q].
- It is a sensitive indicator of availability, utilization and effectiveness of health services (mainly perinatal care).

81. Ans. (a) Population Bed Ratio

Ref: K. Park, 24th ed p-26

Utilization rates is the proportion of people in need of a service who actually receive it in a given time period (usually a year).

- Proportion of infants "fully immunized" against the 9 EPI diseases.
- Proportion of pregnant women having received antenatal care or deliveries by a Skilled Birth Attendant.
- Proportion of population using various methods of family planning.
- Bed-occupancy rate (average daily in-patient census/ average number of beds).
- Average length of stay (days of care rendered/ discharges).
- Bed turnover ratio (discharges/average beds).

Also Know......................

Health policy indicators:

- Proportion of GNP spent on health services
- Proportion of GNP spent on health related activities (water supply, sanitation, housing, nutrition etc.
- Proportion of GNP spent on health services
- Proportion of GNP spent on health related activities (water supply, sanitation, housing, nutrition etc.
- Proportion of total health resources marked for primary health care.
- Degree of equity of distribution of health services, community involvement, organizational framework and managerial process.

Health care delivery indicators → Reflect equity of distribution of health resources across country and provision of health care.

- Doctor-population ratio
- Doctor-nurse ratio
- Population -bed ratio
- Population per health center/sub center

82. Ans. (a) Population per PHC

Ref: K. Park, 24th ed. p 26

DISABILITY RATES

83. Ans. (c) Limitation to perform the basic activities of daily living

Ref: K. Park, 24th ed. p 25

Disability Indicators

Event type indicator: Number of days of restricted activity, Bed disability days, Work loss days.

Person type indicator: Limitation of mobility, Limitation of activity

84. Ans. (d) Disability adjusted life years

Ref: K. Park, 24th ed. p 26

DALY (Disability Adjusted Life Year)

- Measures the burden of disease in a defined population and effectiveness of interventions.
- It is years of life lost to premature death and years lived with disability adjusted for the severity of the disability. It is a composite measure of mortality & disability.
- ***Premature death*** is death before the age to which a dying person could have expected to survive if he/she was a member of a standardized model population with a life expectancy at birth equal to Japan *(longest life expectancy).*

Health Adjusted Life Expectancy (HALE)

- It is the number of years in full health that a newborn can expect to live based on the current morbidity and mortality rates.
- It is based on life expectancy at birth with an adjustment for time spent in poor health.
- HALE has replaced DALE

Disability Free Life Expectancy (DFLE)

- It is the average number years a person can expect to live free of disability based on current mortality & disability rates,.

Quality Adjusted Life Year (QALY)

- It is the number of life years increased by a medical intervention.
- Used to asses cost effectiveness of a medical intervention.
- Measure of burden of disease in both qualitative and quantitative terms.

85. Ans. (a) One lost year of healthy life

Ref: K. Park, 24th ed. p 26

Also Know......................

- One DALY is *"one lost year of healthy life"* and One QALY is "One year of life lived in perfect health"

86. Ans. (d) Disability adjusted life years (DALY)

Ref: 24th ed. p 26

87. Ans. (c) HALE

Ref: K. Park, 24th ed. p 25

Also Know...........................

- HALE is a measure of healthy life expectancy.
- DFLE is a measure of active life expectancy.
- **QALY (Quality Adjusted Life Year)** is number of life years increased by a medical intervention.
- Used to asses cost effectiveness of a medical intervention
- 1 year of life lived in perfect health = 1 QALY

88. Ans. (d) Years lost to premature death and years lived with disability adjusted for severity of disability

Ref: K. Park, 24th ed. p 26

89. Ans. (b) 1 lost year of healthy life

Ref: K. Park, 24th ed. p 26

90. Ans. (c) Measures life expectancy adjusted without disability or free of disability

Ref: K. Park, 21st ed. p-25

Sullivan's index is *expectation of life free from disability*[Q] *or* Disability Free Life Expectancy (DFLEQ) considering current mortality & disability rates.

- **Sullivan's index** = *Life expectancy (at any age) minus Probable duration of bed disability/ Inability to perform major activity.*

Also Know...........................

Summary Measures of Population Health (SMPH) combines data on mortality and non-fatal outcomes.

Summary Measures of Health "Expectancies"

- *Healthy Life Expectancy **(HALE)***
- *Active Life Expectancy **(ALE)***
- *Disability Free Life Expectancy **(DFLE)***
- *Quality Adjusted Life Expectancy **(QALE)***

Summary Measures of Health "Gaps"

- *Years of Potential Life Lost (YPLL) - Years lost to premature death [up to 65 years of age]*
- *Disability Adjusted Life Years (DALY)*

PRIMORDIAL PREVENTION

91. Ans. (a) Primordial prevention

Ref: K. Park, 24th ed. p 45

Primordial prevention is action undertaken to prevent emergence of risk factors conducive to development of disease. In population where it has not yet appeared.

- Primordial prevention is most beneficial in case of chronic diseases (Obesity, Hypertension etc.).

Aim	Establish and Maintain conditions that minimize hazards to health
Action	Prevent emergence of risk factors
Target	Total population or Select (High risk) groups

92. Ans. (b) Create a social security system

Ref: K. Park, 24th ed. p 35

Ottawa Charter for Health Promotion

- It incorporates 5 key action areas in health promotion
  - Building a healthy public policy
  - Creating a supportive environment for health
  - Strengthening community action for health (Community ownership)
  - Development of personal skills
  - Reorientation of health services
- Ottawa charter identified 3 basic strategies for health promotion
  - Advocacy
  - Enabling achieving equity in health
  - Mediating between different interests in society for the pursuit of health

Jakarta declaration on Health Promotion (July 1997)

- It offered a vision and focus for health promotion in the 21st century.
- It focused on evolving approaches to health promotion to meet the changing determinants of health.
- It focused on unlocking the potential for health promotion inherent in many sectors of the society, among local community and within families.
- Poverty was identified as the biggest threat to health.
- Urbanization, social, behavioral, biological changes, new and remerging diseases, mental health problems were identified to require urgent response.

93. Ans. (d) 1 and 4

Ref: K. Park, 24th ed. p 45

Level of prevention	Mode of intervention	Example
Primordial	Individual and Mass education.	Discourage adoption of high risk behaviour in a population where it does not exist. e.g. Smoking, Drinking in societies where it is not prevalent yet.

94. Ans. (a) Primordial Prevention

Ref: Park 24th ed. p-45

95. Ans. (a) Primordial prevention

Ref: K. Park, 24th ed. p 45

Primordial Prevention

- Individual and mass education is the main intervention.
- Primordial prevention is best level of prevention for NCD.
- **Example:** If cigarettes are not available or tobacco is not produced, then we prevent development of conditions that lead to state of pre-pathogenesis (primordial prevention).

96. Ans. (a) Life style changes

Ref: K. Park, 24th ed. p 45

PRIMARY PREVENTION

97. Ans. (d) Encouraging physical activity

Ref: K. Park, 24th ed.p-47

Encouraging physical activity is a life style change that comes under health promotion i.e. primary level of prevention.

Also Know...........................

Health promotion includes:

- Health education
- Environment modification e.g. Safe water, Sanitary latrines, Control of insects and rodents etc.
- Nutritional intervention e.g. Food fortification
- Life style and behavioural changes e.g. Exercise, Meditation.

98. Ans. (a) Health Promotion

Ref: K. Park, 24th ed. p 47

Food fortification is a Nutritional intervention under Health promotion.

99. Ans. (b, c, d) (b) Immunization against specific disease, (c) Specific nutritional diet, (d) Protection from occupational hazard

Ref: Park 24th ed. p 47-48

100. Ans. (c) Pap smear

Ref: K. Park, 24th ed. p 46,48

101. Ans. (a) Measles vaccination

Ref: K. Park, 24th ed. p 46, 47

102. Ans. (b) Specific protection

Ref: K. Park, 24th ed. p 47

Specific protection refers to prophylaxis or preventive measures to prevent the occurrence of a specific disease/ disorder in population at risk of developing the disease/ disorder as predisposing risk factors are already present.

Specific Protection Includes

- Immunization
- Chemoprophylaxis
- Nutrient supplement or Fortification E.g. IFA, Vit A, Iodine
- Protection against occupational hazard, accident, carcinogen etc.
- Avoidance of allergens
- Control of specific environment hazards E.g. Air pollution, noise control, chlorination of water.
- Control of consumer product quality and safety of food and drug.
- Use of helmets and seatbelts to protect against Road Traffic Accident.

103. Ans. (b) Primary prevention

Ref: K. Park, 24th ed p-46

Hand washing to prevent nosocomial infection is a intervention in the early pre pathogenesis phase (when disease process is not initiated, but agent is around. It is thus a primary prevention)

104. Ans. (b) Primary prevention

Ref: K. Park, 24th ed. p 46

Primary prevention is a holistic approach, that relies on measures designed to promote health or to protect against specific disease agents and hazards in the environment.

- Communicable diseases were eliminated in developed countries by raising the standard of living (Primary prevention)

105. Ans. (d) Early Diagnosis

Ref: K. Park, 24th ed. p 46,48

Early Diagnosis and treatment constitute secondary prevention.

106. Ans. (b) Primary prevention

Ref: K. Park, 24th ed. p 46

Primary Prevention

E.g.: In Ischemic Heart Disease –educating and motivating young population not to start smoking, despite availability of cigarettes [risk factors].

- Desks provided with table top are a specific protection to prevent occurrence of neck problem.

107. Ans. (a) Primary Prevention

Ref: K. Park, 24th ed. p 46

Also Know...........................

- Target group in primary and primordial prevention is Healthy individuals.

108. Ans. (a, b, e) (a) Marriage counseling, (b) Health education, (e) Health promotion

Ref: K. Park, 24th ed. p 46

Marriage counseling, Health education & Health promotion are done prior to disease onset & remove the possibility that disease will ever occur- Hence are Primary Prevention.

Also Know...........................

- **Pap smear and Self breast examination meant for *early detection and prompt treatment –secondary prevention*[Q].**

SECONDARY PREVENTION

109. Ans. (c) Secondary prevention

Ref: K. Park, 24th ed. p 46

Secondary prevention is action taken to halt the progress of disease in *early pathogenesis* phase and prevent complications.

Also Know...........................

- Most national health programs act at secondary level of prevention.

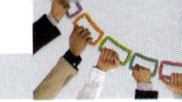

Aim	Reduce the prevalence of disease by shortening duration
Action	Early detection and prompt action
Target	Individuals diagnosed with disease

110. Ans. (c) Reduction of prevalence

Ref: K. Park, 23rd ed. p 42

Intervention	Level of prevention
Reduction of risk factors	Primordial prevention
Reduction of incidence	Primary prevention
Reduction of prevalence	Secondary prevention
Reduction of complication	Tertiary prevention

111. Ans. (a) PAP smear

Ref: K. Park, 24th ed. p 46

Secondary Prevention Involves

Early Diagnosis

- Screening by Pap smear, Self-breast examination, Mammography, Active case search.
- Medical examinations of school children, infants and young children, industrial workers.

Treatment

- DOTS, MDT for leprosy, Dental filling and Tooth extraction.

112. Ans. (b) Secondary prevention

Ref: Park 24th ed. p 46

Fetal cardiac monitoring is a form of Secondary prevention, done for early detection of disease to halt the progress of disease in early pathogenesis phase and prevent complications.

113. Ans. (c) Secondary

Ref: K. Park, 24th ed. p 46

114. Ans. (c) Secondary

Ref: K. Park, 24th ed. p 46

115. Ans. (c) Secondary prevention

Ref: K. Park, 24th ed. p 46

116. Ans. (c) Secondary prevention

Ref: K. Park, 24th ed. p 46

117. Ans. (b) Patients

Ref: K. Park, 24th ed. p 46

TERTIARY PREVENTION

118. Ans. (c) Disability

Ref: K. Park, 24th ed. p 48

Disability is *restriction or lack of ability to perform any activity in a manner or within a range considered normal for a human being for his age, sex, etc. due to impairment.*

Also Know......................

Disease → Impairment → Disability → Handicap

119. Ans. (b) Impairment

Ref: K. Park, 24th ed. p 48

120. Ans. (d) Any of the above

Ref: K. Park, 24th ed. p 48

Impairment is *any loss or abnormality of psychological, physiological or anatomical structure or function.*

Tertiary Prevention

Aim	Reduce the Impact/Complications
Action	Minimize the Impact, Minimize suffering, Maximize potential years of quality life
Target	Patients

121. Ans. (b) Rehabilitation

Ref: http://www.ccdisabilities.nic.in

Indian Disability Evaluation and Assessment Scale (IDEAS) is a scale for measuring and quantifying disability in mental disorders.

Items -

- Self-care: Taking care of body hygiene, grooming, health including bathing, toileting, dressing, eating etc.
- Interpersonal Activities (Social Relationships)
- Communication and Understanding -Spoken/written/non-verbal messages.
- Work: Performing in areas of Employment/Housework/ Education (school/college)

Scores for each item:

0- NO disability (none, absent, negligible)
1- MILD disability (slight, low)
2- MODERATE disability (medium, fair)
3- SEVERE disability (high, extreme)
4- PROFOUND disability (total cannot do)
TOTAL SCORE = Sum of scores of the 4 items

Weightage for Duration of illness (DOI):

DOI: < 2 years: score to be added is 1
2-5 years: add 2.
6-10 years: add 3
> 10 years: add 4

Total Disability score + DOI score = Global **Disability Score**

Percentages:

0 No Disability = 0%
1-6 Mild Disability = <40%
7-13 Moderate Disability = 40-70%
14-19 Severe Disability = 71-99%
20 Profound Disability = 100%
Cut off for welfare measures = 40%

122. Ans. (b) Disease - Impairment – Disability – Handicap

Ref: K. Park, 24th ed. p 48

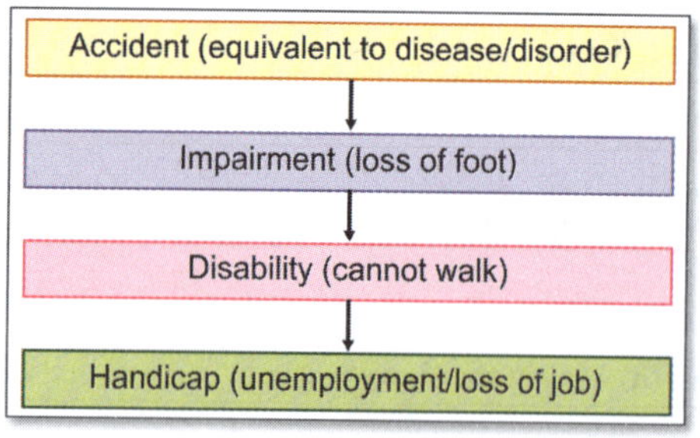

123. Ans. (d) Tertiary prevention

Ref: K. Park, 24th ed. p 46

Disability prevention involves all the levels of prevention:

- Reducing the occurrence of impairment e.g. Polio vaccination (*primary prevention*- most effective).
- Disability limitation by appropriate treatment (*secondary prevention*) and
- Preventing the transition of disability into handicap (*tertiary prevention*).

Tertiary prevention is intervention in the late pathogenesis phase, that reduces/limits impairments, disabilities and handicap.

- *Disability limitation*[Q] means to halt the transition of impairment to disability.
- *Rehabilitation*[Q] is combined and coordinated use of medical, social, educational and vocational measures to enable a handicapped person achieve active participation in mainstream of community life.

Types of Rehabilitation	Purpose	Examples
Physical	Restore function	*Calipers for walking, Artificial limb,* Reconstructive surgery in leprosy, graded exercises in neurological disorders like polio.
Vocational	Restore ability to earn a livelihood	Training and creating job opportunities, Schools for children suffering from PRPP and blindness.
Social	Restore family and social life	Eliminate stigma, Counseling
Psychological	Build confidence and help cope with stress	Counseling, Stress management

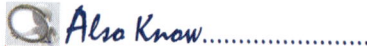

Also Know......................

- *Psychological rehabilitation*[Q] is also known as crisis intervention.

124. Ans. (a) Impairment

Ref: K. Park, 24th ed. p 48

MISCELLANEOUS

125. Ans. (a) Slightly positive

Ref: Hospital Admission: A problem Solving Approach, Sonu Goel, p-356

Turn over Interval is the average period in days a hospital bed remains vacant between one discharge and another admission. It depends on occupancy rate.

- Useful in private sector or paid hospital bed where maximization of revenue is the aim.
- Not of much use in government sector where demand of bed is excessive.
  - Large positive value indicates low demand, defective admission/discharge and underuse of hospital.
  - Large negative values indicate overutilization
  - Slight positive values indicate optimum utilization
  - Slight negative values indicate shortage of bed

Also Know......................

Average daily census is average number of inpatients (excluding newborn) receiving care in a hospital at 12 am (mid night) in a day.

- It represents the average daily load of patients over a given period

$$\text{Average daily census} = \frac{\text{Total No. of patients days in a period excluding newborn}}{\text{No. of days in same period}}$$

Average Length of stay [ALOS] =

$$\frac{\text{Total No. of patient days (sum of daily ALOS = census in a period)}}{\text{Total No. of discharge/deaths during same period}}$$

- In India ALOS is 10–12 days in General hospital (More in medical college and less in district hospital)
- In USA it is 4 to 5 days.
- ALOS is an index of insufficiency (High due to hospital bottleneck)

Percentage of bed occupancy =

$$\frac{\text{Total No. of patient days in a given period}}{\text{Available beds X No. of days in a period}} \times 100$$

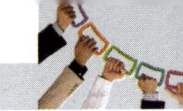

Also Know........................

- 75–85% occupancy means good hospital patient care and hospital economy.
- Higher occupancy means over utilization and lowering of quality of care.
- Low occupancy means over provisioning or wastage of resources.

INFECTIOUS DISEASE EPIDEMIOLOGY

126. Ans. (d) Monitoring

Ref: K. Park, 24th ed. p 44

Monitoring is defined as the performance and analysis of routine measurements aimed at detecting changes in the environment or health status of population. E.g. Growth monitoring, Air quality monitoring

- It is meant for immediate corrective measures if anything goes wrong
- It keeps track of utilization, supplies, equipment, achievements etc
- Monitoring is a specific and essential component of Surveillance.
- It requires careful planning, use of standardized procedures/methods and can be carried out by technicians or automated instrumentation.

Also Know........................

- Surveillance requires professional analysis and sophisticated judgment of data leading to recommendations for control activities.

127. Ans. (b) Passive surveillance

Ref: Disease Control Priorities in Developing Countries. 2nd ed. 2006.

- *Routine health information system is* a **passive** system in which regular reports about diseases and programs are compiled by public health staff members, hospitals, and clinics.

MODERN MEDICINE AND MEDICAL REVOLUTION

128. Ans.(b) Epidemiological work on ...; (c) Work on scurvy...; (e) Chadwick work on ...

Ref: K. Park, 24th ed. p 5, 6, 8, 208

129. Ans. (c) Use of various research finding...

Ref: Evidence-Based Pathology and Laboratory Medicine, Alberto M. Marchevsky, Mark R Wick, p-3

NOTES

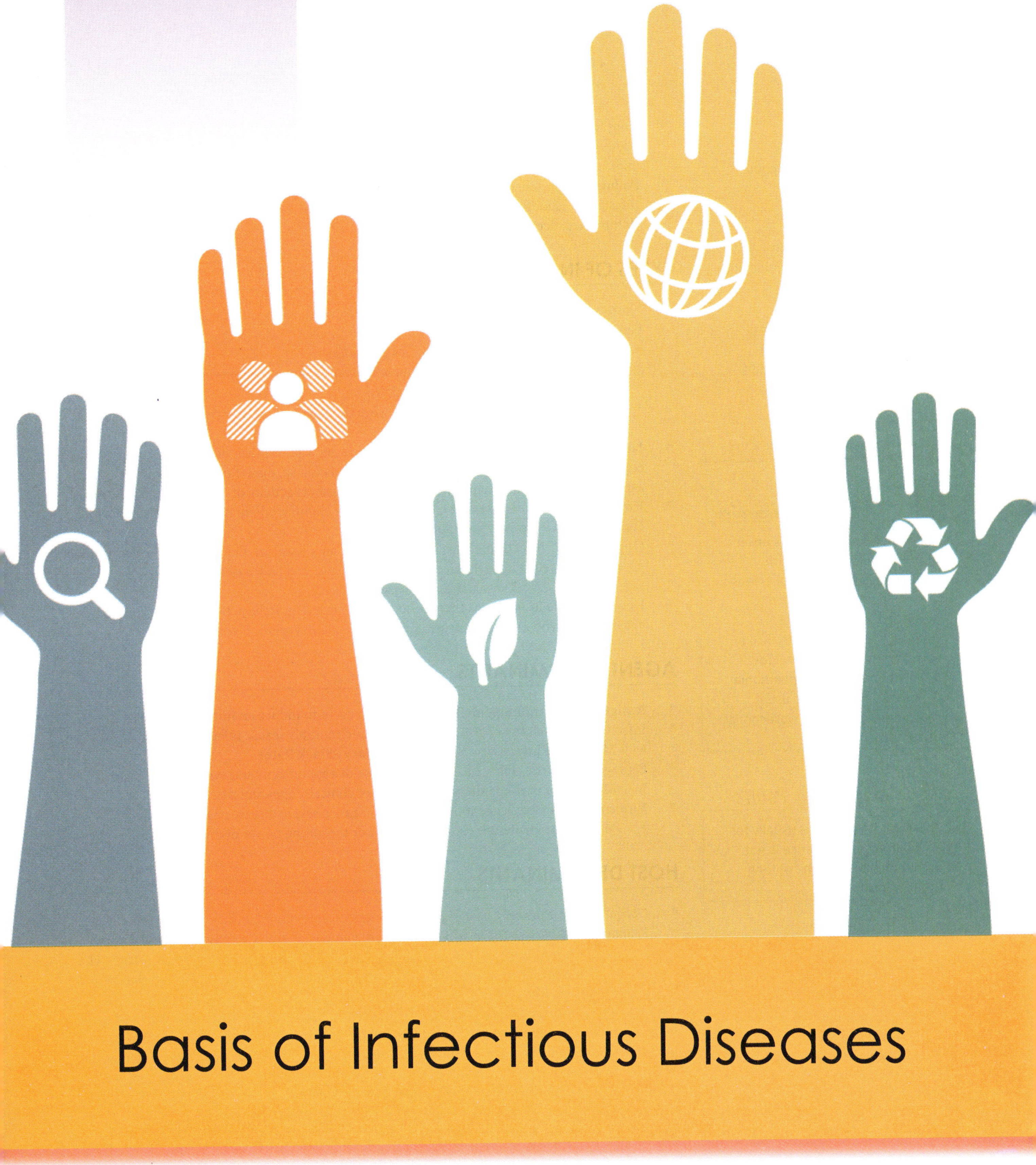

Basis of Infectious Diseases

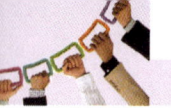

Chapter Outline

21 **Must Remember**

Nosocomial pneumonia is onset of pneumonia features with radiographic or laboratory evidence after 48 hours of admission to hospital or within 48 hours of discharge from the health facility with admission to hospital for sickness unrelated to pneumonia

Staphylococcus is the usual causative organism for nosocomial pneumonia

34 **High Yield Points**

The case fatality rate is usually for acute diseases and hence is not accounting for the time or long duration diseases.

35 **High Yield Points**

In Japanese encephalitis
Man – Dead end host
Pig – Amplifying host
Birds – Maintenance host

INTRODUCTION

- **Infection** is entry and development/multiplication of an infectious agent in the body of man or animal.
  - It does not always cause illness
  - Levels of infection:
    - Colonization,
    - Subclinical,
    - Latent and
    - Manifest/clinical infection
- **Contamination** is presence of an infectious agent on body surface or inanimate articles (clothes, bedding, toy, surgical instruments, dressings, etc.) or substances including water, milk and food
- **Pollution** is presence of offensive (not necessarily infectious) matter in the environment
- **Infestation** is lodgment, development and multiplication of arthropods on body surface or clothing, e.g. lice and itch mite.

TYPES OF INFECTION

- **Nosocomial infection** (Hospital-acquired infection) is an infection that originates in a patient while in a hospital
  - It is not related to patient's primary condition
  - It is neither present, nor incubating at the time of admission or is residual of an infection acquired during a previous admission
  - For example, Infection of surgical wounds, Hepatitis B, urinary tract infections and pneumonias
- **Iatrogenic infection** is any adverse event following a preventive, diagnostic or therapeutic regimen or procedure that results in impairment, handicap, disability or death resulting from a physician's professional activity or from the professional activity of other health professionals
- **Exotic disease** is a disease that is imported into a country, where it was nonexistent before. E.g. Rabies in UK, yellow fever for India
- **Opportunistic infection:** This infection is by an organism that takes the opportunity provided by a defect in host defense to infect the host and hence causes disease. E.g.: *M. tuberculosis*, Herpes simplex, Toxoplasma, etc.
- **Dead - end infection** means there is no portal of exit. E.g. Rabies, Bubonic plague, Tetanus, Trichinosis, Scrub Typhus, Murine typhus, Indian Tick typhus, Hydatid disease.

AGENT DETERMINANTS

- **Antigenicity (Immunogenicity):** Ability of an agent to induce an immune response
- Infectivity is the ability of an agent to invade and multiply (cause infection) in a host
  - **Measure of infectivity: SAR % (Secondary Attack Rate)**
- Pathogenicity is the ability of an agent to cause disease or signs and symptoms of disease
  - **Measure of pathogenicity:** Proportion of clinically apparent cases
- Virulence: Ability of an agent or pathogen to cause a severe disease or fatal disease
  - **Measure of virulence:** Case fatality rate or the killing power of disease.

HOST DETERMINANTS

- *Obligate host* means only host, e.g. man in measles and typhoid fever
- *Primary or definitive hosts* in which the parasite attains maturity or passes its sexual stage
- *Secondary or intermediate* host in which the parasite is in larval or asexual stage. The intermediate host serves only as a site wherein the parasite spends a particular developmental stage of its life cycle

E.g. some tapeworms make use of cows, pigs and fish as intermediate hosts. When any of these animals ingests a tapeworm egg, the egg hatches and the larva moves from the intestine to the muscle of the animal where it forms a cyst. Human ingesting a partially cooked or raw meat containing the cyst may eventually harbor the parasite when the larva moves out of the cyst and grows into its mature or reproductive form and begin to reproduce inside the definitive human host.

Table 1: Parasitic diseases and their primary and secondary hosts

Disease	Primary host	Secondary host
Filaria	Man	Mosquito (Culex)
Malaria	Mosquito (Anopheles)	Man
Tapeworm	Man	Pig (*T. solium*), Cattle (*T. saginata*)
Guinea worm	Man	Cyclops
Hydatid disease	Dog	Sheep, Cattle, Man
Sleeping sickness	Man	Tsetse Fly

SOURCE

It is defined as any person, animal, arthropod, plant, soil or substance (or combination of these) in which an infectious agent lives and multiplies, on which it depends primarily for survival and where it reproduces itself in such manner that it can be transmitted to a susceptible host. E.g. Female anophele mosquito in malaria.

RESERVOIR

Reservoir is a term, often used interchangeably with source. The difference lies in fact of being able to transmit or not. Reservoir is basically any person, place, animal or substance in which the pathogen will live and multiply - (if transmits—it is also a source of infection, otherwise a reservoir only).

Homologous Reservoir

The term homologues reservoir is applied when another member of the same species is the reservoir. E.g. Man is the principal reservoir for some enteric pathogens.

Heterologous Reservoir

The term heterologus is applied when the infection is derived from a reservoir other than man. E.g. Animals and birds infected with salmonella.

* **Human Reservoir** – most important reservoir for infections. It could be presenting as case or carrier.

CASES

A case is defined as a person in the population or study group identified as having the particular disease, health disorders or condition under investigation. Broadly, the presence of infection in a host may be clinical, subclinical or latent.

Clinical Illness

Clinical illness may be mild moderate, typical or atypical, severe or fatal depending upon gradient of involvement.

Subclinical Cases

Subclinical case plays a dominant role in **maintaining chain of infection** in the community.

23 **Must Remember**

Infection	Reservoir	Source
Hookworm	Man	Soil contaminated with infective larvae
Tetanus	Soil	Soil
Anthrax, Coccidioidomycosis and mycetoma	Soil	-

Contd...

36 **High Yield Points**

- *Homologous reservoir* is where another member of the same species is victim, E.g. *V. cholerae*—Man.
- *Heterologous reservoir* is when infection is derived from a reservoir other than man, E.g. animals/birds infected with salmonella.

22 **Must Remember**

The terms reservoir and source are not always synonymous.
E.g. In hook worm infection
Reservoir—man
Source of infection—is the soil contaminated with infective larvae.

37 **High Yield Points**

- **Primary case** is the 1st case of a communicable disease introduced into a population
- **Index case** is the 1st case to come to notice the investigator (not always the primary case)[Q]
- **Secondary cases** are cases developing from contact with primary case[Q]
- **Subclinical infection** occurs in Rubella, Mumps, Polio, Hepatitis A and B, Japanese encephalitis, Influenza, Diphtheria, etc. and have an important role in maintaining endemicity and immunity shown by adults to disease-producing microbes.

23 *Must Remember*

Infection	Reservoir	Source
Typhoid fever	Case or carrier [Man]	Unsafe water and food
Pandemic influenza	Pigs and ducks	-
Chlamydia	Pigeons	-
Histoplasmosis, Ornithosis, arboviruses	Wild birds	-
Tuberculosis	Man	Sputum
HIV/AIDS	Man	Body fluids and secretions
Malaria	Man and Mosquito	Infected blood
Rabies	Dog and other animals	Saliva
Measles	Man	Droplets
Japanese encephalitis	Pig and birds	Infected mosquito
Cholera	Man	Unsafe water and food
Plague	Rodents	Infected flies
KFD	Monkey	Hard Tick

Primary Case

It is the first observed case in the community. It may or may not come to the attention of the investigator

Secondary Case

These are the subsequent cases arising from the primary case within an incubation period

Index Case

It is the first observed case from the community for a specific disease. It may or may not be the primary case

38 *High Yield Points*

- No carrier state for hepatitis A
- Urinary carriers are more dangerous than intestinal carriers
- Pseudo carrier – carriers of avirulent organisms

CARRIER

- Carrier is an infected person/animal harboring an infectious agent, but not developing clinical disease and is a potential source of infection to others
- Carriers are less infectious than cases, but more dangerous (escape diagnosis and may infect susceptible individuals)

Essential elements in a carrier state are:

- Presence in the body of the disease agent
- Absence of recognizable symptoms and signs of disease
- Shedding of the disease agent in discharges or excretions.

24 *Must Remember*

- A carrier is a person with inapparent infection who is capable of transmitting the pathogen to others.
- Asymptomatic or passive or healthy carriers are those who never experience symptoms despite being infected.
- Incubatory carriers are those who can transmit the agent during the incubation period before clinical illness begins.

Table 2: Types of carriers

Carrier by type	Incubatory carrier	Shed infectious agent in incubation period of disease	Measles, Mumps, Polio, Pertussis, Influenza, Diphtheria and Hepatitis B
	Healthy carrier	Continue to shed the infectious agent without suffering from overt disease	Polio, Cholera, Meningococcal meningitis, Salmonellosis and Diphtheria
	Convalescent carrier	Continue to shed the infectious agent during period of convalescence	Typhoid fever, Dysentery (bacillary and amoebic), Cholera, Diphtheria and Pertusis.

Contd...

Carrier by duration	Temporary carrier	Shed infectious agent for short periods	Incubatory/Convalescent or healthy
	Chronic carrier	Excrete infectious agent (intermittently or continuously) for indefinite period	Reintroduce disease into areas free of infection (e.g. Malaria)
Carriers by portal of exit	Urinary carriers, intestinal carriers, respiratory carriers		

- **Healthy carrier:**
  - These are carrier stages emerging from
    - Avirulent strains or
    - Sub clinical cases
  - These are also known as paradoxical carrier or asymptomatic carrier
  - These are important for maintenance of the transmission levels in a community
  - **Example:**
    - Cholera
    - Typhoid
    - Diphtheria
    - Polio
    - Meningitis

DISEASE TRANSMISSION

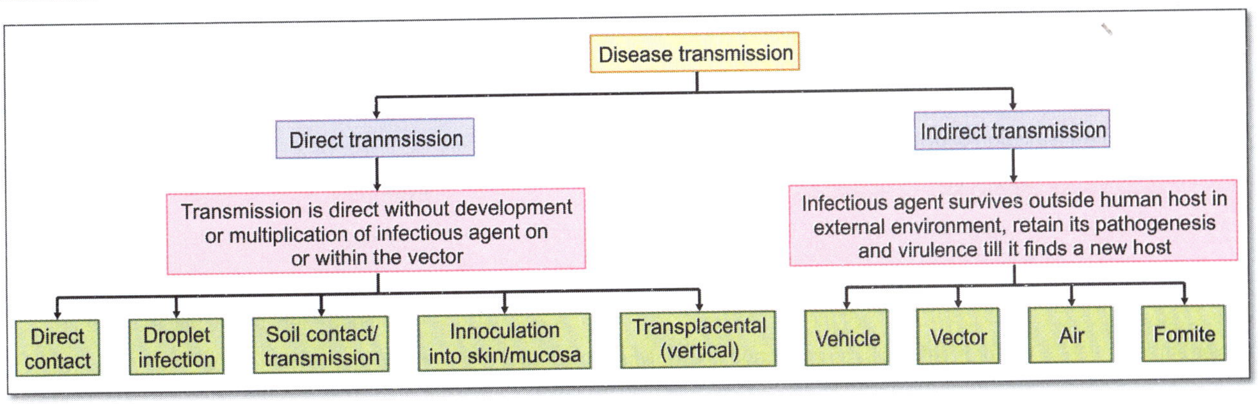

Fig. 1: Disease transmission

Direct Transmission

Table 3: Direct transmission of diseases

	Remarks	Examples
Without multiplication in the vector or the transmitting material		
Direct contact	▪ **Types:** Skin to skin; Mucosa to mucosa; Mucosa to skin ▪ This implies direct, essentially immediate transfer of infectious agents from reservoir to susceptible individual without an intermediate agency.	▪ STD's ▪ AIDS ▪ Leprosy ▪ Leptospirosis ▪ Skin & eye infections.

Contd...

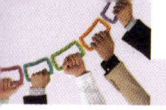

	Remarks	Examples
Droplet infection	▪ Direct projection of spray of droplets of saliva and nasopharyngeal secretions. ▪ Particles of 10mm or > in diameter are filtered off by nose ▪ Those of 5mm or < can penetrate deeply and reach alveoli ▪ Usually limited to distance of 30-60 cm	▪ Respiratory infections ▪ Whooping cough ▪ TB
Contact with soil	By direct exposure of susceptible tissue to disease agent in soil, compost/decaying vegetable matter.	▪ Hookworm larvae ▪ Tetanus ▪ Mycosis
Inoculation into skin/ mucosa	Disease agent may be inoculated directly into skin/mucosa	▪ Rabies virus by dog bite ▪ Hepatitis virus through contaminated needles and syringes
Trans placental/ vertical transmission	Direct transfer from the mother to child. The pathogen/agent may produce malformations in the fetus directly.	▪ TORCH (Toxoplasma gondii, Rubella virus, cytomegalovirus, herpes virus). ▪ Syphilis ▪ Hepatitis B ▪ Coxsackie B ▪ HIV Some of nonliving agents (e.g. Thalidomide, diethylstilbestrol) can also be transmitted vertically.

Indirect Transmission

An "essential requirement" for indirect transmission is that the infectious agent must be capable of surviving outside the human host in external environment and retain its basic properties of pathogenesis and virulence till it finds a new host.

- Flies
- Fingers
- Fomites
- Food
- Fluids/feces

Table 4: Indirect transmission of diseases

	Remarks	Examples
Vehicle transmission	Through agency of water, food (including raw vegetables, milk and its products), ice, blood, serum, plasma or other biological products	▪ By water and food includes: Acute diarrhea, typhoid fever, cholera, polio, hepatitis A, and food poisoning. ▪ By blood: Hepatitis B, malaria, syphilis
Vector-borne	Vector is defined as an arthropod or any living carrier that transports an infectious agent to susceptible individual. It may have: ▪ Mechanical transmission ▪ Biological transmission	▪ Snail: Schistosomiasis ▪ Fish: Tapeworm ▪ Mosquito: Malaria ▪ Ticks: KFD ▪ Sandfly: Kala-azar
Airborne	Droplet nuclei Dust	▪ TB ▪ Varicella ▪ Measles ▪ Influenza
Fomite borne	Fomites are nonliving substances as catheters, pens, paper, stethoscope, etc.	Diarrheal, respiratory Infections
Unclean hands and fingers	—	Diarrheal, respiratory infections

Biological Transmission

- Infectious agent undergoes replication or development or both in vector.
- Three types:
  - *Propagative*: Agent only multiplies in vector, there is no change in form, e.g., Plague bacilli in rat fleas
  - *Cyclopropagative*: Agent changes in form and number, e.g. malaria parasites in mosquito
  - *Cyclodevelopmental*: Agent undergoes only development but no multiplication, e.g. microfilaria in mosquito.
- Transovarian transmission: Infectious agent is transmitted vertically from the infected vector to her progeny.
- Trans-stadial transmission: Transmission of disease agent from one stage of life cycle to another. E.g. Nymph to adult.

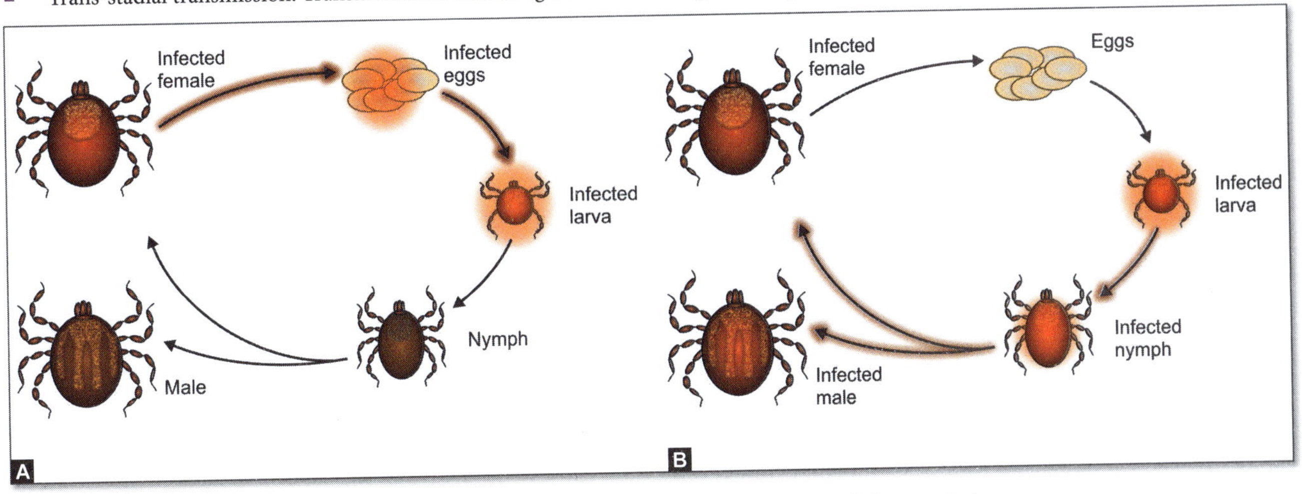

Figs 2A and B: **A.** Transovarial transmission; **B.** Trans-stadial transmission

TIME LINE IN INFECTIONS

Incubation Period

The time interval between invasion by an infectious agent and appearance of the first sign or symptom of the disease in question.

Table 5: Infectious diseases – incubation period

Skin Infections/Rashes		
Disease	**Incubation period**	**Period of communicability**
Chickenpox	10–21	2 days before rash until all sores have crusts (6–7 days)
Fifth disease (Erythema infectiosum)	4–14	7 days before rash until rash begins
Hand, foot, and mouth disease	3–6	Onset of mouth ulcers until fever gone
Impetigo (*Streptococcus or Staphylococcus*)	2–5	Onset of sores until 24 hours on antibiotic
Lice	7	Onset of itch until 1 treatment
Measles	8–12	4 days before rash until 4 days after rash appears
Roseola	9–10	Onset of fever until rash gone (2 days)
Rubella (German measles)	14–21	7 days before rash until 5 days after rash appears
Scabies	30–45	Onset of rash until 1 treatment

Contd...

39 *High Yield Points*

- **Minimum incubation period:** There is minimum incubation period for every disease before which no illness can occur.
- **Median incubation period:** The time required for 50% of the cases to occur following exposure.

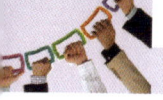

Scarlet fever	3–6	Onset of fever or rash until 24 hours on antibiotic
Shingles (contagious for chicken pox)	14–16	Onset of rash until all sores have crusts (7 days) (Note: No need to isolate if sores can be kept covered.)
Warts	30–180	Minimally contagious
Respiratory infections		
Bronchiolitis	4–6	Onset of cough until 7 days
Colds	2–5	Onset of runny nose until fever gone
Cold sores (Herpes)	2–12	
Coughs (viral) or croup (viral)	2–5	Onset of cough until fever gone
Diphtheria	2–5	Onset of sore throat until 4 days on antibiotic
Influenza	1–2	Onset of symptoms until fever gone
Sore throat, Streptococcus	2–5	Onset of sore throat until 24 hours on antibiotic
Sore throat, viral	2–5	Onset of sore throat until fever gone
Tuberculosis	6–24 months	Until 2 weeks on drugs (Note: Most childhood TB is not contagious)
Whooping cough	7–10	Onset of runny nose until 5 days on antibiotic
Intestinal infections		
Diarrhea, bacterial	1–5	Variable – depends on organism
Diarrhea, Giardia	7–28	Variable – depends on organism
Diarrhea, traveller's	1–6	Variable – depends on organism
Diarrhea, viral (Rotavirus)	1–3	Variable – depends on organism
Hepatitis A	14–50	2 weeks before jaundice begins until jaundice resolved (7 days)
Pinworms	21–28	Minimally contagious, staying home is unnecessary
Vomiting, viral	2–5	Variable – depends on etiology
Other infections		
Infectious mononucleosis	30–50	Onset of fever until fever gone (7 days)
Meningitis, bacterial	2–10	7 days before symptoms until 24 hours on IV antibiotics in hospital
Meningitis, viral	3–6	Onset of symptoms and for 1–2 weeks
Mumps	12–25	Days before swelling until swelling gone (7 days)

Generation Time

The interval of time between receipt of infection by a host and maximal infectivity of that host.

- The incubation period is roughly equal to the generation time. But in certain cases, the time of maximum communicability may precede or follow the incubation period. For example, Mumps, communicability appears to reach its height about 48 hours before the onset of swelling of the salivary glands

Communicable Period

- The time during which an infectious agent may be transferred directly or indirectly from an infected person to another person, from an infected animal to man, or from an infected person to an animal, including arthropods. Communicability may be assessed using the secondary attack rates.

Must Remember

Incubation period can only be applied to infections that result in manifestation of diseases

Generation time is a measure of transmission of infection, whether clinical or subclinical

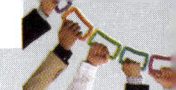

Latent Period

- It is a proxy indicator for the incubation period for the noncommunicable diseases. The time of appearance of first sign and symptoms is usually too much delayed from the time of entry of organism. It is the period from disease initiation to disease detection.

Serial Interval

- It is the time difference between the primary case and the secondary case.
- It is a proxy indicator for the communicability or the generation time of the infectious disease

MEASUREMENTS OF INFECTIOUS DISEASE MORBIDITY

Attack Rates

- These are special incidence rates, usually used for infectious diseases
- They depict the impact of the disease in a population and may be used as yardstick to find the magnitude of epidemic in an area

$$\text{Attack rate} = \frac{\textit{Total number of cases in an area during specified period}}{\textit{Total population at the start of the period}} \times 100$$

- Synonym for:
  - Incidence proportion
  - Risk
  - Probability of having disease (or event)
  - Cumulative incidence
- Attack rates are usually expressed as percentages

Secondary attack rate

$$\text{Secondary attack rate} = \frac{\textit{Total number of cases arising from the primary case within an incubation period}}{\textit{Total number of susceptible contacts}} \times 100$$

Note that the numbers of primary cases are not included in the numerator and the denominator while calculating the secondary attack rates

Advantage:

- To assess the preventive measure as isolation or immunizations
- Asses communicability of a disease of unknown etiology
- Asses the spread of infection in a family, household or contacts within a closed area.

Limitation:

- It is feasible only in diseases which have a manifested disease presentation
- For diseases where the primary case is infective for a short period of time.

Table 6: Measuring disease morbidity

Measure	Numerator	Denominator
Incidence proportion (or attack rate or risk)	Number of new cases of disease during specified time interval	Population at start of time interval
Secondary attack rate	Number of new cases among contacts	Total number of contacts
Incidence rate (or person-time rate)	Number of new cases of disease during specified time interval	Summed person-years of observation or average population during time interval
Point prevalence	Number of current cases (new and preexisting) at a specified point in time	Population at the same specified point in time
Period prevalence	Number of current cases (new and preexisting) over a specified period of time)	Average or mid-interval population

40 High Yield Points

In calculating the secondary attack rates: the primary case is not included in the numerator and the denominator.

41 High Yield Points

Serial interval: The gap in time between the onset of the primary case and the secondary case.

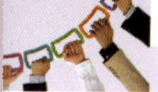

ISOLATION/QUARANTINE

Helps in public health to prevent the disease by prohibiting the exposure of population to people who have or may have a contagious disease

- **Isolation** separates sick people with a contagious disease from people who are not sick.
- **Quarantine** separates and restricts the movement of people who were exposed to a contagious disease to see if they become sick.

Isolation is effective in diphtheria, cholera, pneumonic plague, streptococcal respiratory disease, measles, chicken pox, shigellosis, salmonellosis, influenza, smear +ve TB, pneumonic plague

Isolation may not be effective in mumps (highly infectious before it is diagnosed), typhoid, Hepatitis A (Subclinical infection and carrier state), bubonic plague

Chemical isolation is treatment of cases at their own homes and rendering them noninfectious at earliest—Leprosy, TB and STD

Quarantine It is restriction of movement applicable to healthy persons[Q] and is for the longest incubation period.[Q]

- The concept of quarantine is to prevent of spread of infection based on suspicion that the individual harbours infection and maybe infective. Also applied to a ship, an aircraft, a train, road vehicle etc.
- **Types:** Absolute and Modified (selective partial limitation of freedom of movement, e.g. exclusion of children from school)

Modified quarantine refers to selective partial limitation of movement of contacts of communicable diseases to protect susceptible individuals from contracting disease. Exclusion of children with chickenpox and measles from regular school is an example.

> 26 ***Must Remember***
>
> Isolation can be achieved by "ring immunization" [encircling infected persons with a barrier of immune persons]. It was used in Smallpox eradication.

> 42 ***High Yield Points***
>
> - Isolation – for patients
> - Quarantine – for apparently healthy individuals based on suspicion of disease

DISINFECTION

Disinfectant (Germicide) kills harmful microbe (not spores) and prevent disease transmission. Suitable only for inanimate objects.

Antiseptic kills or inhibits growth of microorganisms on living tissues. A disinfectant in low concentration can act as antiseptic.

Deodorant: A substance which removes foul smell.

Sterilization destroys all forms of life including spores.

Disinfection kills infectious agents outside the body by direct exposure to chemical or physical agents.

Types of Disinfection

- **Concurrent disinfection:** The destruction of the disease agent as soon as it is released from the body. Example disc
- **Terminal disinfection:** After the removal of the patient or the source of infection from the hospital or the medical facility area.
- **Pre-current/prophylactic disinfection:** Disinfection of water with chlorine, pasteurization of milk and hand washing.

Classification of Disinfectants

Class of disinfectant	Subtypes of disinfection
Natural disinfectants	Sunlight, air
Physical disinfectants	Heat, radiation, filtration
Chemical disinfectants	Solid, liquid, gas and other miscellaneous

- **Natural disinfection**
  - Sunlight: By the UV rays, sunlight may have a disinfectant action. The UV rays act by coagulation of the protoplasm of the bacteria
  - **Air:** It destroys the organisms by drying.

- **Physical disinfection**
  - Heat
    - Dry heat – less power of penetration, but may destroy spores, and so maybe used for sterilization (burning)
      - By burning – for ultimate disposal of bandages, swabs, rags. Not recommended on large scale due to environmental hazard
      - Hot air
        - Conventional oven – 160°–180°C deg Celsius x 1 hour – for glassware, powders, oils, Vaseline
        - Infrared oven
        - Microwave ovens – convert radiant energy into heat energy. Useful for
          - Laboratory instruments, media
          - Dental instruments
      - Flaming - For wire loops, needs, microbiological sharps before using
    - Moist heat
      - At temperature below 100°C – for pasteurization of milk, vaccine sterilization
      - Temperature of 100°C (for 20 mins) - for surgical instruments, glass syringes, utensils, linen, gloves
      - Temperature above 100°C
        - Steam – autoclave
          - Most effective sterilizing agent
            - Destroys all life forms
            - Good penetration power
            - Gives of latent heat (absorbed heat for conversion into steam – has longer duration of action)
          - Surgical instruments, OT garments, linen, gloves/masks/gown.
          - Not suitable for plastics
  - Radiation – (gamma rays) – high power of penetration
    - Bandages, plastic syringes, drip sets, cooper T, catheters
    - Effective, but costly method
    - HIV is not inactivated by radiation
- **Chemical disinfection**
  - **Solid disinfectants**
    - Lime – cheap and easily available
      - Dry lime – powder to disinfect surfaces, floors
      - Milk of lime – aqueous solution – walls, in white wash, excreta disinfection
    - Bleaching powder ($CaOCl_2$)
      - It is a chlorinated lime with 33% available chlorine
      - Dose – 2.5 g of bleaching powder is used to disinfect 1000 L of water
      - **Uses:**
        - Water disinfection
        - Bleaching agent in paper and textile industry
        - Deodorant in washrooms, latrines, animal sheds
        - Excreta disinfection
    - Hypochlorite: Powerful liquid bleach. Sodium hypochlorite solution provides 50% available chlorine
    - Potassium permanganate: Good oxidizing agent, but weak disinfectant
      - **Uses:**
        - Disinfect fruits and vegetables
        - Eczema treatment
    - Halazone tablets – contains 25% available chlorine, used at household level
      - Dose: 1 tablet halazone (4 mg of halazone) for 1 L of water with contact time of 30-60 mins
      - Iodophors: release free iodine – which is broad spectrum disinfectant. Example: Povidine iodine
  - **Liquid disinfectants**
    - **Coal tar disinfectant**
      - Phenol: Not effective disinfectant
      - Crude phenol (phenyl) – phenol and cresol mixture – is an effective disinfectant

> **43 High Yield Points**
>
> Hot air is useful for
> - Glassware
> - Vaselines
> - Powders
> - Lab instrument
> - Media

> **44 High Yield Points**
>
> Lime is cheapest disinfectant for
> - Walls
> - Excreta disinfection
> - Cattle sheds
> - Animal houses

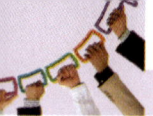

Must Remember
- Dettol-Chloroxylenol
- Hibitane-Chlorhexidine
- Cetavlon-Cetrimide
- Lysol-Saponified cresol

- Characteristic: dark brown oily liquid with characteristic smell
- **Dose:**
  - 10% for feces
  - 5% for mopping floors
- Cresol
  - Pure cresol
    - Characteristic: 10 times powerful than phenol, brown liquid which turns white on contact with liquid
    - Dose: 5-10% for feces and urine
  - Lysol: saponified cresol. Use: disinfect – hands clothes, general disinfectant
  - Izal: Special activity against salmonella. Used to disinfect stools and urine of typhoid patients
  - Cyllin: cresol emulsion. It is cheap and effective disinfectant for drains and latrines
  - Chlorocresol: Used as preservative for injections
- Hexachlorophene – chlorinated phenol
  - Uses: in soaps as antiseptic
- Chloroxylenol (Dettol) - Uses: Wounds and injuries. Active against streptococci, but against gram-negative bacteria
- Chlorhexidine (Hibitane) – used for
  - Hand wash as 0.5% Chlorhexidine
  - Burn creams and lotions as 1% chlorhexidine
  - Mouth washes and neonatal baths

- **Quaternary ammonia compounds**
  - Cetrimide (Cetavlon) – used as surface cleansing cum disinfectant. It has a soapy property and useful for wounds contaminated with dust (road side wounds) to remove dirt, grease, tar, blood
  - Savlon: combination of cetavlon and chlorhexidine – used for dirty wounds and clinical thermometers, plastic instruments
  - Zephiran – all-purpose disinfectant for irrigation of mucosal cavities, storage of surgical instruments, preoperative skin disinfectant
- **Iodine**
  - Broad spectrum germicidal with anti-bacterial, antifungal and anti-viral properties
  - Iodine forms of use
    - Tincture of iodine 2%, povidone-iodine – for wounds
    - Iodine solution for pre-operative antisepsis
    - Mandle's paint for sore throat
    - Tincture iodine add to water for emergency disinfection
- **Hydrogen peroxide**
  - Oxidizing agent – used for cleansing of the suppurative wounds and ulcers
- **Alcohol/Spirit**
  - Pure alcohol does not have disinfectant action.
  - In 60-80% concentration – act as disinfectant
- **Formalin**
  - It is 40% aqueous solution of formaldehyde gas
  - Used for
    - Disinfection of delicate articles as jewelry
    - Preservative for tissues in anatomy/pathology/histopathology

- **Gaseous disinfectant**
  - **Formaldehyde**
    - Obtained by boiling liquid formalin
    - It is highly inflammable, irritating, colorless and toxic gas
    - USES
      - Disinfection of rooms, OTs
      - Disinfection of books, clothes, blankets
  - **Ethylene Oxide**
    - It is highly inflammable, irritating, colorless and toxic gas

- It is not a disinfectant of choice because of hazardous properties
- **Uses:**
  - Disinfection of fabric, rubber, plastic and synthetic material
  - Hospital equipment as electronic, anesthetic, cardiac, diathermic, dental equipment
- **Sulfur dioxide**
  - Highly poisonous gas, lethal to most life forms
  - Used as insecticide and rodenticide

- **Miscellaneous disinfectants**
  - **Metal disinfectants**
    - **Silver –**
      - Exerts germicidal (caustic action) and antiseptic action by release of silver ions after interaction of silver with tissue proteins
      - Uses
        - Silver nitrate applicants for hypertrophied tonsils and aphthous ulcers
        - Bladder and urethra irrigation
        - Prophylaxis of ophthalmia neonatorum, gonococcal infections
        - Water disinfection in Katadyn filters.
    - **Mercury**
      - Release of mercury ions which get absorbed onto the surface of bacteria
      - Not very efficient disinfectant
  - **Disinfectant dyes**
    - Acridine dyes
      - Acriflavine bandages for burn dressings
    - Rosaline dyes
      - Is active against gram positive bacteria and fungi.
      - Maybe used as effective external application for prophylaxis of wound contamination
    - Fluorescein dyes
      - Used to detect corneal ulcers and abrasions

28 Must Remember

- Dettol is not active against gram-negative organisms.
- Cetrimide is cetavlon – soapy feel – used for hand wash
- Savlon – is combination of cetavlon and hibitane – used for OPD clinic instruments as thermometers
- Chlorhexidine (habitant) is powerful skin disinfectant
- Hypochlorite solution is powerful chlorine source and maybe used for water disinfection
- Iodine

Standardization of Disinfectants

- Rideal walker coefficient:
  - The standard for disinfection is taken as **Phenol**
  - The disinfectant properties are compared with phenol using salmonella typhi as the test organism. This is known as Carbolic coefficient or the Rideal walker coefficient (RW)
- Chick Martin coefficient
  - It is an improvisation of the RW coefficient – which gives an estimate for the germicidal action of the disinfectant in presence of organic material as yeast, fungi, excreta

Disinfection Procedures

- Feces and urine
  - Excreta to be collected in non-pervious vessel, equal amount of disinfectant to be added and allowed to stand for 2 hours
  - Disinfectants to be used are
    - 8% bleaching powder (50 gm fresh bleaching powder with 1 L of water)
    - 10% crude phenol (100 mL phenol to 1 L of water)
    - 5% cresol (50 mL to 1 L of water)
    - 10% formalin (100 mL formalin to 1 L of water)
  - Other procedures (in case of non-availability of disinfectants)
    - Excreta with equal amount of milk of lime (1 part of lime in 4 parts of water)
    - Add boiling water to feces – allowed to cool
  - Disinfection of bed pans
    - Steam disinfected followed by 2.5% cresol for 60 mins
    - Field/emergency situation: Burning cotton ball oaked in spirit
- Sputum
  - Receive in gauze/handkerchief - burning – most effective
  - Use 5% cresol with contact time of 1 hr – most effective for large amount sputum disinfection (from spittoons in TB wards)

45 High Yield Points

Disinfectant of choice:

- Feces, vomit: Phenol compounds – phenol, Lysol, 10% crude phenol (best), bleaching powder (household, local level)
- Sputum – burning (at patient level), 5% cresol, autoclave for 20 minutes at 20 lbs pressure
- OT rooms – 1% formaldehyde, chlorinated lime, 2.5% cresol.
- Skin disinfectant – iodine, povidone iodine (iodophor)
- Wounds – hydrogen peroxide (is virucidal, bactericidal, sporicidal, fungicidal), Dettol (Chloroxylenol)
- Cattle sheds, public toilets – lime (cheapest and also odorizer)

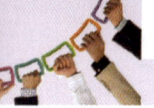

- OT/Isolation rooms
  - Mopping – 10% formalin or 2.5% cresol or 5% phenol – contact time 4 Hrs
  - Fumigation – boiling liquid formalin (500 mL formalin to 1 L water per 30 cu meter of space)
  - Spray of liquid formalin
- Linen/clothes/hospital clothes for patients
  - Soak in 2.5% cresol or 10% formalin or 5% phenol for 1 hr followed by washing with soap and water
- Leather/fur/delicate wool - formaldehyde gas
- Clinical thermometer – surgical spirit
- Paper, books, racks – hot air
- Utensils, crockery – immerse in 10% formalin or 2% Lysol for 10 mins followed by wash
- Needles and syringes
  - **Autoclave:** Hot air oven for 30-60 mins at 160 °C (preferred)
  - Immerse syringe along with needle in disinfectant liquid for 20 minutes

High Level Disinfection

Instruments as laryngoscopes, proctoscopes, vaginal specula should be sterilized before each use or atleast must undergo 'high level disinfection'

- Continuous boiling 20-30 mins – best and most reliable
- Exposure to vapors of ethylene oxide or formaldehyde

HOSPITAL ACQUIRED INFECTIONS (HAI)

Nosocomial infections: these are cross infections occurring in the hospitals, primarily due to the stay in hospital. The symptoms may manifest during the hospital stay (usually after 48 hours of admission) or after discharge. The prevalence of HAI is about 35% in India.

Causes

- Drug Resistance
- Overcrowding in hospitals
- Decreased resistance and higher susceptibility in the vulnerable groups

*Most common cause: staphylococci (55%), gram-negative bacilli (45%) as E. coli, Klebsiella, proteus, pseudomonas, salmonella, shigella

Types of HAI

- Urinary tract infections (most common)
- Lower respiratory tract infections
- Postoperative infections, wound infections
- Systemic infections, septicemia

> 46 *High Yield Points*
>
> Continuous boiling for 30 mins is the most effective form of high level disinfection

Sources of HAI

- From patients own flora
- From another patient
- From environment – air, surface, fomite

Prevention Strategies

- Regular health check for staff
- Care of patients
  - Chamber ward or isolation wards – partition from floor to ceiling with complete isolation of the patient
  - Cubicle wards: Partition extends from floor but not to ceiling, allowing cross ventilation
  - Open wards: General wards. Have highest predisposition for nosocomial infections
- Nursing
  - Barrier nursing – standard pre-exposure prophylaxis and prevention of cross infection by staff nurses

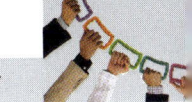

- Task nursing: special nursing staff for special work.
- Administrative planning
  - Formulation of hospital infection control committee consisting of Medical superintendent, head of departments, microbiologist, nursing superintendent, medical record officer and heads from other support services.

DISEASE DETERMINANTS

- The disease magnitude in the community will vary from region to region and with different age groups.
- The disease magnitude as public health problem may be classified as exotic, sporadic, endemic, epidemic or pandemic status

Sporadic	Scattered cases. Not epidemiologically linked in terms of time place or person	▪ Polio ▪ Tetanus ▪ Herpes zoster ▪ Rabies
Endemic	Constant presence of the disease among population, which is epidemiologically linked in time, person or (usually) place.	▪ Hepatitis ▪ Malaria ▪ Dengue ▪ Diarrhea
Epidemic	A rise (usually sudden) in number of cases which is clearly in excess and which is: ▪ More than 80% of expected frequency or ▪ Greater than 2 standard deviation	For any disease
Pandemic	When a disease usually spreads to global level or ▪ When it crosses two **WHO regions** or ▪ Two continents	▪ Influenza ▪ HIV and AIDS ▪ Severe Acute Respiratory Syndrome (SARS) ▪ The 2009 pandemic H1N1 influenza virus, 2014 Ebola Outbreak
Exotic	A disease which is typically **NOT** found in an area and is **ALWAYS** imported from another distinct area, or country	▪ Yellow fever/India ▪ Rabies/UK
Opportunistic	This is infection by an organism that takes the opportunity provided by a defect in host defense to infect the host and hence cause disease	▪ M. Tuberculosis ▪ Herpes simplex ▪ Toxoplasma

Endemic

Is constant presence (usual or expected frequency) of a disease or infectious agent in the population of a given geographic area.

- Infectious agent is not imported from outside.
- Endemic disease may turn into an epidemic if conditions are favorable. (e.g. Hepatitis A, Typhoid)
- Endemic disease may be eliminated if appropriate control or preventive measures are applied
- **Hyper endemic** refers to a persistent intense transmission in an area
- **Holoendemic** means a disease staring early in life and affecting most of the population

47 *High Yield Points*

Epidemic: It is a rise in number of cases, which is clearly in excess, which is:
- More than 80% of the expected frequency. Or
- More than two standard deviation from the average.

Epidemic

Is sudden and unusual occurrence of an illness/health related event in a population clearly *in excess of normal expectancy*. Epidemic threshold = Endemic frequency + 2 Standard Error.

Types of Epidemics

- **Point source epidemics**
  - Single exposure on "point source" epidemic.
    - All cases within one incubation period
    - Epidemic curve rises and falls rapidly
    - No secondary waves
    - Clustering of cases within narrow interval of time, e.g. Bhopal gas tragedy

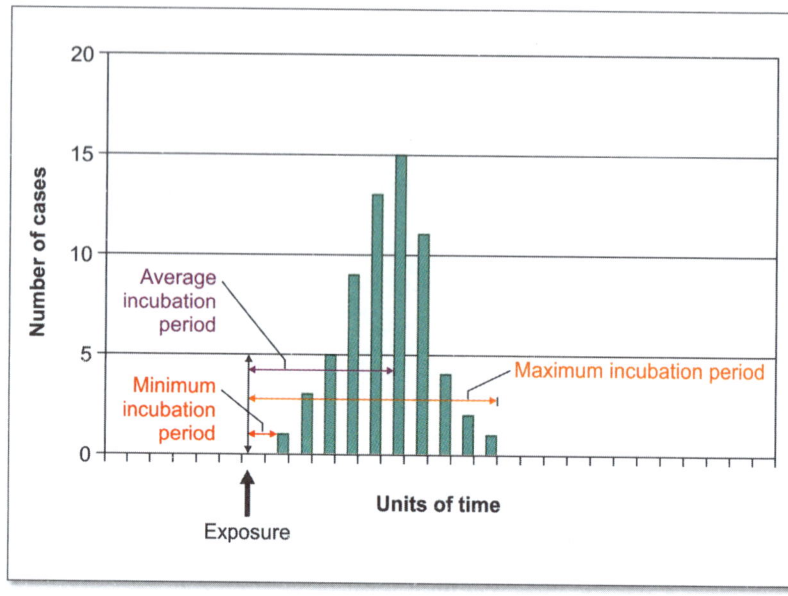

Fig. 3: Point source epidemics with no propagation

  - Continuous or multiple exposure from point source epidemic
    - Multiple exposures, hence leading to many cases over time.
    - Hyperendemicity of disease may be found and is a peculiar feature
    - Secondary waveforms (fluctuations in the disease frequency over long periods of time)

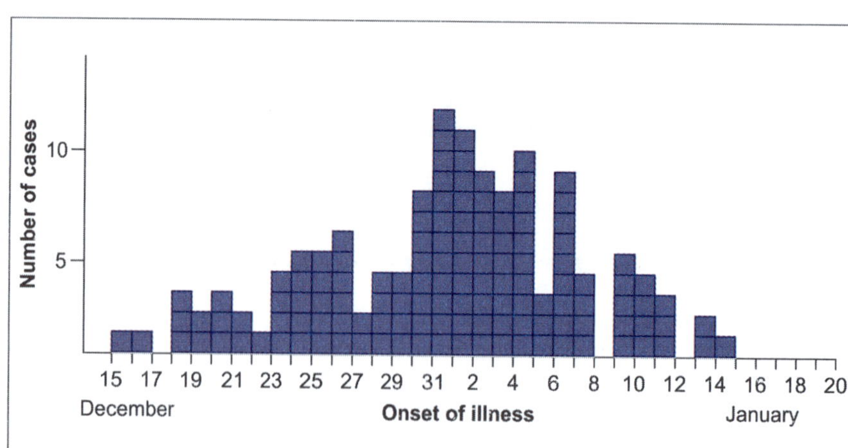

Fig. 4: Continuous or multiple exposure epidemics

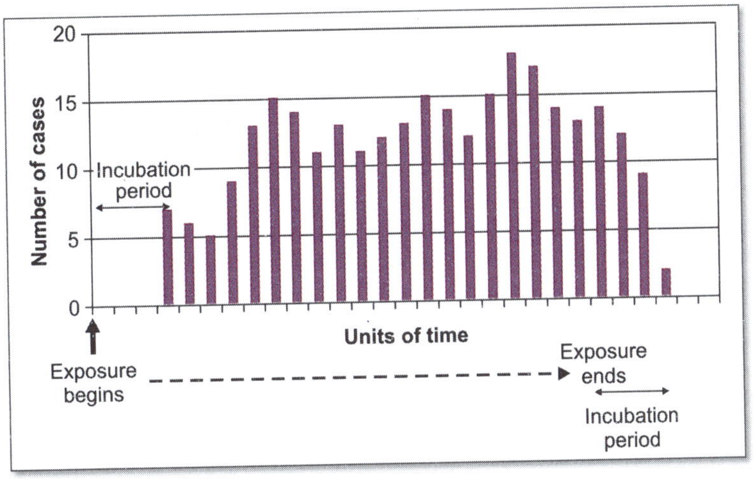

Fig. 5: Continuing source outbreak epidemic

- **Propagated epidemics**
  - Person-to-person
  - Arthropod vector
  - Animal reservoir
    - The disease will 'always' tend to increase in frequency overtime

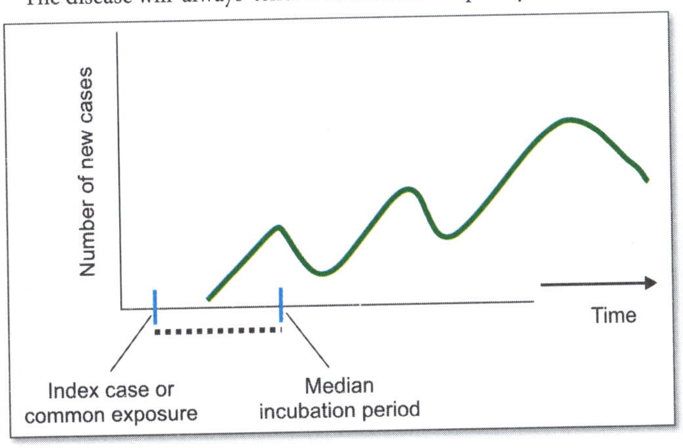

Fig. 6: Epidemic curve—propagated epidemic

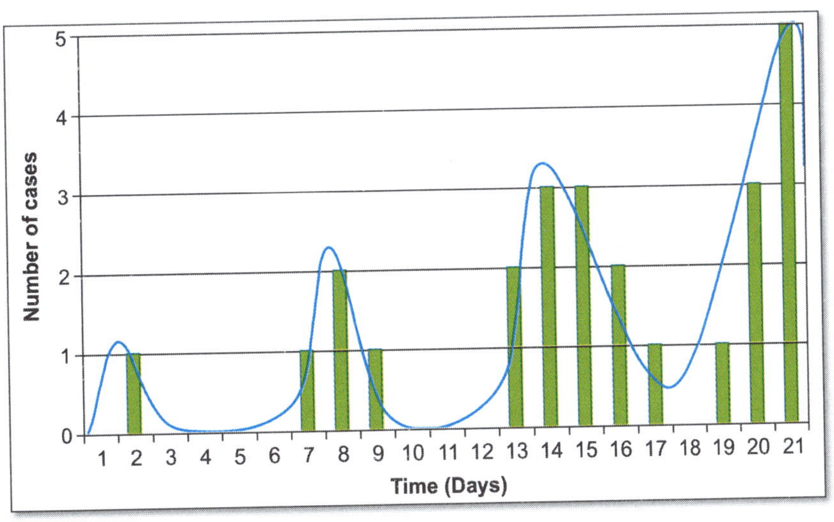

Fig. 7: Person-to-person epidemic

- **Slow (modern) epidemics** – is a slow growing epidemic, the term usually used specifically for noncommunicable disease as diabetes, obesity, cancer and so on.

Time-based Difference of Occurrence of Cases

- **Secular trend:** If the pattern or trend of disease frequency changes only over many years then it is called a secular trend.
- **Cyclic trend:** If the occurrence of disease changes over a short duration of time like a year, it is called a cyclic trend.
- Some diseases change in frequency over seasons and such changes are referred to as seasonal changes – Measles and chicken pox are examples of such diseases.

Summary of Epidemic Curves

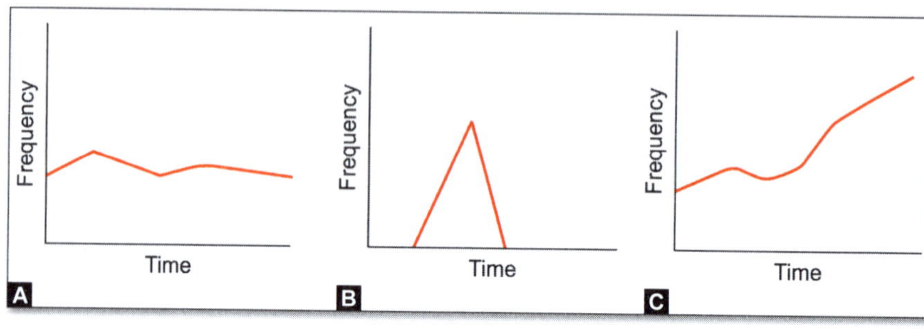

Figs 8A to C: Endemic versus epidemic. **A.** Endemic; **B.** Point epidemic; **C.** Propagating epidemic

Investigation of an Epidemic

- Verification of diagnosis
- Confirmation of existence of an epidemic
- Defining the population at risk
- Rapid search for all cases and their characteristics
- Data analysis – in terms of time, place, person
- Formulation of hypothesis
- Testing of hypothesis
- Evaluation of other social and ecological factors
- Further investigation of population at risk
- Report writing and dissemination of information.

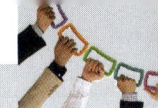

Multiple Choice Questions

1. **Which of the following is not a direct route for transmission of communicable diseases?**
   a. Skin contact
   b. Vertical
   c. Droplet nuclei
   d. Soil contact
2. **Susceptible person developed disease within range of IP after coming in contact with primary case. This is denoted by:** *(Recent Question 2018)*
   a. Secondary attack rate
   b. Case fatality rate
   c. Primary attack rate
   d. Tertiary attack rate
3. **In a case of epidemic, 3 villages are affected simultaneously with typhoid cases. Upon study it is found that one milk man is going to all these 3 villages. Identify the type of epidemic:** *(Recent Question 2017)*
   a. Point source
   b. Common source, propagative
   c. Common source, single exposure
   d. Common source, continuous exposure
4. **Hospital infection is known as:** *(Recent Question 2017)*
   a. Opportunistic infection
   b. Nosocomial infection
   c. Viral infection
   d. Health care infection
5. **In a village with population of 5000, 50 people have a disease and 10 of them died. What is case fatality rate:**
   a. 0.5% b. 1%
   c. 2% d. 20%
6. **The denominator in secondary attack rate:**
   a. Mid-year population
   b. Incidence of disease among exposed
   c. Number of person-weeks months or years of exposure
   d. Incidence of disease among non-exposed
7. **Cyclic trend is seen in:**
   a. Influenza b. Measles
   c. Kala-azar d. Malaria
8. **Specific mortality rate means:** *(Recent Question 2015)*
   a. Mortality are in a specific population during a specified time period
   b. Mortality rate from a specified cause for a population during a specified time period
   c. Percentage of cases of disease who succumb to that disease during a specified time period
   d. Ratio of observed deaths to expected deaths expressed as percentage
9. **The type of epidemic produced by a contaminated source of water is:** *(New Question 2015)*
   a. Common source single exposure epidemic
   b. Common source continuous exposure epidemic
   c. Seasonal trend epidemic
   d. Propagated epidemic
10. **Migration study is done to study the:**
    a. Diseases with long incubation period
    b. Prevalence of disease in a population
    c. Environmental and genetic factors in a disease in population
    d. Sociodemographic reasons for migration of a population
11. **Interval of time between the receipt of infection by a host and maximal infectivity of the host is called:** *(Recent Question 2016)*
    a. Serial interval
    b. Generation time
    c. Minimum incubation period
    d. Communicable period
12. **Infections transmitted from man to animals are known as:**
    a. Anthropozoonoses
    b. Zooanthroponoses
    c. Zoonoses
    d. Metazoonoses
13. **Time interval between receipt of infection and maximum infectivity of host:** *(Recent Question 2016)*
    a. Screening time
    b. Lead time
    c. Serial interval
    d. Generation time
14. **Shortest IP:**
    a. Diptheria b. Influenza
    c. Measles d. Dengue
15. **Generation time:** *(Recent Question 2015)*
    a. Time of infection to time of maximum infectivity
    b. Time of infection to time of clinical diagnosis
    c. Time of clinical diagnosis to resolution
    d. None
16. **The following are the disease frequencies in a population. Based on the number of cases which of the following is the correct match:**
    Disease 1: Number of cases last week 42 this week 43
    Disease 2: Number of cases last week 2 and present week 42
    Disease 3: Number of cases last week 6 and present week 1
    a. Endemic, epidemic, sporadic
    b. Endemic, sporadic, epidemic
    c. Sporadic, endemic, epidemic
    d. Pandemic, endemic, sporadic
17. **Secular trend is demonstrated by:**
    a. Line diagram
    b. Bar graph
    c. Stem-leaf plot
    d. Box and whisker plots
18. **Out of 50 people suffering from cholera in a population of 5000, 10 died. However total deaths are 50. What is the crude death rate:** *(Recent Question 2013)*
    a. 1 per 1000
    b. 5 per 1000
    c. 10 per 1000
    d. 20 per 100

Ans.

1. c
2. a
3. d
4. b
5. d
6. c
7. b
8. b
9. b
10. c
11. b
12. b
13. d
14. b
15. a
16. a
17. a
18. c

Most Recent Questions of 2019-18 are given at the end of MCQs

19. The number of cases among familial or institutional contacts occurring within the accepted incubation period following exposure to a primary case is called:
a. Attack rate b. Secondary attack rate
c. Infectivity d. Communicability

20. Secondary attack rate is measure of:
a. Pathogenicity b. Virulence
c. Morbidity d. Communicability

21. A couple has 4 children, all unvaccinated for measles. A child had measles on 5th Aug 2015. Two other children got measles on 15th Aug, 2015. Secondary Attack Rate is:
a. 0% b. 33%
c. 66% d. 75%

22. A party was attended by 110 people out of which 40 didn't eat fruit salad. From the rest who had salad, 55 developed food poisoning. What is the attack rate?
a. 46% b. 56%
c. 78% d. 50%

23. Measure of communicability of a disease:
a. Case fatality rate b. Secondary attack rate
c. Sullivan index d. Incubation period

24. The denominator in secondary attack rate:
a. Mid-year population
b. Incidence of disease among exposed
c. Incidence of disease among non-exposed
d. Number of person-weeks (months or years) of exposure

25. Specific mortality rate means:
a. Mortality are in a specific population during a specified time period
b. Mortality rate from a specified cause for a population during a specified time period
c. Percentage of cases of disease who succumb to that disease during a specified time period
d. Ratio of observed deaths to expected deaths expressed as percentage

26. The denominator in specific mortality rate is:
a. Number of cases
b. Mid-year population
c. Number of susceptible people in the population
d. Population at risk

27. Case fatality rate indicates: ***(Recent Question 2015)***
a. Infectivity of disease
b. Herd immunity of disease in community
c. Killing power of disease
d. Relative importance of disease in community

28. Hepatitis A epidemic in a community is an example of:
a. Common source, single exposure epidemic
b. Common source, continuous exposure epidemic
c. Propagated epidemic
d. Slow epidemic

29. A gradual progression in number of cases of non-communicable disease as compared to previous year is referred to as: ***(Recent Question 2015)***
a. Cyclic trend b. Periodic trend
c. Seasonal trend d. Secular trend

30. Increased occurrence of Road traffic accidents on weekends is described by which term: ***(Recent Question 2014)***
a. Cyclic trend b. Secular trends
c. Seasonal tends d. Transitional trends

31. The type of epidemic produced by a contaminated source of water is: ***(Recent Question 2014)***
a. Common source single exposure epidemic
b. Common source continuous exposure epidemic
c. Propagated epidemic
d. Seasonal trend epidemic

32. An outbreak of Viral hepatitis A was reported from a town between June and August. Of total cases, 60% occurred in July. Exposure of the community to infection is from:
a. Common single source for a short period
b. Common single source for a prolonged period
c. Multiple sources for a short period
d. Multiple sources for a prolonged period

33. An epidemic of Hepatitis A is an example of:
a. Common source, single exposure epidemic
b. Common source, continuous exposure epidemic
c. Propagated epidemic
d. Slow epidemic

34. All are true for Point source epidemic, except: ***(JIPMER 2014)(AIIMS Nov 2006)***
a. Epidemic curve rises and falls sharply
b. Clustering of cases within a short period of time
c. Person to Person transmission
d. All cases usually develop within one incubation period

35. Influenza pandemic is:
a. Short term fluctuation b. Long term fluctuation
c. Cyclic trend d. Seasonal trend

36. Emporiatrics is a science dealing with:
a. Health of travellers ***(Recent Question 2013)***
b. Occupational health
c. Making, new drugs
d. Genetic disease frequency

37. Pandemic is defined as: ***(Recent Question 2013)***
a. Endemic in small population
b. Endemic in large population
c. Epidemic in small population
d. Epidemic is large population

38. Regarding point source epidemic false statement(s) is/are:
a. Rapid rise and fall ***(Recent Question 2013)***
b. Only infectious disease can cause
c. Explosive
d. Cases occur even after incubation period
e. No secondary wave

39. Migration study is done to study the:
a. Sociodemographic reasons for migration of a population
b. Prevalence of disease in a population
c. Environmental and genetic factors in a disease in population
d. Diseases with long incubation period

40. Interval between the entry of disease agent and the onset of first clinical symptom is: ***(Recent Question 2013)***
a. Incubation period b. Window period
c. Generation time d. External incubation period

41. An outbreak of disease in bird population in called:
a. Enzootic b. Epizootic
c. Epornithic d. Exotic

42. Epornithic is defined as: ***(Recent Question 2013)***
a. Endemic in animals b. Epidemic in animals
c. Endemic in birds d. Epidemic in birds

Ans.

19.	b
20.	d
21.	c
22.	c
23.	b
24.	d
25.	b
26.	b
27.	c
28.	c
29.	d
30.	a
31.	b
32.	d
33.	a
34.	c
35.	c
36.	a
37.	d
38.	b
39.	c
40.	a
41.	c
42.	d

Most Recent Questions of 2019-18 are given at the end of MCQs

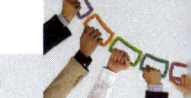

43. A person, animal or object or substance from which an infectious agent passes or is disseminated to the host is called as: ***(Recent Question 2013)***
a. Source b. Reservoir
c. Case d. Carrier

44. The host does not shed the infectious agent which lies dormant within the host without symptoms. This is an example of: ***(Recent Question 2013)***
a. Suspect case
b. Subclinical case
c. Index case
d. Latent infection

45. Interval of time between the receipt of infection by a host and maximal infectivity of the host is called:
a. Serial interval
b. Generation time
c. Communicable period
d. Minimum incubation period

46. All the following are modes of direct transmission, except:
a. Droplet infection b. Droplet nuclei
c. Contact with soil d. Trans placental

47. An example of cyclo-propagative transmission is:
a. Plague b. Malaria
c. Filarial d. Rabies

48. Zoonoses transmitted by invertebrate hosts are called as:
a. Ampixenoses b. Sapro-zoonoses
c. Meta-zoonoses d. Cyclo-zoonoses

49. Nosocomial infections are those which develop:
a. Within 24 hours after hospitalization
b. Within 48 hours of hospitalization
c. After 48 hours of hospitalization
d. After 7 days of hospitalization

50. Hospital infection is known as: ***(Recent Question 2013)***
a. Opportunistic infection
b. Nosocomial infection
c. Viral infection
d. Health care infection

51. Window period is the time taken from:
a. Entry of virus in cell to expulsion of first viral particle
b. Entry of pathogen to time of maximum communicability
c. Entry of pathogen to appearance of first clinical symptom
d. Exposure to laboratory detection of disease

52. Quarantine is not required for cases suffering from which of the following disease? ***(Recent Question 2013)***
a. Avian flu
b. Ebola virus disease
c. Infectious TB
d. Tetanus

53. Organism is multiplying and developing in the host is called: ***(Recent Question 2013)***
a. Cyclopropagative
b. Cyclodevelopmental
c. Developmental
d. Propagative

54. Indirect mode of transmission is:
a. Hand contact b. Via placenta
c. Vector borne d. Dog bite

55. Most common route of spread of nosocomial infection is:
a. Direct contact
b. Indirect contact
c. Droplet transmission
d. Vehicle transmission

56. Serial interval is:
a. Time gap between primary and secondary case
b. Time gap between index and primary case
c. Time taken for a person from receipt of infection to develop maximum infectivity
d. The time taken from infection till a person infects another person

57. First case that comes to notice of a physician is:
a. Primary case b. Secondary case
c. Index case d. Refer case

58. Interval between primary and secondary case is called:
a. Generation time b. Serial interval
c. Incubation period d. Lead time

59. Time interval between receipt of infection by a host and maximum infectivity of that host is known as:
a. Generation time
b. Incubation period
c. Serial interval
d. Secondary attack rate

60. Time between infection and maximum infectivity is known as: ***(Recent Question 2013)***
a. Incubation period
b. Serial interval
c. Generation time
d. Communicable period

61. Chronic carrier state is seen in: ***(Recent Question 2013)***
a. Poliomyelitis b. Measles
c. Malaria d. Tetanus

62. Vectors do not transmit infection by:
a. Ingestion
b. Regurgitation
c. Rubbing of Faeces
d. Contamination with body fluids

63. Most cost effective method of infection control is:
a. Repeated disinfectant use
b. Alcohol based rubbing
c. Prophylactic antibiotic therapy
d. Hand washing

64. Some medicine come with a label of 'store at a cool place only'. At what temperature should these medicines be kept:
a. 8–15°C b. 2–8°C
c. 0°C d. 25–28°C

65. All of the following are correct regarding period of isolation, except: ***(Recent Question 2013)***
a. Measles – Up to 3 days of onset of rash
b. Chicken pox – Up to 6 days of onset of rash
c. Herpes zoster – Up to 6 days of onset of rash
d. Rubella – until 7 days after appearance of rash

66. Isolation is useful for:
a. Hepatitis A b. Diphtheria
c. Typhoid d. Cholera
e. Poliomyelitis

Ans.

43.	a
44.	d
45.	b
46.	b
47.	b
48.	c
49.	c
50.	b
51.	d
52.	d
53.	a
54.	c
55.	a
56.	a
57.	c
58.	b
59.	a
60.	c
61.	c
62.	a
63.	d
64.	a
65.	d
66.	a, b, d, e

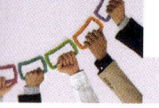

67. **Quarantine period should be:** *(Recent Question 2013)*
   a. Minimum incubation period
   b. Maximum incubation period
   c. Period of communicability
   d. Median incubation period
68. **Application of incubation period is all, except:**
   a. To differentiate primary case from secondary case
   b. To find out time for isolation
   c. To find out time for quarantine
   d. To prevent infection to the contacts of the infected person

ZOONOSES

69. **Metazoonosis include:** *(Recent Question 2013)*
   a. Plague b. Rabies
   c. Schistosomiasis d. Brucellosis
   e. Yellow fever
70. **Plague is:** *(Recent Question 2013)*
   a. Cyclozoonosis b. Direct zoonosis
   c. Saprozoonosis d. Metazoonosis
71. **Zoonotic diseases include:** *(Recent Question 2013)*
   a. Plague b. Rabies
   c. Anthrax d. Tetanus
   e. Brucellosis
72. **Which of the following is an arthropod-borne disease:**
   a. Tetanus b. Q Fever
   c. Scrub typhus d. Rabies
73. **Which of the following is a zoonotic disease?**
   a. Hydatid cyst b. Malaria
   c. Filariasis d. Dengue fever
74. **Zoonotic disease transmitted by arthropods is/are:**
   a. Plague b. Melioidosis
   c. Rabies d. Leishmaniasis
   e. Anthrax
75. **Zoonotic disease of viral etiology include:**
   a. Q fever *(Recent Question 2013)*
   b. Rickettsial disease
   c. Rabies
   d. Rubella
76. **Susceptible persons who developed disease within range of IP after coming in contact with primary case is known as:**
   a. Case fatality rate b. Secondary attack rate
   c. Primary attack rate d. Tertiary attack rate
77. **Which of the following is not an example of direct transmission in communicable diseases?**
   a. Transplacental b. Droplet nuclei
   c. Soil d. STDs
78. **The cycle of yellow fever virus in Aedes is:**
   a. Propagative b. Cyclopropagative
   c. Cyclodevelopmental d. Any of the above
79. **In a village with population of 5000, 50 people have a disease and 10 of them died. What is case fatality rate?**
   a. 1% b. 2%
   c. 0.5% d. 20%

DISABILITY RATES

80. **In a village with population of 5000, 50 people have a disease and 10 of them died. What is case fatality rate?**
   a. 1% b. 2%
   c. 0.5% d. 20%

Most Recent Questions (2019-2018)

81. **A healthy center reports 40 to 50 cases in a week in the community. This week there are 48 cases normally. This is called:** *(AIIMS Nov 2018)*
   a. Epidemic
   b. Sporadic
   c. Endemic
   d. Outbreak
82. **True about Elimination of disease:** *(PGI May 2018)*
   a. This is a stage b/w control and eradication
   b. It has an element of area association
   c. Complete interruption of disease transmission
   d. Incomplete interruption of disease transmission
   e. Agent is absent but vector is present

Ans.

67. b
68. b
69. a, c, e
70. d
71. a, b, c, d
72. c
73. a
74. a, c, d
75. c
76. b
77. b
78. a
79. d
80. d
81. c
82. a, b, d

Answers with Explanations

1. Ans. (c) Droplet nuclei

Direct transmission	Indirect transmission
Direct contact	Vehicle borne
Droplet infection	Vector borne ▪ Mechanical ▪ Biological
Soil contact	Air borne ▪ Droplet nuclei ▪ Dust
Inoculation into skin	Fomite borne
Transplacental	Unclean hands, fingers

2. Ans. (a) Secondary attack rate

3. Ans. (d) Common source, continuous exposure

Ref: K. Park, 24th ed. p 69

4. Ans. (b) Nosocomial infection

Ref: K. Park, 24th ed. p 99

5. Ans. (d) 20%

Ref: K. Park, 24th ed. p 25

CFR = Number of deaths due to a particular case/total cases of the same disease * 100

Hence, CFR = 10/50 * 100

= 20%

6. Ans. (c) Number of person-weeks months or years of exposure

Ref: K. Park, 24th ed. p 105

7. Ans. (b) Measles

Ref: K. Park, 24th ed. p 70

8. Ans. (b) Mortality rate from a specified cause for a population during a specified time period

Ref: K. Park, 24th ed. p 62

9. Ans. (b) Common source continuous exposure epidemic

Ref: K. Park, 24th ed. p 69

10. Ans. (c) Environmental and genetic factors in a disease in population

Ref: K. Park, 24th ed. p 72

11. Ans. (b) Generation time

Ref: K. Park, 24th ed. p 105

12. Ans. (b) Zooanthroponoses

Ref: K. Park, 24th ed. p 99

13. Ans. (d) Generation time

Ref: K. Park, 24th ed. p 105

14. Ans. (b) Influenza

Ref: K. Park, 24th ed. p 164

15. Ans. (a) Time of infection to time of maximum infectivity

Ref: K. Park, 24th ed. p 105

16. Ans. (a) Endemic, epidemic, sporadic

Ref: K. Park, 24th ed. p 98

17. Ans. (a) Line diagram

Ref: K. Park, 24th ed. p 71, 883

Secular trend refers to progressive increase (Lung cancer in developed countries) or decrease (TB, Polio in developed countries) in occurrence of disease over a long period of time (years or decades).

- There is a consistent tendency to move in a particular direction with passage of time.

Line diagram is used to show the trend of events with passage of time and can best demonstrate Secular trend.

18. Ans. (c) 10/1000

Ref: K. Park, 24th ed. p 24

CDR = Total deaths in a population in/mid-year population* 1000

= 50/5000 * 1000

= 10 per 1000

19. Ans. (b) Secondary attack rate

Ref: K. Park, 24th ed. p 105

Secondary attack rate is defined as the number of exposed persons developing the disease within the range of the incubation period following exposure to a primary case.

- It is a special incidence rate
- Primary case is excluded from both numerator and denominator.
- Limitation → applicable to diseases where primary case is infective for a short period only (e.g., measles and chickenpox) and identification of "susceptible" is possible.
- Used to evaluate the effectiveness of control measures such as isolation and immunization.

20. Ans. (d) Communicability

Ref: K. Park, 24th ed. p 105

Communicable period is time during which an infectious agent may be transferred directly or indirectly from an infected person to another person, from an infected animal to man, or from an infected person to an animal, including arthropods

- Communicability of some diseases can be reduced by early diagnosis and treatment.
- Time of maximum communicability may precede or follow the incubation period.
- Secondary attack rate is measure of Communicability

21. Ans. (c) 66%

Ref: K Park, 24th ed. p 105

Secondary attack rate [SAR]

$$= \frac{\text{No. of exposed persons developing the disease within the range of incubation period}}{\text{Total number of exposed susceptible contacts}} \times 100$$

$= 2/3 \times 100 = 66\%$

22. Ans. (c) 78

Ref: K Park, 24th ed. p 66

$$\text{Attack rate} = \frac{\text{Number of new cases of a specific disease in a specified time interval}}{\text{Total population at risk during the same time interval}} \times 100$$

$= 55/70 \times 100 = 78\%$

23. Ans. (b) Secondary attack rate

Ref: K. Park, 24th ed. p 105

Secondary attack rate is a measure of communicability of a disease

Also Know.......................

CFR represents the killing power of a disease[Q] and is closely related to virulence of the organism.[Q]
Sullivan's index is expectation of life free from disability[Q]
***Virulence** is the proportion of clinical cases that develop severe clinical manifestations (including sequelae).*
Pathogenicity of an infectious agent is the ability to induce clinically apparent illness

24. Ans. (d) Number of person-weeks (months or years) of exposure

Ref: K. Park, 24th ed. p 105

Denominator in secondary attack rate is duration of exposure, if the primary case is infective for a longer period of time (e.g., Tuberculosis).

SAR = [Number of contacts developing tuberculosis/Number of person -weeks (months or years) of exposure] × 100

25. Ans. (b) Mortality rate from a specified ...

Ref: K. Park, 24th ed. p 62

Specific Mortality Rate Means

- Mortality from a specific cause **or** disease (e.g., Tuberculosis, Cancer, Accident) in a population during a specified time period.
- Mortality in a specific subgroups (e.g., Age-specific, Sex-specific, Age and Sex specific) of the population during a specified time period

It helps identify etiology and groups "at risk" for preventive action

Also Know.......................

- Specific mortality rates is applicable in countries with a satisfactory civil registration system or high proportion medically certified deaths.

26. Ans. (b) Mid-year population

Ref: K. Park, 24th ed. p 62

27. Ans. (c) Killing power of disease

Ref: K. Park, 24th ed. p 63

Case fatality rate (Ratio) or CFR =

$$\frac{\text{Total number of deaths due to a particular disease}}{\text{Total number of cases of the same disease}} \times 100$$

- CFR represents the killing power of a disease[Q] and is closely related to virulence of the organism.[Q]
- It is expressed in percentage
- In CFR time interval is not specified. [Q]
- CFR is mostly used for acute infectious diseases (e.g., food poisoning, cholera, and measles).[Q]
- CFR for the same disease may vary in different epidemics (Alteration in agent, host and environment)
- CFR= 1- Survival rate.

28. Ans. (c) Propagated epidemic

Ref: K. Park 24th ed. p 70

Propagated Epidemic:- Salient Features

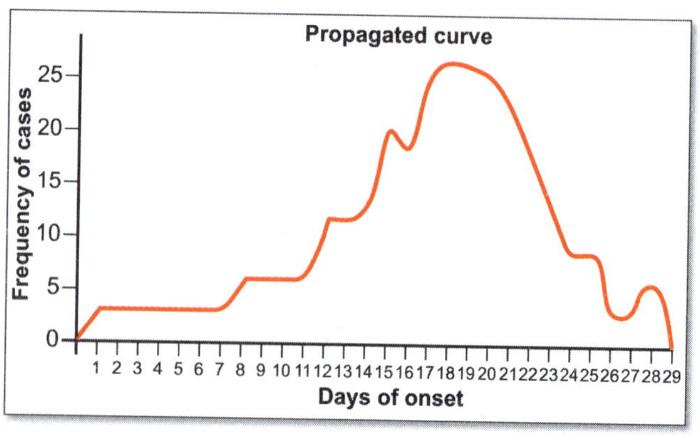

- It is most often of infectious origin involving **person-to-person transmission** of an infectious agent (e.g. epidemics of hepatitis A, Poliomyelitis).

- Epidemic shows a gradual rise, reaches a flat plateau and then declines slowly over a much longer period of time.
- Transmission continues until number of susceptible is depleted or susceptible individuals are no longer exposed to infected persons or intermediary vectors.
- Speed of spread depends upon herd immunity, opportunities for contact and secondary attack rate.

Also Know........................

- Propagated epidemics occur when there is a aggregation of susceptible or new susceptible individuals (e.g., birth, immigrants) are added to population lowering herd immunity.

- **Examples:** Droplet infections like Diphtheria, Mumps, Measles; Vector borne diseases like Malaria, JE and Dengue

29. Ans. (d) Secular trend

Ref: K. Park, 24th ed. p 70

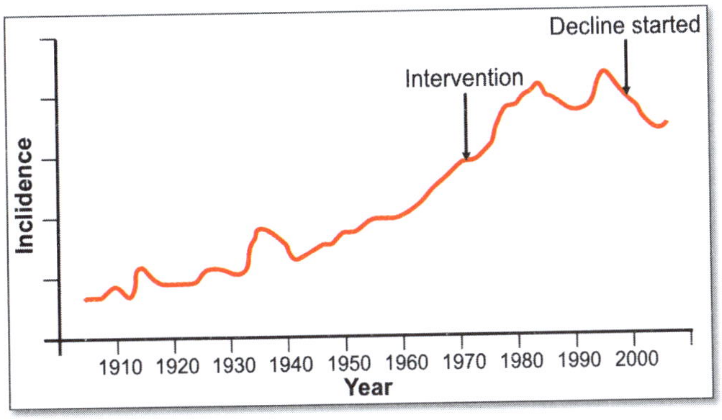

Also Know........................

- Secular trend is characterized by a consistent tendency to change in a particular direction or a definite movement in one direction.

30. Ans. (a) Cyclic trend

Ref: K. Park, 24th ed. p 70

Cyclic trend *refers to* occurrence of a disease/event in cycles spread over short period of time (i.e. Days, Week, Month, Year)

- In case of infectious diseases, it is due to build -up of susceptible in the "herd".
- Measles (every 2-3 years) in pre vaccination era) Rubella (every 6-9 years), Influenza pandemics (7-10 years due to antigenic variations).
- Influenza pandemics occur at intervals of 7 -10 years due to antigenic variations.
- Non-infectious conditions may also show cyclic trend e.g., Road accidents on week-ends (Saturdays).
- Seasonal trend is due to favourable environmental conditions (e.g., Temperature, Humidity, Rainfall etc.).
- Both infectious (Measles, Varicella in early spring, ARI in winter, GI infection in summer) and noninfectious (sunstroke, hay fever, snakebite) disease show seasonal trend.

31. Ans. (b) Common source continuous exposure epidemic

Ref: K. Park, 24th ed. p 69

Common Source Continuous Exposure Epidemic

- Exposure to source is prolonged - continuous, repeated or intermittent.
- Infectious agent persists in the common vehicle for some amount of time.
- Decline of epidemic is either because causative agent is removed or else all "susceptible" have become infected.
- E.g. Contamination of surface/ground or piped water with human excreta, as in infectious hepatitis/cholera, or food borne typhoid fever outbreaks due to carriers or contaminated tinned foods.
- No explosive rise in number of cases. Epidemic curve rises slowly and falls gradually. Peak is not sharp but plateau like
- Epidemics are more extended or irregular beyond one incubation period
- No evidence of secondary cases in contacts of ill persons.

32. Ans. (d) Multiple sources for a prolonged period

Ref: K. Park, 24th ed. p 69

Incubation period of Hepatitis A is 15-45 days. Here the cases were reported over a period of three months (i.e. Beyond one incubation period), hence common source single exposure and exposure for a short period are ruled out.

33. Ans. (a) Common source, continuous exposure epidemic

Ref: K. Park, 24th ed. p 69

Type of epidemic →	Point source epidemic	Continuous epidemic	Propagated epidemic
▪ Example	▪ Bhopal gas tragedy, ▪ Minamata disease Japan ▪ Chernobyl tragedy ▪ Food poisoning	▪ A prostitute and gonorrhea outbreak ▪ A well of contaminated water ▪ Legionnaire's disease (Philadelphia: USA)	▪ Epidemics of hepatitis A ▪ Epidemics of polio

34. Ans. (c) Person to Person transmission

Ref: K. Park, 24th ed. p 69

Epidemic is the sudden and unusual occurrence of cases of a disease or health event in a population in excess of normal expectancy

- Normal expectancy is average number of cases of a disease/ health event in previous 3-5 years in the population of a geographic area.
- If the normal expectancy is Zero- A single case occurrence will be a epidemic E.g. Yellow Fever (New) or Small pox (eradicated disease) in India

Also Know......................

- Epidemic is also measured as number of cases in excess of mean +2SD

Common Source Single (or Point source) Exposure Epidemic

- Exposure to disease agent is brief and simultaneous[Q] (Single one time exposure).
- Epidemic curve shows rapid rise and sharp fall.(one peak with no secondary waves) [Q]
- Epidemic shows clustering of cases in short interval of time (explosive occurrence[Q]).
- All the cases occur within one incubation period of disease.[Q]
- Mostly (not always) due to exposure to an infectious agent.

Common Source Continuous or Repeated Exposure Epidemic (explained earlier)

35. Ans. (c) Cyclic trend

Ref: K. Park, 24th ed. p 70

36. Ans. (a) Health of travelers

Ref: R Sushma et al, Iranian Journal of Public Health, 2012; 41(3): 133

Travel Medicine or Emporiatrics is the branch of medicine that deals with the prevention and management of health problems of international travelers.

- Preventive strategies are chosen without adding unnecessary adverse effects, cost or inconvenience
- It is offered before the travel
- It comprises – medical examination, screening, psychological preparation, provision of a medical kit, first aid training,

37. Ans. (d) Epidemic is large population

Ref: K. Park, 24th ed. p 98

Pandemic is an epidemic affecting a large proportion of population, over a wide geographic area (Entire nation/ continent/globally)

- ***Sporadic is*** *irregular, infrequent or haphazard occurrence of disease from time to time at different places with little or no connection to each other and no recognizable infection source*
- **Epidemic** is sudden and unusual occurrence of an illness/ health related event in a population clearly *in excess of normal expectancy*
- ***Endemic*** *is constant presence (usual or expected frequency) of a disease or infectious agent in the population of a given geographic area*

38. Ans. (b) Only infectious disease can cause (d) Cases occur even after incubation period

Ref: K. Park, 24th ed. p 69

39. Ans. (c) Environmental and genetic factors...

Ref: K. Park, 24th ed. p 72

Migration Studies evaluate the role of possible genetic and environmental factors in occurrence of disease in a population

40. Ans. (a) Incubation period

Ref: K. Park, 24th ed. p 104

Incubation period [IP] *is the time interval between invasion by an infectious agent and appearance of 1st sign/symptom.*[Q]

- *Median incubation period is time required for 50 % of the cases to occur following exposure.*[Q]
- *Factors determining IP are - Generation time of pathogen, Infective dose, Portal of entry and Individual susceptibility.*[Q]
- *Length of the incubation period is characteristic of each disease.*

Also Know......................

- *Latent period is equivalent of incubation period in Non infectious diseases.*[Q]

41. Ans. (c) Epornithic

Ref: K. Park, 24th ed. p 99

- An outbreak (epidemic) of disease in a bird population is referred to as **Epornithic**.
- An outbreak (epidemic) of disease in animal population (likely to affect human) is referred to as **Epizootic**
- Endemic disease in animals (e.g., anthrax, rabies, brucellosis, bovine tuberculosis etc.) is referred to as Enzootic

Also Know......................

- Zoonosis are diseases/infections that are naturally transmitted between vertebrate animal and man. It may be Epizootic or Enzootic.

42. Ans. (d) Epidemic in birds

Ref: K. Park, 24th ed. p 99

43. Ans. (a) Source

Ref: K. Park, 24th ed. p 99

Source is a person, animal, object or substance from which an infectious agent passes or is disseminated to the host

Reservoir is a person, animal, arthropod, plant, soil or substance in which an infectious agent lives and multiplies to be transmitted to a susceptible host.

Also Know......................

- Reservoir is the natural habitat in which the organism metabolizes and replicates. Source may or may not be a part of reservoir.

44. Ans. (d) Latent infection

Ref: K. Park, 24th ed. p 100

Latent infection is a state in which infectious agent lies dormant inside host without symptoms and without demonstrable presence in blood, tissues or body secretions of the host.

- **Example:** Herpes simplex, Brill-Zinsser disease, infections due to slow viruses

45. Ans. (b) Generation time

Ref: K. Park, 24th ed. p 105

Generation time *is the time interval between receipt of infection by a host and maximal infectivity of that host.*

Also Know.....................

- It is equivalent to the incubation period in infection that mostly result in sign and symptoms (not subclinical infection)

46. Ans. (b) Droplet nuclei

Ref: K. Park, 23rd ed. p 96 Refer to Annexure-3.1; 24th ed. p 101

47. Ans. (b) Malaria

Ref: K. Park, 24th ed. p 103

Modes of transmission of arthropod borne disease

- Direct contact: e.g. Scabies,Pediculosis
- Mechanical transmission: e.g. house fly transmitted disease
- Biological
  - **Cyclodevelopmental:** Infectious agent undergoes **o**nly development, no multiplication. E.g. Microfilaria in mosquito, Guinea worm in Cyclops
  - **Cyclopropogative:** Infectiousagent multiplies and also changes in form. E.g. Malaria in mosquito
  - **Propogative:** Infectious agent only multiplies, with no changes in form. E.g. Plague in rat flea, yellow fever in mosquito
- *Transovarian: Infectious agent is transmitted vertically from infected female to her progeny in the vector. E.g. Ticks transmitting Rickettsial disease.*
- *Transstadial: Infectious agent is transmitted from one stage of life cycle to another. E.g. Nymph to adult in ticks.*

48. Ans. (c) Metazoonoses

Ref: K. Park, 24th ed. p 294

Metazoonoses are zoonoses transmitted by invertebrate vectors. The agent multiplies/develops or both in invertebrate host before being transmitted to a vertebrate host after an extrinsic incubation (prepatent) period.

- E.g. Arbovirus infections, plague, schistosomiasis.

Cyclozoonoses are zoonoses that need more than one vertebrate host (But no invertebrate host), to complete developmental cycle of the disease agent.

- E.g. human taeniases, echinococcosis, and pentastomid infections.

Saprozoonoses have both a vertebrate host and a nonanimal developmental site or reservoir (Organic matter, soil, plants)

- E.g. larva migrants, mycoses

Direct zoonoses are transmitted from an infected vertebrate host to a susceptible vertebrate host by direct contact, by a fomite or by a mechanical vector. There is no propagative or developmental change in the agent during transmission.

- E.g. Rabies, trichinosis, and brucellosis.

49. Ans. (c) After 48 hours of hospitalization

Ref: K. Park, 24th ed. p 99

Nosocomial or Hospital acquired infections:

- *Infections acquired during hospital care (i.e. minimum after 48 hours of stay post admission)*
- *Such infection are not present or incubating at admission..*

50. Ans. (b) Nosocomial infection

Ref: K. Park, 24th ed. p 99

51. Ans. (d) Exposure to laboratory detection of disease

Ref: K. Park, 24th ed. p 365

"Window period" is the time period between exposure to infection and the time till the person tests positive on standard antibody blood test.

Also Know.....................

- HIV infected person is infectious in the window period because of the high concentration of virus in the blood.

52. Ans. (d) Tetanus

Ref: K. Park, 23rd ed. p 120-21, CDC http://www.cdc.gov/quarantine; 24th ed p129-30

Quarantine Applies to

- Cholera
- Diphtheria
- Infectious Tuberculosis
- Plague
- Smallpox
- Yellow fever
- Viral hemorrhagic fevers (Marburg, Ebola, and Congo-Crimean)
- SARS (Severe Acute Respiratory Syndromes).

Yellow fever vaccine→India and most countries require a valid certificate of vaccination against yellow fever from travellers coming from infected areas. India requires this even if the traveller has been in transit and vaccination of infants too.

Validity of certificate begins 10 days after the date of vaccination and extends up to 10 years.[Q]

53. Ans. (a) Cyclopropogative

Ref: K. Park, 24th ed. p 103

54. Ans. (c) Vector borne

Ref: K. Park, 24th ed. p 101

Indirect transmission–Infectious agent survives outside human host in external environment, retain its pathogenesis and virulence till it finds a new host

55. Ans. (a) Direct contact

Ref: K. Park, 23rd ed. p 360

56. Ans. (a) Time gap between primary and secondary case

Ref: K. Park, 24th ed. p 105

Serial interval *is the gap in time between onset of primary case and secondary case.*

- *It helps us to calculate the incubation period of disease.*

Also Know........................

- **Primary case** is the first case of disease to occur in a population. It may or may not come to notice of a physician.
- **Secondary case** in one that develops from contact with a primary case

57. Ans. (c) Index case

Ref: K. Park, 24th ed. p 100

58. Ans. (b) Serial interval

Ref: K. Park, 24th ed. p 105

59. Ans. (a) Generation time

Ref: K. Park, 24th ed. p 105

60. Ans. (c) Generation time

Ref: K. Park, 24th ed. p 105

61. Ans. (c) Malaria

Ref: K. Park, 24th ed. p 101

A carrier is an infected person or animal, that harbors a infectious agent in absence of discernible clinical disease and serves as a potential source of infection for others.

Chronic carriers excrete infectious agent (intermittently or continuously) for varying length or indefinite period.

- *Eg. Typhoid fever, Hepatitis B, Dysentery, Cerebrospinal meningitis, Malaria, Gonorrhea*

Also Know........................

- Carriers are more important sources of infection than cases. They often reintroduce disease into infection free areas.

Measles → only source of infection is a case of measles. Carriers are not known to occur
Polio → Sub clinical cases are important. No chronic carriers exist.

Also Know........................

- **Pseudocarrier** - are carriers of avirulent organism

62. Ans. (a) Ingestion

Ref: K. Park, 24th ed. p 103

Vector is an arthropod or carrier (e.g., snail) that serves as a vehicle for transmission of infectious agent to a susceptible host

- *Vector-borne diseases are Malaria, Filaria, JE, Dengue, Chikungunya, Kala-azar*

Also Know........................

Salient features of vector borne transmission:

- Transmission may be mechanical or biological
- Host is infected by biting, regurgitation, scratching-in of infective faeces or contamination with body fluids of vector
- Factors influencing ability of vectors to transmit disease are:
  - Host feeding preferences
  - Infectivity
  - Susceptibility (Ability to get infected)
  - Survival rate of vectors
  - Domesticity, i.e. degree of association with man
  - Suitable environmental factors.

63. Ans. (d) Hand washing

Ref: http://www.un.org/andUnicefwww.unicef.org

Hand washing with soap is among the most effective and inexpensive ways to avert child deaths

- It reduces the risk of diarrhea by 50%, pneumonia by 25% in Under 5 Children and levels of school absenteeism by 20–50%.

October 15 marks Global Handwashing Day

64. Ans. (a) 8-15°C

Ref: Guidelines for the Storage of Essential Medicines and Other Health Commodities, WHO

Storage Guidelines of Essential Medicines

- **Store frozen**: Storage at -20°C (4°F). Frozen storage is normally for longer-term storage at higher-level facilities.
- **Store at 2°-8°C (36°-46°F)**: Products are very heat sensitive but must not be frozen. Usually kept in the 1st and 2nd part of refrigerator (never the freezer). This temperature is appropriate for storing vaccines for a short period of time.
- **Keep cool**: Store between 8°-15°C (45°-59°F).
- **Store at room temperature**: Store at 15°-25°C (59°-77°F).
- **Store at ambient temperature**: Store in a dry, clean, well ventilated area at room temperatures 15° to 25°C (59°-77°F) or up to 30°C, depending on climatic conditions.

65. Ans. (d) Rubella – until 7 days after appearance of rash

Ref: K. Park, 24th ed. p 129

Isolation is separation of infected persons or animals from others in such places and under such conditions for the period of communicability to prevent direct or indirect transmission of infectious agent from those infected to those susceptible or to those who may spread the agent to others.

Disease	Recommended duration of isolation
Chickenpox	Until all lesions have crusted; About 6 days after onset of rash
Measles	From onset of catarrhal stage to 3rd day of rash.
German measles	None

Contd...

Disease	Recommended duration of isolation
Cholera	Until 48 hours after 3 day course of Tetracycline
Diphtheria	Until at least 2 consecutive nose and throat swab, taken 24 hour apart are negative
Shigellosis, Salmonellosis	Until 3 consecutive negative stool cultures
Hepatitis A	3 weeks
Influenza	3 days after onset
Polio	2 weeks for adult, 6 weeks for children
Sputum smear + pulmonary TB	Until 3 weeks of effective chemotherapy
Herpes zoster	6 days after onset of rash
Mumps	Until swelling subsides
Pertussis	4 weeks or until paroxysms cease
Meningococcal meningitis, Streptococcal pharyngitis	Until the first 6 hours of effective antibiotic therapy are completed

66. Ans. (a) Hepatitis A; (b) Diphtheria; (d) Cholera; (e) Poliomyelitis

Ref: K. Park, 24th ed. p 129

67. Ans. (b) Maximum incubation period

Ref: K. Park, 24th ed. p 129

Quarantine is limitation of freedom of movement of a healthy persons or domestic animals exposed to a communicable disease for the longest incubation period to prevent contact with those not so exposed.

- *Quarantine also applies to ship, aircraft, train, road vehicle etc. to prevent spread of disease, reservoirs of disease or vectors of disease.*
- Quarantine measures date from 2nd pandemic of plague in central Asia and Europe in the 14th century.

Also Know......................

- ***Isolation** applies to infected persons/animal, whereas Quarantine applies to healthy people.*

68. Ans. (b) To find out time for isolation

Ref: K. Park, 24th ed. p 104

Importance of Incubation period in epidemiological studies:

- *Tracing source of infection and contacts.*
- *Determining the period of surveillance (or quarantine)*
- *Immunization to prevent clinical illness by. Human immunoglobulins and antisera*
- *Identification of type of epidemic -point source or propagated.*
- *Prognosis: Tetanus, Rabies- shorter the I.P. worse the prognosis.*

ZOONOSES

69. Ans. (a) Plague; (c) Schistosomiasis; (e) Yellow fever

Ref: K. Park, 24th ed. p 294

Classification of zoonoses: Based on type of life cycle of infecting organism.

- ***Direct zoonoses*** is transmitted from an infected vertebrate host to a susceptible vertebrate host by direct contact, contact with a fomite or mechanically. Agent undergoes little or no propagative or developmental change during transmission. E.g. Rabies, trichinosis, and brucellosis.
- ***Cyclozoonoses*** need >1 vertebrate host species, but no invertebrate host, to complete the developmental cycle of the agent. E.g. Human taeniasis, echinococcosis.
- ***Metazoonoses*** are transmitted by invertebrate vectors [Agent multiplies or develops, or both and an extrinsic incubation period exists]. E.g.- Plague, Schistosomiasis.
- ***Saprozoonoses*** have a vertebrate host and a nonanimal developmental site or reservoir (Organic matter (including food), soil, and plants). E.g. larva migrants, mycoses.

70. Ans. (d) Metazoonosis

Ref: K. Park, 24th ed. p 294

71. Ans. (a) Plague; (b) Rabies; (c) Anthrax; (d) Brucellosis

Ref: K. Park, 24th ed. p 99

Types of Zoonoses	Definition	Example
Anthropo-zoonoses	Infections transmitted to man from lower vertebrate animals	Rabies, Plague, Hydatid disease, Anthrax, Brucellosis and Trichinosis
Zooanthroponoses or Reverse zoonoses	Infections transmitted from man to lower vertebrate animals.	Human tuberculosis in cattle
Amphixenoses	Infections maintained in both man and lower vertebrate animal that may be transmitted in either direction.	T. cruzi, and S. japonicum

72. Ans. (c) Scrub typhus

Ref: K. Park 24th ed.p-805

73. Ans. (a) Hydatid cyst

Ref: K. Park, 24th ed. p 99

74. Ans. (a) Plague; (c) Rabies; (d) Leishmaniasis

Ref: K Park, 24th ed. p 294, 310, 321

75. Ans. (c) Rabies

Ref: K. Park, 24th ed. p 294

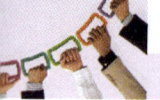

76. Ans. (b) Secondary attack rate

At the MCQ is itself stating, that the persons coming in contact from the 'primary case'.... So the answer is secondary attack rate.
[MRP]
In the outbreak setting, the term **attack rate** is often used as a synonym for risk. It is the risk of getting the disease during a specified period, such as the duration of an outbreak. A variety of attack rates can be calculated.

Overall attack rate is the total number of new cases divided by the total population.

A **secondary attack rate** is sometimes calculated to document the difference between community transmission of illness versus transmission of illness in a household, barracks, or other closed population. It is calculated as:

$$\frac{\text{Number of cases among contacts of primary cases}}{\text{Total number of contacts}} \times 100$$

Often, the total number of contacts in the denominator is calculated as the total population in the households of the primary cases minus the number of primary cases

77. Ans. (b) Droplet nuclei

Option	Mode of transmission	Examples
▪ Transplacental	Direct	TORCH agents, thalidomide, varicella, Hepatitis B
▪ Droplet nuclei	Indirect	Dried reside of droplets – TB chicken pox, influenza and other respiratory infections
▪ Soil	Direct	Hookworm infection, tetanus, mycosis
▪ STDs	Direct	By direct contact – leprosy, STD's, HIV, skin infections, leptospirosis

Modes of Transmission

- Direct transmission
  - Direct contact
  - Droplet infection
  - Contact with soil
  - Inoculation into skin
  - Transplacental
- Indirect Transmission
  - Vehicle borne
  - Vector borne
    - Mechanical—mechanical transport if infection by feet, proboscis or passage though the GI tract of vector
    - Biological—propagative, cyclo-developmental or cyclo-propagative
  - Air borne
    - Dust
    - Droplet nuclei
  - Fomite borne
  - Unclean hands and fingers

78. Ans. (a) Propagative

- *Propagative*-agent merely multiplies in vector but no change in from. e.g. yellow fever, plague
- *Cyclopropagative*-agent changes in form and number. e.g. Malaria parasite, cyclops in guinea worm
- *Cyclodevelopmental*-The disease agent undergoes only development but no multiplication e.g. microfilaria in mosquito

79. Ans. (d) 20%

Ref: K. Park, 24th ed. p 25

$$\text{Case fatality rate (Ratio) or CFR} = \frac{\textit{Total number of deaths due to a particular disease}}{\textit{Total number of cases due to the same disease}} \times 100$$

DISABILITY RATES

80. Ans. (d) 20%

Ref: K. Park, 24th ed. p 25

Case fatality rate (Ratio) or CFR = Total number of deaths due to a particular disease/Total number of cases due to the same disease × 100

81. Ans. (c) Endemic

Epidemic: Sudden rise in number of cases which is clearly in excess and more than 80% or 2 SD of the expected frequency.
Endemic: Persistent presence of the number of the cases in an area
Sporadic: Scattered cases which are not epidemiologically linked

82. Ans. (a) This is a stage b/w control and eradication; (b) It has an element of area association; (d) Incomplete interruption of disease transmission

Option	T/F	Remarks
This is a stage b/w control and eradication	T	Yes correct, elimination is a transitional phase, where with persistence of public health efforts, the disease agent may further cease to exist and hence the disease will enter into eradication phase.
It has an element of area association	T	Yes correct
Complete interruption of disease transmission	F	No, there's not absolute complete interruption of transmission. The transmission may continue to certain permissible levels, but it's certainly not going to cause any major public health problem
Incomplete interruption of disease transmission	T	Yes correct
Agent is absent but vector is present	F	No, the agent exists, but because of transmission interruption, it does not cause any new cases at community level

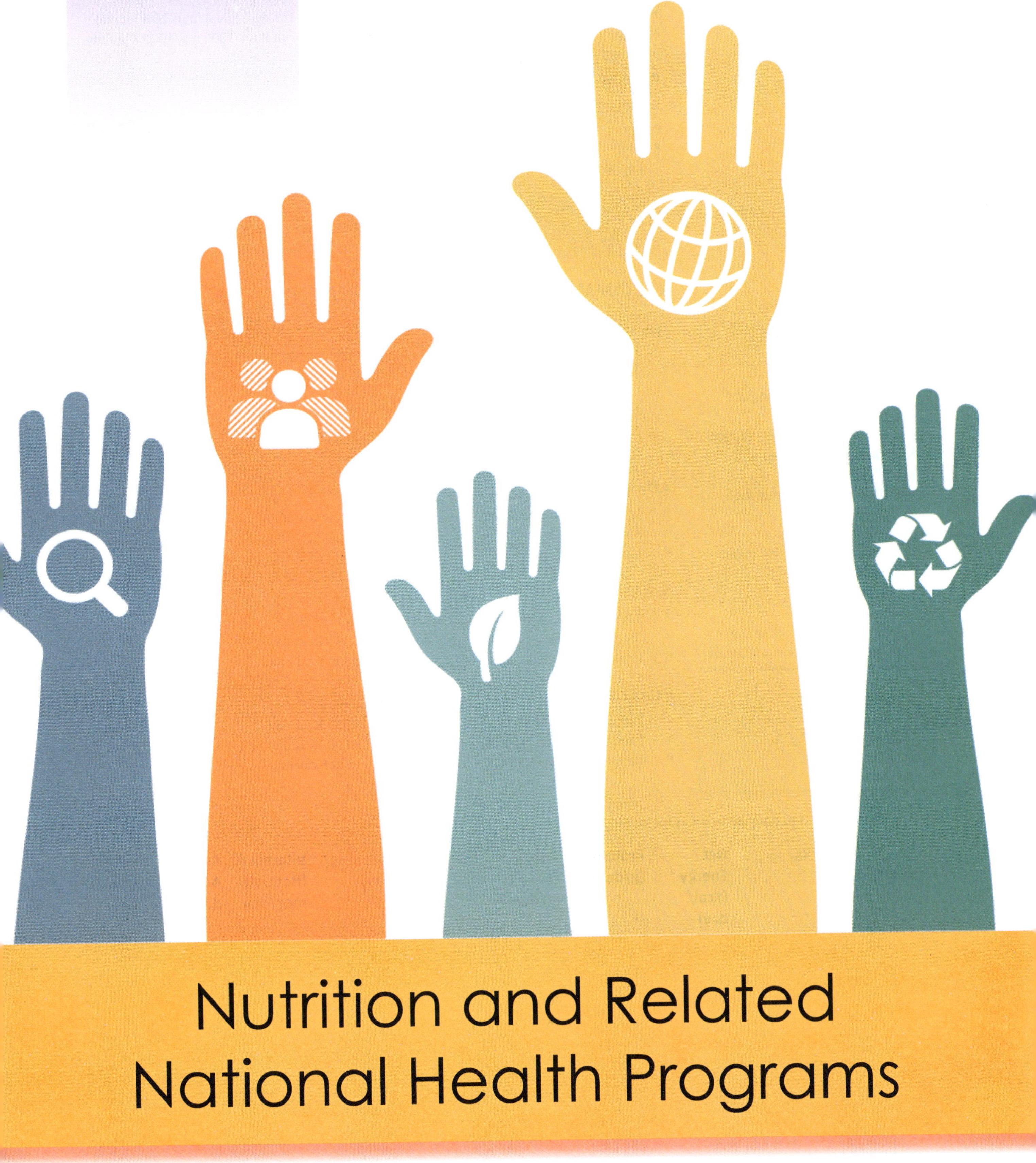

Nutrition and Related National Health Programs

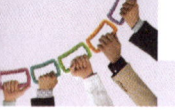

Chapter Outline

48 High Yield Points

- 1 Kcal = 4.184 KJ
- 1 KJ = 0.239 kcal
- 1 MJ = 239 kcal

PHYSIOLOGICAL ENERGY VALUE OF INDIAN FOODS

Carbohydrate	Fats
▪ 4 Kcal/g ▪ 50–70% of total diet ▪ Free sugar should be less than 10% of the total energy intake	▪ 9 Kcal/g ▪ 10–30% of the diet (ideal fat is 20% intake) ▪ Cholesterol intake < 1000 mg/1000 Kcal/day
Proteins	**Fiber**
▪ 4 Kcal/g ▪ 10–15% of the energy intake ▪ Daily requirement is approximately 1 g/kg/day	▪ 2 Kcal/g ▪ Should be the major bulk of the diet ▪ Shorten the transit time of the food and increases the food bulk ▪ Reduce postprandial blood sugars, LDL cholesterol ▪ Reduce the chances of CAD, diverticulitis, irritable bowel syndrome and colon cancer.

RECOMMENDED ENERGY REQUIREMENT

Man and woman in Indianreference

- Man in between 18–29 years of age and weighs 60 kg, height 1.73 m, BMI 20.3
- Woman in between 18–29 years of age, healthy and weighs 55 kg, height 1.61 m, BMI 21.2

General occupation	:	8 hours
Sleep time	:	8 hours
Light activity	:	4–6 hours
Active recreation	:	2 hours

Adult Male

▪ For light work (Sedentary work)	:	2,320 Kcal/day
▪ Moderate work	:	2,730 Kcal/day
▪ Heavy work	:	3,490 Kcal/day

Adult Female

▪ For light work (Sedentary work)	:	1900 Kcal/day
▪ Moderate work	:	2,230 Kcal/day
▪ Heavy work	:	2,850 Kcal/day

Extra Energy

▪ Pregnancy	:	+ 350 Kcal/day
▪ Lactation (First 6 months)	:	+ 600 Kcal/day
▪ Lactation (6–12 months)	:	+520 Kcal/day

Table 1: Recommended daily allowances for Indians —2010

Group [Male = 60 kg, Female = 55 kg]	Net Energy (Kcal/ day)	Protein (g/day)	Visible Fat (g/day)	Calcium (mg/day)	Iron (mg/ day)	Vitamin A (Retinol) mcg/day	Ascorbic Acid (mg/ day)	Folate (mcg/ day)
Sedentary worker male	2,320	60	25	600	17	600	40	200
Moderate worker male	2,730		30					
Heavy worker male	3,490		40					
Sedentary worker female	1,900	55	20	600	21	600	40	200

Contd...

Group [Male = 60 kg, Female = 55 kg]	Net Energy (Kcal/ day)	Protein (g/day)	Visible Fat (g/day)	Calcium (mg/day)	Iron (mg/ day)	Vitamin A (Retinol) mcg/day	Ascorbic Acid (mg/ day)	Folate (mcg/ day)
Moderate worker female	2,230		25					
Heavy worker female	2,850		30					
Pregnant women	+350	78	30	1200	35	800	60	500
Lactating women 0–6 months	+600	74	30	1200	21	950	80	300
Lactating women 6–12 months	+520	68						
Infant [0–6 months]	92 Kcal/ kg/day	1.16 g/ kg/ day	–	500	46 mcg/ kg/ day	350	25	25
Infant [6–12 months]	80 Kcal/ kg/day	1.69 g/ kg/ day	19		05			

Table 2: Calorie coefficient consumption per person

Person	Calorie Coefficient Consumption Unit
Adult male (Sedentary/ Moderate/Heavy worker)	1/1.2/1.6 respectively.
Adult female (Sedentary/ Moderate/Heavy worker)	0.8/0.9/1.2 respectively
Adolescent	1
Children (1–3/3–5 /5–7/7–9 years)	0.4/0.5/0.6/0.7 respectively

PROTEINS

- Complex organic nitrogenous compounds
- Composed of carbon, hydrogen, oxygen, nitrogen, sulfur, phosphorus and iron
- Differ from carbohydrates and fats as it contains 16% of nitrogen
- Essential amino acids (EAA):
  - Cannot be synthesized in body in required amount, so must be obtained from diet.
  - There are nine essential amino acids
    - Leucine
    - Isoleucine
    - Lysine
    - Methionine
    - Phenylalanine
    - Threonine
    - Valine
    - Tryptophan
    - Histidine
- Nonessential amino acids : Synthesized in body. There are six nonessential amino acid.
  - Arginine
  - Asparaginic acid
  - Serine
  - Glutamic acid
  - Proline
  - Glycine
- Animal proteins are rated superior to vegetable proteins because they are biologically complete, i.e. contains all the EAA in amounts required
- Egg proteins are "reference proteins" because of high biological value and digestibility

17 *Good to Remember*

The amino acids are needed for synthesis of tissue proteins.
Essential amino acids (EAA):
- Formation of niacin
- Methionine donor of methyl group
- Formation of new tissues

49 *High Yield Points*

Limiting amino acids:
- Cereals: Threonine + lysine
- Pulses : Methionine + cysteine
- Maize : Tryptophan + lysine

Conditionally essential amino acids: Tyrosine and cysteine for premature babies.

Assessment of Protein

Protein Quality

- Assessed by comparison to "reference protein".
- Following are the methods to assess protein quality
  - **Digestible indispensable amino acid score (DIAAS):****
    - DIAAS% = 100 × [(mg of digestible dietary indispensable amino acid in 1 g of the dietary protein) / (mg of same dietary indispensable amino acid in 1 g of the reference protein)]
    - Currently accepted best to measure protein quality
  - **Protein digestibility corrected amino acid score (PDCAAS):**
    - PDCAAS% = (mg of limiting amino acid in 1 g of test protein / mg of same amino acid in 1 g of reference protein) × fecal true digestibility%
    - PDCAAS value of 1 is highest and 0 is the lowest
  - **Amino acid score (AAS):**
    - AAS = (mg of amino acid per g of test protein / mg of the same amino acid per g of reference protein) ×100
    - The lowest score indicates limiting amino acid
  - **Digestibility coefficient**
    - $\dfrac{\textit{Amount of amino acid absorbed from the food}}{\textit{Amount of protein ingested}}$
    - It is an indicator for the external protein quality of the food product
  - **Biological value**
    - $\dfrac{\textit{Amount of nitrogen retained for body mass}}{\textit{Amount of amino acid absorbed from the food}}$
    - It is an indicator for internal quality of the protein
  - **Net protein utilization (NPU):**
    - NPU = Digestibility coefficient (DC) × Biological value (BV) / 100
    - Or NPU = Nitrogen retained / Protein ingested × 100
    - In calculating the protein quality, 1 g of protein is assumed to be equivalent to 6.25 g of nitrogen.

29 Must Remember

The best indicator for protein quality is:
DIAAS > PDCAAS > NPU

30 Must Remember

NPU
- Egg- 97% (~100%)
- Meat–80%
- Milk–70%

Protein Quantity

- **Protein Energy ratio or %:**
  - PE ratio or % = energy from protein / total energy in diet x 100
- **Protein Efficiency Ratio**
  - PER = weight gain (g) / protein intake (g) × 100
  - PER >2.5 assigned to proteins that are efficient in promoting growth (animal proteins).
  - PER 0.5-2.5 assigned to proteins that are efficient in supporting life but not growth (vegetable proteins).

50 High Yield Points

- Maximum protein energy ratio - Fish
- Maximum NPU - Egg

Requirement

1.0 g protein/kg body weight for an Indian Adult, assuming NPU of 65 for dietary protein.

FATS

Fats and oils are rich sources of energy. They include simple lipids (triglycerides), compound lipids (phospholipids), derived lipids (cholesterol). The fats may further be classified as Saturated or unsaturated fats

Saturated Fatty Acids

- Lauric acid, palmitic acid, stearic acid

Unsaturated Fatty Acids

- Primarily vegetable source of fat
- Further maybe classified as

- Mono-unsaturated fatty (oleic acid)
- Poly-unsaturated fatty acid (linoleic acid, linolenic acid)

Essential Fatty Acids

Those which are not synthesized in the body and are required from food sources
The Essential fatty acids (EFA) and their sources are:

Essential fatty acid	Sources
Linoleic acid (omega 6 fatty acid)	Safflower oil, corn oil, sunflower oil and soybean oil
Arachidonic acid	Meat, eggs and milk
Alpha - Linolenic acid (omega 3 fatty acid)	Flaxseed, canola oil, soybean oil, walnut.
Eicosapentaenoic acid	Fish oil

Functions of EFA

- Maintain integrity of the skin
- EPA and DHA – reduce serum cholesterol
- Maintain enzyme systems, retinal, cerebral cortex complex functions
- Prostaglandin synthesis

Fat Deficiency

Daily requirement of Essential FA – 5 g/day

- Deficiency of EFA
  - Growth retardation, phrynoderma, reproductive failure, sterility, renal hypertension, hemolysis, increased susceptibility to infections
- Omega 6 FA deficiency (linoleic acid, arachidonic acid) - Dermopathy
- Omega 3 FA deficiency (linolenic acid, DHA, EPA) - visual and neurological symptoms
- Saturated fatty acids are present in high quantities in coconut oil, palm oil and butter
- Polyunsaturated fatty acids are present in high quantities in safflower oil, corn oil, sunflower oil, soybean oil, cotton seed oil and margarine

51 *High Yield Points*

- Fat contents among cereals and millet - Bajra [5 g per 100 g grain, highest] > Maize >Jowar > whole Wheat > Ragi > Rice.

Requirements

Daily requirement of fat
Adult – 20–40 g/day
Pregnancy and lactation – 30 g/day

PHVO – Partially Hydrogenated Vegetable Oils

It is a chemical process of converting the vegetable oils into semisolid and solid fat.

Advantage

- More shelf life, easy storage and transport
- Removes excess odor and color

Disadvantage

- Reduced amount of EFA in oils (up to 90% reduction)
- Deficient in fat soluble vitamins (hence all PHVO's are fortified with 2500 IU Vitamin A and 175 IU of vitamin D/100 mL of PHVO.

Refined Oils

It is chemical process to improve the quality of oil by treatment of the vegetable oils with steam and alkali.

Advantage

- Free from free FA, rancid material, Vit A and D.
- Removes excess odor and color

31 **Must Remember**

- Corn has the highest "Glycemic Index" (GI).
- Cornflakes have high glycemic index
- Most fruits have low to moderate glycemic index.
- Melon and grapes have high glycemic index compared to other fruits
- Dates, guava, Indian jujube, acai berry, black berry are lower glycemic index compared to other fruits
- Avocado have high fat content compared to other fruits

- Enhanced taste of oil
- No change in unsaturated content of the oil

Disadvantage

- Deficiency of Vitamin A and D

CARBOHYDRATES

- **Glycemic Index**
  - It measures how fast the food is likely to raise the blood sugar and helps in managing the blood sugar in diabetic patients
  - It indirectly measures effect of foods on blood sugar
  - It indicates area under blood glucose curve.

Table 3: Classification based on the glycemic index

Classification	GI range	Examples
Low GI	55 or less	Whole grains, pasta foods, beans and lentils
Medium GI	56–69	Sucrose, basmati rice, brown rice
High GI	70 or more	Corn flakes, baked potato, white bread, candy bar and syrupy foods

- **Requirement:** 400–500 g/day

MICRONUTRIENTS

- Micronutrient deficiency is also known as hidden hunger
- Most common micronutrient deficiency is iron.

32 **Must Remember**

- **PHVO:** Partially hydrogenated vegetable oil
  - Vanaspati" is hydrogenated vegetable oil (semi solid or solid).
  - During hydrogenation, unsaturated fatty acids are converted into saturated fatty acids and EFA content is reduced. It is fortified with vitamins A (2500 IU) and vitamin D (175 IU per 100 g) by government regulation.

18 **Good to Remember**

- All animals, except **Fish** are good sources of saturated fatty acids
- All plants, except **Coconut** are good sources of unsaturated fatty acids.

VITAMINS

Vitamins are broadly categorized into following two:

- **Fat-soluble vitamins:** A, D, E and K
- **Water-soluble vitamins:** B group and C

Fat-soluble Vitamins

Vitamin A

- **Richest animal source:** Fish liver oil
- **Richest vegetable source:** Red palm oil,* spinach, amaranth
- **First symptom in vitamin A deficiency:** Night blindness
- **First clinical sign of vitamin A deficiency:** Conjunctival xerosis

Requirements

- **Recommended daily allowances (RDA):** 600 mcg for adults, children 7–9 years and adolescents; 350 mcg for infants; 400 children 1–6 years ; 800 mcg for pregnant females.

Vitamin A toxicity

- Repeated **moderately high dose** causes teratogenicity
- **Acute high dose:** Nausea, headache, raised intracranial pressure (pseudotumor cerebri), skin desquamation and hepatomegaly
- **Chronic high dose** causes liver damage and hyperostosis.

Deficiency Disorder

Xerophthalmia

- Refers to all ocular manifestations of vitamin A deficiency
- Most common in children aged 1–3 years
- 5.7% children in India suffer from eye signs of VAD
- ***WHO classification of xerophthalmia:***

- **Primary changes**
  - **X1A** Conjunctival xerosis
  - **X1B** Bitot's spots
  - **X2** Corneal xerosis
  - **X3A** Corneal ulceration / Keratomalacia (<1/3)
  - **X3B** Corneal ulceration / Keratomalacia (>1/3)
- **Secondary changes**
  - **XN** Night blindness (1st symptom)
  - **XF** Fundal changes
  - **XS** Corneal scarring

- **Prevention and Control**
  - **Short-term action**
    - **Treatment:** Administer 2 lakh IU orally on 2 successive days
    - **Prophylactic:** For children <1 year - 1 lakh IU
      For children >1 year- 2 lakh IU every 6 months up to 5 years of age
  - **Medium-term action**
    - Fortification of foods such as *Vanaspati ghee* and toned milk
  - **Long-term action**
    - Change in nutritional habits with inclusion of vitamin A rich foods
    - Breastfeeding for as long as possible
    - Immunization against infectious diseases such as measles
    - Prompt treatment of diarrhea and other associated infections.

Vitamin D

- Nutritionally important and present in two forms:
  - **Calciferol (Vitamin D_2):** Derived from plant source
  - **Cholecalciferol (Vitamin D_3):** Derived from animal source and exposure to UV rays of sunlight.
- **Vitamin D is also considered as kidney hormone.**
- **Richest source:** Fish liver oil

Requirements

- **Daily requirement:** 400 IU (10 mcg) in children, pregnancy and lactation, 100 IU (2.5 mcg) in adults.

Deficiency Disorders

- Rickets in young children (6 months- 2 years)
- Osteomalacia in adults (F>M)

Vitamin D Toxicity

- Large doses cause hypercalcemia (serum CA >10.5 mg %) characterized by nausea, vomiting, constipation, renal failure, metastatic calcification in arteries, kidneys and result in cardiac arrhythmias and renal failure.

Water-soluble Vitamins

Vitamin B1 – Thiamine

- Cereals are the main source in diet of Indian people.
- **Thiamine losses** in the following conditions:
  - Washing and cooking of rice
  - In highly polished rice
  - Prolong storage of fruits and vegetables

Deficiency Disorders

- **Beriberi**
  - **Dry form:** Nerve involvement
  - **Wet form:** Heart involvement

19 Good to Remember

Night blindness is the earliest symptom of xerophthalmia, but is not the primary feature of Vitamin A deficiency

20 Good to Remember

Remember: 2,500 IU of vitamin A and 175 IU of vitamin D is present in 100 mL of Dalda (Vanaspati ghee)

21 Good to Remember

Milk, margarine, Vanaspati and infant foods are artificially fortified with vitamin D.

22 Good to Remember

Vitamin D and B12 have only animal origin sources.

23 Good to Remember

- Magenta red tongue: Riboflavin
- Beefy-red tongue: B12 deficiency
- Strawberry or raspberry tongue: Scarlet fever

- **Infantile beriberi:**
  - Infants 2–4 months
  - Due to breastfeeding by thiamine deficient mother
  - Signs of peripheral neuropathy
- **Wernick's encephalopathy:** In alcoholics and people who fast.

Requirements

- **RDA:** 1–2 mg/day (0.5 mg/1,000 kcal)*

Vitamin B2 – Riboflavin

- Cereals and pulses are **poor source** but because of bulk in which they are consumed, it fulfills the requirement
- **Germination** increases the content in pulses and cereals
- **Angular stomatitis** due to deficiency of vitamin B2
- **RDA:** 0.6 mg/1,000 Kcal*

Vitamin B3 – Niacin

- Differs from other B group vitamins:
  - EAA tryptophan serves as its precursor
  - As water-soluble vitamin, not excreted in urine but metabolized
- Milk is the poor source of niacin but its proteins are rich in tryptophan which is converted in the body into niacin (about 60 mg of tryptophan is required to form 1 mg of niacin).

33 Must Remember

Pellagra

- Due to low tryptophan, which is precursor for niacin formation
- Due to high leucine, which is potent inhibitor of tryptophan metabolism

Deficiency Disorder

- Only dependent on maize or jowar (sorghum) due to excess of leucine interfere in conversion (most common)
- Pellagra- 3 Ds'- disease of poverty
  - Diarrhea
  - Dermatitis
  - Dementia
- **RDA:** 6.0 mg/1000 Kcal*

Vitamin B6 – Pyridoxine

- Patient on Isoniazide treatment (ATT drug) provided with the supplement of 10 mg/day.
- **RDA:**
  - **Adults:** 2.0 mg/day
  - **Pregnancy and lactation:** 2.5 mg/day

24 Good to Remember

Antioxidant properties

Nutrients: Vit. E, Vit. B2, Vit. C, Zinc, Selenium, β-carotene

Non- nutrients: flavonoids, caffeic and ferulic

Enzymes: Superoxide dismutase and catalase superoxides mutase

Vitamin C – Ascorbic Acid

- Most heat sensitive.
- **Amla or Indian gooseberry:** Richest source both fresh and dry form
- Guavas another richest source.
- **Deficiency:** Scurvy
- **RDA:** 40 mg/day for adults.

RDA of Different Vitamins

- Folate
  - Healthy adults 200 mcg/day
  - Pregnancy 500 mcg/day
  - Lactation 300 mcg/day
- Cyanocobalamin
  - Normal adults 1 mcg/day
  - Pregnancy 1.2 mcg/day
  - Lactation 1.5 mcg/day
- Vitamin C
  - Adults, pregnant 40 mcg/day

MINERALS

- **Major minerals:** Calcium, phosphorus, sodium, potassium and magnesium
- **Trace elements:** Iron, iodine, fluorine, zinc, copper, cobalt, chromium, manganese, molybdenum, selenium, nickel, tin, silicon and vanadium
- **Trace contaminants with no known function:** Lead, mercury, barium, boron and aluminum.

> **25 Good to Remember**
>
> Rice is the poorest source of calcium due to presence of phytic acid which leads to poor bioavailability

Iron

- Total daily iron loss of an adult – 1 mg
- Menstruating women- 12.5 mg per 28 days cycle
- Daily recommended iron intake:
  - Adult male = 15 mg/day
  - Adult women = 30 mg/day
  - Pregnancy= 35 mg/day
  - Lactation = 21 mg/day
  - Infants = 46 mcg/kg/day (0–6 m), 05 mg/day (6–12 m)
- **RDA:** 10–30 mg/day in adults, 20–35 mg/day in pregnancy and lactation and adolescent. (Note: females have higher daily requirement of iron due to physiological reasons)
- **Evaluation of iron status**
  - **Hb concentration**
  - **Serum iron concentration:**
    - More useful index than Hb concentration
    - Normal range: 0.80–1.80 mg/L
    - Iron deficiency: below 0.50 mg/L
  - **Serum ferritin:****
    - Most sensitive tool
    - Below 10 mcg/L probably indicate an absence of stored iron
  - **Serum transferrin saturation:**
    - Should be above 16%
    - Normal value- 30%.

> **26 Good to Remember**
>
> - Rice is devoid of vitamin A, D, C and poor source of calcium and iron
> - Rice protein is richer in lysine

Nutritional Anemia

Table 4: Anemia among children and adults

Children age 6–59 months who are anemic (<11.0 g/dL) (%)	55.9	59.4	58.5	69.4
Nonpregnant women age 15–49 years who are anemic (12.0 g/dL) (%)	51.0	54.3	53.1	55.2
Pregnant women age 15–49 years who are anemic (<11.0 g/dL) (%)	45.7	52.1	50.3	57.9
All women age 15–49 years who are anaemic (%)	50.8	54.2	53.0	55.3
Men age 15–49 years who are anaemic (<13.0 g/dL) (%)	18.4	25.2	22.7	24.2

> **27 Good to Remember**
>
> **Anemia cut-off**

	g/dL (venous blood)
Adult males	13
Adult females, nonpregnant	12
Adult females, pregnant	11
Children (6 months- 6 years)	11
Children (6–14 years)	12

- **Interventions:**
  - **Iron and folic acid supplementation:**
    - If Hb is 10–12 g/dL of blood
    - In pregnant women, IFA tablets are given prophylactically containing 100 mg elemental iron (ferrous sulfate) and 500 mcg folic acid for 6 months before delivery and 6 months in postnatal period. **(Start the intervention only in second trimester).**
    - The dosage for children (6 months–2 years) contains 20 mg of elemental iron (60 mg of ferrous sulfate) and 100 mcg folic acid per day for 100 days in a year
    - Children (6–10 years) 30 mg of elemental iron and 250 mcg of folic acid per day for 100 days
    - Adolescents are given same dosage and duration as per adults.
  - **Iron fortification:**
    - Addition of ferrous sulfate with sodium bisulfate or ferric orthophosphate to salt has been done. When consumed for 12–18 months, can reduce the prevalence.

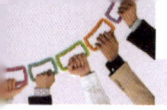

28 Good to Remember

Double fortified salt or two-in-one salt contains both iodine and iron.

Twelve by Twelve Initiative

Motive: Every child across the country should have at least 12 g% Hb by 12 years of age.

Iron Plus Initiative

Under National Iron+ Initiative, the following age groups are covered for lifelong supplementation of iron from the age of 6 months onward:

- Biweekly 20 mg elemental iron and 100 microgram (mcg) folic acid per mL of liquid formulation and age appropriate deworming for preschool children of 6–59 months.
- Weekly supplementation of 45 mg elemental iron and 400 mcg folic acid per child per day for children from 1st to 5th grade in government and government aided schools, and at AWC for out of school children (6–10 years).
- Weekly dose of 60 mg elemental iron and 500 mcg folic acid with biannual deworming in adolescents (10–19 years) under WIFS
- Weekly supplementation for women in reproductive age, pregnant and lactating women

Table 5: IFA supplementation program and service delivery

Age group	Intervention/Dose	Regime	Service delivery
6–60 months	1 mL of IFA syrup containing 20 mg of elemental iron and 100 mcg of folic acid	Biweekly throughout the period 6–80 months of age and deworming for children 12 months and above	Inclusion in MCP card Through ASHA/ANM
5–10 years	Tablets of 45 mg elemental iron and 400 mcg of folic acid	Weekly throughout the period 5–10 years of age and biannual de-worming	In school through teachers and for out-of-school children through Anganwadi centre (AWC)
10–19 years	60 mg elemental iron and 500 mcg of folic acid	Weekly throughout the period 10–19 years of age and biannual de-worming	In school through teachers and for those out-of-school through AWC
Pregnant and lactating women	60 mg elemental iron and 500 mcg of folic acid	1 tablet daily is provided starting from 2nd trimester until delivery and for another 180 days in the postpartum period.	ANC/ANM/ASHA Inclusion in MCP card
Women in reproductive age (WRA) group	60 mg elemental iron and 500 mcg of folic acid	Weekly throughout the reproductive period	Through FHW during house visit for contraceptive distribution

The main objective of providing the iron folic acid tablets is to combat nutritional anemia which is a grave public health problem in India.

Iodine

- Daily requirement of iodine is 150 mcg/day for adult and during pregnancy is 250 mcg/day.
- It is required for synthesis of Thyroid hormones-T4 & T3.
- Sources: Seafood (e.g., Seaweeds, sea fish, salt) Cod liver oil.
  - Seaweeds are the richest source of iodine
  - Potato, onions and cranberries
- About 90% of iodine comes from foods eaten and rest from drinking water (about 1-50 micrograms/L.)
- Iodine content of soil determines its presence in water and locally grown foods
- Daily requirement for adults (>12 years) is 150 micrograms per day. (250 mcg per day during pregnancy)

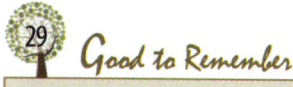

29 Good to Remember

Goitrogens (Cyanoglycoside and Thiocyanate.) are chemicals that interfere with Iodine utilization by thyroid gland leading to goiter.

Brassica group of vegetables (e.g. cabbage cauliflower) may contain goitrogens

Fluorine

- Prolonged ingestion of >1 mg/L fluoride- dental and skeletal fluorosis
- <0.5 mg/L of ingestion—dental caries
- Indicator of dental caries in community: DMF- Index (D = Decayed, M = Mottled, F = Fallen)

- **Recommended level:** 0.5-0.8 mg/L of drinking water
- **Nalgonda technique:**
  - For defluoridation of water
  - Recommended by National Environmental Engineering Research Institute, Nagpur
  - Involves the addition of alum, lime and bleaching powder followed by flocculation, sedimentation and filtration.

Endemic Fluorosis

- This occurs in places with high levels of fluorine in water (3 – 5 mg/L)
- However the Safe limit of fluorine in drinking water in India is – 0.5 to 0.8 mg / dL.
- **Remember:** Dental fluorosis if F2 above 1.5 mg/L
  Skeletal fluorosis if F2 3-6 mg/L
  Crippling (Genu valgum) if F2 above 10 mg/L
- **Intervention**:
  - Change the source of water
  - Nalgonda technique: mentioned above in fluorine
  - Avoid using fluoride toothpaste in endemic areas in children up to 6 years of age.

FOOD PRODUCTS

Cereals

- Provide about 350 Kcal per 100 g (70–80% of total energy intake) and more than 50% of protein intake in typical Indian diet. Cereal proteins are deficient in essential amino acid–Lysine.
- Rice protein content varies from 6% to 9% (Rich in lysine compared to other cereals, hence considered to be of better quality). Rice is a good source of group B vitamins, especially Thiamine.
- Milling leads to loss of Thiamine [up to 75% loss], Riboflavin [60% loss] and protein [15% loss]
- Parboiling (partial cooking in steam) is an ancient Indian technique to preserve nutritive value of rice
- Wheat protein content varies from 9% to 16%.Limiting amino acids are lysine and threonine.
- Maize proteins are deficient in tryptophan and lysine and contain an excess of leucine that interferes in conversion of tryptophan to niacin, aggravating pellagragenic action of maize. It is rich in fat
- Pulses "poor man's meat" contain 20–25% protein (Soybean–40%). Pulse proteins are poor in methionine and cysteine, but rich in lysine. Pulses are rich in minerals and B-group vitamins.

Milk

- Animal milk has three times more protein content than human milk (buffalo > cow > human)
- Animal milk has 10 times more calcium content than human milk (buffalo > cow > human)
- Fat content is more in buffalo milk (it is double in comparison to human milk)
- Milk fat is rich in retinol and vitamin D
- Poor source of vitamin C and iron
- Chief protein is casein; others lactalbumin and lactoglobulin
- Ration of casein to albumin in human milk is 1:1

Pasteurization of Milk

- SNF testing – for assessment of Solid Non Fat in the milk
- Methylene blue reduction test is done to confirm heavy contamination of animal milk (before pasteurization). **
- **Types of pasteurization**
  - **Holder (VAT Method):** 63-66°C for at least 30 minutes, and then quickly cooled to 5°C
  - **High temperature, short time (HTST) method:** Rapidly heated to a temperature of nearly 72°C, is held at that temperature for not less than 15 seconds, and is then rapidly cooled to 4°C.

34 **Must Remember**

Common cooking methods

- ***Parboiling***: The food items are added to boiling water and cooked until they start to soften, then removed before they are fully cooked. Parboiling is usually used to partially cook an item which will then be cooked another way such as braising, grilling or stir-frying.
  Parboiling differs from blanching in that one does not cool the items using cold water or ice after removing them from the boiling water.
- ***Steeping***: Steeping is the soaking in liquid (usually water) of a solid so as to extract flavors or to soften it. The specific process of teas being prepared for drinking by leaving the leaves in heated water to release the flavor and nutrients is known as steeping.

52 **High Yield Points**

Human milk contains more tryptophan, sulfur containing AA (esp. cysteine), linoleic acid, oleic acid, sugar (lactose) and water as compared to animal milk

30 **Good to Remember**

- Types of milk
  - Standard milk : 6% fat
  - Toned milk : 3% fat
  - Double toned milk : 1.5% fat
  - Skimmed milk : <0.5% fat

53 **High Yield Points**

Skimmed milk powder is an important ingredient of 'Hyderabadi mix' - a supplementary food.

- **Ultra high temperature (UHT) method:** Rapid heating to very high temperature of 125°C for few seconds. A second phase of pasteurization takes place under high pressure. UHT is the most modern method and used in large milk production factories
- **Tests of pasteurized milk**
  - Phosphatase test – should be absent in milk
  - Standard plate test - < 30,000 bacterial colony
  - Coliform count – 0/mL

Breast Milk

- Per 100 g or 100 mL contains:
  - 65 Kcal
  - 7.4 g carbohydrate
  - 3.4 g fat
  - 1.1 g protein

Colostrum: First milk after delivery. Usually within first 3 days of delivery, the milk is rich in immunoglobulins (IgA), essential amino acids and maternal antibodies.

Mature milk: is the milk after > 12–16 days after delivery. It is an approximation of complete diet. The mature milk contains almost all nutrients required for adequate growth of a neonate. The initial milk during every feed may be thinner and more watery (foremilk), which becomes more fatty and thick later on in the feeding session (known as hind milk).

31 **Good to Remember**

Difference between Cow Milk and Human Milk

The mature milk grossly resembles a cow milk in terms of energy, nutrients and fat content, however..

- Human milk has only one-third of the protein concentration compared to cow milk
- Human milk contains a lipase enzyme because of which human milk fat is digested easily
- Human milk has almost double the amount of lactose compared to cow milk. Lactose provides an easily digestible source of energy High lactose content helps in myelination in the growing nerve tissue of the baby. Also, part of lactose is converted to lactic acid in the intestine, which prevents growth of undesirable bacteria in the intestine.
- Human milk contains the bifidus factor, which is a nitrogen-containing carbohydrate. Bifidus factor is necessary for the growth of Lactobacillus bifidus, which converts lactose to lactic acid
- Human milk, especially the colostrum, contains large amounts of immunoglobulin A, which is not absorbed but acts in the intestine against certain bacteria (such as *E. coli*) and viruses
- Lysozyme, an enzyme, is present in human milk in concentrations several thousand times that of cow milk. Lysozyme breaks down certain harmful bacteria and also protects against various viruses.

Eggs

- An average egg (60 g) contains:
  - 70 Kcal of energy per egg (100 g of egg yields 145 Kcal of energy)
  - 6 g of protein
  - 6 g of fat
  - 30 mg of Ca
  - 1.8 mg of iron
  - All vitamins except vitamin C

Miscellaneous Points for Nutritive Value of Eggs

- Duck's egg contains—trypsin inhibitor and should not be consumed raw
- Raw egg may transmit salmonellosis
- Egg protein contains avidin which interferes with biotin absorption

Tests for Freshness of Egg

- Candling—fresh egg is translucent and yellow part of the egg is seen floating in white (rotten egg is opaque)
- Floating—fresh egg sinks in 10% saline or normal water. (rotten egg floats)

Fish

- It is rich in proteins (15–25%) of good biological value and amino acid balance, but poor in carbohydrate[Q]
- Fish liver oils (unsaturated fatty acids) are rich source of vitamins A and D.[Q]
- Fish bones are a good source of calcium, phosphorus and fluorides. Sea fish also contains iodine.
- Fish is a poor source of iron (0.7-3 mg/100 g) than meat.
- Diet survey duration may vary from 1 to 21 days, but most commonly it is 7 days or "one dietary cycle".

Features of Fresh Fish

- State of stiffness or rigor mortis
- Bright red gills
- Eyes are clear and prominent

Fish—Public Health Importance

- Intermediate host for *Dibothriocephalus latus*
- Vibrio parahaemolyticus
- Salmonella species

Meat Hygiene

- Floor and walls to be impermeable up to 3 ft
- Food stored overnight in temperature below 5°.

Meat Public Health Importance

- Tapeworm infestation: *T. solium, T. saginata, Trichinella spiralis*
- Bacterial infections: Anthrax, tuberculosis and food poisoning

Alcohol

- Alcohol content in beverage is 5–6% in Beer, 40–45% in Whisky, Rum, Gin and Brandy.
- Alcohol supplies 7 Kcal/mL.

Miscellaneous Facts in Food Products

	Energy	Protein	Fat	Remarks
Ground nuts	567	25	40	Rich in carbohydrates and niacin
Cashew	596	21	45	Rich in iron and carotene
Almond	655	21	60	Rich fat, high energy

	Energy	Remarks
Apple	60	Apple seeds consumed in excess may be neurotoxic to humans
Banana	110	Rich in carbohydrate
Grapes	70	Rich in carbohydrate, calcium
Guava	50	Rich in vitamin C
Papaya	30	Rich in carotene
Dates	300	High fat, iron, and energy
Amla (Indian gooseberry)		Richest source of vitamin C
Hyderabad mix		It is a high energy food product – given in anganwadi centers **Contains:** ▪ Bengal gram ▪ Jaggery ▪ Groundnuts
Amylase rich food		These are highly nutritious, high digestible protein – germinated food products

FOOD ADULTERATION AND INTOXICATION

Any substance which is added to a food product which	decreases the nutritive value or harms the body	Food adulteration	Brick powder – chilly powder Argemone oil/mustard oil Water/honey/milk/juice/chemical/cumin seeds/tea leaves/many food products
	does not alter the nutritive value but increases the shelf life or consumption	Food additive	Preservative/color to many food products
	increases the nutritive value and was not present in food initially	Food fortification	Iodine/salt Vitamins/Vegetable oils
	enhances the nutritive value and was present in lower quantity initially	Food enrichment	

Table 6: Food adulterants

Diseases	Foods	Toxicants	Clinical features
Neurolathyrism (mentioned below)			
Aflatoxicosis (storage fungus)	Food grains (groundnuts* maize and jowar)	Aflatoxins produced by *Aspergillus flavus* and *A. parasiticus*	Liver cirrhosis
Ergotism (field fungus)	Food grains (bajra, rye, sorghum and wheat)	Ergot fungus- *Claviceps purpurea*	Acute cases- Nausea, vomiting, giddiness, drowsiness Chronic cases- Painful cramps and peripheral gangrene
Epidemic dropsy	Mustard oil contaminated with argemone oil	Toxic alkaloid **sanguinarine** in argemone oil	Sudden. Noninflammatory, bilateral swelling of legs with diarrhea, dyspnea and cardiac failure and glaucoma
Endemic ascities	Millets contaminated with weed seeds of crotalaria (Jhunjhunu)	**Pyrrolizidine alkaloids** in weeds	Hepatotoxic
Fusarium toxins	Sorghum	Fungus **Fusarium** incarnatum which produces the toxic metabolites	Nausea, vomiting, diarrhea are predominant features

** Nitric acid paper chromatography test is the most sensitive test to detect argemone oil contamination*

54 High Yield Points

Neurolathyrism risk factors:

- Heavy physical activity
- Male gender
- Young age (15-25 years)
- Micronutrient deficiency (Zn, Cu, Vit C, Vit A)
- Ingestion of the dal beyond critical level of 400 g/day

Lathyrism

- This pulse (**Lathyrus sativus**- khesari dal) contains the toxin **Beta oxalyl amino alanine** (BOAA) that leads to neurolathyrism in humans and osteolathyrism in animals.
- Local names of dal: Teora dal, Lak dal.
- Neurolathyrism is a crippling disease of the nervous system resulting in spastic paralysis of lower limbs (latent stage-no stick-one stick-two stick-crawler stage).
- **Interventions:**
  - Vitamin C prophylaxis (500–1000 mg for a week or so)
  - Removal of toxin by steeping or parboiling
  - Health education
  - Genetic approach
  - Banning of crop

Severity of Neurolathyrism

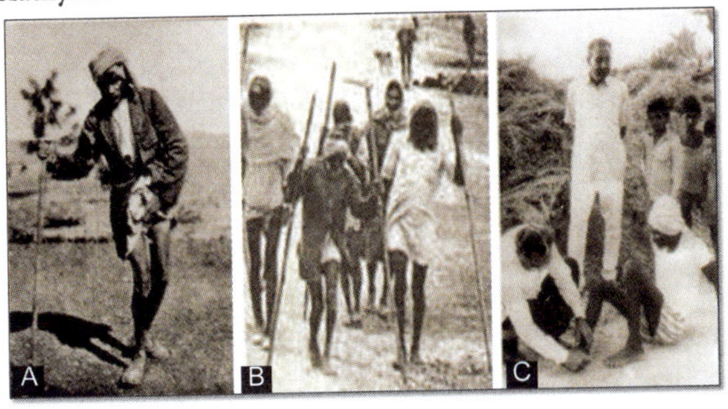

Figs 1A to C: Severity of neurolathyrism (A) One stick stage; (B) Two sticks stage; (c) Crawler stage

NUTRITIONAL DISTURBANCES

Low Birthweight (LBW)

- Defined as one with a birthweight below 2.5 kg (2,500 g) regardless of gestational age.***Preferably measured within in first hour of life, before significant postnatal weight loss has occurred**
- 28% of newborns in India are LBW (NFHS 3).
- Intrauterine growth retardation (IUGR) is the most common reason
- **Leading causes of death** in LBW babies:
  - Atelectasis
  - Malformation
  - Pulmonary hemorrhage
  - Intracranial bleeding secondary to anoxia or birth trauma
  - Pneumonia and other infection.
- **Kangaroo mother care:**
  - Introduced in Columbia in 1979
  - Includes:
    - Skin to skin positioning of a baby on mother's chest
    - Adequate nutrition through breastfeeding
    - Ambulatory care as a result of earlier discharge from hospital
    - Support for the mother and her family in caring for the baby.

Protein Energy Malnutrition (PEM)

- Incidence in preschool children is around 1–2%.
- ***Gomez classification:***
  - It compares the weight of a child with a normal child of the same age. The "normal" reference child is in the 50th centile of Boston standards
  - It is based on weight retardation
  - It is as follows:
    - 90 – 110% of normal: normal nutritional status
    - 75 – 89% of normal: 1st degree, mild malnutrition
    - 60 – 74% of normal: 2nd degree, moderate malnutrition
    - Under 60% of normal: 3rd degree, severe malnutrition
- ***McLaren's classification:***
  - It uses height as the measuring criteria
    - >93% height for expected age – Normal
    - 80–93% height for expected age – Short
    - <80% height for expected age – Dwarf
- ***Waterlow's classification:*** It combines height for age (H/A) and weight for height (W/H)

55 *High Yield Points*

Clinical features:

- Latent: no features.
- Stage I (No stick stage) - Jerky Steps
- Stage II (One stick stage) - Altered gait
- Stage III (Two sticks stage) - Crossed Gait
- Stage IV (Crawler stage) - inability to walk

32 *Good to Remember*

In neurolathyrism:

- Upper motor neuron disorder with symmetrical spastic paralysis.
- Sensation and sphincters are spared.
- The neuronal damages are permanent.

Symptomatic treatment with muscle relaxants help.

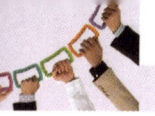

W/H → H/A	> Mean-2SD	< Mean-2SD
> Mean-2SD	Normal	Wasted
<Mean-2SD	Stunted	Wasted and stunted

Table 7: Master chart of classification of protein energy malnutrition

Grade/Degree	(Weight for age in percentage)			Waterlow	
	Gomez	Jelliffe	IAP	Height for age (stunting)	Weight for height (wasting)
Normal	90-110	>90	100-80	>95%	>90%
Mild (1^0)	89-75	90-81	79-70	94-87.5	90-80
Moderate (2^0)	74-60	80-71	69-60	87.4-80	80-70
Severe (3^0)	<60	70-61	59-50	<80	<70
Very severe (4^0)	-	<60	<50	-	-

Table 8: Clinical features of protein energy malnutrition

Features	Marasmus	Kwashiorkor
(Always present)		
Muscle wasting	Obvious	Sometimes hidden by fat and edema
Edema	None	Present mainly in lower limb, face and forearms
Mental changes	Quite and apathetic	Irritable, moaning, apathetic
Fat wasting	Severe loss of subcutaneous fat	Fat often retained but not firm
Weight for height	Very Low	Low but masked by edema
(Sometimes present)		
Hair changes	Seldom	Sparse, silky, easily pulled out, 'flag sign'
Appetite	Good	Poor
Diarrhea	Often	Often
Liver enlargement	Not present	Present due to accumulation of fat
Skin changes	None	Diffuse pigmented skin, "flaky skin dermatosis"
Biochemical		
Plasma/Amino acid ratio	Normal	Elevated
Serum albumin	Normal/slightly decreased	Low (<3 g/100 mL blood)
Urinary urea per g creatinine	Normal/decreased	Low
Hydroxyproline/creatinine ratio	Low	Low

Obesity

Indicators to measure obesity:
- **Broca's index**:** Height (cm) – 100 = expected Weight (in kg)
- **Quetelet's index/[Body mass index** (BMI)] = weight (kg)/ height^2 (m)

Table 9: WHO classification (International classification)

Classification	BMI
Underweight	<18.50
Normal range	18.50–24.99
Overweight	≥25.00
Pre-obese	25.00–29.99
Obese class I	30.00–34.99
Obese class II	35.00–39.99
Obese class III	≥40.00

For many Asian populations, additional trigger points for public health action were identified as:

- 23 kg/m^2 or higher, representing increased risk
- 27·5 kg/m^2 or higher as representing high risk.

For Asian population, the suggested categories are as follows:

1. Less than 18·49 kg/m^2 — underweight
2. 18·5–22.9 kg/m^2 — increasing but acceptable risk
3. 23–27·49 kg/m^2 — increased risk
4. 27·5 kg/m^2 or higher — high risk

- **Corpulence index:**- Actual weight (in kg) / desirable weight (in kg) **(This should not exceed 1.2)**
- **Ponderal index:**- Height (in cm) / Cube root of body weight (kg)
- **Lorentz's formula:**
  Male = [ht (cm) - 100] - [ht (cm) - 150] / 4
  Female = [ht (cm) - 100] - [ht (cm) - 150] / 2
- **Fat fold thickness (skin fold thickness)**
  - Measured by skin callipers
  - Sites: Mid-triceps, biceps, subscapular and suprailliac regions
  - Sum of the above four site measurements should not be less than 40 mm in boys and 50 mm in girls
- **Waist-hip Ratio (WHR)**
  - WHR >1 in men and >0.85 in women indicates abdominal fat.

> **56 High Yield Points**
>
> Overweight is defined as:
> BMI >23
> WHR >1 (males)
> WHR >0.85 (females)

NUTRITION RELATED ACTS

- **Codex:** The "Codex Alimentarius" international food standards, guidelines and codes of practice contribute to the safety, quality and fairness of this international food trade. Consumers can trust the safety and quality of the food products they buy and importers can trust that the food they ordered will be in accordance with their specifications
- **FSSAI:** The Food Safety and Standards Authority of India (FSSAI) has been established under Food Safety and Standards, 2006 which consolidates various acts and orders related to food and nutrition. The FSSAI would provide standards for articles of food and to regulate their manufacture, storage, distribution, sale and import to ensure availability of safe and wholesome food for human consumption
- **BIS:** The Bureau of Indian Standards has evolved from the older organization of the Indian standards institute. It is primarily responsible for providing quality assurance and guidelines for hallmark, service delivery, metals, devices and instruments
- **AGMARK:** It is a certification mark employed on agricultural products in India, assuring that they conform to a set of standards
- **IYCF Substitution Act:** Early initiation of breastfeeding within first hour of birth, exclusive breastfeeding for the first 6 months followed by continued breastfeeding for up to 2 years and beyond with appropriate complementary foods after completion of 6 months is the most appropriate feeding strategy. Prohibits promotion of milk substitutes formula milk for children less than 6 months of age
- **Antyodaya Yojana:** Additional 25 kg food grain are provided to the poorest of poor families at a highly subsidized rate of ₹ 2 per kg for wheat and ₹ 3 per kg for rice.
- **TB poshan Abhiyan:** Support for nutrition to TB patients is provided as cash grant in terms of INR 500 per month to all patients on regular compliance for Anti-Tuberculosis treatment under GoI (Government of India)

> **57 High Yield Points**
>
> All food establishment must adhere to FSSAI for quality of food production and delivery

NUTRITION RELATED NATIONAL HEALTH PROGRAMS

Mid-day Meal Scheme

- Also known as nutritional support to primary education [previous name: National Program of Nutritional Support to Primary Education (NP-NSPE)]
- Objective is to decrease the school dropout rate
- Cooked food is provided every day for promoting school attendance

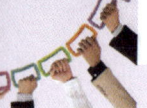

- MDMS promotes school attendance by providing ½ of daily protein requirement and 1/3rd of daily calorie requirement by children
- Recent updates in MDMS is to provide cooked meals to all primary and upper primary (up to class VIII) school children
- **Recent recommendations:**
  - Pulses – 25–30 g
  - Vegetables 65–75 g
  - Fat 7.5 g

Integrated Child Development Scheme (ICDS)

- ***Beneficiaries:*** The beneficiaries under the Scheme are children in the age group of 0–6 years, pregnant women and lactating mothers
- **Objectives:**
  - To improve the nutritional and health status of children in the age group 0–6 years
  - To lay the foundation for proper psychological, physical and social development of the child
  - To reduce the incidence of mortality, morbidity, malnutrition and school dropout
  - To achieve effective coordination of policy and implementation amongst the various departments to promote child development; and
  - To enhance the capability of the mother to look after the normal health and nutritional needs of the child through proper nutrition and health education.
- ***Organization:***
  - One Anganwadi for 800–1,000 population (for AWC in rural / urban projects) Thereafter in multiple of 800
  - Mini-AWC for 150 – 300 population
  - Anganwadi on demand (AOD): Settlement has 40 children under 6 years of age but no AWC
  - One Anganwadi supervisor for 25 Anganwadi
  - One Child development project officer for 100,000 population (one Block)
- ***Benefits***
  - Supplementary nutrition
  - Pre-school, nonformal education
  - Health education and awareness
  - Facilitating immunization
  - Family planning
  - Health check-up, basic health care
  - Referral services to various public health centers
  - Adolescent health, vocational training, food and health program.

58 High Yield Points

The beneficiaries under ICDS are:
- Children 0-6 years
- Pregnant females
- Lactating females
- Adolescent girls

Table 10: Revised nutritional norms

Beneficiaries	Calories	Protein (g)	Cost approved by GOI (source MoWCD, 2017 guidelines)
Children (6 months to 72 months)	500	12–15	₹8
Severely malnourished children (SAM)	800	20–25	₹12.5
Pregnant women and lactating mothers	600	18–20	₹9.5

Kishori Shakti Yojana

Kishori Shakti Yojana (KSY) in ICDS, was started in the year 2000 and is being implemented via ICDS.

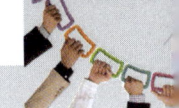

Aim

- To improve the nutritional and health status of adolescent girls (Age 11-18 years).
- Provide literacy and numeracy skills via nonformal education, stimulate desire for more social exposure and knowledge and help improve decision making
- Train and equip to improve home based and vocational skills
- Promote self-development, awareness of health, hygiene, nutrition, family life and child care, literacy and vocational skills and home management.
- Delay marriage to after 18 years or later.
- To gain better understanding of environment related social issues and its impact on lives and to encourage adolescent girls to initiate activities to be productive and useful members of society.

Scheme I → Girl to Girl Approach

- Designed for adolescent girls (Age 11–15 years) belonging to families with income < ₹ 6,400 per annum and school drop outs in urban and rural areas.
- 3 girls are selected per AWC for 6 months duration and are provided supplementary nutrition equivalent to 500 calories and 20 g protein for 6 days a week.
- Learning on preventive health, hygiene, nutrition and family life education by initial 3-day training program and 6 continuing education session of 1 day each month
- These girls act as resource persons for other girls in the neighborhood
- AWC is the focal point of services.

Scheme II → Balika Mandal

- Designed for all adolescent girls (11–18 years, preferable 11–15 years) irrespective of income of family.
- 10% of total AWC in each community development block and urban ICDS area are selected to serve as Balika mandals.
- 20 girls (age 11–18 years) are enrolled for a duration of 6 months in Balika mandal.

Social Welfare Measures under the Anganwadi Scheme

- Under the ***Wheat Based Nutrition Program (WBNP),*** food grains viz., wheat, rice and other coarse grains are allocated at below poverty line (BPL) rates to the States/UTs through the Department of Food & Public Distribution (D/o Food & Public Distribution), for preparation of supplementary food in ICDS
- ***Anganwadi Karyakartri Bima Yojana (AKBY):*** Insurance scheme for accidental death, disability or accidents
- ***Sneha shivir***: Community-based care program for undernourished children less than 6 years of age. It includes
  - During the 12 days, children are fed additional high calorie local foods, provided under ICDS and from contribution of care givers and community. During 12 days, children regain appetite and visible changes are seen as also indicated by gain in weight, a gain of 200–400 g is expected
  - Weight monitoring of the selected children
  - Deworming of these children
  - Ensure IFA and complete immunization for these children
  - 12 days hands-on practice sessions for mothers and care givers to promote improved feeding and child care practices
  - Recording of weight on first day, 12th day and after 18 days
  - Theme based education using IEC on feeding, health, hygiene and psychosocial care on each of the 12 days, using mother child protection card package
  - Health check-up and referral services
  - 18 days home-based practices
  - Repeat of session for each child till child becomes normal
  - Monitoring progress: Child-wise, AWC-wise as well as at the block and district levels.

35 Must Remember

Spectrum of IDD includes

- Goiter (most common)
- Hypothyroidism
- Subnormal intelligence including delayed mile stones, mental deficiency, hearing defects, speech defects
- Squint (Strabismus)
- Nystagmus
- Spasticity (Extrapyramidal type)
- Neuromuscular weakness
- Endemic cretinism
- IUD (Spontaneous abortion, miscarriage)

33 Good to Remember

- **Iodized oil**: Intramuscular injection of iodized oil (mostly poppy-seed oil) which provides a protection for 4 years with 1 mL average dose. NIN, Hyderabad successfully developed the process to produce iodized oil in safflower or saffola oil.
- **Iodized oil oral**: Iodized oil or Sodium Iodate tablets.
- 'Smiling Sun' is a symbol used for Iodized salt

National Iodine Deficiency Disorder Control Program (NIDDCP)

Timeline

- National goiter control program – 1962
- National iodine deficiency disorder control program – 1986

Objectives of Program

- Surveys to assess the magnitude of the iodine deficiency disorders.
- Supply of iodized salt in place of common salt
- Resurvey after every 5 years to assess the extent of iodine deficiency disorders and the impact of iodized salt.
- Laboratory monitoring of iodized salt and urinary iodine excretion
- Health education and publicity.

Control of IDD by:

- **Iodized Salt:**

Moisture	Not more than 6.0% by weight of the sample salt
Sodium chloride	Not less than 96.0% by weight on dry basis
Matter insoluble in water	Not more than 1.0% by weight on dry basis
Matter soluble in water other than sodium chloride	Not more than 3.0% by the weight on dry basis

Iodine content at:

Manufacturing level	Not less than 30 parts per million (ppm) on dry weight basis
Distribution level	Not less than 15 parts per million on dry weight basis

- **IDD Monitoring:** Most sensitive indicator to environmental iodine deficiency is Neonatal hypothyroidism, followed by urinary iodine excretion.
- **Programmatic goal of IDD by 2010:**
  - <5% prevalence of IDD in 10–14 years of age
  - <10% of incidence of IDD
- IDD survey (Goiter Survey)
  - Annual survey to be conducted at district levels
  - Sample size for IDD survey is as under

36 Must Remember

Total sample is calculated as: selection of villages/wards using population proportionate to size (PPS) sampling method

- Sample size = 30 villages/wards. From each village selection is as under:
- 90 children will be selected (45 boys and 45 girls) of age group 6–12 years using the proportionate sample for the enrollment rates in the school
- The examination should be for
  - 100% children to be examined for iodine in house hold salt levels
  - All children to be examined for goiter rate in children (6–12 years age).
    - **Grade 0**- Neither Palpable nor visible—No Goiter
    - **Grade 1**- Goiter palpable but not visible when the neck is in normal position
    - **Grade 2**- A swelling in the neck that is visible when the neck is in a normal position.
  - The Goiter rate (grade 1 and Grade 2) is classified as under:
    - 5–19% goiter rate — IDD is a **Mild** Public health problem
    - 20–29.9% goiter rate — IDD is a **Moderate** Public health problem
    - >30 % goiter rate — IDD is a **Severe** Public health problem
  - 50% children (every alternate child) to be examined for Urinary Iodine Excretion rate (UIE). Median UIE is
    - 50–99 mcg/L — IDD is a **Mild** Public health problem
    - 20–49 mcg/L — IDD is a **Moderate** Public health problem
    - <20 mcg/L — IDD is a **Severe** Public health problem

Indicators to Monitor IDD Control Program

- Impact indicator:
  - Chronic impact indicator – long term indicator – Goiter rate
- Epidemiological indicator/principal impact indicator/most important indicator/sustainability indicator: Urinary iodine levels
- Process indicator: iodine levels in salt (at packaging and at household level)

59 *High Yield Points*

Most common type of goiter – euthyroid goiter
Most common thyroid dysfunction – hypothyroidism (Hashimoto's or autoimmune thyroiditis)
Endemic goiter–Kangra belt (sub-Himalayan region)

34 *Good to Remember*

Ma-kombu and Kizami-kombu are Japanese seaweed (used in salads). It contains 12–24 mg of iodine, which is maximum in any food product. Other iodine-rich sea foods as fish, crabs, octopus contain iodine ranging from 10 mcg to 100 mcg only.

37 *Must Remember*

Iodine-Induced Thyroid Dysfunctions

- Wolff-Chaikoff effect
  - Hypothyroidism
  - Due to: High dose, acute intake of iodine
- Jod-basedow effect
  - Hyperthyroidism
  - Due to: Low dose, chronic intake of iodine

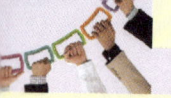

Image-Based Questions

1. Identify the seeds shown in the figure:

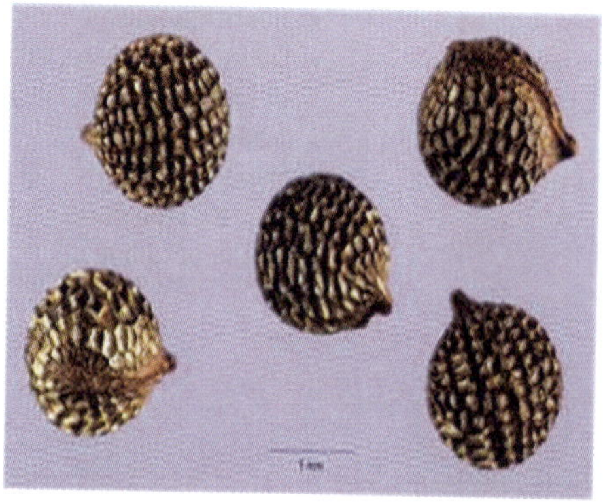

a. Dhatura
b. Argemone
c. Bajra
d. Jowar

2. The item (Jeevan Bindi) shown in the figure is used in:

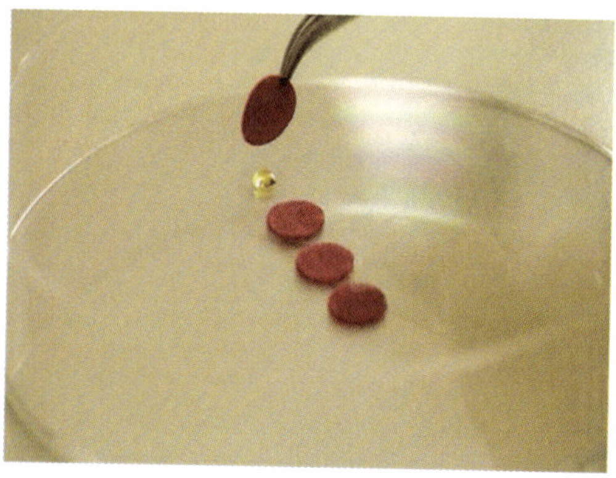

a. Iron deficiency
b. Iodine deficiency
c. Skin sensitivity
d. Folic acid deficiency

3. Identify the item in the figure:

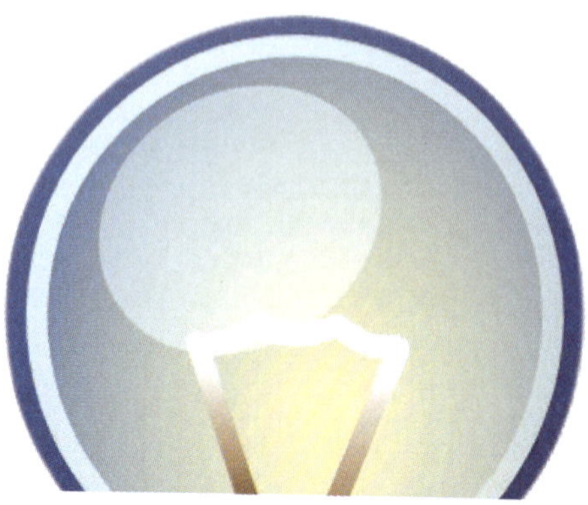

a. Datura
b. Argemone
c. Bajra
d. Jowar

4. Identify the condition depicted in the figure:

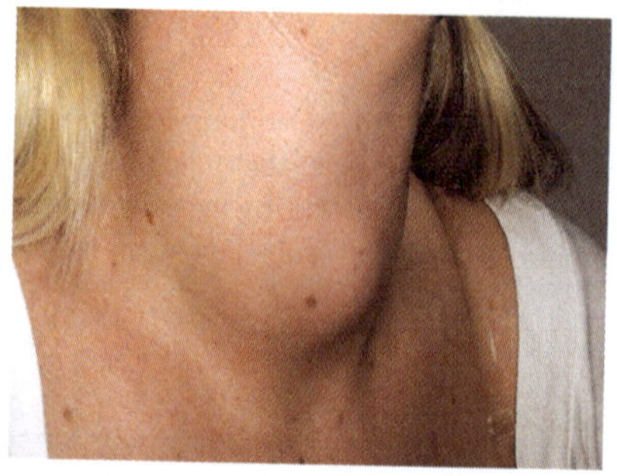

a. Goiter
b. Submandibular lymph node enlargement
c. Ludwig's angina
d. Hyoid bone displacement

5. Identify the cereal in shown in the figure:

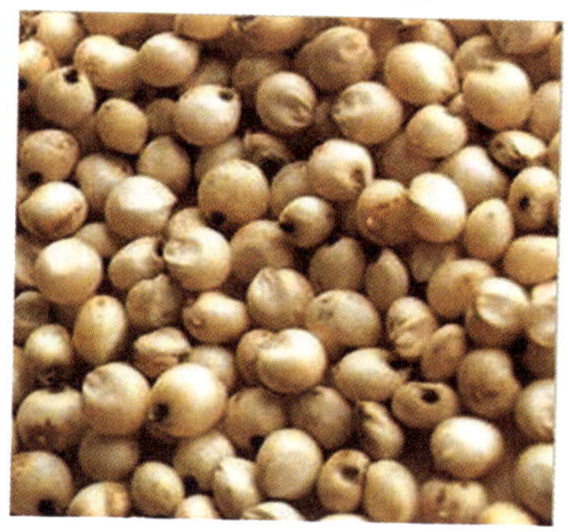

a. Jowar
b. Bajra
c. Soya bean
d. Lentils

6. The logo shown depicts the national program for:

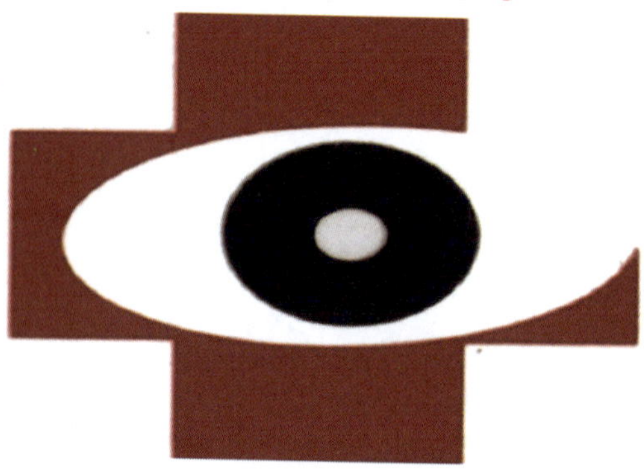

a. Trachoma control
b. Control of Blindness
c. Vitamin A Prophylaxis
d. Vision 20:20

7. The item shown in the figure is:

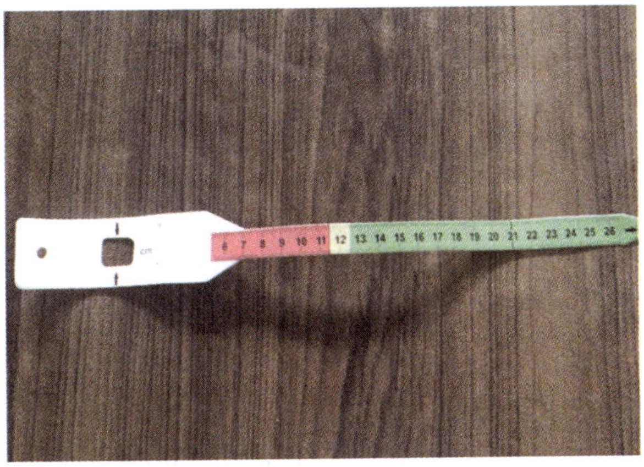

a. Shakir's tape
b. Triage tape
c. Multipurpose tape
d. Wrist tape

8. The symbol shown in figure is used to depict levels of:

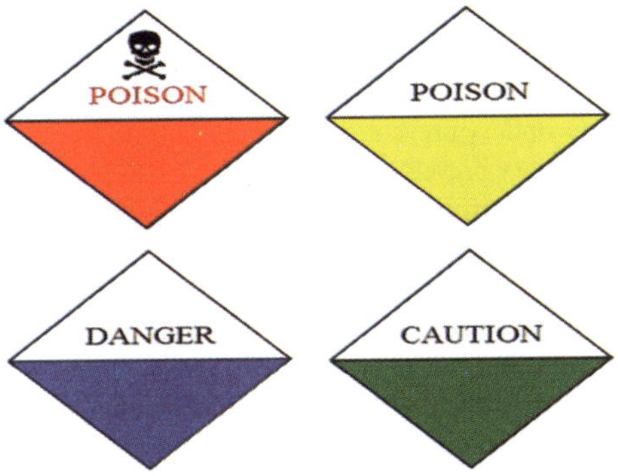

a. Food toxicity in plastics
b. Biomedical waste
c. Pesticide toxicity
d. Cytotoxicity of hospital waste

9. The condition depicted in figure is:

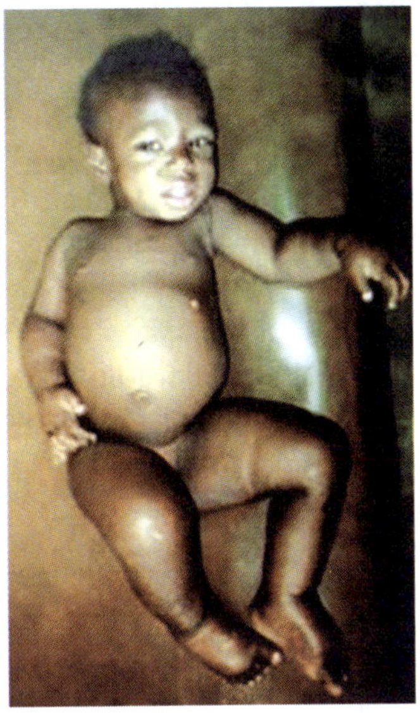

a. Kwashiorkor
b. Marasmus
c. Nephrotic syndrome
d. Epidemic Dropsy

10. The condition depicted in figure is due to:

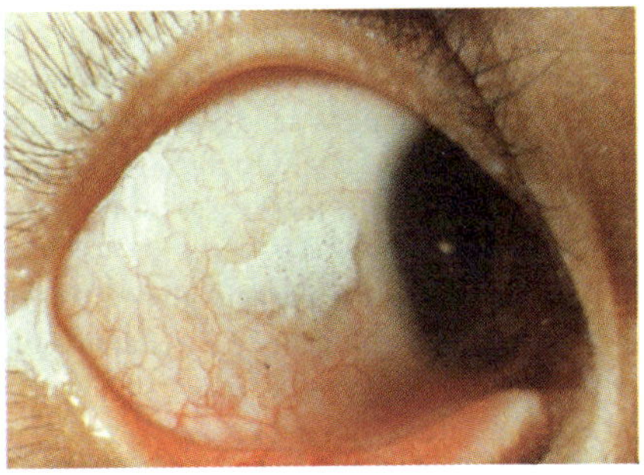

a. Trachoma
b. Vitamin A deficiency
c. Foreign body injury
d. Fat deposits

Answers of Image-Based Questions

1. **Ans. (b)** Argemone
2. **Ans. (b)** Iodine deficiency
3. **Ans. (a)** Datura
4. **Ans. (a)** Goiter
5. **Ans. (a)** Jowar
6. **Ans. (b)** Control of Blindness
7. **Ans. (c)** Multipurpose tape
8. **Ans. (c)** Pesticide toxicity
9. **Ans. (a)** Kwashiorkor
10. **Ans. (b)** Vitamin A deficiency

Multiple Choice Questions

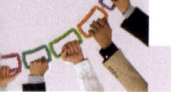

1. Mid-day meal scheme includes provision of *(AIIMS Nov 2017)*
a. 1/3rd Calories, 1/2 Protein
b. 1/2nd Calories, 1/3 Protein
c. 1/2nd Calories, 1/2 Protein
d. 1/3rd Calories, 1/3 Protein

2. A 49 kg primigravida with sedentary lifestyle registers at your clinic. What dietary advice will you give her for the 1st trimester, regarding her calorie intake per day? *(AIIMS Nov 2017)*
a. Extra 300 calories
b. Extra 500 calories
c. Same calories
d. Decrease calories

3. Recommended daily requirement of Iodine for lactating women is: **(Recent Question 2018)**
a. 50–100 µg
b. 100–200 µg
c. 200–300 µg
d. 25–50 µg

4. Which of the following is/are true about National Iron plus initiative: **(PGI May 2017)**
a. Only school going adolescents are covered
b. Adolescents of age group 10-19 yr are covered
c. Preschool children are covered through anganwadi center
d. Biannual deworming through albendazole tablet
e. Screening of target groups for moderate/severe anaemia and referring these cases to an appropriate health facility

5. What is the dose of iron folic acid given till 6-10 years? *(Recent Question 2017)*
a. 20 mg iron with 0.1 mg FA
b. 20 mg iron with 0.2 mg FA
c. 50 mg iron with 0.5 mg FA
d. 100 mg iron with 0.5 mg FA

6. Total calories (kcal/day) required for a Female with sedentary activity: *(Recent Question 2017)*
a. 1900 b. 2200
c. 2500 d. 2800

7. Plant source with highest protein:
a. Black gram b. Dry peas
c. Soybean d. Bengal gram

8. Richest source of linoleic acid:
a. Safflower oil b. Palm oil
c. Sunflower oil d. Corn oil

9. RDA of Vitamin B12 in pregnancy: *(Recent Question 2016)*
a. 1.2 mcg b. 2.5 mcg
c. 0.8 mcg d. 0.2 mcg

10. Total calories (kcal/day) required for a female with moderate activity? *(Recent Question 2016)*
a. 2230 b. 2730
c. 2900 d. 3500

11. Iron required in lactation: *(Recent Question 2016)*
a. 300 µg/day b. 400 µg/day
c. 20 mg/day d. 100 mg/day

12. How many calories are there in 100 mL breast milk?
a. 60–65 b. 67–70
c. 72–78 d. 100–110

13. Epidemic dropsy is caused by this toxin:
a. BOAA b. Sanguinarine
c. Alkaloid d. Ergot

14. Prevention of scurvy using citrus fruits was discovered by: *(Recent Question 2015)*
a. Hippocrates b. James Lind
c. Louis Pasteur d. John Snow

15. Proteins with highest biological value are found in:
a. Legumes b. Cereals
c. Protein of animal source
d. Milk

16. Normal energy requirement for sedentary female is:
a. 1900 Cal/day b. 2200 Cal/day
c. 2600 Cal/day d. 2800 Cal/day

17. Iodized salt in iodine deficiency control program is:
a. Primordial prevention
b. Primary prevention
c. Secondary prevention
d. Tertiary prevention

18. Vitamin A prophylaxis to a child is *(AIIMS May 2010)*
a. Primordial prevention
b. Health protection
c. Specific protection
d. Secondary prevention

19. Village Health Nutrition Day is observed:
a. Every week b. Every month
c. Every 6 month d. Every year

20. Kishori Shakti Yojana has been designed to improve nutritional status of:
a. Adult men b. Adolescent girls
c. Under five children d. Senior citizens

ICDS

21. In Mid-day meal program, the amount of nutrition provided is: *(Recent Question 2015)*
a. 6 g of protein + 450 Kcal of energy
b. 12 g of protein + 600 Kcal of energy
c. 6 g of protein + 600 Kcal of energy
d. 12 g of protein + 450 Kcal of energy

22. Mid-day meal program comes under:
a. Ministry of health and family welfare
b. Ministry of Education
c. Ministry of Social welfare
d. Ministry of Human resource development

23. Integrated child protection scheme is under which ministry
a. Health and family welfare
b. Women and child development
c. Home affairs
d. Labour

Ans.

1.	a
2.	a
3.	c
4.	b, d, e
5.	a
6.	a
7.	c
8.	a
9.	a
10.	a
11.	c
12.	a
13.	b
14.	b
15.	c
16.	a
17.	b
18.	c
19.	b
20.	b
21.	d
22.	b
23.	b

Most Recent Question of 2019-18 is given at the end of MCQs

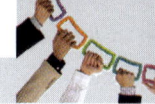

24. **ICDS was launched in:**
a. 1955 b. 1968
c. 1975 d. 2005

25. **Direct cash transfer scheme to adolescent girls is covered under** *(Recent Question 2015)*
a. Indira Gandhi scheme b. Rajiv Gandhi scheme
c. CSSM d. RCH

NIDDCP

26. **Most sensitive indicator of Hypothyroidism in a community is:** *(Recent Question 2014)*
a. T4
b. Neonatal hypothyroidism
c. TSH
d. Median urinary iodine excretion

27. **Minimum level of iodized salt reaching the consumer level according to iodine program should be:**
a. 15 ppm b. 30 ppm
c. 5 ppm d. 20 ppm

MISCELLANEOUS

28. **Food Standards and Safety Authority of India comes under:**
a. Ministry of Agriculture
b. Ministry of Health and Family Welfare
c. Ministry of Consumer Affairs
d. Ministry of Rural development

29. **Diet given to a pregnant lady under ICDS is:**
a. 600 Kcal + 20 g proteins/day
b. 250 Kcal + 12 g proteins/day
c. 300 Kcal + 15 g proteins/day
d. 350 Kcal + 15 g proteins/day

30. **ICDS includes children up to age of years:**
a. 3 b. 4
c. 6 d. 14

31. **Under ICDS calorie supplement for pregnant women:**
a. 300 Cal, 8–10 g of proteins
b. 200 Cal, 6–8 g of proteins
c. 600 Cal, 16–20 g of proteins
d. 500 Cal, 20–25 g of proteins

32. **Late pregnancy calorie requirement is:**
a. 2500 b. 3000
c. 1500 d. 2300

PROTEIN

33. **Which one of the following is the best indicator of protein quality for recommending the dietary protein requirement?**
a. Protein-Efficiency Ratio
b. Biological Value
c. Digestibility Coefficient
d. Net Protein Utilization

34. **Net Protein Utilization is given by the formula:**
a. Weight gained/amount of protein consumed × 100
b. Nitrogen retained by body/Nitrogen intake × 100
c. Nitrogen retained/Nitrogen absorbed × 100
d. Biological value/Digestibility coefficient

35. **Protein constitute__% of body weight in adults:**
a. 10 b. 20
c. 25 d. 30

36. **A biologically complete protein is the one which/whole:**
a. Net protein utilization is 100
b. Amino acid score is 100
c. Contains all amino acids
d. Contains all essential amino acids

37. **ICMR recommends 1.0 g of protein /kg body weight for an Indian adult, assuming a NPU of for dietary proteins:**
a. 55 b. 65
c. 85 d. 100

38. **Energy (kcal/g) released from protein:**
a. 2 b. 4
c. 7 d. 9

39. **The average daily nutrient intake level estimated to meet the requirement of half of the healthy individuals in a particu- lar life stage and gender group is called:**
a. Adequate intake
b. Estimated average requirement
c. Tolerable upper intake level
d. Recommended dietary allowance

40. **Recommended Protein intake of high quality of an Indian adult man according to 2010 Guidelines is:**
a. 0.2 g/kg/day b. 0.83 g/kg/day
c. 1.0 g/kg/day d. 1.2 g/kg/day

FATTY ACID

41. **Highest quantity of PUFA and EFA are present in:**
a. Coconut oil b. Sunflower oil
c. Safflower oil d. Soybean oil

42. **1 kg of adipose tissue is equal to kcal energy**
a. 4400 b. 5500
c. 6600 d. 7700

43. **Not true regarding hydrogenation of fats is**
a. Unsaturated fatty acids are converted into saturated fatty acids
b. EFA content is drastically reduced
c. Partial hydrogenation of PUFA creates trans-fatty acids
d. Trans fatty acids are not atherogenic

44. **Linoleic acid is maximum/highest in:** *(Recent Question 2014)*
a. Groundnut oil
b. Safflower oil
c. Mustard oil
d. Coconut oil

45. **Daily protein requirement of a Neonate (in g/kg body weight) is:** *(Recent Question 2014)*
a. 1.5 g b. 2.5 g
c. 3.5 g d. 4.5 g

46. **Most important essential fatty acid is:** *(Recent Question 2014)*
a. Linoleic acid
b. Linolenic acid
c. Arachidonic acid
d. Eicosapentaenoic acid

47. **Fortification of vanaspati ghee is done with:**
a. Vitamin A b. Iron
c. Iodine d. Calcium

48. **More than 50% PUFA is seen in multiple correct options:**
a. Mustard oil b. Soybean oil
c. Safflower oil d. Corn oil
e. Palm oil

Ans.

24. c
25. b
26. d
27. a
28. b
29. a
30. c
31. c
32. a
33. d
34. b
35. b
36. d
37. b
38. b
39. b
40. b
41. c
42. d
43. d
44. b
45. a
46. a
47. a
48. b, c, d

Most Recent Question of 2019-18 is given at the end of MCQs

VITAMIN A

49. Richest source of vitamin-A: *(Recent Question 2016)*
a. Halibut liver oil b. Carrot
c. Butter d. Margarine

50. Richest source of vitamin A is :
a. Halibut liver oil b. Carrot
c. Pistachio d. Egg

51. Prevalence surveys of vitamin A deficiency is done among:
a. Children 1–3 years
b. Children 6 months to 6 years
c. Adolescents 11–14 years
d. Pregnant women 15–24 years

52. No. of doses for treatment of Vitamin A deficiency:
a. 4 b. 2
c. 3 d. 1

53. Xerophthalmia is a problem in a community if the prevalence of Bitot's spots is more than:
a. 1% b. 0.5%
c. 5% d. 25%

54. Bitot's spots are seen in: *(Recent Question 2016)*
a. Conjunctiva b. Cornea
c. Retina d. Vitreous

55. In xeropthalmia what is X1B: *(Recent Question 2016)*
a. Conjunctival xerosis b. Bitot's spot
c. Corneal xerosis d. Corneal ulcer

56. Xerophthalmia is a problem in a community if the prevalence of Bitot's spots is more than: *(Recent Question 2015)*
a. 1% b. 0.5%
c. 5% d. 25%

57. Incidence of Bitot spots to label it as a public health prob-
a. 0.1% b. 0.5%
c. 1% d. 5%

VITAMIN B1

58. Which of the following is lost on polishing rice?
a. Amino acids b. Vitamins
c. Fiber d. Carbohydrates

59. White polished rice causes deficiency of:
a. Protein b. Tryptophan
c. Riboflavin d. Thiamine

60. RDA of which Vitamin is related to Daily requirement for Proteins: *(Recent Question 2015)*
a. B3 b. B6
c. B1 d. B2

61. Thiamine content is highest in ...... *(Recent Question 2014)*
a. Milled rice b. Whole wheat
c. Gingelly seeds d. Ground nut

NIACIN

62. Pellagra is caused due to deficiency of which vitamin?
a. B2 b. B3
c. B1 d. Folic acid

63. Consumption of which of the following cereal as staple diet is associated with pellagra: *(Recent Question 2014)*
a. Rice b. Wheat
c. Maize d. Bajra

64. Disease characterized by 3 Ds' – Diarrhea, Dermatitis and Dementia occurs due to deficiency of:
a. Vitamin A b. Folic acid
c. Vitamin C d. Niacin

65. Niacin deficiency can result in: *(Recent Question 2015)*
a. Pellagra
b. Anemia
c. Peripheral neurology
d. Beriberi

66. Pellagra in jowar eating population is due to:
a. Niacin in bound form
b. Deficiency of tryptophan
c. Excess of leucine
d. High consumption of milk and milk products

VITAMIN C

67. Vitamin 'C' prophylaxis is helpful in preventing
a. Fluorosis b. Neurolathyrism
c. Iodine deficiency d. Botulism

VITAMIN D

68. Richest source of Vitamin D is: *(Recent Question 2015)*
a. Sunlight b. Shark liver oil
c. Cod liver oil d. Halibut fish liver oil

69. Physiologically most effective form of Vitamin D is:
a. Calciferol
b. Cholecalciferol
c. Ergocalciferol
d. Calcitriol

70. Vitamin D is maximum in: *(Recent Question 2014)*
a. Milk b. Fish fat
c. Eggs d. Cod liver oil

VITAMIN K

71. Daily requirement of Vitamin K: *(Recent Question 2014)*
a. 3 mg/kg b. 0.3 mg/kg
c. 0.03 mg/kg d. 30 mg/kg

ZINC

72. All of the following are a result of Zinc deficiency, except:
a. Sexual infantilism
b. Impaired Immunity
c. Skeletal Abnormalities
d. Increased Appetite

73. Acrodermatitis enteropathica is
a. Inherited disorder of excessive excretion of zinc from body
b. Inherited disorder of impaired uptake of zinc from body
c. Inherited disorder of excessive excretion of copper from body
d. Inherited disorder of impaired uptake of copper from body

CALCIUM

74. RDA of calcium in normal adult male is:
a. 800 mg b. 400 mg
c. 600 mg d. 100 mg

Ans.

49. a
50. a
51. b
52. b
53. b
54. a
55. b
56. b
57. b
58. b
59. d
60. b
61. c
62. b
63. c
64. d
65. a
66. c
67. b
68. d
69. d
70. d
71. c
72. d
73. b
74. c

75. **Daily elemental calcium requirement for an elderly woman is:** *(Recent Question 2014)*
 a. 1200 mg b. 300 mg
 c. 2000 mg d. 2500 mg

IRON AND FOLIC ACID

76. **National Iron Plus Initiative recommends:**
 a. Biweekly IFA to pregnant and Lactating mothers
 b. Biweekly IFA to children 6-60 months
 c. Biweekly IFA to adolescent girls
 d. None
77. **True about National Iron Plus Initiative regarding iron prophylaxis is**
 a. 100 mg Iron + 500 mcg Folic acid tablet weekly for adolescent aged 10-19 years
 b. 20 mg Iron +100 mcg Folic acid syrup weekly for under 5 year children
 c. 45 mg Iron + 400 mcg Folic acid syrup biweekly for children 6-10 year
 d. 100 mg Iron + 500 mcg Folic acid tablet biweekly for adults
78. **False statement regarding folic acid supplementation:**
 a. Fortified in all wheat products in India like as in USA
 b. Preconceptionally given for prevention of neural tube defects
 c. It is present in leafy vegetables, spinach, paneer
 d. Requirement per day in pregnancy is 500 mcg

FLUORINE

79. **The recommended level of fluorides in drinking water in India is:** *(Recent Question 2014)*
 a. 0.5 to 0.8 mg/litre b. 1.0 to 0.5 mg/litre
 c. 1.5 to 1.8 mg/litre d. 2.5 to 2.8 mg/litre
80. **Nalgonda technique is a method of defluoridation of water by adding:** *(Recent Question 2014)*
 a. Bicarbonates b. Lime and alum
 c. Phosphates d. Carbonates
81. **All are true with respect to Fluorosis, except:**
 a. Mottling of dental enamel > 1.5 mg/L
 b. Skeletal fluorosis 3.0-6.0 mg/L
 c. Crippling fluorosis > 10 g/L
 d. None of the above
82. **Skeletal fluorosis is associated with lifetime daily intake of:**
 a. 1.0 – 2.0 mg/L b. 2.0 – 3.0 mg/L
 c. 3.0 – 6.0 mg/L d. 6.0 – 8.0 mg/L
83. **Daily fluorine intake levels associated with development of crippling fluorosis:** *(Recent Question 2014)*
 a. 1.0–1.5 ppm b. 1.5-3.0 ppm
 c. 3.0–6.0 ppm d. >10 ppm

DIETARY FIBER

84. **Desirable intake of dietary fiber per 2000 kcal energy intake is:** *(Recent Question 2013)*
 a. 20 g b 40 g
 c. 60 g d. 100 g
85. **Energy (kcal/g) obtained from fiber:** *(Recent Question 2013)*
 a. 2 b. 4
 c. 7 d. 9
86. **Energy (kcal/g) obtained from alcohol:**
 a. 2 b. 4
 c. 7 d. 9
87. **Rich source of fiber is:**
 a. Spinach b. Ragi
 c. Green Gram d. Wheat
88. **Fiber content is highest in:**
 a. Oat b. Maize
 c. Wheat d. Rice
89. **True about dietary fibres:** *(Recent Question 2013)*
 a. Increase stool transit time
 b. Decrease post prandial glucose
 c. Decrease bile salt reabsorption
 d. Decrease LDL cholesterol
 e. Increases bulk of stool

CEREALS AND MILLETS

90. **Cereals in general are deficient in which of the following amino acids?** *(Recent Question 2013)*
 a. Cysteine b. Methionine
 c. Tryptophan d. Lysine
91. **Correct combination of limiting amino acids in Cereals and Pulses respectively is:** *(Recent Question 2013)*
 a. Lysine and Threonine
 b. Lysine and Tryptophan
 c. Lysine and Methionine
 d. Threonine and Methionine
92. **Tryptophan is deficient in:** *(Recent Question 2013)*
 a. Rice b. Wheat
 c. Maize d. Pulses
93. **All are true regarding nutritive value of rice, except:**
 a. Rice proteins are deficient in lysine
 b. Rice is a good source of group B vitamins
 c. Rice is a poor source of calcium and iron
 d. Outer pericarp and germ contain most of the essential nutrients
94. **Parboiling of rice is the process of:**
 a. Cooking in boiling water
 b. Partial cooking in steam
 c. Milling process
 d. Genetic engineering of rice
95. **Purpose of Parboiling is:**
 a. Milling
 b. Preservation of nutrients
 c. Storage of rice
 d. Polishing
96. **Lysine is deficient in:**
 a. Pulse b. Wheat
 c. Both of the above d. None of the above

PULSES

97. **Limiting amino acid in pulse proteins is:**
 a. Methionine b. Lysine
 c. Threonine d. Tryptophan
98. **For nutritional studies, the following protein is considered as reference proteins:**
 a. Fish protein b. Meat protein
 c. Egg protein d. Vegetable protein

Ans.

75. a
76. b
77. b
78. a
79. a
80. b
81. d
82. c
83. d
84. b
85. a
86. c
87. b
88. b
89. b, c, d, e
90. d
91. c
92. c
93. a
94. b
95. b
96. b
97. a
98. c

Most Recent Question of 2019-18 is given at the end of MCQs

99. Fermentation of Pulses increase the levels of all of the following, except: *(Recent Question 2014)*
a. Niacin b. Vitamin C
c. Thiamine d. Riboflavin

100. Not true regarding pulses is: *(Recent Question 2014)*
a. Pulse proteins are inferior to animal proteins
b. Pulses are poor in methionine and to a lesser extent cysteine
c. Germinating pulses have lower concentration of B and C vitamins
d. In raw state, pulses have anti-nutritional factors like phytates and tannins, which are destroyed by heat

101. An adult male with sedentary life style requires ___g of pulses per day:
a. 40 g b. 60 g
c. 160 g d. 100 g

102. Pulse protein is deficient in which of the following Essential Amino Acid:
a. Lysine b. Methionine
c. Threonine d. Tryptophan

103. What is known as "poor man's meat":
a. Milk b. Pulses
c. Fish d. Egg

104. Pulses are deficient in: *(Recent Question 2013)*
a. Lysine and threonine
b. Lysine and tryptophan
c. Methionine and cysteine
d. Lysine and methionine

EGG

105. Which one of the following is considered as 'Reference Protein'?
a. Meat b. Fish
c. Egg d. Milk

106. Egg is deficient in which vitamin:
a. Vitamin A b. Vitamin B6
c. Vitamin C d. Vitamin D

107. NPU of egg protein is: *(Recent Question 2015)*
a. 65 b. 80
c. 90 d. 100

108. All the following nutrients are present in egg except:
a. Calcium b. Iron
c. Carbohydrate d. Protein

109. Egg has all vitamin, except: *(Recent Question 2014)*
a. B1 b. B6
c. C d. E

110. Out of the following, true about egg is
a. Rich in all vitamin including vitamin C
b. Deficient in essential amino acid
c. 60 g egg has 6 g Fat, 6 g protein and 30 mg Calcium
d. NPU=70

111. Food with maximum cholesterol content:
a. Egg b. Coconut oil
c. Hydrogenated fats d. Ghee

112. Egg has all vitamins, except:
a. B1 b. B6
c. C d. A

MILK

113. The following amino acid is present in lesser quantity in human milk compared to cow's milk:
a. Methionine
b. Tryptophan
c. Cysteine
d. Taurine

114. Quantity of protein in one litre of human milk:
a. 1 g b. 6 g
c. 11 g d. 16 g

115. Quantity of calcium in one litre of cow's milk:
a. 2 g b. 1 g
c. 500 mg d. 250 mg

116. What is the protein content of human breast milk?
a. 3.8 g/100 mL
b. 2.9 g/100 mL
c. 3.2 g/100 mL
d. 1.1 g/100 mL

117. Calcium in human milk is (mg/100 g):
a. 200 b. 100
c. 70 d. 28

118. Human breast milk has more of:
a. Lipids
b. Carbohydrates
c. Proteins
d. Calcium

119. Among the following, which one is the correct sequence with regard to increasing fat content per 100 g/m:
a. Curd (Cow Milk), Human Milk, Cheese, Buffalo milk
b. Human Milk, Buffalo milk, Curd (Cow's Milk), Cheese
c. Human Milk, Curd (Cow's Milk), Buffalo milk, Cheese,
d. Cheese, Human, Curd (Cow's Milk) Buffalo milk,

120. Following tests are used to check the efficiency of pasteurization of milk, except: *(Recent Question 2014)*
a. Phosphatase test
b. Standard plate count
c. Coliform count
d. Methylene blue reduction test

121. Colostrum has in compared to normal milk:
a. Decreased Vitamin A
b. Decrease Na^+
c. Increased proteins
d. Increased calories

122. Which of the following is most deficient in milk?
a. Vitamin K b. Vitamin C
c. Vitamin D d. Vitamin A

123. According to WHO, exclusive breast milk is given up to:
a. 6 months
b. 4 months
c. 8 months
d. 10 months

124. All are true about cow's milk, except:
a. Cow milk contains 80% whey protein and not casein
b. Has more protein than breast milk
c. Has more K^+ and Na^+ than breast milk
d. Has less carbohydrate than mothers milk

Ans.

99. b	100. c
101. a	102. b
103. b	104. c
105. c	106. c
107. d	108. c
109. c	110. c
111. a	112. c
113. a	114. c
115. b	116. d
117. d	118. b
119. c	120. d
121. c	122. a
123. a	124. a

DRY FRUITS

125. Maximum calories are found in which fruit:
- a. Banana
- b. Mango
- c. Orange
- d. Pear

126. Iron is maximum in: *(Recent Question 2014)*
- a. Pista
- b. Cashew nut
- c. Meat
- d. Milk

MISCELLANEOUS

127. Storage temperature of meat in slaughter house should be below what degree Celsius: *(Recent Question 2016)*
- a. 0
- b. 3
- c. 5
- d. 10

128. The base of the food guide pyramid is formed by:
- a. Cereals and pulses
- b. Fruits and vegetables
- c. Milk and milk products
- d. Meat, poultry and fish

129. WHO recommended salt intake is of less than:
- a. 5 g
- b. 6 g
- c. 7 g
- d. 8 g

130. Food standards in India are based on the standards set by:
- a. PFA standards
- b. AGMARK Standards
- c. Codex alimentarius
- d. Bureau of Indian Standards

131. Which of the following formulates food standards for international market? *(Recent Question 2015)*
- a. AGMARK
- b. ISI
- c. PFA
- d. Codex alimentarius

132. Food with Low glycemic index is: *(Recent Question 2015)*
- a. Sucrose
- b. Potato
- c. Wheat bread
- d. Rice

133. Glycemic index is defined as ability of the food item to:
- a. Stimulate the release of glucagon
- b. Raise blood sugar
- c. Stimulate Insulin release
- d. Others

134. A low glycemic index food among the following is:
- a. White bread
- b. Whole grains
- c. Corn flakes
- d. White rice

135. Consider the following statements *(Recent Question 2014)*
1. Ionizing rays are used in food preservation by irradiation.
2. Irradiation does not affect the colour, odour, taste, pH and levels of vitamin in food.

Which of the above statements is/are correct?
- a. 1 Only
- b. 2 Only
- c. Both 1 and 2
- d. Neither 1 nor 2

136. Which of the following are food preservatives?
- a. Lactic acid
- b. Sorbic acid
- c. Sulfurous acid

Choose the correct combination.
- a. 1 and 2 only
- b. 2 and 3 only
- c. None of these
- d. 1, 2 and 3

137. Banana is good source of:
- a. Calcium
- b. Phosphorus
- c. Vitamin B6
- d. Vitamin C
- e. Potassium

138. International food standards include:
- a. BIS standards
- b. Codex alimentarius standards
- c. AgMark standards
- d. FSSAI Act

139. Acute severe malnutrition diagnostic criteria include all, except:
- a. Bipedal edema
- b. Visible severe wasting
- c. Mid arm circumference below 115 mm
- d. Weight for height below 2SD of WHO growth standards 2006

140. Vegans are defined as those who eat:
- a. Both dairy product and egg
- b. Dairy product but not egg
- c. Egg but not dairy product
- d. Neither dairy nor egg

141. Low Glycemic index is for: *(Recent Question 2013)*
- a. Sucrose
- b. Potato
- c. White bread
- d. Fruits

NUTRITIONAL REQUIREMENTS

142. All the following criteria are true for a reference Indian man, except:
- a. Age 18–29 years
- b. Weight 60 kg
- c. Height 1.73 m
- d. BMI 21.2

143. Regarding Indian Reference Woman all are true, except:
- a. Age 18-29 years
- b. Weight 50 kg
- c. Height 1.61m
- d. BMI 21.2

144. For Indian reference male is true:
- a. Weight 60 Kg
- b. Works for 15 hours
- c. Age 20-25 years
- d. Daily exercise

145. True about Indian reference male is:
- a. Age 18-29 years
- b. Weight 65 Kg
- c. Work is mainly sedentary
- d. Works for 10 hrs

146. Indian reference man weighs: *(Recent Question 2013)*
- a. 55 kg
- b. 60 kg
- c. 65 kg
- d. 70 kg

RECOMMENDED DAILY ALLOWANCE

147. Recommended fat in prudent diet:
- a. < 10–15%
- b. < 5–10%
- c. < 15–20%
- d. < 20–30%

148. What is the recommended protein intake for a healthy adult male?
- a. 60 g
- b. 60 g
- c. 1 g/kg body weight of mixed protein
- d. 1 g/kg body weight of egg protein

Ans.

125. a
126. a
127. c
128. a
129. a
130. c
131. d
132. d
133. b
134. b
135. a
136. d
137. c, e
138. b
139. d
140. d
141. d
142. d
143. b
144. a
145. a
146. b
147. d
148. c

Most Recent Question of 2019-18 is given at the end of MCQs

149. Energy required for an Indian reference man, engaged in sedentary work is: *(Recent Question 2013)*
a. 2320 Kcal b. 2420 Kcal
c. 2850 Kcal d. 2730 Kcal

150. Recommended calorie and protein intake respectively for the age group 0-6 months:
a. 500 kcal and 1.16 g/kg/day
b. 600 kcal and 1.16 g/kg/day
c. 500 kcal and 1.69 g/kg/day
d. 600 kcal and 1.69 g/kg/day

RDA IN PREGNANCY AND LACTATION

151. Energy requirement in late pregnancy for a moderate worker is: *(Recent Question 2013)*
a. 2500 Cal b. 1400 Cal
c. 1000 Cal d. 500 Cal

152. Extra calories required in 5th month of pregnancy:
a. 150 Kcal b. 200 Kcal
c. 300 Kcal d. 350 Cal

153. The extra calories per day recommended for a pregnant woman is: *(Recent Question 2013)*
a. 300 b. 330
c. 350 d. 360

154. Total iron requirement in pregnancy:
a. 1000 mg b. 35 mg
c. 500 mg d. 800 mg

155. Recommended iodine dose in pregnancy is:
a. 15 mcg b. 100 mcg
c. 150 mcg d. 250 mcg

156. Extra calories per day in lactating mothers in first six months:
a. 300 b. 500
c. 600 d. 1000

157. Recommended Dietary allowance in pregnancy are:
a. + 100-300 Kcal b. 30 mg Iron
c. 4 mg Folic acid
d. 2500 mg Magnesium
e. 270 mcg iodine

RDA CALCIUM

158. Adult nonpregnant female requires, calcium per day:
a. 400 mg b. 600 mg
c. 800 mg d. 1000 mg

159. Nutrient requirement that decreases during lactation compared to pregnancy is:
a. Vitamin C b. Vitamin B12
c. Calcium d. Iron

160. Recommended dose of folic acid in pregnancy is:
a. 200 mcg/day b. 300 mcg/day
c. 400 mcg/day d. 500 mcg/day

161. RDA of calcium in normal adult male is:
a. 800 mg b. 400 mg
c. 1200 mg d. 600 mg

162. Daily calcium requirement of infants is:
a. 300 mg b. 500 mg
c. 600 mg d. 1200 mg

RDA PROTEIN

163. In 13-15 year female child, recommended daily protein in- take (g/kg/day) is: *(Recent Question 2013)*
a. 0.68 b. 0.95
c. 1 d. 1.33

RDA IODINE

164. A sensitive indicator of environmental iodine deficiency and an effective indicator for monitoring the impact of a program: *(Recent Question 2013)*
a. Neonatal hypothyroidism
b. Prevalence of goiter
c. Prevalence of cretinism
d. Urinary iodine excretion

165. In India, the level of iodization is fixed at:
a. Not less than 30 ppm at production point and at consumer level
b. Not less than 15 ppm at production point and at consumer level
c. Not less than 30 ppm at production point and not less than 15 ppm at consumer level
d. Not less than 50 ppm at production point and not less than 25 ppm at consumer level

166. Trace elements constitute what percentage of body weight:
a. 0.001% b. 0.01%
c. 0.1/% d. 1%

167. Two in one salt is common salt fortified with:
a. Iron and iodine
b. Zinc and iodine
c. Vitamin A and iodine
d. Vitamin B12 and iodine

168. Daily requirement of iodine in adults is:
a. 50 mcg b. 100 mcg
c. 150 mcg d. 200 mcg

169. Iodine comes in iodine salt, Requirement in humans at consumer level: *(Recent Question 2013)*
a. 5 PPM b. 15 PPM
c. 25 PPM
d. 35 PPM

RDA VITAMIN A

170. Vitamin A deficiency in 18 months old child what is recommended dose:
a. 200 IU b. 2,000 IU
c. 200,000 IU d. 20,000 IU

171. Vitamin A requirement in infant is:
a. 350 mcg b. 600 mcg
c. 800 mcg d. 1000 mcg

ASSESSMENT OF NUTRITIONAL STATUS

172. Assessment of malnutrition is/are done by all, except: *(Recent Question 2013)*
a. Creatinine-height index
b. Transferrin saturation
c. Folate concentration
d. Albumin concentration
e. None of above

Ans.
149. a
150. a
151. a
152. d
153. c
154. a
155. d
156. c
157. e
158. b
159. d
160. d
161. d
162. b
163. c
164. a
165. c
166. b
167. a
168. c
169. b
170. c
171. a
172. e

Most Recent Question of 2019-18 is given at the end of MCQs

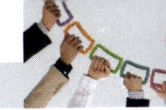

FOOD SURVEILLANCE/HYGIENE/TOXICANTS/ ADULTERATION EPIDEMIC DROPSY

173. Epidemic dropsy is caused by this toxin:
a. BOAA
b. Sanguinarine
c. Alkaloid
d. Ergot

174. A person after consuming an allegedly adulterated food developed bilateral swelling of legs, diarrhoea, glaucoma, cardiac failure. The toxin most likely to cause these symptoms is: *(Recent Question 2013)*
a. Aflatoxin
b. Pyrrolizidine
c. Sanguinarine
d. β-oxalyl-amino-alanine

175. Most sensitive for sanguinarine is:
a. $FeCl_3$
b. Paper chromatography
c. HCl
d. Nitric acid

176. Epidemic dropsy is caused by: *(Recent Question 2013)*
a. Sanguinarine
b. BOAA
c. Pyruvic Acid
d. Mustard oil

177. Argemone oil contamination of mustard oil can be detected by: *(Recent Question 2013)*
a. Phosphorus test
b. Nitric acid test
c. Coliform test
d. Methylene blue test

178. Cause of epidemic dropsy is:
a. Pyrrolizidine
b. Sanguinarine
c. Fusarium toxin
d. BOAA

179. Epidemic dropsy is caused by:
a. Sanguinarine
b. BOAA
c. Pyruvic Acid
d. Mustard oil

ENDEMIC ASCITIS

180. Endemic ascites is caused by: *(Recent Question 2013)*
a. Argemone Mexicana seed
b. Khesari dal
c. Jhunjhunia seeds
d. Ergot poisoning
e. Aspergillus flavus

181. Endemic ascites is associated with which of the following:
a. Pyrrolizidine
b. Aflatoxin
c. Sanguinarine
d. Beta Oxalyl Amino Alanine (BOAA)

LATHYRISM

182. The toxin in the pulse lathyrus Sativus can be removed by the following method: *(Recent Question 2013)*
a. Milling
b. Steeping
c. Nalgonda technique
d. Polishing

183. Lathyrism is due to excessive consumption of:
a. Khesari dal
b. Aflatoxin
c. Ergotoxin
d. Contaminated mustard oil

184. The toxin implicated in lathyrism:
a. Aflatoxin
b. Pyrrolizidine
c. Sanguinarine
d. Beta-oxalyl-amino-alanine

185. Lathyrism results due to: *(Recent Question 2013)*
a. Aflatoxin
b. BOAA
c. Pyruvic acid
d. Sanguinarine

ERGOTISM

186. Ergot infested grains can be easily removed by:
a. Floating in 20% salt water
b. Steeping method
c. Parboiling method
d. Nalgonda technique

187. Ergotism is due to toxic alkaloids produced by fungus:
a. Trichophyton
b. Claviceps purpura
c. Fusarium species
d. Absidia

MILK STERILIZATION AND ADULTERATION

188. The following test is not done on pasteurized milk:
a. Methylene blue reduction test
b. Phosphatase test
c. Standard plate count
d. Coliform count

189. Among the following milk borne disease:
1. Brucellosis
2. Salmoneilosis
3. Listeriosis
4. CBS

Which ones can be controlled by Pasteurization?
a. Brucellosis only
b. 2 and 3
c. Salmoneilosis only
d. All the above

190. Pasteurization of milk is achieved by boiling at:
a. 65° for 30 min
b. 72° for 10 sec
c. 100° for 20 sec
d. 136° for 30 sec

191. Test performed for checking pasteurisation of milk is:
a. Catalase test
b. Oxidase test
c. Phosphatase test
d. Methylene blue test

LEVELS OF HEALTH CARE

192. As per ICDS scheme, 1 Anganwadi centre should cover a population of: *(Recent Question 2013)*
a. 1000-1500
b. 2000-25000
c. 400-800
d. 100-200

193. Iodine requirement in pregnant women in mcg/mL:
a. 200
b. 150
c. 250
d. 100

194. Pasteurization of milk is done at:
a. 73°C for 20 minutes
b. 72°C for 30 seconds
c. 63°C for 30 seconds
d. 63°C for 30 minutes

195. Number of children to be evaluated for assessment of NIDDCP is:
a. 2700 children in a block
b. 2700 children in a village
c. 2700 children in a district
d. 2700 children in a taluk

Most Recent Question (2019-2018)

196. The meal provided in mid-day meals program should supply every day: *(AIIMS Nov 2018)*
a. One-third of energy requirement and half of the protein requirement
b. Half of energy requirement and one-third of the protein requirement
c. Half of energy requirement and half of the protein requirement
d. One third of energy requirement and one-third of the protein requirement

Ans.

173. b
174. c
175. b
176. a
177. b
178. b
179. a
180. c
181. a
182. b
183. a
184. d
185. b
186. a
187. b
188. a
189. d
190. a
191. c
192. c
193. c
194. d
195. c
196. a

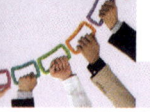

Answers with Explanations

1. Ans. (a) 1/3rd Calories, 1/2 Protein

Mid-day Meal Scheme

In 1925, a Mid-day Meal Program was introduced for disadvantaged children in Madras Municipal Corporation. Later other states as kerala, Gujarat, Pondicherry also started the scheme. Further by 1977, the program was spread to cover all blocks in the country. Salient features:

- It is under the ministry of HRD, department of school education and literacy
- The scheme guidelines envisage to provide cooked mid-day meal with 450 calories and 12 g of protein to every child at primary level and 700 calories and 20 g of protein at upper primary level.
- This energy and protein requirement for a primary child comes from cooking 100 g of rice/flour, 20 g pulses and 50 g vegetables and 5 g oil, and for an upper primary child it comes from 150 g of rice/flour, 30 g of pulses and 75 g of vegetables and 7.5 g of oil.
- Free supply of food grains @ 100 grams per child per school day at Primary and @ 150 grams per child per school day at Upper Primary.
- Provision for essentials for implementation of program as grant for stores, kitchen space and kitchen appliances.
- The program focusses on engaging females as cook-cum-helper, community participation for value addition, role of mothers for supervision and improvement of quality of food.

Revised cooking cost per child per school day w.e.f. 1.07.2016

Stage	Total cost	Central-state sharing			
		Non-NER states (60:40)		NER-States, UTs (90:10)	
		Central	State	Central	State
		Central	State	Central	State
Primary	₹4.13	₹2.48	₹1.65	₹3.72	₹0.41
Upper primary	₹6.18	₹3.71	₹2.47	₹5.56	₹0.62

2. Ans. (a) Extra 300 calories

Ref: park 24th, pg 672

Energy requirements of Indians at different ages (2010)

Age group	Category	Body weight	Requirement	
			(kcal/d)*	(kcal/kg/day)
Man	Sedentary work	60	2,320	39
	Moderate work	60	2,730	46
	Heavy work	60	3,490	58
Woman	Sedentary work	55	1,900	35
	Moderate work	55	2,230	41
	Heavy work	55	2,850	52
	Pregnant woman	55 + GWG	+350	
	Lactation	55 + WG	+600	
			+520	
Infants	0–6 months	5.4	500	92
	6–12 months	8.4	670	80
Children	1–3 years	12.9	1,060	82
	4–6 years	18.1	1,350	75
	7–9 years	25.1	1,690	67
Boys	10–12 years	34.3	2,190	64
Girls	10–12 years	35.0	2,010	57
Boys	13–15 years	47.6	2,750	58
Girls	13–15 years	46.6	2,330	50
Boys	16–17 years	55.4	3,020	55
Girls	16–17 years	52.1	2,440	47

a. Rounded off to the nearest 10 kcal/d

b. GWG-Gestational weight gain. Energy need in pregnancy should be adjusted for actual body weight, observed weight gain, and activity pattern for the population.

c. WG-Gestational weight gain remaining after delivery

Note: The current estimate of energy requirement of infants is 11–20 per cent lower than the 1988 estimates

3. **Ans. (c) 200–300 μg**

4. **Ans. (b) Adolescents of age group 10-19 yr are covered; (d) Biannual deworming through albendazole tablet (e) Screening of target groups for moderate/severe...**

5. **Ans. (a) 20 mg iron with 0.1 mg FA**

Ref: K. Park, 624; National Iron Plus Initiative, Guidelines, mohfw.nic.in

6. **Ans. (a) 1900**

Ref: K. Park, 24th ed. p 672

7. **Ans. (c) Soybean**

Ref: K. Park, 24th ed. p 666

8. **Ans. (a) Safflower oil**

Ref: K. Park, 24th ed. p 649

9. **Ans. (a) 1.2 mcg**

Ref: K. Park, 24th ed. p 658

RDA of Cyanocobalamin

- Normal adults 1 mcg/day
- Pregnancy 1.2 mcg/day
- Lactation 1.5 mcg/day

10. **Ans. (a) 2230**

Ref: K. Park, 24th ed. p 672

11. **Ans. (c) 20 mg/day**

Ref: K. Park, 24th ed. p 674

12. **Ans. (a) 60–65**

Ref: K. Park, 24th ed. p 668

13. **Ans. (b) Sanguinarine**

Ref: K. Park, 24th ed. p 695

14. **Ans. (b) James Lind**

Ref: K. Park, 24th ed. p 6

15. **Ans. (c) Protein of animal source**

Ref: K Park 24th ed. p 668

16. **Ans. (a) 1900 Cal/day**

Ref: K. Park, 24th ed. p 672

17. **Ans. (b) Primary prevention**

Ref: K. Park, 24th ed. p 46

18. **Ans. (c) Specific protection**

Ref: K. Park, 24th ed. p 47

19. **Ans. (b) Every month**

Ref: K. Park, 24th ed p- 936

20. **Ans. (b) Adolescent girls**

Ref: K. Park, 24th ed. p 629

Kishori Shakti Yojana (KSY) in ICDS, was started in the year 2000

Refer to Notes for Details

ICDS

21. **Ans. (d) 12 g of protein + 450 kcal of energy**

Ref: K. Park, 24th ed. p 698

Mid-day Meal Program [1962]

- Objective
  - To enhance school enrolment, retention and attendance of children.[Q]
  - To provide nutritional support to school children
- **Important goals** → Reorientation of eating habits, Incorporating nutrition education in curriculum, Encourage use of local available food, Improve school attendance and educational performance of pupil
- **Mid-day meal** should supply at least 1/3rd of total energy requirement and 1/2 of the protein need[Q]

Latest Updates

- Since, 2004- Hot cooked meal has been introduced
- Presently it covers all school going children in primary and upper primary classes (up to 14 year) in Govt., Govt. aided, local body schools.
- Children in primary class (Std. I –V) –are provided 450 Calories and 12 g protein+adequate micronutrient per day
- Children in upper primary classes (up to 14 year)-are provided 700 Calories and 20 g protein +adequate micronutrient per day
- Mid-day meal is provided in summer vacation in drought affected area
- Food Corporation of India has to maintain continuous availability of food grains.

22. **Ans. (b) Ministry of Education**

Ref: K. Park, 24th ed. p 698

Program	Ministry
Special Nutrition Program	Ministry of Social Welfare
Mid-day meal scheme	Ministry of Human Resource Development
ICDS	Ministry of Social Welfare
Balwadi Nutrition Program	Ministry of Social Welfare
IDD Control Program	Ministry of Health and Family Welfare
Mid-day meal program	Ministry of Education

Contd...

Program	Ministry
Vitamin A Prophylaxis Program	Ministry of Health and Family Welfare
Prophylaxis against Nutritional Anaemia	Ministry of Health and Family Welfare

23. Ans. (b) Women and child development

Ref: Revised Integrated Child Protection scheme (ICPS; 24th ed. p Ministry of Women and Child Development, Government of India

ICPS is a Government (Ministry of Women and Child Development) and Civil Society Partnership to reach out to all children (including those in difficult circumstances) under the direction and responsibility of Central and State Government

- It works to create protective environment for children in the country.
- It has strong lateral linkages and complementary systems for vigilance, detection and response.
- The scheme visualizes a structure for providing services as well as monitoring and supervising the effective functioning of child protection system

24. Ans. (c) 1975

Ref: K. Park, 24th ed. p

Integrated Child Development Services (ICDS)
Refer to Notes

25. Ans. (b) Rajiv Gandhi scheme

Ref: DK Taneja, Health Policies and Programs in India,13th ed. p- 369. Welfare schemes for Adolescent girls in India

Rajiv Gandhi Scheme for empowerment of adolescent Girls - SABLA is implemented via ICDS Scheme .

Services under SABLA

- Nutrition provision (Hot cooked food or Take home ration). For 14-18 year –All girls, 11-14 year – Out of school girl
- Iron and Folic Acid (IF(a) supplementation
- Health check-up and Referral services
- Nutrition and Health Education (NH(e)
- Counseling/Guidance on family welfare, ARSH, child care practices and home management
- Life Skill Education and accessing public services
- 16-18 year -Vocational training for girls aged 16 and above under National Skill Development Program (NSDP)

NIDDCP

26. Ans. (d) Median urinary iodine excretion

Ref: K. Park 24th ed. p 663

Indicators for IDD Control Program

- Prevalence of goiter
- Prevalence of cretinism
- Urinary iodine excretion (**Recommended for use in surveillance**)
- Serum Thyroxine (T_4) and Thyrotropic hormone (TSH).
- Prevalence of neonatal hypothyroidism [Sensitive indicator of environmental Iodine deficiency and monitoring the impact of a program)[Q]

Criteria for classifying IDD as a significant public health problem

Indicator	Mild	Moderate	Severe
Prevalence of goiter (%)	5 – 19.9	20—29.9	≥ 30
Median Urinary Iodine Excretion [mcg/L]	50 – 99	20 - 49	< 20

27. Ans. (a) 15 ppm

Ref: K. Park, 24th ed. p 681

Iodized Salt

- Most widely used prophylactic public health measure against endemic goiter.[Q]
- In India, level of iodization fixed under PFA act is not less than 30 ppm of Iodine at production point and not less than 15 ppm of iodine at the consumer level [Q]

MISCELLANEOUS

28. Ans. (b) Ministry of Health and Family Welfare

Ref: www.fssai.gov.in

29. Ans. (a) 600 Kcal + 20 g proteins/day

Ref: DK Taneja, Health Policy and Programs in India, 13th ed. p-367. K Park, 23rd ed. p 591

As per the latest revision in rates (2012), Supplementary Nutrition norms are:

Beneficiary	Calorie/ day	Protein/ day	Revised rates/ beneficiary
Pregnant and Lactating Women	600	18–20 g	₹ 7/day
Severely Malnourished Child (6-72 month)	800	20–25 g	₹ 9/day
Child (6-72 month)	500	12–15 g	₹ 6/day

- Child < 3 year, Pregnant and Lactating Women are given take home rations
- Supplementary nutrition is provided for 300 days a year or 25 days in a month
- Child 3-6 year are provided 2 meals – 1 hot cooked meal and 1 Ready to eat snacks

30. Ans. (c) 6

Ref: K Park, 24th ed. p 628

ICDS Scheme was started in the year 1975, with following objectives

- To improve health and nutritional status of children 0-6 years of age
- To lay foundations for Psychological, Physical and Social development of the child
- To cut down mortality, morbidity, malnutrition and school drop-out
- To achieve coordination between various departments working for the promotion of child development
- To increase capability of mother and cater nutritional needs of child through proper nutrition and health education.

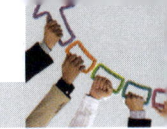

Services under ICDS	Beneficiary
Health check-up	Pregnant and Lactating women, Children (6–72 month)
Supplementary nutrition	Pregnant and Lactating women, Children (6–72 month), Adolescent girls (11–18 yr)
Nutrition and health education	Pregnant and Lactating women, Women aged 15–45 year, Adolescent girls (11–18 yr)
Referral	Children (6–72 month)
Non formal education	Children in age group 3-6 years
Immunization	Pregnant women (TT), Children (6–72 month)

31. Ans. (c) 600 cal, 16-20 g of proteins

Ref: K. Park, 24th ed. p 628

32. Ans. (a) 2500

Ref: K. Park, 24th ed. p 672

Recommended Daily Energy Requirements

Group	Category	Net energy [Kcal/day]	Protein [g/day]	Visible fat [g/day]
Male [60 kg]	Sedentary work	2320	60	25
	Moderate work	2730		30
	Heavy work	3490		40
Female [55 kg]	Sedentary work	1900	55	20
	Moderate work	2230		25
	Heavy work	2850		30

Recommended Additional Daily Allowances (Pregnancy and lactation)

Group	Energy (kcal/ day)	Protein *(g/ day)	Fat (g/day)	Calcium (mg/day)**	Iron (mg/ day)	Vit A (retinol) mcg / day***	Folate mcg/ day****
Pregnancy	+ 350	78 (i.e. +23)	30	1200 (i.e. RDA +600)	RDA of 21mg/ day + 14 mg/ day	800 (i.e. RDA +200	500 (i.e. RDA +300)
Lactation [0-6 month]	+ 600	74 (i.e. +19)	30	1200 (i.e. RDA +600)	RDA of 21mg/ day	950 (i.e. RDA +350)	300 (i.e. RDA +100
Lactation [6-12 month]	+ 520	68 (i.e. +13)					

** RDA = 1 g/ kg body weight/day, **RDA= 600 mg/day, ***RDA= 600mcg/ day, ****RDA= 200 mcg/day So, pregnant woman with moderate work requires 2580Kcal/day (2230+350)*

PROTEIN

33. Ans. (d) Net Protein Utilization

Ref: K. Park, 24th ed. p 672

Protein quality of any food item is assessed by comparing it to a "***Reference protein***" (Egg protein). Methods used are:

- **Amino acid** (or chemical) **score:**
  - It is concentration of each essential amino acid in test protein expressed as a percentage of that amino acid in
  - Amino acid score = $\dfrac{\text{Number of mg of one amino acid per g of protein}}{\text{Number of mg of the same amino acid per g of egg protein}} \times 100$
  - Amino acid score is between 50-60 for starch and 70-80 for animal foods
- **Net protein utilization (NPU):**
  - In calculating protein quality, 1 g of protein is assumed to be equivalent to 6.25 g of Nitrogen
  - *If NPU is low, protein requirement is high and vice versa.* NPU of protein in Indian diets is 50 - 80.

Protein quantity *of any food item is assessed by PE Ratio (Protein Energy Ratio)*

- *PE Ratio is the percentage of total energy in diet supplied by protein content of food.*[Q]

Also Know...................

- *NPU is a better indicator of protein quality compared to amino acid score.*[Q] DIASS is regarded as the best indicator.

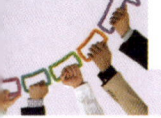

34. Ans. (b) Nitrogen retained by body/Nitrogen intake) × 100

Ref: K. Park, 24th ed. p 672

NPU is the proportion of ingested protein retained in the body under specified conditions for maintenance and/or growth of tissues.

$$NPU = \frac{\text{Nitrogen retained by the body}}{\text{Nitrogen intake}} \times 100$$

$$\text{or} \quad \frac{\text{Biological value} \times \text{Digestibility coefficient}}{\text{Nitrogen intake}}$$

35. Ans. (b) 20

Ref: K. Park, 24th ed. p 647

36. Ans. (d) Contains all essential amino acids

Ref: K. Park, 24th ed. p 647

Biologically complete protein is one that contains all essential amino acids in amounts in accordance to human needs.

Also Know......................

- *Animal proteins are rated superior to vegetable proteins because they are "biologically complete".*[Q]

37. Ans. (b) 65

Ref: K. Park, 24th ed. p 648

38. Ans. (b) 4

Ref: K. Park, 24th ed. p 672

Energy (kcal/g) obtained from dietary sources:
- Proteins - 4 kcal/g (or 17 kJ)
- Fat - 9 kcal/g (or 37 kJ)
- Carbohydrate - 4 kcal/g (or 17 kJ)
- Dietary Fiber -2 kcal/g (or 17 kJ)

Also Know......................

- Cereals constitute about 80% of our diet and provide 50-80% of daily energy requirement

39. Ans. (b) Estimated average requirement

Ref: K. Park, 24th ed. p 670

Estimated Average Requirement (EAR) is the average daily nutrient intake level estimated to meet the requirement of half of the healthy individuals in a particular life stage and gender group.
- Daily safe level = Estimated average requirement + 1.96 SD of protein requirement

40. Ans. (b) 0.83 g/kg/day

Ref: K. Park, 24th ed. p 670

Daily safe level of protein intake = Estimated average requirement + 1.96 SD of protein requirement = 0.83 g/kg/day
- Quality of protein adjustment, makes RDA = 1 g/kg/day

FATTY ACID

41. Ans. (c) Safflower oil

Ref: K. Park, 24th ed. p 672

Fatty Acids

- **Saturated fatty acids** (Lauric, Palmitic and Stearic acids) are mainly found in animal fats.
  - *Exception* is coconut and palm oils
  - ***Richest source are*** → Coconut oil > Palm oil > Butter/ Ghee > Cotton seed oil >Palmolein.[Q]
- ***Unsaturated fatty acids*** are Mono Unsaturated Fatty Acid (MUFA) [e.g., oleic acid] and Poly Unsaturated Fatty Acids (PUFA) [e.g. Linoleic acid and α-Linolenic acid]
  - **Richest source of MUFA** are → Mustard, Rape seed, Groundnut oil > Palm oil> Butter > Sunflower oil and Corn oilQ
  - **Richest source of PUFA** (mostly found in vegetable oils, *exception* is fish oil)
  - Linoleic (n-6) → Safflower oil (75%) > Sunflower oil > Corn oil > Soya bean oil > Cotton seed oil
  - a-Linolenic acid (n=3) → Rapeseed, Mustard, Soybean

42. Ans. (d) 7700

Ref: K. Park, 24th ed. p 648

Adipose tissue constitutes 10%-15% of body weight. 1 Kg of adipose tissue corresponds to 7700 kcal of energy.

43. Ans. (d) Trans fatty acids are not atherogenic

Ref: K. Park, 24th ed. p 650

Hydrogenation is a process in which under conditions of optimum temperature and pressure, in the presence of a catalyst, the vegetable liquid oils are converted into semi – solid/solid fat known as "Vanaspati".
- During hydrogenation, unsaturated fatty acids are converted into saturated acids
- EFA content is drastically reduced.
- Partial hydrogenation results in formation of Trans fatty acids.

Also Know......................

- Trans fatty acid is atherogenic (↑LDL and ↓HDL) and increases risk of Coronary Heart Disease. It takes years for the body to flush it out.
- Vanaspati lacks fat-soluble vitamins, hence is fortified with 2500 IU of vitamin A and 175 IU of vitamin D per 100 g.
- Refined oils –There is no change in unsaturated fatty acid content, free fatty acids and rancid materials are removed and quality and taste of oils improves.

44. Ans. (b) Safflower oil

Ref: K. Park, 24th ed. p 649

45. **Ans. (a) 2.5 g**

Ref: Textbook of community Medicine, R Bhalawar, 1st ed. p-343

Daily Energy and Protein Requirement of Infant

- 0–3 month → 115 Kcal/Kg body weight Energy and 2.30 g/Kg body weight proteins (In terms of milk protein)
- 3–6 month → 99 Kcal/Kg body weight Energy and 1.85 g/Kg body weight proteins (In terms of milk protein)
- 6-9 month → 95 Kcal/Kg body weight Energy and 1.65 g/Kg body weight proteins (In terms of milk protein)
- 9–12 month → 101Kcal/Kg body weight Energy and 1.50 g/Kg body weight proteins (In terms of milk protein)

46. **Ans. (a) Linoleic Acid**

Ref: K. Park, 24th ed. p 648

Essential fatty acids (EFA) are fatty acids that *cannot be synthesized by humans and are derived only from food.*[Q]

- *Most important EFA is Linoleic acid*[Q] [Base for production of other EFA (e.g., Linolenic and Arachidonic acids)]
- Linoleic acid is found in abundance in vegetable oils

Also Know......................

- Not all polyunsaturated fatty acids are essential fatty acids.

47. **Ans. (a) Vitamin A**

Ref: K.Park, 24th ed. p 696

Food Fortification

"The process whereby nutrients are added to foods (in relatively small quantities) to maintain or improve the quality of the diet of a group, a community, or a population."

Examples

Fluoridation of water → Prevention of dental caries
Iodization of salt → Prevention of endemic goiter
Fortification of vanaspati, milk with vitamins A and D.
Twin fortification of salt with iodine and iron.

Characteristics of Food and Nutrient for Successful Fortification

- Food item to be fortified must be consumed consistently on a regular basis in diet.
- Quantity of nutrient added must provide an effective supplement for low consumers of the food
- Nutrient should not be hazardous for the amount added for those who consume more
- There should not be any noticeable change in taste, smell, appearance, or consistency
- Cost of fortification must not be high
- Adequate system of surveillance and control

48. **Ans. (b) Soybean oil, (c) Safflower oil, (d) Corn oil**

Ref: K. Park, 24th ed. p 649

Richest source of PUFA (mostly found in vegetable oils, *exception* is fish oil)

- Linoleic (n–6) → Safflower oil (75%) > Sunflower oil > Corn oil > Soya bean oil > Cotton seed oil
- a-Linolenic acid (n = 3) → Rapeseed, Mustard, Soyabean

VITAMIN A

49. **Ans. (a) Halibut liver oil**

Ref: K. Park, 24th ed. p 653

Sources of Vitamin A

- Animal food (Contain preformed vitamin A or Retinol) → Liver, Eggs, Butter, Cheese, Whole milk, Fish and Meat.
- Plant food (Contain provitamin or carotenes) → Green leafy vegetables (Spinach and Amaranth), Carrots, Yellow fruits and vegetables (e.g., Papaya, Mango, Pumpkin)
- Fortified food- Vanaspati, Milk

Also Know......................

- Fish liver oil (used as nutritional supplement) is the richest natural source of Vitamin A.
- Green leafy vegetables is the cheapest source (Darker the green leaves higher the carotene content)

50. **Ans. (a) Halibut liver oil**

Ref: K. Park, 24th ed. p 653

51. **Ans. (b) Children 6 months to 6 year**

Ref: K. Park, 24th ed. p 654

Refer to Notes

52. **Ans. (b) 2**

Ref: K. Park, 24th ed. p 654

Treatment of Vitamin A Deficiency

Early treatment can reverse all early stages of Xerophthalmia.

- *Administration of massive dose (2, 00, 000 IU or 110 mg) of Retinol palmitate orally on 2 successive days*[Q]
- *All children with corneal ulcers should receive vitamin A whether or not a deficiency is suspected.*

53. **Ans. (b) 0.5%**

Ref: K. Park 24th ed. p 654

54. **Ans. (a) Conjunctiva**

Ref: K park 24th ed. p 654

Bitot's spots are pearly white or yellowish, triangular foamy spots on bulbar conjunctiva on either side of cornea (frequently bilateral)

55. **Ans. (b) Bitot's spot**

Ref: Mahajan and Gupta, Textbook of PSM, 4th ed., p-418

56. **Ans. (b) 0.5%**

Ref: K. Park, 24th ed. p 654

57. **Ans. (b) 0.5%**

Ref: K. Park, 24th ed p 654

VITAMIN B1

58. Ans. (b) Vitamins

Ref: K. Park, 24th ed. p 656

Milling (Polishing) of rice results in loss of Vitamin B1.

- *Washing, Cooking practices (Toast or use of baking Soda), prolonged storage of fruits/vegetables also results in loss of Vitamin B1.*

59. Ans. (d) Thiamine

Ref: K. Park, 24th ed. p 656

60. Ans. (b) B6

Ref: K. Park, 24th ed. p 658

Pyridoxine (vitamin B6) plays an important role in the metabolism of amino acids, fats and carbohydrate.

- Source → Milk, Liver, Meat, Egg yolk, Fish, Whole grain cereals, Legumes and Vegetables.
- Deficiency results in peripheral neuritis. Patients receiving INH are often provided a supplement of pyridoxine
- Riboflavin deficiency impairs the optimal utilization of pyridoxine.
- Requirements of adults vary directly with protein intake. Adults may need 2 mg/day; during pregnancy and lactation, 2.5 mg/day. Balanced diets usually contain pyridoxine [deficiency is rare].

61. Ans. (c) Gingelly seeds

Ref: K. Park, 24th ed. p 656

Thiamine (Vitamin B_1) is a water soluble vitamin *essential for utilisation of carbohydrates.*[Q]

RDA is *0.5 mg per 1000 kcal of energy intake.*

Thiamine deficiency leads to:

Beriberi

- *Dry Beriberi:* Nerve involvement (*peripheral neuritis*)[Q]
- *Wet Beriberi:* Heart involvement (cardiac beriberi)[Q]
- *Infantile beriberi:* in infants (2-4 month) breast-fed by a Thiamine-deficient mother.[Q]

Wernicke's encephalopathy [characterised by ophthalmoplegia, polyneuritis, ataxia and mental deterioration] occurs in alcoholics and sometimes in people who fast.

Thiamine (Vitamin B) Source

- Whole grain cereals (wheat and rice), g, yeast, pulses, oil seeds and nuts are important source of Vitamin B1
- Gingelly seeds [Til] and Groundnut are richest source of vitamin B[Q]
- Meat, fish, eggs, vegetables and fruits contain smaller amounts.
- Milk is an good source of thiamine for infants, provided mothers Thiamine status is satisfactory.
- Major source of thiamine in Indian diet is cereals [contribute 60–85% of the total supply].

NIACIN

62. Ans. (b) B3

Ref: K. Park, 24th ed. p 657

Nutrient	Richest Sources
Vitamin A	Halibut Liver Oil
Vitamin B1	Gingelly seeds
Vitamin B2	Sheep liver
Vitamin C	Amla (Indian Gooseberry)
Vitamin D	Halibut Liver Oil
Calcium	Ragi
Iron	Pistachio
Linoleic acid	Safflower oil
Linolenic acid	Flaxseed oil
Eicosapentaenoic acid	Fish

63. Ans. (c) Maize

Ref: K. Park, 24th ed. p 657

Jowar/Maize predominant diets result in amino acid imbalance → Excess of Leucine, that interferes in conversion of Tryptophan to Niacin resulting in deficiency (Pellagra)

- It occurs in Telangana, where people eat Jowar, consume very less milk or other food of animal origin

64. Ans. (d) Niacin

Ref: K. Park, 24th ed. p 657

Niacin *deficiency results in* **Pellagra,** characterised by **3 D's** - ***Diarrhoea, Dermatitis*** [bilaterally symmetrical and on body surfaces exposed to sunlight] and **Dementia**[Q]

- Glossitis, Stomatitis and Mental changes (depression, irritability and delirium) may also occur.
- **Prevention-**Mixed diet containing milk and/or meat and avoid total dependence on maize or sorghum
- **Requirement–RDA** is 6.6 mg/1000 kcal of energy intake

Also Know......................

- Casal's necklace-refers to skin lesions on neck in Pellagra

65. Ans. (a) Pellagra

Ref: K. Park, 24th ed. p 657

Vitamin Deficiency Disorders

Type of Vitamin	Vitamin	Deficiency
Fat Soluble Vitamin	A	Xerophthalmia
	D	Rickets and Osteomalacia
	E	Haemolytic anaemia in newborn
	K	Haemorrhagic disease in newborn

Contd...

Type of Vitamin	Vitamin	Deficiency
Water Soluble Vitamin	B1 [Thiamine]	Beri-Beri
	B2 [Riboflavin]	Ariboflavinosis
	B3 [Niacin]	Pellagra [3D]
	B5 [Pantothenic Acid]	Burning Feet Syndrome
	B6 [Pyridoxine]	Peripheral neuritis
	B7 [Biotin]	Dermatitis, Enteritis
	B9[Folic Acid]	Megaloblastic Anaemia, Neural Tube defect
	B12	Megaloblastic [pernicious] anaemia
	C	Scurvy

66. Ans. (c) Excess of leucine

Ref: K. Park, 24th ed. p 657

VITAMIN C

67. Ans. (b) Neurolathyrism

Ref: K. Park, 24th ed. p 682

Lathyrism [Neurolathyrism] is a *gradual onset spastic paralysis of lower limbs* [Q], occurring *in adults consuming the pulse, Lathyrus sativus [Khesari dal] in large quantities.*

- ***Toxin present in Lathyrus seeds is Beta Oxalyl Amino Alanine (BOAA)***[Q]

Recommended Interventions

- Vitamin C Prophylaxis-500–1000 mg per day for a week and generous amounts in athyrogenic diet.
- PFA Act has banned Lathyrus in all forms i.e. whole, split and flour
- Removal of toxin- (a). Steeping method (b) Parboiling
- Education on dangers of consuming Khesari dal and need to remove toxin before consumption
- Genetic approach-Selective propagation and cultivation of strains with very low levels of toxin (0.1 %).
- Socio- economic upliftment

VITAMIN D

68. Ans. (d) Halibut fish liver oil

Ref: K. Park, 24th ed. p 655

Fish liver oils are the richest source of vitamin D. (Used as supplements)

- Halibut fish liver oil (Maximum Vit D) > Cod liver oil> Shark liver oil

Vitamin C (ascorbic acid) is a water-soluble vitamin. [most sensitive of all vitamins to heat.]

Functions

- Collagen formation.
- Facilitate absorption of iron from vegetarian diet (Reducing ferric iron to ferrous iron).
- Inhibition of nitrosamine formation by the intestinal mucosa.
- Prevents common cold and protects against infection.

Dietary sources

- Fresh fruit, Green leafy vegetable, Germinating pulses
- Amla [Indian gooseberry] is one of the richest sources of vitamin C.[Q]
- Guavas and Sitaphal are also rich source.
- Milk, Egg, Cereals and Dry fruits are poor sources of vitamin C.

Deficiency results in Scurvy

- ***Estimated requirement*** is 40 mg/day for adults.

69. Ans. (d) Calcitriol

Ref: Committee to Review Dietary Reference Intakes for Vitamin D and Calcium Food and Nutrition Board

Vitamin D2 (Ergocalciferol) and Vitamin D3 (Cholecalciferol) synthesized in human skin from 7-dehydrocholesterol and intake of animal-based foods are biologically inactive until they undergo hydroxylation reactions in liver (25-hydroxyvitamin D) and kidney to form Calcitriol (1, 25-dihydroxyvitamin D).

Also Know......................

- Vitamin D3 (Cholecalciferol) is more potent compared to Vitamin D2 in all primate species.

70. Ans. (d) Cod liver oil

Ref: K. Park, 24th ed. p 655

Source of Vitamin D

- Exposure to sunlight (synthesized in body by action of UV rays on 7-dehydrocholesterol in skin).
- Food of animal origin [Liver, egg yolk, butter/cheese, Milk, Fish fat].
- Human milk has water soluble vitamin D sulphate for infants.
- Fortified food [Milk, margarine, vanaspati and infant foods].

Also Know......................

- Fish liver oils are the richest source of vitamin D.

VITAMIN K

71. Ans. (c) 0.03 mg/kg,

Ref: K. Park, 24th ed. p 656

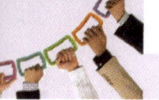

Vitamin K

- **Source:**
  - Vitamin K1-Fresh green vegetables (particularly dark green) and fruits, cow's milk.
  - Vitamin K2 -Synthesized by intestinal bacteria
- **Role**-Stimulate production and/or release of coagulation factors.
- **Deficiency**-Prolonged blood clotting time (Low level of prothrombin in blood).
- **RDA** is about 0.03 mg/kg for adult.
- **High risk group**-Newborn infants.
- **Prophylaxis**-Single intramuscular dose of Vitamin K (0.1-0.2 mg of Menadione Sodium Bisulfite)
- Long-term administration of antibiotics > 1 week may temporarily suppress normal intestinal flora.

ZINC

72. Ans. (d) Increased Appetite

Ref: K. Park, 24th ed. p 663

Zinc deficiency results in

- Growth retardation, short stature, failure to thrive and sexual infantilism in adolescents
- Loss of taste andd ecreased appetite
- Impaired immunity and delayed wound healing
- In pregnancy spontaneous abortion, congenital malformation (anencephaly), LBW, IUGR and preterm delivery

Also Know......................

- Zinc is needed for metabolism of glucides and proteins and synthesis of insulin by pancreas
- It acts as an antioxidant.
- Low zinc level in blood is seen in Liver disease, Pernicious anaemia, Thalassaemia and Myocardial infarction.
- Zinc + ORS significantly reduce duration/severity of acute and persistent diarrhea and increase survival.
- Zinc supplementation may reduce incidence of clinical attacks of malaria in children
- Source → Animal food (meat, milk and fish). Bio-availability in vegetables is low.
- Suggested daily intake for → Adult male is 15 mg/day, female is 12 mg/day, children is 10 mg/day and infants is 5 mg. Growing children, pregnant and lactating women need more.

73. Ans. (b) Inherited disorder of impaired...

Ref: Nelson textbook of pediatrics, 18th ed., Nutritional derma- tosis, p- 670

Acrodermatitis enteropathica – is a rare genetic disorder

- ***Clinical features*** – Diarrhoea, Inflammatory rash around mouth/anus, hair loss
- It is due to malabsorption of Zinc via intestinal cells.

CALCIUM

74. Ans (c) 600 mg

Ref: K. Park, 24th ed. p 674 Dietary Supplement Fact Sheet, National Institute of Health. http://ods.od.nih.gov/factsheets/Calcium-HealthProfessional/

Calcium

- Good source are green leafy vegetables (cheapest), milk and milk products (e.g. Cheese, Curd, Skimmed milk, Butter milk), nuts/oil seeds and fish 1 litre of cow's milk provides about 1200 mg of calcium and human milk about 300 mg.[Q]
- Among Cereals–Ragi, Bengal gram (whole), Rajmah and Soyabean are good source.
- Rice and wheat are poor in calcium
- Calcium is drinking water may provide up to 200 mg/day.
- **Among fruits:** Sitaphal is a good source.
- About 20-30 % of dietary calcium is normally absorbed.
- *Absorption is enhanced by vitamin D*[Q]
- Absorption is decreased by phytate [Cereals], oxalate [Green leafy vegetable] and fatty acid in diet.
- Calcium absorption is also regulated to some extent by body need.
- **Deficiency** results in Rickets and Osteomalacia

75. Ans. (a) 1200 mg

Ref: K. Park, 24th ed. p 674 Dietary Supplement Fact Sheet, National Institute of Health. http://ods.od.nih.gov/factsheets/Calcium-HealthProfessional/)

As per dietary supplement factsheet, NIH (USA) – Recommended Daily Allowance for Calcium among elderly people is as follows.

Age (in years)	Male	Female
51–70 years	1,000 mg	1,200 mg
71 year and above	1,200 mg	1,200 mg

RDA of Calcium in Indians (ICMR-NIN, Dietary Guideline for Indians)

Group	Calcium mg/day
Adult Man	600
Adult Woman	600
Pregnant Woman	1200
Lactating Woman	1200
Infant	500
Children (1–9 year)	600
Adolescents (10–19 year)	800

It does state that elderly need more of calcium, iron, zinc, vitamin A and antioxidants for healthy ageing.

IRON AND FOLIC ACID

76. Ans. (b) Biweekly IFA to children 6-60 months

Ref: National Iron Plus Initiative, Guidelines, mohfw.nic.in

77. Ans. (a) 100 mg Iron + 500 mcg Folic acid…

Ref: National Iron Plus Initiative, Guidelines, mohfw.nic.in

78. Ans. (a) Fortified in all wheat products in…

Ref: K. Park, 24th ed. p 658

FLUORINE

79. Ans. (a) 0.5 to 0.8 mg/litre

Ref: K. Park, 24th ed. p 663

Fluorine *is essential for normal mineralization of bones and formation of dental enamel.*

- *Major source* → Drinking water, Sea fish, cheese and tea.
- **Recommended** fluoride concentration in drinking water is 0.5 to 0.8 mg/L.[Q] [In temperate countries, with low water intake 1- 2 mg/L is acceptable]

80. Ans. (b) Lime and alum

Ref: K. Park, 24th ed. p 682

Nalgonda technique developed by National Environmental Engineering Research Institute, Nagpur is a technique for defluoridation of water.

- It involves addition of lime and alum in sequence followed by flocculation, sedimentation and filtration.
- It can be used for household defluoridation of water

Also Know……………………

- **Other Interventions:** Change of drinking water source (Fluoride level *0.5 to 0.8 mg/L*)[Q], No Fluoride supplements and avoiding fluoride toothpaste for children up to 6 years of age in areas of endemic fluorosis

81. Ans. (d) None of the above

Ref: K. Park, 24th ed. p 682

Endemic fluorosis is reported in Andhra Pradesh (Nellore, Nalgonda and Prakasam), Punjab, Haryana, Karnataka, Kerala and Tamil Nadu

- ***Toxic manifestation*** *comprise*:
  - **Dental fluorosis:** "mottling" of dental enamel. [Fluoride ingestion > 1.5 mg/L in first 7 years of life (years of tooth calcification)]
  - **Skeletal fluorosis** (lifetime daily intake of 3–6 mg/L or more) and Crippling fluorosis and permanent disability. (Daily intake in excess of 10 mg/L),
  - **Genu valgum:** In people whose staple food is sorghum (Jowar) that promotes higher retention of ingested fluoride.

82. Ans. (c) 3.0–6.0 mg/L

Ref: K. Park, 24th ed. p 682

83. Ans. (d) > 10 ppm

Ref: K. Park, 24th ed. p 682

DIETARY FIBER

84. Ans. (b) 40 g

Ref: K. Park, 24th ed. p 652

- Desirable **daily intake** of dietary fiber is about 40 g per 2000 kcal consumed[Q].
- Intake >60 g per day can reduce the nutrient absorption and cause bowel irritation.

85. Ans. (a) 2

Ref: K. Park, 24th ed. p 672

Energy (kcal/g) obtained from Dietary Fiber -2 kcal/g (or 17 kJ)

- 70% fiber in conventional food is fermentable.

86. Ans. (c) 7

Ref: K. Park, 23 ed. p-631; 24th ed. p 669

Alcohol yields about 7 kcal energy per g.

Alcohol content in alcoholic beverages range from 5–6 % in beers to 40–45 % in whisky, rum, gin and brandy

87. Ans. (b) Ragi

Ref: K.Park, 24th ed. p 652

Cereals are major source of dietary fiber, followed by protein

Chick pea> Ragi > Wheat, Bajra, Maiza> Lentil pea, Pigeaon Pea, Green gram

88. Ans. (b) Maize

Ref: K.Park, 24th ed. p 652

Although Wheat has higher amount of Total Dietary Fiber, but Soluble fiber is more. Hence the answer is Maize

89. Ans. (b) Decrease post prandial glucose, (c) Decrease bile salt reabsorption, (d) Decrease LDL cholesterol, (e) Increase in bulk of stool

Ref: K. Park, 24th ed. p 652 Textbook of PSM, Gupta and Mahajan, 4rd ed., p-393

Dietary fiber comprise carbohydrates (Pectin, cellulose, hemicelluloses) and non carbo hydrates (lignin) in plant food resistant to endogenous digestive enzymes of human gastro-intestinal tract.

- It increases volume and softens consistency of stool.[Low fiber diet leads to constipation]
- It decreases the glycemic response [rise in post prandial glucose] to an oral carbohydrate meal.
- It lowers risk of atherosclerosis (Decreasing total serum cholesterol and LDL and increasing HDL) and CHD

- It has a protective role against cancer, especially cancer colon, stomach, breast, prostate.
- It has a role in weight reduction.[Q]
- It has a role in management of Irritable Bowel Syndrome and recurrent diverticulitis

CEREALS AND MILLETS

90. Ans. (d) Lysine

Ref: K. Park, 23rd ed. p 627

Limiting amino acids in Cereals

- *Wheat* → Lysine and Threonine.[Q]
- *Maize* → Lysine and Tryptophan.[Q]
- *Sorghum* → Lysine and Threonine

Also Know......................

- ***Rice protein** is rich in Lysine compared to other cereal proteins*[Q]. Hence, considered superior cereal protein.[Q]

91. Ans. (c) Lysine and Methionine

Ref: K. Park, 24th ed. p 664-66

Cereal are deficient in lysine and threonine[Q]; *Pulse in methionine.*[Q]

Also Know......................

- ***Supplementary action of proteins*** → If 2 or more vegetarian foods are consumed together (rice-dal), their proteins supplement one another and provide a protein comparable to animal protein

92. Ans. (c) Maize

Ref: K. Park, 24th ed. p 664

Excess of Leucine in Maize and Sorghum interferes in conversion of Tryptophan to Niacin, aggravating pellagragenic action of maize

- Maize is the 3rd (next to rice and wheat) most consumed cereal worldwide.
- Yellow variety has significant amount of carotenoid pigments.
- Maize is rich in fat.
- Opaque-2 gene incorporation into maize has led to improvement in quality of protein.
- Pellagra in Telangana and Marathwada regions, is due to Sorghum predominance in diet consumed

93. Ans. (a) Rice proteins are deficient in lysine

Ref: K. Park, 24th ed. p 664

Rice

- Protein content varies from 6-9%
- Rice protein is of better quality (rich in lysine) compared to other cereals
- Rice is a good source of group B vitamins (Especially Thiamine), but is devoid of Vitamins A, D and C
- Rice is a poor source of calcium and iron
  - Milling leads to loss of Thiamine [up to 75% loss], Riboflavin [60% loss] and protein [15% loss].
  - Washing in large quantities of water leads to loss of up to 60% of water- soluble vitamins and minerals.

94. Ans. (b) Partial cooking in steam

Ref: K. Park, 24th ed. p 665

Parboiling ***is an ancient Indian technique to preserve nutritive value of Rice.***
Central Food Technological Research Institute
Mysore recommends hot soaking process for parboiling

Parboiling

- Unhusked rice is soaked in hot water (65°C–70°C) for 3–4 hours, followed by drainage of water and steaming for 5–10 min, drying and milling
- In process of steaming, vitamins and minerals in the outer aleurone layer are driven into the inner endosperm and are not lost on subsequent milling
- During drying, germ gets attached more firmly to the grain and hardens the rice grain making it more resistant to insect invasion and suitable for storage.
- Starch also gets gelatinized which improves the keeping quality of rice
- Disadvantage - Bad odour.
- **Consumption of under-milled or "parboiled" rice is advocated in place of withe polished rice.**

95. Ans. (b) Preservation of Nutrients

Ref: K. Park, 24th ed. p 665

96. Ans. (b) Wheat

Ref: K. Park, 24th ed. p 664

- ***Limiting amino acids in cereals is Lysine and Threonine.***[Q]
- ***Limiting amino acids in pulses** is Methionine and Cysteine.*

Also Know......................

- ***Rice protein** is rich in Lysine compared to other cereal proteins*[Q]. Hence, considered superior protein.[Q]

PULSES

97. Ans. (a) Methionine

Ref: K. Park, 24th ed. p 666

98. Ans. (c) Egg protein

Ref: K. Park, 24th ed. p 668 Egg protein is considered as the "reference protein".[Q]

- *Quality of a protein is assessed by comparison to egg protein*
- Egg proteins have high Biological value of 94, Digestibility and NPU of 100

99. Ans. (b) Vitamin C

Ref: K. Park, 24th ed. p 666

Fermentation enhances the levels of riboflavin, thiamine and niacin in pulses.

- Germinating pulses are rich in Vitamin C and B (Dry pulses do not contain vitamin C)

100. Ans. (c) Germinating pulses have lower...

Ref: K. Park, 24th ed. p 666

101. Ans. (a) 40 g

Ref: K. Park, 24th ed. p 700

102. Ans. (b) Methionine

Ref: K. Park, 24th ed. p 666

Pulses (*Poor man's meat*)

- Pulses contain 20–25 % protein [more than eggs, fish or meat and cereals]
- *Pulse proteins are inferior to animal proteins.*[Q]
- *Pulse proteins are poor in methionine and to a lesser extent in cysteine, but are rich in lysine.*[Q]
- Pulses are rich in minerals and group B vitamins (Riboflavin and Thiamine).

Also Know......................

- Soyabean contains highest amount of protein (40%), fat (20 %) and minerals (4%) among pulses.[Q]
- Proteins quality is also superior (NPU=55)
- Limiting amino acid is methionine.[Q]
- Phytates and Tannins in raw pulse decrease bio availability of nutrients to body (Anti nutritional factors)

103. Ans. (b) Pulses

Ref: K. Park, 24th ed. p 666

104. Ans. (c) Methionine and Cysteine

Ref: K. Park, 24th ed. p 666

EGG

105. Ans. (c) Egg

Ref: K. Park, 24th ed. p 668

Egg protein is "***reference protein***" because of high biological value and digestibility. **NPU = 100**

- Egg proteins have all 9 essential amino acids in right proportions

106. Ans. (c) Vitamin C

Ref: K Park 24th ed. p 668

A 60 g egg contains 6 g of protein, 6 g of fat, 30 mg of calcium and 1.5 mg of iron.

- It supplies about 70 kcal of energy.
- **Egg** *contains all nutrients except carbohydrate and vitamin C.*

High cholesterol (250 mg/egg) in egg is a risk for CHD

107. Ans. (d) 100

Ref: K Park 24th ed. p 668

Egg proteins have high Biological value of 94, Digestibility and NPU of 100

108. Ans. (c) Carbohydrate

Ref: K Park 24th ed. p 668

109. Ans. (c) C

Ref: K Park 24th ed p- 668

110. Ans. (c) 60 g egg has 6 g Fat, 6 g protein ...

Ref: K. Park, 24th ed-668

111. Ans. (a) Egg

Ref: S Lal, Textbook of PSM, 4st ed., p-591, K. Park, 24th ed. p 668

Sources of Cholesterol

- Endogenous- Synthesized by body tissues, e.g. Liver
- Exogenous – Richest source are egg yolk (250 mg/egg), > whole milk dairy products and organ meat.

Also Know......................

Cholesterol is not found in food of plant origin.

- Normal level is 150-250 mg/100 mL or less.
- Safe level is 200mg/100 mL or less
- Ideal ratio of Saturated fatty acid, MUFA and PUFA is 1:1.5:1

112. Ans. (c) C

Ref: K Park 24th ed. p 668

MILK

113. Ans. (a) Methionine

Ref: K. Park, 24th ed. p 574

Human milk has more of Cysteine and Taurine (considered indespensable) compared to cow's milk.

- Human milk has lesser quantity of Methionine compared to cow's milk.

114. Ans. (c) 11 g

Ref: K. Park, 24th ed. p 574-75

Protein content of cow milk is 3 times more than human milk.

- Cow's Milk has 33 g protein/L (28 g Casein and 5 g Soluble protein), whereas human milk has 11 g protein/L (4 g Casein and 7 g Soluble protein)
- Soluble protein content of human milk is more (Lactalbumin -3.5 g, Lactotransferrin 1-2 g, Immunoglobulin 1-2 g, Lysozyme-0.5 g). Beta-Lactalbumin is found in cow milk (not human milk)
- Human milk is also rich in Lactose, Linoleic acid

115. Ans. (b) 1 g

Ref: K. Park, 24th ed. p 574-75

- Cow's Milk has higher amount of Calcium and Phosphorous -1 g/L each.
- Human milk has higher amount of Iron, Vitamin C and D

116. Ans. (d) 1.1 g/100 mL

Ref: K. Park, 24th ed. p 668

Nutritive value of milk (per 100 g)

	Human	Cow	Buffalo	Goat
Lactose (g)	7.4	4.4	5.1	4.6
Protein (g)	1.1	3.2	4.3	3.3
Fat (g)	3.4	4.1	6.5	4.5
Calories (Kcal)	65	67	117	72
Iron (mg)	–	0.2	0.2	0.3
Calcium (mg)	28	120	210	170
Vitamin C (mg)	3	2	1	1
Water (g)	88	87	81	86.8

117. Ans. (d) 28

Ref: K. Park, 24th ed. p 668

Calcium Content in Human Milk is less compared to other source of animal milk, however it is better absorbed

118. Ans. (b) Carbohydrates

Ref: K. Park, 24th ed. p 668

119. Ans. (c) Human Milk, Curd (Cow's Milk)...

Ref: K. Park, 24th ed-668

Also Know......................

- **Normal adult male [Moderate work]:** Milk requirement per day is 200 g
- **Normal adult female [Moderate work]:** Milk requirement per day is 150 g

120. Ans. (d) Methylene blue reduction test

Ref: K. Park, 24th ed. p 693

Tests of Pasteurized Milk are

- Phosphatase test-(widely used to check efficiency of pasteurization)
- Standard plate count
- Coliform count

121. Ans. (c) Increased protein

Ref: Community Medicine and Recent Advances, 3rd ed., p-184

Colostrum

- It is rich in proteins, Vitamin A and K, Immunoglobulin's (IgA)
- It contains low amounts of carbohydrates, fat and potassium than normal milk.
- It has growth factors [that stimulate development of gut]

122. Ans. (a) Vitamin K

Ref: K. Park, 24th ed. p 574,668

All milk are deficient in vitamin C. (However, human milk has more vitamin C compared to other milk)

Human milk lacks adequate amount of Vitamin K (Human milk – 15 μg/L, Cow milk – 60 μg/L)

Also Know......................

- Vitamin K – Green leafy vegetables, fruits, cheese, egg yolk, liver are rich source.

Tomato

- Contain "moderate" amount of oxalate 50 mg/100 g serving.
- Ripe tomato contain higher oxalate.
- Sources of oxalic acid: Rhubarb, Lemon, Strawberries, Green leafy vegetables [Spinach, Beet greens], amaranth, raw parsley, roasted peanuts, tea, whole grains.
- Lycopene (in tomato) is most efficient biological antioxidant and reduces risk of cancer.

123. Ans. (a) 6 months

Ref: K. Park, 24th ed. p 573

WHO and UNICEF's global recommendations for optimal Infant and Young Child Feeding (IYCF) comprises of:

- Exclusive breastfeeding for 6 months
- Nutritionally adequate and safe complementary feeding starting from the age of 6 months
- Continued breastfeeding up to 2 years of age or beyond

124. Ans. (a) Cow milk contains 80% whey...

Ref: K. Park, 24th ed. p 574

Milk is the best and most complete of all foods.

Proteins: [Buffalo > Goat > Cow > HUMAN]

- Animal milks contain 3 times as much protein as human milk.[Q]
- Casein is the chief protein. Lactalbumin and Lactoglobulin are other important protein.
- Milk proteins contain all essential amino acids.
- Human milk has higher amount of Tryptophan, Taurine and Cystein (Sulphur containing amino acids).

Fat: [Buffalo > Goat > Cow > HUMAN]

- Fat content is less in human milk (3.4%) compared to Buffalo milk (8.8%).
- Human milk contains a higher percentage of linoleic acid and oleic acid.
- Milk fat is a good source of retinol and vitamin D.

Sugar: [HUMAN > Buffalo > Goat > Cow]

- Carbohydrate in all milks is lactose. Human milk contains more Lactose than animal milks.

Minerals:

- Milk contains all known minerals - calcium, phosphorus, sodium, potassium, etc.
- *Milk is rich in calcium; but is a poor source of iron*[Q]
- Iron in breast milk, however has high bioavailability.
- Human milk is rich in copper, selenium and cobalt but contains less sodium.

- Calcium/Phosphorus ratio is high, so that the uptake of calcium is better.

Nutritive Value of Milk [Value per 100 g]

- Calcium (in mg): Buffalo milk (210) > Goat milk (170) >Cow milk (120) > HUMAN milk (28)
- Iron (in mg): Goat milk (0.3) > Buffalo milk (0.2) and Cow milk (0.2) > HUMAN milk
- Minerals (g): Buffalo milk, Goat milk and Cow milk (0.8) > HUMAN milk (0.1)
- Vitamin C (in mg): HUMAN milk (3) > Cow milk (2) >Buffalo milk and Goat milk (1).

Vitamins: Milk is a good source of all vitamins except vitamin C.

DRY FRUITS

125. Ans. (a) Banana

Ref: K. Park, 24th ed. p 667

- Fresh Fruits have low energy value [Exception Calories/100 g edible portion –Banana and Custard Apple (104), Mango (74) and Grapes (71)]

126. Ans. (a) Pista

Ref: Textbook of Public health and community medicine, 1st ed. p 748

- Dry fruits are good sources of calcium and iron. Pistachio has maximum iron (7.7 mg/100 g and carotene 144 micro g). Almond and cashew nuts are moderate sources of iron and proteins.
- Milk contains almost all known minerals except iron. It is rich in calcium.
- Meat contains about 2 to 4 mg/100 g of Iron

Also Know......................

- **Nuts** are a good source of fats, vitamins and proteins.

MISCELLANEOUS

127. Ans. (c) 5

Ref: K. Park, 24th ed. p 693

Minimum Standards for **Slaughter Houses** [Model Public Health Act (1955)]

- Location: Away from residential areas
- Structure: Impervious and easy to clean floors and walls (up to 3 feet)
- Waste Disposal: Separate collection, Not to be discharged into public sewers
- Water supply: Independent, adequate and continuous
- Facilities for Antemortem and postmortem examination. Animals or meat found unfit for human consumption should be destroyed or denatured.
- Storage of meat: Fly-proof and rat-proof rooms, Temperature <5°C (for overnight storage)
- Transportation of meat: Fly-proof covered vans.
- Animals other than those to be slaughtered should not be allowed inside the shed

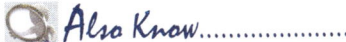

Also Know......................

- Diseases transmitted by consumption of unwholesome meat are Tape worm infestations (T. Solium, T. saginata), Anthrax, Actinomycosis, Tuberculosis, Food poisoning.

128. Ans. (a) Cereals and pulses

Ref: K. Park, 24th ed. p 676

Food Guide Pyramid

- It emphasizes on consumption of 5 major food groups
- Base of the pyramid is of Cereals and Pulses group. Maximum 6-11 serving/day is recommended
- Apex is formed by fat/oil and sweets, to be consumed sparingly

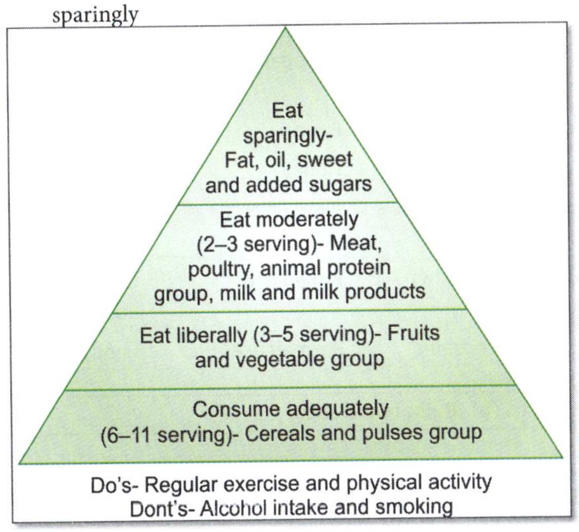

129. Ans. (a) 5 g

Ref: K. Park, 24th ed. p 675

WHO recommendation for ***Prudent diet*** comprises reduction of *salt intake to < 5 g/day.*

130. Ans. (c) Codex alimentarius

Ref: K. Park, 24th ed. p 697

Codex Alimentarius Commission

- It formulates food standards for international market.
- It is a principal organ of joint FAO/WHO Food standards Program
- Food standards in India are also based on standards of Codex Alimentarius Commission

PFA standards were set under PFA Act (1954), by ***Central Committee for Food Standards.*** It prescribes a minimum level of quality of foodstuffs attainable under Indian conditions.

Note: PFA is now replaced with FSSAI Act - Food Safety and Standards Authority of India (2006)

Also Know......................

- **AGMARK** (Directorate of Marketing and Inspection, Govt. of India) and **ISI** (Bureau of Indian Standards) express degrees of excellence above PFA standards. [Not Mandatory].

131. Ans. (d) Codex alimentarius

Ref: K Park 24th ed. p 697

132. Ans. (d) Rice

Ref: K. Park, 24th ed. p 651 Dietary Guidelines for Indians, - A Manual. ed., 2011, NIN, Hyderabad.p-111

Glycemic Index of a food is the area under the 2 hour post prandial blood Glucose response curve (AUC) following intake of 50 g test carbohydratye, as a proportion of AUC of the standard (Glucose or white bread)

Low [GI ≤ 55]	Medium [56-69]	High [≥ 70]
Milk	Soft Drink	Glucose
Apple, Banana	Popcorn	Cornflakes
Soya Bean	Chappathi	White/Brown Bread
Lentil	Banana	White Rice
Barley	Honey	Potato boiled
Ice cream	Pineapple	Water Melon (Raw)
Mango (Raw)	Brown rice	Oat/Rice/Millet Porridge
Whole grains	Basmati rice	Candy bar

133. Ans. (b) Raise blood sugar

Ref: K. Park, 24th ed. p 651)

134. Ans. (b) Whole grains

Ref: K. Park, 24th ed. p 651-52; Dietary Guidelines for Indians, - A; Manual. 2 ed., 2011, NIN, Hyderabad.p-111;

135. Ans. (a) 1 Only

Ref: Textbook of community Medicine, R Bhalawar, 1st ed. p-368

Irradiation is a modern method of food preservation

- Food is exposed to radioactive rays, High intensity X-ray or Electron beams
- **Advantage:**-No exposure to chemicals, Food is preserved in packaged form, Minimal person to food contact, Shelf life of food like strawberries, potatoes, onions etc is increased.
- **Disadvantage**: Change in colour and Texture.

136. Ans. (d) 1, 2 and 3

Ref: K. Park, 24th ed. p 695 and The Prevention of Food Adulteration Act and Rules (as on 1.10.2004) http://www.fssai.gov.in/

"Preservative" is a substance which when added to food, inhibits, retards or arrests the process of fermentation, acidification or decomposition of food.

- Class I: Common salt, Sugar, Dextrose, Glucose 1[Syrup], Spices, Vinegar or acetic acid, Honey and edible vegetable oils
- Class II: Benzoic acid, Sulfurous acid, Sorbic acid, Propionic acid and salts, Nitrates or Nitrites of Sodium or Potassium, Calcium or Sodium Propionates, Lactic acid, Nisin, Methyl or propyl Parahydroxy-benzoate, Sodium diacetate, Sodium, potassium and calcium salts of lactic acid

Also Know......................

- Use of more than one Class II preservative is prohibited

Food additives are non-nutritious substances added intentionally to food in small quantity, to improve its appearance, flavour, texture or storage properties. It also includes components of packing materials which may find their way into food

- Food additives are classified into two categories:
- Category I-Include colouring agents (e.g., saffron, turmeric), flavouring agents (e.g., vanilla essence), sweeteners (e.g., saccharin), acidity imparting agents (e.g., citric acid, acetic acid) and preservatives considered safe for human consumption.
- Category II-Include contaminants during packing, processing, farming practices (insecticides) and environmental conditions.
- Uncontrolled or indiscriminate use of food additives may pose health hazards among consumers
- In India-Prevention of Food Adulteration Act and Fruit Products Order govern rules and regulations of food additives.

137. Ans. (c) Vitamin B6, (e) Potassium

Ref: Suryakanta, Community Medicine Recent Advances, 3rd ed., p-173, Encyclopedia of human nutrition, 2nd ed., p-515

Fresh fruits are poor source of iron, calcium and phosphorous. Banana is a rich source of potassium (next only to dry apricots)

Also Know......................

- Citrus fruits (Lemon, Orange, Amla) and Guava are rich in Vitamin C
- Dry fruits have fair amount of calcium and iron compared to fresh fruits.

Mineral	Dry Fruit	Fresh Fruit
Calcium	Almonds > Dates > Ground	nut>Raisin
		Amla > Orange
Iron	Raisins > Dates	Sitaphal
Carotene		Papaya >
		Orange > Mango

138. Ans. (b) Codex alimentarius standards

Ref: K. Park, 24th ed. p 697

139. Ans. (d) Weight for height below 2SD of WHO growth standards 2006

Ref: Mahajan and Gupta, Textbook of PSM, 4thed, p-415

Severe malnutrition has two extreme forms, viz Marasmus (More common and Less serious) and Kwashiorkor.

WHO defines Severe Acute Malnutrition (SAM) as

- Mid-upper arm circumference (MUAC) < 11.5 cm (Age 6–59 months)
- Weight-for-Height *z*-score < –3

- Presence of bilateral pedal edema in children with kwashiorkor

SAM can also be diagnosed by assessing children for visible severe wasting (muscle wasting in gluteal region), loss of subcutaneous fat or prominence of bony structures (thorax).

Also Know........................

- Chronic malnutrition manifests as stunting
- Marasmus is characterised by loss of weight, wasting of muscles and loss of subcutaneous fat-"wise, old man" appearance.
- Kwashiorkor (seen in toddlers- 1 to 3 years age) is characterised by edema.-"moonface" appearance. Marasmic kwashiorkor (a mixed syndrome) is characterised by body weight less than 60% in presence of edema.

140. Ans. (d) Neither dairy nor egg

Ref – Slella Lucia, Fitness Nutrition for Special Dietary Needs, p-71

A vegetarian is someone who lives on a diet of grains, pulses, legumes, nuts, seeds, vegetables, fruits, fungi, algae, yeast and/or some other non-animal-based foods (e.g. salt) with, or without, dairy products, honey and/or eggs.

A vegetarian does not eat foods that consist of, or have been produced with the aid of products consisting of or created from, any part of the body of a living or dead animal (eg. meat, poultry, fish, shellfish, etc.).

Types of Vegetarians

- Lacto-ovo-vegetarians: Eat both dairy products and eggs (Most Common)
- Lacto-vegetarians: Eat dairy products but avoid eggs.
- Ovo-vegetarian: Eats eggs but not dairy products.
- Vegans: Do not eat dairy products, eggs, or any other products which are derived from animals.
- Pollotarian: Avoids all other meat but does intake poultry and fowl. They do not eat seafood, fish or red meat
- Pescatarian (Pescetarian): They restrict all of their meat consumption, besides seafood and fish.
- The Flexitarian: Eats mainly plant-based and only occasionally consume meat products.

141. Ans. (d) Fruits

Ref: K. Park, 24th ed. p 652; Dietary Guidelines for Indians, - A Manual. 2nd ed., 2011, NIN, Hyderabad.p-111

NUTRITIONAL REQUIREMENTS

142. Ans. (d) BMI 21.2

Ref: K. Park, 24th edp-670

Reference Indian Male		Reference Indian Female
Age	18 - 29 years free from disease	18 - 29 years. Non pregnant non lactating and free from disease
Weight	60 kg	55 Kg
Height	1.73	1.6 m
BMI	20.3	21.2
Employment	Involves 8 hours of moderate activity.	Involves 8 hours of moderate activity.
When not at works pends	8 hours in bed, 4-6 hours sitting/ moving around and 2 hours in walking, active recreation or household duties	8 hours in bed, 4-6 hours sitting/ moving around and 2 hours in walking, active recreation or household duties

Energy intake recommendation are formulated for a "Reference man"

143. Ans. (b) Weight 50 kg

Ref: K. Park, 24 p-670

144. Ans. (a) Weight 60 Kg

Ref: K. Park, 24 p-670

145. Ans. (a) Age 18-29 yrs

Ref: K. Park, 24th p-670

146. Ans. (b) 60 kg

Ref: K. Park, 24th ed. p 670

RECOMMENDED DAILY ALLOWANCE

147. Ans. (d) < 20-30%

Ref: K. Park, 24th ed. p 672

WHO Recommendation for Prudent Diet Comprises

- Protein intake of approximately 15-20% of the daily energy intake[Q]
- Dietary fat restricted to 15-30 % of total daily energy intake[Q]
- Saturated fats restricted to not more than 10 % of total *energy intake.*[Q]
- *Avoidance of excessive consumption of refined carbohydrate*
- *Restricted intake of food* rich in energy (Fats and Alcohol)
- *Salt intake reduced to an average of not more than 5g per* day.[Q]
- Junk foods [Colas, ketchups etc that supply empty calories] should be reduced.

Above recommendations do not apply in following conditions → special needs of growth, pregnancy, lactation, physical activity and medical disorders (e.g., diabetes).

148. Ans. (c) 1 g/kg body weight of mixed protein

Ref: K. Park, 24th ed. p 672

Refer to Annexure 2

149. Ans. (a) 2320 Cal

Ref: K. Park, 24th ed -672

150. Ans. (a) 500 kcal and 1.16 g/kg/day

Ref: K. Park, 24th ed. p 674

RDA IN PREGNANCY AND LACTATION

151. Ans. (a) 2500 Cal

Ref: K. Park, 24th ed. p 672

Refer to Annexure 2

152. Ans. (d) 350 Cal

Ref: K. Park, 24th ed. p 672

153. Ans. (c) 350

Ref: K. Park, 24th ed. p 672

154. Ans. (a) 1000 mg

Ref: K. Park, 24th ed. p 674

Nils Milman. Oral Iron Prophylaxis in Pregnancy: Not Too Little and Not Too Much! Hindawi Publishing Corporation Journal of Pregnancy Volume 2012.

- In pregnancy, Total demand for absorbed iron is approximately 1240 mg (Obligatory iron loss = 230 mg.

155. Ans. (d) 250 mcg

Ref: K. Park, 24th ed. p 662

Recent recommendation of WHO on Iodine uptake in pregnancy is 250 mcg/day.

156. Ans. (c) 600

Ref: K. Park, 24th ed. p 674

157. Ans. (e) 270 mcg iodine

Ref: K. Park, 24th ed. p 674

RDA CALCIUM

158. Ans. (b) 600 mg

Ref: K. Park, 24th ed. p 674

159. Ans. (d) Iron

Ref: K. Park, 24th ed. p 674

160. Ans. (d) 500 mcg/day

Ref: K. Park, 24th ed. p 658

161. Ans. (d) 600 mg

Ref: K. Park, 24th ed. p 660

As per new guidelines, RDA of Calcium for adult male and female is 600 mg. The requirement doubles in pregnancy and lactation in females [RDA =1200 mg]

162. Ans. (b) 500 mg

Ref: K. Park, 24th ed. p 674

RDA PROTEIN

163. Ans. (c) 1

Ref: K. Park, 24th ed. p 674; Dietary Guidelines for Indians, - A Manual. 2nd ed., 2011, NIN, Hyderabad

Recommended Daily Allowances for Infants and Children

Age Groups	Boys						Girls					
	Weight (Kg)	Energy (kcal)	Protein (g)	Fat (g)	Calcium (mg)	Iron (mg)	Weight (Kg)	Energy (kcal)	Protein (g)	Fat (g)	Calcium (mg)	Iron (mg)
0-6 month	5.4	92/Kg	1.16/Kg		500	46μg/kg	Similar as Boys					
6-12 month	8.4	80/Kg	1.69/Kg	19	500	5						
1-3 year	13	1060	16.7	27	600	9						
4-6 year	18	1350	20.1	25	600	13						
7-9 year	25	1690	29.5	30	600	16						
10-12 year	34	2190	39.9	35	800	21	35	2010	40.4	35	800	27
13-15 year	47.6	2750	54.3	45	800	32	46.6	2330	51.9	40	800	27
16-17 year	55.4	3020	61.5	50	800	28	52	2440	55.5	35	800	26

Recommended daily protein intake (g/kg/day) in girl 13-15 year = 51.9/46.6 = 1.11

RDA IODINE

164. Ans. (a) Neonatal hypothyroidism

Ref: K. Park, 24th ed. p 662-63

Also Know......................

Indicators for Epidemiological Assessment of Iodine Deficiency:

- Prevalence of goiter
- Prevalence of cretinism
- Urinary iodine excretion [recommended for use in surveillance]
- Serum levels of T4 and TSH [Serum T4 is more sensitive indicator of thyroid insufficiency than T3]
- Prevalence of neonatal hypothyroidism [A sensitive indicator of environmental iodine deficiency]

165. Ans. (c) Not less than 30 ppm at production...

Ref: K. Park, 24th ed. p 681

***Iodization of salt** is the most widely used prophylactic public health measure against endemic goiter.*

In India under the Prevention of Food Adulteration (PFA) Act the level of iodization is fixed at

- *Not less than 30 ppm at the production point*[Q]
- *Not less than 15 ppm of iodine at the consumer level.*[Q]

Also Know......................

- "Two-in-one" salt → developed by NIN Hyderabad is common salt fortified with iron and iodine.
- It contains 40 mcg Iodine and 1 mg Iron per gram of salt

166. Ans. (b) 0.01%

Ref: BR Thirunavalli, Textbook of Community Medicine, 3rd edition, p-667

- *Macrominerals* constitute>0.01% of body weight. These are Calcium, Phosphorous, Sodium, Potassium, Manganese.
- Microminerals or Trace elements constitute ≤0.01% of body weight. 14 trace elements vital for human growth. are Iron, Iodine, Fluorine, Zinc, Copper, Chromium, Selenium, Manganese, Cobalt, Nickel, Molybdenum, Vanadium, Silicon, Arsenic.

Selenium Deficiency Causes

Keshan disease [a cardiomyopathy endemic in china] and Kashin beck disease [Endemic osteoarthritis]

167. Ans. (a) Iron and iodine

Ref: Dietary Guidelines for Indians-A Manual, ICMR, NIN, Hyderabad, p-62

Also Know......................

- DEC Medicated Salt (1g-4g DEC per kg salt) is used in mass treatment of Filariasis for 6-9 month

168. Ans. (c) 150 mcg

Ref: K. Park, 24th ed. p 662

- Daily requirement for adults is → 150 micrograms per day. [250 mcg per day during pregnancy]

Latest Updates

Indicators for IDD Elimination

- Proportion of households consuming effectively iodised salt (>90%)
- Urinary iodine excretion: Proportion below 100 mcg/L (<50%) and proportion below 50 mcg/L (<20%)
- Thyroid size: Proportion of school children 6–12 years age with enlarged thyroid, by palpation or ultrasound (<5%)

169. Ans. (b) 15 ppm

Ref: K. Park, 24th ed. p 681

RDA VITAMIN A

170. Ans. (c) 200, 000 IU

Ref: K. Park, 24th ed. p 654

Vitamin A Deficiency

- ***Treatment***: Early treatment can reverse all early stages of Xerophthalmia.
  - *Administration of massive dose (2, 00, 000 IU or 110 mg) of Retinol palmitate orally on 2 successive days*[Q]
  - *All children with corneal ulcers should receive vitamin A whether or not a deficiency is suspected.*
- **Prevention**
  - **Long term measure:** Intensive nutrition education and community participation for
  - Regular and adequate intake of foods rich in vitamin A.
  - Reducing frequency and severity of contributory factors, e.g. PEM, RTI, diarrhoea and measles.
  - **Short term measure:** Community based intervention [Evolved by NIN, Hyderabad]
  - *Administer 200,000 IU of vitamin A in oil (Retinol palmitate) orally every 6 months to preschool children (1 year to 5 years)*[Q]
  - *Administer a dose of 100, 000 IU to children between 6 months and one year of age* [Q]
  - **Medium term**
  - Fortification of food

171. Ans. (a) 350 mcg

Ref: K. Park, 24th ed. p 654

Daily Intake of Vitamin A Recommended by ICMR (2010)

- Adults (Man and Woman) and Adolescents – 13-19 years → 600 mcg Retinol
- Pregnancy → 800 mcg Retinol
- Lactation → 950 mcg Retinol.
- Infants-0 to 12 months → 350 mcg Retinol.
- Children
  - 1 to 6 years → 400 mcg Retinol.
  - 7 to 12 → 600 mcg Retinol.

ASSESSMENT OF NUTRITIONAL STATUS

172. Ans. (e) None of above

Ref: Harrison's 16thed, p 415

Assessment of malnutrition: [by Lab tests → Harrison-Chapter 72. Malnutrition and Nutritional Assessment]

- **Marasmus** → Creatinine-Height Index <60% standard
- **Kwashiorkor** → Serum albumin <2.8 g/dL, Serum transferrin (<150 mg/dL), Total iron-binding capacity <200 g/dl. Lymphocyte count < 1500/L (in adults and older children) and energy is also seen.

Serum Biochemical Tests Used in Nutritional Surveys

Nutrient	Method	Normal value
Protein	Creatinine height index [*Harrison's 16thed, Pg 415*]	< 60 % of standard signals Marasmus
	Serum Transferrin	20 g/L
	Serum Albumin	35 g/L
	Thyroid binding prealbumin	250 mg/L
Folate	Serum folate	6 mcg/mL
	Red cell folate	160 mcg/mL
Vitamin A	Serums retinol	20 mcg/dl
Vitamin B_{12}	Serum vitamin B_{12} concentration	160 mg/L

FOOD SURVEILLANCE/HYGIENE/TOXICANTS/ ADULTERATION EPIDEMIC DROPSY

173. Ans. (b) Sanguinarine

Ref: K. Park, 24th edp-695

174. Ans. (c) Sanguinarine

Ref: K. Park, 24th edp-695

Epidemic Dropsy is characterised by sudden onset of non-inflammatory, bilateral swelling of legs, often with diarrhoea, dyspnoea, cardiac failure and death. Some patients may develop glaucoma.

- It occurs due to ***consumption of*** *Mustard oil contaminated with Argemone oil (containing toxic alkaloid -**Sanguinarine**Q)*
- All age group are affected, except breast-fed infants
- Mortality varies from 5-50%

Also Know........................

- Sanguinarine interferes with oxidation of pyruvic acid and leads to accumulation of pyruvic acid in blood

175. Ans. (b) Paper chromatography

Ref: K. Park, 24th ed. p 695

Tests to detect argemone oil in edible oils and fats are

- Nitric acid test
- Paper Chromatography test (Most sensitive → can detect argemone oil up to 0.0001 %)

Also Know........................

- Argemone oil is orange in colour with an acrid odour

176. Ans. (a) Sanguinarine

Ref: K. Park, 24th ed. p 695

177. Ans. (b) Nitric acid test

Ref: K. Park, 24th ed. p 695

178. Ans. (b) Sanguinarine

Ref: K. Park, 24th ed. p 695

179. Ans. (a) Sanguinarine

Ref: K. Park, 24th ed. p 695

ENDEMIC ASCITIS

180. Ans. (c) Jhunjhunia seeds

Ref: K. Park, 24th ed. p 695

Endemic ascites is due to a hepatotoxin (*Pyrrolizidine alkaloid*Q) in seeds of Crotolaria (Jhunjhunia-a weed) that contaminate millet seeds

- Clinical features → Rapid development of ascitis and jaundice with high mortality.
- **Prevention** → Education, Deweeding of Crotalaria plant, Sieving to separate seeds of Crotalaria

181. Ans. (a) Pyrrolizidine

Ref: K. Park, 24th ed. p 695

LATHYRISM

182. Ans. (b) Steeping

Ref: K. Park, 24th ed 683

Methods of Toxin Removal from Lathyrus Sativus

- Steeping Method: Pulse is soaked in hot boiled water for 2 hours, after which the soaked water is drained off. The pulse is then washed again with clean water and is dried in the sun.
  - Advantage – It can be practiced at home.
  - Drawback -Loss of vitamins and minerals.
- Parboiling: Better method suitable for large scale operation. Pulse is soaked in lime water overnight followed by boiling, washed with clean water and dried.

183. Ans. (a) Khesari dal

Ref: K. Park, 24th ed. p 682

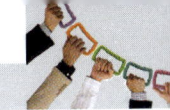

184. Ans. (d) Beta-oxalyl-amino-alanine

Ref: K. Park, 24th ed. p 682

185. Ans. (b) BOAA

Ref: K. Park, 24th ed. p 682

Lathyrism [Neurolathyrism] *is a gradual onset spastic paralysis of lower limbs*[Q], *occurringin adults consuming the pulse, Lathyrus sativus [Khesari dal] in large quantities (Diet with >30% Khesari dal consumed over 2-6 month)*

- *Toxin present in Lathyrus seeds is* ***Beta Oxalyl Amino Alanine (BOAA)Q***
- Stages – Latent → No stick stage → 1 Stick stage → 2 Stick stage → Crawler stage

ERGOTISM

186. Ans. (a) Floating in 20% salt water

Ref: K. Park, 24th ed. p 695

Ergotism is caused by consumption of ergot [Fungus-Claviceps fusiformis] infested food grain (Bajra, Rye, Sorghum, Wheat).

- Symptoms are nausea, vomiting, giddiness and drowsiness extending for 24 -48 hr. Rarely fatal.
- Painful cramps in limbs & peripheral gangrene occurs due to consumption of fungus infested grain over a long period.
- Upper safe limit for ergot alkaloids is 0.05 mg per 100 g of food material.
- Ergot infested grains can be removed by floating them in 20 % salt water, hand-picking or air floatation
- Ergotis a field fungus and food grains get infested during flowering.

187. Ans. (b) Claviceps Purpura

Ref: K. Park, 23 ed. p-658; 24th ed. p 695

MILK STERILIZATION AND ADULTERATION

188. Ans. (a) Methylene blue reduction test

Ref: K. Park, 24th ed. p 693

Tests Performed on Pasteurised Milk

- ***Phosphatase test*** *-to test the efficiency of pasteurization.*[Q]
  - "Phosphatase" in raw milk is destroyed on pasteurization.

Its presence is indicator of inadequate pasteurization or addition of raw milk

- ***Standard Plate Count*** is used to determine bacteriological quality of pasteurized milk [Limit -30, 000 bacterial count/ mL of pasteurized milk]
- ***Coliform Count-****Presence* of coliform in milk indicates improper pasteurization or post pasteurization contamination.

Also Know......................

- ***Methylene blue reduction test***[Q] is done on milk accepted for pasteurization. Positive test confirms heavy contamination with microorganisms.

189. Ans. (d) All the above

Ref: U.S. Food and Drug Administrationwww.fda.gov/Food/Resources For You/Consumers/ucm

Pasteurization kills harmful organisms responsible for the following diseases

- Listeriosis
- Typhoid fever
- Tuberculosis
- Diphtheria
- Brucellosis.

Also Know......................

- There is no difference in the nutritional values of pasteurized and unpasteurized milk.
- Pasteurized milk contains low levels of nonpathogenic bacteria that can cause food spoilage, so pasteurized milk must be kept in refrigerator.

190. Ans. (a) 65°C for 30 minutes

Ref: K. Park, 23rd ed. p 655

Methods of Pasteurization of Milk[Q]

- *Holder (Vat) Method*:
  - Milk is kept at 63-66°C for at least 30 minutes and then quickly cooled to 5°C.
  - Ideal for small and rural communities.
- HTST or "High Temperature and Short Time Method"
  - Milk is rapidly heated to 720C, is kept at this temperature for not less than 15 seconds and then rapidly cooled to 4°C.
  - Recommended for large scale pasteurization
- *UHT or "ultra - high temperature method."*
  - Milk is rapidly heated usually in 2 stages (2nd stage is under pressure) to 125 deg C, for a few seconds only. It is then rapidly cooled and bottled as quickly as possible.

191. Ans. (c) Phosphatase test

Ref: K. Park, 24th ed. p 693

LEVELS OF HEALTH CARE

192. Ans. (c) 400-800

Ref: K. Park, 24th ed. p 936

Revised population norm for AWC and Mini AWC [Aim – cover all habitations by SC/ST /Minorities]

Urban/Rural project →

- 1 AWC for 400-800 population, 2 AWC for 800-1600 population and 3 AWC for 1600-2400 population. Thereafter 1 AWC for multiples of 800 population.[Q]
- Mini AWC → 1 mini AWC for 150–400 population.[Q]
- Tribal/Riverine/Desert/Hilly and other difficult areas:
  - 1 AWC for 300–800 population[Q]
  - 1 Mini AWC for 150–300 population[Q]

193. Ans. (c) 250

Daily Requirement of Iodine

- 12 years - 150 mcg/day for adult
- Pregnancy - 250 mcg/day.
- Lactation 250- 290 mcg/day

194. Ans. (d) 63°C for 30 seconds

Reference: Park 25th ed 711,

VAT method – 63-66°C for at least 30 mins, cooled to 5°C
HTST – high temperature, short time – 72°C for at least 15 seconds then rapid cooling to 4°C
UHT – Ultra high temperature – heating to 125°C for few seconds and then rapid cooling along with putting milk under high pressure. This is the most modern and best method for pasteurization.

195. Ans. (c) 2700 children in each district

In the IDD survey, 30 clusters are selected with 90 children are selected from each cluster.

Equal proportion of boys and girls, with proportionate sample from school and from outside school (based on the school enrollment ratio) is selected and the variables collected are:

- Urinary iodine excretion rate
- Goiter rate
- Iodine in household salt levels

The IDD (iodine deficiency disorder) survey is conducted as annual survey

196. Ans. (a) One-third of energy requirement and half of the protein requirement

Mid-Day Meal Scheme

- Objective is to decrease the school dropout rate
- Cooked food is provided every day for promoting school attendance
- MDMS promotes school attendance by providing ½ of daily protein requirement and 1/3rd of daily calorie requirement by children

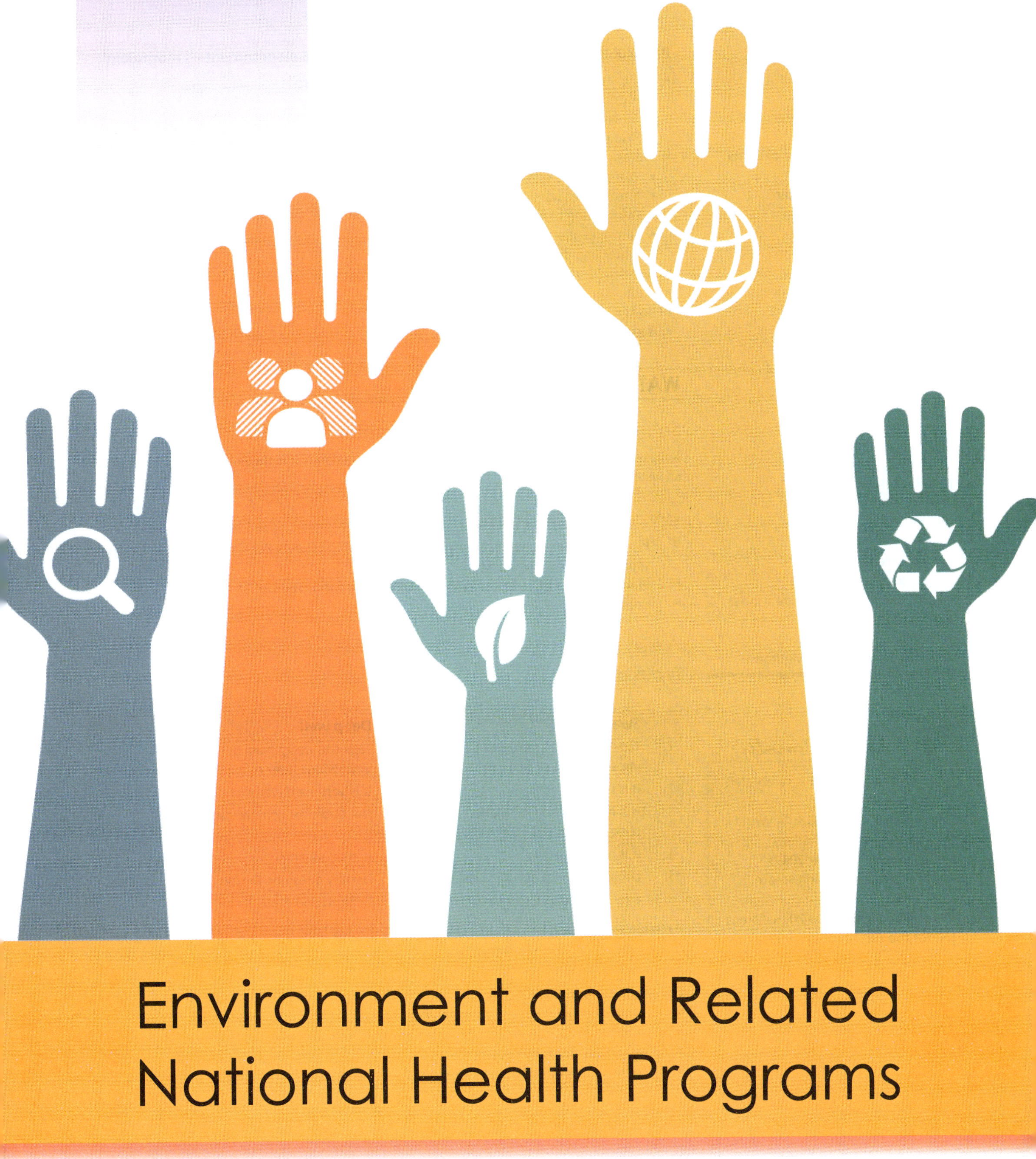

Environment and Related National Health Programs

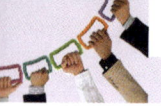

Chapter Outline

35 Good to Remember

- **World Earth Day:** It is celebrated on 22nd April.
- **Theme for year 2018:** "A World without Plastic Pollution"
- **Theme for the year 2017:** "Environmental and Climate Literacy"
- **Theme for the year 2016 :**"Trees for the Earth. Let us get planting".

ENVIRONMENT

Anything not internal is external…and anything external is environment.

Definition: The natural world, as a whole or in a particular geographical area, especially as affected by human activity.

The environment can be divided into:

Physical environment	Biological environment—Entomology
▪ Air • Air pollution • Air comfort • Humidity ▪ Water • Water quality criteria • Hardness of water • Disinfection of water—chlorination • Filtration of water • Water and disease ▪ Noise ▪ Light ▪ House ▪ Radiation	▪ Mosquito ▪ Housefly ▪ Ticks ▪ Rodents ▪ Louse ▪ Flea ▪ Mite

WATER

Source and Characteristics of Water Supply

Rain water is very soft water with traces of solids (0.0005%). It is the purest and prime source of all water.[Q]

Norms of Water Supply

- Piped water supply only (No sewer system)-70 LPCD (Liters Per Capita in Day) piped water supply + Sewer –135 LPCD
- Piped water supply + Sewer (Metropolitan/Mega City)- 150 LPCD
- Public Stand post - 40 LPCD

Wells

Types of Wells

	Swallow well	Deep well
1.	Taps the water from above the first impervious layer of earth	Taps the water from below the first impervious layer of earth
2.	It is hard-water	It is very hard water
3.	It is liable for contamination (from the cone of filtration)	Not liable for contamination
4.	It is not safe water	It is safe water
5.	Usually dries up during summer	Usually does not dry even during summer
6.	Easy and cheap to construct	Difficult and costly to construct

Artesian well: It is a kind of deep well, in which the water table is at a higher level than the surface of the earth, because of the slope of the impervious layer. So, when a bore taps the water, it comes out like a fountain because of the pressure.

Criteria for a sanitary well:

- *Located within 60 meters (not more than 100 meters) of human dwellings*
- *Located of at least more than 15 meters of site of probable contamination*
- *Appropriate depth of 6 meters*
- *Parapet wall around the well of approx. 1 meter above the ground level*

- *Concrete platform of 1 meter around the well, with slope to periphery, away from the cone of filtration*
- *Preferably covered well, fitted with pump or machine to lift water*
- *Cleanliness around the area*

Disinfection of Well

The various steps of disinfection of wells are:

- Finding the volume of water in the well:
  - Formula to be used is: $(3.14 \times d^2 \times h)$
- Estimating the quantity of bleaching powder required – Using Horrock's Apparatus

Method for estimating the chlorine demand using Horrock's Apparatus:

Preparation of stock (standard) chlorine solution: One level spoonful (2 g) of bleaching powder is taken in the black-cup and made into a thin paste by adding little water. Then more of water is added gradually by stirring till the level reaches the white circular mark. It is stirred well and allowed to settle, so that calcium of the bleaching powder settles down. This is the stock chlorine solution.

- All the six white cups are now filled with water from the well, to be tested up to a cm below the brim.
- With the help of the pipette, one drop of standard chlorine solution is added to first white cup, two drops to second cup, three drops to third cup, so on and six drops to sixth cup.
- The water in each cup is stirred well with separate stirrers for each cup.
- Wait for 30 minutes for process of chlorination to happen
- 3 drops of Starch-iodide indicator is added (Starch-cadmium/potassium-iodide) for all the six cups and stirred again.
- Development of blue color indicates the presence of free residual chlorine. The intensity of the blue color is directly proportional to the quantity of free residual chlorine in the water
- The first cup which develops this color gives an estimate of the amount of bleaching powder needed to disinfect 455 L of the sample water.

Example

Blue color in which cup	Amount of bleaching powder	
1st cup	2 g	1 spoonful of bleaching powder for 455 Liters of water
2nd cup	4 g	2 spoonful of bleaching powder
3rd cup	6 g	3 spoonful of bleaching powder
4th cup	8 g	4 spoonful of bleaching powder
5th cup	10 g	5 spoonful of bleaching powder and so on...

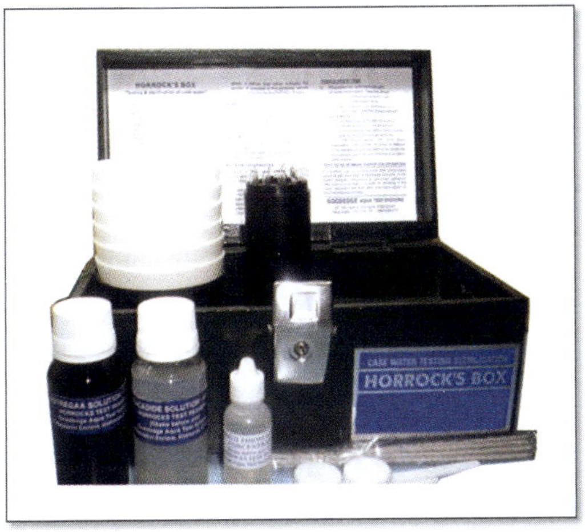

Fig. 1: Horrock's apparatus

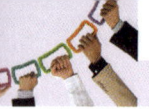

- Preparation of the **chlorine solution** for the water in the well
  - After estimating the total amount of bleaching powder required for the total amount of water in the well, the estimated amount of bleaching powder is taken in a bucket and made into a thin paste by adding little water.
  - Then more of water is added till the bucket is three-fourths full. It is stirred well and allowed to sediment for 1 minute, so that lime settles down. The supernatant chlorine solution is transferred to another bucket and the chalk or lime is discarded and not poured into the well, as it increases the hardness of well-water.
- Delivery of the chlorine solution: The bucket with the chlorine solution is lowered into the well, below the surface of the water and agitated vertically and horizontally, so that chlorine solution mixes with the well water uniformly.
- Contact period of minimum '1 hour'
- Orthotolidine test: To verify whether water has been properly chlorinated or not, orthotolidine test is done. If free residual chlorine level is less than 0.5 ppm after contact period of one hour, the chlorination procedure should be repeated.

Laboratory Examination of Water

The Water Quality may be assessed as per the:

1. Physical parameters (discussed below)
2. Chemical parameters (discussed below)
3. Bacteriological examination (discussed below)
4. Virologic examination: Virologic examination of water: water maybe at risk for Enteroviruses, reoviruses and adenoviruses. The WHO recommends upper limit for viruses as 1 PFU (Plaque forming unit) per litre of water.
5. Radiological examination: Radioactivity in drinking water should be within safe limits and as low as reasonably possible. WHO guideline values:
   - Gross alpha activity: 3 pCi/L
   - Gross beta activity: 30 pCi/L (note: 1 pc = 2.22 radioactive disintegrations per minute)

1. **Physical Parameters**: those which affect the physical or aesthetic quality of water. These include:
   - Turbidity: 5 NTU Nephelometric Turbidity Unit (NTU) (measured by Jackson Candle Turbidimeter)
   - Color: <15 True Color Units (TCU) or < 5 hazel units
   - Odour: The recommended threshold odour number is <3 (when one part of water is added to two parts of odour free water, odour should be barely detectable)
2. **Chemical examination of water:**
   - Toxic substances: include Arsenic cyanide, lead, cadmium, barium, beryllium, cobalt, molybdenum, thiocyanate, tin, uranium. The WHO recommends the upper limit for the chemicals to be below 0.01 ppm
   - Substances affecting after prolonged exposure as
     - Fluorides: The optimum concentration for drinking purpose is 0.5 to 0.8 mg/L (ppm) but the permissible upper limit is 1.5 mg/L (1.5 ppm).
     - PAH – Polynuclear aromatic hydrocarbons (example - benzene, benzpyrene, benzopyrelene, benzofluoranthene)
   - Substances affecting the potability of water: these can be summarised in the table below:

Table 1: Acceptable Chemical Quality of potable water – recommended upper limits

Substances	Prescribed upper limit
▪ Optimum – pH	7.5 (range of pH = 7 to 8)
▪ Total dissolved solids (affecting turbidity)	1000 mg/L (< 600 mg/L is very safe)
▪ Total hardness	3 mEq/L (1 to 3 mEq/L of $CaCO_3$) (50 to 150 mg of $CaCO_3$/L)
▪ Iron	0.3 mg/L
▪ Calcium	75 mg/L

Contd...

Substances	Prescribed upper limit
▪ Magnesium	30 mg/L
▪ Sulfate	200 mg/L
▪ Chlorides	200 mg/L
▪ Zinc	5 mg/L
▪ Copper	0.05 mg/L
▪ Manganese	0.05 mg/L
▪ Phenolic substances	0.001 mg/L
▪ Ammonia	1.5 mg/L

- Chemical indicators of water pollution
  - Chlorides: The standard prescribed limit of chloride for drinking purpose is 200 mg/litre. The maximum permissible limit is 600 mg/liter. Above 250 mg/L, the water becomes salty and becomes undesirable. Excess NaCl causes cardiovascular disease.
  - Free and saline ammonia: may indicate sewage contamination
    - Recommended levels: 0.05 ppm (mg/L)
  - Albuminoid ammonia (Organic ammonia) – indicator for presence of organic matter.
    - Recommended levels should be < 0.1 ppm in drinking water.
  - Nitrites – should be absent in drinking water. The presence of nitrites will indicate active biological life forms in water
  - Nitrates -indicate biological oxidation process. The presence may indicate old contamination in water.
    - Recommended levels < 1 ppm

Table 2: Water quality criteria

Physical parameters	Odor, color, taste, turbidity
Inorganic constituents	**Chlorides:** Standard is 200 mg/L (Maximum permissible is 600 mg/L) **Hardness:** Moderately hard (1–3 mEq/L or 50–150 mg/L)
	H_2S: Taste and Odour threshold in water is 0.05-0.1 mg/L **Acceptable pH** is 6.5–8.5.
Chemical aspect	Arsenic – Recommended maximum concentration (mg/L) is 0.01 Lead-0.01, Cadmium-0.003, Chromium-0.05, Cyanide-0.07, Fluoride <1.5 ppm, NO_3: NO_2 = 50/3
Microbiological aspects	Drinking water should be free of any pathogenic bacteria, virus, protozoa or infective stage of helminth

3. **Biological Quality of Water**

Bacteriological indicators of fecal contamination of water:

- ***Primary indicator*: Coliform group of organisms (*E. coli*)**
- *Presumptive Coliform Count* (Multiple Tube Technique) yields the probable number of Coliform bacilli per 100 mL of water (using McCrady's table).

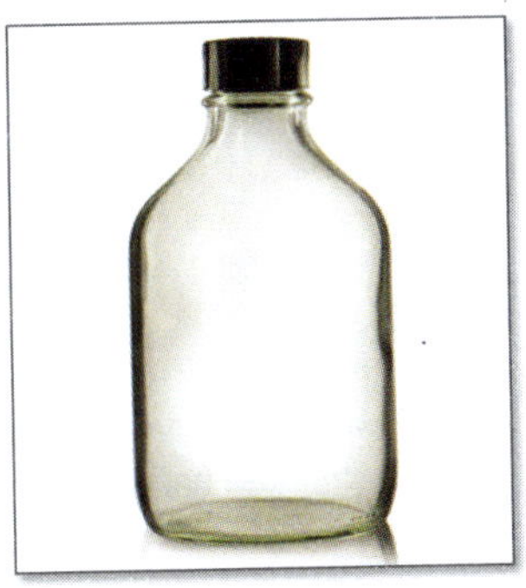

Fig. 2: Clear Winchester Bottle for Collecting Water Sample.

Interpretation of the results of disinfected water

- No coliforms in 100 cc of water—Excellent water
- 1–3 coliforms in 100 cc of water—Satisfactory water
- 4–10 coliforms in 100 cc of water—Suspicious water
- More than 10 coliform in 100 cc of water—Unsatisfactory water

- *Supplementary indicator*: Fecal streptococci (Recent) and spores of *clostridium perfringens* (Remote)
- Sulfite reduction method: Volumes of water mixed with melted medium is incubated at 37°C for 2 days. Development of black colonies indicates contamination with Cl. perfringens.
- *Eijkman's test*: It is used to confirm type of Coliform organism (Fecal/Nonfecal) by incubating tubes at 37°C and 44°C). *E. coli* grow at 44°C while the other coliforms do not.
- *NOAEL (No observed adverse effect level)*: It is the highest concentration of a chemical in drinking water that causes no detectable adverse health effect.
- *LOAEL (Lowest observed adverse effect level):* It is the lowest observed concentration of a substance at which there is a detectable adverse health effect. An additional uncertainty factor used with LOAEL.
- *TDI (Tolerable daily intake):* It is the amount of a substance (chemical contaminant) in food or drinking water, in mg/kg or µg/kg of body weight that can be ingested daily over a lifetime without appreciable health risk.
- *ADI (Acceptable daily intake):* It is established for food additives and pesticide residues that occur in food for necessary technological purposes or plant protection reasons.

36 Good to Remember

WHO Criteria for Water

- Guideline value for Nitrate (NO_3) in water is 50 mg/L.
- Nitrite (NO) is 3 mg/L[Q].
- If both are present:

(Concentration of Nitrate/Guideline value) + (Concentration of Nitrite/ Guideline value) ≤ 1

37 Good to Remember

$$\text{TDI} = \frac{\text{NOAEL or LOAEL}}{\text{Uncertainty factor}}$$

$$\text{Guideline value} = \frac{\text{TDI} \times \text{Body weight} \times \text{Fraction of TDI allocated to drinking water}}{\text{Daily drinking water consumption}}$$

Hardness of Water

- It is the soap-destroying power of water.[Q]
- It is measured in "milli equivalents/L" (mEq/L). 1 mEq/L of hardness producing ion is equal to 50 mg $CaCO_3$ (50 ppm) in 1 L of water.
- Drinking water should be moderately hard.

Disadvantages of hard water

- Consumes more soap and detergents.[Q]
- Causes furring or scaling of boilers[Q], more fuel consumption, loss of efficiency and may cause boiler explosions.
- Adversely affects cooking
- Fabrics do not have a long life
- Not suitable for many industries
- Shortens life of pipes and fixtures.[Q]

60 High Yield Points

Softening is recommended when hardness exceeds 3 mEq/L (150 mg/L).[Q]

Table 3: Classification of hardness in water[Q]

Classification	Level of hardness (mEq/L)
Soft	Less than 1 (<50 mg/L)
Moderately hard	1–3 (50–150 mg/L)
Hard	3–6 (150–300 mg/L)
Very hard	Over 6 (>300 mg/L)

61 High Yield Points

- Drinking water should be moderately hard.[Q]
- Softening is recommended when hardness exceeds 3 mEq/L.[Q]

Methods for Treatment of Hard Water

Table 4: Causes and treatment for hardness in water

Hardness	Causes	Treatment options
Carbonate or *Temporary hardness*	Calcium and Magnesium bicarbonates[Q]	Boiling of water, Addition of lime or Sodium carbonate and Permutit process
Non-carbonate or Permanent hardness	Calcium and Magnesium sulfates, chlorides and nitrates.[Q]	Addition of Sodium carbonate and Permutit process

- **Boiling:** Boing of water, evaporates CO_2, precipitating the carbonates and making the water soft. This can only be done for household water supply at domestic level and not at community level.

- **Adding Lime:** Water + calcium hydroxide, absorbs the CO_2 and precipitates insoluble calcium carbonates, making the water as soft
- **Addition of Sodium carbonate (soda ash):** Treatment for permanent and temporary hardness
- **Permutit process (also called as sodium zeolite - Na_2Z):** Zeolite consists of sodium, aluminium and silica. When this is added to hard water, the Ca and Mg ions exchange with NaZ and forms Ca and Mg permutit and the water is softened to zero hardness. As Zero hard water is corrosive to pipe system, the soft water is again mixed with raw water to achieve a desired hardness level. This treats temporary hardness and the permanent hardness.

Disinfection of Water

Chlorination

- Kills bacteria, but does not kill spores/certain virus (e.g., polio, hepatitis) except in high doses.[Q]
- Disinfecting action of chlorine is mainly due to hypochlorous acid.[Q] (at a pH of around 7).
- Minimum recommended concentration of free chlorine is 0.5 mg/L for one hour.[Q]
- Free residual chlorine provides a margin of safety against subsequent microbial contamination during storage and distribution-*Residual Effect*

Principles of Chlorination

- Water should be clear and free from turbidity.
- *Chlorine demand* [Difference between amount of chlorine added to water and amount of residual chlorine remaining at the end of a specific period of contact (usually 1 hour), at a given temperature and pH of the water] should be estimated.
- Secondary Properties of Chlorine:
  - Oxidizes iron, manganese and hydrogen sulfide
  - Destroys some taste and odor-producing constituents
  - Controls algae and slime organisms
  - Aids coagulation.
- *Dose of chlorine*: Chlorine demand of specific water + free residual chlorine of 0.5 mg/L.
- *Methods of chlorination*: Chlorine gas (1st choice), Chloramine and Perchloron.[Q]

Tests for Chlorination of Water

- *Orthotolidine (OT) Test*: Measures free chlorine (within 10 seconds) and free + combined chlorine (15-20 minutes) in water.[Q]
- *Orthotolidine Arsenite (OTA) Test:* Measures free and combined chlorine residuals separately.[Q] Errors due to interfering substances (nitrites, iron and manganese) in OT test is overcome by OTA test.

Bleaching Powder or Chlorinated Lime ($CaOCl_2$)

- It contains about 33% of "available chlorine".[Q]
- It is an unstable compound and rapidly loses chlorine on exposure to air, light and moisture.
- It should be stored in a dark, cool, dry place in a closed container resistant to corrosion and chlorine content of stocks should be frequently checked.

Filtration of Water

Purification of Water on Smaller Scale

Ozone

It is a powerful oxidizing and strong virucidal agent. It eliminates undesirable odor, taste, color and removes all chlorine from water. Dose for potable water treatment varies from 0.2 to 1.5 mg/L.

UV Irradiation

A film of water, up to 120 mm thick, is exposed to one or several quartz mercury vapor arc lamps emitting UV radiation at a wavelength 200 to 295 mm.

38 Must Remember

- Chlorine demand - Horrock's apparatus
- Chlorine estimation - chloroscope (orthotolidine test)

62 High Yield Points

- Disinfectant action of chlorine is after the breakpoint chlorination
- The main disinfectant action is by the Hypochlorous ions

38 Good to Remember

- *Chlorine demand* [Q] is the amount of chlorine needed to destroy bacteria and to oxidize all the organic matter and ammoniacal substances present in the water.
- *Break-point chlorination* [Q] is the point at which the chlorine demand of the water is met. If further chlorine is added free chlorine ($HOCl^-$ and OCl^-) begins to appear in the water in proportion to the added dose of chlorine
- *Stabilized bleach* is bleaching powder mixed with excess of lime, it retains its strength.

39 Must Remember

Disadvantage of Ozone and UV irradiation is no residual effect.[Q]

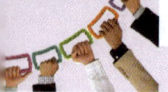

Chemical Disinfection

- Bleaching powder
  - Contains 33% free chlorine
  - Chlorine solution -4 kg bleaching powder with 25% free chlorine mixed in 20 liters of water will yield ready to use 5% chlorine solution for water disinfection
  - Advantage: maybe used for disinfection of small community water supply
- High test hypochlorite (Perchloron) – contains 65% free chlorine
- Chlorine tablets –0.5 g tablet for 20 liters of water
- Iodine
  - It may be used for emergency disinfection of water.
  - 2 drops of 2% ethanol iodine solution, with contact time for 30 minutes
  - Disadvantage: higher costs, thyroid dysfunctions, bad taste, color and odor
  - Iodine tablets are available as: Nesfield's tablets and Bursoline's tablets

Mechanical Filtrations

- Katadyn filters:
  - Oligodynamic action: Silver ions are released from the silver catalyst coat of the candle, which absorb the oxygen of the water and destroys the bacteria.
  - Not very effective for removal of microorganisms
- Domestic filters (aqua guards)
  - It filters, i.e. traps the dirt, mud and such other turbid impurities.
  - It removes the organic impurities (thereby removes the color and odor)
  - It inactivates the pathogens by U-V treatment in the U-V chamber
- Reverse osmosis filtration system: it is a multistage system consisting of 5 stage filtration process.
  - Stage 1: 5μ sediment filter. This removes sand, silt, dust and rust particles (i.e. suspended impurities)
  - Stage 2: Activated carbon block filter. Removes chlorine, organic matter, colors and bleaches (Removes chemical impurities).
  - Stage 3: Gag filter. Removes harmful chemicals and color, taste and odor producing substances (Removes bad taste, color and odor).
  - Stage 4: Reverse osmosis composite membrane with 0.0001 mm pore. Removes dissolved salts, organics, germs, bacteria, virus, compound metals and minerals. Allows only water molecules to pass through. The last stage may be combined with taste enhancers as well.

Purification of Water on a Large Scale

Storage

- 90% of suspended impurities settle down in 24 hour, total bacterial count drops by 90% in 5-7 days.[Q]
- Optimum period of storage of river water is about 10–14 days.[Q]
- Purification occurs by sedimentation, aerobic oxidation and drop in bacterial count

Filtration

Slow sand filter

Slow sand filters are almost obsolete nowadays. Components of a slow sand filter are:

- Supernatant raw water column
- A bed of graded sand and graded gravel
- An under-drainage system
- A system of filter control valves.

The main functioning part of the slow sand filter is slimy, greenish, jelly like layer, known as 'Vital layer', 'Zoogleal layer', 'Schmutzdecke' or 'Biological layer', which is composed of algae, planktons, fungi and diatoms. It is this layer which purifies the water by chemical and biological processes.

Advantages of slow sand filters	Disadvantages of slow sand filters
▪ Simple to construct, easy to operate	▪ Filters occupy large area
▪ Cheaper to construct than rapid sand filters	▪ Rate of filtration is slow (0.1 to 0.4 m^3/hour/sq m area)
▪ Physical, chemical and bacteriological quality of filtered water is very high (99.9% of bacteria are removed).	▪ Not very efficient in removing colloidal matters and color
	▪ Some standard of efficiency cannot be maintained from the beginning to the end of filter-run
	▪ The long period of about 18 hours, required for filtration of water may result in an anaerobic condition, depletion of oxygen and establishment of undesirable conditions at the bottom of the filter.

Rapid sand filters

Also known as 'mechanical filters'. It involves pretreatment of water with 'alum' and no pre-treatment requirement to store water, it can directly deal with raw, flowing water.

There are two types of rapid sand filters:

- Paterson's gravity type: water gets filtered through the sand-bed under its own weight.
- Candy's pressure type: water is passed through the bed under pressure, which is higher than the atmosphere pressure.

Advantages of rapid sand filters	Disadvantages of rapid sand filters
▪ Preliminary storage is not necessary	▪ The water requires preliminary treatment
▪ Can deal with raw water directly	▪ It requires the services of skilled persons
▪ Filters occupy less space	▪ The troubles that can occur are formation of mud-balls, cracking of filter-bed, air-binding, loss of sand and displacement of gravel
▪ Filtration is continuous and rapid	
▪ Cleaning is easy	
▪ Cheap and efficient filters	
▪ Suitable for turbid waters	

Table 5: Characteristics of rapid and slow sand filter

Characteristics	Rapid sand filter	Slow sand filter
Space	Occupies very little space	Occupies large area
Rate of Filtration[Q]	200 mgad	2-3 mgad
Effective size of sand[Q]	0.4-0.7 mm	0.2-0.3 mm
Preliminary treatment	Chemical coagulation and sedimentation	Plain sedimentation
Loss of head allowed	6-8 feet	4 feet
Washing	By back-washing	By scraping sand bed
Operation	Highly skilled	Less skilled
Removal of turbidity	Good	Good
Removal of bacteria[Q]	98-99%	99.9-99.99%
Ideal for	Cities	Small towns
Removal of color	Good	Fair

Note: Disinfection is a supplement, not a substitute to sand filtration

Water and Disease

Table 6: Types of disease caused due to water

Types of disease	Cause	Disease
Waterborne Disease[Q]	Water contaminated by humans, animals and chemical wastes	Diarrhea, Cholera, Typhoid, Dysentery, Polio, Hepatitis A and E
Water-Based Disease[Q]	Due to intermediate hosts in Water (aquatic hosts)	Snails-Schistosomiasis Cyclops- Dracunculiasis (Guinea worm disease)
Water-Scarce Disease or Water-washed disease[Q]	Scarcity of water and consequent poor hygiene	Trachoma, Salmonellosis and Worm infestation, Conjunctivitis, Bacillary and amoebic dysentery, Skin sepsis, Lice infestation, Scabies.
Water-Related Vector borne Disease	Mosquitoes and TseTse fly	Malaria, Filaria, Dengue, JE, Sleeping sickness

AIR

Air Pollution

- **Primary pollutants:** Emitted as such (SO_2, NO_2, CFC, CO, Ammonia, Hydrocarbons, Lead, Cadmium, Copper, Nickel, Particulate matter)
- **Secondary pollutants:** Formed as a result of interaction among primary pollutants (Ozone, Peroxyacetyl nitrate)
- SO_2 is considered as the best indicator of air pollution in urban and industrial areas. It is monitored in all air pollution surveys.
- The recommended level for SO_2 in 24 hours exposure is <20 mcg/m^3
- Carbon monoxide is the most common and widely distributed air pollutant
- Ozone gas recommended level is <100 mcg/m^3 for 8 hours mean exposure

Monitoring of Air Pollution

- Sulphur dioxide – best indicator[Q]
- Soiling (smoke) index – a specified amount of air is filtered through a filter paper and the stain is measured by photoelectric meter.
- Grit (dust) index: to check for deposit of dust, grit and small particulate matter
- Coefficient of haze – assessment of smoke, aerosols and fine particulate matter in air.
- Air pollution Index – a composite index which takes into account multiple air pollutants with defined upper limits

Table 7: Indoor air pollutants and their sources

Indoor air pollutants	Sources	Remarks
Carbon dioxide	Combustion, respiration	Major effect on climate change and global warming
Nitrogen dioxide	Gas cookers, cigarettes	COPD, bronchitis
Nitric oxide	Coal burning, road traffic, electricity production	Bronchitis, asthma, COPD
Respirable particles	Tobacco smoke, Stove, Aerosol spray	Pneumoconiosis is the main health hazard
Formaldehyde	Particle board, carpet adhesives, insulation	Short term effect- burning and watery eyes Long term effects- Carcinogenic
Asbestos	Insulation, fireproofing	Asbestosis
Carbon monoxide	Combustion equipment, stove, gas heaters	Carboxyhemoglobin formation, impaired cognitive functions, impairment of higher thinking, sleep impairment
Sulfur dioxide	Coal combustion	▪ Asthma, pulmonary function derangement, respiratory diseases, chronic bronchitis ▪ Also responsible for 'acid rain'

Contd...

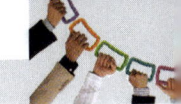

Indoor air pollutants	Sources	Remarks
Ozone	Electric arcing, UV light sources	Chronic lung diseases
Radon	Building material	Lung cancer
Other organic vapours (Benzene, Toluene)	Solvents, adhesives, resin products, aerosol sprays	Risk of lung cancers
Hydrocarbons	Incineration, coal burning, petroleum burning	Responsible for 'photochemical smog'
Lead	Burning of material containing lead – leaded fuels, stripping lead paints, smelting, recycling	Plumbism

Air Comfort

- **Cooling power of air:** The cooling power of air determines the capacity of the ambient atmosphere to dissipate the metabolic heat generated by the humans.
  - It includes an adjustment for air temperature, air humidity, air velocity and is a good field measure for ventilation and air quality
  - It is measured by the Kata thermometer (see Figure)
- **Heat stress index** (HSI): It is the ratio of the evaporation required to maintain heat balance to the maximum evaporation which could be attained in the particular environment, expressed as percentage
  - The HSI is related to strain, in terms of body sweating
  - HSI range from 0 – 100

Table 8: Heat stress index values

0 -	No thermal stress
10–30	Moderate to mild heat strain
40–60	Severe heat strain
70–90	Very severe heat strain
100	Upper limit of heat tolerance

- **Effective temperature**: Includes indices as air temperature, humidity and air flow.
  - It is a measure for heat stress index
- **Corrected effective temperature**:
  - C.E.T. scale is an improvement over Effective Temperature Index and considers 4 factors namely

Parameter	Instrument used to measure
i. Air temperature	Thermometer
ii. Velocity	Anemometer (see Fig. 4)
iii. Humidity	Hygrometer (see Fig. 5), Psychrometer (see Figs 6A and B)
iv. Mean radiant heat	Globe thermometer (see Fig. 7)

  - Corrected Effective Temperature (CET) and Effective Temperature Index are often used as indices for warmth.
    i. 34°C – reasonable efficiency
    ii. 38.6°C – upper limit for tolerance
- **Predictable 4 hours sweat rate:** Air comfort is measured using McArdle's rate (predictable 4 hours sweat rate)
  - The Predicted Four-hour Sweat Rate (P4SR) may classify the thermal comfort levels as:
    i. Comfort zone - 1–3 L
    ii. Just tolerable - 3–4.5 L
    iii. Intolerable - 4.5 L
- **Comfort Zone:** It is the range of corrected effective temperature in which the individual or the worker in an industry, feels comfortable. The criteria of comfort zone are:[Q]
  - Corrected effective temperature—25 to 27°C (77–80°F)
  - Relative Humidity—30 to 65 percent
  - Dry kata—6 and above
  - Wet kata—20 and above
  - Predicted four hours sweat rate (P4SR)—1 to 3 L

P4SR is applicable only in that situation where sweating occurs.

Table 9: Subjective feeling of occupant at various temperatures

Corrected effective temperature	Subjective feeling of occupant
69°F or 20°C	Pleasant and cool
69–76°F or 20–25°C	Comfortable and cool
77–80°F or 25–27°C	Comfortable
81–82°F or 27–28°C	Hot and uncomfortable
≥83°F or ≥28°C +	Extremely hot
≥86°F or ≥30°C	Intolerably hot

Instruments and Devices in Air Quality and Meteorology

Kata Thermometer (See Fig. 3)

- Used for measuring
  - Cooling power of air
  - Velocity of air
- Composition:
  - Two alcohol thermometers each with a bulb of 1.8 cm diameter and 4 cm length
  - The bulb of one is covered with a wet muslin cloth and is known as wet kata thermometer and the other one is left as it is and is known as dry kata thermometer.
- Procedure:
  - The bulbs of both the kata's are immersed in warm water till the temperature rises above 130°C
  - The bulb of the dry kata thermometer is wiped to dry
  - The muslin cloth over the wet kata is moistened
  - The kata thermometers are suspended in air and the time required for the temperature to fall from 100°C to 95°C is noted for both the kata thermometers.

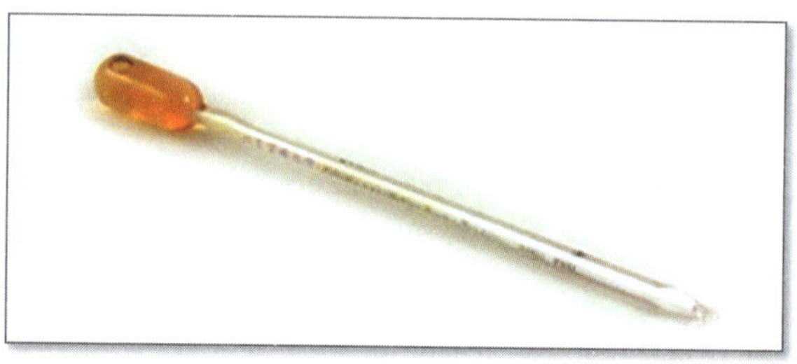

Fig. 3: Kata Thermometer

- Anemometer
  - Used to measure the wind velocity

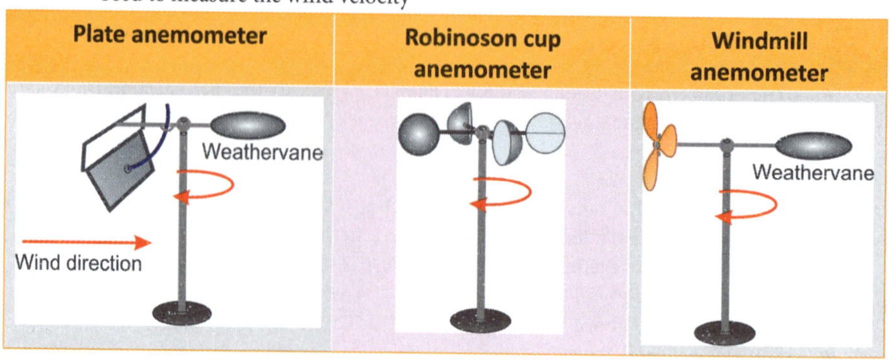

Fig. 4: Anemometer

- Dry and wet bulb hygrometer
  - Used to measure the air humidity

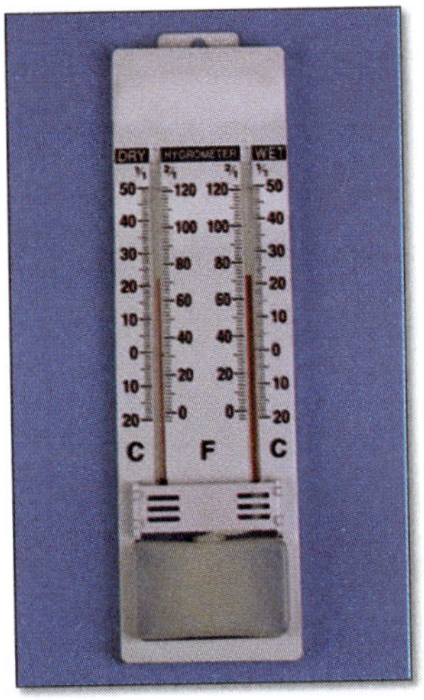

Fig. 5: Dry and wet bulb hygrometer

- Sling psychrometer
  - Used to measure the relative air humidity
- Aassman psychrometer
  - Used to measure the relative air humidity

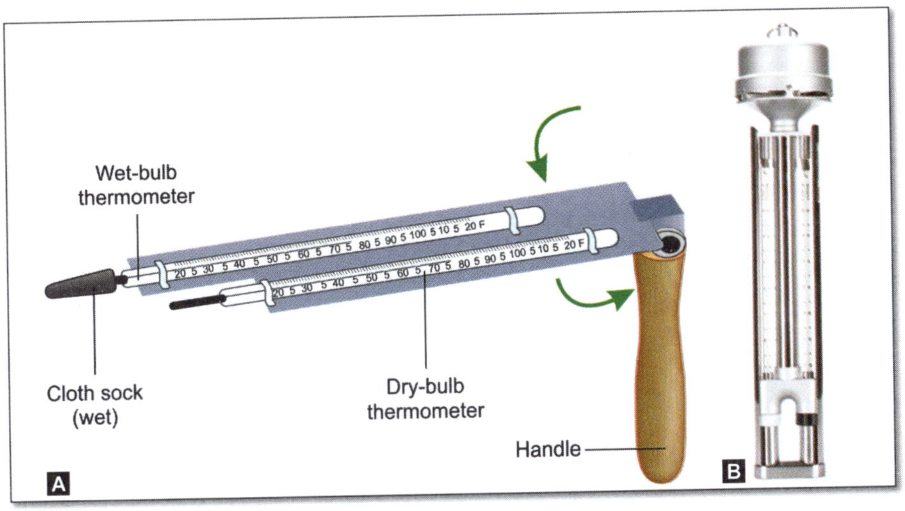

Figs 6A and B. **A.** Sling psychrometer; **B.** Aassman psychrometer

- Globe thermometer
  - Used to measure the radiant heat or transferred heat

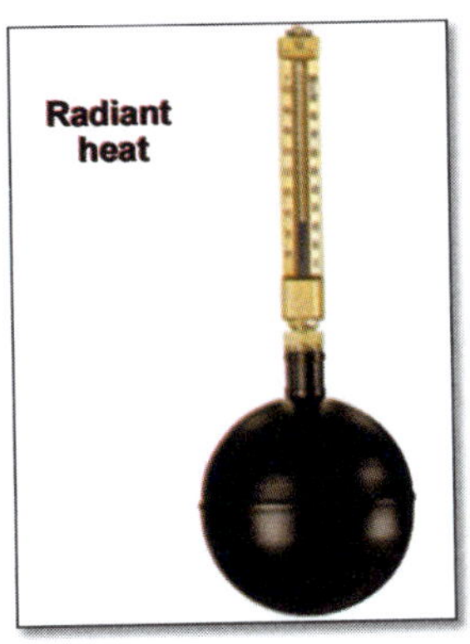

Fig. 7: Globe thermometer

- Barometer
  - Used to measure the atmospheric pressure.

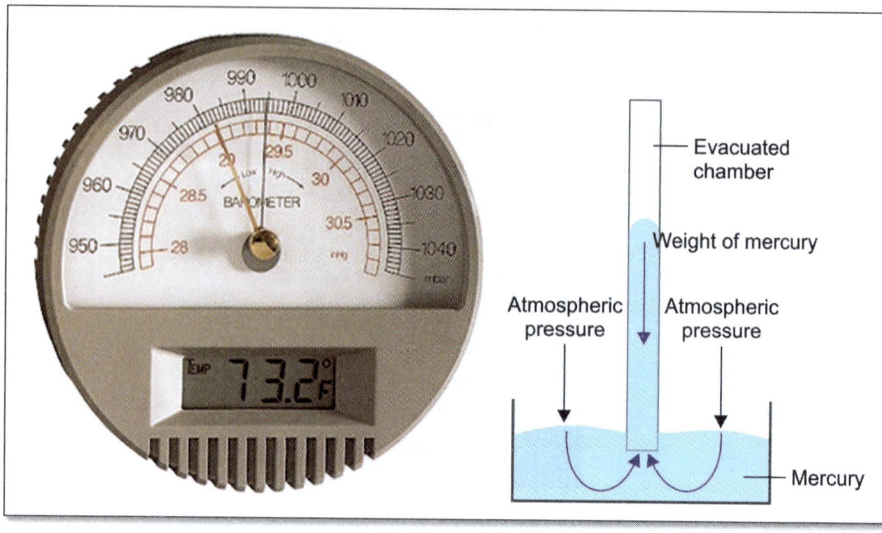

Fig. 8: Barometer

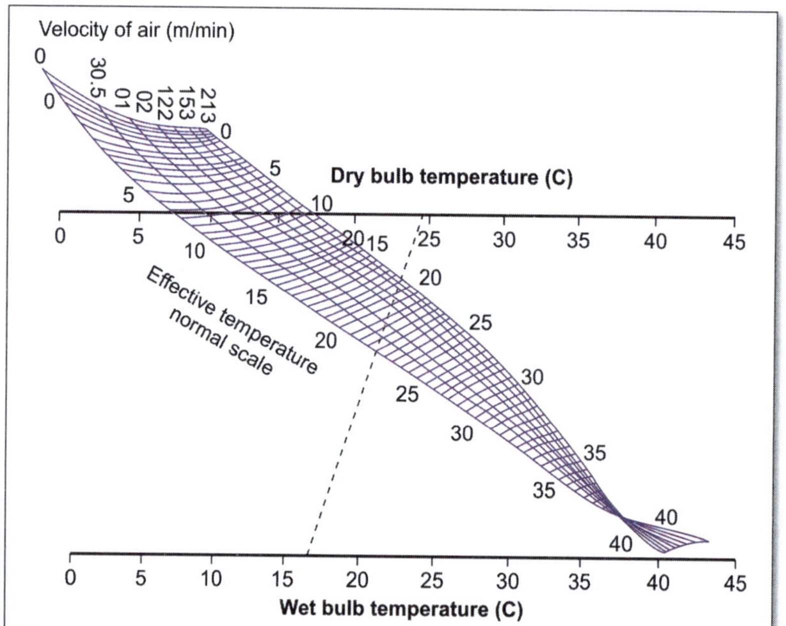

Fig. 9: Chart showing the graphical presentation of the corrected effective temperature

Humidity

- **Absolute humidity** is weight of water vapor in a unit volume of air. It is expressed as g/m^3 of air. Absolute humidity is weight of water vapor in a unit volume of air. It is expressed as g/m^3 of air.
- **Relative humidity** (RH)(used more commonly) is ratio of amount of water vapor present in air to the maximum amount of water vapor required for saturation at that particular temperature and pressure.

$$RH = \frac{\textit{Water vapor content}}{\textit{Water vapor capacity}}$$

RH = (Actual vapor pressure/Saturation vapor pressure) × 100

- RH of air is expressed in percentage
- RH < 35% = unpleasant = skin crack, dry flake or itch, dry nasal mucosa /predisposition to persistent infection *viz.* sore-throat, cough
- 50% RH means that air contains ½ the amount of water vapor needed for saturation.
- RH > 65% - unpleasant – sticky skin
- Air with RH more than 100% is said to be supersaturated.

RH of air can be changed in 2 ways
- Change in water vapor content of air
- Change in temperature of air with water vapor content remaining same. (RH increases on cooling and decreases on warming of air)

Dew point: It is the temperature to which air has to be cooled (without any change in air pressure or moisture content) for saturation to occur.

Frost point: When determined with respect to a flat surface of ice, it is called frost point. It is used to predict the formation of dew, frost, fog and even minimum temperature.

High dew point indicates high water content and low dew point indicates low water vapor content.

> 39 **Good to Remember**
>
> Instruments used to measure relative humidity[Q]
> - Dry and wet bulb hygrometer (see Fig. 5)
> - Sling or whirling psychrometer (see Fig. 6A)
> - Aassman psychrometer (see Fig. 6B)

Ventilation

Types of Ventilation

- **Natural ventilation:** Wind (Perflation, aspiration), diffusion, movement of air as a result of difference in temperature
- **Mechanical ventilation**
- **Exhaust ventilation:**
  - Air is extracted out by exhaust fans creating a vacuum that induces fresh air to enter via window, door etc.
  - Ideal for large halls and auditorium for removal of vitiated air.
  - Used in industries to remove dusts, fumes, concentrated contaminants at source
- **Plenum ventilation: (limited utility)**
  - Fresh air is blown into the room by centrifugal fans so as to create a positive pressure and displace vitiated air.
  - Used in air-conditioned buildings and factories. Air is delivered through ducts at desired points.
- **Balanced ventilation:** It is a combination of exhaust and plenum ventilation (Blowing fan must balance exhaust fan)
- **Air conditioning:** Air is filtered, excess humidity is removed, heating/cooling of air occurs, some percent of fresh air is mixed.

HOUSING, NOISE, LIGHT, RADIATION ENVIRONMENT

Noise

Loudness of noise is measured in decibels (dB). A daily exposure up to 85 dB is the limit people can tolerate without substantial damage to their hearing. [Q]
- Noise threshold for pain is 140 dB [Q]
- Human ear can hear frequencies from about 20 to 20,000 Hz
- Vibrations <20 Hz are infra-audible and >20,000 Hz are ultrasonic

> 40 **Must Remember**
>
> **Noise levels**
>
> | | |
> |---|---|
> | Normal conversation | 60–65 dB |
> | Whispering | 20–30 dB |
> | Heavy street traffic | 60–80 dB |
> | Boiler factories | 120 dB |
> | Jet take off | 150 dB |

Auditory Effects of Noise Exposure

- Auditory fatigue occurs in 90 dB region and at 4000 Hz
- Deafness
  - Deafness (In frequency range 4,000 to 6,000 Hz)
  - Permanent deafness (Repeated or continuous exposure to noise around 100 decibels)
  - Rupture of Tympanic membrane-Exposure to noise above 160 dB[Q]

Nonauditory Effects

- Interference with speech (300-500 Hz). Speech sound level must exceed SIL (Speech Interference Level) by about 12 dB

- Annoyance (psychological response) and reduced efficiency
- Physiological: Rise in blood pressure, intracranial pressure, heart rate, breathing rate and an increase in sweating.

Light

Measurement of Day Light

- The daylight factor in a building may be determined by daylight factor meter.
- Recommended value: rooms – 8%, kitchen 10%

$$\text{Daylight factor} = \frac{\textit{Instantaneous illumination indoors}}{\textit{Simultaneous occurring illumination outdoors}} \times 100$$

Table 10: Units of measurement of light

		Recommended units
Luminous intensity	Power of light source	Candela/candle power
Luminous flux	Flow of light	Lumens
Illumination	Amount of light reaching the surface	Lux
Brightness/luminance	Amount of light re-emitted by the surface	Lambert
Daylight measure		Day light factor

63 High Yield Points

Standards for lighting

- Casual reading : 100 Lux
- Office work : 400 Lux
- Fine work : 1000–2000 Lux
- Watch making : 2000–3000 Lux

Artificial Lighting

Two types of artificial illumination are done:

1. Fluorescent lamps 5% light + 95% heat
2. Filament lamps 21% light + 79% heat

- *Direct*: 99 to 100% of the light is projected directly towards the working area. It is efficient, economical, but tends to cast sharp shadows
- *Semi-direct*: 10 to 40% of light is projected upwards so that it is reflected back on the object.
- *Indirect*: 90 to 100% of the light is projected towards the ceiling and walls.
- *Semi-indirect*: Here, 60 to 90% of the light is directed upwards, and the rest downwards.
- *Direct indirect*: Here, light is distributed equally, No one system can be recommended.
- A good sun screen ointment should have a *Sun protection factor (SPF)* of at least 15, to be able protect against both UVA and UVB rays, when going out in the sun.

House

Standards

- Walls: 9 inch brick wall, plastered
- Roof: 10 ft
- Floor –
    - Height of the plinth should be at least 2-3 feet
    - Floor area:
        - >70-90 – one person*
        - >110 sq.ft. – 2 persons*
        - Baby under 1 year not counted, child 1-10 years counted as half unit
          * otherwise known as overcrowding (Refer to topic on overcrowding discussed below)
- Window
    - To be placed at height < 3 ft.
    - 1/5th of floor area
    - Combined door and window to be 2/5th of floor area
      ** Cattle shed – at least 25 meters away*

Overcrowding

Where a higher than normal number of persons are living in a single dwelling unit, so that it may pose a risk for serious health related issues.

The following criteria may be used for defining overcrowding in a dwelling:

- Person criteria for overcrowding: if
  - 1 room >2 persons
  - 2 rooms >3 persons
  - 3 rooms >5 persons and so on..
- Floor space criteria: Adequate floor space area counts as-
  - 50-70 sq ft ½ person (children age 1-10 years are counted as ½ unit person)
  - 70-90 sq ft 1 person (age > 10 years)
  - 90-100 sq ft 1 ½ persons
  - 110 sq ft or more 2 persons and so on…
- Gender criteria: 2 persons of different gender, age more than 9 years (not husband and wife) are sharing a single room, it is overcrowding.

Radiation

Natural Sources

- Cosmic rays
  - Normal living altitude : 30–35 mrad/year
  - Jet pilots : 300 mrad/year
- Terrestrial radiation : Average humans – 50 mrad/year
- Internal radiation : 25–50 mrad/year

Man-made Sources

- Skin dose to the patient from a single X-ray film : 0.02–0.3 Rad
- Radioactive fallout : C_{14}, I_{131}, Cs_{137}, Sr_{90} (most dangerous ones)

Types of Radiation

- Ionizing radiation
  - Electromagnetic radiations
  - Corpuscular radiations
    - Alpha rays are more harmful (10 times more than X-rays)
    - Gamma rays and alpha rays have short wave length and deep penetrations
- Nonionizing radiation (longer wave lengths)
  - Ultraviolet (UV) radiation
  - Visible light, Infrared radiation
  - Microwave radiation
  - Radio frequency radiation

Radiation Effects

- <5 Rad : No immediate effect
- 5-50 Rad : Slight blood changes
- 50-150 Rad : Blood changes + nausea vomiting, fatigue
- 150-1100 Rad : Severe blood changes,
  1. Approx. 2 weeks later a few may die
  2. Within 60 days, approx. 50% will die
  3. Bone marrow transplant is the management in case of severe exposures
- 1100 – 2000 Rad : Death within 14 days
- > 2000 Rad : Death is certain and almost immediate. Medical therapy may only prolong suffering.

High Yield Points

- Permissible doses from man-made radiation source is up to 5 Rads
- Routine fluoroscopy gives approx. 4 Rads

Prevention

- Lead apron with at least 0.5 mm Lead
- Radiation badge to show the cumulative radiation dose

ENTOMOLOGY

The phylum arthropoda consists of three important classes— Class Insecta, Arachnida and Crustacea. **Arthropods of medical importance are:**

	Insecta	Arachnida	Crustacea
Body shape	Cylindrical	Circular or oval	Pear shaped
Body division	Head, thorax and abdomen	Cephalothorax and abdomen	Cephalothorax and abdomen
Antennae in head	1–pair	Absent	2–pairs
Wings	Some are winged, some are wingless	Absent	Absent
Legs	3–pairs	4–pairs	5–pairs
Living	On land	On land	In water
Examples	Winged ▪ Mosquitoes ▪ Flies Wingless ▪ Fleas ▪ Lice ▪ Bugs	▪ Ticks ▪ Mites ▪ Spiders* ▪ Scorpions*	▪ Cyclops ▪ Crabs* ▪ Lobsters* ▪ Prawns*

**These do not transmit any disease*

Class Insecta: Mosquito

General Features of Mosquito

- There are two broad tribes of mosquitos:
  - Tribe *anopheline* – contains genus *anopheles*
    - About 45 species of anopheles mosquitoes are found in India:
    - *An. fluviatilis* and *An. minimus* in foot-hill regions
    - *An. sundaicus* and *An. stephensi* in coastal regions, urban cities
    - *An. culicifacies* and *An. philippinensis* in plains, rural areas
    - *Anopheles fluviatilis* is highly anthropophilic
  - Tribe *culicini* – genus *Culex, aedes, Mansonia*
    - *Culex fatigans* is vector of Bancroftian filariasis in India[Q]. It is highly anthrophilic, enters houses at dusk and reaches maximum density by midnight (peak biting time).
    - Aedes: *Aedes aegypti, Aedes vittatus, Aedes albopictus*
    - Most abundant during rainy season, Important vector with public health importance
    - Mansonia: *M. annulifera, M. uniformis, M. indiana, M. longipalpis*
- Males survive of plant juices, whereas female mosquitoes are hematophagous
- Life span of mosquito is about 14 days, males are short-lived.
- Under favorable it takes 7-10 days to complete the life cycle
- Relative humidity of 60% and temperature of 20-30 degree is optimum for mosquito
- Both high and low temperatures are fatal

Table 11: Features of mosquitoes

Tribe	Tribe Anophelini	Tribe culicini		
Genus	**Anopheles**	**Aedes**	**Culex**	**Mansonia**
Water breeding habitat	Clean, stagnant water	Artificial, stored water	Dirty polluted water	Large water body with aquatic vegetations (pistia plant and water hyacinths)
Egg type	Single egg, boat shaped	Single egg, cigar shaped, barrel shaped	Cluster egg	Star shaped, cluster under the leaves

Contd...

Tribe	Tribe Anophelini	Tribe culicini		
Genus	**Anopheles**	**Aedes**	**Culex**	**Mansonia**
Larva type	Surface feeder	Siphon present	Siphon present	Siphon present
Flight range	2-3 km	100-200 meters	11-13 km	500 meters – 2 km
Peak biting	Morning and evening, Non painful bite	Day time 2 hours before sunset and 2 hours after sunrise, painful bite	Night time, painful bite	Twilight and late evening, non painful bite
Sitting posture	Landing position, inclined at 45 deg to surface	Parallel to ground, with hunch back posture	Hunch back posture	Long legs with hunch back posture
Identifying feature	▪ Tail in air ▪ Spotted wings ▪ No noise in flying	▪ Legs and body is banded ▪ Also called as tiger mosquito ▪ Unspotted wings	▪ Strong, unspotted wings ▪ Buzzing sound ▪ Brownish color	▪ Unspotted wings, banded legs ▪ Pepper powder thrown on white background ▪ No sound while flying

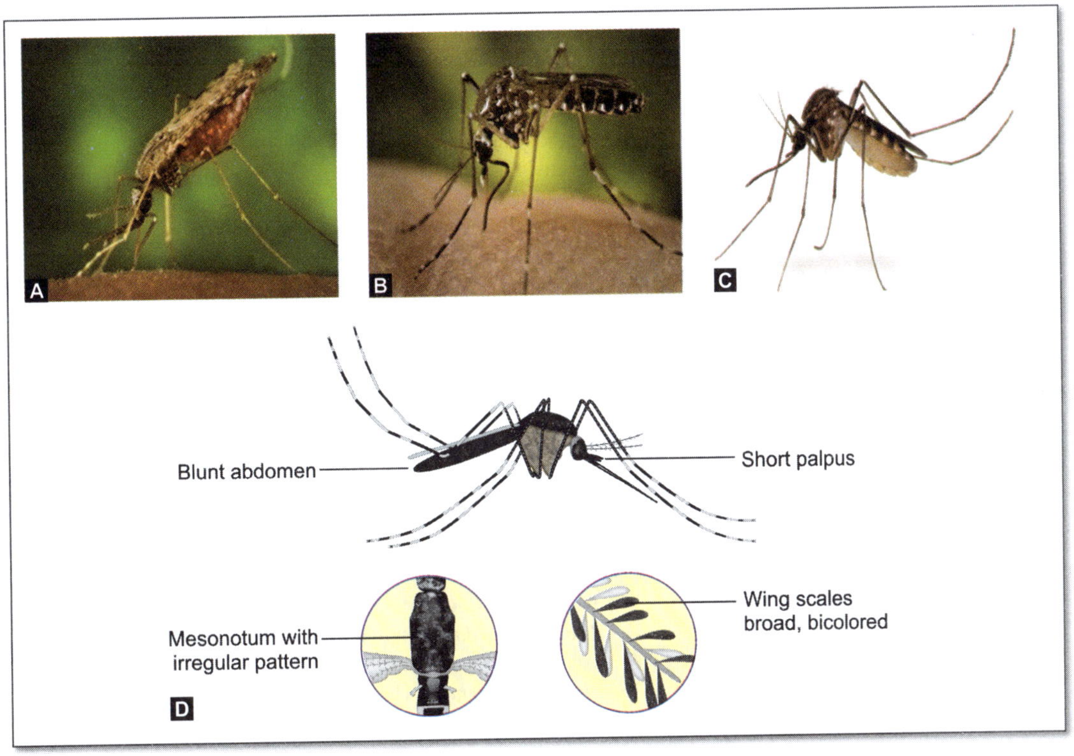

Figs 10A to D: **A.** Anopheles; **B.** Aedes; **C.** Culex; **D.** Mansonia

Table 12: Mosquito-borne diseases

Mosquitoes	Diseases caused
Anopheles	Malaria, Filaria (not in India)
Culex	Bancroftian filariasis, Japanese encephalitis, West Nile fever, Viral arthritis
Aedes	Dengue, hemorrhagic fever, Chikungunya fever, Chikungunya hemorrhagic fever, Rift valley fever, Filaria and Yellow fever (not in India)
Mansonoides	Malayan (Brugian) filariasis, Chikungunya fever

Mosquito Control Measures

- Anti-larval measures: Environmental Control, Chemical Control and Biological Control
- Anti-adult measures: Residual Sprays, Space Sprays, Genetic Control
- Protection against mosquito bites: Mosquito Net, Screening, Repellents

Experts recommend "integrated approach" that combines one or more methods, to obtain maximum results with minimum inputs and also prevent environmental pollution with toxic chemicals and development of insecticide resistance.

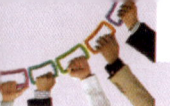

- Anti-larval measures:
  - Environmental Control or Source reduction–
    - Minor engineering methods (filling, leveling, drainage), water management (intermittent irrigation), rendering water unsuitable for mosquito breeding (Changing salinity of water).
    - Aedes mosquito: remove artificial water containers
    - Culex: Disposal of sewage, dirty water. Remove domestic and peri-domestic sources of water collections
    - Anopheles: filling of road side water collections, open ditches
    - Mansonia: removal of plants in water – use herbicides
  - Chemical Control
    - Mineral oil
      - Dose: 40-90 L/Hectare, once a week on all breeding places.
      - Disadvantages: renders water unfit for drinking; it kills fish.
    - Paris green: (copper acetoacetate) – contains 50% arsenious oxide
      - Emerald green, micro crystalline powder and is a stomach poison
      - Dose: 2% dust spray @ 1 kg paris green/hectare of water surface
    - Synthetic insecticides (Fenthion, Chlorpyrifos, and Abate) – these are organophosphorus compounds
      - Abate (Temephos):
        1. Brown viscous liquid soluble in petroleum compounds
        2. Good larvicide, poor adulticide
        3. May also be used for control of *An. stephensi* in wells
      - Fenthion
        1. Colorless, oily liquid, insoluble in water. It has a garlic odor
        2. It is a stomach poison with high effectivity for *Culex* larvae
      - Dose:

Abate (Temephos)	50-100 g/hectare or as 1 ppm for wells
Malathion	500 g/hectare
Fenthion	100 g/hectare

*organochlorine compounds as DDT, HCH is not recommended because of long residual effects.

  - Biological Control
    - Larvivorous fish
      - *Gambusia affinis*
      - *Lebistes reticulatus* (Barbados Millions)
      - *Apolocheilus panchax*
    - *Toxorhynchites splendens* (Predator Mosquito) for *Aedes aegypti*
- Anti-Adult measures

The adulticides may be of two varieties:

  - Residual sprays: These chemicals have a residual lasting effect.
  - Space sprays: Include the fumigants with minimal residual action

As per the chemical composition of the adulticides, they may be classified as:

  - Organochlorous compounds
    - **DDT** (Dichloro-Diphenyl-Trichloroethane) (was) the adulticide of choice. But now with accumulation in the food chain and emergence of DDT resistance, DDT is being less commonly used.
      1. DDT contains 70–80% of para-para isomer (most active fraction of DDT).[Q]
      2. DDT is a contact poison and acts on the nervous system of insects.
      3. Residual action is for about 18 months and has no repellent action on insects.[Q]

Must Remember

- DDT residual spray → 5% suspension is applied at 100-200 mg/foot to kill Adult mosquitoes.[Q]
- As a dust, DDT is used in 5 to 10% strength for the control of lice, fleas, ticks and bugs.
- In aerosol or space sprays, DDT is one of the main constituents.

4. Not recommended for larvicidal operations due to long residual effect, water contamination and increased risk of developing resistance in vector mosquitoes.
5. In areas where DDT resistance is encountered- Malathion (100-200 mg/Sq. ft every 3 month or as ULV), Propoxur (OMS-33), Lindane are recommended.[Q]

- **Benzene Hexa-Chloride** - BHC
  1. White, light brown colored powder with a musty smell, irritating to the eyes, nose and throat.
  2. Pure HCH contains 99% of lindane or gamma HCH. Gamma isomer of the HCH (Hexa-chloro-cyclohexane) is most effective form. It is more toxic and effective than DDT
  3. Kills insects by direct contact
- Dose

DDT	1-2 g/m^2	6-12 months
Malathion	2 g/m^2	3 months
OMS-33	2 g/m^2	3 months
BHC	20-25 mg/ft^2	3 months

- Organophosphorus compounds
  - **Malathion:**
    1. Yellow or brown colored liquid (or powder) with an unpleasant smell.
    2. It is a contact poison and is more effective than DDT but least toxic of all Organochlorous compounds
    3. Dose: 100-200 mg per sq ft every 3 months for good insecticidal action
  - **Parathion:** It is a contact and stomach poison with fumigant action. It is highly effective and toxic insecticide
  - **Diazinon:** Colorless liquid, with moderate toxicity. Used as fumigant
  - **Dichlorvos:** Pleasant smelling, colorless liquid soluble in water and organic solvents. It may be used as fumigant or is mixed with wax and solid chemicals for tablet formulations
- Carbamates
  - **Propoxur:** It is a broad-spectrum insecticide. It is insoluble in water but soluble in organic solvents. It is generally used to kill variety of household insects and arthropods. Maybe used in DDT resistant areas
  - **Carbaryl:** General broad-spectrum insecticide. Carbaryl is quite effective against ticks, fleas, bugs and cockroaches.
- Plant insecticides
  - **Pyrethrum and pyrethroids:** These are potent space sprays and lack residual effect.
    1. They are extracts of pyrethrum or chrysanthemum cinerariifolium flower.
    2. The active components are Pyrethrum I and II ; and Cinerins I and II – all are nerve poison. The ready to spray solution is formulated as dusts, aerosols, emulsions, solutions, mosquito coils and fumigant mats.
    3. Dose: 1 oz (30 g) of spray solution per 1000 cu ft of the space
  - **Rotenone and rotenoids:** Derived from the roots of leguminous plants of Derris and Lonchocarpus genus. They kill by paralysis of insects. Also active for ticks, mite, lice and flea.

- Personal protection
  - Mosquito nets
    - Size of hole in net – not more than 0.0475 inch in any diameter
    - Number of holes -150 holes per square inch of the net
  - Insecticide Treated Bed Nets (ITBN)
    - Use synthetic pyrethroids- Deltamethrin (2.5% mg/m^2) or Cyfluthrin (5%-50 mg/m^2). Retreatment is needed after 6 months.
    - Long-lasting Insecticidal Nets: Use a chemical binder along with synthetic pyrethroids. Effective for 3 years or >20 wash.
  - Screen of doors, windows:
    - The aperture size should be measuring 0.04 to 0.05 sq. inch in diameter

- Mosquito repellents:
  - Effective for 1-3 hours - oil of citronella
  - Effective for 4-5 hours - vanishing cream of Dimethyl phthalate, Diethyltoluamide (DEET), Dimethyl carbate, Ethyl hexanediol, Indolone, etc.
- Genetic control: novel technique for mosquito control.
  - Sterilization techniques
  - Male hybridization- chromosomal aberrations technique
- GIS-remote sensing – is a novel technique to asses for the land use, monitoring vector density and entomological surveillance

Housefly

General features:

- Species of public health importance are:
  - *Musca domestica, M vicina, M. Nebulo. M. Sorbens*
- They are regarded as the most important index for insanitation
- In Males – eyes are close together, while in females – eyes are wide apart
- Breeding habits: excreta (horse > human > other animals – in order of preference)

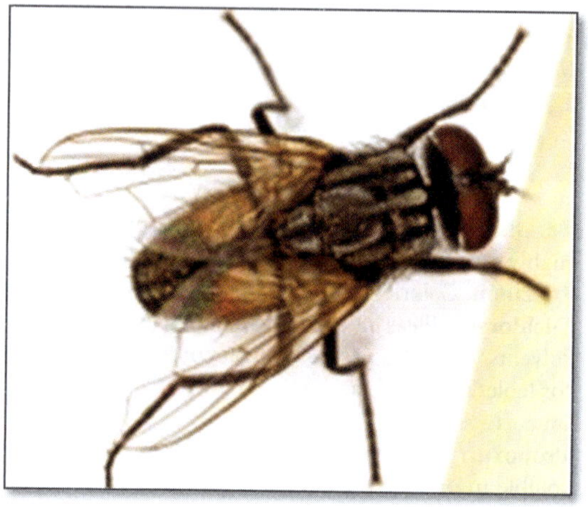

Fig. 11: Housefly

- Mode of transmission
  - Mechanical transmission – by feet and hairy legs
  - Vomit drops – regurgitated stomach contents from excreta meal
  - Defecation on food or wound surface
- Control
  - Elimination of breeding places and appropriate sanitation
  - Insecticide – DDT (5%), methoxychlor (5%), lindane (0.5%), chlordane (2.5%)
  - Baits: combined with malathion, Dichlorvos, ronnel are used.
  - Fly papers – composed of resins, ground nuts, Vaseline base

Sandfly

General features:

- Small insect (smaller than a mosquito), measuring 2 mm
- It is winged, long legged, hairy insect and they hop (rather than flying!) and the flight (hopping) range is about 50 to 70 meters.
- Only the females bite, which is painful and particularly during night time.
- It takes about 30 to 45 days for the completion of the life cycle and the adult lives for about 2 weeks.
- Public health importance:
  - *Phlebotomus argentipes* — Kala-azar
  - *Phlebotomus papatasi* — Sandfly fever, Oriental sore, Chandipura encephalitis
  - *Phlebotomus sergenti* — Oriental sore
  - *S. punjabensis* — Sandfly fever
  - Lutzomyia versa crum — Oroya fever, Carrion's disease

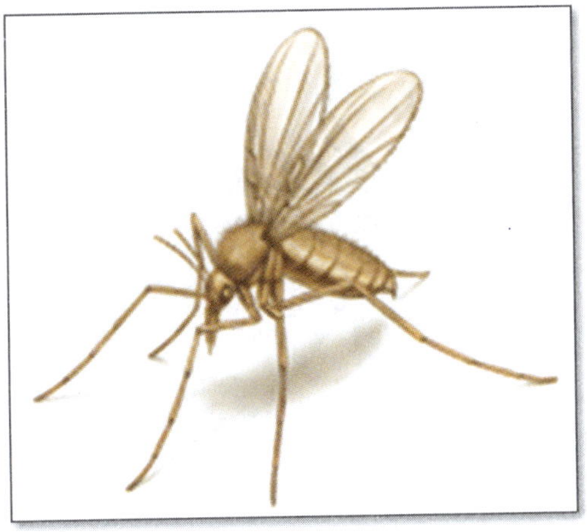

Fig. 12: Sandfly

- Control
  - Insecticides 1-2 /m^2 of DDT
  - Sanitation: Removal of shrubs within 50 meters of human dwelling. Keep area clean, fill up cracks and crevices in walls and floors

Lice

General characteristics:

- Louse is dorsoventrally flattened, Small wingless ectoparasites, and human lice feed exclusively on human blood. The infestation is called as pediculosis
- They are of three types:
  - Head louse (Pediculus humanus capitis),
  - Body louse (Pediculus humanus corporis)
  - Public louse (Pthirus pubis)
- The life cycle occurs in three stages, namely egg, nymph and adult and the metamorphosis is incomplete. The life cycle is completes in around 15-17 days. The adult louse life span is 30–50 days
- Public health importance:
  - Epidemic typhus caused by *Rickettsia prowazeki*
  - Relapsing fever caused by *Borrelia recurrentis*
  - Trench fever caused by *Rickettsia quintana*
  - Dermatitis: The bites by the lice cause considerable irritation and often itching. The secondary infection due to scratching can result in dermatitis.
- Mode of transmission: direct or indirect contact

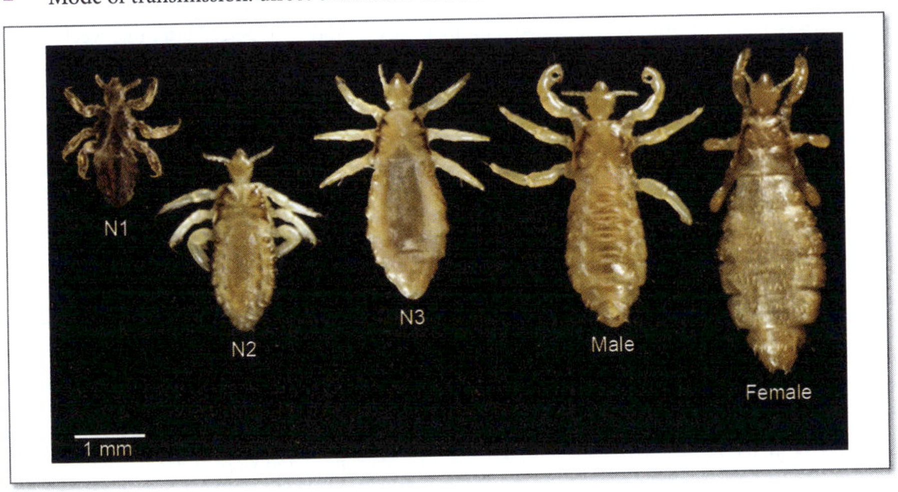

Fig. 13: Body louse

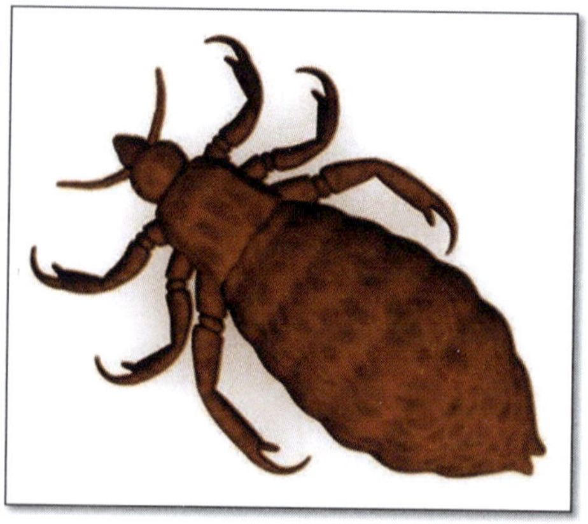

Fig. 14: Louse

CRAB Louse

- Also known as pubic louse or pthirus pubis. It is found in pubic or perianal region
- Small size of body, head impacted in the thorax

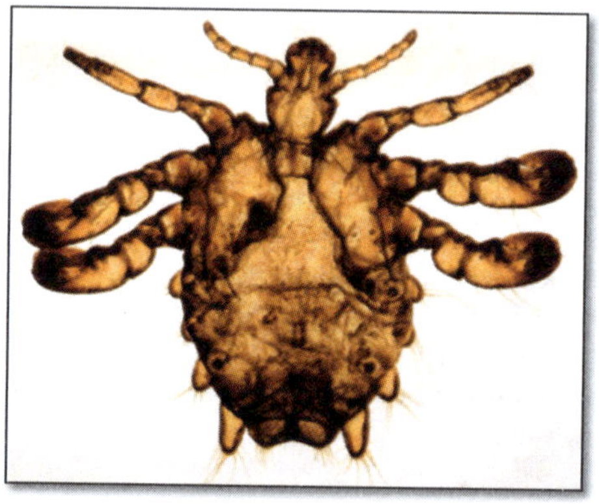

Fig. 15: Pubic louse

Control of Lice

- For head and crab lice: Application of 0.5% malathion lotion followed by head bath after one day. Malathion destroys lice and nits also.
- For body louse: Dusting with 1% malathion powder over the chest, axilla and to the inner surface of the cloths, socks and also into the trousers. May be repeated after one week.
- Personal Hygiene

Flea

General Features

- Small bilaterally compressed, hard skinned, brown colored, wingless insects, found as blood sucking ectoparasites on the body of warm-blooded hosts and birds
- If the chief host is not available, the fleas attack the other hosts called as secondary hosts.
- Various species of flea are:

• Rat fleas (oriental)	Xenopsylla astia, Xenopsylla brasiliensis, Xenopsylla cheopis
• Rat fleas (Temperate zone)	Nosopsylla fasciatus (Europe), Nosopsylla niligiriensis (India)
• Human flea	Pulex irritans
• Cats/Dogs	Ctenocephalides canis, Ctenocephalides felis
• Sand flea	Tunga penetrans (recorded in western parts of India, not frequently found)

- Public health importance of Fleas
  - Plague (bubonic plague)
  - Endemic (murine) typhus
  - Chiggerosis
  - Hymenolepis diminuta
- Control of FLEA
  - Insecticidal control
    - DDT dust spray (10%)
    - Malathion powder (5%) - usually used as 20-30g / rat burrow
    - Cyanogas fumigation - highly toxic gas
  - Repellents as Diethyltoluamide, Benzyl benzoate
  - Rodent control

Rat Flea

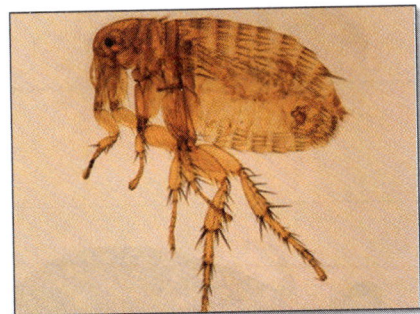

Fig. 16: Rat flea

- Morphology: Rat flea is a bilaterally compressed, wingless insect, having bristles over the body, directed backwards. Body is divisible into head, thorax and abdomen
- Life cycle: The life cycle of the rat flea occurs in four stages – egg, larva, pupa and adult, thus undergoing a process of complete metamorphosis
- Breeding places: Dust collections with organic matter and moisture as in burrows of the rats, cracks and crevices in the floor
- Mode of transmission
  - Shows a propagative mode of biological transmission (pathogen undergoes multiplication inside the body of the vector). A partial blocked flea is more dangerous to spread plague rather than a blocked flea
  - By defecation: the pathogen is found in the feces. When the host scratches over the flea-bitten area, humans get the infection through the contamination of abrasions or wounds. This is mechanism of transmission for murine typhus caused by Rickettsia mooseri
- Flea indices
  - General flea index (GFI)
    - It is the average number of fleas of all species, found per rodent.
    - GFI = Total no. of fleas of all species collected/Total no. of rodents collected.
    - Normal GFI = 3-5
  - Specific flea index (SFI)
    - It is the average number of fleas of each species found per rodent.
    - SFI = Total no. of fleas of each species collected/Total no. of rodents collected
    - Cheopis index of more than 1.0 indicates impending plague outbreak and need for corrective measures.
  - Percentage incidence of flea species: It is the percentage of fleas of each species found per rodent.
  - Rodent infestation rate: It is the percentage of rodents infested with fleas of all species.

Ticks (Class Arachnida)

These are of two families:

- Ixodidae (hard ticks)
- Argasidae (soft ticks)

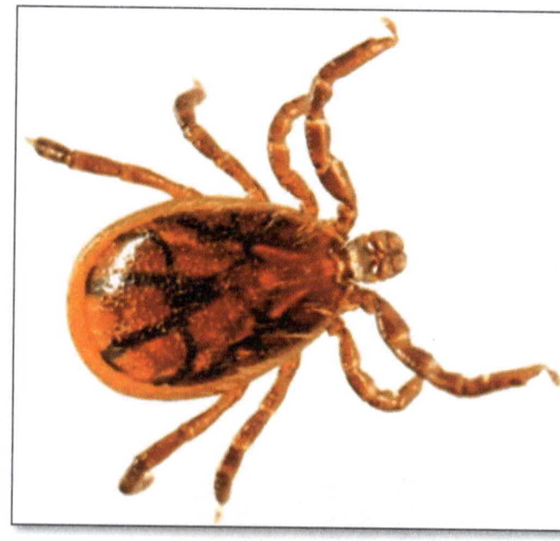

Fig. 17: Hard tick

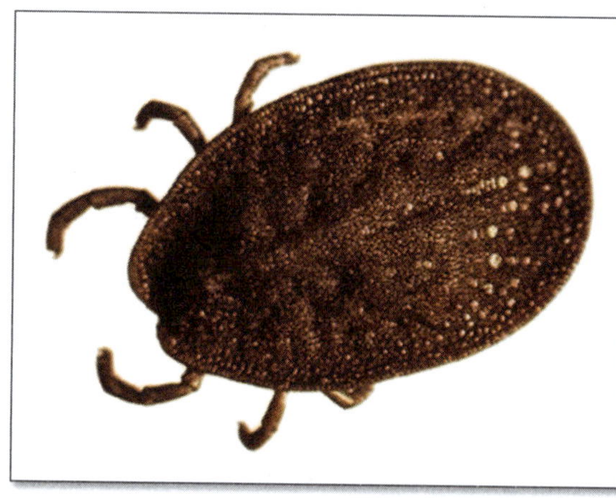

Fig. 18: Soft tick

Head ticks	Soft ticks
▪ They belong to the family ixodidae	▪ They belong to the family argasidae
▪ Capitulum is anterior in position	▪ Capitulum is ventral in position
▪ Scutum is present	▪ Scutum is absent
▪ Dorsally sexual dimorphism is well marked, i.e. scutum covers the entire dorsal surface in male and covers only a small portion in the female	▪ Sexual dimorphism is absent dorsally
▪ Spiracles exist behind the fourth pair of legs	▪ Spiracles exist between the third and the fourth pair of legs
▪ Festoons are present in some hard ticks	▪ Festoons are absent
▪ They cannot resist starvation. So they are always found on the body of the host (Day and night) (like lice)	▪ They can resist starvation for months. Therefore they are found on the body of the host only while feeding blood (i.e. only during night times) (like bedbugs)
▪ They require continuous blood meal	▪ They require intermittent blood meal

Contd...

Head ticks	Soft ticks
▪ They are always found on the body of their hosts	▪ They are found in cracks and crevices during day time and on the body of the host during night times
▪ Gravid female lays hundreds or thousands of eggs at one sitting	▪ Eggs are laid in batches of 20–100 over a long period of time
▪ Nymphal stage is one	▪ Nymphal stage are five
▪ Important species are *Dermacentor andersoni, Haemphysalis spinigera*	▪ Important specimen is *Ornithodoros moubata*
▪ Diseases transmitted are tick typhus, (Africa) tick paralysis, tularemia, viral encephalitis, Hemorrhagic fever (KFD) Human babesiosis. Rocky Mountain Spotted fever (USA), Q-fever (in US and Australia)	▪ Disease transmitted is Endemic Relapsing fever, caused by *Borrelia duttonii*, a spirochete

Mites

Trombiculid Mite

- The adult mites are spider like arthropods, the body consists of one unit only, having shape of the figure '8'. It measures about 1 to 2 mm and the whole body is covered with profuse hairs.
- Adult trombiculid mite does not bite. It is free living. It feeds on vegetable juice. The larval stage is the biting stage.
- When the larva bites the rodent infected with Rickettsia orientalis, the pathogens pass through the nymph stage, adult stage and to the eggs and larvae of next generation and larvae thus transmit the disease. This method of transmission is called 'Transovarian transmission.' Man gets the infection accidentally when bitten by the infected larva.

Vector (larva of ..)	Disease	Microorganism
Trombiculid (Leptotrombidium) akamushi	Tsutsugamushi disease	Rickettsia orientalis
Tr. (Lepto) akamushi and deliensis	Scrub typhus	Rickettsia Orientalis

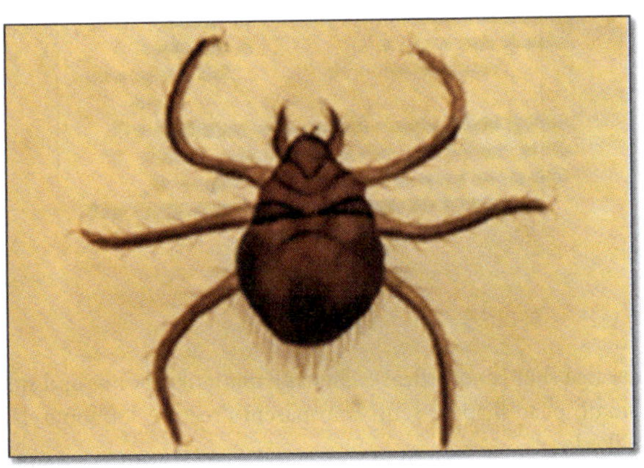

Fig. 19: Trombiculid mite

Itch Mite

General features:

- Small, globular and saccular creature, measuring about 0.2 to 0.4 mm in size, the females being larger than the males, body resembling like that of tortoise, round above and flat below

- The itch mite passes through the stages of egg → larva → nymph → adult. The entire life cycle takes about 10 to 14 days. The metamorphosis is incomplete. The life span of a mite is 1-2 months
- This Parasite causes "Scabies" or "Itch". The female mite comes into contact with the human skin and makes burrows in upper layers of epidermis at the rate of 2-3 mm per day, lays eggs along the sides of the skin in the burrows (known as ovigerous tunnels) and later dies. There is itching which is due to secretion of acrid fluid. The secondary infection resulting from itching, may destroy the parasites. Hence under such conditions, it is difficult to find them
- Mode of transmission: close contact, contaminated clothes, fomites
- Control of scabies:
  - Treat all members of the household–Blanket treatment for scabies
  - Benzyl benzoate (25%) is effective sarcopticidal agent. Apply to whole body below the chin including soles of feet and allow to dry. Application to be repeated after 12 hours and after further 12 hours, bath is given with all clothes to be changed and washed in hot water.
  - HCH – 0.5 – 1% of gamma HCH (lindane) mixed in coconut oil, applied at interval of 2-3 days
  - Other effective sarcopticides are

◆ Permethrin ointment	single application
◆ Crotamiton ointment	twice application
◆ Tetmosol (5%) solution	thrice application
◆ Sulfur (10%) ointment	four times application

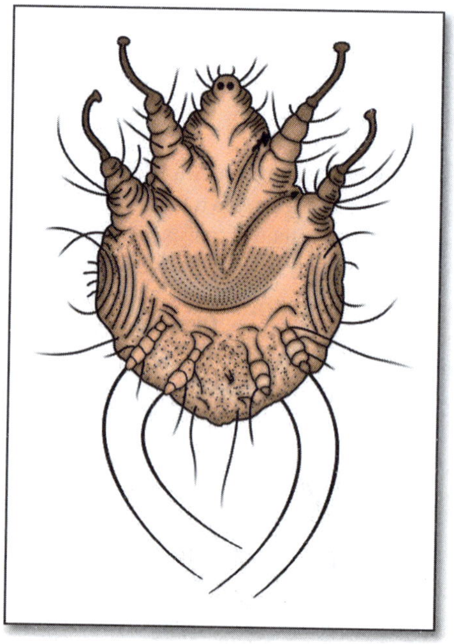

Fig. 20: Itch mite

Cyclops

Also known as Water flea (but is not a flea!). They inhabit tanks, ponds and step-wells.

- Cyclops is a small, pear shaped, semi-transparent creature, of about 1 mm size and just visible to the naked eye
- There is a small, pigmented, single eye with a pair of antennae on sides
- Life cycle:
  - Eggs are dispersed in water, which hatch after 2-3 days.
  - The first stage of larva is called as 'Nauplius' which further develops into a 'metanauplius' which further develops into an adult cyclops.
  - Life cycle is complete in about 15 days, showing incomplete meta-morphosis. Adults have a maximum life span of 3 months.

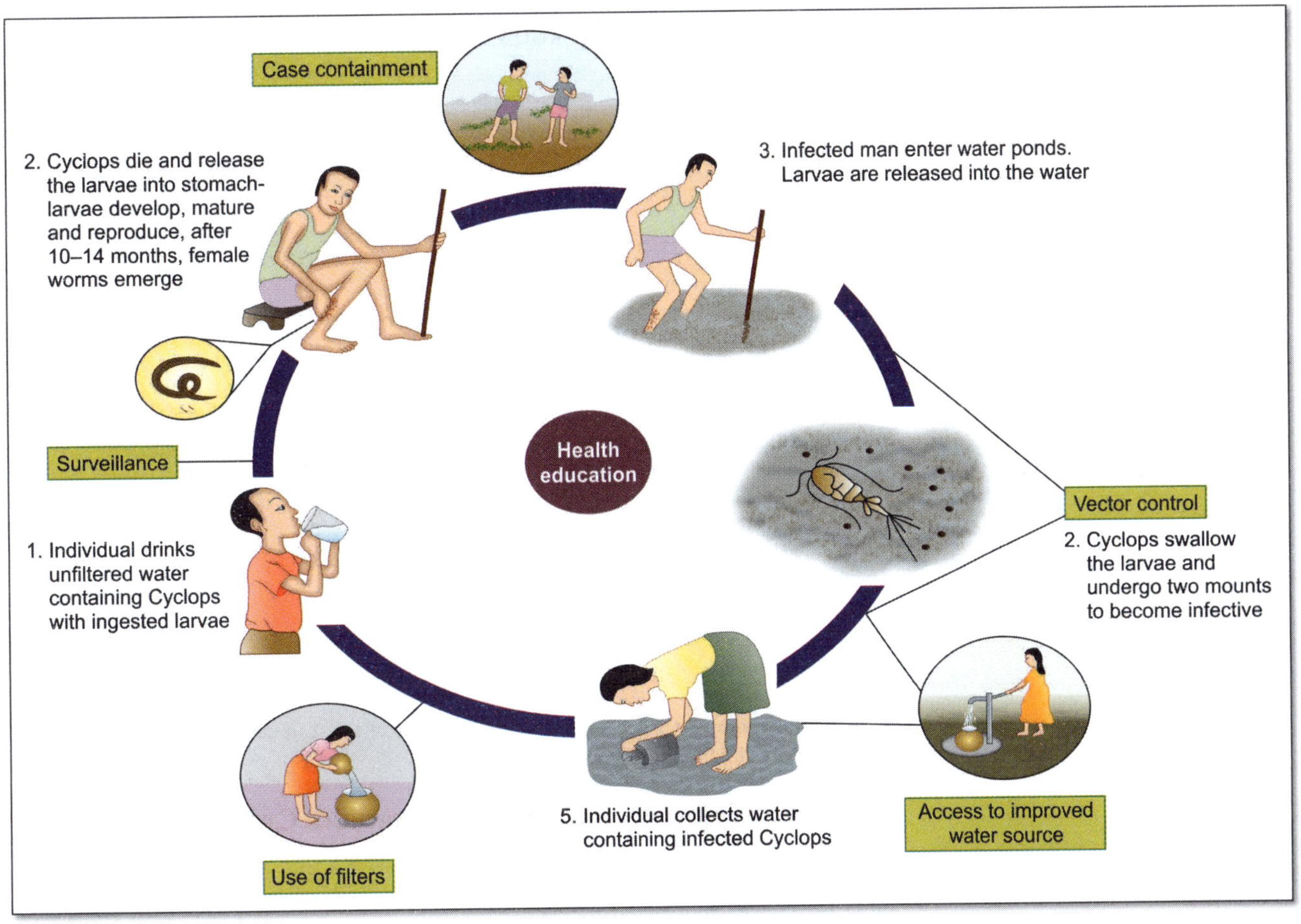

Case containment
2. Cyclops die and release the larvae into stomach- larvae develop, mature and reproduce, after 10–14 months, female worms emerge
3. Infected man enter water ponds. Larvae are released into the water
Surveillance
Health education
Vector control
2. Cyclops swallow the larvae and undergo two mounts to become infective
1. Individual drinks unfiltered water containing Cyclops with ingested larvae
5. Individual collects water containing infected Cyclops
Access to improved water source
Use of filters

Fig. 21: Life cycle of cyclops

- Public health importance:
  - Dracunculiasis or guinea worm disease
  - Fish tape worm – Diphyllobothrium latum infestation (rare in India)
- Control measures for cyclops:
  - Physical measures
    - Boiling
    - Straining
  - Chemical measures
    - Chlorination @ 5 ppm
    - Lime water @ 1 g/L of water
    - Abate @ 1ppm to water
  - Biological measures. Use of cyclopsivorous (feed on cyclops) fish such as
    - Ambassis ranga (glass fish)
    - Etroplus maculatus (orange chromide)
    - Trichogaster fasciata
    - Barbel and gambusia fish

Rodents

Domestic rodents

- Rattus rattus
- Rattus norvegicus
- Mus musculus

Wild rodents

- Tatera indica
- Bandicota bengalensis
- Bandicota indica

Diseases Associated with Rodents

Bacterial → Plague, Tularaemia, Salmonellosis
Viral → Lassa fever, Hemorrhagic fever, Encephalitis
Rickettsial → Scrub typhus, Murine typhus, Rickettsial pox
Parasitic → Hymenolepis diminuta, Leishmaniasis, Amoebiasis, Trichinosis, Chagas disease
Others → Rat bite fever, Leptospirosis, Histoplasmosis, Ring worm etc.

Mode of Transmission

- Rat bite (e.g., Rat bite fever) or
- Contamination of food or water (e.g. Salmonellosis, Leptospirosis) or
- Via Rat fleas (e.g., Plague and Typhus)

Antirodent Measures

- **Sanitation:** Proper storage of food, Proper collection and disposal of garbage, Construction of rat-proof buildings, Elimination of rat burrows.
- **Trapping:** Number of traps recommended to be laid is at least 5% of the human population. 'Wonder trap' developed by Haffkine Institute, Mumbai can trap as many as 25 rats at a time.
- **Rodenticides:**
  - **Single dose:** Red squill; Norbormide, Zinc phosphide, Sodium fluoroacetate, Fluoroacetamide; Strychnine
  - **Multiple dose:** Warfarin, Diphacinone, Coumaryl
- **Fumigation:** Cyanogas (extensively used in India), Carbon disulfide, Methyl bromide, Sulfur dioxide, etc.
- **Chemosterilants:** (Experimental stage) A chemical that can cause temporary/permanent sterility in either or both sex.

Insecticides and Rodenticides – Chemical Control

Insecticides

Table 13: Classification of insecticides

Classification		Insecticides
Stomach poison		Paris green, Sodium fluoride
Fumigants		Hydrogen cyanide, Methyl bromide, Sulfur dioxide, Carbon disulfate
Contact poison (Natural)		Pyrethrum, Rotenone, Derris, Nicotine and Mineral oil
Contact poison (Synthetic)	Organochlorine	DDT, HCH(BHC), Lindane, Chlordane, Heptachlor, Methoxychlor, Dieldrin, Aldrin, Toxaphene, Kepone and Mirex
	Organophosphorus	Chlorthion, Malathion, Diazinon, Parathion, Methyl Parathion, Fenthion, Fenitrothion, Dioxathion, Dichlorvos, Chlorpyrifos, Ronnel, Gardona
	Carbamates	Carbaryl, Propoxur, Dimetilan, Pyrolan
Repellents		Benzyl benzoate, Indalone, Meta diethyltoluamide, Dimethyl phthalate
Synthetic pyrethroids		Resmethrin, Bioresmethrin, Polythnin, Tetramethrin, Resethrin, Proparthin[Q] and Prothrin

The details of the individual insecticides have been discussed in the topic of Mosquito control measures in this chapter.

Rodenticides

Those requiring ordinary care

- Red squill
- Norbormide
- Zinc phosphide

Requires maximum precautions
- Strychnine
- Sodium fluoroacetamide

Hazardous for general use
- Arsenic trioxide
- Phosphorus
- Gophacide
- ANTU

Commonly used rodenticides in India are:

Barium carbonate
- White tasteless powder
- Mixed with wheat/rice flour as baits for rats

Zinc phosphide
- Mixed in wheat / rice flour as rodenticide baits
- Recommended for use in India

Insecticide Resistance

It is the ability of the strain of insects to tolerance doses of toxicants which would prove lethal to the majority of individuals in the normal population of the same species.
- Resistance to DDT and its analogues as methoxychlor
- Resistance to HCH – dieldrin group and its analogues

Insecticide Formulations

- Solution
  - Solid insecticide (solute) is mixed with liquid (solvent) to make a solution
  - Best for walls, roofs, outdoor sprays (on adsorbent surfaces)
- Suspension:
  - Suspending agent is added to the immiscible mixture, which keeps the insecticide particles uniformly dispersed in the liquid medium
  - Best for adsorbent surface as walls where residual effect is required
- Emulsion:
  - Suitable emulsifying agent is added to the water so that the oily insecticide is dispersed uniformly through the medium of water in the form of minute oily droplets
  - Best for non-adsorbent surfaces as cement walls with paint/distemper, wooden surfaces
- Dust:
  - A fine powder of solid insecticide and an inert diluent like chalk powder, limestone powder, Kieselguhr, bentonite, clay.
  - For treatment of rubbish dumps and manure pits
- Granules
  - These are insecticide carriers. Insecticidal granules are prepared by impregnating the coarse particles, such as sand, pyrophyllite or vermiculite with an insecticide
  - Used for outdoor use and have a sustained and prolonged effect of the insecticide, along with side effect of longer duration of action may lead to adverse toxic effects as well

Insecticide Equipments

- Sprays
  - *Stirr-up pump sprayer*: It is a manual spray method. The insecticide is delivered under hydraulic pressure with the help of a plunger pump
  - *Knapsack sprayer*: Sprayer is fitted on the back of the worker with the help of two straps. Insecticide comes out under pressure of compressed air
  - *Power operated sprayer*: used for insecticide spray of large area. Uses motorized engine sprayer mounted on a small vehicle
- Duster: Different types of dusters are the plunger type, the bellow type, the rotary crank type and the power duster are available. This equipment contains an agitator and insecticide powder for dusting

Toxicity of Insecticides

- Organochlorous compounds: DDT and related chemical are nerve poisons –

- Nervous excitability, tremors, convulsions
- DDT < HCH < Dieldrin (5-8 times toxic than DDT) with respect to toxicity
- Treatment: phenobarbitone, stomach wash outs, purgatives

- Organophosphorus and carbamates – these chemicals act by nerve impulse inhibition by inhibiting the cholinesterase enzyme and leads to accumulation of ACh.
  - Effects of toxicity are: Headache, giddiness, cold sweating, salivation, uncontrolled urination and defecation, loss of consciousness, respiratory paralysis, coma, death
  - Treatment:
    - Atropine is antidote. It is given at rate of 1-2 mg IM, repeat at 30 minutes interval.
    - 2 PAM iodine, 2 PAM chloride and P2S
- Pyrethrins and Pyrethroids
  - Contact: Due to their irritant property, they cause conjunctival congestion, irritation of nose, throat
  - Ingestion may cause nausea, vomiting and other intestinal disturbances.

WASTE

Waste disposal is largely the domain of sanitarians, public health engineers and department of public water works and sewage disposal in various municipal limits across country.

Sanitation Barrier

Transmission of all endemic diseases in our country can be prevented and controlled by simple understanding of the "Prevention" of contamination of physical environment by constructing a sanitation barrier. This barrier will safeguard from the Six F's as shown in image below

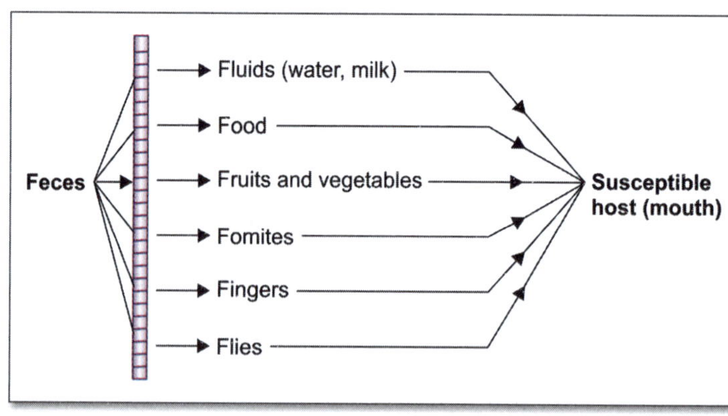

This Topic will be dealt under three broad heading as:

- Refuse – types and disposal methods
- Human Excreta disposal
- Sewage treatment system

Refuse

Refuse could be collected from various sources as streets, household, industries and so on. The methods for refuse disposal are:

- Dumping – most hazardous and most insanitary method
  - Sanitary landfills – also known as controlled tipping. (most satisfactory where suitable land is available.[Q])
  - **Trench method:**
    - Dumping in a trench 2-3 meters deep and 5-10 meters wide.
    - Trench would require an area of 1 acre per year for a population of 100,000
  - Ramp method – in sloping terrain
  - Area method – the depressions in earth as ponds or clay pits are used for filling with refuse. After about one week of burial of refuse, temperature rises to about 60°C, killing all the pathogens followed by decomposition process. After another 2 to 3 weeks, it cools down. Within 4 to 6 months, all the organic matter are decomposed into innocuous mass – this is known as 'made-up' soil and maybe used as manure in the land

- Composting: Method of combined disposal of refuse and night soil or sludge.
  - Bangalore method – anaerobic method. Also known as *hot fermentation process*. It is layering of night soils with refuse in a 3 ft deep trench and covering with excavated earth.
  - Mechanical composting – aerobic method. It is a mechanized process in many developed parts of the world as well as in India. The refuse is pulverized and mixed with night soil. Later the matter is mechanically incubated. It is faster and improvised version of the Bangalore method.
- Other methods as burial, incineration or manure pits may also be used.

Excreta Disposal

A sanitary latrine is the one which fulfils the following criteria:
- The night soil should not contaminate the ground or surface water.
- It should not pollute the soil.
- It should not be accessible to house flies, rodents and animals like pigs, dogs, cattle, etc.
- It should not create nuisance by sight and smell.
- It should be cheap, easy to construct and acceptable to the people.
  Most important prerequisite in sanitary latrine is ***water seal***.

Types are:
- Bore Hole Latrine
  - Dimensions: 30-40 cm diameter, depth of around 6 meters
  - Serves a family of around 6 people for a year
  - Should be located 15 meters away from the water source
- Pit latrine (or dug well)
  - Dimensions: 75 cm diameter, depth of around 4 meters
  - Serves a family of around 5 people for 5 years
- Water seal latrines
  - These have a pipe-bend (trap) below the squatting plate, which holds the water. This is known as water seal. It prevents any fly nuisance, or foul odor.
  - Types:
    - Direct type: Pit is directly underneath the squatting plate
    - Indirect type: Pit is away from squatting plate.
  - Types:
    - RCA type – Research cum Action project in environmental sanitation, mostly used
    - PRAI – Planning Research and Action Institute, direct type, cheaper than RCA type.
    - ICMR type – Indian Council of Medical Research, direct type.
    - VIP latrines – (Ventilated improved - VIP) indirect type, contains a vent with fly screen.
- Septic Tank latrine
  - Consist of a tank (~ 200 Liters capacity) into which the sewage and sullage of house is drained.
  - The tank should be cleaned every 5 years, for a family of 5-6 members.
- Aqua privy
  - The sewage is directed into a tank filled with water with drop pipe from the latrine seat
  - The night soil undergoes purification by anaerobic digestion
  - A capacity of 1 cu. meter of aqua privy is recommended for a family of 5 to 6 members for about 5 to 6 years.
- Chemical closet
  - Metal tank consisting of disinfectant is placed below the pan of the latrine
  - Disinfectant used - caustic soda and phenol and covered with a layer of crude oil.
  - Used in isolated houses, boats, aircrafts, motor caravans etc
- Temporary latrine
  - Shallow trench latrine
    - 30 cm wide x 1.5 meters deep x 3 meters long – applicable for 100 individuals
  - Deep trench latrine
    - 90 cm wide x 2.5 meters deep
- Bio-gas plant – uses human, animal excreta

Sewage Treatment

Sewage:

- The average amount of sewage which flows through the sewage system in 24 hrs is called as "Dry weather flow"
- 1 gm of sewage contains –
  - 1000 million E. coli
  - 0-100 million fecal streptococci
  - 1-10 million spores of Cl. Perfringens
- Average adult – excretes 100 grams of feces

Table 14: Strength of sewage

Strength of Sewage	Weak	Strong
BOD (Biological Oxygen Demand)	100 mg/L	300 mg/L and above
Suspended solids	100 mg/L	500 mg/L

Methods of Sewage Disposal

Modern sewage treatment plant: Treatment of sewage is done in two stages.

- **Stage 1: Primary treatment**: Solids are separated by screening, sedimentation and anaerobic digestion.[Q]
  - Sewage after screening flows through the Grit or Detritus chamber (10–20 m long) at a constant velocity of 1 feet/sec, with detention of 30–60 seconds. Heavy solids (i.e. sand and gravel) settle down
  - Sewage then enters the primary sedimentation tank and flows very slowly (1–2 feet/min) and spends 6-8 hours in the tank. 50–70% of solids settle down, Coliform are reduced by 30–40% and microorganisms in sewage break down complex organic solids into simpler soluble substances and ammonia.
  - Sewage with organic trade wastes, is treated with chemicals (lime, aluminium Sulfate and ferrous Sulfate) that precipitate the animal protein
  - Organic matter which settles down is called ***sludge*** and is removed by mechanical devices.
- **Stage 2: Secondary treatment**- Effluent is subjected to aerobic oxidation. [Q] *(Trickling Filter or Activated Sludge process)*
  - *Biofiltration process: Trickling filter* – the sewage passes through a filter composed of zoogleal layer over a stone/ gravel bed. It is cheap and efficient process of oxidation of sewage
  - *Bio-aeration process – Activated sludge process*
    - Is a modern method of sewage treatment.
    - It involves mixing of the sewage with activated sludge and further into an aeration chamber
- **Stage 3**: The effluent collected from the secondary treatment is directed to another secondary sedimentation tank, where it is stored for 3-4 hours and desludging is done periodically.

Other Methods of Sewage Disposal

- Sea outfall
- River outfall
- Land treatment (sewage farming – for fodder grass, potato cultivation)
- Oxidation pond/Waste stabilization pond (Redox pond, Sewage lagoons)
- Oxidation ditches / aerated lagoons.

NATIONAL WATER SUPPLY AND SANITATION PROGRAMME

- Initiated in 1954 with the object of providing safe water supply and adequate drainage facilities for the entire urban and rural population of the country.
- In 1972 a special programme known as the ***Accelerated Rural Water Supply Programme*** was started as a supplement to the national water supply and sanitation programme.

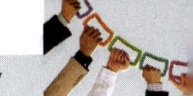

- During the Fifth Plan, rural water supply was included in the Minimum Needs Programme of the State Plans.
- International Drinking Water Supply and Sanitation Decade Programme started in 1981.
- The stipulated norm of water supply is 40 L of safe drinking water per capita per day, and at least one hand pump/spot-source for every 250 persons.
- Information, education and communication is an integral part of rural sanitation programme to adopt proper environmental sanitation practices including disposal of garbage, refuse and waste water, and to convert all existing dry latrines into low cost sanitary latrines.

Must Remember

A "*problem village*" is the one where no source of safe water is available within a distance of 1.6 km, or where water is available at a depth of more than 15 meters, or where water source has excess salinity, iron, fluorides and other toxic elements, or where water is exposed to the risk of cholera.

SWACHH BHARAT MISSION

To accelerate the efforts to achieve universal sanitation coverage and to put focus on safe sanitation, the Prime Minister of India launched the Swachh Bharat Mission on 2nd October, 2014.

The mission aims to achieve a Swachh Bharat by 2nd October, 2019, as a fitting tribute to Mahatma Gandhi on his 150th birth anniversary. Swachh Bharat, in rural areas shall mean improving the levels of cleanliness through Solid and Liquid Waste Management activities and making Gram Panchayats Open Defecation Free (ODF), clean and sanitized. ODF would mean the termination of fecal-oral transmission, defined by, no visible feces found in the environment/ village and every household as well as public/community institution(s) using safe technology option for disposal of feces, as defined by the Ministry.

THE MINISTRY OF DRINKING WATER AND SANITATION (MDWS)

- The Ministry of Drinking Water and Sanitation, Government of India, is headed by the Cabinet Minister, Drinking Water and Sanitation.
- It is the Nodal Ministry for the overall policy, planning, funding and coordination of two flagship programs of the Government of India, namely, the National Rural Drinking Water Program (NRDWP) for rural drinking water supply and the Swachh Bharat Mission (Gramin) [SBM (G)] for sanitation in the country.

Image-Based Questions

1. The arthropod shown in figure is responsible for transmission of:

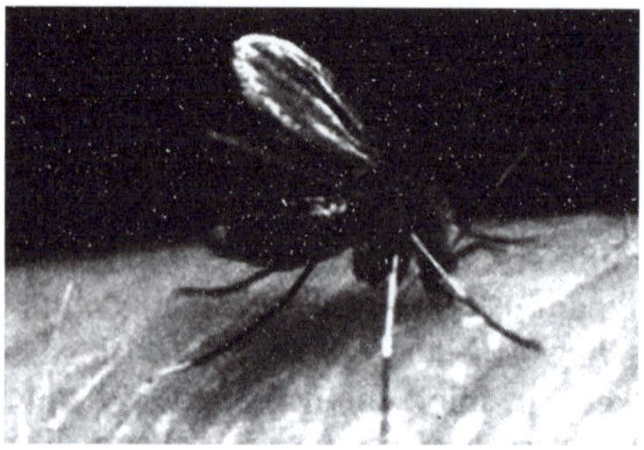

a. Filaria
b. Leishmaniasis
c. Yellow fever
d. Malaria

2. The transmission depicted in figure is of:

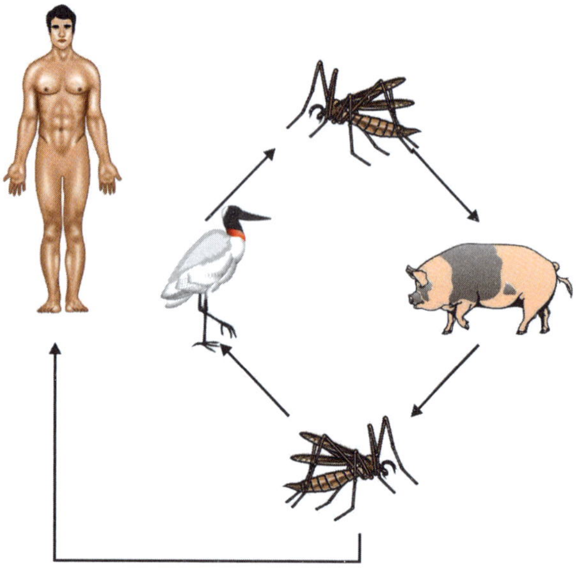

a. Dengue
b. Japanese encephalitis
c. Kyasanur forest disease
d. Ebola

3. The life cycle shown in figure is of:

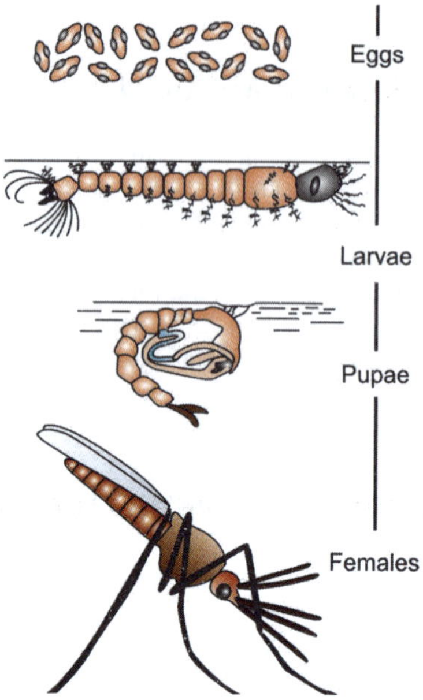

a. Culex
b. Aedes
c. Mansonoides
d. Anopheles

4. Disease transmitted by the vector shown in figure is:

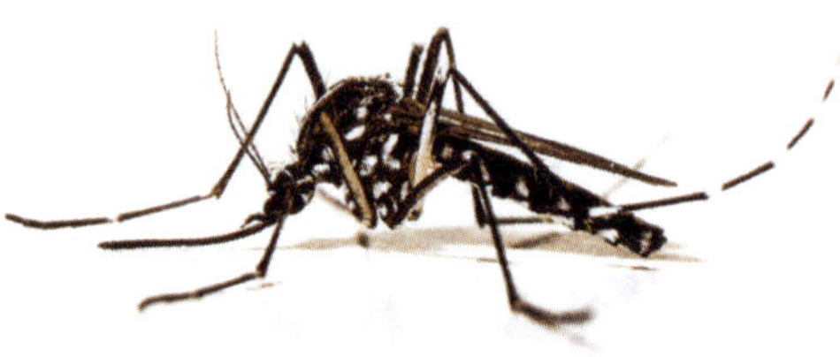

a. Japanese encephalitis
b. Malaria
c. Visceral leishmaniasis
d. Dengue

5. Larva shown in figure belongs to which species:

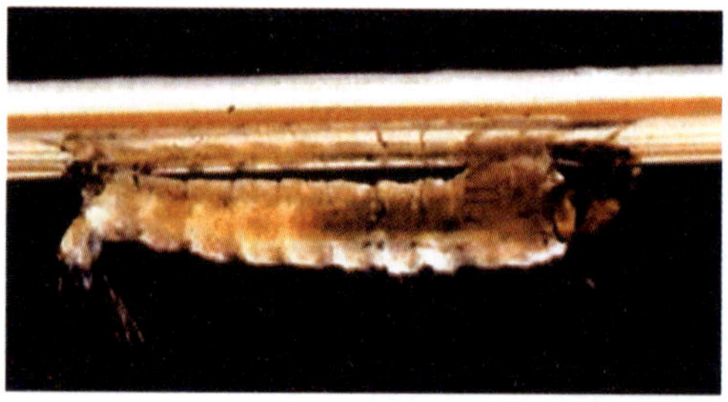

a. Anopheles
b. Culex
c. Aedes
d. Mansonia

6. The instrument in the figure is used to measure:

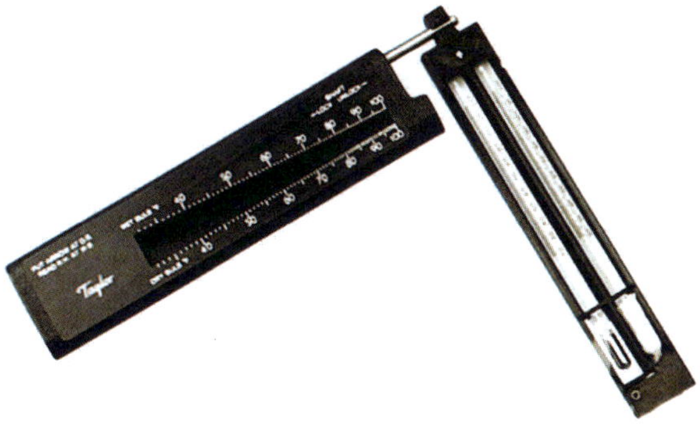

a. Air velocity
b. Mean radiant temperature
c. Humidity
d. Cooling power of air

7. Identify the instrument shown in figure:

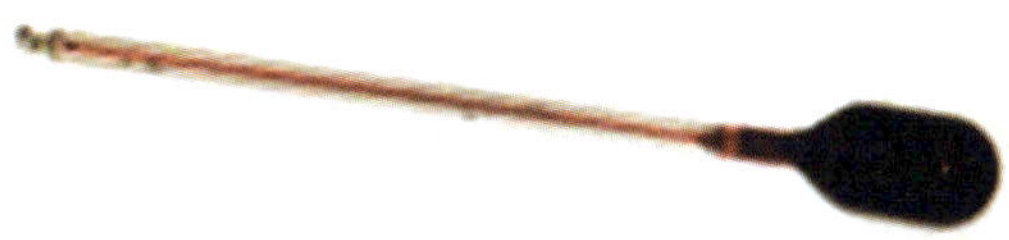

a. Globe thermometer
b. Kata thermometer
c. Wet bulb thermometer
d. Dry bulb thermometer

8. Identify the instrument in figure:

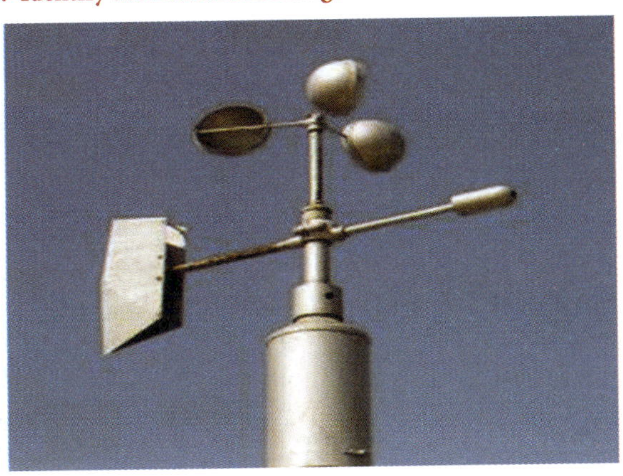

a. Anemometer
b. Assmann Psychrometer
c. Lightening conductor
d. Rain gauge

9. Identify the vector in figure:

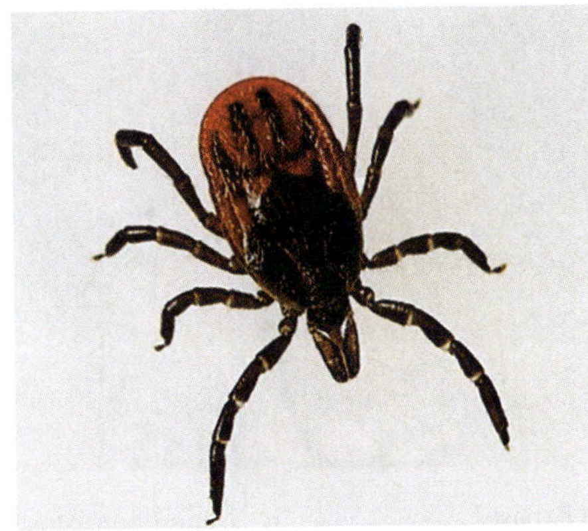

a. Hard tick
b. Soft tick
c. Louse
d. Mite

10. Identify the vector in figure:

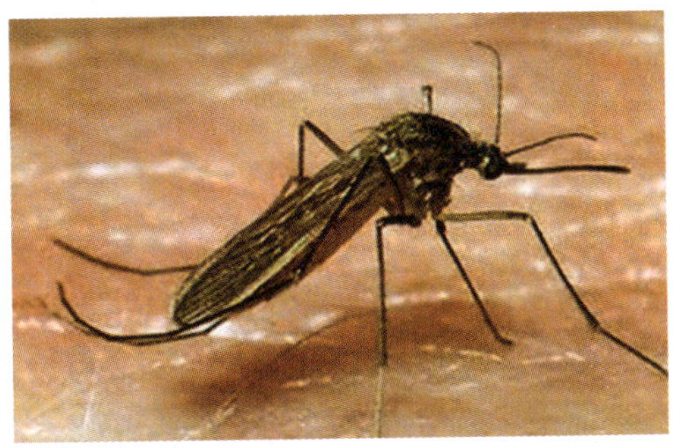

a. Culex mosquito
b. Mansonia mosquito
c. Anopheles mosquito
d. Aedes mosquito

11. Identify the use of instrument in figure:

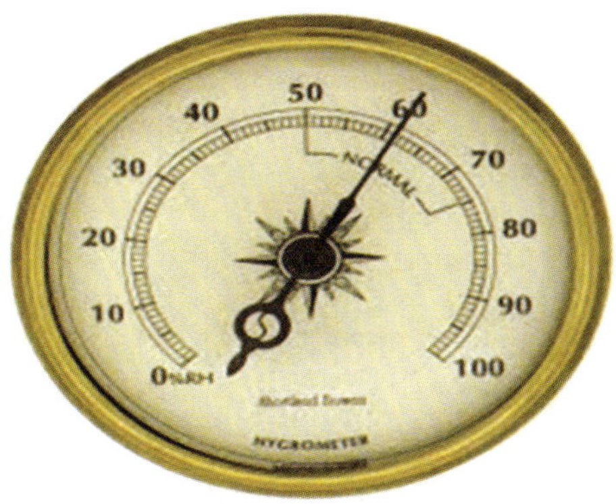

a. Relative air humidity
b. Average rainfall
c. Pressure in autoclave
d. Hydroclave temperature

12. Identify the condition in figure:

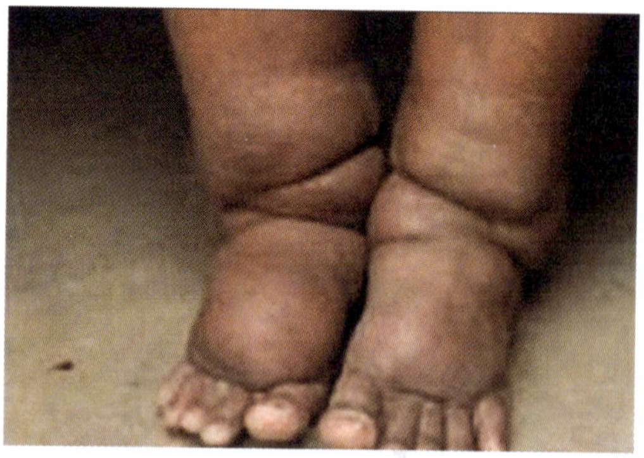

a. Filariasis
b. Neurofibromatosis
c. Leprosy
d. Yaws

13. Identify the vector in figure:

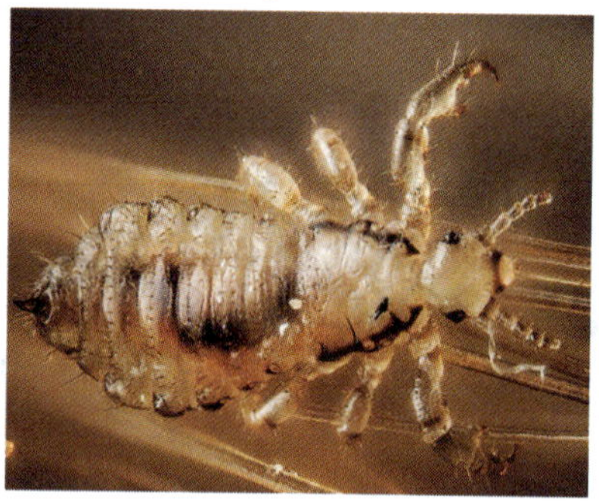

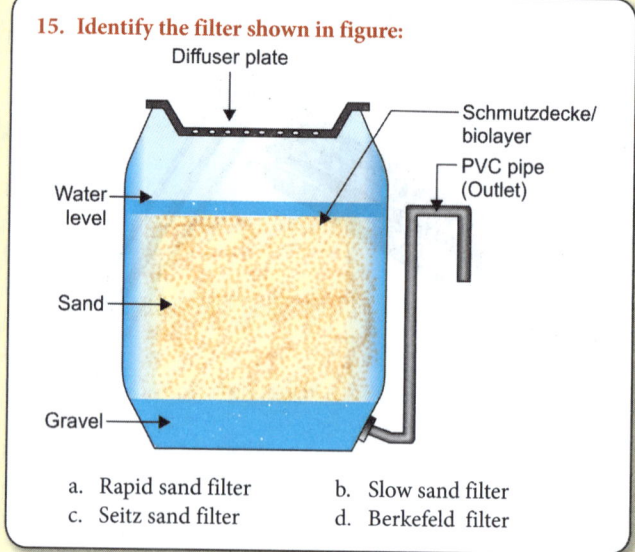

a. Louse
b. Soft ticks
c. Cule mosquito
d. Sandfly

14. Identify the national programme depicted by the symbol in figure:

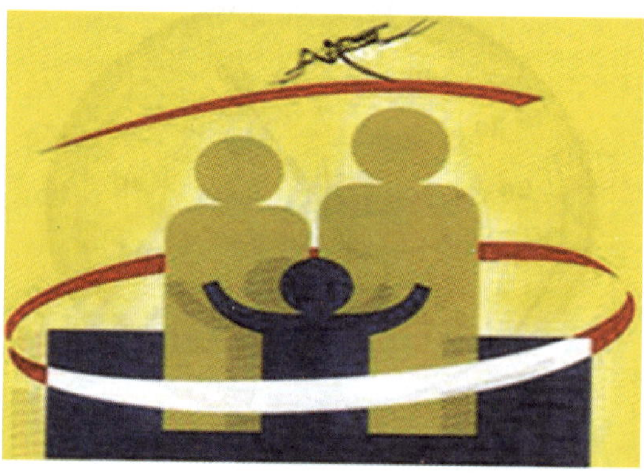

a. NLEP
b. NVBDCP
c. NMEP
d. IDSP

15. Identify the filter shown in figure:

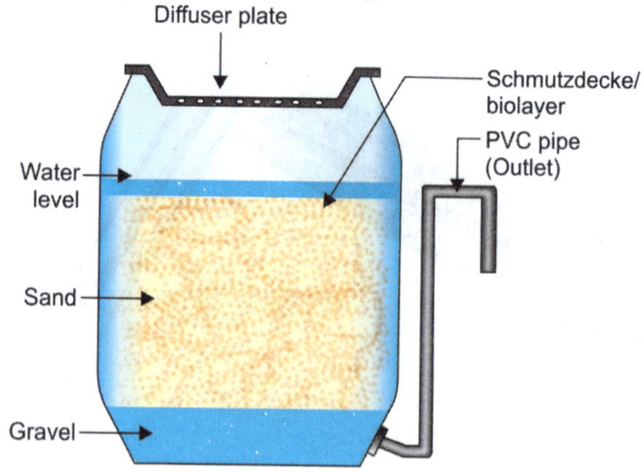

a. Rapid sand filter
b. Slow sand filter
c. Seitz sand filter
d. Berkefeld filter

16. Instrument shown in figure is used for measuring:

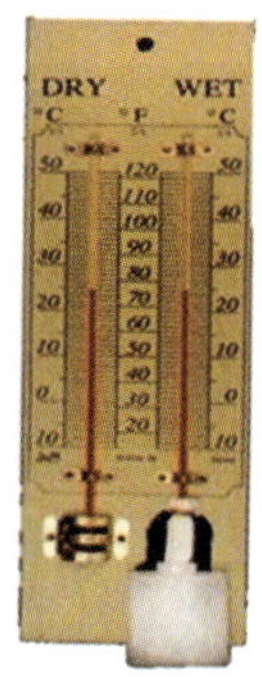

a. Humidity
b. Temperature
c. Pressure
d. Wind velocity

17. Identify the lesion shown in figure:

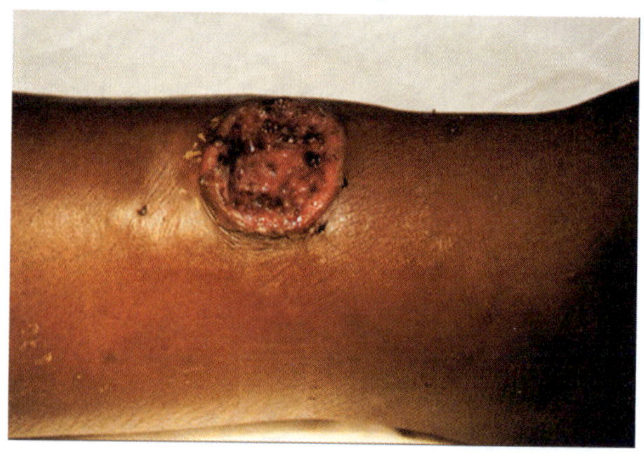

a. Primary yaws
b. Chancroid
c. Syphilis
d. Neurofibromatosis

Answers of Image-Based Questions

1. **Ans. (b)** Leishmaniasis
2. **Ans. (b)** Japanese encephalitis
3. **Ans. (d)** Anopheles
4. **Ans. (d)** Dengue
5. **Ans. (a)** Anopheles
6. **Ans. (c)** Humidity
7. **Ans. (b)** Kata thermometer
8. **Ans. (a)** Anemometer
9. **Ans. (a)** Hard Tick
10. **Ans. (a)** Culex mosquito
11. **Ans. (a)** Relative air humidity
12. **Ans. (a)** Filariasis
13. **Ans. (a)** Louse
14. **Ans. (b)** NVBDCP
15. **Ans. (b)** Slow sand filter
16. **Ans. (a)** Humidity
17. **Ans. (a)** Primary yaws

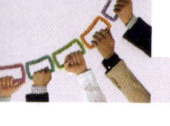

Multiple Choice Questions

1. **Hardness of water occurs due to the presence of all of the following except:** *(Recent Question 2018)*
   a. $CaCO_3$ b. $BaCO_3$
   c. $MgCO_3$ d. $MgCl_2$
2. **Disinfecting action of chlorine in chlorination of water is mainly due to:** *(AIIMS May 2017)*
   a. Hypochlorite ion b. Chloride ion
   c. Sodium chloride d. Hypochlorous acid
3. **Greenhouse gas includes:**
   a. CO_2, ozone, methane b. Only ozone
   c. Ozone, methane only d. Methane, CO
4. **Depth of water in a RCA latrine:** *(Recent Question 2017)*
   a. 9 cm b. 5 cm
   c. 3 cm d. 2 cm
5. **Kyasanur forest disease is transmitted by:**
   a. Soft tick b. Hard tick
   c. Louse d. Sandfly
   e. Flea
6. **Malaria parasite was discovered by?** *(Recent Question 2013)*
   a. Robert Koch b. Louis Pasteur
   c. Laveran d. Ronald Ross
7. **Who discovered transmission of malaria by anopheline mosquitoes?** *(Recent Question 2013)*
   a. Ronald Ross b. Laveran
   c. Müller d. Pamana
8. **Which of the following scientist pointed towards the association between environment and health?**
   a. James Lind b. Hippocrates
   c. David Marley d. John Snow
9. **Microenvironment indicates** *(Recent Question 2015)*
   a. Place where microbial organisms multiply
   b. Place which is inaccessible for humans
   c. Individuals housing, occupation and social environment
   d. Individuals way of living, Life-style, personal habits

MISCELLANEOUS

10. **All of the following are true about Swajaldhara programme except** *(Recent Question 2015)*
   a. Community led participatory program
   b. All water supply is maintained and managed by State Government
   c. Provision of drinking water in rural areas
   d. Encouragement of water harvesting practices
11. **All the following are features of problem village except**
   a. No source of safe water within a distance of 1.6 km
   b. Water is available at a depth of >15 m
   c. Water source has excess salinity, iron, fluorides and other toxic elements
   d. Water is exposed to the risk of dracunculiasis
12. **Per capita water requirement for all domestic purposes is**
   a. 25 L
   b. 50 L
   c. 100 L
   d. 150 L
13. **WHO recommends the following system of water distribution**
   a. Intermittent and low pressure
   b. Intermittent and high pressure
   c. Continuous and low pressure
   d. Continuous and high pressure

PURIFICATION OF WATER – FILTRATION

14. **Regarding purification of water all are true except:**
   a. Multiple tube method is used for sampling
   b. E. coil can be tested by Indole test
   c. Clostridial infection indicates recent infection
   d. Level of residual chlorine should be 0.5 mg/L
   e. Softening of water is recommended after 3 mEq/L of hardness
15. **Which one of the following methods is used for the estimation of the chlorine demand of water?**
   a. Chlorometer b. Horrock's apparatus
   c. Berkefeld filter d. Double pot method
16. **All are true about bleaching powder except**
   a. Has 33% available chlorine
   b. Is a stable compound
   c. Has a rapid and brief action
   d. Is used for disinfection of wells
17. **Orthotolidine test is used to determine:**
   a. Nitrates in water
   b. Nitrates chlorine in water
   c. Free and combined chlorine in water
   d. Ammonia content in water
18. **All of the following are true about break point chlorination, EXCEPT**
   a. Free chlorine is retained in water after break point chlorination
   b. Chlorine demand is the amount needed to kill bacteria, oxidize organic matter and neutralize ammonia
   c. 1 ppm free chlorine should be present in water after break point has reached
   d. Contact period of 1 hour is necessary
19. **According to WHO, what is minimum bacteriological standard for drinking water:**
   a. All samples should be free from coliform
   b 3 consecutive samples of water should not contain any coliform
   c. 3 Coliform in 100ml water is acceptable.
   d. 1 Coliform in 100 water is acceptable
20. **During water analysis in a hostel, amoebic cysts were seen. The best method to purify this water would be**
   a. Iodine b. Boiling
   c. U.V. Rays d. Chlorination
21. **All of the following are water borne diseases EXCEPT:**
   a. Leptospirosis
   b. Schistosomiases
   c. Fish tape worm disease
   d. Brucellosis

Ans.

1. b
2. d
3. a
4. d
5. a, b
6. c
7. a
8. b
9. d
10. b
11. d
12. d
13. d
14. a, c
15. b
16. b
17. c
18. c
19. a
20. b
21. d

Most Recent Questions of 2019-18 are given at the end of MCQs

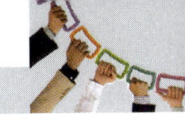

22. All are indicators of faecal pollution of water except:
a. E. coli
b. Streptococcal faecalis
c. Clostridium welchii
d. Clostridium botulinum

23. The importance of fluoridation of water is that it:
a. Cause disinfection of water
b. Prevent dental fluorosis
c. Prevent dental caries
d. Help in absorption of calcium and phosphate in body

24. In a remote area of the country a gastroenteritis epidemic broke out. A community shallow well was suspected to be the cause. The doctor in charge of PHC had no other facility to check the quality of water except physical examination of water. Which one of the following is a physical parameter that would indicate water pollution
a. Chemical oxygen demand
b. NO_2
c. Biological oxygen demand
d. Turbidity

25. Which of the following is Not surface water
a. River b. Ponds
c. Lake d. Spring

26. Bleaching powder is produced by the action of chlorine on
a. Lime b. Sodium
c. Potassium d. Calcium

27. Presence of spore of clostridium perfringens in the absence of coliform group in water is suggestive of:
a. Fecal contamination of recent origin
b. Fecal contamination of remote origin
c. No fecal contamination of water
d. Non fecal contamination of water

28. For controlling an outbreak of cholera all of the following are recommended Except:
a. Chlorination of drinking water
b. Early diagnosis and treatment of case
c. Proper disposal of excreta
d. Mass chemoprophylaxis

29. The best step to interrupt transmission of amoebiasis in community is:
a. Filtration of drinking water
b. Chlorination of drinking water
c. Mass chemoprophylaxis
d. Storage of drinks water

30. In water fit for drinking the number of coliform /100 ml of water should be
a. 0 b. 5-10
c. 10-15 d. 15-20

31. The most common precipitant used for purification of water is
a. Aluminum sulfate b. Lead nitrate
c. Copper sulfate d. Silver oxide

32. The most hazard free and cost effective Chemical disinfectant for drinking water is:
a. Ozonation
b. Chlorination
c. UV radiation
d. Silver treatment

33. Temporary hardness of water is due to the presence of:
a. Ca and Mg bicarbonate
b. Ca^{++} and Mg^{++} free ions
c. Ca and Mg sulfate
d. Ca and Mg chloride

34. Salt concentration in sea water is
a. 1.5% b. 2%
c. 3.5% d. 5%

35. Which one of the following is not a water borne disease?
a. Poliomyelitis b. Giardiasis
c. Roundworm d. Kala-Azar

36. The sum of HOCL and HCL in water is called:
a. Free residual chlorine
b. Chlorine demand of water
c. Chloramines
d. Chemical Chlorine-demand

37. For disinfecting large bodies of water, chlorine is applied in the form of
a. Bleaching powder b. Perchloran
c. Chloramines d. Chlorine gas

38. Permutit water softener is suitable for removal of:
a. Hardness of water
b. Microorganisms from water
c. Dissolved organic solvents
d. Dissolved inorganic solvents

39. Bacteriological indicators of water contamination are all except
a. E. coli b. Streptococcus faecalis
c. Cl. Perfringens d. Salmonella typhi

40. The available chorine content in bleaching powder is:
a. 5-10% b. 35-70%
c. 20% d. 33%

41. Zero hardness of water can be achieved by:
a. Base exchange process
b. Sodium carbonate addition
c. Lime addition
d. Boiling

42. The concentration of free residual chlorine in water required for effective disinfection is:
a. 0.4 ppm b. 0.1 ppm
c. 0.5 ppm d. 0.6 ppm

43. The ratio of chlorine and ammonia in chloramines is:
a. 4:1 b. 10:1
c. 2:1 d. 3:5

44. Bleaching powder used for disinfection of drinking water:
a. Chlorine gas
b. Calcium hypochlorite ($CaOCl_2$)
c. Sodium hypochlorite
d. Chloramines
e. Carbon dioxide

45. Purest form of water available in nature in form of:
a. Springs b. Ponds
c. Rain d. Lakes

46. Drinking water should be:
a. Soft water
b. Hard water
c. Moderately hard water
d. Very hard water

Ans.
22. d
23. c
24. d
25. d
26. a
27. b
28. d
29. a
30. a
31. a
32. b
33. a
34. c
35. d
36. a
37. d
38. a
39. d
40. d
41. a
42. c
43. a
44. b
45. c
46. c

Most Recent Questions of 2019-18 are given at the end of MCQs

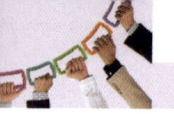

47. The presence of nitrates in water indicates:
a. Temporary hardness of water
b. Permanent hardness of water
c. Recent faecal pollution
d. Past faecal pollution

48. Water whose quality is such that it can be used for drinking purposes is known as:
a. Clean water
b. Potable water
c. Fresh water
d. Distilled water

49. Presence of excess of nitrates in water can give rise to:
a. Blue baby syndrome b. Dental caries
c. Minimal disease d. Goiter

50. The method implied for cleaning a rapid sand filter is called:
a. Ripening b. Back washing
c. Scraping d. Under drainage

51. The distance between a well and a potential source of contamination should be less than:
a. 5 meters b. 10 meters
c. 15 meters d. 20 meters

52. Copper sulfate is added to swimming pool water to destroy:
a. Bactria b. Viruses
c. Protozoa d. Algae and fungi

53. Water washed disease includes:
a. Infant methemoglobinemia
b. Trachoma
c. Cholera
d. Endemic goitre

54. Optimum level of fluoride in drinking water recommended on international basis is
a. Less than 0.5 ppm b. 0.5 to 0.8 ppm
c. 2 ppm d. 0.1 ppm

55. Consider the following statements regarding drinking water samples:
1. No sample should contain coliform organisms
2. No sample should contain B. coli
3. No two successive samples should contain coliform organisms
4, No two successive samples should contain E. coli

Which of the above criterion/criteria is/are included in the standards prescribed by WHO for drinking water?
a. 1 only b. 1 and 2
c. 2 and 3 d. I and 4

56. Contact time for chlorination
a. 4 hrs b. 1 hr
c. 11/2 hr d. 2 hrs

57. The minimum recommended concentration of free chlorine level in water is
a. 10 mg/dL
b. 0.5 mg/dL
c. 0.05 mg/dL
d. 0.1 mg/dL

58. Regarding chlorination of the water
a. It has residual effect
b. It is a substitute to sand filtration
c. It cannot control algae and slime organisms
d. Even if pH value exceeds 8.5, it is reliable as a disinfectant

59. Which of the following is true, regarding trickling filter:
a. It has biological zoogleal layer
b. It acts purely as a mechanical filter
c. It is used for primary treatment of sewage
d. It needs rest pauses for cleaning

60. The slow sand filter has following advantage over rapid sand filter
a. Achieves better bacteriological purity
b. Occupies less area
c. Removes turbidity
d. Rapid in action

61. Effective size of sand in rapid sand filter is
a. 0.2 mm b. 0.5 mm
c. 0.8 mm d. 0.1 mm

62. Vital layer in slow sand filter is seen
a. Top of water
b. On the sand bed
c. Near filter valves
d. In the bottom of the sand bed

63. All of the following are the correct procedures for the chlorination of a well except
a. The volume of water is estimated
b. The chlorine demand of the well water is estimated
c. Bleaching powder is dissolved in water and immediately added to the well
d. A contact period of one hour is allowed

64. Action of Bleaching powder is due to release of
a. Free Chlorine b. Lime
c. Hydrochloric acid d. Hydrogen ions

65. For recent fecal pollution of water, confirmatory evidence is provided by the presence of
a. Streptococci b. Klebsiella
c. Clostridium perfringens d. E. coil

66. Hardness of water is expressed as milliequivalent per liter (mEq/L), one unit of which is equivalent to which of the following?
a. 20 mg $CaCO_3$ (20 ppm)
b. 30 mg $CaCO_3$ (30 ppm)
c. 40 mg $CaCO_3$ (40 ppm)
d. 50 mg $CaCO_3$ (50 ppm)

67. Hardness of water has a beneficial effect against which one of the following?
a. Renal diseases
b. Metabolic diseases
c. Cerebrovascular diseases
d. Cardiovascular diseases

68. Water sample which is likely to contain chlorine, will affect the result of bacteriological analysis of water. Which one of the following, if added in small amount in the test tube will help overcome it?
a. Potassium nitrate b. Copper sulfate
c. Calcium hypochlorite d. Sodium thiosulfate

69. Which of the following is not true about WHO standards recommended for drinking water:
a. Hardness of water below 300 mg/litre
b. Lead below 0.01 mg/litre
c. Nitrates below 0.1 mg/litre
d. Nitrites below 3 mg/litre

Ans.

47.	d
48.	b
49.	a
50.	b
51.	c
52.	d
53.	b
54.	b
55.	b
56.	b
57.	b
58.	a
59.	a
60.	a
61.	b
62.	b
63.	c
64.	a
65.	a
66.	d
67.	d
68.	d
69.	c

70. Which of the following is not true about chlorination of water?
a. Contact period of at least 6 hours is essential
b. Recommended residual free chlorine levels is 0.5 mg/litre for one hour
c. Water should be free from turbidity
d. Chlorine demand of water should be estimated

71. Which of the following is false regarding orthotolidine test:
a. Yellow color
b. Red color in ten seconds
c. 0.1 ml of reagent is used for one ml of water
d. Free chlorine is estimated

72. Which of the following is true about chlorination?
a. Orthotolidine test measures free chlorine
b. Acts best when pH is around 7
c. Kills bacteria, viruses and spores
d. Disinfecting action is mainly due to hypochlorite ions

73. Following an earthquake, the public health department took measures to prevent outbreak of cholera. Advisable residual chlorine level in water should be
a. 0.3 b. 0.5
c. 0.7 d. 0.9

74. Residual chlorine is determined by which of the following method:
a. Horrock's test b. Berkefeld filter
c. Superchlorination d. Orthotolidine test

75. Normal fluoride level for drinking purposes is .... mg per liter:
a. 0.08-0.5 b. 0.5-0.8
c. 1-1.75 d. 1.5-3.5

76. Commensal bacteria (coliforms) provide most reliable evidence of fecal contamination of water because
a. They occur in great abundance in water and therefore easily detectable
b. They survive in water for comparatively longer period
c. They are easily identified by sample culture method
d. They are never present in portable water

PURIFICATION OF WATER–FILTRATION

77. Essential part of Chamberland type filter is the candle, which is made up of? *(Recent Question 2015)*
a. Infusorial earth b. Porcelain
c. Kieselgur d. Latex

78. Schmutzdecke in a slow sand filter is situated at
a. Above the sand bed
b. Top layers of sand bed
c. Bottom layers of sand bed
d. Below the sand bed

79. Effective diameter of sand grains in slow sand filter
a. 0.2 to 0.3 mm b. 0.4 to 0.7 mm
c. 0.8 to 1.0 mm d. 1.0 to 1.5 mm

80. Ripening of slow sand filter indicates
a. The filter is in optimum functioning capacity
b. Cessation of the function of filter
c. Formation of vital layer
d. Running such plant is not beneficial

81. Rate of filtration in rapid sand filters
a. 15 to 30 $m^3/m^2/hour$ b. 5 to 15 $m^3/m^2/hour$
c. 1 to 4 $m^3/m^2/hour$ d. 0.1 to 0.4 $m^3/m^2/hour$

82. Cleaning of slow sand filter is done by
a. Backwashing b. Bleaching powder
c. Scraping d. Front washing

83. Seitz filter is? *(Recent Question 2015)*
a. Membrane filter
b. Asbestos filter
c. Candle filter
d. Polyester filter

84. True about slow sand filter is: *(Recent Question 2014)*
a. Occupies less space
b. More expensive
c. Requires longer duration
d. Sand size 0.4 - 0.7 mm

85. The vital layer in a slow sand filter is:
a. Sand bed
b. Under drainage
c. Zoological layer
d. Supernatant

86. Feature of slow filter (with respect to fast filter) is/are: *(Recent Question 2015)*
a. Occupies less space
b. Highly skilled operation
c. Poor bacterial quality
d. Take more time for purification
e. Size of sand is smaller

PURIFICATION OF WATER – CHLORINATION RESIDUAL CHLORINE

87. The disinfecting action of chlorine is mainly due to
a. Hypochlorous acid
b. Free chlorine
c. Hypochlorite ion
d. Hydrochloric acid

88. The major action in chlorination is due to *(Recent Question 2014)*
a. Hypochlorous acid
b. Hypoch1orous ion
c. Hypochlorite ion
d. None

89. The minimum recommended concentration of free residual chlorine in water for routine chlorination is
a. 0.1 mg/L for a contact period of 1 hour
b. 0.5 mg/L for a contact period of 1 hour
c. 0.5 mg/L for a contact period of ½ hour
d. 1.0 mg/L for a contact period of 1 hour

90. A 0.5 g chlorine tablet will be sufficient to disinfect how many litres of water *(Recent Question 2014)*
a. 1 L b. 5 L
c. 10 L d. 20 L

91. Color produced in orthotolidine test after 5 minutes is due to action of? *(Recent Question 2014)*
a. Dissolved solids
b. Free chlorine
c. Combined chlorine
d. Free and combined chlorine

92. Minimum recommended level of residual chloride in water after treatment in post-epidemic period is
a. 0.2 mg/L
b. 0.5 mg/L
c. 5 g/L
d. 10 g/L

Ans.

70.	a
71.	b
72.	b
73.	c
74.	d
75.	b
76.	d
77.	b
78.	b
79.	a
80.	c
81.	b
82.	c
83.	b
84.	c
85.	c
86.	d, e
87.	a
88.	a
89.	b
90.	d
91.	d
92.	b

Most Recent Questions of 2019-18 are given at the end of MCQs

93. Method of choice for purification of highly polluted water on a large scale is *(Recent Question 2013)*
a. Superchlorination followed by dechlorination
b. Boiling
c. Chlorination
d. UV treatment

94. Minimum contact period for chlorination:
a. 30 minutes b. 1 hour
c. 2 hours d. 5 hours

95. Disinfecting action of chlorine due to:
a. Hypochlorous acid *(Recent Question 2013)*
b. Hypochlorite ion
c. Hydrochloric acid
d. Both hypochlorous acid and hypochlorite ion

96. Orthotolidine test is used to detect:
a. Free residual chlorine
b. Bound chlorine
c. Free and combined chlorine
d. Chlorine demand

97. Orthotolidine test is used to detect:
a. Nitrates in water *(Recent Question 2013)*
b. Nitrites in water
c. Chlorine in water
d. Ammonia content in water

98. Horrock's apparatus determines chlorine demand of water, with a holding level of: *(Recent Question 2013)*
a. 1.0 mg/L b. 1.5 mg/L
c. 2.0 mg/L d. 0.5 mg/L

99. Horrock's apparatus contains which of the following as an indicator
a. Bleaching powder b. Soda lime
c. Potassium permagnate d. Starch Iodide

100. Which one of the following methods is used for the estimation of chlorine demand of water?
a. Chlorometer b. Horrock's apparatus
c. Berkefeld filter d. Double pot method

101. Nalgonda technique for deflouridation is in what sequence:
a. Lime + Alum
b. Soda + Alum
c. Alum + Soda
d. Alum + Lime

102. Following is a process of deflouridation of water:
a. Nalgonda technique
b. Soaking
c. S and filter
d. Parboiling

103. All the following are true regarding deep well except
a. Taps water from below the first impervious layer
b. Soft water
c. Pure water
d. Provides a source of constant supply even in summer

104. Permanent hardness can be removed by
a. Boiling
b. Addition of sodium carbonate
c. Addition of lime
d. Permutit process

105. Hardness of water is not caused by *(Recent Question 2013)*
a. Calcium bicarbonate b. Magnesium bicarbonate
c. Sodium bicarbonate d. Calcium sulfate

106. Softening is recommended when hardness of water is more than: *(Recent Question 2013)*
a. 50 mg/L
b. 75 mg/L
c. 100 mg/L
d. 150 mg/L

107. If hardness level of water is 50-150 mg/L, the water is defined as –
a. Soft
b. Moderately hard
c. Hard
d. Very hard

108. Hardness of drinking water should be
a. >3 mEq/L b. <1 mEq/L
c. 1-3 mEq/L d. 3 -6 mEq/L

WATER QUALITY STANDARDS AND BACTERIOLOGICAL INDICATORS OF WATER CONTAMINATION

109. The following organisms are indicative of fecal pollution of water except: *(Recent Question 2013)*
a. Clostridium perfringens
b. E. coli
c. Fecal streptococci
d. Halophilic vibrio

110. Fecal contamination of water is evaluated by
a. Klebsiella b. E coli
c. Proteus d. Staphylococci

111. To avoid bacterial contamination, a sanitary well should be located not less than from the likely sources of contamination *(Recent Question 2013)*
a. 5 m b. 15 m
c. 25 m d. 50 m

112. Coliform test is for: *(Recent Question 2013)*
a. Air pollution b. Water contamination
c. Sound pollution d. None

113. Not an indicator for fecal contamination of water:
a. Staphylococcus b. Streptococcus
c. E. coli d. Clostridium perfringens

114. Confirmatory test for coliform count is :
a. Eijkman test b. Casoni's test
c. Nitrate test d. Urease test

115. Bacterial indicator of recent contamination of water is:
a. Clostridium perfringens *(Recent Question 2013)*
b. E. coli
c. Clostridium welchii
d. Fecal streptococci

116. Fecal contamination of drinking water is known by:
a. Klebsiella
b. E. coli
c. Proteus
d. Coagulase negative staphylococci

117. Which of the following is used as an indicator for recent fecal contamination of water: *(Recent Question 2013)*
a. E coli
b. Corynebacterium diphtheriae
c. Pseudomonas
d. Streptococci

Ans.

93. a
94. b
95. a
96. c
97. c
98. d
99. d
100. b
101. a
102. a
103. b
104. b
105. c
106. d
107. b
108. c
109. d
110. b
111. d
112. b
113. a
114. a
115. d
116. b
117. d

Most Recent Questions of 2019-18 are given at the end of MCQs

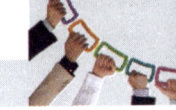

118. **Not an indicator for fecal contamination of water is**
a. E. coli
b. Staphylococcus
c. Streptococcus
d. Clostridium perfringens

119. **All of the following about purification of water are true except?**
a. Clostridiums pores indicates recent contamination of water
b. Coliforms may be detected by Multiple Tube Method and Indole production
c. Sodium thiosulfate is added to neutralize certain contaminants
d. Coliforms must not be detectable in any 100 mL sample of drinking water

120. **Guideline value for color of drinking water is up to:**
a. 1 TCU b. 5 TCU
c. 15 TCU d. 25 TCU

121. **Water with total dissolved solids (TDS) concentrations below mg/L is acceptable** *(Recent Question 2013)*
a. 100 b. 200
c. 500 d. 1000

122. **Optimum concentration of fluoride in drinking water** *(Recent Question 2013)*
a. 0.1 – 0.5 ppm
b. 0.5 – 0.8 ppm
c. 1.0 – 1.5 ppm
d. 1.5 – 2.0 ppm

123. **True statement regarding swimming pool sanitation is**
a. pH is to be kept between 7.4 – 7.8
b. It is equipped with rapid sand filters and filtering should be continuous, so that all water is refiltered in <2 hours
c. 50% of water is replaced by fresh water daily
d. 5 ppm of free chlorine residual provides adequate protection against bacterial and viral agents

124. **Recent contamination of water is indicated by which of the following** *(Recent Question 2013)*
a. Nitrates b. Nitrites
c. Ammonia d. Chlorides

125. **Criteria for drinking water quality recommended by WHO includes all except:** *(Recent Question 2013)*
a. Color < 5 TCU b. pH 6.5 – 8.5
c. Chloride 200-600 mg/l d. Zinc <4 mg/l

126. **Most undesirable mineral in water is**
a. Iron b. Copper
c. Zinc d. Lead

127. **Maximum permissible chloride level is:**
a. 200 mg/L
b. 300 mg/L
c. 500 mg/L
d. 600 mg/L

AIR

128. **Psychrometer is used for measuring-**
a. Air velocity
b. Core temperature
c. Humidity
d. Height from sea level

129. **All are indicators for air pollution except;**
a. CO_2
b. SO_2
c. Soiling Index
d. Smoke Index

130. **Soiling index is used for-**
a. Air pollution
b. Water pollution
c. Faecal contamination
d. Milk contamination

131. **The most harmful gas responsible for the destruction of ozone is:** *(2014)*
a. NO_2
b. SO_2
c. CO_2
d. CFCs

132. **The most abundant hydrocarbon pollutant of the air is:**
a. Methane b. Benzene
c. Terpene d. Ammonia
e. Hydrogen sulfide

133. **The most abundant greenhouse gas is:**
a. CFC's
b. CO_2
c. CO
d. CH_4

134. **Acid rain is caused by all except:**
a. Water
b. Carbonic acid
c. Sulfuric acid
d. Hydrochloric acid

135. **Which of the following is not an indicator for determining general level of air pollution-**
a. Smoke index
b. Sulfur dioxide
c. Suspended particle
d. Carbon-monoxide

136. **Anemometer is used to measure:**
a. Humidity b. Air velocity
c. Air temperature d. Air pollution

137. **Kata meter is used to measure**
a. Maximum temperature b. Minimum temperature
c. Cooling power of air d. Radiant heat

138. **Auditory fatigue occurs at:**
a. 2000 Hz b. 3000 Hz
c. 4000 Hz d. 8000 Hz

139. **Which is not primary air pollutant:**
a. Smoke and dust b. SO_2
c. Ozone d. NO_2

140. **Corrosive effect on building is caused by:**
a. Ozone depletion
b. Green house effect
c. Acid rain
d. Excessive industrialization

141. **All are indicators of air pollution Except:**
a. CO_2 b. SO_2
c. Soiling index d. Smoke index

142. **Oxide not emitted by automobiles is-**
a. Carbon dioxide b. Carbon monoxide
c. Nitrogen oxides d. Hydrocarbons

Ans.
118. b
119. a
120. c
121. d
122. b
123. a
124. c
125. a
126. d
127. d
128. c
129. a
130. a
131. d
132. a
133. b
134. d
135. d
136. b
137. c
138. c
139. a
140. c
141. a
142. a

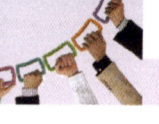

143. The best indicator for determining the general level of air pollution in an urban area is
a. Sulfur dioxide
b. Carbon dioxide
c. Hydrogen
d. Nitrogen

144. The maximum ozone concentration in polluted atmosphere is dependent on the concentration and ratio of nitrogen oxides and which one of the following?
a. Carbon monoxide
b. Lead
c. Volatile organic compounds
d. Sulfur dioxide

145. Kata thermometer is used to measure:
a. Cooling power of air b. Maximum temperature
c. Minimum temperature d. Body temperature

146. As per WHO recommended standards for floor space, a space of 90-100 sq.ft. can accommodate
a. 1 adult
b. 2 adult
c. 1 adult, 1 child of 8 years and 1 child of 2 years
d. 1 adult, 1 child of 6 years and a 6 month old infant

147. Indoor air pollution does not cause:
a. Chronic lung disease
b. Pregnancy problems
c. Childhood pneumonia
d. Neurodevelopment problems

148. Which of the following does not cause indoor air pollution?
a. Carbon Monoxide
b. Nitrogen dioxide
c. Radon
d. Mercury vapor

149. Which of the following is non natural gas causing green-house effect? *(Recent Question 2013)*
a. Carbon Dioxide b. Methane
c. Ozone d. CFCs

150. Greenhouse gas includes *(Recent Question 2013)*
a. CO_2, Ozone, Methane b. Only ozone
c. Ozone, methane only d. Methane, CO

151. Global warming true is
a. CO_2 is a major greenhouse gas
b. Stratosphere ozone layer is harmful
c. CFC increases Stratosphere ozone layer
d. Kyoto protocol called for 20% reduction in Greenhouse emissions

152. Gas used as an indicator of air pollution is
a. SO_2 b. CO_2
c. Ozone d. CO

153. Soiling index is used to measure:
a. Noise pollution
b. Water pollution
c. Air pollution
d. Soil pollution

154. Soling index is a measure of: *(Recent Question 2015)*
a. Soil pollution
b. Water pollution
c. Noise pollution
d. Air pollution

155. Which agency monitors air quality in India:
a. Central Research Institute
b. Ministry of Health and Family Welfare
c. National Environmental Engineering Research Institute
d. Central Pollution Control Board

156. Which of the following is not associated with heat stress?
a. Cramps
b. Numbness
c. Hyperpyrexia
d. Syncope

157. The effective temperature of 'comfort zone' is:
a. 69–76°F
b. 77–80°F
c. 83–85°F
d. 86–90°F

158. Air velocity is measured by:
a. Hygrometer
b. Psychrometer
c. Anemometer
d. Wet bulb thermometer

159. Number of air changes in a drawing room per hour should be at least: *(Recent Question 2014)*
a. 2–3
b. 3–4
c. 4–5
d. 5–6

160. Kata thermometer measures: *(Recent Question 2014)*
a. Air temperature only
b. Air temperature and humidity
c. Air temperature, humidity and air movement
d. Air velocity only

LIGHT

161. Luminous flux is measured in?
a. Lux b. Lumen
c. Candela d. Lambert

162. Luminous Intensity is measured in terms of (SI Unit)
a. Candela b. Lux
c. Coulomb d. Lumen

163. Daylight factor in living room should be:
a. 8% b. 6%
c. 10% d. 15%

NOISE

164. Acceptable noise level is
a. 50-60 dB b. 40-50 dB
c. 20-30 dB d. 70-85 dB

165. Auditory fatigue appears at
a. 65 dB b. 85 dB
c. 90 dB d. 100 dB

166. Normal human ear can hear frequencies from about
a. 10 to 10,000 Hz b. 20 to 20,000 Hz
c. 20 to 30,000 Hz d. 10 to 40,000 Hz

167. Recommended maximum level of noise exposure, up to which people can tolerate without substantial damage to their hearing *(Recent Question 2014)*
a. 150 dB b. 120 dB
c. 85 dB d. 80 dB

Ans.
143. a
144. c
145. a
146. d
147. d
148. d
149. d
150. a
151. a
152. a
153. c
154. d
155. d
156. b
157. b
158. c
159. a
160. c
161. b
162. a
163. a
164. d
165. c
166. b
167. c

168. **Acceptable noise level in class room**
 a. 20–30 dB b. 30–40 dB
 c. 40–50 dB d. 10–20 dB

169. **The 'acceptable' noise level is:** *(Recent Question 2014)*
 a. 85 dB b. 90 dB
 c. 95 dB d. 100 dB

170. **Acceptable' noise level is:**
 a. 95 dB b. 90 dB
 c. 85 dB d. 100 dB

RADIATION

171. **What is the maximum permissible level of occupational exposure to ionising radiation per year to the whole body of an individual as set by the International Commission of Radiological Protection?**
 a. 2 rad b. 3 rad
 c. 5 rad d. 8 rad

172. **Unit of absorbed radiation is:** *(Recent Question 2013)*
 a. Roentgen
 b. Rad
 c. Rem
 d. Sievert

173. **The following radiation unit measures the degree of potential danger to health**
 a. Rem
 b. Rad
 c. Roentgen
 d. Becquerel

174. **Acceptable safe dose of radiation during pregnancy is:**
 a. 1 rad b. 2 rad
 c. 5 rad d. 0.5 rad

175. **Thickness of lead apron to prevent radiation exposure is:**
 a. 0.1 mm b. 0.2 mm
 c. 0.5 mm d. 1 mm

176. **10 days rule is related to:** *(Recent Question 2013)*
 a. Sewage disposal
 b. Air quality
 c. Water quality
 d. Radiation protection in pregnancy

AIR VELOCITY/ HUMIDITY

177. **In sling psychrometer, the desirable speed is?**
 a. 5 m/s b. 50 m/s
 c. 75 m/s d. 100 m/s

178. **Cooling power of air is measured by**
 a. Kata thermometer b. Anemometer
 c. Sling psychrometer d. Hygrometer

HOUSING & VENTILATION

179. **All of the following are causes of discomfort in overcrowded & poorly ventilated room except**
 a. Increased CO_2 b. Increased humidity
 c. Increased temperature d. Decreased air exchange

180. **Caisson disease is associated with:**
 a. Mountain climbing
 b. Deep sea diving
 c. Flying
 d. Space travel

181. **To facilitate cross-ventilation in educational institutions, the recommended combined space for doors and windows as a percentage of floor space is**
 a. 10% b. 15%
 c. 25% d. 35%

182. **What is the basic minimum illumination required for satisfactory vision?**
 a. 10–15 foot candles b. 15–20 foot candles
 c. 20–25 foot candles d. 25–30 foot candles

WASTE DISPOSAL

183. **Which method of disposal of wastes is not safe but good for soil building?**
 a. Dumping
 b. Controlled tipping
 c. Composting
 d. Burial

184. **All are true about oxidation pond as method of sewage disposal, except—**
 a. Cheap method
 b. Mixed aerobic - anaerobic decay
 c. Suitable for large community
 d. Algae is a source of oxygen

185. **The biological oxygen demand indicates:**
 a. Organic matter
 b. Bacterial content
 c. Anaerobic bacteria
 d. Chemicals

186. **Biochemical oxygen demand (B.O.D) is determined by;**
 a. Organic matter and bacteria
 b. Oxygen content
 c. Algae content in water
 d. Agriculture fertilizer content in water

187. **Anaerobic decomposition of organic matter leads to production of:**
 a. CO_2 and H_2O
 b. H_2S and NH_3
 c. Ozone and dioxin
 d. CH_4 and CO_2

188. **The most cost effective method for disposal of human excreta for Rural area is:**
 a. Sewage farming b. Dumping into river
 c. Trench burial d. Water carriage system

189. **The leakage of hazardous material from composting site into sub soil water can be prevented by:**
 a. Burning the waste in the dump
 b. Lining the wall of the pit with an impervious material
 c. Pouring of chemical into it
 d. Covering it with soil and lime
 e. Making it 300 feet away from a water body

190. **Biomagnification and bioaccumulation is a property shown by:**
 a. Simple biodegradable waste
 b. Fat soluble complex biodegradable and nondegradable waste
 c. Water soluble complex biodegradable and non degradable waste
 d. Organic waste

Ans.

168. b
169. a
170. c
171. c
172. b
173. a
174. c
175. c
176. d
177. a
178. a
179. a
180. b
181. c
182. b
183. c
184. c
185. a
186. a
187. d
188. c
189. b
190. b

Most Recent Questions of 2019-18 are given at the end of MCQs

191. Presence of 250-300 hookworm eggs per gram of feces indicates that:
a. The infection is not of much significance
b. It is a minor public health problem
c. It is a potential danger for the community
d. It is an important public health problem
e. It is a host parasite balance stage

192. 'Sanitation barrier' implies:
a. Segregation of faeces b. Elimination of flies
c. Water pollution d. Personal hygiene

193. The heart of the activated sludge process is:
a. Primary sedimentation tank
b. Sludge digester
c. Aeration tank
d. Final settling tank

194. Oxidation pond is a method used for:
a. Solid waste disposal b. Sewage treatment
c. Water purification d. Sullage disposal

195. Kitchen refuse is also known as:
a. Sullage b. Sludge
c. Garbage d. Sewerage

196. Sewage is defined as:
a. Discarded waste arising from man's activities
b. Waste matter arising from preparation, cooking and consumption of food
c. Waste water from community containing solid and liquid excreta
d. Waste water which does not contain human excreta

197. Biological oxygen demand gives an indication of:
a. E. coli b. Anaerobic bacteria
c. Organic matter d. Oxygen content

198. According to WHO, the most insanitary method of waste disposal *(Recent Question 2013)*
a. Dumping b. Burial
c. Composting d. Incineration

199. Most satisfactory method of waste disposal when suitable land is available is: *(Recent Question 2013)*
a. Sanitary land fill b. Manure pits
c. Incineration d. Composting

200. Sullage consists of: *(Recent Question 2013)*
a. Solid vegetable waste material
b. Inorganic waste
c. Waste containing human excreta
d. Waste water from kitchen

EXCRETA DISPOSAL

201. Dry weather flow is:
a. The average humidity recorded on a peak summer day
b. Minimum rainfall measured during peak rainy season
c. The average amount of sewage that flows through the sewerage system in 24 hrs
d. Average maximum and minimum temperature in a given year

202. Sanitary toilets result in decreased incidence of all except:
a. Diarrhea
b. Polio
c. Malaria
d. Cholera

203. % of population with access to adequate sanitation in India
a. 34%
b. 40%
c. 72%
d. 92%

204. True about Septic tank is/are: *(PGI Pattern)*
a. Treatment of household sewage
b. Suitable in presence of public sewage system
c. Aerobic oxidation occurs outside septic tank
d. Retention period 6 hours
e. Anaerobic digestion inside septic tank

205. True about sewage is/are *(PGI Pattern)*
a. Does not contain human excreta
b. Strength measured by biological oxygen demand
c. BOD >100 mg/L is strong sewage
d. Composed of 90% water
e. Dry weather flow is measured for 24 hours period

206. Percentage of bleaching powder used to disinfect feces
a. 2% b. 5%
c. 10% d. 15%

207. Sanitary toilets can decrease incidence of all except
a. Diarrhea b. Poliomyelitis
c. Malaria d. Cholera

208. If waste water contains toxic substances, organic load is measured by: *(Recent Question 2014)*
a. Biological oxygen demand
b. Chemical oxygen demand
c. Suspended solid
d. None

209. The heart of activated sludge process is :
a. Aeration tank
b. Primary sedimentation
c. Digestion tank
d. Secondary sedimentation tank

210. All of the following are methods of sewage disposal except
a. River outfall
b. Land treatment
c. Oxidation ponds
d. Bangalore method (Composting)

ENTOMOLOGY

211. Which of the following is not included in class insecta:
a. Ticks b. House fly
c. Reduviid bug d. Rat flea

212. All are true about Aedes aegypti except-
a. Eggs can survive without water for more than 7-8 days
b. Transmits dengue
c. Bites repeatedly
D. Incubation period in mosquito is 8-10 days

213. Flying range of Aedes aegypti is-
a. 100 meters b. 200 meters
c. 300 meters d. 400 meters

214. Which of the following is not spread by Aedes mosquito?
a. Dengue fever
b. Chikungunya
c. Japanese encephalitis
d. Yellow fever

Ans.
191. b
192. a
193. c
194. b
195. c
196. c
197. c
198. a
199. a
200. d
201. c
202. c
203. b
204. a,c e
205. b,e
206. b
207. c
208. b
209. a
210. d
211. a
212. a
213. a
214. c

Most Recent Questions of 2019-18 are given at the end of MCQs

215. All of the following have a common vector except:
a. Dengue fever b. Yellow fever
c. Kala Azar d. Japanese encephalitis

216. Name the disease transmitted by Aedes aegypti in India
a. Yellow fever b. Dengue
c. Scrub typhus d. Filariasis

217. Culex mosquito is associated with the transmission of which disease in India
a. Malaria b. Brugian Filariasis
c. Dengue **d. Japanese encephalitis**

218. Life span of a mosquito ranges
a. Between 7 and 15 days b. Between 15 and 30 days
c. Between 8 and 34 days d. More than 34 days

219. Match list I (Arthropod) with list II (Disease transmitted) and select the correct answer using the codes given below the lists:

List I (Arthropod)	List II (Disease transmitted)
A. Mosquito	1. Sleeping sickness
B. Rat flea	2. Onchocerciasis
C. Black fly	3. Viral encephalitis
D. Tsetse fly	4. Bubonic plague

Codes:
a. A3 B2 C4 D1 b. A3 B4 C2 D1
c. A1 B2 C3 D4 d. A1 B4 C2 D3

220. Which of the following viral infections is transmitted by tick?
a. Japanese encephalitis
b. Dengue fever
c. Kyasanur forest disease (KFD)
d. Yellow fever

221. Which one of the following is transmitted by soft tick?
a. Tick typhus b. Tularemia
c. Relapsing fever d. Colorado tick fever

222. Tick transmits all, EXCEPT:
a. Tularemia
b. Kyasanur forest disease
c. Japanese encephalitis
d. Tick typhus

223. Which of the following is transmitted by hard tick?
a. Oriental sore
b. Human babesiosis
c. Leishmaniasis
d. Oroya fever

224. Scabies is classified as which type of water related disease:
a. Water borne
b. Water based
c. Water washed
d. Water dispersed

225. Mites are the vectors of the following diseases except:
a. Scabies
b. Scrub typhus
c. Rickettsialpox
d. Kyasanur forest disease

226. Rat flea transmits all of the following except:
a. Plague
b. Epidemic typhus
c. Hymenolepiasis
d. Endemic typhus

227. Vector for Kala-azar is:
a. Flea b. Tsetse fly
c. Sand fly d. Mosquito

228. Rickettsia typhi is transmitted by:
a. Mite b. Tick
c. Louse d. Rat flea

229. The concentration of abate recommended for killing Cyclops is..........mg/L:
a. 2 b. 1
c. 5 d. 0.5

230. The average life of a Cyclops is:
a. 1 month b. 2 months
c. 3 months d. 4 months

231. Urban malaria is due to: *(Recent Question 2013)*
a. Anopheles stephensi
b. Anopheles culicifacies
c. Aedes
d. Culex vishnui

232. Vector for Japanese encephalitis is
a. Mansonia
b. Anopheles
c. Aedes
d. Culex

233. Disease transmitted by Mansonoides mosquitoes is?
a. Japanese encephalitis
b. Rift Valley fever
c. West Nile fever
d. Chikungunya fever

234. The following mosquito is referred to as tiger mosquito
a. Mansonia
b. Anopheles
c. Aedes
d. Culex

235. The following mosquitoes are called nuisance mosquitoes
a. Mansonia
b. Anopheles
c. Aedes
d. Culex

236. Under the WHO, international health regulations (IHR), all international airports and seaports are kept free form all types of mosquitoes for a distance of around the perimeter of the ports *(Recent Question 2013)*
a. 100 m
b. 400 m
c. 500 m
d. 1000 m

237. Mansonia mosquito is a vector for all of the following, except: *(Recent Question 2013)*
a. Malaria b. Brugian filariasis
c. Chikungunya fever d. St. Louis encephalitis

238. Cigar shaped eggs are seen in which of the following:
a. Aedes b. Culex
c. Anopheles d. Mansonia

239. All the following are true about anopheles mosquitoes except: *(Recent Question 2013)*
a. Eggs are laid singly
b. Larva has siphon tube
c. Larva rests parallel to water surface
d. Adults are inclined at an angle to surface at rest

Ans.
215. c
216. b
217. d
218. c
219. b
220. c
221. c
222. c
223. b
224. c
225. d
226. b
227. c
228. d
229. b
230. c
231. a
232. d
233. d
234. c
235. d
236. b
237. a
238. a
239. b

240. Not a feature of anopheles is
a. Spotted wings
b. Siphon tube seen in larvae
c. Boat shaped eggs
d. Rest at an angle, inclined to the surface

241. The following statement is true about Culex larva:
a. It has siphon tube
b. Long palmate hair present
c. Rest parallel to water surface
d. None

242. Which of the following is NOT a feature of the vector for Malaria:
a. Adult has spotted wings
b. Larva has siphon tube
c. Eggs are boat-shaped with lateral floats
d. It rests with body inclined at an angle to surface of skin

243. Features of anopheles mosquito are:
a. Have stripes on wings
b. Larva rest at an angle to water surface
c. Adults rest at an angle to surface of skin
d. Eggs are laid in clusters
e. Larva does not have a siphon tube

244. Japanese encephalitis is transmitted by:
a. Mosquito
b. Tick
c. Mite
d. Rat flea

245. Urban malaria is transmitted by: *(Recent Question 2013)*
a. Anopheles culicifacies
b. Anopheles stephensi
c. Anopheles fluviatilis
d. Anopheles minimus

246. Range of flight of Aedes mosquito is:
a. 1 km b. Less than 100 m
c. 400 m d. 10 km

247. The distance from airport or seaport which has to be kept free from Aedes mosquitoes is: *(Recent Question 2013)*
a. 400 m b. 500 m
c. 1 km d. 100 m

248. Mosquito net hole diameter is:
a. 0.02 inch b. 0.0475 inch
c. 0.5 inch d. 0.9 inch

249. Disease(s) transmitted by Aedes aegypti incude:
a. Yellow fever
b. Dengue
c. Chikungunya fever
d. West Nile fever
e. Rift Valley fever

250. Most efficient antilarval measure to prevent urban malaria is: *(Recent Question 2013)*
a. Clean drainage and sewage system
b. Covered overhead tanks
c. Filling of cesspools and ditches
d. Cover pits

251. Chikungunya is transmitted by: *(Recent Question 2013)*
a. Aedes
b. Culex
c. Mansonoides
d. Anopheles

252. Regarding anopheles mosquito true is all except:
a. Eggs are laid singly on water
b. Larva do not have siphon tube
c. Wings are spotted
d. Pupa don't have siphon tube

253. Not true about Aedes mosquito:
a. Are recurrent day-time biters
b. Eggs cannot survive more than one week without water
c. Transmits dengue fever
d. Takes 7–8 days to develop the parasite and transmit disease

254. Spread by mosquitoes is:
a. Dengue
b. Kala-azar
c. Trypanosomiasis
d. Listeriosis
e. Trench fever

255. Vector for epidemic typhus is
a. Mite
b. Flea
c. Louse
d. Tick

256. Ixodidae tick transmits *(Recent Question 2013)*
a. Lyme disease
b. Scrub typhus
c. Rickettsialpox
d. Plague

257. True about hard tick *(Recent Question 2013)*
a. Have four stages in life cycle
b. Female lays thousands of eggs
c. Larval stage is known as seed ticks
d. All of the above

258. Transovarian transmission is seen is:
a. Rickettsial disease
b. Malaria
c. Filariasis
d. None

259. Transovarian transmission is seen in:
a. Ticks
b. Louse
c. Flea
d. None

260. Disease(s) spread by ticks include:
a. Epidemic typhus
b. Endemic typhus
c. Scrub typhus
d. RMSF
e. Crimean-Congo fever

261. Disease transmitted by hard ticks includes all except:
a. Viral encephalitis
b. Oriental sore
c. Tick paralysis
d. Tularemia

262. Trombiculid mite transmits
a. Scrub typhus b. Endemic typhus
c. Scabies d. Relapsing fever

263. Reduviid bug transmits which of the following diseases
a. Relapsing fever b. Lyme's disease
c. Chagas disease d. Scrub typhus

Ans.

240. b
241. a
242. b
243. c,e
244. a
245. b
246. b
247. a
248. b
249. a,b, c,e
250. c
251. a
252. d
253. b
254. a
255. c
256. a
257. d
258. a
259. a
260. d,e
261. b
262. a
263. c

Most Recent Questions of 2019-18 are given at the end of MCQs

264. **Scrub typhus is transmitted by:** *(Recent Question 2013)*
a. Mite b. Tick
c. Flea d. Louse

265. **Average number of mites found on the body in a person suffering from scabies is:**
a. 1–2 b. 5–10
c. 10–15 d. 15–20

266. **All of the following statements about scrub typhus are true, Except** *(Recent Question 2013)*
a. Caused by O. tsutsugamushi
b. Mites act as reservoirs
c. Transmitted when adult mites feed on hosts
d. Tetracycline is the drug of choice

267. **Scabies is transmitted by** *(Recent Question 2013)*
a. Mite
b. Tick
c. Louse
d. Rat flea

268. **Louse transmitted disease(s) is/are:**
a. Trench fever
b. Q fever
c. KFD
d. Epidemic typhus
e. Pediculosis

269. **Disease(s) transmitted by louse include:**
a. Epidemic typhus
b. Scrub typhus
c. Relapsing fever
d. Q fever
e. Trench fever

270. **Cyclodevelopment stage is seen in:**
a. Malaria b. Filaria
c. Plague d. Cholera

271. **Cyclo propagative cycle is seen in:**
a. Malaria b. Plague
c. Cholera d. Filarial

272. **Plague undergoes:**
a. Transovarian cycle b. Propagative cycle
c. Cyclodevelopment d. Cyclopropagative

273. **Sandfly can fly up to............**
a. 50 yards b. 100 yards
c. 200 yards d. 300 yards

274. **Phlebotomus argentipes is killed by:**
a. Pyrethrum b. DDT
c. Malathion d. None of the above

INSECTICIDES

275. **Malathion spray is effective for:**
a. One month
b. Two months
c. Three months
d. Four months

276. **Which of the following is an organophosphorus poison:** *(PGI Pattern)*
a. Abate
b. DDT
c. Propoxur
d. Malathion e. Pyrethrum

277. **DDT is a**
a. CNS poison
b. Stomach poison
c. Contact poison
d. Suffocating agent

278. **Match list I (Insecticides) with list II (Characteristics) and select the correct answer using the codes given below the list:**

List I (Insecticides)	List II (Characteristics)
A. Derris	1. Synthetic contact poison
B. Gardona	2. Natural contact poison
C. Sodium fluorocetate	3. Fumigant
D. Methyl bromide	4. Stomach poison

Codes:
a. A-3 B-1 C-4 D-2 b. A-2, B-1, C-4, D-3
c. A2 B4 C1 D3 d. A3 B4 C1 D2

279. **Which of the following insecticide is of plant origin?**
a. Paris green
b. Propoxur
c. Malathion
d. Pyrethrum

280. **Dose of malathion used for residual insecticidal action is:**
a. 100-200 mg/square foot
b. 25-50 mg/square foot
c. 10-20 mg/square foot
d. 500-1000 mg/square foot

281. **All are true about DDT except?**
a. It is a contact poison
b. Causes immediate death
c. Residues can be found up to 18 Months
d. Synergistic action with permethrin
e. Shows biomagnification effect

282. **Diethyltoluamide is a:** *(Recent Question 2013)*
a. Stomach poison
b. Contact poison
c. Repellent
d. Fumigant

283. **Removing pistia plants and water hyacinthians effective anti-larval measure against which species of mosquito:**
a. Anopheles
b. Aedes
c. Culex
d. Mansonia

284. **Paris green mainly kills larva of** *(Recent Question 2013)*
a. Anopheles
b. Aedes
c. Culex
d. Mansonia

285. **Average duration of effectiveness of DDT when sprayed at a dose of 1–2 g/m²:** *(Recent Question 2013)*
a. 1 – 3 months
b. 3 – 6 months
c. 6 – 12 months
d. 1 – 2 years

286. **Pyrethrum is a:**
a. Contact poison
b. Stomach poison
c. Nerve poison
d. Space poison

Ans.
264. a
265. d
266. c
267. a
268. a,d,e
269. a,c,d
270. b
271. a
272. b
273. a
274. b
275. c
276. a,d
277. c
278. b
279. d
280. a
281. b,d
282. c
283. d
284. a
285. c
286. c

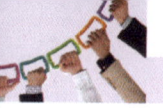

287. Which of the following is not an aryl phosphate?
a. TIK 20
b. Malathion
c. Parathion
d. Folidol

288. Most hazardous pesticide Color coding is:
a. Red
b. Green
c. Yellow
d. Black

289. Fenthion is: *(Recent Question 2013)*
a. Space spray
b. Residual spray
c. Stomach poison
d. Fumigant

290. Which of the following is not a Synthetic Pyrethroid Compound: *(Recent Question 2013)*
a. DDT
b. Permethrin
c. Proparthin
d. Cypermethrin

291. All are water borne diseases except:
a. Typhoid
b. Fish tape worm
c. HAV
d. Cholera

292. Reduviid bug acts as vector for transmission of
a. Chagas disease
b. Lyme disease
c. Relapsing fever
d. Scrub typhus

293. Best way to control houseflies: *(Recent Question 2013)*
a. Eliminate breeding places
b. Insecticide spray
c. Bed Net use
d. Paris green

294. All of the following methods are antilarval measures except:
a. Intermittent irrigation
b. Fumigation
a. Gambusia affinis
d. Malathion

295. Paris green is useful for killing:
a. Anopheline larvae only
b. Culicine larvae only
c. Adult mosquitoes
d. None

296. Paris green is chemical insecticide for:
a. Sandfly
b. Anopheline mosquito
c. House fly
d. Aedes Mosquito

297. Which of the following is a stomach poison?
a. Mineral oils
b. Gardona
c. Sodium fluoride
d. DDT

Most Recent Questions (2019–2018)

298. Permanent Hardness of water is not due to: *(Recent Question 2019)*
a. Calcium Sulfate
b. Calcium Chloride
c. Magnesium Nitrates
d. Magnesium Bicarbonate

299. Chlorine disinfection of water is due to which ions? *(Recent Question 2019)*
a. Hypochlorite ions
b. Hydrogen ions
c. Hypochlorous acid
d. Hydrochloric acid

300. Under the water supply program, which of the following statement is false: *(Recent Question 2019)*
a. At least 1 hand pump (safe water spot) for 250 population
b. At least 40 liters PCD in rural area
c. At least 140 L in urban areas with sewage
d. It is a problem village, if there is no safe water within 1 km

301. Which engineered water purification system is the most effective for elimination of *cryptosporidium parvum?* *(Recent Question 2019)*
a. Flocculation
b. Disinfection
c. Boiling
d. Filtration

302. Breteau index is defined as: *(JIPMER Nov 2018)*
a. Number of Aedes mosquito per man hour
b. Number of Aedes larva/container
c. Number of container with Aedes larva/number of houses checked
d. Number of aedes mosquitos within 400 meters of an area

303. Maximum permissible sound in city for residential purpose is *(JIPMER Nov 2018)*
a. 45 dB
b. 55 dB
c. 65 dB
d. 85 dB

304. True about Tsetse fly *(JIPMER Nov 2018)*
a. Lay single egg
b. Lay egg in cluster near water/marsh areas
c. It does not fly
d. Fast reproduction rate of less than 10 days

305. How much land is required for a population of 10000, to have a deep trench: *(Recent Question 2019)*
a. 1 acre
b. 2 acre
c. 3 acre
d. 5 acre

Ans.

287. b
288. a
289. b
290. a
291. b
292. a
293. a
294. b
295. a
296. b
297. c
298. c
299. c
300. d
301. d
302. c
303. b
304. a
305. a

Answers with Explanations

1. Ans. (b) $BaCO_3$

Hardness is suallay due to calcium and magnesium salts. Temporary hardness is due to carbonates an bi carbonates, while the permanent hardness is due to sulphates, phosphates of calcium or magnesium

2. Ans. (d) Hypochlorous acid

3. Ans. (a) CO_2, ozone, methane

Ref: K. Park, 24th ed. p 785; 23rd ed. p 748; Inventory of US greenhouse gas emissions and sinks, 1990-1994 By United States Environmental Protection Agency

4. Ans. (d) 2 cm

Ref: K. Park, 24th ed. p 796

5. Ans. (a) Soft tick; (b) Hard tick

Ref: K. Park, 24th ed. p 817

Public Health Importance

Hard ticks transmit the following disease:
- Tick typhus (Rocky mountain spotted fever)
- Viral encephalitis (e.g., Russian spring-summer encephalitis)
- Viral fevers (e.g., Colorado tick fever)
- Viral hemorrhagic fevers (e.g., KFD in India)
- Tularaemia
- Tick paralysis, and
- Human babesiosis

Soft ticks transmit:
- Q fever
- Relapsing fever, and
- KFD

6. Ans. (c) Laveran

Ref: History of the discovery of the malaria parasites and their vectors. Francis EG Cox. Parasites and Vectors 2010, p-3-5

Milestones in Malaria Cure

- Hippocrates—1st to describe clinical manifestation and relate it with time/place of residence.
- Laveran, a French army surgeon (Noble Prize in 1907)—Discovered malaria parasite in blood of malaria patient (1880).
- Ronald Ross (Noble Prize in 1902)—Discovered transmission of malaria parasite by mosquito (1898).
- Hans Andersag—Discovered Chloroquine (1934).
- Paul Hermann Müller (1945)—Discovered Insecticide DDT.

7. Ans. (a) Ronald Ross

Ref: K. Park, 24th ed. p 6

8. Ans (b) Hippocrates

Ref: K. Park, 24th ed. p 3

Hippocrates also known as Father of Medicine[Q] is considered the 1st true epidemiologist.[Q]

Hippocrates in his book "Air, Water and Places" was the first Scientist to relate environment with health.

9. Ans. (d) Individuals way of living, Life style, personal habits

Ref: K. Park, 24th ed. p 19

Microenvironment

- It is also called as domestic environment.
- It includes an individual's way of living and lifestyle e.g. eating habits, personal habits like smoking, drinking etc.

MISCELLANEOUS

10. Ans. (b) All water supply is maintained and managed by State Government

Ref: K. Park, 24th ed. p 500

Swajaldhara – launched on 25th Dec 2002 is a community led participatory program aimed to
- Provide safe drinking water in rural areas, with full ownership of the community
- Build awareness on management of drinking water projects, including better hygienic practices
- Encourage water conservation practices along with rain water harvesting

11. Ans. (d) Water is exposed to the risk of dracunculiasis

Ref: K. Park, 24th ed. p 500

Accelerated Rural Water Supply Programme, 1972 defined Problem Village as village with -
- No available source of safe drinking water within a distance of 1.6 km or
- Water is available at a depth of more than 15 metres or
- Water has excess salinity, iron, fluorides and other toxic elements or
- Water is exposed to risk of cholera.

12. Ans. (d) 150 L

Ref: K. Park, 24th ed. p 743

Water Requirements

- *Physiological-Drinking water for survival is about 2L/ Person/ Day*[Q]
- *Urban domestic purposes - 150-200 L per capita per day is considered adequate.*[Q]
- Rural area -40 L of water per capita per day is the target

13. Ans. (d) Continuous and high pressure

Ref: K. Park, 24th ed. p 765

WHO does not recommend intermittent and low pressure service water distribution system

Types of Water Distribution System

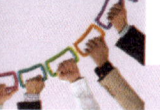

Type	Advantage	Disadvantage
Intermittent supply — *Water is supplied only during fixed hours*	▪ Saves wastage of water	▪ Non availability of water in emergency ▪ Likelihood of contamination from improper storage practices ▪ Empty water pipes result in a negative pressure, leading to back-siphoning (Bacteria, foul gases may be sucked in via leaky joints) ▪ Outbreaks of Typhoid, Relapsing fever etc reported
Continuous supply-*Water is delivered 24 hours*	▪ Water is available in emergency, No need to store, Less likely to be contaminated	▪ Misuse and Wastage
Dual water supply (Kolkata)- *Separate set of pipes for supply of filtered water for personal* use and unfiltered water for flushing toilets, washing roads etc.	▪ Saves wastage of water	▪ People may mistake *unfiltered water for filtered water* ▪ Possibility of cross-connection exists.

Also Know........................

- Water supply in most Indian cities is Intermittent

PURIFICATION OF WATER – FILTRATION

14. Ans. (a) Multiple tube method is used for sampling; (c) Clostridial infection indicates recent infection

▪ Multiple tube method is used for sampling	No it is used to test for coliforms
▪ E. coil can be tested by Indole test	Yes, correct. Other indole positive organisms are H. Influenza, Proteus, shigella
▪ Clostridial infection indicates recent infection	No, it indicates remote or old water contamination
▪ Level of residual chlorine should be 0.5 mg/L	Yes correct
▪ Softening of water is recommended after 3 mEq/L of hardness	Yes, 1-3 mEq is recommended water for use. It is known as moderately hard water.

Contd...

15. Ans. (b) Horrock's apparatus

Horrock's apparatus is used for chlorine demand
Chlorine estimation – by Chloroscope or Chlorometer
Chlorine estimation is done using Orthotolidine test

16. Ans. (b) Is a stable compound

No, bleaching powder or chlorinated lime is an unstable compound. It rapidly releases chlorine into the air

17. Ans. (c) Free and combined chlorine in water

18. Ans. (c) 1 ppm free chlorine should be present in water after break point has reached

The recommended level is 0.5 ppm of free chlorine after achieving break point chlorination

19. Ans. (a) All samples should be free from coliform

20. Ans. (b) Boiling

Chlorination, as expected is NOT the correct answer here. Chlorination is effective for most pathogens, however, it has no effect on the spores ova, cysts and certain viruses like poliovirus, hepatitis A virus, except in high concentration.

Iodine can be used for emergency disinfection, but altered odor, color alongside effect on thyroid function may not be a suitable choice

As far as UV rays is concerned, the viruses, bacterial spores, and the amoebic cysts required about 3 to 4 times, 9 times, and 15 times, respectively, the dose required for E. coli disinfection. The E. histolytica cysts are relatively resistant to disinfection of water with chlorine.

Boiling is a very effective procedure, but only applicable for smaller water supplies. It kills all bacteria, spores, cysts. Drinking boiled or bottled water is advised in such cases.

Filtration and boiling are recommended methods for water purification rather than chemical methods

21. Ans. d. Brucellosis

It is a zoonotic disease

22. Ans. (d) Clostridium botulinum

Clostridium botulinum is a Gram-positive, rod-shaped, anaerobic, spore-forming, motile bacterium with the ability to produce the neurotoxin botulinum. It is a food borne infection

23. Ans. (c) Prevent dental caries

24. Ans. (d) Turbidity

Chemical and biological oxygen demand are bacteriological indicators of water.

NO_2 is chemical indicator.

The physical parameters are: color, odor, turbidity, temperature

25. Ans. (d) Spring

26. Ans. (a) Lime

27. Ans. (b) Fecal contamination of remote origin

Faecal streptococci or nitrite—Indicator for recent contamination
Cl. perfringens or nitrates—Indicator for remote or old contamination

28. Ans. (d) Mass chemoprophylaxis

Mass chemoprophylaxis is not advised for the total community/cholera has healthy carriers, chronic carriers and mass chemoprophylaxis is not effective for preventing a single case of cholera

29. Ans. (a) Filtration of drinking water

Ref: K.Park (Page 220)

Filtration and boiling are recommended methods for water purification rather than chemical methods

30. Ans. (a) 0

31. Ans. (a) Aluminum sulfate

32. Ans. (b) Chlorination

33. Ans. (a) Ca and Mg bicarbonate

34. Ans. (c) 3.5%

This means that for every 1 litre of seawater there are 35 grams of salts are dissolved in it.

35. Ans. (d) Kala-Azar

Kala-azar is a vector borne disease

36. Ans. (a) Free residual chlorine

37. Ans. (d) Chlorine gas

In public health water supply systems, chlorination is done by a permanent supply of chlorine gas and further storage before supply to community

38. Ans. (a) Hardness of water

It is a method for removal of hardness of water. It uses sodium zeolite and removes both permanent and temporary

39. Ans. (d) Salmonella typhi

40. Ans. (d) 33%

41. Ans. (a) Base exchange process

Synonyms are ion exchange process or base exchange process or zeolite softening. When sodium zeolite is added to hard water, the Ca and Mg ions exchange with Na_2Z and forms Ca and Mg permutit and the water is softened to zero hardness

42. Ans. (c) 0.5 ppm

The best answer here should be 0.5 ppm as the MCQ is asking for minimum levels.

The recommended chlorine levels in impending outbreak is 0.7 ppm

43. Ans. (a) 4:1

The formation of chloramine consists of adding ammonia in the presence of free chlorine in a ratio of about 3 – 5 parts free chlorine to 1 part of ammonia.

44. Ans. (b) Calcium hypochlorite ($CaOCl_2$)

45. Ans. (c) Rain

46. Ans. (c) Moderately hard water

47. Ans. (d) Past faecal pollution

48. Ans. (b) Potable water

49. Ans. (a) Blue baby syndrome

Blue baby syndrome could be due to methemoglobinemia potentially caused by nitrates in drinking water

50. Ans. (b) Back washing

For rapid sand filter: backwashing is done almost daily or multiple times a day and requires a skilled operator

51. Ans. (c) 15 meters

52. Ans. (d) Algae and fungi

Algae are particular problems in swimming pools and need persistent preventive measures.
Green algae–susceptible to chemical treatment – super chlorination
Mustard algae–resistant to chemical treatment, amenable to copper based ($CuSO_4$) algicide.
Black algae–needs more stringent measures with wire brushes and superchlorination
A pool concentration of 0.3 ppm – 0.6 ppm is usually considered "algae control" typical level. Any level above this will likely turn the hair green.
Other algicide is: potassium tetraborate. This chemical, when added to the pool water in proper dosage, prevents algae from converting carbon dioxide into the fuel it needs for growth. It is quite effective.

53. Ans. (b) Trachoma

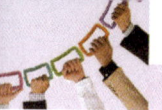

Water washed diseases are due to lack of hygiene and sanitation. It may include trachoma, dermatitis, scabies, pediculosis

54. Ans. (b) 0.5 to 0.8 ppm

- Fluoride concentration of 0.5 to 0.8 ppm in drinking water is considered optimum (a concentration of 1 ppm is regarded as optimum in temperate climate because the consumption of water is low).
- The recommended maximum limit in drinking water is 1—2 mg/L.

55. Ans. (b) 1 and 2

Guidelines for drinking water by WHO has the following variables:

- Acceptability aspect,
- Microbiological aspect,
- Chemical aspect, and
- Radiological aspect.
  - Microbiological aspects – refers to bacteriological quality of drinking water.
  - Virologic aspects: Drinking water should be free from any virus infections for man. To inactivate virus, disinfections with 0.5 mg/L of free chlorine residual after contact period of at least 1 hour at pH 8.0.

56. Ans. (b) 1 hr

Principles of chlorination:

- Water to be chlorinated should be clear and free from turbidity as it may decrease the effect of chlorination
- Estimate chlorine demand (by Horrock's apparatus)
- Add the estimated required chlorine by bleaching powder or perchloron or high test hypochlorite solution of chlorine gas
- Estimate the amount of residual chlorine remaining at the end of a specific period of contact (usually 60 minutes), at a given temperature and pH of the water".
- Chlorine estimation is to be done – orthotolidine test in a chloroscope, should be more than 0.5 ppm after minimum contact period of one hour

57. Ans. (b) 0.5 mg/dl

58. Ans. (a) It has residual effect

- Chlorination is one of the greatest advances in water purification. It is supplement, not a substitute to sand filtration
- Chlorine kills pathogenic bacteria, but is has no effect on spores and certain viruses (E.g., polio, viral hepatitis) except in high doses.

59. Ans. (a) It has biological zoogleal layer

Trickling filter method is used for treating effluent from the primary sedimentation tank. Trickling filters has a zoogleal layer over the surface and down through the filter. Zoogleal layer is a very complex biological growth consisting of fungi and bacteria of many kinds. Trickling filters do not need rest pauses, because wind blows freely through the beds supplying the oxygen needed by the zoogleal flora. The action of the tricking filter is purely biological one, and not the mechanical one as suggested by the name.

60. Ans. (a) Achieves better bacteriological purity

61. Ans. (b) 0.5 mm

Rapid sand filters:

- Rapid sand filters are of two types.
  - Gravity type (e.g. Paterson's filter)
  - Pressure type (E.g. candy's filter).
- Both the types are in use
- Each unit of Filter bed has a surface of about 80 to 90 m^2 (about 900 sq. feet).
- Sand is the filtering medium. The "effective size" of the sand particles is between 0.4-0.7 mm. The depth of the sand bed is usually about 1 metre. Below the sand bed is a layer of graded gravel, 30 to 40 cm deep.
- The depth of the water on the top of the sand bed is 1.0 to 1.5 m (5-6 feet). The under-drains at the bottom of the filter beds collect the filtered water. The rate of filtration is 5-15 m^3/ m^2/hour

62. Ans. (b) On the sand bed

Vital layer: When the filter is newly laid, it acts merely as a mechanical strainer, and cannot truly be considered as "biological".

- But very soon, the surface of the sand bed gets covered with a slimy growth known as "Schmutzdecke", vital layer, zoogleal layer or biological layer.
- This layer is slimy and gelatinous and consists of threadlike algae and numerous forms of life including plankton, diatoms and bacteria.
- The formation of vital layer is known as "ripening" of the filter. It may take several days for the vital layer to form fully, and when fully formed it extends for '2 to 3 cm 'into the top portion of the sand bed.

63. Ans. (c) Bleaching powder is dissolved in water and immediately added to the well

Dissolve bleaching powder in water: The bleaching powder required for disinfecting the well is placed in a bucket (not more than 100 g in one bucket of water) and made into a thick paste.

- More water is added till the bucket is nearly three-fourths full
- The content are stirred well, and allowed to sediment for 5 to 10 minutes when lime settles down.
- The supernatant solution which is chlorine solution is transferred to another bucket, and the chalk or lime is discarded.

64. Ans. (a) Free Chlorine

Bleaching powder:

- When freshly made, bleaching powder contains about 33% of "available chlorine". It is, however, an unstable compound.

- On exposure to air, light and moisture, it rapidly loses its chlorine content.
  But when mixed with excess of lime, it retains its strength; this is called "stabilized bleach'
- Chlorine controls algae and slime - organisms.

65. Ans. (a) Streptococci

- The primary bacterial indicator of fecal pollution—coliform (typical example of fecal group of E. coil and of the nonfecal group of Klebsiella aerogenes).
- For recent fecal pollution—fecal streptococci.
- For remote contamination—Clostridium perfringens (in absence of coliform).

66. Ans. (d) 50 mg $CaCO_3$ (50 ppm)

67. Ans. (d) Cardiovascular diseases

There is an inverse statistical association between the hardness of drinking water and the death rate from cardiovascular disease.

68. Ans. (d) Sodium thiosulfate

Explanation:
If water to be sampled contains or is likely to contain chlorine, a small quantity of sodium thiosulfate (0.1 mL of 3% solution or crystal of the salt) should be added to the bottle before sterilization.

69. Ans. (c) Nitrates below 0.1 mg/litre

The maximum recommended concentration of nitrates in drinking water is below 50 mg/lit.

Constituents	Recommended maximum concentration in drinking water (mg/L)
Lead	0.01
Nitrate	50
Nitrite	3
Manganese	0.5
Fluoride	1.5
Hardness	300

70. Ans. (a) Contact period of at least 6 hours is essential

- To kill bacteria and viruses, a minimum residual free chlorine concentration of 0.5 mg/L. For a contact period of at least one hour is essential.
- Bacterial spores protozoal cysts and helminthic ova are resistant to chlorination (except at high doses of chlorine).

71. Ans. (b) Red color in ten seconds

Orthotolidine Test is done by adding 0.1 ml of the reagent to one ml of water. The yellow color produced is matched against color discs. It is essential to take the reading within ten seconds after the addition of the reagent to estimate free chlorine in water. The color that is produced after a lapse of fifteen to twenty minutes is due to the action of both free and combined chlorine.

72. Ans. (b) Acts best when pH is around 7

- Chlorine acts best as a disinfectant when the pH of water is around 7 because of the predominance of hypochlorous acid, the form which is mainly responsible for the disinfecting action of chlorine.

73. Ans. (c) 0.7

Chlorination of water is first priority of ensuring water quality in emergency situations. Since the risk of epidemics in such situation is high, residual chlorine level desirable is little higher. Normally the chlorination level for a water source is 0.5 mg/L.

74. Ans. (d) Orthotolidine test

Both free and combined chlorine in water can be determined by orthotolidine test. In this test 0.1 ml of reagent (analytical grade O-tolidine dissolved in 10% solution of HCL) is added to 1 ml of water. The yellow color produced is matched against suitable standards or color discs. It is essential to take the reading within 10 seconds after the addition of reagent to estimate free chlorine in water, because the color produced after a lapse of 15-20 minutes is due to action of both free and combined chlorine.

75. Ans. (b) 0.5-0.8

Fluorine is the most abundant element in nature. About 96% of the fluoride in the body is found in bones and teeth. Fluorine is essential for the normal mineralization of bones and formation of dental enamel. The major source of fluorine to man is drinking water and in most parts of India the fluoride content of drinking water is about 0.5 mg per liter. In fluorosis-endemic areas it may be as high as 3 to 12 mg per liter. Fluorides also occur in traces in many foods but some foods such as sea fish, cheese and tea are rich in fluorides. Fluorine is a double-edged sword because prolonged ingestion of fluorides through drinking water in excess of the daily requirement is associated with dental and skeletal fluorosis; and inadequate intake with dental carries. The recommended level of fluorides in drinking water in India is accepted as 0.5 to 0.8 mg per liter.

76. Ans. (d) They are never present in portable water

Ref: K. Park page 669

77. Ans. (b) Porcelain

Ref: K. Park, 24th ed. p 754

Type of Filter	Candle
Chamberland filter	Porcelain
Berkefeld filter	Kieselguhr (Infusorial earth)
Katadyn filter	Candle is coated with silver catalyst (Kills bacteria by "oligodynamic" action of the silver ions)

Pasteur Chamberl and Type Filter

- Consists of porous tubes or bougies of unglazed porcelain screwed to a tap
- It is mechanical filter

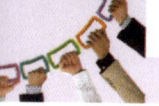

- It is slow acting
- It can separate suspended particle and bacteria but not virus

78. Ans. (b) Top layers of sand bed

Ref: K. Park, 23r d ed. p-712; 24th ed. p 749

Elements of a Slow Sand Filter (Top to Bottom)

- Supernatant raw water about *1 to 1.5 metre depth.*[Q]
  - Provides a constant head of water to overcome resistance of filter bed and promote downward flow of water through the sand bed.
  - Waiting period is 3-12 hours. *Partial purification occurs by sedimentation, oxidation and particle agglomeration.*
- ***"Schmutzdecke"*** *or* ***Vital layer*** extends for 2–3 cm into top portion of the sand bed
  - *It removes organic matter and bacteria, oxidizes ammoniacal nitrogen into nitrates and yields bacteria-free water*[Q]
- Sand Bed (*0.2–0.3 mm diameter* free from clay and organic matter about 1 m thick)
  - As water percolates through the sand bed, it gets purified by *mechanical straining, sedimentation, adsorption, oxidation and bacterial action.*[Q]
- Layer of graded gravel (30–40 cm deep)- It supports the Sand bed
- **Under-drainage system** of porous/ perforated pipes at bottom of filter bed. It provides outlet for filtered water and supports the filter medium.
- **Filter control valves** incorporated in the outlet - pipes maintain a constant rate of filtration.

Also Know.......................

- Venturimeter measures bed resistance (loss of head) If it exceeds 1.3 m it is uneconomical to run the filter.

79. Ans. (a) 0.2 to 0.3 mm

Ref: K. Park, 24th ed. p 751

Effective size of sand in Rapid sand filter is 0.4–0.7 mm and *Slow sand filter* ***is*** 0.2–0.3 mm.

80. Ans. (c) Formation of vital layer

Ref: K. Park, 24th ed. p 749

"Schmutzdecke" *or* ***Vital/zoogleal/biological layer*** is a slimy gelatinous layer of algae, plankton, diatoms and bacteria in a slow sand filter.

- *It is referred to as* ***"heart"*** *of slow sand filter.*[Q] It extends for about 2-3 cm into top portion of the sand bed
- Its formation is known as "***ripening***" of filter.[Q]

81. Ans. (b) 5 to 15 m³/ m²/ hour

Ref: K. Park, 24th ed. p 750

Rate of Filtration of Water

- Rapid sand filter is **5 to 15 m**^{3}*/hour/ m*^{2} *of sand bed surface.*[Q]
- *Slow sand filter is 0.1 to 0.4 m*^{3}*/hour/m*^{2} *of sand bed surface.*[Q]

82. Ans. (c) Scraping

Ref: K. Park, 24th ed. p 750

Filter Cleaning

- Slow sand filter it is done by Scraping off the top portion of the sand bed (1-2 cm)
- Rapid sand filter it is done by back-washing with water or compressed air

83. Ans. (b) Asbestos filter

Ref: F.J. Baker, R.E. Silverton, Introduction to Medical Laboratory Technology

Seitz filter is made of Asbestos disc supported in a metal mount, attached to a vacuum flask by a silicone rubber bung

- Type K has largest pores
- Type EK has smallest pores

84. Ans. (c) Requires longer duration

Ref: K. Park, 24th ed. p 751

Refer to Notes

85. Ans. (c) Zoological layer

Ref: K. Park, 24th ed. p 749

86. Ans. (d, e) (d) Take more time for purification; (e) Size of sand is smaller

Ref: K. Park, 24th ed. p 750

Slow Sand Filter

- **Advantages:** Cheaper, easy to operate (less skilled), No pre-treatment of water needed, better removal of bacteria.
- Disadvantages- Slow, large area needed

PURIFICATION OF WATER – CHLORINATION RESIDUAL CHLORINE

87. Ans. (a) Hypochlorous acid

Ref: K. Park, 24th ed. p 751 Disinfecting action of chlorine is mainly due to hypochlorous acid[Q]

Disinfecting action of chlorine is mainly due to hypochlorous acid[Q] (Small extent due to Hypochlorite ions).

- Hence it acts best at pH of around 7[Q] It is unreliable when pH value exceeds 8.5

88. Ans. (a) Hypochlorous acid

Ref: K. Park, 24th ed. p 751

89. Ans. (b) 0.5 mg/L for a contact period of 1 hour

Ref: K. Park, 24th ed. p 752

Minimum recommended concentration of free chlorine is 0.5 mg/L of water at the end of 1 hour contact.[Q]

90. Ans. (d) 20 L

Ref: K. Park, 24th ed. p 754

91. (d) Free and combined chlorine

Ref: K. Park, 24th ed p752

Tests for Chlorination of Water

- **Orthotolidine (OT) Test**- measures *free chlorine (**within 10 seconds**) and free + combined chlorine (**15-20 minutes**) in water.*[Q]
- **Orthotolidine Arsenite (OTA) Test** measures *free and combined chlorine residuals separately.*[Q] Errors due to interfering substances (nitrites, iron and manganese) in OT test is overcome by OTA test

92. Ans. (b) 0.5 mg/L

Ref: Textbook of Community Medicine, Rajvir Bhalawar, 1st ed., p-713, WHO Factsheet on Chlorine Monitoring.

Water source	Residual chlorine after treatment
Clear piped water at all points	0.5-1 mg/L
Protected tube wells, ring wells, clear rain water	2 mg/L
Tanker filling site	2 mg/L
Unprotected wells and cloudy water (filtered before purifying)	5 mg/L

Minimum recommended level of residual chloride in water after treatment is 0.5 mg/L after 30 minutes contact time

93. Ans. (a) Super chlorination followed by dechlorination

Ref: K. Park, 24th ed. p 752

Super chlorination comprises addition of large doses of chlorine to water and removal of excess of chlorine after disinfection.

- It is *applicable to heavily polluted water*[Q]

Also Know........................

Methods of chlorination

- Chlorine gas (1st choice *for disinfection of urban water supplies*[Q] - cheap, quick, efficient and easy to apply)
- Chloramine (slower action, but gives a more persistent residual chlorine)
- Perchloron (60–70% of available chlorine).[Q]

94. Ans. (b) 1 hour

Ref: K. Park, 24th ed. p 752

95. Ans. (a) Hypochlorous acid

Ref: K. Park, 24th ed. p 751

96. Ans. (c) Free and combined chlorine

Ref: K. Park, 24th ed. p 752

97. Ans. (c) Chlorine in water

Ref: K. Park, 24th ed. p 752

98. Ans. (d) 0.5 mg/L

Ref: K. Park, 24th ed. p 766

Horrock's apparatus is used to estimate the ***chlorine demand*** of water and to find out the ***dose of bleaching powder*** required for disinfection of water.

Steps

- A stock solution is made by taking a level spoonful (2 g) of bleaching powder and water in the black cup.
- 6 white cups are filled with water to be tested, up to about a cm below the brim and then one drop of stock solution is added to the 1st cup, 2 drops to the 2nd cup, 3 drops to the 3rd cup, and so on.
- 3 drops of **starch -iodide indicator** is added to each of the white cups and stirred again.
- *Development of blue color indicates the presence of free residual chlorine.*
- The 1st cup which shows distinct blue color is noted. Supposing the 3rd cup shows blue Color, then 3 level spoonful's or 6 g of bleaching powder would be required to disinfect 455 L of water

Also Know........................

- ***Berkefeld filter*** is used for filtration of water on small scale
- ***Double pot method*** devised by NEERI, ensures a constant dosage of chlorine to well water during an emergency
- **Chloroscope** is used for measuring residual chlorine level

99. Ans. (d) Starch Iodide

Ref: K. Park, 24th ed. p 766

Starch-iodide is the indicator used in Horrock's apparatus. It develops a blue Color in presence of free residual chlorine.

100. Ans. (b) Horrock's apparatus

Ref: K. Park, 24th ed. p 765

101. Ans. (a) Lime + Alum

Ref: S Lal, Textbook of Community Medicine, 4th ed. p-258

Nalgonda technique devised by National Environment Engineering Research Institute, Nagpur is used for defluoridation of water.

- It involves addition of lime, bleaching powder and alum in sequence followed by flocculation, sedimentation and filtration.

102. Ans. (a) Nalgonda technique

Ref: S Lal, Textbook of Community Medicine, 4th ed., p-258

103. Ans. (b) Soft water

Ref: K. Park, 24th ed. p 746

104. Ans. (b) Addition of sodium carbonate

Ref: K. Park, 24th ed. p 764

Hardness	Cause	Treatment option
Carbonate or Temporary hardness	Calcium and Magnesium bicarbonates[Q]	Boiling of water, Addition of lime or Sodium carbonate and Permutit process
Non-carbonate or Permanent hardness	Calcium and Magnesium sulfates, chlorides and nitrates.[Q]	Addition of Sodium carbonate and Permutit process

105. Ans. (c) Sodium bicarbonate

Ref: K. Park, 24th ed. p 764

106. Ans. (d) 150 mg/L

Ref: K. Park, 24th ed. p 764

- Drinking water should be moderately hard. *Softening is recommended when hardness exceeds 3 mEq/L (150 mg/L).*[Q]

107. Ans. (b) Moderately hard

Ref: K. Park, 24th ed. p 764

108. Ans. (c) 1-3 mEq/L

Ref: K. Park, 24th ed. p 764

WATER QUALITY STANDARDS AND BACTERIOLOGICAL INDICATORS OF WATER CONTAMINATION

109. Ans. (d) Halophilic vibrio

Ref: K. Park, 24th ed. p 757

Bacteriological indicators of water contamination (*fecal contamination*):

- ***Primary indicator:*** Coliform group of organisms (E. coli)
- ***Supplementary indicator:*** Fecal streptococci and *Spores of CI perfringens*

110. Ans. (b) E. coli

Ref: K. Park, 24th ed. p 757

111. Ans. (d) 15 m

Ref: K. Park, 24th ed. p 746

Sanitary well is a properly located, well-constructed well that is protected against contamination and yields a supply of safe water

- It is located at a higher elevation (≥15 m or 50 feet) from a likely sources of contamination, Its location is such that no user has to carry water for >100 m.
- It is lined with bricks or stones set in cement up to a depth of ≥6 m or 20 feet. Lining is extended 60-90 cm (2-3 feet) above the ground level.
- It has a parapet wall ≥ 70-75 cm height above ground.
- It has a concrete platform round the well extending ≥ 1 m in all directions with a gentle slope outwards
- It has a drain along the edges of the platform that carries off spilled water to a public drain or soakage pit constructed well beyond "cone of filtration" (area of drainage) of the well.
- The top is closed by a cement concrete cover.
- Water is lifted using a hand pump

Also Know......................

- Strict cleanliness in the vicinity of the well is the responsibility of the consumers for success of Sanitary well.

112. Ans. (b) Water contamination

Ref: K. Park, 24th ed. p 757

113. Ans. (a) Staphylococcus

Ref: Park 23/e, p 721, 22/e, p 674

114. Ans. (a) Eijkman test

Ref: Mahajan and Gupta, Textbook of Preventive and Social Medicine, 4th ed., p-58

- **Presumptive coliform count (multiple tube technique)** yields the probable number of Coliform bacilli per 100 mL of water (using McCrady's table).
- **Eijkman's test** is used to confirm type of Coliform organism (Fecal/Nonfecal) by incubating tubes at 37°C and 44°C.
- E. coli grow at 44°C while the other coliforms do not.

115. Ans. (d) Fecal streptococci

Ref: K. Park, 24th ed. p 758

- ***Spores of CI perfringens*** *in absence of coliform group suggests remote fecal contamination.*[Q]
- **Fecal streptococci** *in water suggest recent fecal contamination.*[Q]

116. Ans. (b) E. coli

Ref: K. Park, 24th ed. p 757

All coliforms organisms are assumed to be of fecal origin unless a non fecal origin is proved.[Q]

Reasons for choosing coliform organisms as indicators of fecal pollution:

- They are constantly present in abundance in human intestine. An average person excretes 200-400 billion per day.
- They are foreign to potable waters.
- They are easily detected by culture methods - as small as 1 bacteria in 100 mL of water.
- They survive longer

Frequency of collection of water samples for bacteriological confirmation – 2 successive samples should be collected at least 1 month apart (if population served is <20000), 14 days apart (if population served is 20001-50,000), 4 days apart (population served is 50001-1 Lakh) and 1 day (if population served is > 1 Lakh)

117. Ans. (d) Streptococci

Ref: K. Park, 24th ed. p 758

118. Ans. (b) Staphylococcus

Ref: K. Park, 24th ed. p 757-58

119. Ans. (a) Clostridium spores indicates recent…

Ref: K. Park, 24th ed. p 757

Spores of ***Cl. perfringens*** in natural water *in absence of coliform group suggest remote fecal contamination.*[Q]
Fecal streptococci *in water suggest recent fecal contamination.*[Q]

- In any *100 mL* drinking water *sample, E. coli or thermo tolerant Coliform bacteria must not be detectable.*
- In case of large supplies (many samples are examined) *E. coli or thermo tolerant Coliform bacteria* must not be present in 95% of samples taken throughout any 12 month period or Not more than 5% samples should have any coliforms.
- In rural areas *Coliform bacteria are not acceptable indicators of sanitary quality of water supply, particularly in tropical areas.*[Q]

120. Ans. (c) 15 TCU

Ref: K. Park, 24th ed p758

WHO Criteria for Drinking Water Quality

Refer to Notes

121. Ans. (d) 1000

Ref: K. Park, 24th ed. p 758

Water is unpalatable at TDS > 1200 mg/ L. TDS < 1000 mg/L is acceptable

122. Ans. (b) 0.5 – 0.8 ppm

Ref: K. Park, 24th ed. p 663

Acceptable fluoride concentration in drinking water is 0.5 to 0.8 mg/L.[Q] (In temperate countries, with low water intake acceptable level is 1–2 mg/ L.)
Maximum recommend concentration is 1.5 mg/L

123. Ans. (a) pH is to be kept between 7.4 – 7.8…

Ref: K. Park, 23rd ed. p 728

***Sanitation measures* for swimming pool**–(Bacteriological quality of water should be close to standards for drinking water)

- Recommended area per swimmer is 2.2 square meter (24 sq. ft.)
- Rules and regulations governing use of pool should be displayed in prominent places.
- Entry of persons suffering from skin, eye, ear and upper respiratory tract or other communicable disease is restricted.
- All bathers need to be strictly instructed to empty the bladder and if necessary use the toilet
- A cleansing shower bath in nude with soap and water is required before entering the pool
- Spitting, spouting of water, blowing the nose are prohibited
- Shower rooms, walk ways and pool decks must be properly disinfected.
- ***Swimming pools must be equipped with rapid sand filters***[Q] *All water must be refiltered in less than 6 hours and Up to 15 % of water should be replaced by fresh water every day*[Q] (To remove solutes ammonia, albuminoid, organic and nitrate nitrogen derived from the bathers).
- *Chlorination is the most widely used method for pool disinfection.*[Q] *1 mg/L (1 ppm) of free residual chlorine must be maintained at all times to provide adequate protection against bacteria and virus.*[Q]
- The pH of water must be kept between 7.4-7.8

Also Know……………………

- ***Health hazards associated with swimming pools are:***
- Fungal (Epidermophyton/Trichophyton-Athlete's foot) and Viral (HPV → plantar warts) infection of skin.
- Infections of the eye, ear, upper respiratory tract and Intestinal infections
- Accidents

124. Ans. (c) Ammonia

Ref: Mahajan and Gupta, Textbook of Preventive and Social Medicine, 4th ed., p-59, Ref: K. Park, 24th ed. p 756

Ammonia is formed by decomposition of organic matter and its presence indicates organic or sewage pollution of recent origin.

- Maximum acceptable level is of 0.005 mg/l.

Nitrate and Nitrite are naturally occurring ions and part of nitrogen cycle.

125. Ans. (a) Color < 5 TCU

Ref: K. Park, 24th ed. p 756

The standard limits for chloride is 200 mg/L, while the upper permissible limits are 600 mg/L
Zinc levels should be below 5mg/L

126. Ans. (d) Lead

Ref: K. Park, 24th ed. p 757

Lead (Toxicant and possible human carcinogen) is the mineral most undesirable in water

- *Susceptible individuals are Infants, children up to six years of* age, and pregnant women
- *Lead interferes with calcium metabolism, is toxic to both* central and peripheral nervous system
- *Health-based guideline value of lead is 0.01mg/L.*

127. Ans. (d) 600 mg/L

Ref: K. Park, 24th ed. p 756

Standard prescribed for chloride in water is 200 mg/L. and Maximum permissible level is 600 mg/L.[Q]

AIR

128. Ans. (c) Humidity

129. Ans. (a) CO_2

CO_2 is a good indicator for climate change and global warming for Air pollution – gasses as Carbon monoxide, sulphur dioxide are the indicators.

130. Ans. (a) Air pollution

131. Ans. (d) CFCs

132. Ans. (a) Methane

133. Ans. (b) CO_2

134. Ans. (d) Hydrochloric acid

The main component of acid rain is sulphuric acid mixed with water and other acids. It is not containing the HCl (hydrochloric acid)

135. Ans. (d) Carbon-monoxide

Air pollution indices are:
- Sulphur dioxide index
- Soiling index
- Suspended particulate matter
- Air pollution index
- Coefficient of haze

Carbon monoxide is a widely distributed pollutant gas, but is not an indicator for air pollution.

136. Ans. (b) Air velocity

137. Ans. (c) Cooling power of air

138. Ans. (c) 4000 Hz or 90 db

139. Ans. (a) Smoke and dust

Smoke, dust are considered as secondary air pollutants. Primary air pollutants are the gasses - CO, CO_2, H_2S, CH_4, NO_2, SO_2

140. Ans. (c) Acid rain

141. Ans. (a) CO_2

Because it is a natural constituent of air

142. Ans. (a) Carbon dioxide

- The main sources of air pollution are:
- Automobiles:
  Motor vehicles are a major source of air pollution throughout the urban areas.
- They emit hydrocarbons, carbon monoxide, lead, nitrogen oxides and particulate matter. In strong sunlight, certain of these hydrocarbons and oxides of nitrogen maybe converted in the atmosphere into "photochemical" pollutants of oxidizing nature. In addition, diesel engines, when misused or badly adjusted are capable of emitting black smoke and malodorous fumes
- Carbon dioxide: This is not commonly regarded as automobile pollutant.
  Carbon dioxide is a natural constituent of the air.

143. Ans. (a) Sulphur dioxide

- Best indicators of air pollution are sulphur dioxide, smoke, suspended particles.

144. Ans. (c) Volatile organic compounds

145. Ans. (a) Cooling power of air

Kata thermometer is a device consisting of two thermometers, one a dry bulb and the other a wet bulb. Both thermometers are heated to 43.3°C and the time required for each thermometer to fall from 37.8° to 32.2°C is noted. The dry bulb gives the cooling power by radiation and convection, the wet bulb by radiation, convection, and evaporation.

146. Ans. (d) 1 adult, 1 child of 6 years and a 6 month old infant

Ref: K. Park, 24th ed. p 789

Overcrowding is a condition in which more number of people are living within a single dwelling than there is space for, so that movement is restricted, privacy secluded, hygiene impossible, rest and sleep difficult

Accepted standards with respect to overcrowding

Persons per room	Floor space	Sex separation
▪ 1 room – 2 persons ▪ 2 rooms – 3 persons ▪ 3 rooms – 5 persons ▪ 4 rooms - 7 persons ▪ 5 or more rooms –10 persons (additional 2 for nil each further room)	▪ 110 sq.ft. or more -2 persons ▪ 90-100 sq.ft. - 11/2 persons ▪ 70-90 sq.ft. - 1 person ▪ 50-70 sq.ft. - 1/2 person ▪ < 50 sq.ft –Nil ▪ Infant is not counted ▪ Children aged 1 to 10 are counted as half a unit.	▪ Overcrowding exists if 2 persons over 9 years of age, not husband and wife, of opposite gender are obliged to sleep in the same room

$$\text{Degree of overcrowding} = \frac{\text{No. persons in the household}}{\text{No. of rooms in the dwelling}}$$

Risks associated with overcrowding– Spread of infectious diseases (TB, Influenza and Diphtheria), irritability, frustration, lack of sleep, anxiety, violence and mental disorders. Children are more affected.

147. Ans. (d) Neurodevelopment problems

Ref: K. Park, 24th ed. p 772-73

Indoor air pollution

- Rural people in developing countries are most exposed to indoor air pollution (2/3rd of global exposure to particulates.)
- Women and young children exposed to high levels of indoor air pollution suffer more

Latest Updates

Hazards of Indoor air pollution

- 4.3 million premature deaths occur per year from illness due to indoor air pollution. (Pneumonia-12%, Stroke-34%, Ischemic heart disease-26%, COPD- 22% and Lung cancer-6%).
- Risk of childhood pneumonia is doubled
- Low birth weight/Still birth, Tuberculosis, Cataract, Nasopharyngeal and Laryngeal cancers.

148. Ans. (d) Mercury vapor

Ref: K. Park, 24th ed. p 773

149. Ans. (d) CFCs

Ref: Global change of planet earth OECD, Wikepedia, K Park, 24th ed. p 785

Global warming is increase in average global surface temperature brought about by emission of greenhouse gases into the atmosphere. It is expected to contribute to

- Rise in global surface temperature to *about 30°C by 2030*, resulting in a *rise in sea level of 0.1-0.3 m by 2050*
- Increase in occurrence of extreme climatic events (cyclones, heat waves, draughts), impaired grain production and emergence of vector borne diseases in new areas.

Major greenhouse gases in earth's atmosphere and their direct contribution to greenhouse effect are

- Water vapor (36–72%)
- Carbon dioxide (9–26%)
- Methane (4–9%)
- Ozone (3–7%)–Beneficial cuts down UV transmission
- Other greenhouse gases include Nitrous oxide, Sulfur hydrofluorocarbons (CFC) and perfluorocarbons.

Also Know......................

Kyoto Protocol is an international agreement linked to United Nations Framework Convention on Climate Change

- It came into force on 16 February 2005
- It sets binding targets for 37 industrialized countries and European community for reducing greenhouse gas emissions (CO_2, Methane, CFC, PFC, SF6, Nitrous oxide) by an average of 5% against 1990 levels over 2008- 2012.
- Protocol places a heavier burden on developed nations under principle of "common but differentiated responsibilities."
- 182 Parties of the Convention have ratified its Protocol to date.
- **Marrakesh Accords 2001** are detailed rules for implementation of the protocol
- Countries must meet their targets primarily through national measures or by way of market- based mechanisms i.e. *Carbon trading* the "***carbon market***", clean development mechanism and Joint implementation.

150. Ans. (a) CO_2, Ozone, Methane

Ref: K. Park, 24th ed. p 785

151. Ans. (a) CO_2 is a major greenhouse gas

Ref: K. Park, 24th ed. p 785

- *Major greenhouse gases* in earth's atmosphere are Water vapor, carbon dioxide, Methane, Ozone and Nitrous oxide.
- Ozone layer in stratosphere absorbs harmful UV–B radiation from sun.
- Ozone Hole (reduction in Ozone concentrations in Stratosphere) appears in winter over Antarctica
- ***Montreal Protocol*** stipulates that production and consumption of compounds that deplete ozone in the stratosphere such as CFC, Halons, Carbon tetrachloride, Methyl chloroform etc. are to be phased out.
- In India ***Ozone Depleting Substances (Regulation) Rules 2000*** set up under the Environmental Protection Act 1986 control the production, emission and consumption of Ozone depleting substances.
- **Green peace** is an NGO working against environmental degradation.

Also Know......................

- Heat island phenomenon – Cities are warmer than surrounding rural areas resulting in longer and more severe heat waves.

152. Ans. (a) SO_2

Ref: K. Park, 24th ed p 773

***Indicators of Air Pollution* (monitored on a daily basis over several sites)**

- **SO_2** (Sulfur dioxide) in urban and industrial areas.

Guideline value is 500 microgram/m^3 in 10 minutes (Time weighted average).

- *Smoke or* ***Soiling index***[Q].
- Suspended Particulate Matter.

Latest Updates

Particulate matter is a complex mixture of solid and liquid particles (organic and inorganic).

- It comprises of Sulfate, Nitrate, Ammonia, Sodium chloride, Black carbon, Mineral dust and water.
- PM10 is suspended particulate matter less than 10 µm in aerodynamic diameter. It enters the thoracic region.
- PM 2.5 (Fine fraction of PM10) has very high chances of deposition in smaller airways and alveoli.

Also Know......................

- ***Coefficient of haze*** is used in USA in assessing the amount of smoke or other aerosol in air.
- ***Air Pollution Index*** (API) used in USA = 10 x SO concentration*+2x Carbon monoxide concentration*+^{2} 2 x Coefficient of haze. It is alarming when the value API rises from its value of about 12-50 or more. *(ppm by volume).

153. Ans. (c) Air pollution

Ref: K. Park, 24th ed. p 773

Smoke or ***Soiling index*** is an index of air pollution and it is expressed in micrograms/m^3 of air over a period of time.

- A known volume of air is filtered through white filter paper under specified conditions and the stain is measured by photoelectric meter.

154. Ans. (d) Air pollution

Ref: K. Park, 24th ed. p 773

155. Ans. (d) Central Pollution Control Board

Ref: K. Park, 24th ed. p 774

National Air Quality Monitoring Programme, sponsored by Central Pollution Control Board (CPCB) monitors **air pollution in India** (since 1990). Common pollutants monitored are:

- Suspended Particulate Matter (SPM),
- Concentration ratio of < P10 fraction (Human Respirable Particles)
- Secondary pollutants (Chromium, copper, nickel, arsenic, lead, Sulfate, nitrate, ammonia, for the assessment of dry deposition of air pollutants

156. Ans. (b) Numbness

Ref: K. Park, 24th ed. p 784

Heat stress is the amount of heat that must be dissipated from the body, for it to remain in thermal equilibrium.

Effects of Heat Stress

Heat stroke: It is a triad very high body temperature [110 F (43.3°C)], CNS dysfunction (convulsions, partial/complete loss of consciousness) and Anhidrosis (absent or diminished sweating and dry hot skin)

- Attributed to failure of the heat regulating mechanism.
- Outcome is often fatal (CFR = 40%)
- Treatment→ Rapidly cooling of body with ice water bath [Bring rectal temperature <102°F (38.9°C)] Further treatment is supportive.

Heat hyperpyrexia: (Temperature > 106°F)

- Attributed to failure of the heat regulating mechanism of body without features of heat stroke. It may proceed to heat stroke.

Heat Exhaustion

- *Attributed to imbalance or inadequate replacement of water and salts lost in perspiration due to heat.*[Q]
- It occurs on exposure to high temperature for several days.
- Body temperature may be normal or moderately elevated [<102°F (38.9°C)]
- Treatment → Normalizing fluid and electrolyte balance. ***Heat cramps*** (Painful and spasmodic contractions of the skeletal muscles)
- Occur in persons doing heavy muscular work in high temperature and humidity.
- Occurs due to loss of sodium and chlorides from the body.

Heat Syncope

- Occurs due to pooling of blood in lower limbs due to dilatation of blood vessels, resulting in reduced cardiac output, Blood pressure and impaired supply to brain
- On exposure to heat for long hours (soldiers standing for parades in the sun) -Face turns pale, blood pressure falls and patient collapses suddenly. There is no rise in body temperature.
- Treatment –Lie down in the shade with the head slightly down; recovery occurs within 5 to 10 minutes.

Also Know........................

- *Acclimatization to heat* takes 10 - 14 days.

157. Ans. (b) 77-80°F

Ref: Suryakanta, Community Medicine with Recent advances, 3rd ed., p-48

Comfort Zone Criteria

- Corrected effective temperature →25–27°C or 77–80°F
- Relative humidity → 30–65%
- Dry kata → 6 and above
- Wet kata → 20 and above
- Predicted 4 hours sweat rate → 1-3 L

158. Ans. (c) Anemometer

Ref: K. Park, 24th p-787

- *Kata thermometer was originally devised for measuring the "cooling power" of the air.*[Q]
- *Now it is largely used as an anemometer for recording low air velocities.*[Q] It is to be done in open space at a height of 10 m.

Also Know......................

- Wind speed of 0.5 m/s is described as Complete calm, 1.3 m/s as Slight breeze, 10 m/s as Strong wind, 15–20 m/s as Storm, 25–30 m/s as Gale and> 30–50 m/s as Hurricane.

159. Ans. (a) 2-3

Ref: K. Park, 24th ed. p 776

Standards of Ventilation

- Cubic Space: 300 to 3,000 c.ft. per hour per person
- Air Change per hour: (More important than cubic space)- Living rooms 2 or 3,Work rooms/Assemblies 4 to 6.
  - More frequent air change (>6 times in one hour) may produce a drought.
  - Number of air changes per hour = Total hourly air supply to room / cubic capacity of the room.
- Floor Space per person-Optimum is 50 to 100 sq. ft. (Heights in excess of 10-12 feet are ineffective for ventilation)

Minimum Housing Standards

- Site–At a higher level from surroundings, with independent access to a street, away from vector breeding places and areas with dust, smoke, smell, excessive noise and traffic, pleasant surroundings and dry and safe soil, subsoil water should be below 10 feet

- Set back (Open space all-round the house for adequate lighting and ventilation) should be minimum 1/3rd and 2/3rd of total area in urban and rural area respectively. Rural houses should have ample verandah space
- Minimum No. of living room should be 2. Minimum 500 c.ft./capita of air space (preferably 1000 c.ft.)
- Floor should be impervious, easily washable, smooth, free from cracks and crevices, damp-proof, height of the plinth 2 to 3 feet Floor area minimum 120sq.ft for occupancy by > 1 person and 100 sq.ft for 1 person.
- Windows- 2 window per living room (Height < 3 feet above floor) with one opening directly to an open space.
- Wall- Strong (≥30 cm thick), plastered on both sides, smooth and colored (cream or white), weather resistant and with low heat capacity.
- Roof ≥10 feet in the absence of air-conditioning and with low heat transmittance coefficient.
- Lighting- Daylight factor >1 % over half the floor area.
- Ventilation - Window area 1/5th of the floor area and Door + window area combined 2/5th of the floor area.
- Separate kitchen, Bathroom with water supply and drainage
- Cattle shed (Rural area) should be 8 to 10 meters away from the living house and open on all sides, with area of 3 m^2 per cattle

Also Know......................

- Made soil - Ground leveled by dumping refuse is unsatisfactory for building purposes for at least 20 to 25 years.

160. Ans. (c) Air temperature, humidity and air movement

Ref: K. Park, 24th ed. p 784

Also Know......................

- *Cooling power of air has 3 determinants-* Air temperature, Humidity and Movement of air
- A wet Kata reading of >20 and dry Kata reading of >6 indicate thermal comfort

LIGHT

161. Ans. (b) Lumen

Ref: K. Park, 24th ed. p 777

Also Know......................

Measurement of light

- **Luminous intensity** refers to "power" of a light source, radiating in all directions and is measured as candelas or candle power
- **Luminous flux** is the flow of light related to a unit of solid angle measured in lumens.
- **Illumination or illuminance** is the amount of light reaching a surface measured in lux per unit area.
- **Brightness or luminance** is the amount of light reflected from a surface measured in lamberts.

162. Ans. (a) Candela

Ref: K. Park, 24th ed. p 777

163. Ans. (a) 8%

Ref: K. Park, 24th ed. p 777-78

Daylight Factor (D.F.) is the ratio of illumination at a given point to illumination at a point exposed simultaneously to whole hemisphere of the sky (taken as 500 foot candles) excluding direct sunlight.

$$D.F = \frac{\text{Instantaneous illumination indoors}}{\text{Simultaneous illumination outdoors}} \times 100$$

- In living rooms a DF of at least 8% and in kitchens DF of about 10% is recommended.

NOISE

164. Ans. (d) 70-85 dB

165. Ans. (c) 90 dB

166. Ans. (b) 20 to 20,000 Hz

- The human ear can hear frequencies from about 20 to 20,000 Hz.

167. Ans. (c) 85 dB

Ref: K. Park, 24th ed. p 779

Daily exposure of up to 85 dB is the limit people can tolerate without substantial loss to their hearing.

Also Know......................

- Acceptable levels of noise in dB at work places- Hospital wards-20–35, Class room/Library – 30–40, Lab – 40–50, Factory workshops and Restaurants-40–60, Offices- 35- 45, Living room -40, Bed room -25.

168. Ans. (b) 30–40 dB

Ref: K. Park, 24th ed. p 779

169. Ans. (a) 85 dB

Ref: K. Park, 24th ed. p 779

Acceptable loudness of noise *that people can tolerate without substantial damage to their hearing is 85 dB.*

Also Know......................

- Phone is a psychoacoustic index of loudness. It takes into consideration intensity and frequency.

170. Ans. (c) 85 dB

Ref: K. Park, 24th ed. p 778

RADIATION

171. Ans. (c) 5 rad

According to ICRP, additional permissible dose of radiation to man in a source should not be more than 5rem a year.

Remember the following important points commonly asked in examination:

- Amount of radiation received from outer space and background radiation is about 0.1 RAD a year.
- Skin dose of radiation from a single x-ray film varies roughly from 0.02 to 3 RAD.
- Alpha particles are 10 times as harmful as x-rays, beta particles or gamma rays.
- Gamma ray has tissue penetration power of about 50 cm (maximum besides some cosmic rays).
- Alpha particles cannot penetrate lead.
- Lead apron 0.5 mm thick reduces the intensity of scattered X-rays over 90%.

172. Ans. (b) Rad

Ref: K. Park, 24th ed. p 781

Unit of Absorbed Radiation is Rad

- *Amount of radiation received from outer space and background radiation* is about 0.1 rad a year.
- *Additional permissible dose from man-made sources should not exceed 5 Rad a year.*[Q]

173. Ans. (a) Rem

Ref: K. Park, 24th ed. p 781

Radiation potency is measured in terms of

- **Roentgen**: (Unit of exposure)-It is the amount of radiation absorbed in air at a given point (No. of ions produced in 1 mL of air). It is being replaced by Coulomb per kilogram (C/kg).

1 Roentgen = 2.58×10^{-4} C/kg

- **Rad**:(Unit of absorbed dose). It is the amount of radioactive energy absorbed per gram of tissue/material. It is being replaced by Gray (Gy) (dose of ionizing radiation that impart 1 Joule of energy to 1 kg of absorbing material). 1 Rad = 0.01 Gy
- Rem:(Degree of potential danger to health): It is the product of the absorbed dose and modifying factors. It is being replaced by Sievert (Sv). 1 Sv = 100 rem

Also Know......................

- **Becquerel** (Bq) is the unit of activity of a radioactive material (i.e. number of nuclear disintegration per unit of time). 1 Bq = 1 disintegration per second. 1 Bq = 27 picocuries.

174. Ans. (c) 5 rad

Ref: Kevin S. Toppenberg. Safety of Radiographic Imaging During Pregnancy. Am Fam Physician. 1999 Apr 1; 59 (7) : 1813-1818.

The accepted cumulative dose of ionizing radiation during pregnancy is 5 rad

- Non-urgent radiation exposure should be delayed in pregnancy.
- 10 to 17 weeks is the most sensitive period of gestation (8 to 15 weeks after conception) for radiation exposure
- Fetal malformations most commonly caused by high-dose radiation are CNS changes, especially microcephaly and mental retardation.

175. Ans. (c) 0.5 mm

Ref: K. Park, 24th p-782

Among workers associated with X-ray procedures **lead shields and lead rubber aprons (0.5 mm thick)** reduce intensity of scattered exposure over 90%.

176. Ans. (d) Radiation protection in pregnancy

Ref: National Radiation Protection Board. Board statement on diagnostic medical exposure to ionizing radiation during pregnancy and estimate of late radiation risks to the UK population. Document NRPB. 1993;4:1–14.

'Ten day rule' was postulated by ICRP for woman in reproductive age group.

- It states that whenever possible, one should confine the radiological examination of the lower abdomen and pelvis to the 10-day interval following the onset of menstruation
- There is growing evidence that a strict adherence to the "ten-day rule" may be unnecessarily restrictive.
- Failure to implant or death of the conceptus is common, whereas malformations are unlikely or very rare.
- Applied more often when relatively high radiation dose examinations(>10 mGy to fetus) such as pelvic CT, diagnostic fluoroscopy of the abdomen and pelvis is to be done

28-day Rule

- Radiological examination if so justified, can be carried throughout the cycle until a period is missed (Possible pregnancy)
- In case of a missed period, every care should be taken to explore other methods using non-radiological examinations
- Applied more of ten when examinations that deliver low radiation dose to the uterus are used-Non-contrast X-rays of the proximal thigh, pelvis and abdomen and examinations at remote sites (Head and neck, upper and lower limbs except upper thigh and chest)

AIR VELOCITY/HUMIDITY

177. Ans. (a) 5 m/s

Ref: K. Park, 24th ed. p 786

Sling psychrometer is used to measure *Relative humidity*

- It has 2 mercury thermometers (wet and dry) mounted side by side, on a wooden frame with a handle.
- Wet bulb is moistened with water and instrument is whirled standing with back to the sun, for 15 seconds (4 revolution/sec) to obtain air speed of about 5 m/sec. Reading of wet bulb is noted.
- Instrument is again whirled for 10 seconds and the wet bulb reading is noted. This is repeated till 2 successive readings of the wet bulb are identical. The reading of the dry bulb is then noted.

Also Know.......................

Dry and wet bulb hygrometer is *most widely used to measure relative humidity*[Q]

- Difference in Dry Bulb Temperature (DBT) and Wet bulb Temperature (WBT-usually lower) yields relative humidity using psychometric chart or slide rule. For accurate reading of WBT, air must pass over bulb at a speed of 800 ft/min

Assmann Psychrometer is also used to measure *Relative humidity*

- It is portable, Air is drawn at a speed more than 5 m/sec by a clock-work fan.
- Bulbs are protected from solar radiation so that it can be used even in strong sunshine.

178. Ans. (a) Kata thermometer

Ref: K. Park, 24th ed. p 787 Kata thermometer was originally devised to measure the "cooling power" of the air.[Q]

HOUSING & VENTILATION

179. Ans. (a) Increased CO_2

180. Ans. (b) Deep sea diving

Decompression sickness (DCS) or bends or caisson disease:

It is due to nitrogen bubbles (gas embolism) which form in the blood supply while fast ascent from a deep sea diving or flying in unpressurized aircraft at high altitude

Features:

Mild DCS (most common): itching, headache, dizziness and body aches

Moderate DCS:

- Joint pains involving large joints – elbow, hips, knee, shoulders
- Hypertension
- Persistent dry cough

Severe DCS:

All previous symptoms + neurological features as confusion, hearing loss, altered sensorium, convulsions

181. Ans. (c) 25%.

182. Ans. (b) 15-20 foot candles

SEWAGE AND WASTE DISPOSAL

183. Ans. (c) Composting

Method of disposal of wastes:

- Dumping: Refuse is dumped in low lying areas. Not very good measure for waste disposal
- Controlled tipping (sanitary landfill): is the most satisfactory method of refuse disposal but only where suitable land is available.
- Composting: it is a method of combined disposal of refuse and night soil or sludge. It is a process of nature whereby organic matter breaks down into humus, which has an important role as manure for the soil.
- Incineration: Refuse can be disposed hygienically by burning or incineration. It is a method of choice where land is not available
- Burial: Suitable for small temporary arrangement.

184. Ans. (c) Suitable for large community

This is also called 'sewage lagoon'. It is so called because in this lagoon (pond) the sewage organic matters are oxidized into inorganic substances including CO_2, Ammonia and water and thus the sewage is purified.

The organic matter is oxidised by bacteria. The algae, with the help of sunlight, carry out photosynthesis, by utilizing CO_2, water and inorganic materials and liberate oxygen. Thus, oxygen required by the aerobic bacteria for oxidation, is obtained mainly from the algae and secondary source from the atmosphere.

There is both aerobic digestion and anaerobic putrefaction of the sewage.

These ponds are suitable for small community supplies.

185. Ans. (a) Organic matter

- Biochemical oxygen demand (BOD) is the amount of dissolved oxygen required by the living organisms in the sewage, during 5 days incubation at 20°C for aerobic oxidation of the organic matter.
- Weak sewage - < 100 mgms/L (or ppm)
- Moderate sewage: 100-300 mgms/L (or ppm)
- Strong sewage > 300 mgms/L (or ppm)

186. Ans. (a) Organic matter and bacteria

187. Ans. (d) CH_4 and CO_2

188. Ans. (c) Trench burial

Sewage farming is not the 'most' cost effective method as it involves higher risk of soil contamination, food contamination and may involve higher costs of treatment of diseases, if they may occur. Fodder grass, potatoes may be grown in sewage farming.

River dumping is 'not' sanitary methods for sewage disposal.

Water carriage system is undoubtly the best, but involves higher costs, which may (presently) not be applicable to the rural parts of our country.

Trench burial is cost effective method for sanitary disposal.

189. Ans. (b) Lining the wall of the pit with an impervious material

190. Ans. (b) Fat soluble complex biodegradable and nondegradable waste

Bio-accumulation, Bio-concentration and Bio-magnification are three different concepts. **Bio-accumulation** occurs within a trophic level and is increase in concentration of a substance in our bodies through food and environment.

Bioconcentration occurs within a trophic level through absorption from water

Biomagnification occurs across different trophic levels in a food chain

Features for bio-magnification to occur

- In order for biomagnification to occur, the pollutant must be: long-lived, mobile, soluble in fats, biologically active. E.g. DDT.
- If a pollutant is short-lived, it will be broken down before it can become dangerous.
- If the pollutant is soluble in water, it will be excreted by the organism. Pollutants that dissolve in fats, however, may be retained for a long time.
- It is traditional to measure the amount of pollutants in fatty tissues of organisms such as fish.

May happen with heavy metals, insecticides, or few non-biodegradable pharmaceutical drugs which tend to build up in the environment

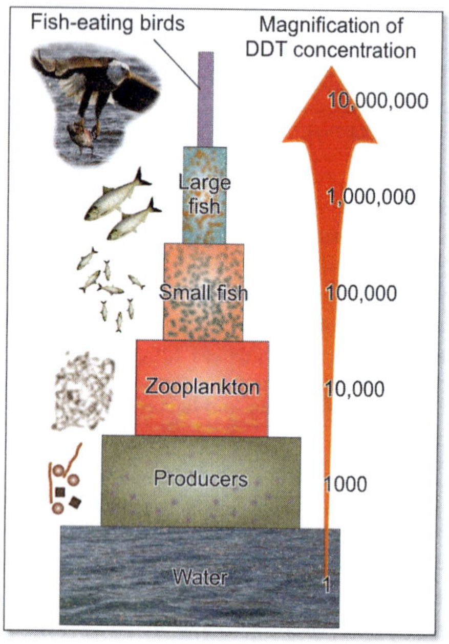

191. Ans. (b) It is a minor public health problem

Ref: K.Park Page 221)

Chandler's index is used to identify the importance of hookworm infestation as a public health problem in a community. It is calculated based on average number of hookworm eggs/gram of stool.

Average no. of hookworm (eggs/gm of stool)	Significance of hookworm infestation
<200	Not much significance
200-250	Potential danger
250-300	Minor public health problem
>300	Major public health problem

192. Ans. (a) Segregation of faeces

Sanitation barrier is a barrier created by provision of a sanitary latrine in order to prevent contamination of channels such as soil, flies, finger, water, water and food with faeces

193. Ans. (c) Aeration tank

194. Ans. (b) Sewage treatment

195. Ans. (c) Garbage

Category	Type of waste	Also called as
Kitchen waste	Organic waste	Garbage
Household waste	Inorganic waste	Rubbish
Powder waste	–	Ash
Faecal matter	Organic waste	Sewage
Waste water	–	Sullage

196. Ans. (c) Waste water from community containing solid and liquid excreta

Sewage is defined as waste water from community containing solid and liquid excreta.

"Sullage" is waste water from the community which does not contain human excreta e.g., waste water from kitchens and bathrooms.

197. Ans. (c) Organic matter

The strength of sewage is expressed in terms of biological oxygen demand. It is defined as the amount of oxygen absorbed by a sample of sewage during a specified period, generally 5 days, at a specified temperature, generally 20°C for the aerobic destruction or use of organic matter by living organisms.

198. Ans. (a) Dumping

Ref: K. Park, 24th ed. p 791

199. Ans. (a) Sanitary land fill

Ref: K. Park, 24th ed. p 791

Controlled tipping or Sanitary landfill is the most satisfactory method of refuse disposal where suitable land is available.[Q]

- Trench method- Trench (2–3 m deep and 4–12 m wide) is dug; Refuse is compacted and covered with excavated earth. About 1 acre land per year is needed for 10,000 populations. It is used where level ground is available.
- Ramp method used where the terrain is moderately sloping. Some excavation is done to secure covering material.
- Area method is used to fill and depressions, disused quarries and clay pits. Refuse is deposited, packed and consolidated in uniform layers 2-2.5 m (6-8 ft.) deep and each layer is sealed on its exposed surface with a mud cover 30 cm thick.
    - Disadvantage à supplemental earth from outside sources is required.
- Normally it takes 4 to 6 months for complete decomposition of organic matter into an innocuous mass.

- Tipping of refuse in water should not be done (nuisance from odors due to decomposition of organic matter)

Also Know.......................

- *Modified sanitary landfill-* Compaction and covering are accomplished once or twice a week.

200. Ans. (d) Waste water from kitchen

Ref: K. Park, 24 edp-799

Sullage (Gray Water) is waste water that does not contain human excreta (E.g., Waste water from kitchens and bathrooms).[Q]

- Gobar gas plant is ideal to dispose sullage

EXCRETA DISPOSAL

201. Ans. (c) The average amount of sewage that…

Ref: K. Park, 24th ed. p 799

Dry weather flow is the *average amount of sewage that flows through sewer system in 24 hours*[Q]

202. Ans. (c) Malaria

Ref: K. Park, 24th ed. p 793

Sanitation barrier to break the disease transmission comprises

- Segregation of feces
- Protection of water supplies
- Protection of foods
- Personal hygiene
- Control of flies.

Also Know.......................

- Sanitary latrine serves as the most effective Sanitation barrier for disease transmitted by Water, Finger, Flies, Soil and Food.

Malaria is mosquito borne disease, hence Sanitary latrine has no role, whereas Diarrhea, polio, cholera are water borne.

Also Know.......................

- ***Water Seal or Trap****-It is a bent pipe 7.5 cm in diameter that holds water and is connected to pan. It prevents the access of flies to fecal matter and nuisance of smell in sanitary latrine. Its depth is 2 cm in RCA latrine.*

203. Ans. (b) 40%

Ref: http://data.worldbank.org/indicator

Percentage of population with access to improved sanitation facilities as per World Bank data 2015 is 40%.

Also Know.......................

- Improved sanitation facilities include flush/pour flush (to piped sewer system, septic tank, pit latrine), ventilated improved pit (VIP) latrine, pit latrine with slab, and composting toilet.

204. Ans. (a) Treatment of household sewage; (c) Aerobic oxidation occurs outside septic tank; (e) Anaerobic digestion occurs inside septic tank

Ref: K. Park, 24th ed. p 797

Septic tank *is a water-tight masonry tank into which household sewage is admitted for treatment.*

- *Suitable for individual dwelling, small group of houses, institutions with adequate water supply but no access to public sewer system.*[Q]
- *Not recommended for large communities.*[Q]
- *It* can be double chambered or single chambered
- Recommended capacity for household septic tanks is 20-30 gallons (2.5-5 c.ft./ person). M*inimum capacity of 500 gallon.*[Q]
- Length is usually twice the breadth and Depth is 1.5-2 m with liquid depth of only 1.2 m and minimum air space of 30 cm
- Bottom is sloping towards the inlet end. There is an-inlet and outlet pipe, which are submerged.
- Septic tank is covered by a concrete slab of suitable thickness and provided with a manhole.
- Septic tanks are designed to allow a retention period of 24 hours.

Working of a septic tank -2 stages are involved in the purification of sewage.

- 1st stage → (Anaerobic digestion) takes place in septic tank proper.
  - Solids settle down ("sludge") and lighter solids (grease, fat) rise to surface to form "scum".
  - Solids are broken down into simple chemical compounds (stable and inoffensive) by anaerobic bacteria and fungi
- 2nd stage → (Aerobic oxidation) takes place in the sub-soil
  - Effluent coming out of outlet pipe is allowed to percolate into the subsoil, where aerobic bacteria oxidize organic matter into stable end-products, i.e., nitrates, carbon dioxide and water.

205. Ans. (b) Strength measured by biological oxygen demand; (e) Dry weather flow is measured for 24 hours period

Ref: K. Park, 24th ed. p 799

Sewage is waste water from a community, containing solid and liquid excreta.[Q]

Sewage contains 99.9% water and 0.1% Solids (organic and inorganic)

Strength of sewage	Weak	Strong
BOD	100 mg/L	300 mg/L and above
Suspended solids	100 mg/L	500 mg/L

206. Ans. (b) 5%

Ref: K. Park, 24th ed. p 138

Bleaching powder contains about 33 % available chlorine

- It has a rapid but brief action.
- A 5 % solution is used to disinfect feces and urine with a contact period of one hour.
- It is used to disinfect water and as a deodorant

- Drawback-Unstable compound (loses chlorine content on storage).

207. Ans. (c) Malaria

Ref: Park's textbook of PSM 23/e, p 757, 24th ed. p 794

Sanitary disposal of excreta reduces incidence of faeco-oral diseases (Diarrhea, intestinal worm infestations, Schistosomiasis, Polio, Cholera), Skin and eye infection, Guinea worm disease etc.

208. Ans. (b) Chemical oxygen demand

Ref: K. Park, 24th ed. p 800

***"Strength" of sewage** is expressed in terms of:*

- ***Biochemical oxygen demand*** **(BOD)** *is the amount of oxygen absorbed by a sample of sewage in a specified period (5 day), at a specified temperature (20°C) for aerobic destruction of organic matter by living organisms.*
  - BOD ranges from 1 mg/L for natural water to 300 mg/L for untreated domestic sewage.
- **Chemical oxygen demand (COD)** is the oxygen equivalent of that portion of organic matter in a sample which is susceptible to oxidation by a strong chemical oxidizer.
  - If wastes contain toxic substances, COD is the only practical method for determining the organic load.
- **Suspended solids**: Amount in domestic sewage varies from 100 to 500 p.p.m. (mg/L).

209. Ans. (a) Aeration tank

Ref: K. Park, 23 ed. p-764; 24th ed. p 801

Secondary Sewage Treatment Comprises

- Trickling filter (A bed of crushed stones, 1–2 m (4–8 ft.) deep and 2 to 30 m (6–100 ft.) in diameter) are best suited for small towns as they are cheaper to install and easier to operate
  - Effluent is sprinkled uniformly on the surface of bed by a revolving device (hollow pipes with row of holes).
  - As the effluent percolates through filter bed, it gets oxidized by bacterial flora in zoogleal layer (algae, fungi, protozoa and bacteria).
  - The oxidized sewage is then led into the secondary sedimentation tanks or humus tanks.
- **Activated Sludge process:** (Activated sludge is a rich culture of aerobic bacteria)requires less space and is ideal for big cities
  - Effluent from primary sedimentation tank is mixed with activated sludge drawn from the final settling tank
  - Mixture is aerated in the aeration tank for 6-8 hours (Mechanical agitation or Diffuse aeration (compressed air blown from the bottom of aeration tank)
  - *Aeration tank (**Heart of activated sludge process**)*- Organic matter is oxidized into carbon dioxide, nitrates and water by aerobic bacteria.

Also Know......................

Modern method of Sewage treatment: has 2 stages.

- Primary treatment → Screening, Sedimentation and anaerobic digestion
- Secondary treatment → Effluent is subjected to aerobic oxidation.

210. Ans. (d) Bangalore method (Composting)

Ref: K. Park, 24th ed. p 802

Methods of Sewage Disposal

- **Modern sewage treatment plant**
- **Sea and river outfall**-Purification is by dilution and oxidation.
  - Drawback → offensive solid matter may be washed back to shore and create public nuisance.
- **Land treatment (sewage farming)** *practiced if sufficient (1 acre land per 100-300 persons) and suitable land (porous soil) is available.*[Q]
  - Land is laid into ridges and furrows and sewage is fed into furrows. Crops/Fodder/Trees that do not come in contact with sewage and likely to be eaten raw are grown on the ridges.
    - A competent agricultural expert is needed.
    - During rainy season, it may not be possible to operate sewage farms.
    - Badly managed farms stink "***sewage sickness***" due to lack of sufficient aeration and rest pauses to land.
- **Oxidation/ Waste stabilization pond** (Redox pond, Sewage lagoons) -Both sewage and industrial wastes are treated. 1st large scale installation in India was at Bhilai. Sewage purification is by a combination of aerobic and anaerobic bacteria.
  - It is an open, shallow pool 1-1.5 m deep with an inlet and outlet. Ideal for purifying sewage from small communities.
  - It must have
    - Algae → Utilize the carbon dioxide, water and inorganic minerals for their growth and liberate oxygen under influence of sunlight.
    - Certain Bacteria → Oxidize organic matter in sewage to simple chemical compounds like carbon dioxide, ammonia and water.
    - Sun light
  - Cloudy weather lowers the efficiency.
  - Effluent can be used to grow vegetable /crop or discharged into river after appropriate treatment.
  - Mosquito breeding is avoided by keeping weed growth in nearby of oxidation ponds to a minimum and water line free from marginal vegetation.
  - No Odor nuisance if properly managed
- Oxidation ditches/aerated lagoons.
  - Make use of mechanical rotors for extended aeration.
  - To treat wastes of a population of 5,000 to 20,000 an oxidation ditch requires 1 acre of land and 2.5 acres for an aerated lagoon.

ENTOMOLOGY

211. Ans. (a) Ticks

Ticks belong to the suborder Metastigmata in the order Acari, class Arachnida, phylum Arthropoda. Tick is the common name for members of a group of large mite-like arachnids parasitic on mammals, birds, and reptiles. All ticks are bloodsucking parasites. Ticks are found in most parts of the world but are generally limited to those habitats frequented by their hosts namely, woods, tall grass, and shrubby vegetation-where they climb onto plants and wait to jump on a passing host.

212. Ans. (a) Eggs can survive without water for more than 7-8 days

Eggs are usually laid on the surface, 100 – 200 at a time and lasts for 1-2 days in a favourable climate

Gonotrophic cycle: moment of blood meal until the eggs are laid.

213. Ans. (a) 100 meters

214. Ans. (c) Japanese encephalitis

215. Ans. (c) Kala Azar

All are mosquito borne, except kala-azar – which is sand fly borne disease

216. Ans. (b) Dengue

Both yellow fever and dengue are transmitted by the Aedes mosquito. However, yellow fever is exotic for India

217. Ans. (d) Japanese encephalitis

Culex transmits: bancroftian filariasis, Japanese encephalitis, west Nile fever, viral arthritis

Burgian filariasis is transmitted by the Mansonia mosquito

218. Ans. (c) Between 8 and 34 days

Under favorable conditions of temperature and food supply, the life cycle from the egg to adult is completed in 7—10 days. Normally, an adult mosquito lives for about 2 weeks. Normal life span of mosquitoes varies from 8—34 days.

219. Ans. (b) A-3, B-4, C-2, D-1

220. Ans. (c) Kyasanur forest disease (KFD)

221. Ans. (c) Relapsing fevers

222. Ans. (c) Japanese encephalitis

- Japanese encephalitis is transmitted by culicine mosquitoes.
- Diseases transmitted by ticks:

Hard ticks transmit
- Tick typhus (Rocky Mountain spotted fever)
- Tularemia
- Kyasanur forest disease
- Tick paralysis
- Human babesiosis
- Colorado tick fever
- Viral encephalitis

Soft ticks transmit
- Q fever
- Kyasanur forest disease
- Relapsing fever
- Kyasanur forest disease is transmitted by a wide variety of ticks including hard as well as soft ticks.

223. Ans. (b) Human babesiosis

- Babesiosis is a protozoan disease of animals that is transmitted by ticks. Humans are infected incidentally and initially develop a nonspecific febrile illness.
- Babesia microti and Babesia divergens cause most human infections.
- Ixodid (or hard-bodied) ticks, in particular, Ixodes dammini (Ixodes scapularis or deer tick) and Ixodes Ricinus (castor bean tick), are the vectors of the parasite.

224. Ans. (c) Water washed

225. Ans. (d) Kyasanur forest disease

Itch mite: scabies

Trombiculid mite: scrub typhus, rickettsialpox

KFD is caused by tick (both hard and soft tick)

226. Ans. (b) Epidemic typhus

Rat flea transmits:
- Bubonic plague
- Endemic typhus
- Chiggerosis
- Hymenolepis diminuta

*Epidemic tyhphus is a louse born disease

227. Ans. (c) Sand fly

228. Ans. (d) Rat flea

Rickettsia typhi (old name R. mooseri) is etiologic agent for murine or the endemic typhus

Rickettsia typhi is maintained in mammalian host/flea cycles, with rats (Rattus rattus and Rattus norvegicus) and the Oriental Rat FLEA (Xenopsylla cheopis) as the classic zoonotic niche. Fleas acquire R. typhi from rickettsemic rats and carry the organisms for the rest of their lives. Nonimmune rats and humans get infected when Rickettsia laden flea faeces are "scratched" into pruritic bite lesions. Less frequently, the flea bite itself transmits the organisms. Another possible route of transmission is the inhalation of aerosols of flea faeces.

229. Ans. (b) 1

Cyclops may be controlled by the using physical, chemical or biological methods:

Physical Methods
- Straining of water through a piece of fine cloth is sufficient to remove Cyclops.
- Boiling: Cyclops is readily killed by heat at 60 degree C.

Chemical Methods
- Chlorine destroys Cyclops and larvae of guinea worm in strength of 5 ppm.

- Lime at a dosage of 4 gram per gallon of water is very efficient for killing Cyclops.
- Abate: organophosphorus insecticide, abate (OMS-786) has been found effective in killing Cyclops at a concentration of 1 mg/L

Biological Method

Certain kinds of small fish such as barbel fish and gambusia fish have been found to feed on Cyclops.

230. Ans. (c) 3 months

Cyclops or water flea is a crustacean found in collections of fresh water. The average life of a Cyclops is about 3 months. Cyclops is the intermediate host of guinea worm disease. Man acquires infestation by drinking water containing infected Cyclops.

231. Ans. (a) Anopheles stephensi

Ref: Mahajan and Gupta, Textbook of Preventive and Social Medicine, 4th ed., p 309

Urban malaria is transmitted by A. stephensi (Breed in wells, cisterns and other fresh water collections)

Also Know......................

- Breeding habitats- Anopheles (Clean water), Culex (Dirty water), Aedes (Artificial collection), Mansonia (Water body with aquatic plants).

232. Ans. (d) Culex

Ref: K. Park, 24th ed. p 809

Mosquito-borne diseases[Q]	
Anopheles	Malaria, Filaria (not in India)
Culex	Bancroftian Filariasis, Japanese encephalitis, West Nile fever, Viral arthritis
Aedes	Dengue, Dengue hemorrhagic fever, Chikungunya fever, Chikungunya hemorrhagic fever, Rift valley fever. Filaria and Yellow fever (not in India)
Manso-noides	Malayan (Brugian) filariasis, Chikungunya fever

Also Know......................

- Culex vishnui, Culex tritaeniorhynchus, Culex gelidus transmit Japanese encephalitis. Culex quinquefasciatus-transmit Bancroftian Filariasis

233. Ans. (d) Chikungunya fever

Ref: K. Park, 24th ed. p 809

234. Ans. (c) Aedes

Ref: K. Park, 24th ed. p 808

Aedes mosquitoes are referred to as Tiger mosquito because of striped and banded pattern of legs.

235. Ans. (d) Culex

Ref: K. Park, 24th ed. p 808

236. Ans. (b) 400 m

Ref: K. Park, 24th ed. p 808

As per WHO International Health Regulations (IHR), all international airports and seaports are to be kept free from all types of mosquitoes for a distance of 400 m around the perimeter of the ports

Also Know......................

- **Aedes aegypti Index**-is the ratio of number of houses in a limited well defined area on the premises of which actual breeding of Aedes aegypti is found to the total number of houses examined in that area.
- **Aedes aegypti Index** is kept zero at all ports.

237. Ans. (a) Malaria

Ref: K. Park, 23rd ed. p 772, Refer to notes; 24th ed. p 809

238. Ans. (a) Aedes

Ref: K. Park, 23 ed. p-769; 24th ed. p 806

Mosquito	Characteristic of Eggs
Culex	Eggs are laid in clusters or rafts (100-250)
Anopheles	Eggs are laid singly, are boat shaped and have lateral floats
Mansonia	Eggs are laid in star shaped clusters underneath leaves of aquatic plants (Pistia)
Aedes	Eggs are cigar shaped and single

239. Ans. (b) Larva has siphon tube

Ref: K. Park, 24th ed. p 808

No siphon tube found in larva of **anopheles mosquitoes**

	Anopheline (Anopheles) Mosquito	Culicini (Culex/Aedes/ Mansonia) Mosquito
Eggs	Eggs are boat-shaped with lateral floats and laid singly.	Eggs are oval-shaped (Without lateral floats) and are laid in clusters or rafts of 100-250 eggs. Mansonia eggs are laid in star shape cluster. Exception-**Aedes eggs are laid singly**.
Larvae	Siphon tube is absent and larvae rest parallel to water surface. Palmate hairs are present on abdominal segments.	Siphon tube is present and Larvae remain suspended upside down at an angle to water surface. There are no palmate hairs. (Mansonia larva is attached to rootlets of aquatic plants)

Contd...

	Anopheline (Anopheles) Mosquito	Culicini (Culex/Aedes/ Mansonia) Mosquito
Pupae	Siphon tube is present and is broad and short in length	Siphon tube is present and is narrow and longer in length
Adults	Rest with body inclined at an angle to surface; wings are spotted and Palpi are long in both sexes	Rest with a hunch back; wings are not spotted and Palpi are short in female

240. Ans. (b) Siphon tube seen in larvae

Ref: K. Park, 24th ed. p 806

241. Ans. (a) It has siphon tube

Ref: K. Park, 24thed p-808

242. Ans. (b) Larva has siphon tube

Ref: K. Park, 24th ed. p 808

243. Ans. (c) Adults rest at an angle to surface of skin; (e) Larva does not have a siphon tube

Ref: K. Park, 24th ed. p 806

244. Ans. (a) Mosquito

Ref: K. Park, 24th ed. p 809

Culex (**Nuisance**) mosquito transmits Bancroftian filariasis, Japanese encephalitis, West Nile fever, Viral arthritis.

- *They breed profusely in dirty water collections (stagnant drains, cesspools, septic tanks, burrow pits etc.)*[Q]

245. Ans. (b) Anopheles stephensi

Ref: Mahajan and Gupta, Textbook of Preventive and Social Medicine, 4th ed., p-309

246. Ans. (b) Less than 100 m

Ref: K. Park, 24th ed. p 808

Vector	Flight range
A dirus, A annularis and A fluviatilis	1 km
A culicifacies and A stephensi	2 km
A sundaicus	8-10 km
Culex	11 km
Aedes	100 m (110 yards)

247. Ans. (a) 400 m

Ref: K. Park, 24th ed. p 808

248. Ans. (b) 0.0475 inch

Ref: K. Park, 24th ed. p 810

Specifications for Mosquito net for Malaria protection

- Ideally white in color.
- The top as well as the sides of the net should be of netting.
- Best pattern is rectangular net.
- No hole or rent in the net.
- Size of the openings in the net should not exceed 0.0475 inch in any diameter.
- Number of holes in one square inch is usually 150.

Also Know...

- Screening of buildings: Ideally of copper or bronze gauze having 16 meshes per inch. The aperture should not be larger than 0.0475 inch in any diameter.
- Protection against Sand flies– Very fine screening or mosquito nets (10 to 12 mesh/cm, aperture size not more than 0.85 mm).

249. Ans. (a) Yellow fever; (b) Dengue; (c) Chikungunya fever; (e) Rift Valley fever

Ref: K. Park, 23rd ed.p-772; Refer to Notes; 24th ed. p 809

250. Ans. (c) Filling of cess pools and ditches

Ref: K. Park, 24th ed. p 433

Major recommendation for Urban malaria vector control are as follows:

- Larvicide -Chemical and biological (costly and need to be done frequently)
- Environmental source reduction (most efficient)
- Personal protection –ITN/LLIN, Screening of houses
- Focal Insecticide Residual spray

251. Ans. (a) Aedes

Ref: K. Park, 24th ed. p 809

252. Ans. (d) Pupa do not have siphon tube

Ref: K. Park, 24th ed. p 808

253. Ans. (b) Eggs cannot survive more than one week without water

Ref: K. Park, 24th ed. p 808

Aedes Mosquito or "Tiger Mosquito"

- It transmits Dengue, Dengue hemorrhagic fever, Chikungunya fever; Chikungunya hemorrhagic fever, Rift valley fever, Yellow fever (not in India) and Filaria (not in India)
- It *breeds in stagnant artificial collection of water* (discarded tins, broken bottles *etc) in and around human dwellings*[Q] and are most abundant during rainy season.
- *Aedes aegypti is the first proven vector of a viral disease-Yellow fever.*
- Aedes eggs are cigar-shaped and laid singly.
- *Eggs can withstand long periods of dessication up to 1 year*[Q]

- *Aedes females are fearless biters and bite repeatedly during day time.*[Q]
- Extrinsic incubation period is of 8-10 days.

254. Ans. (a) Dengue

Ref: K. Park, 24th ed. p 809

255. Ans. (c) Louse

Ref: K. Park, 24th ed. p 814

Refer to Theory

256. Ans. (a) Lyme disease

Ref: K. Park, 24th ed. p 817https://www.cdc.gov/lyme/

Lyme Disease

Causative agent: *Borrelia burgdorferi (Bacteria)*
Transmission: *Bite of Infected blacklegged ticks.*
Symptoms: *Fever, headache, fatigue, and a characteristic skin rash called erythema migrans. If left untreated, joints, the heart, and the nervous system may be involved*
Diagnosis: *Symptoms, physical findings (e.g., rash), and possibility of exposure to infected ticks.*
Prevention: *Using insect repellent, removing ticks promptly, applying pesticides, and reducing tick habitat.*

257. Ans. (d) All of the above

Ref: K. Park, 24th ed. p 817

TICK –(**Life history: It has 4** stages -Egg, Larva, Nymph and Adult)

- **EGG:** Hard ticks lay hundreds or even thousands of eggs at one time, after which the female dies. Soft ticks lay eggs in batches of 20 -100 over a long period. Eggs are deposited on the ground and hatch in 1 to 3 weeks.
- **Larva (3 to 13 days):** It has 3 pairs of legs. It lies in grass/ herb and attaches to a suitable host. After a blood meal, it drops off and moults to become a nymph.
- **Nymph:** It has 4 pairs of legs, but no genital pore. Nymphs feed on blood. Soft ticks has 5 nymphal stages
- **Adult:** Oval shaped (no distinct head, thorax and abdomen), 4 pairs of legs, no antennae.
  - Hard ticks have a chitinous shield (scutum) covers entire back in male and only a small part in front in female
  - Scutum is absent in soft ticks.
  - Hard ticks "head" lies at anterior end; soft ticks have a head on underside
  - Males are smaller than females.
  - Hard ticks feed both night and day (always found on host), whereas soft ticks feed at night (hide in cracks and crevices in day)
  - Hard tick cannot withstand starvation, whereas soft tick can withstand starvation for several months.

Soft tick Ornithodoros moubata transmits relapsing fever.

258. Ans. (a) Rickettsial disease

Ref: K. Park, 24th ed. p 817-18

Mite (Scrub typhus, Rickettsial pox) and Tick (Indian tick typhus, Rocky Mountain spotted fever) act as arthropod reservoir for Rickettesial disease by maintaining Rickettsiae via transovarial transmission

- Transovarial transmission has also been demonstrated for Dengue virus in mosquito

Also Know......................

- **Transovarian transmission**- Infectious agent is passed vertically to succeeding generations
- **Transstadial transmission**- Infection is transmitted from one stage of lifecycle to another (Nymph to adult). E.g. Tick

259. Ans. (a) Ticks

Ref: K. Park, 24t ed p-818

260. Ans. (d) RMSF; (e) Crimean Congo fever

Ref: K. Park, 24th ed. p 817

261. Ans. (b) Oriental sore

Ref: K. Park, 24th ed. p 817

262. Ans. (a) Scrub typhus

Ref: K. Park, 24th ed. p 818

Arthropod	Disease transmitted
Trombiculid mite	Scrub typhus, Rickettsialpox
Itch-mite	Scabies

263. Ans. (c) Chagas disease

Ref: K. Park, 24th ed. p 817

264. Ans. (a) Mite

Ref: K. Park, 24th ed. p 818

265. Ans. (d) 15–20

Ref: Medical Entomology Department, University of Sydney and Westmead Hospital, Australia(http://medent.usyd.edu.au/ fact/scabies.html

Sarcoptes scabiei is aparasitic mite that lives within the subcutaneous tissues of skin on humans causing "scabies"

- A fertilized female mite can only initiate successful scabies infections.
- During an infection, number of mites increase rapidly, then drop off, leaving infected persons with a relatively stable mite population of 15-20 females.

266. Ans. (c) Transmitted when adult mites feed on hosts

Ref: K. Park, 24th ed. p 317

Scrub typhus is the most widespread rickettsial disease in man caused by *Rickettsia tsutsugamushi.*[Q]

- *Reservoir of infection is the trombiculid mite*[Q]
- Infection is maintained in nature transovarially from one generation of mite to the next.
- Nymphal and adult stages of mite are free-living in soil
- *Larval stage acts both as a reservoir and vector for infecting humans and rodents.*[Q]

- Mode of transmission – Bite of infected larval mites. No direct person to person transmission.[Q]
- The transmission cycle:
  - Mite →Rats and mice → Mite → Rats and mice
  - Mite →Rats and mice → Mite → Man
- Incubation period -10–12 days (vary from 6 to 21 days)
- **Eschar** a punched out ulcer covered with a blackened scab at site of mite bite is characteristic feature[Q].
- Weil Felix reaction is strongly positive with the Proteus strain OXK.
- Control measures –
  - **Treatment:** Tetracycline (Drug of choice).[Q]
  - **Vector control:** Clearing vegetation where rats and mice live; application of insecticides (Lindane or chlordane) to ground and vegetation
  - **Personal prophylaxis:** Impregnating clothes and blankets with miticidal chemicals (Benzyl benzoate) and application of mite repellents (Diethyltoluamide) to exposed skin

267. Ans. (a) Mite

Ref: K. Park, 24th ed. p 818

Scabies is a familial or household infection transmitted by itch mite (Sarcoptes scabiei) (1st disease of man with known cause)

- Mode of spread
  - *Close contact with an infected person*
  - *Contaminated clothes*
- It classically affects the hands and wrist (63%), extensor aspect of elbows (10.9%). Axilla, buttocks, lower abdomen, feet, ankles, palms are common sites in infants. It may affect breasts in women and genitals in men.
- Main diagnostic features →
  - Itching (worse at night), Follicular lesions at affected site, Secondary infection (papules and pustules)
  - Other members of the household are also affected
- Confirmation of diagnosis is by searching for the parasite in the skin debris under microscope.
- Drug of choice -5% Permethrin

268. Ans. (a) Trench fever; (d) Epidemic typhus; (e) Pediculosis

Ref: K. Park, 24th ed. p 814

- Louse transmits Epidemic typhus, Relapsing fever, Trench fever and Pediculosis

269. Ans. (a) Epidemic typhus; (c) Relapsing fever; (d) Trench fever

Ref: K. Park, 24th ed. p 814

- Louse transmits Epidemic typhus, Relapsing fever, Trench fever and Pediculosis
- Q Fever is not transmitted via any arthropod. Mode of transmission of Q fever is
  - Inhalation of infected dust
  - Abrasions
  - Conjunctiva
  - Ingestion of contaminated food
- Scrub typhus is transmitted by Trombiculid Mite.

270. Ans. (b) Filaria

Ref: K. Park, 24th ed. p 103

Types of Biological Transmission

- **Propagative:** Disease agent undergoes no cyclical change, but multiplies in body of vector. e.g. Plague bacilli in rat fleas.
- **Cyclopropagative:** Disease agent undergoes cyclical change and multiplies in the body of vector e.g. Malaria parasite in anopheles mosquito
- **Cyclo developmental:** Disease agent undergoes only cyclical change in vector e.g. Filaria parasite in culex mosquito, Guinea worm embryo in cyclops

271. Ans. (a) Malaria

Ref: K. Park, 23ed. p-98; 24th ed. p 103

272. Ans. (b) Propogative cycle

Ref: K. Park, 24th ed. p 103

273. Ans. (a) 50 yards

Ref: K. Park, 24th ed. p 813

- Sand Fly are nocturnal pest. They hop (do not fly) and their movement is confined to within 50 yards of breeding places.
- *They infest dwellings during night and take shelter during day in holes and crevices in walls, holes in trees, dark rooms.*[Q]

274. Ans. (b) DDT

Ref: K. Park, 24th ed. p 813

Control Measures for Sand Fly

- **Insecticide spraying** in human dwellings, cattle sheds and other places walls up to a height of 4-6 feet
  - Single application of DDT 1-2 g/m^2 (Effective for 1-2 years) or Lindane 0.25 g/m^2 (Effective for 3 months)
- **Sanitation**: Removal of shrubs and vegetation within 50 yards of human dwellings, filling up cracks and crevices in walls and floors, location of cattle sheds and poultry at a fair distance from human habitations.

Also Know......................

- Sand Fly are smaller in size (compared to mosquito), sit upright, have lanceolate (Flame shaped) wings, long leg (2 times the body length) and hairy body.
- Only Female sandfly need blood meal for oviposition (every 3-4 days)

INSECTICIDES AND DISINFECTION

275. Ans. (c) Three months

Malathion is used in the doses of 100-200 m square foot for every three months. It has least toxicity of all organophosphorus compounds.

276. Ans. (a) Abate; (d) Malathion

Classification of insecticides is:

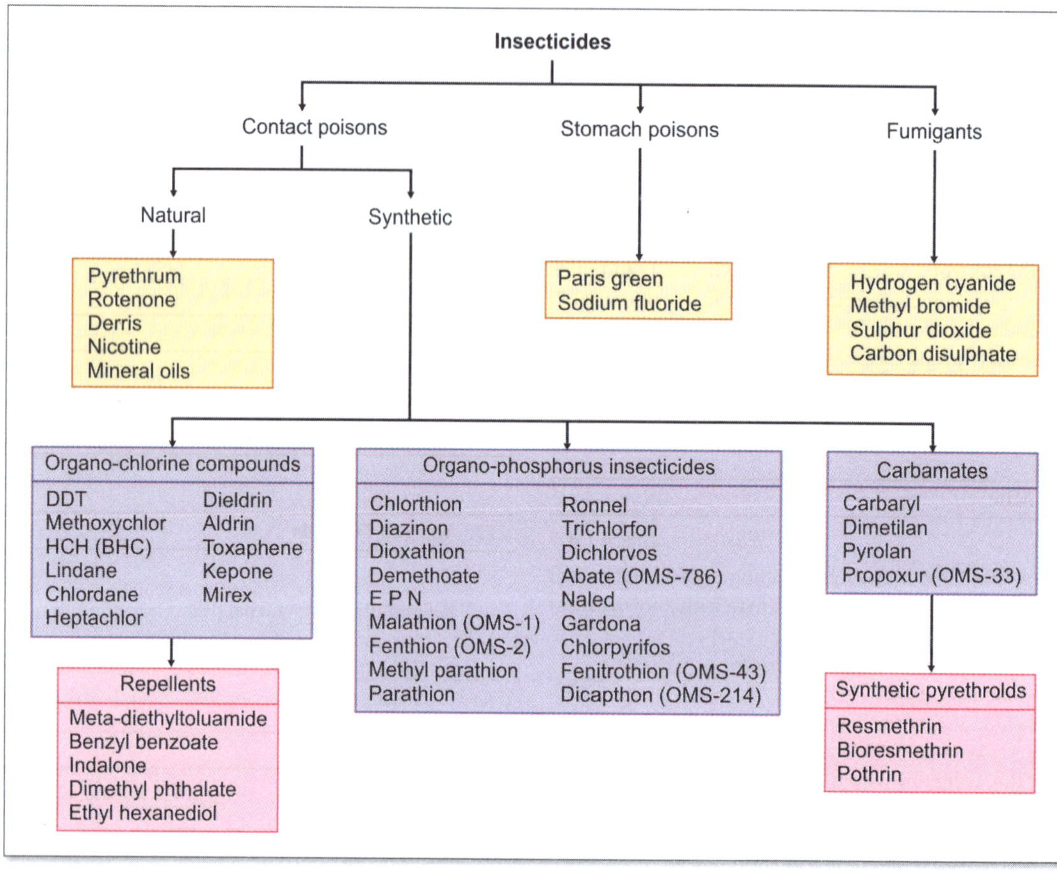

277. Ans. (c) Contact poison

DDT is a contact poison. DDT dissolves in the body of the mosquito through the cuticle and legs. It causes paralysis of the legs and wings, further leading to convulsions and finally the death of mosquito.

278. Ans. (b) A-2, B-1, C-4, D-3

- Rotenone is derived from the roots of the plant *Derris elliptica*.
- Gardona is a synthetic insecticide used for worms and insects in fields. It is used as a 3% dust.
- Sodium fluorocetate is a component in the rat poison, though it's the dose which makes it a poison.
- Methyl bromide is used as a fumigant and pesticide.

279. Ans. (d) Pyrethrum

Pyrethrum is extracted from the flowers of Chrysanthemum cinerariifolium. It is an excellent space spray.

280. Ans. (a) 100-200 mg / square foot

- Dose of malathion used for residual insecticidal action is 100-200 mg/square foot area.
- Dose of DDT used for residual insecticidal action is also 100-200 mg. per square foot area

281. Ans. (b) Causes immediate death; (d) Synergistic action with permethrin

As far as DDT is concerned in this MCQ, lets talk about a few salient facts about DDT

- DDT is white amorphous powder, insoluble in water.
- Mechanism of action – It does not have a repellent action. It is contact poison, causes paralysis, convulsions and death. It takes a few hours to kill the insect (action is not immediate)
- Dosage 100-200 mg/sq foot area
- Has biomagnification effect in the food chain and environment
- Drawback – prolonged residual action (of as long as up to 2 years)

Now if we talk about Insecticide resistance: DDT (and its analogues) are known to have significant amount of resistance. There is also evidence of cross resistance between the organochlorous compounds (i.e. DDT, HCH etc) and the carbamates or pyrethroids. Hence, it does not seem to be a synergistic effect of DDT with pyrethrum, where in fact, may be presence of cross-resistance between the two groups of insecticides.

282. Ans. (c) Repellent

Ref: K. Park, 24th ed. p 820

283. Ans. (d) Mansonia

Red: 24th ed. p 808

Mansonia mosquito larvae attach themselves to underneath of *aquatic plants (*Pistia and Water hyacinth) *and destroying aquatic plants by herbicides is* an effective anti- larval measure *against Mansonia*[Q]

284. Ans. (a) Anopheles

Ref: K. Park, 24th ed. p 822

Paris green: (Copper acetoarsenite) is a stomach poison.

- A good sample of Paris green must contain 50% arsenious oxide.
- It kills Anopheles larvae (Surface-feeders).
- Bottom-feeding larvae are killed when Paris green is applied as a special granular formulation.
- It is applied as 2% dust by hand blowers or rotary blowers (Dose = 1 kg/ hectare of water surface). Does not harm fish, man or domestic animals at this concentration.

285. Ans. (c) 6 – 12 months

Ref: K. Park, 24th ed. p 821

Residual spray insecticides	Dose (g/m²)	Duration of effectiveness (Month)
DDT	1–2	6–12
BHC (Lindane)	0.5	3
Dieldrin	0.5	6–12
Malathion	2	3
OMS-33 (Propoxur)	2	3

286. Ans. (c) Nerve poison

Ref: K. Park, 24th ed. p 821

Pyrethrum is an insecticide of vegetable origin (extracted from flowers of Chrysanthemum Cinerariaefolium), cultivated in Kashmir and Nilgiris.

Active principle in Pyrethrum extract is *Pyrethrin a nerve toxin.*

- Dose is 1 oz of spray solution (containing 0.1% of Pyrethrin) per 1,000 C. ft. of space.
- The doors and windows are kept closed for half an hour.
- Effective in reducing number of mosquitoes but the reduction is only temporary since it has no residual action.
- Most space sprays contain pyrethrum and DDT or other synthetic insecticides, added for synergistic action.

287. Ans. (b) Malathion

Ref: Sharma, Concise Textbook of Forensic Medicine and Toxicology, p-254

Aryl Phosphates

- Parathion, (folidol)
- Paraoxon
- Methyl parathion (metacide)
- Chlorthion
- Diazinon (diazinon, tik 20)

Alkyl phosphate – HETP, TEPP, OMPA, malathion, systox, dipterex

288. Ans. (a) Red

Ref: Insecticides Rules, 1971. Central Insecticides Board, India

Toxicity status of pesticides are mandatory on pesticide containers in India since 1971.

Label Color	Level of toxicity	*Oral lethal dose* (mg/ kg body weight of test animal)	Listed chemicals
Red	Extremely toxic	1–50	Monocrotophos, Zinc Phosphide, Ethyl Mercury Acetate
Yellow label	Highly toxic	51–500	Endosulfan, Carbaryl, Quinalphos
Blue label	Moderately toxic	501–5000	Malathion, Thiram, Glyphosate
Green label	Slightly toxic	More than 5000	Mancozeb, Oxyfluorfen, Mosquito repellent oils

289. Ans. (b) Residual spray

Ref: K. Park, 24th ed. p 821

290. Ans. (a) DDT

Ref: K. Park, 24th ed. p 822;

291. Ans. (b) Fish tape worm

Ref: K. Park, 24th ed. p 747

Refer to Theory

292. Ans. (a) Chagas disease

Ref: K. Park, 24th ed. p 817

Reduviid bugs (Cone-nose bugs) transmit Trypanosoma cruzi, the causative agent of Chagas disease.

Reduviid bugs live in cracks, fissures in human dwellings and in animal habitations and nests

Control - Residual spray of HCH (0.5 g/m² or dieldrin 1 g/m²)

293. Ans. (a) Eliminate breeding places

Ref: K. Park, 24th ed. p 811

294. Ans. (b) Fumigation

Anti-larval measures are:

- Environmental (source reduction) measures
- Chemical measures
  - Mineral oils
  - Paris green

- Synthetic insecticides (organophosphorus compounds)
  - Abate
  - Malathion
  - Fenthion
- Biological measures – as fishes, bacillus thuringiensis

295. Ans. (a) Anopheline larvae only

Paris Green kills mainly the anopheles larvae because they are surface feeder. Bottom feeding larvae are also killed when Paris green is applied as a special granular formation.

296. Ans. (b) Anopheline mosquito

Paris Green is a stomach poison. Till the introduction of DDT, Paris green was widely used in the control of Anopheline Larvae, by spraying as a 2 % dust over breeding places once a week. The use of Paris green was principally responsible for the eradication of A. gambiae from Brazil in 1940, and the near eradication of the same species in Egypt in 1944.

297. Ans. (c) Sodium fluoride

Paris green and sodium fluoride are stomach poisons.

298. Ans. (c) Magnesium Nitrates

The hardness of water is classified as carbonate or non-carbonate
- Carbonate hardness – called as temporary hardness – is due to calcium and magnesium bicarbonates
- Non - Carbonates – called as permanent hardness – due to calcium and magnesium sulfate, chlorides and nitrates.

The drinking water should be moderately hard. Softening is recommended for hardness more than 3 mEq/L (which corresponds to 150 mg/L of calcium carbonate)

299. Ans. (c) Hypochlorous acid

The mechanism of action for chlorination is:
- Formation of chloramines
- Destruction of chloramines into
  - Residual organochlorous compounds
  - Free radical production (responsible for disinfection action of chlorine)
    - Hypochlorous ions (main element for destruction of pathogenic bacteria)
    - Hypochlorite ions (minor effect)
  - Free and residual chlorine in water

The presence of free and residual chlorine in water is indicative of effective chlorination and disinfectant action of chlorine. The estimated free chlorine levels in water should be more than > 0.5 ppm

300. Ans. (d) It is a problem village, if there is no safe water within 1 km

Rural water supply is 40 L, and 140 liters for urban water supply But a problem village (or area) is one which does not have a safe water supply within 1.6 Kms (and not 1 km)

301. Ans. (d) Filtration

- Slow sand, rapid granular or membrane filtration is the most effective water treatment method to remove cryptosporidium cysts, as they are destroyed by disinfection.
- Flocculation and sedimentation do not remove cysts.
- Boiling is 'not' an engineered water sanitation process but of course is one of the simplest methods to avoid to some extent cryptosporidium parvum infections. The water intended for drinking should be boiled for at least 1 min
- Filtration also does not provide absolute protection as in some cases high water turbidity may hamper the filtration process to remove the parasite.

302. Ans. (c) Number of container with Aedes larva / number of houses checked

Larval survey for Dengue: a house to house survey is done and the household water containers are checked for presence of any aedes larva inside them. The following indicators are assessed by the district epidemiologist:

- House index = $\frac{\text{number of houses positive for aedes larva}}{\text{number of houses checked}} \times 100$
- Container index = $\frac{\text{number of artificial containers positive for aedes larva}}{\text{number of containers checked}} \times 100$
- Breteau index = $\frac{\text{number of artificial containers positive for aedes larva}}{\text{number of houses checked}} \times 100$

303. Ans. (b) 55 dB

Zone	Permissible noise level standards in the daytime (dB)	Permissible noise level standards at night (dB)
Industrial Zone	75	70
Commercial Zone	65	55
Residential Zone	55	45
Silent zone	50	40

304. Ans. (a) Lay single egg

Tsetse Fly:

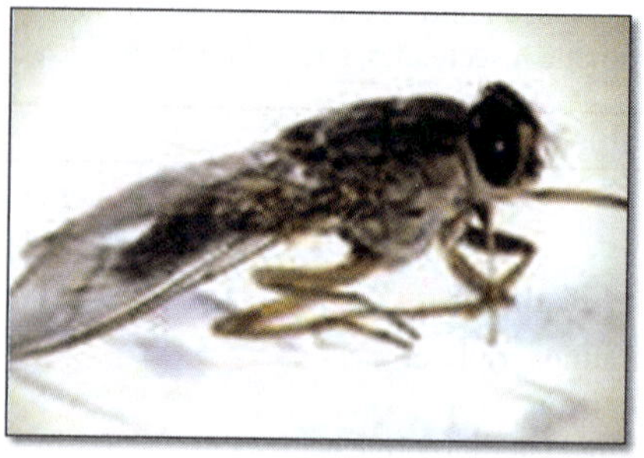

General features:

- Size 6–14 mm
- Typical feature:
  - Fold their wings completely when they are resting so that one wing rests directly on top of the other over their abdomen
  - Long proboscis which extends directly forward and is attached by a distinct bulb to the bottom of their head
- These maybe found in patches alongside rivers, dense tropical forests, arid terrain

Life cycle:

- Has a typical parental investment in offspring and relatively slower rate of reproduction
- Female tsetse mate just once. After 7 - 9 days she produces a single egg which develops into a larva within her uterus
- About nine days later, the mother produces a larva which burrows into the ground where it pupates.
- The mother continues to produce a single larva at roughly nine day intervals for her entire life.
- Eggs hatch in the female and after larval development, the deposited larvae pupates immediately.
- The pupal stage lasts about 3 weeks.
- The adult fly emerges from the pupa in the ground after about 30 days
- Over a period of 12-14 days it matures, mates and, if it is a female, deposits its first larva.
- Thus 50 days elapse between the emergence of one female fly and the subsequent emergence of the first of its progeny

Cause the disease – trypanosomiasis

Trypanosomiasis

Pathogen:

- *Trypanosoma brucei gambiense*
  - Causing acute disease
  - Lasting from weeks to months
- *Trypanosoma brucei rhodesiense*
  - Case chronic long term disease
  - Lasting from months to years
- Fever
- Swollen lymph nodes
- Headaches
- Somnolence
- Abnormal behaviour
- Loss of consciousness
- Coma

The main feature is:

- Sleep disturbances (hence the name)
- Deep sensory disturbances,
- Abnormal tone and mobility, ataxia,
- Psychiatric disorders, seizures, coma and ultimately death

Management:

- DOC: NECT – (nifurtimox & eflornithine) combination drug is given
- Approved drugs: registered drugs for treatment are:
  - Pentamidine
  - Suramin
  - Melarsoprol (available for late stage of T.b. rhodesiense or advanced disease)
  - Eflornithine (most effective for T.b.gambiense infection)
- Nifurtimox, (not approved) is used in combination under special authorizations

Note: trypanosoma cruzi is pathogen for chagas disease, predominant in South America

305. Ans. (a) 1 acre

Ref: Park 25th Ed. Pg 814

Controlled tipping (also called as sanitary landfills) is the most suitable method for refuse disposal where the suitable land is available.

Features of Controlled Tipping

- Based on chemical, physical and bacteriological changes in the buried refuse
- Increase in temperature over 60 °C with 7 days and kills all pathogen
- Rise in temperature hastens the decomposition process, takes 4-6 months for complete decomposition

Three methods of controlled tipping are possible:

- **Trench method**
  - Long trench – 10 ft deep, 30 ft wide
  - Refuse is compacted and covered with earth
  - Estimate 1 acre land for 10,000 population per year
- Ramp method – in sloping land
- Area method – for filling land depressions and pits.

NOTES

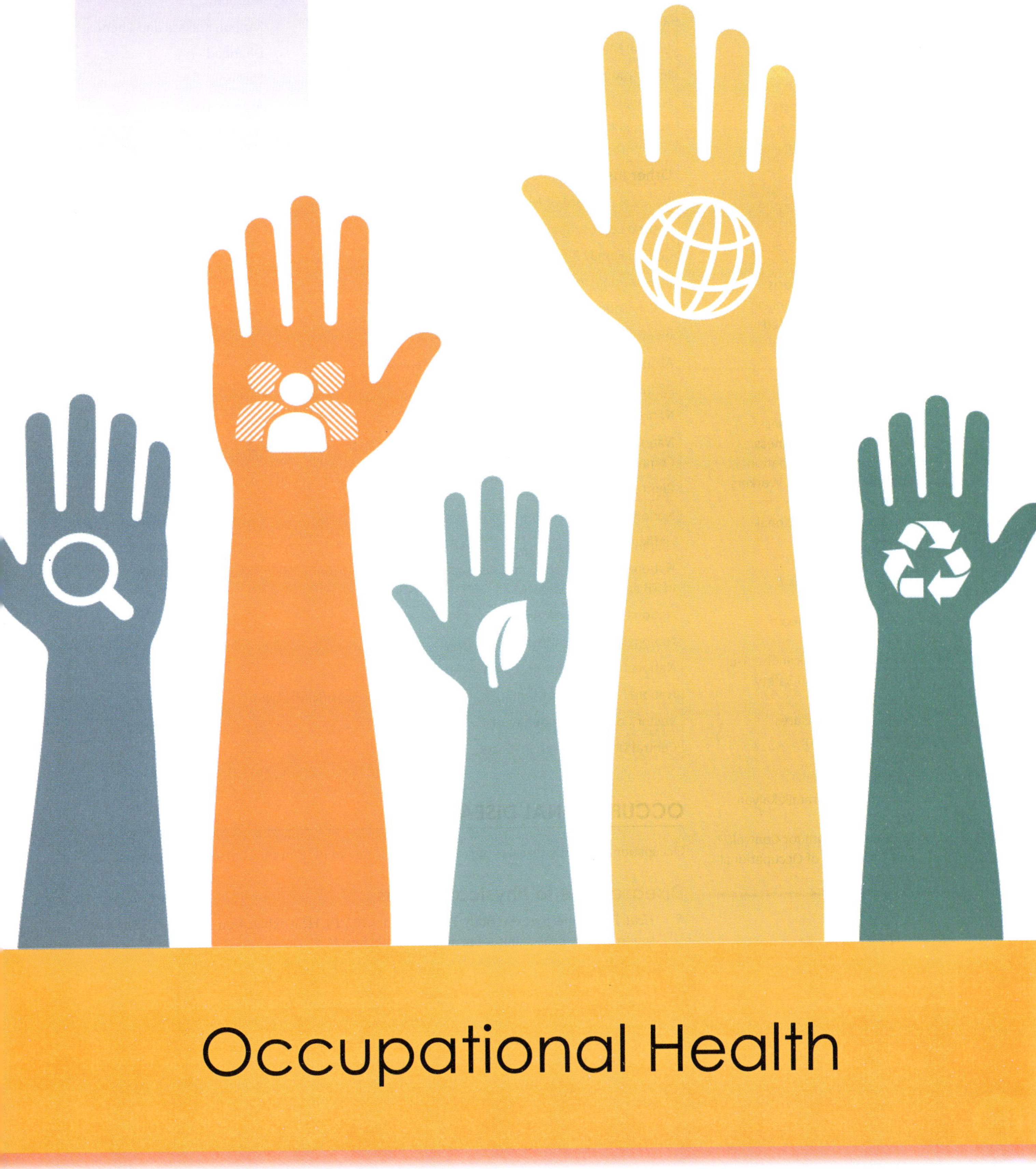

Occupational Health

Chapter Outline

- Occupational Health Research Institutes
- Occupational Diseases - Classification
  - Physical Agents
  - Chemical Agents
  - Biological Agents
  - Occupational Cancers
  - Occupational Dermatosis
  - Psychological Origin
- Thermal Injuries
  - Heat Injury
  - Cold Injury
- Pneumoconiosis
  - Silicosis
  - Asbestosis
  - Other Pneumoconiosis
- Occupation Related Cancers
- Other Occupation Related Diseases
  - Caplan
  - Metal Fume Fever
  - Plumbism
  - Decompression Sickness
  - Acute Mountain Sickness
  - Miscellaneous Occupational Hazards Agricultural Workers
    - Accidents
- Prevention of Occupational Diseases
  - Health
  - Sickness Absenteeism
  - Medical Measures
    - Preplacement Health Examination
    - Periodical Medical Check-up
    - Notification and Safety Audit
  - Engineering Measures
- Acts and Legislations
  - Factory Act
  - ESI Act
  - Rajiv Gandhi Shramik Kalyan Yojna
  - National Program for Control and Treatment of Occupational Diseases

65 High Yield Points

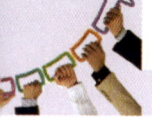

Bernardino Ramazzini is considered the Father of occupational medicine

OCCUPATIONAL HEALTH RESEARCH INSTITUTES

Institutes	Location
Central Labor Institute	Mumbai
Regional Labor Institutes	Kanpur, Kolkata and Chennai
Central Mining and Research Station, CSIR	Dhanbad
Industrial Toxicology Research Centre	Lucknow
National Institute of Occupational Health	Ahmedabad
National Environmental Engineering Research Institute	Nagpur

Other Institutes	Location
National Institute of Nutrition	Hyderabad
Central Leprosy Teaching and Research Institute	Chengalpattu
Central Family Planning Institute	New Delhi
International Institute for Population Studies	Mumbai
Indian Council of Medical Research	New Delhi
Blood Group Reference Centre	Mumbai
All India Institute of Hygiene and Public Health	Kolkata
All India Institute of Mental Health	Bengaluru
National Tuberculosis Institute	Bengaluru
National Centre for Diseases Control (Formerly National Institute of Communicable Diseases)	New Delhi
Central Research Institute	Kasauli
National Institute of Health and Family Welfare	New Delhi
Haffkine Institute	Mumbai
National Institute of TB and Respiratory Diseases (Formerly LRS Institute of TB and Allied Diseases)	New Delhi
National Institute of Virology	Pune
National JALMA Institute for Leprosy	Agra
National Institute for Research in Tuberculosis	Chennai
National Institute of Mental Health and Neurosciences (NIMHANS)	Bengaluru
Vector Control Research Centre	Puducherry
Central Drug Research Institute	Lucknow

OCCUPATIONAL DISEASES

Occupational hazards/diseases are conditions arising out of or in the course of employment

Diseases due to Physical Agents

- *Heat*: Heat hyperpyrexia (Body Temperature <102°F), Heat exhaustion (>106°F), Heat stroke (up to 110°F), heat cramps, burns and prickly heat.[Q]
- *Cold*: Trench foot, Frost bite, chilblains[Q]
- *Light*: Occupational cataract, miner's nystagmus
- *Pressure*: Caisson disease (Decompression Sickness occurs due to Nitrogen, Helium, Oxygen and combinations), Air embolism
- *Noise*: Occupational deafness
- *Radiation*: Cancer, Leukemia, Welder's flash[Q] (conjunctivitis and keratitis due to UV rays exposure in arc welding), Aplastic anemia, Pancytopenia, Genetic changes, etc.

- *Mechanical factors*: Injuries, Accident, Burns
- *Vibration:* Neurogenic damage, White fingers, Hand Arm Vibration syndrome (HAVS) or Raynaud's phenomenon

Diseases due to Chemical Agents

- *Gases*: CO_2, CO, HCN, CS_2, NH_3, H_2S, HCl, SO_2 gas poisoning.
- *Dusts (Pneumoconiosis)*[Q]
  - Pneumoconiosis is a lung disease occurring after a variable period of exposure to dust particles of size 0.5 to 5 micron.
- *Metals and compounds*: Toxic hazards from Lead, Mercury, Cadmium, Manganese, Beryllium, Arsenic and Chromium
- *Chemicals*: Acids, Alkali and Pesticides
- *Solvents*: Carbon bisulfide, Benzene, Trichloroethylene, Chloroform, etc.

Diseases due to Biological Agents

- Brucellosis, Leptospirosis, Anthrax, Actinomycosis, Hydatidosis, Psittacosis, Tetanus, Encephalitis, fungal infections, etc.

Occupational Cancers

- Skin cancer, lung cancer, bladder cancer, leukemia

Occupational Dermatosis

- Dermatitis, Eczema
  - Important Causes:
    - Physical: Heat, cold, moisture, friction, pressure, X-rays Chemical -acids, alkalies, dyes, solvents, grease, tar, pitch, chlorinated phenols.
    - Biological: Virus, bacteria, fungi and other parasites. Plant products—leaves, vegetables, fruits, flowers, vegetable dust.

Prevention of Occupational Dermatitis

- Pre placement medical examination.
- Personal Protection - protective clothing, long leather gloves, aprons and boots.
- Personal hygiene
- Periodic inspection/medical check-up

Diseases of Psychological Origin

Industrial neurosis, Hypertension, Peptic ulcer

THERMAL INJURIES

Heat Injury

Heat Stroke

- Mechanism: Failure of heat regulating mechanism
- Characterized by
  - Very high body temperature (>110°F)
  - Delirium, convulsion or loss of consciousness
  - Dry and hot skin
  - Sweating is absent or diminished
- High case fatality (~40%)
- Management – rapid cooling of body in ice water bath

Heat Hyperpyrexia

Mechanism: Impaired heat regulating function of the body
Characterized by temperature >106°F
Milder form of heat stroke

Heat Exhaustion

- Mechanism: Imbalance of body water and salt levels, due to thermal stress
- Body temperature usually <102°F
- Management: Fluid and electrolyte replacement

Heat Cramps

- Mechanism: Loss of serum sodium and chloride levels
- Due to heavy physical work in hot environment, may lead to painful spasmodic muscular contractions
- Related occupation: Soldiers, physical laborer

Heat Syncope

- Mechanism: Vasodilatation and pooling of blood in lower limbs with inadequate cardiac filling
- Characterized by
  - Sudden paleness
  - Hypotension
  - Collapse
  - No rise in body temperature
- Management – recovery within 10–15 minutes, lie in shade with slight lowering of head.
- Related occupations: Long standing in sun, soldiers, security guards, field workers

Heat Stress Index

It is the percentage of heat storage capacity of the individual

Heat stress % age	Interpretation
0	No thermal loss
10–30	Mid – moderate heat stress
40–60	Severe heat stress
70–90	Very severe heat stress
100	Maximum tolerable

Cold Injury

Acute Transient Inflammatory Reaction

- Mechanism–initial vasoconstriction followed by vasodilation (called as hunting phenomenon)
- Characterized by:
  - Pain numbness and loss of sensation
- Management–removal of cold stress

Trench Foot

- Mechanism: Acute transient vasoconstriction followed by intense vasodilation, transudation, hemoconcentration, platelet conglomeration
- Characterized by:
  - Swelling, numbness of tissue
  - Anesthetic waxy white with cyanotic areas
  - Tissue edema and gangrene
- Related occupation: Field workers, farmers, soldiers in snow terrains, prolonged standing in cold water/snow

Frostbite

- Mechanism: Freezing of tissue and formation of ice crystals in tissue
- Characterized by:
  - Pale, dull opaque skin
  - Blister formation after removal of stressor
  - Necrosis, gangrene of affected part
- **Management:** Rewarming in water at 42°C for 20 minutes

Cold Stress Severity Grading

Stages	Condition of fingers	Work and social interference
00	No tingling, numbness, or blanching of fingers	No complaints
OT	Intermittent tingling	No interference with activities
ON	Intermittent numbness	"
TN	Intermittent tingling and numbness	"
01	Blanching of fingertip with or without tingling and/or numbness	"
02	Blanching of one or more fingers beyond tips, usually during winter	Possible interference with nonwork activities; no interference at work
03	Extensive blanching of fingers; during summer and winter	Definite interference at work, at home and with social activities; restriction of hobbies
04	Extensive blanching of most fingers; during summer and winter	Occupation usually changed because of severity of signs and symptoms

Must Remember

Indicator for

- Heat injury – heat stress index
- Cold injuries – cold stress severity grading

PNEUMOCONIOSIS

Pneumoconiosis are collective group of diseases primarily due to long term dust exposure. Prolonged dust exposure causes local inflammatory reaction in the lung parenchyma, principally leading to fibrosis and usually restrictive type of lung disease along with other complications.

Dust Particle Size as Health Hazard for Pneumoconiosis

Particle size	Behaviour
>10 micron	Settle down by gravity
5–10 micron	Arrested in upper respiratory tract
3–5 micron	Deposited in mid respiratory tract
1–3 micron	Entered alveoli & settle there
<1 micron	Brownian movement

High Yield Points

Dust particle size ranging from 0.5 microns up to 5 microns is a potential health hazard predisposing to variety of lung disease - pneumoconiosis

Table 1: Pneumoconiosis caused by the dust originated from the specific industries

Dust		Industries
Inorganic (mineral) dusts		
Silica	Silicosis	Sand stone industry, granite industry, pottery and ceramic industry, gold, mica and steel industry
Asbestos	Asbestosis	Asbestos cement factory, fireproof textiles
Iron	Siderosis	Iron ores and mines, iron and steel industry
Coal dust	Anthracosis	Coal mines
Aluminum	Aluminosis	Aluminum industries
Barium	Baritosis	Photography, printing, barium diagnostic works
Stone	Lithosis	Stone industries
Organic (soluble) dust		
Cotton dust	Byssinosis	Textile industries
Sugar cane dust (Bagasse)	Bagassosis	Cane sugar factories, paper and card- board factories
Tobacco dust	Tobaccosis	Tobacco factories (Beedi, Cigar and Cigarette)
Moldy hay (Grain dust)	Farmers lung	Agricultural industry

Must Remember

Factors influencing pneumoconiosis

- Concentration of dust in air
- Composition of the dust
- Size of dust particle
- Duration of exposure
- Individual susceptibility (health status)

High Yield Points

Silicosis, Anthracosis, Byssinosis, Asbestosis are among the 29 notifiable diseases under Factory Act, 1948

X-ray Appearance in Pneumoconiosis

- Ground glass: Asbestosis
- Black lung (Multiple nodular opacities): Anthracosis
- Mottling: Bagassosis
- Fine nodular opacity: Farmers lung
- Snow storm: Silicosis (characteristic HRCT pattern "crazy paving")

Silicosis

General Features

- Silicosis is a notifiable disease under Factories Act, 1948 & Mines Act, 1952
- Silicosis patients are more prone to pulmonary TB.
- In most of cases we can see combination of silicosis and pulmonary tuberculosis in same patient.
- X-ray chest shows "snowstorm appearance" of the lung, usually in the upper 2/3rd of lung fields.
- Maximum permissible level of silica exposure is 40 micrograms per cubic meters for 10 hours for 35 years.
- There is no effective treatment as fibrotic changes cannot be reversed.

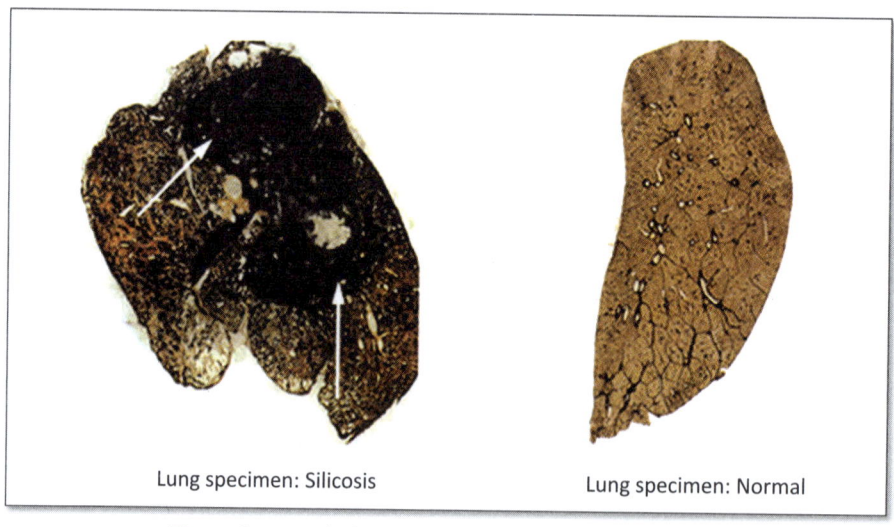

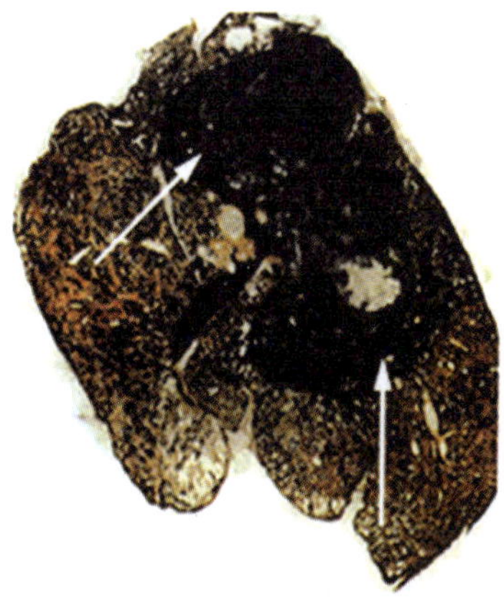

Lung specimen: Silicosis

Lung specimen: Normal

Fig. 1: Lung pathology in silicosis showing black nodules

Clinical Symptoms

- **First stage:** Patient notices **mild dyspnea** (i.e. dyspnea on exertion) which gradually increases. Clinical signs – little unproductive cough. Working capacity is slightly affected.
- **Second stage:** Marked by **dyspnea which impairs patient ability** to work and clinical signs of bronchial breathing, dullness on percussion and scattered rhonchi.
- **Third stage:** Patient is **totally in capacitated** with signs of right heart failure.

Asbestosis

General Features

- X-ray of chest shows "Ground glass appearance" in lower 2/3rd of lung fields
- Sputum shows 'asbestos bodies' which are asbestos fibers coated with fibrin.
- Once established, disease is progressive even after removal of worker from contact.

Clinical Features

- Dyspnea is first symptom which gradually increases in severity
- Cough—initially absent but later becomes more common
- In chronic cases clubbing of fingers, cardiac distress and cyanosis appear.

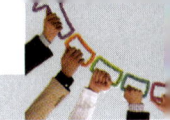

Table 2: Types of asbestos

Chrysolite	Serpentine family	White asbestos	Most common used	Roof, ceiling, wall, floor, ducts, appliances
Amosite	Amphibole family	Brown	In construction	Cement sheets, pipe insulations, ceiling tiles
Crocidolite	Amphibole family	Blue	Not very commonly used	Insulation of steam engines, coating spray on plastics, cement products
Anthophyllite	Amphibole family	Dull gray	Noncommercial use, Limited use	Thermal insulation
Tremolite and actinolite	Amphibole family	Different colors	Not used commercially	As contaminants in other varieties of asbestos

Note: The mineral families of asbestos are classified as:

- **Serpentine asbestos**:
  - Made of curly fibers
  - More than 95% of asbestos used is of this type
- **Amphibole asbestos**
  - Needle shaped fibers
  - Studies suggest "lesser" exposure to amphibole type for causing pneumoconiosis or malignancy in asbestosis.

Hence, some authors have concluded amphibole to be a dangerous type, whereas in reality as asbestos are dangerous. However, most countries have banned the amphibole type, but continuing use of serpentine type

Table 3: A brief about silicosis and asbestosis

	Silicosis	**Asbestosis**
Due to	Silica dust	Asbestos fiber
Industry	Construction, foundry, stone cutting, tunnel, glass factory	Heat insulators, construction, airplanes, cement roofs, fire proofing industry
Involvement	Upper zone of lungs	Lower zones of the lungs
Pathology	Bilateral nodular fibrosis	Diffuse fibrosis with/without inflammation
	Radiological signs are ≫ clinical signs	Clinical signs ≫ radiological signs
X-ray picture	Snow storm appearance of lungs	Ground glass appearance of lungs
	Prone to Tuberculosis	Prone to malignancy – most commonly seen is bronchial cancers

Other Pneumoconiosis

Anthracosis or Coal Miners Pneumoconiosis

- Frist phase: Simple pneumoconiosis, with little ventilatory impairment (Requires about 12 years of exposure)
- Second phase: Progressive Massive Fibrosis (develops without further exposure), severe respiratory disability and premature death
- Risk of death among coal miners is nearly twice that of the general population

45 ***Must Remember***

Effect of asbestosis on lung pathology

- Fibrosis of lung with/without pleural fibrosis;
- Hyaline pleural plaque formation
- Malignant mesothelioma
- Bronchial carcinoma

- *It is notifiable disease as per Indian Mines Act of 1952, Factory Act 1948 and compensable in Workmen's Compensation (Amendment) Act of 1959.*[Q]

Bagassosis

- Occupational disease of the lung caused by inhalation of fibrous residue of sugarcane (bagasse)
- Causative agent is *Thermoactinomyces sacchari*
- Bagasse contains a percentage of silica, innumerable fungal spores and microorganism
- Bagasse dust blocks bronchioles thus leading to bronchitis and bronchopneumonia
- Lung pathology: Mottled appearance of lung
- Prevention:
  - **Dust control:** Wet process, enclosed apparatus and moisture content (>20%)
  - **Personal protection:** Masks, respirators, etc.
  - **Medical control:** Examination and check-ups
  - **Bagasse control:** Spraying with 2% propionic acid (fungicide).

Byssinosis

- Byssinosis is due to inhalation of cotton fiber dust over long periods of time
- Commonly seen in workers of textile industries
- Symptoms
  - Chronic cough and
  - Progressive dyspnea.
- Later it leads to chronic bronchitis and emphysema
- Prevention: Dust control

Farmer's Lung

- Due to inhalation of Moldy hay or Grain dust
- Causative agent: Thermophilic actinomycete/Micropolyspora faeni
- Seen during winter when grain dust has moisture content over 30%, which is favorable for growth of fungus
- Acute illness is characterized by general respiratory symptoms and physical signs
- Repeated attacks cause pulmonary fibrosis and inevitable pulmonary damage and cor pulmonale.

OCCUPATION RELATED CANCERS

Skin Cancer

(Nearly 75% of occupational cancers)

- Squamous cell carcinoma is the most common.
- Caused by exposure to coal tar, X-rays, oils/dyes in gas workers, coke oven workers, tar distillers, oil refiners, dye makers, road makers and industries using mineral oil, pitch, tar and related compounds.
- **Carcinogens for skin cancer:**
  - Anthracene, Coal tar, soot, pitch, Oils and dyes, UV rays, X-rays

Lung Cancer

- It is a hazard in gas industry, asbestos industry, nickel and chromium work, arsenic roasting plants and in mining of radioactive substances (e.g. uranium)
- Carcinogens:
  - Arsenic, beryllium and isopropyl oil
  - Chromium, cobalt, tobacco, coal tar, nickel
- >90% lung cancers are attributed to tobacco smoking, air pollution and occupational exposure.

Cancer Bladder

- Caused by aromatic amines in dye-stuff and dyeing industry, rubber, gas and electric cable industries[Q]
- Carcinogens:
  - Beta-naphthalene, benzidine, auramine, aromatic amines, hemotoxins

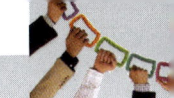

Leukemia

- Exposure to benzol, roentgen rays and radioactive substances.
- Carcinogens:
  - Ionizing radiations (X-rays, Gamma rays), radioactive isotopes

Table 4: Carcinogens and predisposing cancers

Predisposing agents	Cancers
Benzene, Ethylene Oxide	Leukemia
Beryllium, Cadmium, Chromium, Radon, Silica, Ionizing radiation, PAH, Nickel	Lung
Asbestos	Mesothelioma
Arsenic	Skin, Lung, Liver cancer
Benzidine	Bladder
PAH	Skin, Scrotum and Lung
Vinyl Chloride	Liver
Wood dust, Nickel, Chromium	Nasal Sinus

68 *High Yield Points*

Notable Cancers

- Chimney sweeper's cancer – cancer scrotum
- Mule spinners cancer – cancer scrotum (due to a special oil – 'shale oil' used in wool spinning)

Not occupational cancers are:

- Bladder cancer due to Schistosoma haematobium
- Dhoti cancer – due to mechanical irritation of skin on waist due to dhoti cloth

Control Measures for Industrial Cancer

- Elimination/control of industrial carcinogens: Well-designed building or machinery, closed system of production
- Medical examination of workers at regular interval
- Inspection of factories
- Notification
- Licensing of establishments
- Personal hygiene measures
- Education of workers and management
- Research

OTHER OCCUPATION RELATED DISEASES

Caplan's Syndrome

- It is combination of rheumatoid arthritis and pneumoconiosis with intrapulmonary nodules
- Caplan's syndrome occurs usually in pneumoconiosis related to mining dust (coal, asbestos and silica). The condition occurs in miners (especially those working in anthracite coal mines), asbestosis, silicosis and other pneumoconiosis.
- Other associations: Genetic predisposition and smoking.

Plumbism

Source

- Industrial:
  - Manufacture of storage batteries, printing, paint, ship building, glass manufacture, potteries, lead pipe, dyes, etc.
- Non-industrial:
  - Air pollution (gasoline) from automobile exhausts
  - Drinking water through lead pipes
  - Accidental ingestion of lead paints from wooden toys by children
- Most common **route of exposure**: Inhalation > ingestion > contact

Pathogenesis

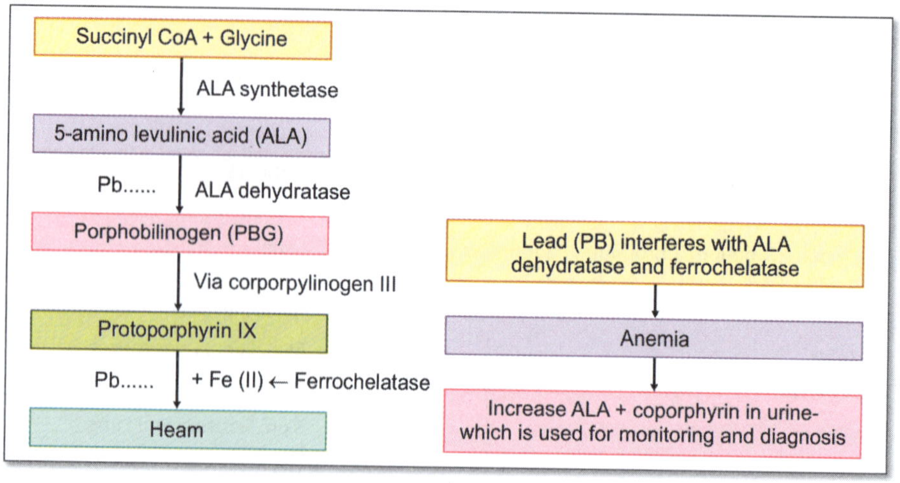

Clinical Presentation

- Burtonian line (blue discoloration on gums)
- Abdominal colic (also known as painter's colic)
- Anemia, fatigue and loss of appetite
- Neurological manifestations:
  - Wrist drops
  - Foot drops
  - Peripheral motor neuropathy
  - Generalized pain
- Encephalopathy

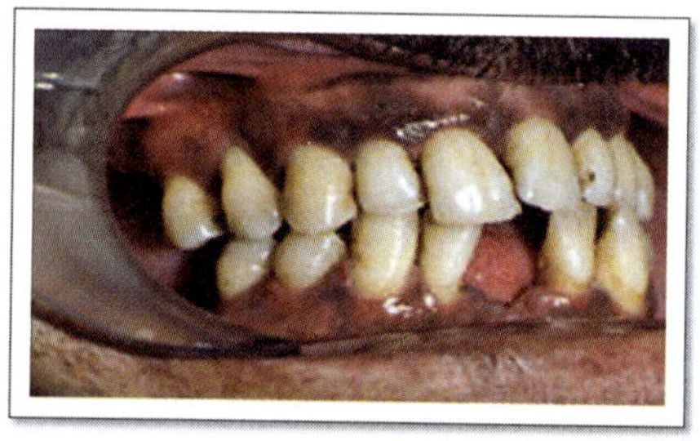

Fig. 2: Burtonian line—blue line on gums

Diagnosis

Laboratory investigations indicative of plumbism
- Hemoglobin – low
- Microcytic hypochromic RBC on PBS
- Basophilic stippling of RBCs
- Low reticulocyte count.

Diagnostic and confirmatory indicator

Initial investigation is:
- Free erythrocyte protoporphyrin (FEP) levels are good indicator of lead toxicity
- Urinary ALA levels may also be done

Confirmatory/diagnostic
- Blood lead levels (BLL)
  - Normal is <10 mcg/dL
  - Anything more than 10 mcg/dL should be dealt with caution and needs removal of lead, management and follow-ups

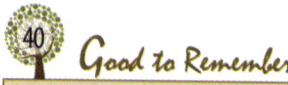

40 Good to Remember

EDTA cannot cross the blood brain barrier and hence will not help in case of lead toxicity related medical emergencies involving encephalopathies. Dimercaperol can cross blood brain barrier and hence should be given before Ca Na_2 EDTA to have its effect of chelation in the brain.

Table 5: Blood lead levels at different stages

Stages	Blood lead levels	Remarks
Stage I	10–14 mcg/dL	No further treatment, health education and follow ups
Stage II	14–20 mcg/dL	Treat if levels persist for more than three months
Stage III	20–44 mcg/dL	Complete medical evaluation. Chelate recommended only in case of organ involvement
Stage IV	45–69 mcg/dL	Complete medical evaluation and Chelation recommended in most cases
Stage V	> 70 mcg/dL	Chelation and management of lead toxicity is recommended with or without symptoms

Table 6: Levels of lead in normal and dangerous level in humans

Parameter	Normal levels	Dangerous levels
Blood lead	<10 mcg per 100 mL	> 45 mcg per 100 mL
Urinary lead	0.2 – 0.8 mg per litre	> 0.8 mg per litre
Urinary Aminolevulinic Acid (ALA)	6 mg per litre	60 mg per litre
Urinary coproporphyrin	< 150 mcg per litre	> 250 mcg per litre

Treatment

Blood lead levels >70 mcg/dL require urgent chelation and treatment

- Succimer – oral water soluble agent
- Dimercaprol (BAL) parental chelator. Agent of first choice in lead encephalopathy
  - With high BLLs (i.e. >100 µg/dL), it is used in conjunction with $CaNa_2$ EDTA
- Ca Na_2 EDTA (calcium disodium EDTA) not recommended for use as single chelation based therapy
- D penicillamine: Second line chelation therapy.

Metal Fume Fever

- It is temporary disease resulting from inhalation of fresh metallic oxide fumes of zinc and magnesium
- **Features:**
  - Rise in body temperature
  - Sweating, chills
  - Dryness of throat, cough, breathlessness
- It does not cause permanent changes and recovery takes place within 24 hours
- Occupation at risk: metal welders, galvanizing, heavy metal molting factories

Decompression Sickness

- Decompression sickness is a disorder in which nitrogen dissolved in the blood and tissues by high pressure forms bubbles as pressure decreases.
- **Mechanism:** The air is composed of oxygen and nitrogen molecules. Now while normal breathing, the oxygen molecules are consumed but nitrogen molecules may accumulate in blood and tissues. So, when a diver ascent from high pressure zone to low pressure zone, the excess nitrogen already accumulated in the blood may not be directly exhaled and thus form bubbles – to block the blood supply to vital organs and tissues. This may lead to characteristic pain in muscles, joints, tendons, sudden weakness and dizziness.
  - Type I decompression sickness tends to be mild and affects primarily the joints, skin, and lymphatic vessels.
  - Type II decompression sickness, which may be life-threatening, often affects vital organ systems, including the brain and spinal cord, the respiratory system, and the circulatory system.
- **Occupations at risk:** Deep sea divers
- **Management:** 100% hyperbaric oxygen (oxygen first aid)
- Prevention–
  - Use of decompression chambers
  - Slow ascent with safety stops before resurfacing
  - Resurfacing rate at no more than 10mts/min with 'decompression stops'

Acute Mountain Sickness

- Mechanism: exposure to low partial pressure of oxygen and subsequent alkalosis
- Typically occurs after ascent of more than 2500 meters
- **Features:**
  - Intense headache with fatigue, peripheral edema, epistaxis, dyspnea

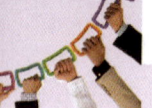

- **Complication:**
  - High altitude pulmonary edema (HAPE)—due to vasoconstriction in the pulmonary circulation due to ventilation-perfusion mismatch and maintain the cardiac output
  - High altitude cerebral edema (HACE)—due to local vasodilation in response to hypoxia
- **Prevention:**
  - Altitude pre-acclimatization
  - Ascent not more than 300 m/min

Miscellaneous Occupational Hazards

Agricultural Workers

Farming and agriculture sector take a major role in India's GDP. Various diseases may be predisposed due to farming and agriculture as

- Zoonotic diseases
  - Tetanus, anthrax, Q-fever
- Accidents
  - Insect bites, snake bites, animal bites
- Toxic hazards
  - Use of fertilizers, pesticides may expose the farming community to various chemical intoxications
- **Other hazards:**
  - Physical hazards – due to heat, prolonged sun exposure or cold exposure
  - Respiratory diseases- due to work with grains, husk, tobacco plants, cotton seeds
  - Psychological stress – due to financial burdens, low crop productivity, climatic changes

Accidents

- 98% of accidents are preventable
- Human factors predisposing to accidents are:
  - Unskilled workers – lack of training and experience
  - Young age groups
  - Long working hours
- Environmental factors
  - Unsafe machines
  - Unsafe temperature, illumination and lack of space

PREVENTION OF OCCUPATIONAL DISEASES

Ergonomics: Application of psychological, medical and engineering principles for making the work place more suitable for enhancing proficiency of the workers and maintenance of health of the workers.

Emporiatrics: Application of psychological and medical understanding for protecting health and preventing disease in people with different external environments due to more than usual long distance traveling.

Sickness Absenteeism

- This is an index of health status of the workers in industry.
- Cause:
  - Economic (Entitlement to sick leave)
  - Social (Family obligations e.g. Wedding)
  - Medical
  - Nonoccupational (nutritional disorders, alcoholism and drug addiction, etc).

Sickness Absenteeism Rate (SAR)

$$\frac{\text{Number of workers remaining absent during a year}}{\text{Total no. of workers}} \times 100$$

- Incidence of SAR in India is 15–20% or 8–10 days/person/year (High SAR is indicator of poor health status of workers and industry)

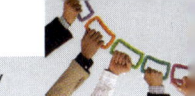

- Control comprises of good management practices, pre placement exam and ergonomics.
- Preplacement examination is done at the time of employment to place the right man in the right job. It serves as a useful benchmark for future comparison.

Medical Measures to Prevent Occupational Disease Burden

Preplacement Health Examination

- Should include X-rays, physical examination, ECG, vision testing, routine urine and blood examination
- Usually considered as primary prevention
  - In case of screening of disease before employment in food handling industry – would fit into the category of primary prevention – as objective is to find disease in the food handlers "to prevent spread of disease in other individuals – who might be at risk due to consumption of the food"

Table 7: Diseases to be screened in case of special industries

Industries	Diseases to be screened for employment
Lead	Anemia, Hypertension, Nephritis and Peptic ulcer
Dyes	Asthma, skin, bladder and kidney diseases and Precancerous lesions
Solvents	Liver and Kidney disease, Dermatitis and Alcoholism
Silica	Pulmonary TB (Healed or active), Chronic lung disease
Radium and X-rays	Blood disorder
Food handlers	For communicable diseases, hepatitis, typhoid, contagious diseases

Periodical Medical Check-up of Workers

- It fits into the category of secondary prevention (objective is to find the earliest possible point of occupation-related health issues)
- Frequency and content depend upon the type of occupational exposure
  - Usually done on annual basis
  - Monthly in case of exposure to lead, toxic dyes, radium, etc.
  - Daily if chemicals like dichromate are handled.

Notification of Diseases

- Inclusion of acts and legislations for early notification of disease and implementation of preventive measures
  - Mines act – 3 diseases
  - Dock act – 8 diseases
  - Factories act – 22 diseases

Safety Audit

Safety audit is a comprehensive study of the safety of a particular workplace. It is carried out at three levels

- *Level - I*: Internal audit inspection by Safety Officers from within the factory once in every 3 months.
- *Level - II*: Audit inspection by a group of 3 officers of the factory in concerned group, 6 monthly.
- *Level - III*: Annual audit inspection by the Regional Controller of Safety.

Engineering Measures

- Extensive use of Ergonomics – to study efficiency of people in an environment
- Better building designs and architecture
  - Illumination
  - Ventilation
  - Thermal control
  - Dust control

- Hygiene and house keeping
- Substitution of harmful chemical with less toxic chemicals

Table 8: Common substitutions to prevent occupational exposure

Harmful substance	Harmless Substitute substance
Yellow (White phosphorous)	Phosphorous sesquisulfide (prevents "phossy jaw")
Lead paints	Zinc or Iron paints
Mercury salts	Silver salts
Benzene	Acetone
Sandstone	Carborundum

ACTS AND LEGISLATIONS

Factory Act, 1948

- Factory is defined as an establishment employing 10 or more workers where power is used, and 20 or more workers where power is not used
- There is no distinction between perennial and seasonal factories
- 'Worker' includes contract labor employed in the manufacturing process
- The Act applies to the whole of India except the State of Jammu and Kashmir.[Q]

Prescribed Work Hours

- Maximum 48 hours per week, not more than 9 hours per day with rest of at least 1/2 hour after 5 hours of continuous work
- For adolescents, maximum hours of work is $4^{1/2}$ per day
- Total hours of work in a week including overtime shall not exceed 60 hours. (Maximum permissible)
- Spread over period of work (including rest intervals) of an employee in a factory is 12 hours.

Employment Regulations

- Employment of children below age of 14 completed years is prohibited[Q]
- Employment of women and children is restricted in certain dangerous occupations
- Adolescent (15–18 years) is allowed to work only between 6 A.M.-7 P.M after medical certification by "Certifying Surgeons" as fit for work.
- Leave with wage 1 day per 15 day of work (maximum accumulated up to 30 day in adult and 40 day in children)

Health and Welfare Provisions

- Minimum 500 Cu.ft of space for each worker (space 14 ft above ground level not taken into account). For factories installed before the 1948 Act, a minimum of 350 Cu.ft of space is prescribed.
- Safety provisions like casing of new machinery, devices for cutting off the power, lifts, cranes etc.
- Empowers state governments to prescribe maximum weights which may be lifted or carried by men, women and children.

> **46 Must Remember**
> - 1 Safety Officers in every factory wherein 1,000 or more workers are employed.[Q]
> - 1 Canteen in every factory wherein more than 250 workers are employed.[Q]
> - 1 Creche in every factory wherein more than 30 women workers are employed.[Q]
> - 1 Welfare Officer in every factory, wherein 500 or more workers are employed.
> - 1 Chief Inspector of Factories and additional Chief Inspectors as thought fit to enforce the provisions.

ESI Act, 1948

ESI scheme constituted under the ESI (Employee State Insurance) Act, 1948 is s a self-financing health insurance scheme administered by "Employees State Insurance Corporation" (ESIC)
ESI Act applies to the following establishments:

- Small factories employing 10 or more persons, whether power is used in manufacturing or not
- Shops, Hotels/Restaurants, Cinemas/Theaters
- Road-Motor transport and Newspaper establishments
- Private medical and educational institutions employing 20 or more persons in some states
- Now extended to agricultural or commercial establishment

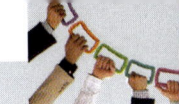

- With effect from 06.09.2016, the Act covers all employees—manual, clerical, supervisory and technical getting up to ₹21000 per month
- It covers all states except Manipur, Sikkim, Mizoram, Arunachal Pradesh and Union Territory of Delhi and Chandigarh
- **ESIC** runs on contributions by employees, employers and grants from Central/State Governments.
- Employer contributes 4.75% of total wage bill
- Employee contributes 1. 75% of wages. Employee with wages up to ₹100/day are exempted
- State Government and ESIC share of expenditure on medical care is 1/8th and 7/8th of total cost respectively

Benefits to Employees

- Medical benefit: Primary, Secondary and Tertiary medical care including hospitalization, OPD, drugs/dressings, emergency services, pathological/radiological tests, etc. free of cost to insured person and his family members in case of sickness, employment injury and maternity with no cap on individual expenditure
- Sickness benefit: 91 days at 70% of average daily wages. Insured worker is required to contribute for 78 days in a contribution period of 6 months
- Extended sickness benefit: Sickness benefit is extendable up to 2 years in the case of 34 malignant and long-term diseases at an enhanced rate of 80% of wages
- Enhanced sickness benefit (or medical benefit) at full wages for 14 days for tubectomy and 7 days for vasectomy
- Maternity benefit at full wages for 24 week (under Pradhan Mantri Surakshit Matritva Abhiyan)
- Disablement benefit comprises of cash payment and Free medical treatment
- Temporary disablement benefit is at 90% of wages as long as disability lasts. From 1st day of entering insurable employment and irrespective of having paid any contribution
- Permanent disablement benefit at 90% of wages in the form of monthly payment based on loss of earning capacity determined by a medical board.

Dependent's Benefit

- In case of death as a result of employment injury, dependents of an insured person are eligible for monthly cash payments, up to the rate of 90% of wages, shared by dependent.
- Eligible son/daughter can avail the benefit up to the age of 18 year and benefit is withdrawn if the daughter marries earlier
  - *Funeral expenses* – Cash payment on death of an insured person (Maximum INR 10,000).
  - *Rehabilitation:* On payment of ₹10/month, insured person and his family continue to get medical treatment after permanent disablement or retirement.
  - *Confinement expenses:* An insured Woman or an insured person in respect of his wife in case confinement occurs at a place where necessary medical facilities under ESI Scheme are not available

Benefits to Employers

- Exemption from the applicability of Workmen's Compensation Act 1923 and Maternity Benefit Act 1961.
- Exemption from payment of medical allowance to employees/dependents or arranging for their medical care
- Rebate under Income Tax Act on contribution deposited in the ESI Account.
- Healthy work-force.

Rajiv Gandhi Shramik Kalyan Yojana (2005)

An Insured Person who becomes unemployed after being insured three or more years, due to closure of factory/establishment, retrenchment or permanent invalidity of not less than 40% out of nonemployment injury is entitled to:

- Unemployment Allowance equal to 50% of wage for a maximum period of 1 year.
- Medical care for self and family from ESI Hospitals/Dispensaries during the period insured Person gets unemployment allowance.

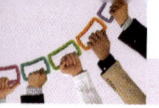

- Vocational Training for upgrading skills - Expenditure on fee/traveling allowance borne by ESIC.
- Allowance can be availed in one spell or in different spells of not less than 1 month.

ESIC-2 *(2ND Generation Reforms Agenda in ESI, launched on 20th July 2015 by Honorable Prime Minister Shri Narendra Modi)*

Agenda-1-Extending Coverage

- Cover all states/UT not yet covered (Arunachal Pradesh, Mizoram, Manipur, Andaman and Nicobar) by 31st December 2015.
- Cover all the construction workers under ESIC by 31st December 2015
- Open health scheme for select groups of unorganized workers (e.g. Rickshaw pullers, Auto rickshaw drivers) in select urban/metropolitan area by 30th November 2015.
- Setting up state ESI Corporation/Society in all states/UT as subsidiary of ESI Corporation by 31st March 2016

Agenda-2-Reforms in Health Services

- Online availability of electronic health record of ESI beneficiaries
- Abhiyan Indradhanush (Use of bed sheets of specified color daily-VIBGYOR pattern)
- Upgradation of ESI dispensaries to 6 bedded hospitals as per IPHS Standards in a phased manner
- Medical helpline -1800-11-3839 for emergency and seeking guidance
- Special OPD for elderly and differently abled patients between 3 pm and 5 pm
- Cancer detection /Treatment, Cardiology, Dialysis and Pathological Test facilities by 31st December 2015

Agenda-3- Improving Patient/Attendant Care

- Queue management system, Reception counters, Behavioral training of staff, Proper and attractive signage's, feedback system for indoor patient
- Pregnant mother and newborn tracking in Insured persons families for safe delivery and complete immunization.
- One Mother and Child care hospital with higher facility in every state by 31st March 2016.
- Facilities for YOGA, Telemedicine and AYUSH

National Program for Control and Treatment of Occupational Diseases

- Launched by Ministry of Health and Family Welfare, Government of India in1998-99.
- National Institute of Occupational Health, Ahmedabad is the nodal agency.

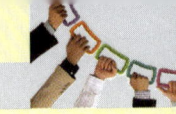

Image-Based Questions

1. The picture shown is related to:

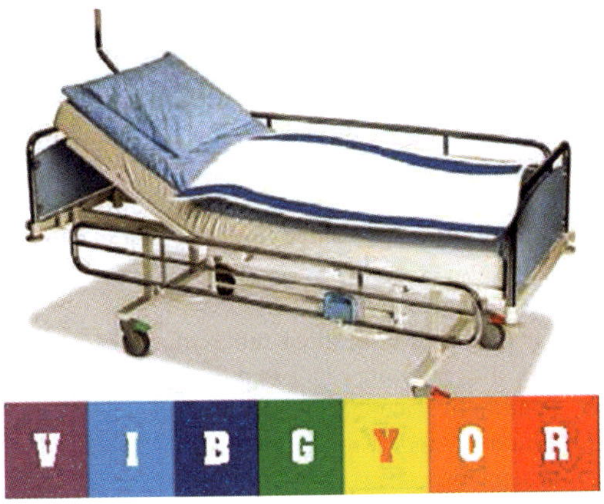

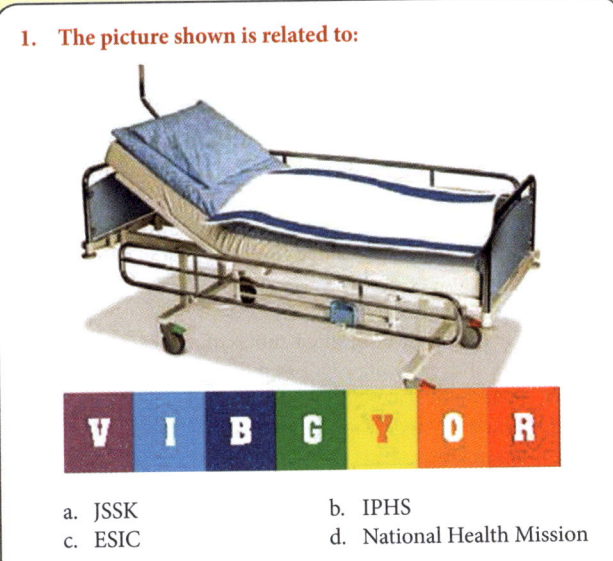

a. JSSK
b. IPHS
c. ESIC
d. National Health Mission

2. Identify the compound in the image:

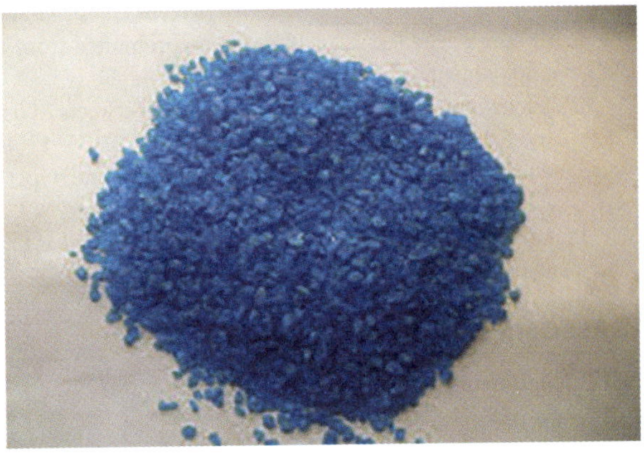

a. Rhodamine blue
b. Copper sulfate
c. Barium powder
d. $MgSO_4$ granules

3. Identify the most probable diagnosis of the X-ray shown:

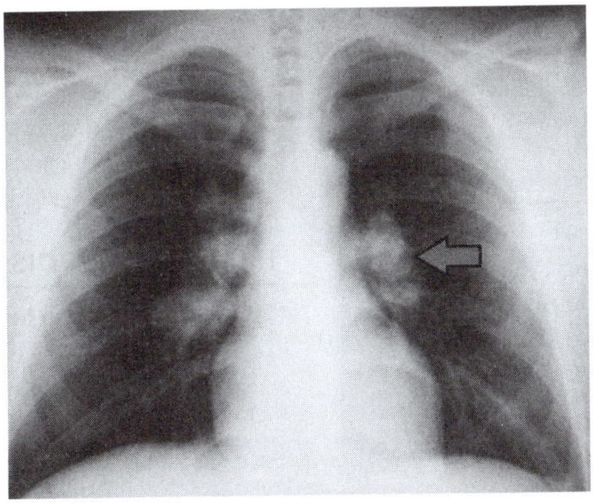

a. Silicosis
b. Asbestosis
c. Pneumoconiosis
d. Pneumonia

Answers of Image-Based Questions

1. **Ans. (c)** ESIC
2. **Ans. (b)** Copper sulfate
3. **Ans. (a)** Silicosis

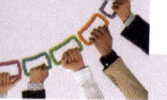

Multiple Choice Questions

1. **Which of the following is true under Factories Act of 1976?** *(Recent Question 2018)*
   a. Children aged less than 14 years are prohibited from any employment.
   b. Adolescents aged 15–18 years can work between 7.00 pm and 6.00 am.
   c. Women and children can be employed in all types of works.
   d. Adolescents of 16 years need not be duly certified as fit for work by certifying surgeon.

BAGASSOSIS

2. **Inhalation of sugarcane dust results in:**
   a. Bagassosis b. Byssinosis
   c. Tobaccosis d. Farmer's lung
3. **Bagassosis is caused by dust of:** *(Recent Question 2017)*
   a. Jute b. Cotton
   c. Sugar cane d. Textiles
4. **Thermoactinomyces Sacchari is causative agent for:**
   a. Bagassosis b. Siderosis
   c. Byssinosis d. Anthracosis

BYSSINOSIS

5. **Byssinosis is seen in:** *(Recent Question 2017)*
   a. Cement factories b. Textile industries
   c. Iron factories d. Grain fields

FARMERS LUNG

6. **Micropolyspora faeni causes:**
   a. Bagassosis b. Farmer's lung
   c. Suberosis d. Sequousis
7. **Main cause of Farmer's lung is** *(Recent Question 2016)*
   a. Pneumococcus
   b. Mycobacterium Tuberculosis
   c. Micropolyspora faeni
   d. Staphylococcus aureus

ASBESTOSIS

8. **Most common manifestation of asbestos exposure comprises of:**
   a. Pleural plaques
   b. Pulmonary fibrosis
   c. Pleural effusion
   d. Lung nodules
9. **Size of respirable dusts is:**
   a. <0.5 microns b. <1 microns
   c. <5 microns d. 5–15 microns

SILICOSIS

10. **Silicosis was first reported in:** *(Recent Question 2016)*
    a. USA b. Russia
    c. Africa d. India
11. **Silicosis was first identified in which mine in India:**
    a. Kolar b. Bokaro
    c. Shimoga d. Bellary
12. **Most commonly implicated form of silica in silicosis:**
    a. Amorphous b. Quartz
    c. Cristobalite d. Tridymite
13. **All are true regarding silico-tuberculosis, except:**
    a. Silicotics are more prone to pulmonary tuberculosis
    b. Sputum in silico-TB usually show tubercle bacilli
    c. Children and women of silico-TB do not develop tuberculosis
    d. Postmortem on silicotuberculotics failed to prove the existence of tuberculosis disease
14. **True about silicosis:** *(PGI Pattern)*
    a. Caused by exposure of silica oxide
    b. Severe exposure- whole lung lavage may helpful in alleviating symptoms
    c. Fibrosis of upper lung
    d. Fibrotic change can be reversed after stopping exposure
    e. More risk of TB and lung cancer
15. **True regarding sickness benefit as per ESI Act 1948:**
    a. Payable for maximum of period of 91 days
    b. Extended benefit is payable for 309 days
    c. Benefit is 30% of average daily wage
    d. Viral fever is an indicator for extended benefit

HEAVY METAL POISONING

16. **Most common heavy metal poisoning in the world:**
    a. Lead b. Arsenic
    c. Mercury d. Cadmium
17. **The following is the minimum blood level of lead to be associated with clinical manifestations:**
    a. 50 µg/100 mL b. 70 µg/100 mL
    c. 90 µg/100 mL d. 110 µg/100 mL

OCCUPATIONAL CANCER AND OTHER DISORDERS

18. **Occupational cancer involve following organs, except:**
    a. Lung b. Breast
    c. Bladder d. Liver
19. **Contribution of State according to ESI Act:**
    a. 4.75%
    b. 1.75%
    c. 12.5%
    d. 20%

Ans.

1. a
2. a
3. c
4. a
5. b
6. b
7. c
8. a
9. c
10. d
11. a
12. b
13. b
14. a, c, e
15. a
16. a
17. b
18. b
19. c

Most Recent Question of 2019-18 is given at the end of MCQs

20. Chimney sweeps Cancer is also known as:
a. Carcinoma Scrotum
b. Carcinoma urinary bladder
c. Carcinoma testis
d. Carcinoma penis

21. Most common occupational cancer is:
a. Skin cancer
b. Lung cancer
c. Bladder cancer
d. Brain cancer

22. All the following are characteristic features of occupational cancers, except: *(Recent Question 2016)*
a. The period between exposure and development of the disease may be as long as 10–25 years
b. The disease may develop even after the cessation of exposure
c. The average incidence is earlier than that for cancer in general
d. The localization of the tumors is variable in any one occupation

23. Benzene occupational exposure may lead to: *(Recent Question 2016)*
a. Lung cancer
b. Leukaemia
c. COPD
d. Neurofibromas

24. Occupational exposure that may cause sterility in females:
a. Aniline b. Lead
c. Radon d. Nickel

FACTORY ACT

25. Minimum area per person mandatory under the factory act: *(Recent Question 2016)*
a. 100 cu. ft b. 200 cu. ft
c. 500 cu. ft d. 1000 cu. ft

26. Notification of occupational diseases is required in all of the following legislations, except:
a. ESI Act b. Mines Act
c. Factories Act d. Labor Act

27. True regarding the factories Act, 1948:
a. A minimum of 1000 cu. ft. per worker has been prescribed
b. Appointment of safety officers where 500 or more employees are employed
c. Creches where more than 30 women are employed
d. Maximum 42 hrs work per week, not exceeding 8 hrs per day

ESI ACT

28. ESIC chairman is: *(Recent Question 2015)*
a. Prime Minister
b. Union Minister Labor
c. Union Minister Health and Family Welfare
d. Union minister for Human Resource Development

29. Ergonomics means
a. Fitting job to worker
b. Study of human behavior
c. Study of social mobility
d. Study of health of female workers

30. Ergonomics means *(Recent Question 2015)*
a. Fitting the job to the worker
b. Fitting the worker to the job
c. Industrial hygiene
d. Industrial health

31. Chairman of ESI corporation is:
a. Union health minister
b. Union minister of labor
c. Union minister of law
d. Union minister of finance

32. A Family Dispensary under ESI Act, is opened for ___ number of insured family units *(Recent Question 2014)*
a. 500 b. 1000
c. 1500 d. 2000

33. Under the ESI scheme, the employer's contribution is:
a. 1.75% b. 2.75%
c. 3.75% d. 4.75%

34. In ESI Act, 1948 the employer's contribution is 4.75% of the:
a. Total wages b. Yearly profit
c. Cost of company d. Total welfare cost

35. All are true regarding cash benefit under ESI scheme, except: *(Recent Question 2014)*
a. Standard sickness benefit at 50% of wages
b. Extended sickness benefit at 50% of wages
c. Temporary disablement benefit at 60% of wages
d. Dependent's benefit at 70% wages

36. All of the following are benefits of ESI Act, except:
a. Medical benefit
b. Rehabilitation allowance
c. Sickness benefit
d. Nutritional allowance

37. Standard sickness benefit under ESI scheme is given for a period of:
a. 30 days b. 42 days
c. 91 days d. 120 days

38. Amount payable as enhanced sickness benefit under the ESI scheme for persons undergoing sterilization operation is: *(Recent Question 2014)*
a. 50% of wages
b. 75% of wages
c. 90% of wages
d. 100% of wages

39. The maximum period for which an insured person shall be entitled to draw unemployment allowance:
a. 6 months b. 9 months
c. 12 months d. 15 months

40. All the following are true regarding Rajiv Gandhi Shramik Kalian Yojana, except: *(Recent Question 2013)*
a. Launched by ESI in the year 2005
b. Comes under the ministry of labor and employment
c. Provides unemployment allowance
d. Only persons who have contributed to the scheme for 5 years or more are eligible

41. True about ESI Act 1948 is: *(Recent Question 2013)*
a. Applicable on educational institution also
b. Employers contribution is 1.75%
c. Maternity benefit for 3 months
d. Beneficiaries are those having income with >15,000/month

Ans.

20. a
21. a
22. d
23. b
24. c
25. c
26. a
27. c
28. b
29. a
30. a
31. b
32. b
33. d
34. a
35. None
36. d
37. c
38. d
39. c
40. d
41. a

Most Recent Question of 2019-18 is given at the end of MCQs

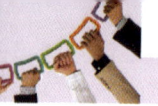

42. False about ESI in India is:
a. Centre contribute 7/8 and state contribute 1/8 part on expenditure
b. A worker with income less than 70/- per day has to pay only 300/- per month
c. Funeral expenses is 50,000/-
d. Medical benefit include full medical care

43. True about ESI Act is: ***(Recent Question 2013)***
a. Funeral charges up to ₹50,000
b. State government share is 1/8 and ESI Corporation is 7/8
c. Employee contribute 8.75% and employee 3.75%
d. Maximum limit for each family member is ₹30,000

44. Regarding ESI all are correct statement except:
a. Abhiyan Indradhanush is under the ESI
b. Full wage compensation is paid for vasectomy and tubectomy
c. The centre government also contributes as 12.5% of the expense for ESI
d. It is applicable for all workers with salary upto 21,000 INR per month

45. Which of the following is/are not true of ESI act, 1948?
a. Involves those working in restaurants
b. 100% wages in temporary disability
c. Extended sickness benefit 91 days
d. Workers pay 1.75% of income
e. Run by central government

46. Sickness benefit under ESI Act extended into:
a. 91 days
b. 61 days
c. 1 year
d. 2 year

47. Rajiv Gandhi Shramik Kalyan Yojana is a part of:
a. National Rural Employment Guarantee Scheme
b. Employee's State Insurance Scheme
c. Pradhan Mantri Jan Dhan Yojana
d. Pradhan Mantri Suraksha Bima Yojana

48. Which of the following statement regarding Factory Act is correct
a. Child age less than 18 years cannot be employed
b. Child age less than 14 years cannot be employed in dangerous work
c. Working hours should not be more than 40 hours per week for adults
d. Working hours are 6 hours per day for children

Most Recent Question (2019-2018)

49. In ESI scheme which of the following benefits is/are given by cash: ***(PGI May 2018)***
a. Maternity benefit
b. Funeral expense
c. Dependent benefit
d. Sickness benefit
e. Medical benefit

Ans.

42. b, c
43. b
44. c
45. b, c, e
46. a
47. b
48. b
49. b

Answers with Explanations

1. Ans. (a) Children aged less than 14 years are prohibited from any employment

BAGASSOSIS

2. Ans. (a) Bagassosis

Ref: K. Park, 24th ed. p 844

Bagassosis is an occupational disease of the lung *caused by inhalation of bagasse or sugar-cane dust.*[Q]

- Thermophilic actinomycete *(Thermoactinomyces sacchari)*[Q] is the causative agent.

Preventive measures comprise:

- **Dust control:** Wet process, enclosed apparatus, exhaust ventilation etc.
- **Personal protection:** Masks or respirators with mechanical filters or with oxygen or air supply.
- **Medical control:** Initial and periodical medical check-ups of workers.
- **Bagasse control:** Keeping moisture content above 20 % and spraying bagasse with 2 % propionic acid.

Also Know

- *Hazardous effects of dusts on lungs depend upon* (a) chemical composition (b) fineness (c) concentration of dust (d) period of exposure(e) health status of exposed person

3. Ans. (c) Sugar cane

Ref: K. Park, 24th ed. p 844

4. Ans. (a) Bagassosis

Ref: K. Park, 24th ed. p 844

BYSSINOSIS

5. Ans. (b) Textile industries

Ref: K. Park, 24th ed. p 843

Byssinosis *is due to inhalation of cotton dust over a long period of time.*[Q]

- It affects 7-8% of workers in Textile industry
- Aerobacter Cloacae is a possible cause (contaminates cotton fibres in hot and humid climate)
- Characterized by acute symptoms of tightness in chest and altered respiratory function, within hours after beginning exposure, *especially on Mondays or after holidays*. Hence called "***Monday fever***".[Q]
- Continued exposure over several years can lead to irreversible impairment (chronic cough, progressive dyspnoea, emphysema)

FARMERS LUNG

6. Ans. (b) Farmers lung

Ref: K. Park, 23rd ed. p 807

7. Ans. (c) Micropolyspora faeni

Ref: K. Park, 24th ed. p 844

Farmer's lung *is due to the inhalation of mouldy hay or grain dust.*[Q]

- Thermophilic actinomycetes "***Micropolyspora faeni***" is the main cause [Q]
- Acute illness is characterised by general and respiratory symptoms and physical signs.
- Repeated attacks can cause pulmonary fibrosis, inevitable pulmonary damage and corpulmonale.

ASBESTOSIS

8. Ans. (a) Pleural plaques

Ref: K. Park, 24th ed. p 844

Asbestosis results from prolonged inhalation (minimum 5-10 year) of Asbestos dust (silicates of Mg, Fe, Ca, Na and Al –generated in manufacture of asbestos cement, fireproof textiles, roof tiling, brake lining, and gaskets).

It is characterized by

- Pulmonary fibrosis (*Peri-bronchial, diffuse and basal*[Q])
- Respiratory insufficiency (dyspnoea out of proportion to clinical signs), clubbing, cardiac distress, cyanosis and death
- Carcinoma of bronchus, Mesothelioma (Pleura and Peritoneum) and Cancer of GI tract.
- Sputum shows 'asbestos bodies'.
- X-ray of chest shows a ***ground-glass appearance***[Q] in the lower 2/3rd of the lung fields.
- ***Most common manifestation*** – Pleural plaques (thickening and calcification of parietal pleura)[Q]
- ***Most common site of calcification*** – Along the lower lung fields, diaphragm and the cardiac border[Q]

Also Know

- Crocidolite and Amphibole variety of Asbestos exposure is most dangerous.

Pulmonary fibrosis in

- Asbestosis is peri-bronchial, diffuse and basal.[Q]
- Silicosis is nodular and present in upper part of the lungs[Q]

Asbestosis is a progressive disease (once established it progresses even after removal of exposure).

Preventive Measures

- Use of safer types of asbestos (chrysotile and amosite)
- Substitution—Other insulants: Glass fibre, mineral wool, calcium silicate, plastic foams.
- Rigorous dust control

- Periodic examination of workers; biological monitoring (clinical, X-ray, lung function)
- Continuing research.

9. Ans. (c) <5 microns

Ref: K. Park, 24th ed. p 843

SILICOSIS

10. Ans. (d) India

Ref: K. Park, 24th ed. p 843

Silicosis was first reported from Kolar Gold Mines, Mysore, India in 1947

11. Ans. (a) Kolar

Ref: K. Park, 24th ed. p 843

12. Ans. (b) Quartz

Ref: K. Park, 24th ed. p 843

***Silicosis** is caused by inhalation of dust containing free silica as Quartz (Silicon dioxide -SiO2)*[Q]

- It occurs in mining industry (coal, mica, gold, silver, lead, zinc etc), pottery, ceramic industry, sand blasting, metal grinding, building, construction work, rock mining, iron and steel industry.
- It is a notifiable disease under the Factories Act 1948 and the Mines Act 1952
- *Incidence depends upon*
  - Chemical composition of dust (Higher the concentration of free silica greater the hazard)
  - ***Size of the particles** (**0.5 to 3 micron are most dangerous**)*[Q]
  - Duration of exposure (longer the duration, greater the risk)
  - Individual susceptibility.
- *Incubation period* is few months to 6 years of exposure.

Clinical Features

- Early manifestations-irritant cough, dyspnoea on exertion and pain in chest.
- Advanced disease-impairment of Total Lung Capacity (TLC)

Dense bilateral "nodular" fibrosis[Q] **in the upper 2/3rd of lung** (nodules 3–4 mm in diameter)

"***Snow-storm***" appearance in chest X-ray.[Q]

No effective treatment exists and fibrotic changes already taken place cannot be reversed.

Control Measures

- Rigorous dust control (substitution, complete enclosure, isolation, hydro blasting, good house-keeping)
- Personal protective measures
- Regular physical examination of workers.

Also Know......................

Maximum permissible level of Silica exposure is 40 μg/m³ for 10 hour a day (or 40 hrs a week) for 35 years

13. Ans. (b) Sputum in silico-TB usually show...

Ref: K. Park, 24th ed. p 843

Silicotuberculosis

- Silicosis is progressive and Silicotics are prone to pulmonary TB[Q]
- Sputum rarely shows tubercle bacilli
- Post-mortem on silicotuberculotics have not confirmed existence of tuberculosis.
- Radiological appearance in the two conditions is similar

14. Ans. (a) Caused by exposure of silica oxide; (c) Fibrosis of upper lung; (e) More risk of TB and lung cancer

Ref: K. Park, 23rd ed. p 806; 24th ed p 843, European Medical Journal,, Therapeutic effect of whole lung lavage on pneumoconiosis, 2016, p 98

15. Ans. (a) Payable for maximum of period of 91 days

Ref: http://www.esic.nic.in

Comment:
Option A: Correct
Option B: Incorrect, it is till 2 years
Option C: Incorrect, it is up to 70% of the wage
Option D: Incorrect

HEAVY METAL POISONING

16. Ans. (a) Lead

Ref: K. Park, 24th ed. p 844-45

Lead poisoning (Plumbism/ Painters Colic/ Saturnism) is common heavy metal poisoning worldwide

Source of Lead Poisoning

- ***Occupational***:[Q] Manufacture of storage batteries, glass, ship building, printing and potteries, rubber.
- ***Non-occupational***:[Q] Gasoline, drinking water from lead pipes, lead paint on window sills or toys.

Also Know......................

Modes of Occupational Lead Poisoning
- *Inhalation of fumes & dust of lead or its compounds. (Most common)*
- *Ingestion*
- *Skin absorption*

Clinical picture: Facial pallor is the earliest and most consistent sign

- Inorganic lead exposure → Abdominal colic, Obstinate constipation, Loss of appetite, Blue line on gums of upper jaw (Burtonian Line), Punctate basophilia and stippling of RBC, Anemia (Microcytic hypochronic), Lead palsy (*Wrist drop and foot drop*), Lead encephalopathy [Q]
- Organic lead compounds → Affect CNS- insomnia, headache, mental confusion, delirium, etc.

Treatment: EDTA

17. Ans. (b) 70 mcg/100 mL blood

Ref: K. Park, 24th ed. p 845

Laboratory Parameters for Lead Poisoning Diagnosis

- ***Coproporphyrin in Urine (CPU)*** more than 150 microgram/L indicates lead exposure (**Screening test**)
- ***Aminolevulinic Acid (ALA) in urine*** of more than 5 mg/ L indicates lead absorption.
- ***Lead in urine*** more than 0.8 mg/L indicates lead exposure (**quantitative indicator**)
- **Lead in blood** more than 70 microgram/100 ml is associated with clinical symptoms (quantitative indicator)
- ***Basophilic stippling of RBC*** is a sensitive parameter of hematological response.
- ***In Lead exposure:*** Number of subjects with blood lead level >70 mg/ml and Urinary ALA >10 mg/L is important than Average level of Lead in blood.

OCCUPATIONAL CANCER AND OTHER DISORDERS

18. Ans. (b) Breast

Ref: K. Park, 24th ed. p 845

Occupational cancer can involve all 4 options (Lung/Bladder/ Liver/Breast), but breast cancer is least likely and hence the answer.

19. Ans. (c) 12.5%

Ref: K. Park, 24th ed p-853

ESIC runs on contributions by employees, employers and grants from Central/State Governments)

- Employer contributes 4.75% of total wage bill
- Employee contributes 1.75% of wages. Employee with wages below ₹70 are exempted
- State Govt. and ESIC share of expenditure on medical care is 1/8th and 7/8th of total cost respectively
- 1/8th or 12.5% of the total expense shared by state government. The remaining 87.5% (7/8th) is shared by the Centre Government.

20. Ans. (a) Carcinoma scrotum

Ref: K. Park, 24th ed p-845

Cancer of the scrotum in chimney sweeps was brought to notice by Percival Pott

- About 75% occupational cancers are skin cancer.
- They are a result of exposure to coal tar, X-rays, certain oils and dyes among gas workers, coke oven workers, tar distillers, oil refiners, dye-stuff makers, road makers and in industries associated with the use of mineral oil, pitch, tar and related compounds

21. Ans. (a) Skin cancer

Ref: K. Park, 24th ed. p 846

Sites most commonly affected in Occupational Cancer are skin, lungs, bladder and blood-forming organs[Q].

22. Ans. (d) The localization of the tumors is...

Ref: K. Park, 24th ed. p 845

Also Know.......................

Characteristics of occupational cancer:

- Appear after prolonged exposure i.e. 10 to 25 years
- Disease may develop even after the cessation of exposure
- Average age incidence is earlier than that for cancer in general
- Localization of tumour is remarkably constant in anyone occupation.
- Personal hygiene is important in prevention.

23. Ans. (b) Leukaemia

Ref: K. Park, 24th ed. p 845

Type of carcinoma	Predisposing occupational exposure
Lung	Arsenic, Beryllium, Cadmium, Chromium, Asbestos, Silica, Radon, Nickel, Aromatic hydrocarbons
Liver	Vinyl chloride, Arsenic
Bladder	Benzidine, Auramine, β Naphthylamines, Para amino-diphenyl, Magenta
Leukemia	Benzene, Ethylene oxide, Roentgen rays and Radio-active substances.
Skin	Arsenic, Ionising radiation, Polycyclic aromatic hydrocarbons

24. Ans. (c) Radon

Ref: K. Park, 24th ed. p 846

Ionizing radiations - X-rays and radioactive isotopes (e.g. Cobalt 60, Phosphorus 32) can lead to genetic changes, malformation, cancer, leukaemia, depilation, ulceration, sterility and in extreme cases death

- Maximum permissible level of occupational exposure set by International Commission of Radiological Protection is 5 rem per year to the whole body.

Also Know.......................

- ***Acute radiation syndrome*** occurs due to accidental irradiation of whole body with 1 gray of penetrating radiation in a single exposure or over 1–2 days. Characterized by cell damage and death in exposed tissue.

FACTORY ACT

25. Ans. (c) 500 cu. ft

Ref: K. Park, 24th ed. p 852

26. Ans. (a) ESI Act

Ref: K. Park, 24th ed. p 852

Occupational diseases are notifiable under the following Laws and Regulations

- Factories Act, 1976 (22 diseases)
- Mines Act, 1952 (3 diseases)
- Dock Laborers Act, 1948 (8 diseases)

Objective of Notification

- To initiate prevention and protection measures and reduce incidence of ill health
- To investigate working conditions and circumstances suspected to cause occupational diseases

27. Ans. (c) Creches where more than 30 women are employed

Ref: K. Park, 24th ed. p 852

Health and Welfare Provisions in Factory Act, 1948

- Minimum 500Cu.ft of space for each worker (space 14 ft above ground level not taken into account). For factories installed before the 1948 Act, a minimum of 350 Cu.ft of space is prescribed.
- ***1 Safety Officers*** per 1,000 workers[Q]
- 1 Canteen in every factory where more than 250 workers are employed.[Q]
- ***1 Creches*** in every factory where more than 30 women workers are employed.[Q]
- ***1 Welfare Officer*** in every factory where 500 or more workers are employed.
- Chief Inspector of Factories and additional Chief Inspectors as thought fit to enforce the provisions.
- Safety provisions like casing of new machinery, devices for cutting off the power, lifts, cranes etc.
- Empowers state governments to prescribe maximum weights which may be lifted or carried by men, women and children.

ESI ACT

28. Ans. (b) Union Minister of Labor

Ref: K. Park, 24th ed. p 853

29. Ans. (a) Fitting job to worker

Ref: K. Park, 24th ed. p 840

30. Ans. (a) Fitting the job to the worker

Ref: K. Park, 24th ed. p 840

Ergonomics ("ergon" meaning work and "nomos" meaning law) means fitting the job to the worker. It involves

- Designing of machines, tools, equipment and manufacturing processes, lay-out of the places of work, methods of work and environment
- Objective is to achieve greater efficiency of both man and machine (By best mutual adjustment of man and his work).

Also Know......................

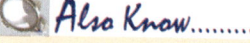

Ergonomics was coined in Stockholm in 1961 at International Ergonomics Association Conference

31. Ans. (b) Union minister of labor

Ref: K. Park, 24th ed. p 853

The Employees' State Insurance Corporation (ESIC) is a statutory body constituted under the administrative control of Ministry of Labor and Employment, Government of India.

Also Know......................

ESIC was inaugurated in Kanpur on 24th February 1952 (ESIC Day) by Pandit Jawahar Lal Nehru (1st honorary insured person of the Scheme). Today it is one of the Largest social security scheme in Southeast Asia

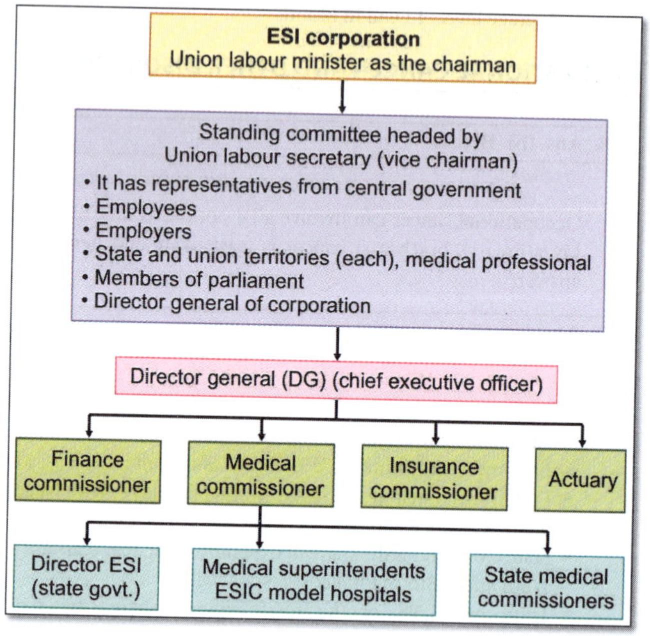

Medical Benefit Council (Advisory Body)

- Director General of Health Services
- Deputy Director General of Health Services
- Medical Commissioner of the ESIC
- One member from each state, 3 representatives of employees, 3 of the employers
- Member from medical profession (Minimum one woman)

32. Ans. (b) 1000

Ref: K. Park, 24th ed. p 853. S Lal, Textbook of Community Medicine, 4th ed

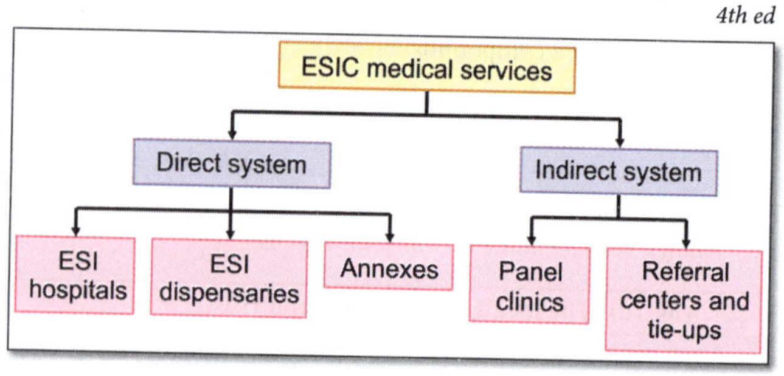

A full-time dispensary (with medical and para-medical personnel) is established as per following norms

- **1 Doctor dispensary** in areas with 1,000 or more Insured person family units
- ***2 Doctor dispensary*** in areas with 3,000 Insured person family units
- ***3 Doctor dispensary*** in areas with 5,000 Insured person family units
- ***5 Doctor dispensary*** in areas with 10,000 Insured person family units

33. Ans. (d) 4.75%

Ref: K. Park, 24th ed. p 853

34. Ans. (a) Total wages

Ref: K. Park, 24th ed. p 853

35. Ans. None

Ref: http://www.esic.nic.in/

Refer to theory

36. Ans. (d) Nutritional allowance

Ref: K. Park, 24th ed. p 853

37. Ans. (c) 91 days

Ref: K. Park, 24th ed. p 854 http://www.esic.nic.in/

- **Standard Sickness benefit** is available for 91 days at 70% of average daily wages

38. Ans. (d) 100% of wages

Ref: K. Park, 24th ed. p 854 http://www.esic.nic.in/

- **Enhanced sickness benefit** is payable at full wages for 14 days for tubectomy and 7 days for vasectomy

39. Ans. (c) 12 months

Ref: K. Park, 24th ed. p 854 http://www.esic.nic.in/

Refer to theory

40. Ans. (d) Only persons who have contributed...

Ref: K. Park, 24th ed. p 853 http://www.esic.nic.in/

41. Ans. (a) Applicable on educational...

Ref: K. Park, 24th ed. p 853

Refer to theory

Act covers all employees manual, clerical

42. Ans. (b) A worker with income less than 70/- per...; (c) Funeral expenses is 50,000/-

Ref: K. Park, 24th ed. p 855

43. Ans. (b) State government share is 1/8 and ESI Corporation is 7/8

Ref: K. Park, 24th ed. p 853

44. Ans. (c) The centre government also contributes as 12.5% of the expense for ESI

Ref: K. Park, 24th ed. p 853

The state ESIC contributes 12.5% (1/8th) of the expense, while the remaining of 87.5% (7/8th) is contributed by the centre government

45. Ans. (b) 100% wages in temporary disability; (c) Extended sickness benefit 91 days; (e) Run by central government

Ref: K. Park, 24th ed. p 854

46. Ans. (a) 91 days

Ref: K. Park, 24th ed. p 854

- Sickness benefit for 91 days
- Extended sickness benefit up to 2 years

47. Ans. (b) Employee's State Insurance Scheme

Ref: K. Park, 23rd ed. p 818 http://www.esic.nic.in/;

Rajiv Gandhi Shramik Kalyan Yojana (2005) comes under the ESI Scheme

48. Ans. (b) Child age less than 14 years cannot be employed in dangerous work

Children age less than 14 years can not be employed as per the factories act

- Article 24 Prohibition of employment of children in factories, etc.: No child below the age of fourteen years shall be employed to work in any factory or mine or engaged in any other hazardous employment.
- The permissible working hours are 48 hours/week with an overtime of 2 hours per day.
- Article 39 contain principles to safeguard health and strength of men, women and children of tender age to avoid any kind of abuse forced by economic necessity unsuited to age or strength.

49. Ans. (b) Funeral expense

Option	T/F	Remarks
Maternity benefit	F	No, it is not in cash. The benefit is in terms of leave from work for the female
Funeral expense	T	Yes, it is cash paid to the grieved family members
Dependent benefit	F	No, it is in form of free/reimbursed treatment for the dependent
Sickness benefit	F	No, it not in direct cash, but some amount of salary (depending on the sickness) is paid as wages compensation
Medical benefit	F	No, it is not in direct cash, but some proportion of wage compensation

NOTES

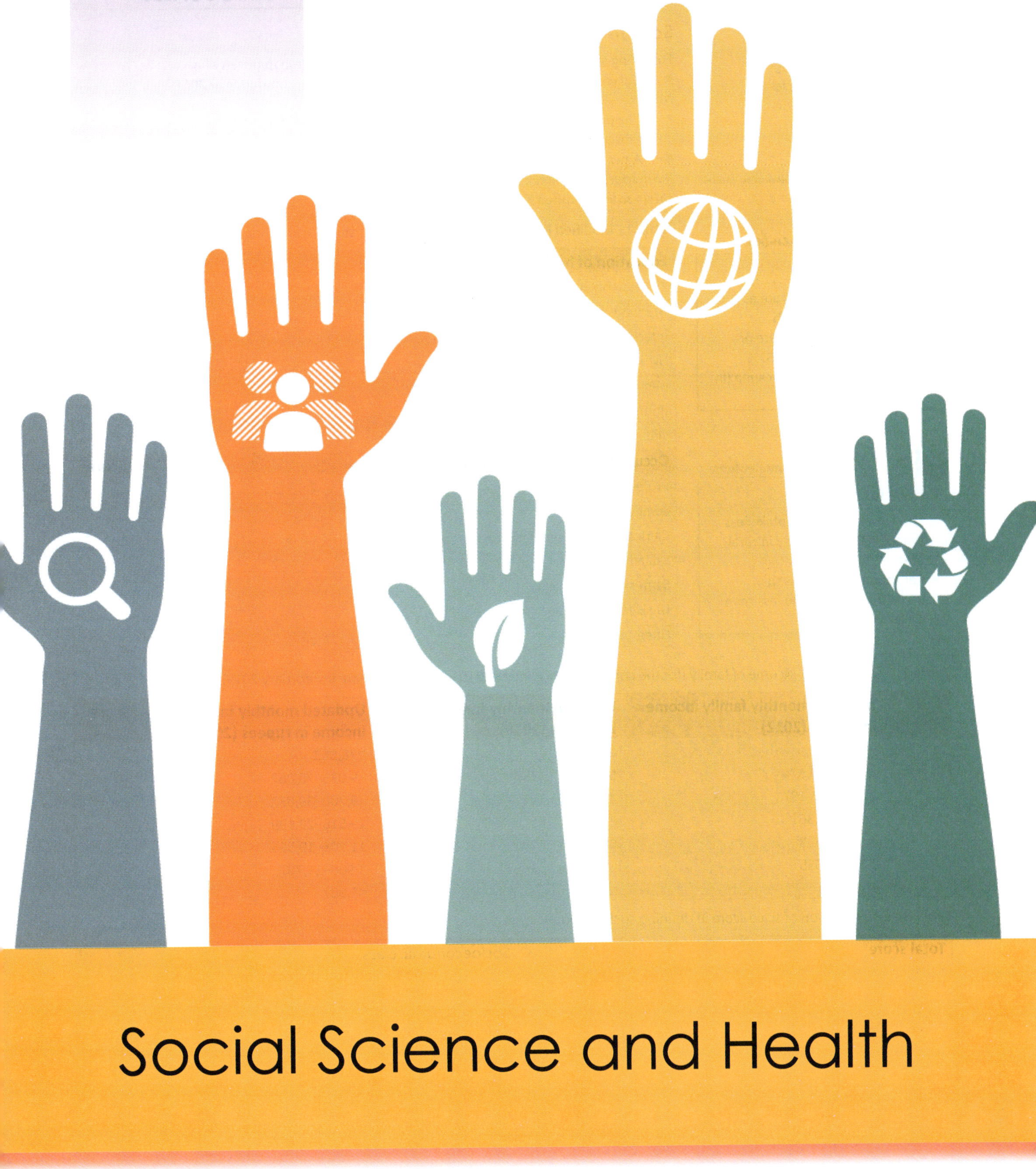

Social Science and Health

Chapter Outline

41 **Good to Remember**

Facts from India

- Public health expenditure as percent of GDP – 1.25%
- Out of pocket expenditure on health (private sector)–67%
- Health expenditure per capita (in US $).75 US $

47 **Must Remember**

Criteria for BPL family

- Food intake – calorie intake less than 2,400 Kcal per day in rural area
- Per capita income less than 32 INR/day (rural) and less than 47 INR/day (urban)

Louis Blanc set forth socialist principle "from each according to his abilities, to each according to his needs"

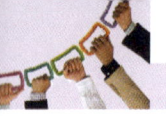

HEALTH ECONOMICS AND SOCIOECONOMIC SCALES

Socioeconomic Classification

Following are the development of socioeconomic classification in poverty line

- Current norms for BPL were proposed by - Rangarajan committee in ***2014***

Note:

- The previous guidelines on methodology and estimation for cutoff for poverty in India were formulated by Tendulkar committee in 2009.
- A per WHO if per capita income < 1.9 US $ per day then it comes under poverty

Rural scale: Udai Pareek , Modified BG Prasad, Shirpurkar, Radhuka

Urban scale: Modified Kuppuswamy Scale, Shrivastava, Jalota, Kulshrestha, Gaurs

Table 1: Modified Kuppuswamy socioeconomic status scale (India)

Education of head of family	Score
Professional degree or honors	7
Graduate or postgraduate	6
Intermediate or post-high school diploma	5
High School Certificate	4
Middle school certificate	3
Primary school certificate	2
Illiterate	1
Occupation of head of family	**Score**
Professional	10
Semi-professional	6
Clerical, shop-owner, farmer	5
Skilled worker	4
Semi-skilled worker	3
Unskilled worker	2
Unemployed	1

Table 2: Total monthly income of family (for the consumer price index 2019 with inflation rate in February 2019)

S. No.	Updated monthly family income in rupees (2012)	Updated monthly family income in rupees (2018)	Updated monthly family income in rupees (2019)	Score
1.	≥30,375	≥126,360	≥78,063	12
2.	15,188–30,374	63,182–126,359	39,033–78,062	10
3.	11,362–15,187	47,266–63,181	29,200–39,032	6
4.	7,594–11,361	31,59147,265	19,516–29,199	4
5.	4,556–7,593	18,953–31,590	11,708–19,515	3
6.	1,521–4,555	6,327–18,952	3,908–11,707	2
7.	≤1,520	≤6,326	≤3,907	1

Table 3: Interpretation of scale score in defining socioeconomic class

Total score	Socioeconomic class
26–29	Upper (I)
16–25	Upper middle (II)
11–15 middle	Lower-middle (III)
5–10 lower	Upper-lower (IV)
<5	Lower (V)

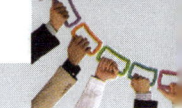

Table 4: Modified Pareek rural socioeconomic status scale

- **Caste:** SC (1), Lower caste (2), Artisan caste (3), Agriculture caste (4), Prestige caste (5), Dominant caste (6).
- **Occupation of head of family:** None (0), Labourer (1) Caste occupation (2), Business (3), Independent profession (4), Cultivation (5), Service (6)
- **Education of head of family:** Illiterate (0), Can read only (1), Can read/write (2), Primary (3) Middle (4), High school (5), Graduate and above (6)
- **Land holding:** No land (0), less than 1 acre (1), 1-5 acre (2), 5-10 acre (3), 10-15 acre (4), 15-20 acre (5), >20 acre (6)
- **Social participation of head of family:** None (0), Member of one organization (like Panchayat, Nambardar, etc.) (1), Member of >1 organization (2), Office holder in such organization (3), Wider public leader (6)
- Family members up to 5(1), Above 5(2)
- **Level of housing:** No house (1), Kutcha house (2), Mixed house (3), Pucca house (4), Mansion (6)
- **Farm power:** No. drought (buffalo/cow) animal (1), 1-2 drought animal (2), 3-4 drought animals (3), 5-6 drought animals or tractor (6)
- **Material possession:** Bullock cart (1), Cycle (1), Radio (1), Chairs (1), Improved agriculture equipment (2), none (0)

**Figures in ( ) brackets indicate scores*

Table 5: Socioeconomic class (Pareek scale)

Socioeconomic class (Pareek scale)	Class
Scale score more than 43	Class-I
33–42	Class-II
24–32	Class-III
13–23	Class-IV
Less than 13	Class-V

Table 6: BG Prasad socioeconomic scale

Socioeconomic class	Original classification (1960)–based on per capita family income in rupees	Updated based on per capita family income in rupees method P Kumar
Class-I	100 and above	6254 and above
Class-II	50–99	3127–6253
Class-III	30–49	1876–3126
Class-IV	15–29	938–1875
Class-V	<15	<937

SOCIAL SCIENCE AND SOCIOLOGY

Basic Definitions

- ***Social science*** is a discipline concerned with scientific examination of human behavior. It comprises of *economics, political science, sociology, social psychology and social anthropology.*
- *Sociology, social psychology and social anthropology* deal directly with human behavior hence are referred to as Behavioral sciences.
- **Sociology** (science of society) is concerned with organization/structure of social groups. (Types, Variation, Process by which intactness of social structure in maintained). It deals with study of behavior/relationship of man in a society or group of humans.
- *Medical Sociology* is a specialized field of sociology dealing with study of health, health behavior and medical institutions.
- ***Social psychology*** is largely a study of attitudes
- Sociology has emerged from Economics (Parent discipline).
- ***Social Diagnosis of illness/pathology*** is made by sociomedical surveys
- **Economics** deals with human relationships in the specific context of production, distribution, consumption and ownership of scarce resources, goods and services
- **Political Science** is the study of the system of laws and institutions which constitute government of whole societies

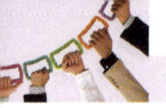

42 Good to Remember

Sociometry is a quantitative method for *measuring social relationships* developed by psychotherapist Jacob L Moreno. It is inquiry into the evolution and organization of groups and position of individuals within them.

69 High Yield Points

- **Opinions** are views held by people on a point of dispute. They are temporary, provisional and subjective in nature.
- **Beliefs** are permanent, stable, almost unchanging and subjective in nature.
- **Attitudes** are relatively enduring organization of beliefs around an object, subject or concept that predispose one to respond in some preferential manner. It is objective in nature. These are usually basic to an individual and do not change easily
  It has three components: Cognitive (Knowledge element), Affective (Feeling element) and Psychomotor (Tendency to action).
  Attitudes are more or less permanent ways of behaving acquired by social interaction.

48 Must Remember

Social medicine is the study of socioeconomic, cultural, environmental, genetic and psychological factors that impact health

- **Social psychology** is the study of effect of social environment on individual psychology. It is concerned with how and why perceptions, thoughts, opinions, attitudes and behavior vary in different groups and societies.

Anthropology is study of physical, social and cultural history of man. It is closest to being a total study of man

- Physical anthropology is study of human evolution, racial differences, inheritance of body traits, growth and decay
- Social anthropology is study of development and various types of social life
- Cultural anthropology is study of total ways of life of contemporary primitive man (thought, feeling and action).
- Linguistic anthropology is the study of process of communication (verbal/nonverbal, language) in humans
- **State medicine** is provision of free medical service to the people at Government expense.[Q]
- **Socialized medicine** is provision of medical service and professional education by the State (like state medicine), but the programed is operated and regulated by professional groups (not by Government)
  - It eliminates competition among physicians for clients
  - It ensures social equity (Universal coverage by health services)
  - It ensures free medical care to the patients supported by the State
  - **Limitation:** Does not ensure utilization of health services

Concepts in Sociology

- **Society** is an organization of member agents having a social relationship between the individuals. Society regulates the behavior of individual by law and customs.
- **Community** as defined by WHO, community is social group determined by geographical boundaries and/or common values and interests. Members know and interact with each other.
- **Social structure** pattern of inter-relations between the individuals. Social structure comprises of major institutions, groups, power structure and status hierarchy.
- **Social Institutions** organized pattern of behavior wherein persons participate in order to further group interest. E.g. School, hospital, religious institutions as temples, political parties etc.
- **Role** can be either "given" by virtue of age, sex and birth status or "acquired" by virtue of education. E.g. A man plays the role of husband, son, father, employee, friend, etc.
- **Socialism** system of production and distribution based on social ownership for raising living standard of working class.

Capitalism and Socialism

Table 7: Comparison between capitalism and socialism

Capitalism	Socialism
Capitalism is private ownership of means of production and aims at maximum private profit at the expense of the working masses	Socialism is a system of production and distribution based on social ownership for raising living standard of working class
Motto of capitalism is ***'all for each'*** *and* ***'each for each'***	*Motto of socialism is* ***'all for all'*** *and* ***'each for all'.***

Terminologies in Sociology

- **Socialization**: **Socialization**[Q] is a process by which an individual gradually acquires cultural beliefs, customs, traditions and prejudices and becomes member of a social group, e.g. Children going to school, internship training of doctors
- **Customs (folkways mores):** Customs are conventions - practice promoted by convenience of society or the individual that guide laws. It may further be classified into:
  - **Folkways** are customary ways of behavior enforced by informal social controls (gossip and ridicule) and not by fear of being penalized. Their origin is usually unplanned and obscure.
  - **Mores** are socially acceptable ways of behavior that involve moral standards.
- **Social Control Mechanisms:** Done by rules—formal and informal. Laws and enactments of parliament are social control mechanisms. Informal social pressures help in determining the behavior of a person.

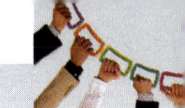

- **Culture**: **Culture**[Q] is learned behavior acquired socially and transmitted from one generation to another.
- **Acculturation** is "culture contact" between people with different types of culture (due to trade, industrialization, propagation of religion etc.). It leads to diffusion of culture (good and bad aspects) in bilateral directions.
- **Standard of living:** Depends upon
  - Level of national income
  - Total amount of goods and services country is able to produce
  - Population size
  - Level of education
  - General price level
  - Distribution of national income
- **Dynamics of social change:** Income level, birth and death rates of a country, migration from rural to urban areas are some of the factors determining about the changes in social structure.
- **Social stress:** Generally seen in transitional societies due to new opportunities and frustrations arising due to societal changes. E.g. Rapid population expansion putting younger population in greater competition for the available limited resources.
- **Social problems:** Poverty, crime, drug abuse, divorce, housing, population growth and disease are common social problems.
- **Social pathology** is systematic study of human disease in relation to social conditions and disease process outside the human body. It includes substance abuse, violence, abuses of women and children, crime, terrorism, corruption, criminality, discrimination, isolation, stigmatization and human rights violations.
- **Social surveys** are used to disclose and know about the existing social pathologies. E.g. social epidemiological studies.
- **Case study** method of exploring and analyzing the life of a social unit. It aims to determine the factors that account for complex behavior patterns of unit and relationships.
- **Field study** concerned with the depth of knowledge involving observation of people *in situ*.
- **Communication** refers to a social process with flow of information, circulation of knowledge and ideas and propagation of thoughts.
- **Social defense**:
  - Social defense covers preventive, therapeutic and rehabilitative services for protection of society from antisocial, criminal or deviant conduct of man by creating conditions in community conducive for a healthy and wholesome growth
  - It includes measures relating to prevention and control of juvenile delinquency, eradication of beggary, social and moral hygiene programs, welfare of prisoners, prison reforms, elimination of prostitution, control of alcoholism, drug addiction, gambling and suicides.
  - National Institute of Social Defense (under Department of Social Welfare) is at New Delhi.

    Self-defense is mechanisms employed by an individual when faced with problems, difficulties or failures, to achieve health, happiness or success.
  - It includes—rationalization, projection, compensation, escape mechanism, displacement and regression.
- **Temporary social groups:**
  - Crowd – a group of individuals coming together by a common interest
  - Mob — an emotionally charged up crowd, usually with a leader
  - Herd – A crowd with a leader, the members follow the group without any questions.
- **Permanent spatial groups**
  - Band – most elementary community comprising of few families living together
  - Village – small collection of people permanently settled with cultural values
  - Town/city – large, dense and permanent settlement of socially heterogenous groups. A size of more than 100,000 in an area is usually called as a city
  - State – an ecological social group based on based on defined geographical boundary, usually with common culture, language and code of conducts.
- **Social security** is "security that society furnishes through appropriate organization, against certain risks like poverty, disability, unemployment, etc. to which its members are exposed".

70 *High Yield Points*

Crowd, Mob, Herd

- **Crowd:** A group of individuals coming together by a common interest
- **Mob:** An emotionally charged up crowd (usually with a leader)
- **Herd:** An emotional crowd with a dictator type leader

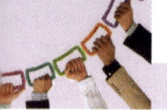

High Yield Points

Unit of study in Sociology is Group and in Psychology is Individual.

PSYCHOLOGY

It is a study of human behavior. Branches of psychology are:

- Normal psychology
- Abnormal psychology
- Social psychology
- Child psychology
- Applied psychology
- Medical psychology etc.

Intelligence: It is the ability to see meaningful relationships between things.

Intelligence Quotient (IQ):

$$IQ = \frac{\text{Mental age}}{\text{Chronological age}} \times 100$$

When mental age is same as chronological age, the IQ is 100.

Table 8: Levels of intelligence and IQ ranges

Levels of Intelligence	IQ Ranges
Idiot	0-24
Imbecile	25-49
Moron	50-69
Borderline	70-79
Low normal	80-89
Normal	90-109
Superior	110-119
Very Superior	120-139
Near genius	140 & over

As per DSM-V classification, IQ less than 70 is approximation of 2 standard deviations below the normal population and is considered as ***intellectual disability.***

Table 9: Intellectual disabilities and IQ ranges

IQ Ranges	Intellectual disabilities
50-69	Mild
36-49	Moderate
20-35	Severe
<20	Profound

THE FAMILY

- **Family** is a group of individuals related biologically or by marriage or adoption, living together and eating from a common kitchen.
- **Household** consists of all people who occupy a housing unit regardless of relationship. A household may consist of a person living alone or multiple unrelated individuals or families living together. Number of households is determined by the number of kitchens in a housing premise.

Table 10: Primary and secondary relationships

Primary relationship	Secondary relationship
Spontaneous, continuous and informal	Formal, Nonspontaneous
Permanent	Temporary
No starts and ends date	Starts and ends at specific date
Relation comes first	Motive comes first- then relation
Emotional bonding	No emotional bonding
Nontransferable	Transferable
Examples: Family, friends	Example – Business

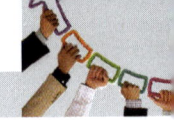

Family Cycle

Table 11: Family cycle

Phases	Beginning	End
Formation	Marriage	Birth of first child
Extension	Birth of first child	Birth of last child
Complete extension	Birth of last child	1st child leaves home
Contraction	1st child leaves home	Last child has left home of parents
Completed contraction	Last child has left home of parents	Spouse dies
Dissolution	Spouse dies	Death of survivor

Types of Families

- **Nuclear family**—consists of married couple and their dependent children, occupying the same dwelling space.
  New families- recent terminology. It is applied to those under 10 years of duration and consists of parents and children. It is important for family planning.
- **Joint/extended family**—common in India. It consists of a number of married couples and their children living together in the same household. Characteristics of a joint family:
  - All the men are related to each other by blood and the females are their wives, sisters or daughters.
  - All the property is held in common.
  - Senior male member of the family holds the authority.
- **Three generation family**—consists of a household representing three generations. Members of three generations related to each other by direct descent live together.
- **Broken family:** It is the one where the parents have separated or where death of one or both parents has occurred.
- **Problem family:** In these families, the home life is highly unsatisfactory usually due to relationship problems, poverty, illness or mental and emotional problems.
- **Motivation:** Goal-oriented behavior
- **Propaganda:** A process which is information centered

SOCIAL SECURITY

- Social security for Industrial workers in India is provided by Workmen's Compensation Act, 1923, Central Maternity Benefit Act, 1961, Employees State Insurance Act, 1948, Family Pension Scheme, 1971
- Social security for civil servants (Central and State Govt.) includes Pension, Gratuity, Provident fund and family pension schemes
- Social security for general public comprises of Insurance schemes (LIC, PPF)
- First social security act was enacted in Germany in 1881 for industrial workers
- Bismarck was instrumental in introduction of social insurance in Germany in1883
- Sweden is the only country where entire population is under social security schemes
- Social security also includes social insurance (Contributory benefit) and social assistance (Noncontributory benefit)
- Risks covered by social security are sickness, unemployment, maternity, old age and death.

Social safety net is a collection of services provided by the state or NGO, that includes welfare, unemployment benefit, universal healthcare, homeless shelters, subsidized services so as to prevent individuals from falling into poverty beyond a certain level.

Social distancing is actions taken by health officials to stop or slow down the of a highly contagious disease. E.g. pandemic influenza. It includes stopping large groups of people coming together, closing buildings and cancelling events

Social therapy is holistic development centered therapeutic and support services (Education, legislation, individual and group counseling, motivation, providing services on equity basis). It addresses and supports the total social, emotional and educational needs of young and the entire family.

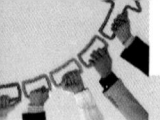

Social assistance implies provision of relief to individuals at critical times without having received any contribution from them.

Social environment includes all the things which arise out of social relationships as customs, traditions, social conduct, rituals, way of life, habits, diet and almost everything including health, which may be influenced by social environment

Social stratification: Horizontal division of society into several socioeconomic scales or strata. Each layer of the society will have a set of lifestyle and cutlers unique to its strata.

- Field study is concerned with depth of knowledge and involve observation of people in situ
- Case study *attempts to collect a large amount of information from a small number of units*
- Survey collects a small amount of information from a large number of units. It is concerned with the breadth of knowledge.

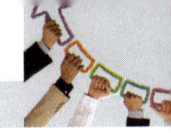

Multiple Choice Questions

1. The term 'Social Medicine' was coined by: *(Recent Question 2015)*
a. Rene Sand b. Jules Guerin
c. John Ryle d. Alfred Grotjahn

2. Socialization of medicine leads to all, except:
a. Ensures complete utilization of services by all people.
b. Free medical care supported by the State
c. Eliminates competition among physicians in search of clients
d. Ensures social equity, universal coverage of health services.

3. COPRA recognizes how many rights to the consumer:
a. 3 b. 4
c. 5 d. 6

4. An organized group of people with social relationship:
a. Community b. Association
c. Society d. Family

5. The study of physical, social and cultural history of man is called: *(Recent Question 2017)*
a. Sociology
b. Social medicine
c. Social psychology
d. Anthropology

6. The study which deals with cultural component in the ecology of health and disease: *(Recent Question 2017)*
a. Physical anthropology
b. Social anthropology
c. Medical anthropology
d. Cultural anthropology

7. Study of physical, social, and culture history of man is known as: *(Recent Question 2016)*
a. Social science b. Anthropology
c. Acculturation d. Sociology

8. As per Maslow's hierarchy of needs, the correct sequence from base to top of pyramid is:
a. Physiological, safety, belonging, self-esteem, actualisation
b. Actualization, physiological, safety, belonging, self-esteem
c. Safety, actualization, belonging, self-esteem, physiological need
d. Safety, physiological, belonging, self-esteem, actualization

9. According to Maslow's hierarchy of needs, following is at the top of pyramid: *(Recent Question 2016)*
a. Physical needs b. Self-actualization
c. Safety d. Esteem recognition

10. Social psychology is:
a. Human relationships and behavior
b. Psychology of individuals in society
c. Culture history of man
d. None

11. Which of the following is associated with emotional valence and is most likely to be influenced by motivation:
a. Attitude b. Belief
c. Practice d. Knowledge

12. Sociology is *(Recent Question 2013)*
a. Study of human relationship
b. Study of human behavior
c. Both
d. None

13. Social pathology is *(Recent Question 2013)*
a. Change in disease pattern due to change in lifestyle
b. Study of social problems which cause disease in population
c. Conflicts arising from new opportunity in transitional societies
d. Study of human relationships and behavior

14. Movement across socioeconomic levels is termed as:
a. Social equality b. Social upliftment
c. Social mobility d. Social insurance

15. Socially acquired learned behavior is:
a. Custom b. Culture
c. Habit d. Attitude

16. Acculturation means: *(Recent Question 2014)*
a. Culture contact
b. Study of various cultures
c. Culture history of health and disease
d. None of the above

17. Acculturation means: *(Recent Question 2014)*
a. Culture contact
b. Study of the various cultures
c. Cultural history of health and science
d. None of the above

18. Which is the transfer point of civilization and a bridge between generations?
a. School b. Orphanage
c. Family d. Recreational club

19. Arrange the following stages of family cycle in chronological sequence: *(Recent Question 2013)*
a. Formation, extension, complete extension, dissolution, contraction, complete contraction
b. Formation, extension, contraction, complete extension, complete contraction, dissolution
c. Formation, contraction, complete contraction, extension, complete extension, dissolution
d. Formation, extension, complete extension, contraction, complete contraction, dissolution

20. Nuclear family consist of *(Recent Question 2013)*
a. Husband, wife and son
b. Husband, wife and dependent children
c. Husband and wife only
d. Father mother husband and wife

21. All of the following are scales used for assess socio-economic status of populations, except?
a. Udai Pareek scale
b. Likert scale
c. BG Prasad scale
d. Modified Kuppuswamy scale

Ans.

1. b
2. a
3. d
4. c
5. d
6. c
7. b
8. a
9. b
10. b
11. c
12. c
13. b
14. c
15. b
16. a
17. a
18. c
19. d
20. b
21. b

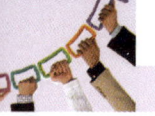

22. Total score of upper middle socioeconomic class in Kuppuswamy's SES scale ranges from?

a. 4–20 b. 15–20
c. 15–25 d. 16–25

23. Which of the following is a socioeconomic scale for urban areas? ***(Recent Question 2013)***

a. Udai Pareek scale
b. Radhukar scale
c. Modified Kuppuswamy scale
d. Shirpurkar scale

24. Upper class score in Kuppuswamy Socioeconomic status scale is:

a. 5–10 b. 11–15
c. 16–25 d. 26–29

25. All of the following are taken into consideration in kuppuswamy scale, except: ***(Recent Question 2013)***

a. Education status
b. Occupation status
c. Living/housing conditions
d. Per capita income

26. Following statement is/are true about women empowerment? ***(Recent Question 2013)***

a. Power over resources
b. Involvement in political decision making
c. Involvement in economic decision making
d. Improved standard of living
e. Increased life expectancy

27. Which of the following is best suited for the role of social worker? ***(Recent Question 2013)***

a. Health professional involved in physiotherapy
b. Health professional involved in making strategies, interpersonal skills, adjustment with family
c. A person involved in finding jobs and economic support for disabled
d. Health professional involved in treatment of patients

28. Current Govt. (public) expenditure on health as percentage of GDP is: ***(Recent Question 2013)***

a. 1.2 b. 12
c. 5 d. 0.12

29. The poverty line is defined as an expenditure required for a daily calorie intake of: ***(Recent Question 2013)***

a. 2400 per person in urban areas
b. 3200 per person in rural areas
c. 3200 per person in urban areas
d. 2400 per person in rural areas

30. Maximum number of students in a school classroom is:

a. 30 b. 35
c. 40 d. 50

31. The reason behind setting up of the "Nirbhaya Fund" by the Govt. is:

a. Provision of free education
b. Ensuring safety for women
c. Promotion of financial literacy
d. Promotion of Self Help Groups

Ans.

22. d
23. c
24. d
25. c
26. a, b, c
27. b
28. a
29. d
30. c
31. b

Answers with Explanations

1. Ans. (b) Jules Guerin

Ref: K. Park, 24th p 52

Social Medicine is the study of impact of social, cultural, economical, psychological, environmental and genetic factors on health.

Also Know.......................

- The term *'Social Medicine'* was introduced by **Jules Guerin** (French physician).
- **Neumann (1847) and Virchow (1848)** were pioneers of social medicine.
- **Alfred Grotjahn** revived social medicine & stressed on importance of social factors in disease etiology (*Social Pathology).*
- **Rene Sand** founded the *Belgian Social Medicine Association* in 1912.
- **John Ryle** was the *1st professor of Social Medicine at Oxford University in* ***1942***
- Russia was the 1st country to socialize medicine completely[Q].

2. Ans. (a) Ensures complete utilisation of...

Ref: K. Park, 24th ed. p 10

Advantages of Socialized Medicine

- It eliminates competition among physicians for clients.
- It ensures social equity (Universal coverage by health services).
- It ensures free medical care to the patient supported by the State.

Limitation—Does not ensure utilization of health services. [It requires "community participation" or "Health by the People"].

Also Know.......................

- Community participation is the process by which individuals and families assume responsibility for their own health and welfare and for those of the community, and develop the capacity to contribute to their health and the community's development. It implies community is involved in planning, organization and management of their own health services.

3. Ans. (d) 6

Ref: Textbook of community medicine, Gupta and Mahajan, 4th ed. p-140

COPRA (Consumer Protection Act, 1986) is a piece of comprehensive legislation and recognizes 6 rights of the consumer namely

- Right to safety
- Right to be informed
- Right to choose
- Right to be heard
- Right to seek redressal
- Right to consumer education.

Also Know.......................

- SARDA Act – Child Marriage Restraint Act 1929 –(Named after Rai Sahib Har Bilas Sarda, British India Legislatur(e) - Age of marriage was fixed for girls at 14 years and boys at 18 years all across India.

4. Ans. (c) Society

Ref: K. Park, 24th ed. p 707

Society is an organized group of individuals, in a network of social relationships and compulsions that propel, direct and constrain individual efforts.

- It controls and regulates individual behavior both by law and customs.
- Society is dynamic (changes over time and place).
- Individuals in society are allocated roles
  - Ascribed role → given by virtue of sex, age and birth status
  - Achieved role → acquired by virtue of education or otherwise.
- Public health is influenced by society and society by public health.

Also Know.......................

Community is a social group determined by geographical boundaries and/or common values and interests.

- It functions within a social structure (a complex of institutions, groups, power structure and status hierarchy) and exhibits certain norms and values.
- Thee individual belongs to society through his family and community

Social institutions are organized complex pattern of behavior in which a number of persons participate in order to further group interest.

- E.g. Family, school, church, club, hospital, political parties, professional associations and panchayat
- Within each institution, the rights and duties of the members are defined.

Association is a group of individuals united for a specific purpose based on utilitarian interest. E.g. Junior Doctors Association.

5. Ans. (d) Anthropology

Ref: K. Park, 24th ed. p 707

Anthropology is study of physical, social and cultural history of man. It *comes nearest to being a total study of man*[Q]

6. Ans. (c) Medical anthropology

Ref: K. Park, 24th ed. p 707

Medical anthropology is concerned with the cultural component in the ecology of health and disease.

7. Ans. (b) Anthropology

Ref: K. Park, 24th ed. p 707

8. Ans. (a) Physiological, safety, belonging…

Ref: Sunder Lal. Textbook of Community Medicine. 4th ed. p-36-37

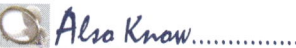

Also Know…………………..

Maslow's Hierarchy of needs designates categories of needs & their strengths.

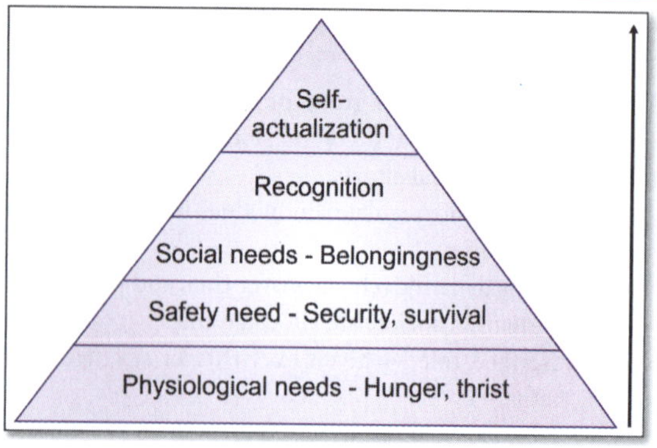

Physiological needs are at the bottom of the pyramid and are of top priority. Once it is satisfied the next higher needs take priority.

9. Ans. (b) Self-actualization

Ref: Sunderlal. Textbook of Community Medicine. 4th ed. p-36-37

10. Ans. (b) Psychology of individuals in society

Ref: K. Park, 24th ed. p 707

Social psychology is concerned with the psychology of individuals living in human society or groups.

- It emphasizes on understanding the basis of perception, thought, opinion, attitudes, general motivation and learning in individuals and how these vary in human societies and groups.

11. Ans. (c) Practice

Ref: K. Park, 24th ed. p 712-714

Emotion valence refers to positive (Intrinsic attractiveness E.g. Joy) and negative (Aversiveness – E.g. Anger, Fear) character of an emotion.

- Attitudes, Beliefs and Practice/Habit are associated with emotional valence.
- Knowledge is not associated with emotional valence

Habit or Practice is an accustomed way good (promotes health) or bad (Ruins health) of doing things.

- Habits are modifiable; Cultivation of good habits is desirable.

Affect valence refers to positive and negative character of emotional experience (how good or bad an emotion feels).

Also Know…………………..

FEAR is the most common emotion of man

12. Ans. (c) Both

Ref: K. Park, 24th ed. p 707

Sociology is concerned with organization/structure of social groups (kinds, variation in social structure; process by which intactness of social structure in maintained).

- It is the study of human relationships and behavior in a society or group of human beings.
- It seeks to understand the effects on the individual of ways in which other individuals think and act.

13. Ans. (b) Study of social problems which…

Ref: K. Park, 24th ed. p 710

Social Pathology is a systematic study of human disease in relation to social conditions.

- Social pathology includes substance abuse, violence, abuses of women and children, crime, terrorism, corruption, criminality, discrimination, isolation, stigmatisation and human rights violations.
- Social pathology is uncovered by "social surveys" or socio-medical surveys
- Cause of Social Pathology include
  - Social Problems (Poverty and destitution, illiteracy and ignorance, lower status of women, child neglect and child abuse, child labour, drug abuse, juvenile delinquency)
  - Social conditions (housing, environmental sanitation, crime and corruption, stress, suicide)
  - Social circumstances (stigma, social isolation, vulnerable populations).

14. Ans. (c) Social mobility

Ref: K. Park, 24th ed. p 725

Social Mobility[Q] is movement across socioeconomic levels of a family or group over time on basis of their achievements in a system of social hierarchy.

Closed class society	Open class society
There is little social mobility, i.e., people cannot change their caste or religion E.g. Indian society	Unrestricted movement in the social ladder, on the basis of achievement or gaining wealth.
It is difficult to make reforms without meeting resistance of the people.	More progressive as people according to their ability can go up the social ladder.

Social upliftment is betterment of previously disadvantaged sections of the society.

15. Ans. (b) Culture

Ref: K. Park, 24th ed. p 709

Culture is *socially acquired learned behaviour*[Q] transmitted from one generation to another via formal and informal learning

- It lays down norms of behavior and provides mechanism which secures for an individual his personal and social survival.
- Cultural factors are important in relation to personal hygiene, nutrition, immunization, seeking early medical care, family planning etc.

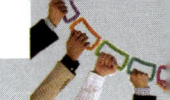

16. Ans. (a) Culture contact

Ref: K. Park, 24th ed. p 709

Acculturation is "culture contact" resulting from trade, industrialization, propagation of religion etc.

- Diffusion of culture (good and bad aspects) occurs both ways.
- Introduction of scientific medicine, change in food habits of people is brought about by culture contact.
- Radio, TV & Cinema are important mediums shaping the cultural-behavior patterns of people.

17. Ans. (a) Culture contact

Ref: K. Park, 24th ed. p 709

18. Ans. (c) Family

Ref: K. Park, 24th ed. p 721

Functions of Family

- *To provide a clean and decent residence*
- *Division of labour*
- *Reproduction and bringing up of children*
- *Socialization: Family acts as a bridge between generation and is the transfer point of civilization. Attitude behavior, eating, dressing, cleanliness are all transmitted via family*
- *Economic functions: Inheritance, ownership and/or control of property*
- *Social care or Status in a society to its members*

19. Ans. (d) Formation, extension, complete...

Ref: K. Park, 24th ed. p 719-720

Family is a group of individuals related biologically or by marriage or adoption, living together and eating from a common kitchen.

- **Family of origin**-family into which one is born
- **Family of procreation**-family which one sets up after marriage

A Normal Family Cycle has Six Phases

- Formation - [Marriage to Birth of first child]
- Extension –[Birth of first child- Birth of last child]
- Complete extension- [Birth of last child- 1st child leaves home]
- Contraction- [1st child leaves home -Last child leaves home of parents]
- Completed contraction-[Last child has left home of parents - 1st spouse dies]
- Dissolution- [1st spouse dies-Death of survivor]

Also Know......................

- **Household** is a group of biologically unrelated people living together and having meals from a common kitchen unless work prevents any of them from doing so. E.g. Boarding houses, mess, hostels, jails, ashrams etc.

20. Ans. (b) Husband, wife and dependent...

Ref: K. Park, 24th ed. p 720-721

Types of Families

- **Nuclear** (Elementary) family comprises of husband, wife and unmarried children (dependent) residing under same roof.
  - Husband usually plays a dominant role in the household.
  - Greater burden in terms of responsibilities for child rearing [in absence of grandparents, uncles etc.]
  - Husband-wife relationship is more intimate in the nuclear family than in the joint family.
- **Conjugal** family is a nuclear family where relations with extended kin is voluntary and emotional and not by duty or obligation.
- **Joint family** (lateral extension of nuclear family) comprises families of siblings living together. [E.g. Married man with his family + unmarried sister or brother living together].
  - It has a common family purse.
  - All authority is vested in a senior male member.
  - Familial relations enjoy primacy over marital relations
- **Extended family** (linear extension of a nuclear family) consists of husband, wife and their married children living together.
- **3 Generation family**- Households with representatives of three generation.
- ***New family***[Q] is a family under 10 years duration, consisting of parents and children. important in relation to family planning
- ***Broken family***[Q] is one where parents have separated or death has occurred of one or both the parents
  - Separation of child from father (paternal separation) or from both parents (dual-parental separation)
  - Children may display in later years psychopathic behavior, immature personality and even retardation of growth, speech and intellect.
  - Children from these families may drift away to prostitution, crime and vagrancy.
- ***Problem family***[Q] is one that lags behind the rest of the community (Standards of life is poor & parents are unable to meet the physical and emotional needs of their children. The home life is utterly unsatisfactory.
  - Underlying factors are of personality/relationship, backwardness, poverty, illness, mental and emotional instability, character defects and marital disharmony.
  - These families are recognized as problems in social pathology
  - Children reared in such an environment are victims of prostitution, crime and vagrancy.
  - May be found in all social classes but are *more common in the lower social classes.*
  - Health visitor, Health inspector, Social worker, Medical officer can render useful service in rehabilitating such families in a community.

Communal family is a family where there is steady enlargement of the freedom of wives and even children and where all its members play a part in its management.

Also Know......................

- Most common type of "joint family" found in India is a joint extended family.

21. Ans (b) Likert scale

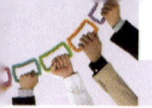

Ref: Mahajan and Gupta, Textbook of PSM, 4th Ed, p 133

Likert scales are used to record the level of agreement or disagreement with a particular statement.

Likert scales are always symmetrical (odd number of choices allowing the neutral option or even number of choices without a neutral option

22. Ans. (d) 16-25

Ref: K. Parks, 24th ed. p 727

23. Ans. (c) Modified Kuppuswamy scale

Ref: K. Park, 24th ed. p 726

24. Ans. (d) 26-29

Ref: K. Park, 24th ed. p 726-27

25. Ans. (c) Living/housing conditions

Ref: K. Park, 24th ed. p 726-27

26. Ans. (a) Power over resources; (b) Involvement in...; (c) Involment in economic

Ref: K. Park, 21st ed. p-19

Gender Empowerment Measures [GEM] is an index reflecting gender inequalities in human development has 3 Dimensions

- Political participation and decision making
- Economic participation and decision making
- Power over economic resources

27. Ans. (b) Health professional involved in...

Ref: Obvious by the nature of job- Reasoning

28. Ans. (a) 1.2

Ref: DK Taneja, Health policies and programs in India, 13th ed. p-1)

- Gross National Income (GNI) is gross income generated from within the country and also received from abroad. It is expressed either at "current prices" or "constant prices"
- ***GNI per capita US*** $ is national currency converted to current US Dollars using the Work Bank Atlas Method. [using a 3 year average of exchange rates]
- **Gross Domestic Product (GDP)** is gross income generated within a country. It excludes income received from abroad.
- **Net National Product (NNP)** - GNP minus the capital we consume (e.g., equipment, machinery etc.) in the production process. NNP is market value of all final goods and services after providing for depreciation.
- **Net Domestic Product (NDP)** - It is the GDP minus the value of depreciation on fixed assets.
- **Purchasing Power Parity (PPP)** is number of units of a country's currency required to buy the same amount of goods and services in the domestic market as one dollar would buy in the USA.

Also Know......................

- India's per capita GNP in 2010 is estimated at $ 3560 (PPP). [4th largest country in terms of GNP (PPP) $2.5 tm, preceded by the USA ($ 9.98 tm), China ($ 5.4 tm) and Japan ($ 3.5 tm)].

- **Gross domestic savings:** It is excess of current income over current expenditure.

29. Ans. (d) 2400 per person in rural areas

Ref: K. Park, 24th ed. p 739

"***Poverty line***" is defined as expenditure required for a daily Calorie intake of 2,400 per person in rural areas and 2,100 in urban areas.

- This expenditure is estimated at ₹ 228.9 per capita per month in rural area and ₹ 264.1 in urban area (at 1993-94 prices)

Also Know......................

- Per capita income in India (2012-13) was ₹68,748 at current prices.

30. Ans. (c) 40

Ref: Guidelines for School Infrastructure and Strengthening, MOHRD, GOI, December 2014

Guidelines for School Infrastructure

- Class Room- Pupil Ratio: 1:40 (Minimum ratio :1:25)
- Class Room size: As per State norm, or plinth area of 66 sq. m.

31. Ans. (b) Ensuring safety for women

Nirbhaya Fund

- Being administered by Department of Economic Affairs, Ministry of Finance
- To be used for projects for women safety and security
- Ministry of Women and Child Development is the nodal ministry.

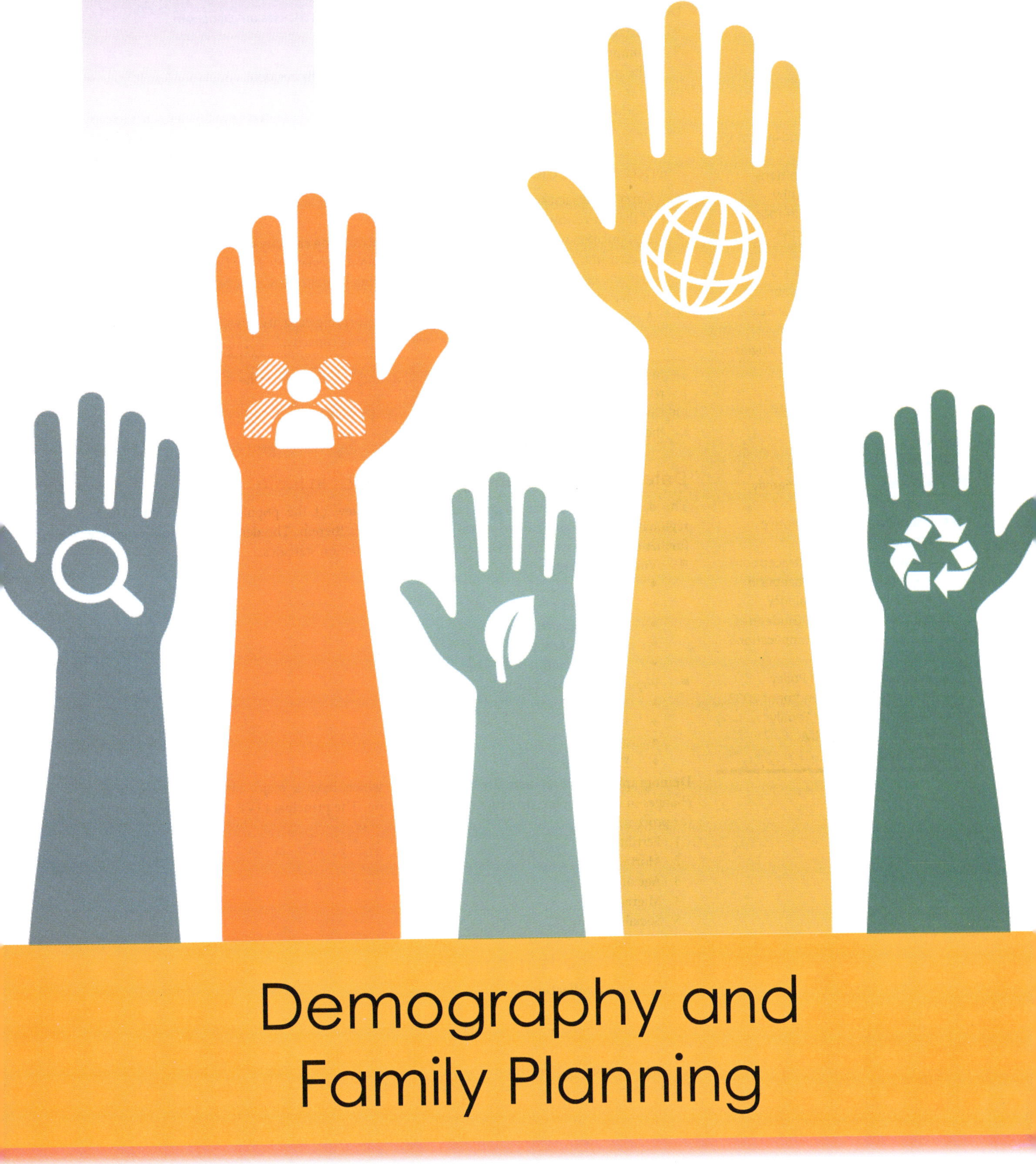

Demography and Family Planning

Chapter Outline

DEMOGRAPHY

INTRODUCTION

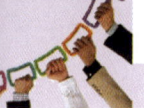

Demography is the scientific study of human population. It focuses on changes in
- Size of population (growth or decline)
- Composition of population

The mid-year population estimates relate to the usually resident population on 30 June of each year.

World Population day is an annual event, observed on July 11 every year, which seeks to raise awareness of global population issue

Trends in Population Growth

- Carrying capacity is the maximum population size of a particular species, that a given part of the environment can maintain indefinitely.
- A population which has grown larger than the carrying capacity of its environment degrades its environment (uses resources faster than they are regenerated) and produces waste (faster than the environment can absorb without being degraded). Such a population is said to be in "overshoot".
- A population can only temporarily overshoot carrying capacity. It will subsequently decline in number, to return to a level at or below carrying capacity.

> - In 1999 world population touched 6 billion and in 2014 it became 7 million (Expected to reach 8 billion by 2025).
> - On 11th May 2000, India's population crossed 1 billion (Projected to reach 1.53 billion by the year 2050)

Determinants of Demographic Trends in India

The demographic characteristics provide an overview of the population size, composition, regional and geographic distribution and the changes therein. The demographic indicators are further divide into two types–vital statistics and population statistics.
- Vital statistics include:
  - Birth rate
  - Death rate
  - Natural growth rate
  - Life expectancy at birth
  - Mortality and fertility rates
- Population statistics include:
  - Population size
  - Sex ratio
  - Density
  - Dependency ratio

Demographic process–these are the variables which have a major attribution towards the changes in demographic structure of the population. The principal FIVE demographic variables (or process) are:
1. Fertility
2. Mortality
3. Age of marriage
4. Migration
5. Social mobility

Survey Methods in India

Sources of data collection–
- Census
- National Sample Survey–sample registration system
- Registration of vital events
- Ad hoc demographic studies
- Census

Types of data collection

De facto system: Data collection is done based on the place, where the individual is found. It was followed in India till 1931.

De Jure system: Data collection is done based on the place of the permanent residence of the individual. It is being followed since the 1941 census till date.

72 *High Yield Points*

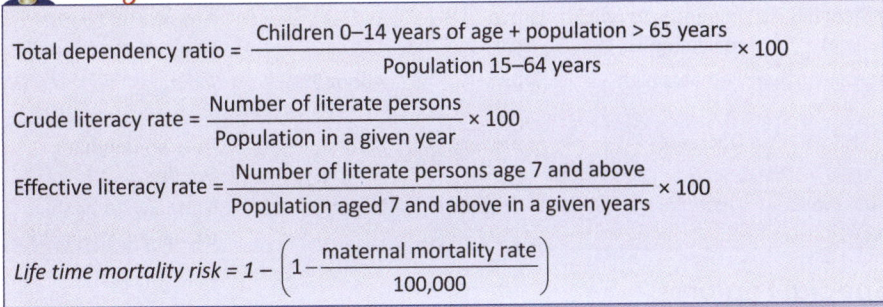

$$\text{Total dependency ratio} = \frac{\text{Children 0–14 years of age + population > 65 years}}{\text{Population 15–64 years}} \times 100$$

$$\text{Crude literacy rate} = \frac{\text{Number of literate persons}}{\text{Population in a given year}} \times 100$$

$$\text{Effective literacy rate} = \frac{\text{Number of literate persons age 7 and above}}{\text{Population aged 7 and above in a given years}} \times 100$$

$$\textit{Life time mortality risk} = 1 - \left(1 - \frac{\text{maternal mortality rate}}{100{,}000}\right)$$

DEMOGRAPHIC CYCLE

Definitions and Terminologies

The demographic cycle (or stages) denotes the changes a country or a defined population will undergo as overall development takes place over time. There are 5 broad stages in the demographic life cycle of a country.

Demographic transition is change in population trend/size from a condition where both Birth Rate and Death Rate are high to a condition where both are low. Before and after demographic transition population size is relatively stable.

Demographic dividend or bonus or gift is rise in economic growth rate due to rising share of working age people in a population. It usually occurs when fertility rate and dependency ratio declines. It is evident from stage III onwards.

Demographic window is the period when the proportion of children and youth under 15 years falls below 30% and the proportion of people 65 years and older is still below 15%. Proportion of working age group population is prominent.

Demographic trap: The country's economic gains are used up to support the needs of the exploding population instead of economic and social development. It is due to decline in death raters but a persistently higher birthrate, which may yield a rapidly expanding population and further a difficulty to decline the birth rate, usually noticed in stage II.

Demographic burden is increase in the total dependency ratio during any time, mostly caused by increased old age dependency ratio. It is inevitable consequence of demographic transition.

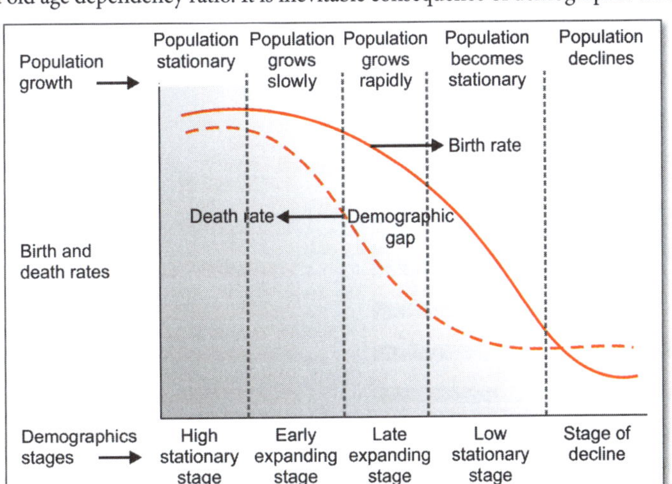

Fig. 1: The demographic cycle

49 **Must Remember**

The mid-year population estimates relate to the usually resident population on 30 June of each year. World Population day is an annual event, observed on July 11 every year, which seeks to raise awareness of global population issue

73 *High Yield Points*

Vital statistics include:

- Birth rate
- Death rate
- Natural growth rate
- Life expectancy at birth

Mortality and fertility rates

Population statistics include:

- Population size
- Sex ratio
- Density
- Dependency ratio

50 **Must Remember**

Annual Growth Rate[Q] = (Crude Birth Rate – Crude Death Rate)/10
AGR (2016-2017) 1.19 ~ 1.2% (India is in rapid growth phase)

51 **Must Remember**

Adult sex ratio in India – 991, sex ratio at birth in India is 919

52 **Must Remember**

Total fertility rate (TFR) gives the approximate magnitude of "Completed family size"[Q]. TFR is a period measure constructed by summing the age-specific fertility rates and multiplying by length of the age groups used.

Characteristics

The characteristics of the stages in the demographic cycle have been summarized in the table given below:

Table 2: Demographic cycle

Stage	Birth rate (BR)	Death rate (DR)	Demographic gap	Population	Annual growth rate	Countries experiencing
I (*High stationary*[Q])	High	High	–	Stationary	<1%	India till 1920
II (*Early expanding*[Q])	High	Decreases (Starts to decline)	Increases to reach maximum[Q]	Grows	1–2%	African and South Asian countries
III (*Late expanding*[Q])	Decreases(*Starts to decline*[Q])	Decreases further	Remains high	Grows	About 2%	*India*
IV (*Low stationary*)	Low	Low	Decreases	Stationary	Zero	Austria, Denmark, Sweden
V (*Declining*)	Lower than DR	Low but more than BR	*Negative*[Q]	Decreases	Negative	Germany, Hungary, UK, Japan, Spain, Italy

Special Features

Stage II
- Population growth rates are usually the maximum
- Demographic gap starts increasing
- Demographic gap is maximum towards end of stage II
- Demographic trap is observed in stage II (country would stay in Stage II for longer time, because of increasing population and difficulty to decline the Birth rates)

Stage III
- India is in stage III (since 2011 census)
- Demographic gap starts decreasing from this stage onwards
- Demographic dividend (or gifts or bonus) is observed from stage III onwards

Stage V
- Birth rates may be lower than death rates in later part of stage V
- The population will show declining trend and negative growth
- Demographic liability (higher number of older population compared to younger population) may be observed in this phase

74 High Yield Points

India is in the late expanding (stage III) of the demographic cycle[Q]

POPULATION PYRAMIDS

It is a graphical presentation of the age and gender distribution in format of horizontal bar diagram. The horizontal axis will represent the gender, while the vertical axis represents the age distribution.

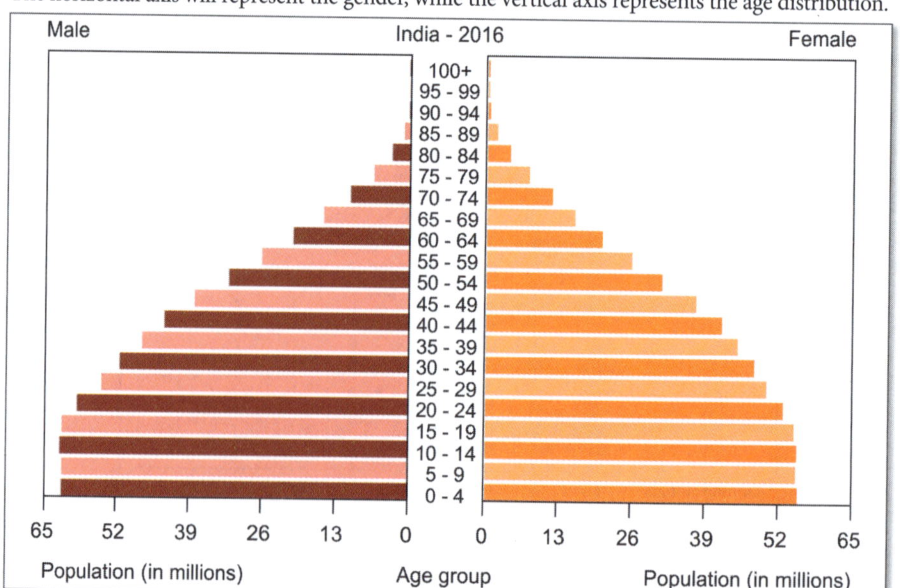

Fig. 2: Age pyramid

The age pyramids maybe further classified based on the fertility rates and age composition of the population.

- Developing countries – the features are as follows:
  - Will show a typical pyramid type of distribution
  - Also known as expanding type or broad base type of age pyramid
  - It is due to higher fertility rates and high death rates
- Advanced or developed countries – the features are
  - It has a narrow base and will show constrictions on the either extremes of age
  - Also known as broad belly or constricting type of age pyramid
  - It is due to low death rates and very low birth rates, where the birth rates may be lower than the death rates
- Stable population
  - Usually is a cylindrical type, with slight constriction in the upper extreme of age due to biological phenomenon of death rates

The different age pyramids from different countries have been shown below for more understanding of the concept.

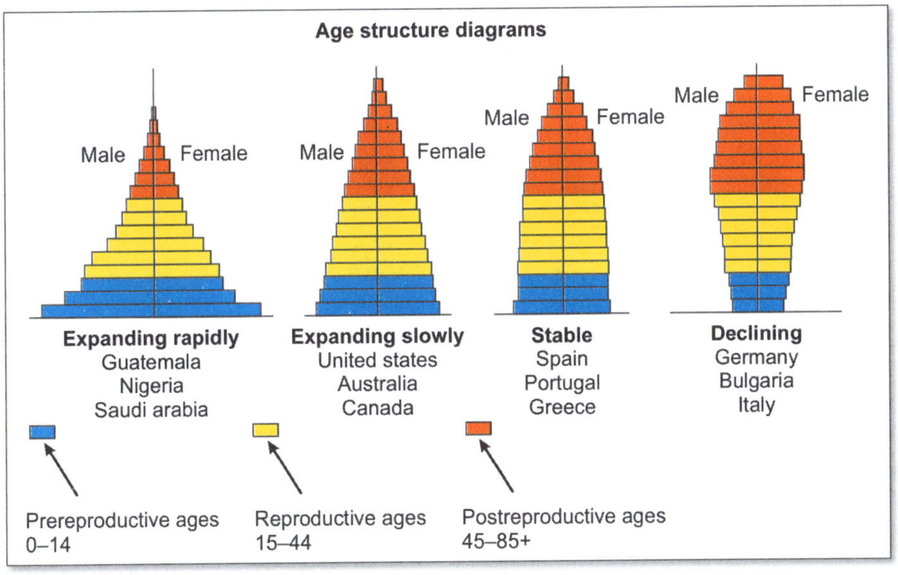

Fig. 3: Age pyramid from different countries

Dependency Ratio

$$\text{Total dependency ratio} = \frac{\text{Children age 0-14 years + population more than 65 years of age}}{\text{Population 15-64 years of age}} \times 100$$

For India (Jan 2018)

- Young dependency ratio = 41.115%
- Old dependency ratio = 9.386%
- Total dependency ratio = 50.55%

Source: Demographic profile India 2018

POPULATION DYNAMICS–DEMOGRAPHIC RATES

Demographic Indicators (Update 2018-2019)

Table 1: Demographic indicators in India

Indicators	Data	Source
Population (2016)	1329 million (17.5% of World population) most populated state - UP	Census 2011

Contd...

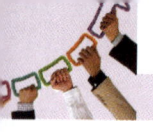

Indicators	Data	Source
Urban population (2011)	377.1 million (31.8%)	Census 2011
Rural population	833.1 million (68.8%)	Census 2011
Annual growth rate (2011)	1.19%	Institute of population studies, NFHS 4
Decadal growth rate (2011)	17.64% Highest in India –Dadra and N. Haveli, Lowest- Nagaland	Census 2011
Total dependency ratio	50.55	India profile 2018
Young age dependency ratio Old age dependency ratio	41.12 9.4	India profile 2018
Life expectancy at birth (2015)	Overall: 67.5 years Male = 67, Female = 70 Highest in world- Japan (Male = 80, Female = 86) and Switzerland (Male = 81, Female = 85)	Population reference bureau 2018
Literacy rate (2011) (Age more than 15 and can read and write)	71.2%	Census 2011
Population < 15 years	27.0	SRS 2016-18
Population >60 years	8.3	SRS 2016-18
CBR – crude birth rate	20.4	SRS 2016-18
GFR – general fertility rate	74.4	SRS 2016-18
CDR- crude death rate	6.4	SRS 2016-18
IMR – infant mortality rate	34	SRS 2016-18
IMR Madhya Pradesh	47 (Max)	SRS 2016-18
IMR Kerala	10 (Minimum)	SRS 2016-18
U5MR – under five mortality rate	39	SRS 2016-18
MMR – maternal mortality ratio	130	SRS 2018
Maternal mortality rate	8.8	SRS 2018
Lifetime mortality risk*	0.3 %	SRS 2018
Sex ratio adults	991	NFHS 4
Sex ratio at birth	919	NFHS 4
Registered births	79.7	NFHS 4
Female literacy (15-49 years)	68.4	NFHS 4
Male literacy (15-49 years)	85.7	NFHS 4
TFR – total fertility rate	2.2	NFHS 4
Any contraceptive method used 15-49 years	53.5	NFHS 4

* The life time mortality risk is defined as the probability that at least one women of reproductive age (15-49) will die due to child birth or puerperium assuming that chance of death is uniformly distributed across the entire reproductive span and has been worked out using the following formula

Demographic Indicators

- **Crude birth rate** is the number of live births per 1000 estimated mid-year population (on 1st July)[Q], in a given year.
- **Crude death rate** is the number of deaths per 1000 estimated mid-year population (on 1st July) Q, in a given year.
  - Crude death rate (CDR) is simplest measure of mortality.
  - Disadvantage – CDR cannot be used to compare death rates of different communities (As population composition and Age-specific death rates may vary indifferent populations).
- **Sex ratio:** It is the number of females per 1000 males.
  - **Female deficit syndrome** – is an adverse sequel of poor political legislations, gender preferences and gender inequality which leads to an unstable population and further complications at ecological level
- **Juvenile or child sex ratio (CSR)** is the number of female children 0–6 year per 1000 male children 0–6 year age.

Annual Growth Rate

It is the average increment (or growth) of the population in a year.

Table 3: Annual growth rate and population doubling time

Rate/phase	(Annual growth rate = CBR-CDR)	Population doubling time
Stationary	No growth	
Slow growth	< 0.5	>139 years
Moderate growth	0.5–1	139–70
Rapid growth	1–1.5	70–47
Very rapid	1.5–2	47–35
Explosive or population explosion[Q]	>2	35–18

Rule of 70–Doubling time of a population can be estimated by dividing 70 by the annual (exponential) percentage growth rate. A population growing at 1% will double in 70 year and the one growing at 2% will take 35 years
- 70/% Growth rate = Doubling time
- 70/ Doubling time = % Growth rate

Fertility Indicators

General Fertility Rate (GFR)

- It is number of live births per 1000 women in the reproductive age-group in a given year.
- It is a general indicator for the fertility trends in a country

Related indicators:
- **General marital fertility rate (GMFR)** is number of live births per 1000 married women in the reproductive age group in a year.
- **Age-specific fertility rate** is the number of live births in a year per 1000 women in any specified age-group.
- **Age-specific marital fertility rate** is number of live births in a year per 1000 married women in any specified age group.

75 *High Yield Points*
- TFR = Proxy indicator for family size
- NRR = Best indicator for population growth monitoring

76 *High Yield Points*

Targets:
- NRR = 1 (Replacement level) and
- TFR = 2.1

43 *Good to Remember*
- Life expectancy at birth is highest in Japan (Male 80 years and Female 87 years)
- Among South East Asian countries—Life expectancy at birth is highest in Thailand followed by Sri Lanka > Bangladesh > India > Nepal > Pakistan > Myanmar

- **Total fertility rate (TFR)**
  - It is the average number of children a female will bear during her entire reproductive period, assuming the age specific fertility pattern.
  - It is the widely accepted measure for impact of the family planning program and also a proxy indicator for the family size in an area.
  - The target for TFR is 2.1
  - The TFR for India is 2.2 (NFHS-4)
- **Gross reproduction rate (GRR)**
  - It is an average number of girls to be born to a woman if she experiences the current fertility pattern throughout her reproductive span (15–44 or 49 years), assuming no mortality.
  - GRR is thus equivalent to TFR for female children only.[Q]
- **Net reproduction rate (NRR)**
  - Average number of girls which a newborn girl child will bear during her entire life, assuming the age specific fertility and mortality patterns.
  - It is a sensitive indicator for family planning services implementation in a country and thus is the best measure for growth of a population

Interpretation and Public Health Importance of NRR

- **Replacement-level fertility:** It is the average number of children a woman would need to have to reproduce herself by bearing a daughter who survives to childbearing age. It corresponds to a NRR of 1, which also corresponds to TFR = 2.1. If replacement level fertility is sustained over a sufficiently long period, each generation will exactly replace itself in the absence of migration.
- **Below-replacement fertility:** Total fertility levels below 2.1 children per woman. (Population aging increases and size eventually decreases)
- **Very low fertility:** Total fertility levels below 1.3 children per woman.
- **Very high fertility:** Total fertility levels above 5 children per woman.
- *Percentage of births of order 3 and above is a direct measure of fertility.* (High percent of birth of order ≥3 indicates weak impact of the family welfare program).

Formulae and Definitions of Demography Rates

- Crude birth rate (CBR) $= \dfrac{\textit{Number of live births during the year}}{\textit{mid-year population}} \times 1000$

- Crude death rate (CBR) $= \dfrac{\textit{Number of deaths during the year}}{\textit{mid-year population}} \times 1000$

- General fertility rate (GFR) $= \dfrac{\textit{Number of live births in a year}}{\textit{mid-year female population in age group 15-49 years}} \times 1000$

- General marital fertility rate (GMFR)

$$= \frac{\textit{Number of live births in a year}}{\textit{mid-year married female population in age group 15-49 years}} \times 1000$$

- Age specific fertility rate (ASFR)

$$= \frac{\textit{Number of live births in a particular age-group}}{\textit{mid-year female population of the same age group}} \times 1000$$

- Age specific marital fertility rate (ASMFR)

$$= \frac{\textit{Number of live births in a particular age-group}}{\textit{mid-year married female population of the same age group}} \times 1000$$

- Total fertility rate (TFR) $= \dfrac{5 \times \sum_{19-49}^{15-49} ASFR}{1000}$

- Total marital fertility rate (TMFR) $= \dfrac{5 \times \sum_{15-19}^{45-49} ASMFR}{1000}$

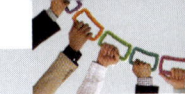

- Gross reproduction rate (GRR) = $\dfrac{5 \times \Sigma_{15-19}^{45-49} \text{ASFR for female live births}}{1000}$
- Infant mortality rate (IMR) = $\dfrac{\text{Number of infant deaths during the year}}{\text{number of live births during the same year}} \times 1000$
- Neonatal mortality rate (NnMR)
  $$= \frac{\text{Number of infant deaths age <29 days during the year}}{\text{number of live births during the same year}} \times 1000$$
- Early neonatal mortality rate (E-NnMR)
  $$= \frac{\text{Number of infant deaths age <7 days during the year}}{\text{number of live births during the same year}} \times 1000$$
- Late neonatal mortality rate (L-NnMR)
  $$= \frac{\text{Number of infant deaths age 7 days to < 29 days during the year}}{\text{number of live births during the same year}} \times 1000$$
- Post neonatal mortality rate (P-NnMR)
  $$= \frac{\text{Number of infant deaths age 29 days to <1 year during the year}}{\text{number of live births during the same year}} \times 1000$$
- Peri-natal mortality rate (PnMR)
  $$= \frac{\text{Number of still births and infant deaths of <7 days during the year}}{\text{number of still births and live births during the same year}} \times 1000$$
- Still birth rate (SBR)
  $$= \frac{\text{Number of still births during the year}}{\text{number of still births and live births during the same year}} \times 1000$$

Other Related Indicators

- **Child-woman ratio** is the number of children 0–4 years of age per 1000 women of child-bearing age (15–44 or 49 years).
- **Pregnancy rate** is the ratio of number of pregnancies in a year to married women in the ages 15–44 (or 49) years.
- **Abortion rate** is number of all types of abortions, per 1000 women of child-bearing age.
- **Abortion ratio** is ratio of number of abortions during a particular time period to number of live births over the same period.
- **Marriage rate** is the number of marriages in the year per 1000 midyear population.

VARIABLES IN DEMOGRAPHY

Population Concentration

- **Centralization:** People living together due to activities like industrialization, plantation etc.
- **Segregation:** People living together due to socio cultural habits.
- **Net migration** = Immigration – Emigration.

$$\textit{Migration rate} = \frac{\textit{Number of immigrants}}{\textit{Total population}} \times 100$$

Settlement Hierarchy

- **Isolated dwelling** – less than 10 families in a small area
- **Small village** (hamlets) – a few 100 population, usually less than 600
- **Village**–with a panchayat, usually ranging from 1000 – 2000 population
- **Town**–population of 1,000 to 20,000, with a jurisdiction and local governing body (municipality)
- **City** or Large town - a large town has a population of 20,000 to 100,000 – with a municipal corporation

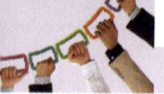

- **Block:** It is an administrative compartmentalization of 100,000 population in each block
- **Mega city** are cities with a population of 10 million or more and population density of at least 2000 person/km^2 e.g. Mumbai, Kolkata and Delhi.
- **Urban community** means a population >5000, population density of at least 390/km^2 or 1000 per square mile and at least 75% adult male population is engaged in nonagricultural occupation.

Life Expectancy

It is the expectation of life at a given age is the average number of years which a person of that age may expect to live, according to the mortality pattern prevalent in that country.

- Life expectancy is one of the *best indicators* of country's level of development and of overall health status of its population.
- India has a life expectancy of 67.5 years and targets to achieve the life expectancy of 70 years by 2025
- Life expectancy is an important determinant in calculating the human development index for international comparisons

Miscellaneous Indicators in Demography

Table 4: Miscellaneous indicators in demography

Indicators	Basic formulae	Use	Common applications
Indicators commonly used in emergencies			
Crude mortality rate (CMR, or death rate)	Deaths due to any cause, in any age group/(population at risk x period of time)	Rate of occurrence (incidence of death in the general population)	Usually expressed as deaths per 10,000 people per day; always presented
Age-specific mortality rate (or death rate)	Deaths in age group/(population in age group at risk x period of time for those within the age range)	Rate of occurrence of death in a given age group	Most common is under 5 mortality rate (U5MR): Deaths among children <5 years per 10,000 children <5 years per day
Group-specific mortality rate	Deaths among members of a given sub-group/(population belonging to the group at risk x period of time)	Rate of occurrence of death in a given group	Usually calculated for especially vulnerable groups, such as IDPs, orphans, etc.
Period-specific mortality rate	Deaths during sub-period/(population at risk during sub-period x duration of sub-period)	Rate of occurrence of death during a specific sub-period within the crisis	Monthly MR, MR during epidemic period, MR before/after displacement
Cause-specific mortality rate	Deaths due to a given cause/(population at risk x period of time)	Rate of occurrence of death due to a given cause in the general population	MR due to intentional injury: MR due to disease causing epidemic
Proportionate mortality	Deaths due to a given cause/total deaths	Proportion of all deaths that are attributable to a given cause	Usually expressed as a percentage; can be calculated in the general population or among people dying in a health facility
Case-fatality rate (or rate) or CFR	Deaths due to a given cause (disease)/total cases of given disease	Probability of dying as a result of a given disease/cause of ill health (lethality of a given disease)	Can be calculated for a given disease/cause, or when evaluating the situation in a whole hospitalization ward
Excess mortality rate (and total number of excess deaths)	Observed MR—expected noncrisis MR (x population at risk x period of time)	Rate of occurrence of death attributable to crisis conditions	Fundamental and objective indicator of crisis severity
Indicators less commonly used in emergencies, but prominent in long-term development settings			
Neonatal mortality ratio (or rate)	Deaths among neonates <28 days old/live births	Probability of dying before age 28 days	Usually calculated for a given year (i.e. on an annual basis), and out of 1,000 live births

Contd...

Indicators	Basic formulae	Use	Common applications
Infant mortality ratio (or rate)	Deaths among children <1 year old over one year/live births	Probability of dying before age 1 years	
Under 5 mortality ratio (or rate); also known as child mortality ratio (or rate)	Deaths among children <5 years/live births	Probability of dying before age 5 year	
Maternal mortality ratio	Deaths while pregnant or within 42 days of pregnancy termination, due to pregnancy related causes/live births	Probability of dying as a result of one's pregnancy	Usually calculated for a given year (i.e. on an annual basis), and out of 100,000 live births

SOURCES OF DATA COLLECTION

The basis for health planning, providing accessible health care and implementation of all national health programs is dependent on assessment of the demographic demand and the related dynamics. It is important to assess the quantum of services to be provided and plan for the same. The various sources for collection of data for analysis of the population growth is listed as below:

- **Civil registration system:**
  - It is under the central births and death registration act 1969
  - All births and deaths are registered within 21 days of the event
- **SRS** – sample registration system
  - Started from 1960's
  - It is a 6 monthly registration system conducted at the national and the state level
  - The main components of SRS are:
    - Base-line survey of the sample units to obtain usual resident population of the sample areas
    - Continuous (longitudinal) enumeration of vital events pertaining to usual resident population by the enumerator
    - Independent retrospective half-yearly surveys for recording births and deaths which occurred during the half-year under reference and up-dating the House list, Household schedule and the list of women in the reproductive age group along with their pregnancy status by the Supervisor;
    - Matching of events recorded during continuous enumeration and those listed in course of half-yearly survey
    - Field verification of unmatched and partially matched events.
    - Filling of Verbal Autopsy Forms for finalized deaths.
  - It is a major source of data for
    - Mortality rates - infant mortality, neonatal mortality, crude death, maternal mortality rates
    - Birth rates, natural growth rates
- **NFHS** – national family health survey
  - The major objective of NFHS is
    - Obtain essential data on health and related aspects
    - Assess the emerging health and family welfare issues
  - The survey provides state and national information for India on fertility, infant and child mortality, the practice of family planning, maternal and child health, reproductive health, nutrition, anaemia, utilization and quality of health and family planning services
  - Last round was done as NFHS -4 in 2015-2016, with data published in 2017-2018
- **Census**
  - It is the main and core source of data undertaken by almost every country in the world
  - 1st census was done in India in 1881
  - The last census was done in 2011
  - Disability was also accounted and measured in the census in India from year 1981 onwards

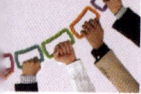

Must Remember

Example 1

Death of a person due to chronic pancreatitis

Part I

- Acute exacerbation of chronic pancreatitis
- Chronic pancreatitis
- Chronic alcoholism

Part II

- Diabetes mellitus

Example 2

Death of a person due to pneumonia

Part I

- Bronchopneumonia
- Fracture of neck of femur (Lt)

Part II

- Essential hypertension

INTERNATIONAL DEATH CERTIFICATE

	Cause of death	Approximate interval between onset and death
I. Disease or condition directly leading to death*	(a)....................................... due to (or as a consequence of)	....
Antecedent causes Morbid conditions, if any, giving rise to the above cause, stating the underlying condition last	(b)....................................... due to (or as a consequence of)	....
	(c)....................................... due to (or as a consequence of)	....
	(d).......................................	....
II. Other significant conditions contributing to the death, but not related to the disease or condition causing it	....	....
	....	....

**This does not mean the mode of dying, e.g. heart failure, respiratory failure. It means the disease, injury, or complication that caused death*

Part I: Cause of Death—One cause is to be entered on each line.

Underlying cause is to be filled on the lowest line. It is the condition that started the sequence of events which lead to immediate cause of death from normal health to immediate cause of death.

- **Immediate cause of death:** Disease or injury or complication that precedes death. Mode of dying, e.g., heart failure, respiratory failure should not be entered.
- **Due to (or as a consequence of):** If immediate cause occurred as a consequence of another condition it should be entered here. Antecedent condition might have just prepared the ground for immediate cause of death, even after a long interval.
- Morbid condition leading to the underlying condition.

Part II

- All diseases or conditions, which were not directly related to the disease directly causing death, though might have unfavorably influenced the morbid process.

Interval between Onset and Death

Exact period from onset of morbid condition and the date of death is to be mentioned. In cases where period is not known, approximate period—"from birth", "several years" or "Unknown" is to be filled.

Accident, Suicide, Homicide

Explain briefly the circumstances or cause of accident. In case of medico-legal cases pending investigations should be mentioned there.

Female Death

If women are of child bearing age group (15–49 years), information on pregnancy and delivery is to be given even though the pregnancy may have nothing to do with occurrence of death.

FAMILY PLANNING

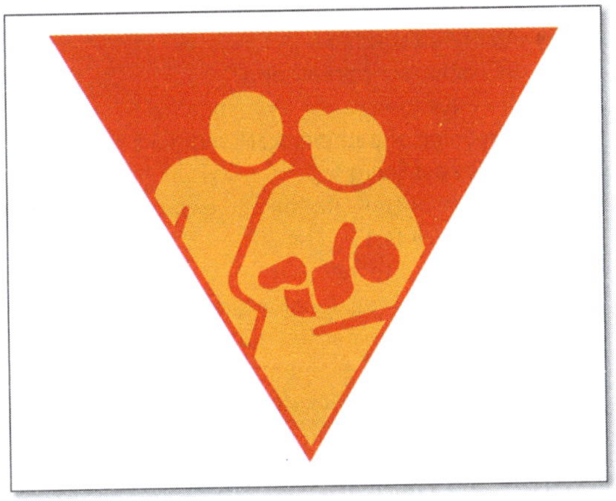

Fig. 4: Logo for family planning

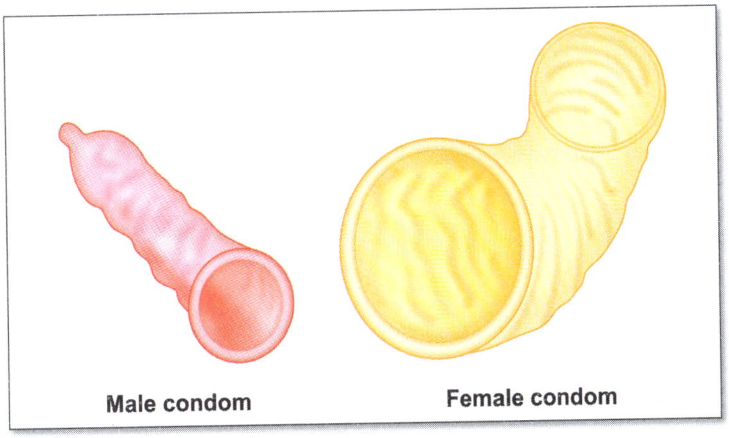

Fig. 5: Male condom and Female Condom

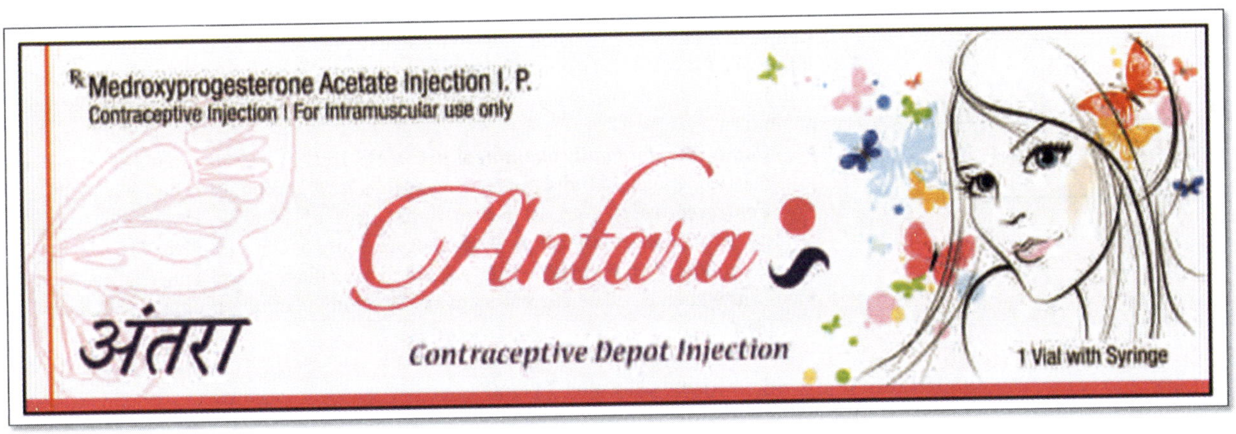

Fig. 6: Antra (I/M injection)

INTRODUCTION AND TERMINOLOGIES

- A family is called as a *planned family* when:
  - Birth of the 1st child is delayed till the mother is over 20 years of age.
  - There is at least 3 years gap between 2 children.
  - Family size is limited.

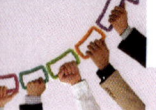

Table 5: Family planning services

- Proper spacing and limitation of births
  - Advice on sterility
  - Education for parenthood
  - Sex education
  - Screening of pathological conditions related to reproductive system e.g. Cervical cancer
- Genetic counseling
  - Premarital consultation and examination
  - Pregnancy test
- Marriage counseling
- Preparation of couple for arrival of 1st child
  - Services for unmarried mothers
  - Teaching home economics and nutrition
  - Provide adoption services

Selected Definitions

Eligible Couples

- **Eligible couple (EC)**[Q] is a newly married couple wherein the wife is in the reproductive age (15 to 45 years).
- There are 15–18% eligible couple in India
- Eligible couple are the targets for providing any method of effective contraception

Target Couples

- **Target couple**[Q] is a couple having 2–3 living children or have completed family.
- They are the targets for providing methods of permanent family planning – sterilization methods

Couple Protection Rate

- **Couple protection rate (CPR)**[Q] is the percentage of eligible couples protected against childbirth by one or other approved methods of family planning.
- Percentage of eligible couple using one or other contraception is **54%** (NFHS IV)
- States with ***low CPR*** → Bihar, UP, Assam, Rajasthan, West Bengal & J&K. Minimum – Meghalaya and Maximum – Himachal Pradesh (NFHS III).
- Sterilization contributes to about >60% of effectively protected couples[Q].
- CPR is an indicator of prevalence of contraceptive practice in the community.
- ***Effective CPR*** is percentage of eligible couples protected against childbirth by one or other approved method of family planning taking into consideration effectiveness of contraceptive method
  - ***Unmet need for family planning*** as per DLHS-III (2007–08) is about 20.5% in currently married women in India (for spacing birth is 7.2% and Limiting births is 13.3%).
  - ***Contraceptive efficacy*** is measured in terms of number of unwanted pregnancy occurring in a specified period of exposure or use of contraceptive.
  - ***Pearl Index***[Q] and Life table analysis is used to evaluate contraceptive efficacy.
  - "Three theme" - The current focus of the family planning program is "Three Theme plan"
    - Son or daughter – 'two will do'
    - Second child after 3 years
    - Universal immunization

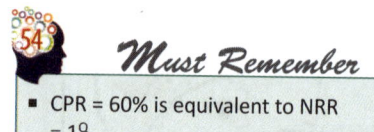

Must Remember

- CPR = 60% is equivalent to NRR = 1[Q]

CONTRACEPTIVE METHODS

The methods of contraception may be divided into temporary methods or permanent methods (sterilization)

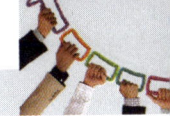

Table 6: Methods of contraception

Spacing methods	Terminal methods
▪ Barrier methods (Physical/Chemical/ Combined) ▪ Intrauterine devices ▪ Hormonal methods ▪ Postconceptional methods ▪ Miscellaneous	▪ Male sterilization (Vasectomy) ▪ Female sterilization (Tubectomy)

Table 7: Classification of contraceptive methods

Physiological	Barrier methods
▪ Withdrawal/coitus interruptus ▪ Rhythm method/calendar/mucus/ symptothermal ▪ Lactational amenorrhea ▪ Chance – no method used ▪ Abstinence of all sexual activity	▪ Condom alone ▪ Spermicide alone ▪ Sponge – Parous • Nulliparous ▪ Diaphragm with spermicide ▪ Female condom ▪ Cervical cap – Parous • Nulliparous
Hormonal	**Intrauterine devices**
▪ OCP ▪ Nuvarng^{R} ▪ Transdermal (Ortho Evra^{R}) ▪ Depo-Provera^{R} ▪ Progestin-only pill (Micronor^{R}) ▪ Mirena^{R} IUS ▪ Jaydess^{R} IUS	▪ Inert IUD ▪ CuT ▪ Hormonal IUD
Surgical	**Emergency postcoital contraception (EPC)**
▪ Tubal ligation ▪ Vasectomy	▪ Yuzpe method ▪ 'Plan B' levonorgestrel only ▪ Postcoital IUD ▪ Ella

Natural Methods of Contraception

Safe Period (Rhythm/Calendar) Method

It is based on the fact that ovulation occurs between 12 and 16 days before onset of menstruation. First described by Ogino in 1930.

Days on which conception is likely to occur are calculated as follows:

- Shortest cycle minus 18 days gives the first day of the fertile period.
- Longest cycle minus 10 days gives the last day of the fertile period.
- If calculations are not possible, couple is advised to avoid intercourse from 8th to 22nd day of menstrual cycle, counting from the first day of the menstrual period.

Drawbacks

- Menstrual cycles are not always regular. Requires educated and responsible couples with high degree of motivation and cooperation.
- Compulsory abstinence of sexual intercourse for nearly 15 days of a month.
- Not applicable during postnatal period.
- High failure rate of 9 per 100 woman-years

Basal Body Temperature Method (BBT)

- Based on identification of rise in BBT at time of ovulation (due to high progesterone level)
- Rise of temperature is very small 0.3–0.5°C. Temperature is measured preferably before getting out of bed in morning.

Drawbacks

- Abstinence is necessary for the entire preovulatory period.

Cervical Mucus Method/Billings Method/Ovulation Method

- Based on observation of changes in the characteristics of cervical mucus.
- At the time of ovulation cervical mucus becomes watery clear resembling raw egg white, smooth, slippery and profuse. Postovulation it becomes thick and less in quantity.
- Woman should be able to distinguish between different types of mucus.

Drawbacks

- High degree of motivation.
- Appropriateness in developing countries is an issue.

Symptothermal Method

- Combines the BBT, cervical mucus and calendar techniques for identifying fertile period. Hence more effective.

Lactational Amenorrhea Method

- Prolongs postpartum amenorrhea and provides some degree of protection against pregnancy.
- This method is effective when:
  - The mother practices exclusive breastfeeding (i.e. frequent feeding during day and night as during the first six months after delivery).
  - The menstrual periods have not returned.
  - Child is less than six months of age.
  - As the breastfeeding decreases after the weaning, the prolactin level also decreases, reducing the natural contraceptive effect of breastfeeding. Thus, this method is very effective up to first six months.

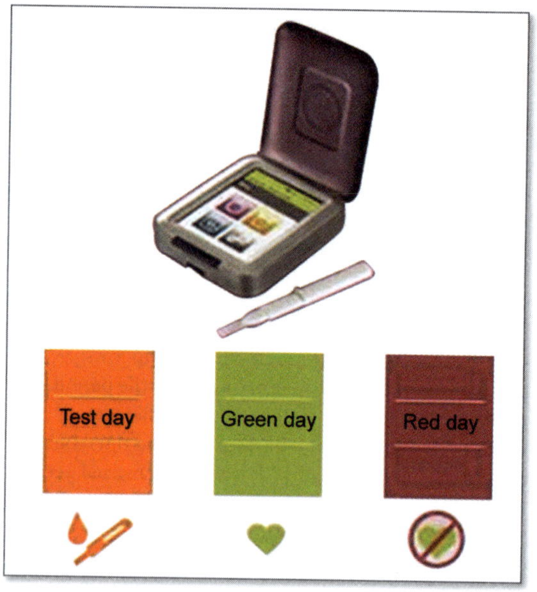

Fig. 7: Persona contraception monitor to know the contraceptive status

Other Methods

Coitus Interruptus and Sexual Abstinence

Persona Contraception Monitor

- It works by monitoring hormones (estrogen and luteinizing hormone) that directly control the cycle and takes into account both egg and sperm survival times.

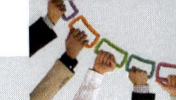

- Test Sticks collect hormones from 1st urine of the day and process it into information on the monitor.
- Monitor tells the contraceptive status-
  - Red day (Unsafe period) → One is at risk of becoming pregnant.
  - Green day (Safe period) → Free to have intercourse without a contraceptive.
  - Yellow (Uncertain)

Persona is 94% reliable when used as per instructions.

Cycle of Beads

- It is based on standard days approach for providing contraception.

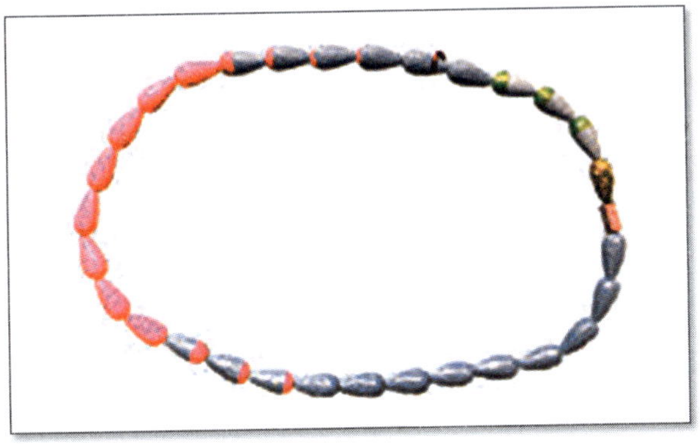

Fig. 8: Cycle of beads used to calculate contraception day

Barrier Methods of Contraception

- Prevent live sperm from meeting the ovum.
- Conventional contraceptives are methods that require action at the time of sexual intercourse E.g., Condoms, Spermicides

Physical Methods

Male Condom

- (Most commonly used[Q])
  - Failure rates 2–14 per 100 women-years.
  - Condom is a safe, easy to use and cheap contraceptive most widely used by males worldwide[Q].
  - **Advantages:**
    - *Contraceptive*: Absence of side effects associated with pill and IUD
    - *Non-contraceptive*[Q]: Protection against HIV and RTI/STI infection
  - **Disadvantage:** Require a high degree of motivation on the part of the user.
  - Number of condom needed for effective protection in a year is 72[Q]

Female Condom

- Failure rates during 1st year use 5–21 per 100 women-years.
- Female Condom (FEMIDOM) (invented by Lasse Hessel) is made of Polyurethane/Nitrile or Latex with 2 rings (outer and inner).
- **Advantage:** Controlled by women, prevents pregnancy and STD/HIV, reusable, compatible with oil lubricants.
- **Disadvantage:** Cost, motivation on part of women, covers skin around external genitals. It has a higher failure rate than male condom.

Diaphragm or Dutch Cap

- Barrier contraceptive (invented by a German physician in 1882) used along with spermicides.
  - It is a shallow cup 5–10 cm (2–4 inches) in diameter, made of synthetic rubber or plastic with a stiff but flexible rim around the edge.

44 **Good to Remember**

Molecular condom is used to prevent HIV infection. It turns into a gel like coating when inserted into vagina. On exposure to semen it returns to liquid form and releases an antiviral drug for HIV prevention

- It is inserted into the vagina to cover the entrance to the uterus, before sexual intercourse and must remain in place for not less than 6 hours after sexual intercourse.
- It is held in position partly by the spring tension and partly by the vaginal muscle tone
- **Advantage:** Nil side effects, low failure rate when used with spermicide (6 to 12 per 100 women-years)
- **Disadvantage:** Initial guidance and practice required, privacy is desired for practice washing and storing the diaphragm—hence not popular in India. There is a Remote Risk of Toxic Shock syndrome
- **Precaution:** It must be ensured that the diaphragm fits properly (Correct size) and is not damaged.

> Diaphragm is not recommended in the National Family Welfare Program

Vaginal Sponge

- Failure rate in parous women is 20–40 per 100 women-years and in nulliparous women 9–20 per 100 women-years.
- *Today* is a small polyurethane foam sponge (5 cm × 2.5 cm), saturated with spermicide, nonoxynol-9.[Q]
- It is wet with water and then inserted into vagina prior to intercourse (to cover the cervix) and is left in its place for about 6 hours post ejaculation.
- It is removed within 24 hours of insertion
- **Disadvantage:** High failure rate, no protection against HIV/STD, increased risk of UTI and risk of toxic shock syndrome.

Chemical Methods

Spermicides are "surface-active agents" that attach to spermatozoa and inhibit oxygen uptake and kill sperms. Available as:

- **Foams:** Foam tablets, foam aerosols
- **Creams, jellies and pastes:** squeezed from a tube
- **Suppositories:** inserted manually
- **Soluble films:** C-film inserted manually

Intrauterine Devices

- IUD is made of polyethylene or other polymers (Nontoxic, Non-tissue reactive and durable) and contains a small amount of Barium Sulfate to allow for X-ray observation.[Q]
- IUD has attached thread or "tail" of fine nylon, that projects into vagina after insertion (a reassurance to user that the IUD is in its place) and makes it easy to remove IUD when desired.

Classification

Table 8: Intrauterine devices and their mechanism of action

Types of IUD	Examples	Mechanism of action
1st Generation (Non-medicated)	Lippes loop, Gräfenberg's ring (ring of silver wire)	▪ Foreign-body reaction (cellular and biochemical changes in endometrium and uterine fluids, Impair viability of gamete and reduce its chances of fertilization)
2nd Generation (Medicated - release metal ions (copper))	Copper T-200,T Cu-220, T Cu-380 A, Nova T, ML-Cu-250, ML-Cu-375	▪ Copper enhances Foreign-body reaction ▪ Alters biochemical composition of cervical mucus and prevent sperm from entering the cervix. ▪ Affect sperm motility, capacitation and survival

Contd...

Types of IUD	Examples	Mechanism of action
3rd Generation (Medicated - release hormone)	Progestasert, Levanova (LNG)	▪ Increase the viscosity of the cervical mucus and prevent sperm from entering the cervix. ▪ Maintain high levels of progesterone and relatively low levels of estrogen in endometrium → sustaining an endometrium unfavorable to implantation

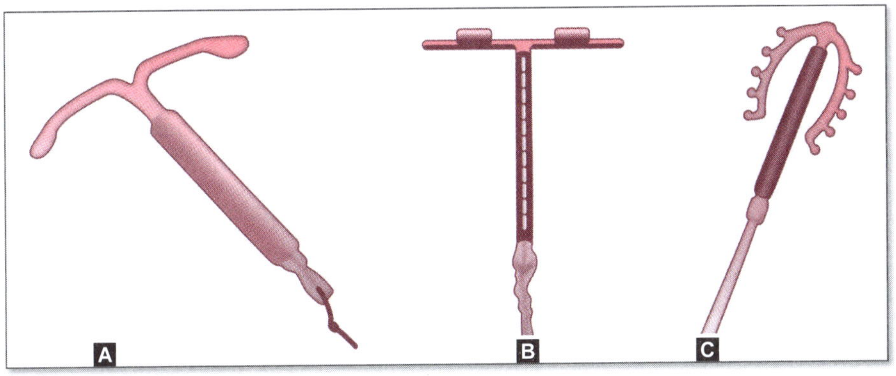

Figs 9A to C: Intrauterine devices. **A.** Mirena; **B.** Copper T; **C.** Multiload

Advantages of Copper Devices

- Low expulsion rate
- Lower incidence of side-effects, e.g., pain and bleeding
- Easier to fit and better tolerated by nulliparous women
- Increased contraceptive effectiveness
- Effective postcoital contraceptives, if inserted within 3–5 days of unprotected-intercourse.

Table 9: Advantages of intrauterine device

Contraceptive advantage	Noncontraceptive advantage
▪ Effective method (Average pregnancy rate after 1 year of about 3–5 per 100 typical users) ▪ Relatively inexpensive, because of its long life ▪ IUD use is independent at the time of intercourse ▪ Relatively high continuation rates	▪ Prevents Synechiolysis (Asherman's syndrome) ▪ Reduces risk of endometrial cancer ▪ Reduced incidence of anemia
▪ No systemic metabolic effects associated with oral pills ▪ Does not interfere with lactation ▪ IUDs should preferably be used in settings where follow-up facilities are available	▪ Used to treat menorrhagia ▪ Hormone replacement therapy

Effectiveness of 2nd generation copper IUD is directly related to the amount of copper surface area.[Q] *Numbers included in names of devices refer to surface area (in sq. mm) of copper on the device.*

Nova T and T Cu-380 Ag have *a silver core* over which the copper wire is wrapped.

Side Effects and Complications of IUD Insertion

- **Bleeding:** Most common complaint (Accounts for 10–20% of all IUD removals).[Q]
  - Management-Reassurance and IFA (Ferrous Sulfate 200 mg) TDS or removal
- **Pain:** 2nd major side-effect leading to IUD removal[Q] (15-40% of IUD removals)–Usually disappears by 3 month. More in Nullipara
- Pelvic infection or pelvic inflammatory disease (PID)– 2 to 8 times more likely in IUD users than nonusers[Q] and in ones with multiple sexual partners.[Q]
  - ***Risk of PID*** appears to be the highest in the first few months after IUD insertion
  - Introduction of bacteria occurs during IUD insertion or by organisms ascending the IUD tail.

- **Organism responsible:** Gardnerella, Anaerobic streptococci, Bacteroides, Coliform bacilli and Actinomyces.
- **Clinical features:** Vaginal discharge, pelvic pain and tenderness, abnormal bleeding, chills and fever.
- Even one or two episodes of PID can cause permanent infertility (blocking fallopian tubes).
- PID if diagnosed, it should be treated promptly with broad-spectrum antibiotics.

▪ **Uterine perforation:** 1: 150 to 1: 9000 insertions.
- More frequent when insertions are performed between 48 hours and 6 weeks postpartum.
- May be completely asymptomatic or cause intestinal obstruction, peritoneal adhesions etc.
- Conclusive diagnosis of perforation is usually made by a pelvic X-ray.

▪ **Pregnancy:** Failure rate in the first year is approximately 3% (Varies in different IUDs).
- Ectopic pregnancy–(0.2 per 1000 women-year in Levonorgestrel IUD and Cu-T 380A. In progesterone IUD it is higher about 6.8)
- Women at high risk are those with previous PID, tubal pregnancy or ectopic pregnancy.

▪ **Expulsion:** Expulsion rates vary between 12% and 20%. Expulsion can be partial or complete.
- It usually occurs in the first few weeks following insertion or during menstruation.
- It is common among young nulliparous women and women with a postpartum insertion.
- Expulsion rates are somewhat lower for copper than for inert devices.

Table 10: Contraindications of intrauterine device

Absolute	Relative
▪ Suspected pregnancy ▪ Pelvic inflammatory disease ▪ Vaginal bleeding of undiagnosed etiology ▪ Cancer of cervix, uterus or adnexa and other pelvic tumors ▪ Previous ectopic pregnancy	▪ Anemia ▪ Menorrhagia ▪ History of PID since last pregnancy ▪ Purulent cervical discharge ▪ Distortions of uterine cavity due to congenital malformations, fibroids ▪ Unmotivated person

Approved Period of Use

- Inert IUDs (Lippes Loop) may be left in place as long as required, if there are no side-effects.
- Copper devices and hormone-releasing IUD need periodic replacement- CuT-380A -10 years[Q], Cu T-200- 4 years, Nova T -5 years[Q], Progesterone IUD- every year[Q], Levonorgestrel IUD- 7 years.

> **High Yield Points**
>
> **IUD expulsion rate:** Lowest- Progestasert, Highest- Lippes loop
> **IUD removal rate:** Lowest- Progestasert, Highest- Levonorgestrel
> **IUD pregnancy rate:** Lowest- Levonorgestrel, Highest-Lippes loop

Ideal IUD Candidate

Ideal IUD candidate is a woman:

- Who has borne at least one child (IUD is not a method of first choice for nulliparous women)
- Who has no history of pelvic disease
- Who has normal menstrual periods
- Who is willing to check the IUD tail
- Who has access to follow-up and treatment of potential problems, and
- Who is in a monogamous relationship (multiple partners increase the risk of PID) and possible infertility.

Timing of IUD Insertion

- During menstruation or within 5–10 days of beginning of menstruation (Ideal)
- **Postpartum:** Within 1 week of delivery and before discharge.[Q] High risk of perforation and expulsion.
- **Postpuerperal:** (Preferable) 6–8 weeks postdelivery.[Q] Can be clubbed with follow-up examination of mother and child.
- **Postabortion:** After a legally induced 1st trimester abortion or after 1st menstrual period following spontaneous abortion
- **Postcoital:** Within 3–5 days of unprotected intercourse (Emergency contraception[Q])

Hormonal Methods

Oral Contraceptive Pills (OCPs)–Combined Pill

MALA-N and MALA-D are low-dose combined oral contraceptive pills

- They are monophasic OCP containing Levonorgestrel 0.15 mg and Ethinylestradiol 0.03 mg[Q]
- Mala-D is a package of 28 pills (21 OCP and 7 brown film coated Ferrous fumarate tablets). It is available to the consumer under social marketing scheme at a price of ₹3 per strip.
- Mala-N is supplied free of cost through all PHCs, CHC/Sub Center, Urban family welfare centers, etc.

Table 11: Oral contraceptive pills (action and dosage)

Methods	Physiological role	Progestin	Estrogen
Combined pill	Fixed dose of both estrogen and progestin, while synergize to inhibit ovulation, the progestin ensures prompt bleeding at end of a cycle	▪ Norgestrel 0.3 mg ▪ Norgestrel 0.5 mg ▪ Levonorgestrel 0.25 mg ▪ Desogestrel 0.15 mg	▪ Ethinylestradiol 30 µg ▪ Ethinylestradiol 50 µg ▪ Ethinylestradiol 50 µg ▪ Ethinylestradiol 20 µg
Phased pill	▪ Triphasic regimens, estrogen dose fixed, progestin dose increased from first phase to third phase ▪ Women >35 years with no withdrawal bleeding	▪ Levonorgestrel 50–75 µg ▪ Norethindrone 0.5–0.75 mg	▪ Ethinylestradiol 30–40 µg ▪ Ethinylestradiol 35–35 µg
Postcoital pill (Emergency pill)	For women not taking any contraception (but does not want pregnancy)	Levonorgestrel 0.25 mg Levonorgestrel 0.75 mg	Ethinylestadiol 50 µg
MIni pills	Devised to eliminate estrogen, low dose of progestin is suggested, menstrual cycle tends to become irregular and ovulation occurs in 20–30% persons	Norethindrone 0.35 mg	Norgestrel 75 µg

Current recommendation by NHM for emergency contraception: ***i-Pill*–single dose 1.5 mg levonorgestrel** to be taken as early as possible best with 72 hrs of unprotected intercourse

Low dose OCP contain 30-35 mcg of synthetic estrogen and 0.5 to 1 mg of progesterone

Very low dose OCP contain 20 mcg of ethinylestradiol and 0.15 mg Desogestrel. Loestrin 1/20, Femilon.

Triphasic pill (Triquilar) is an oral contraceptive pill with varying strength of estrogen and progesterone administered in 3 phases.

Table 12: Doses of oral contraceptive pills

Ethinylestradiol (mcg)	Levonorgestrel (mcg)	Days
30	50	6 (1st phase)
40	75	5 (2nd phase)
30	125	10 (3rd phase)

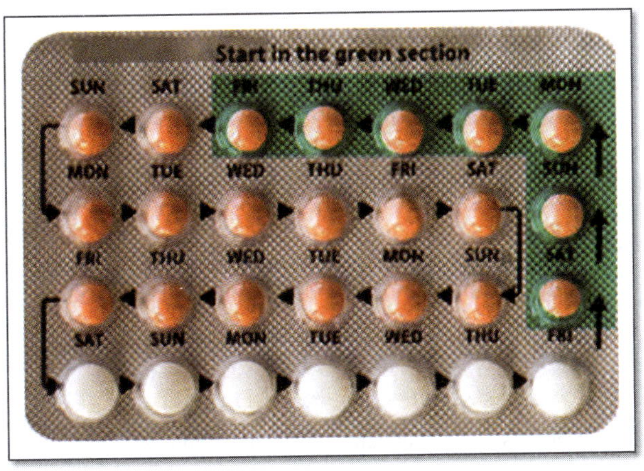

Fig. 10: Doses of oral contraceptive pills

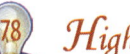

> **78 High Yield Points**
>
> The current NHM 2018 recommendation for emergency contraception is: single dose levonorgestrel tablet, 1.5 mg (iPill) to be taken as early as possible, best within 72 hours of unprotected intercourse

Beneficial Effects of OCP

- Almost 100% effective in preventing unplanned pregnancy.[Q]
- **Noncontraceptive health benefits[Q]:** Protects against:
  - Benign breast disorders (Fibrocystic disease and Fibroadenoma)
  - Ovarian cysts
  - Iron deficiency anemia (Decreased blood loss or Menorrhagia)
  - Osteoporosis
  - Pelvic inflammatory disease
  - Ectopic pregnancy
  - Ovarian cancer (Reduces risk by 40% compared to nonusers)
  - Endometrial cancer (Reduces risk by 50% compared to nonusers)
  - Used in case of dysfunctional uterine bleeding (DUB), irregular menstrual cycles, Dysmenorrhea.

Adverse Effects of Oral Contraceptive

- **Cardiovascular (Due to Estrogen dose):** Myocardial infarction, cerebral thrombosis and venous thrombosis (with or without pulmonary embolus). Risk increases with age and smoking.
- **Carcinogenesis:** Increased risk of cervical cancer
- **Metabolic (Due to progestogen dose):** Elevated BP, alteration in serum lipids (Fall in HDL), blood clotting and altered carbohydrate metabolism (elevations of blood glucose and plasma insulin.)
  - **Liver:** Hepatocellular adenoma and gallbladder disease.
  - Cholestatic Jaundice in some pill users.
  - **Lactation:** High estrogen affects quantity and constituents of breast milk. Less frequently cause premature cessation of lactation.
- Slight delay in conception following discontinuation.
- **Ectopic pregnancies:** (More likely with Progestogen only pills).
- **Other unwanted effects:** Breast tenderness, weight gain, headache, migraine, bleeding disturbances (Break-through bleeding/spotting in early cycles. No withdrawal bleeding at end of a cycle.)

45 Good to Remember

- **Social marketing scheme** – Condom and OCP are provided at subsidized rates (70–85 %) by agency of Social Marketing Organization (SMO) through diverse outlet.
- Deluxe Nirodh – ₹3 per pack of 5 pieces
- Combined OCP (0.03 mg of Ethinylestradiol + 0.15 mg of Levonorgestrel[Q])- Mala D at ₹3 per strip (21 OCP + 7 Iron tab + 60 mg Ferrous fumarate)[Q]

Absolute Contraindication of OCP

- Cancer of the breast and genitals
- Liver disease
- Previous or present history of thromboembolism
- Cardiac abnormalities
- Congenital hyperlipidemia
- Undiagnosed abnormal uterine bleeding

Special Problems Requiring Medical Surveillance for OCP

- Age over 40 years
- Smoking and age over 35 years
- Mild hypertension
- Chronic renal disease
- Epilepsy
- Migraine
- Nursing mothers in the first 6 months
- Diabetes mellitus
- Gallbladder disease
- History of infrequent bleeding, amenorrhea, etc.

Injectables and Implants

Depot Medroxyprogesterone Acetate (DMPA)—ANTRA

Dose: 150 mg every 3 months by deep intramuscular injection into Gluteus maximus muscle.[Q]

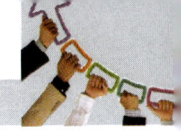

Administration: Initial injection during first 5 days of menstrual period and then at regular intervals (maybe given 2 weeks early or late)

- **Mechanism of action**
  - Suppression of ovulation.[Q]
  - Indirect effect on endometrium
  - Direct action on fallopian tubes and production of cervical mucus.
- **Adverse effects**
  - Weight gain
  - Irregular menstrual bleeding
  - Increased incidence of ectopic pregnancy
  - Increased risk of ovarian cyst
  - Prolonged anovulation and infertility after discontinuation of use
  - Osteoporosis
- **Advantages**
  - Can be used by lactating mothers, as it does not affect the quality and quantity of breast milk.[Q]
  - Requires a minimum of motivation or none at all.
  - Recommended in Multipara >35 years who have completed their families.[Q]
- **Contraindications**
  - Breast and genital cancers
  - Undiagnosed abnormal uterine bleeding
  - Suspected malignancy
  - High BP (Systolic ≥ 160 or diastolic ≥ 100)
  - History of stroke, heart attack
  - Certain conditions of heart, blood vessel and liver
  - Deep vein thrombosis
  - Women breastfeeding a baby <6 weeks.

DMPA- SC 104 mg

- New lower dose formulation of DMPA (Depo-sub[Q] provera 104)
- **Dose:** 104 mg every 3 months, subcutaneous injection in upper thigh or abdomen.

Norethisterone Enantate (NET-EN)

It has slightly higher pregnancy rate compared to DMPA

- **Dose:** 200 mg every 60 days, intra muscular injection.
- **Mechanism of action:** Suppression of ovulation and thickening of cervical mucus
- **Advantage:** Effective, Long acting and Reversible.
- **Adverse effect:** Disruption of normal menstrual cycle, amenorrhea

Subdermal Implant

Norplant

Developed by the population council, New York

- Consist of 6 silastic (silicone rubber) capsules containing 35 mg each of Levonorgestrel.[Q]
- **Norplant-2** – Recent device, Levonorgestrel in 2 small rods, (75 mg) easy to insert and remove
- **Site of insertion:** Beneath skin of the forearm or upper arm
- Effective contraception for 5 years
- **Major disadvantage:** Irregular menstrual bleeding and surgical procedure for insertion/removal.

Implanon

- It is a single flexible rod 4 cm long and 2 mm in diameter placed subdermally.
- It contains 68 mg of 3-keto Desogestrel (Etonogestrel), 67 ugm of hormone is released daily initially, decreasing to 30 ugm after 2 years.
- It suppresses ovulation for 2.5 years and provides effective contraception for at least 3 years. Concentrations that inhibit ovulation are achieved within 8 hours of insertion.
- Ideal for obese women. (Etonogestrel concentration is not affected by body weight unlike Levonorgestrel)
- Contraceptive efficacy (Pearl Index of 0.01) surpasses Norplant and Sterilization.

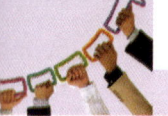

Newer Birth Control Measures

Combined injectable contraceptive: Contain a progesterone and estrogen
Mechanism of action: Suppression of ovulation and thickening of cervical mucus+ unfavorable endometrium (Due to progesterone)
Administration: Monthly injection (Plus Minus 3 days) e.g. – Cyclofem, Cyclo-Provera and Mesigyna
Combined hormonal contraceptive ring: Contain a progesterone and estrogen
MOA: Suppression of ovulation
Administered once monthly (Once inserted into vagina, it is removed after 3rd week, followed by a gap of 1 week)
Contraceptive transdermal patch: It releases ethinyl estradiol and norelgestromin. 1 patch lasts 7 days (3 to be applied consecutively with a gap of 1 week). Mechanism and effectiveness similar to OCP (Inhibits ovulation)
Birth control vaccine: 3 type of vaccine are under research- Anti-hCG vaccine, Anti zona vaccine and Anti sperm vaccine

NonHormonal Methods

Centchroman (Chhaya)

- It is a nonhormonal and nonsteroidal, long acting weekly contraceptive
- Each tablet has 30 mg of Centchroman (Methoxychroman hydrochloride).
- Chemical formulation is – ormiloxifene
- Mechanism of action: selective estrogen receptor modulator
- Only anti implantation agent (Interferes with nidation) approved for clinical use worldwide.
- **Schedule:** Start on 1st day of menstrual cycle, then twice a week 3 days apart for 3 months, then once a week as long contraception is required.
- **In case of missed dose:** It should be taken as soon as possible within 2 days of missing and normal schedule is followed. If missed by >2 days but within 7 days normal schedule is continued with condom till next period.
- **Contraindication:** Lactation (1st 6 month), Hepatic dysfunction, PCOD, Cervical hyperplasia and hypersensitivity.
- **Noncontraceptive Benefit:** Treatment of dysfunctional uterine bleeding (DUB).

Menstrual Regulation

- Aspiration of uterine contents in 6–14 days of a missed period, before pregnancy test can confirm pregnancy.

Menstrual Induction

- Normal progesterone prostaglandin balance is disturbed by intrauterine application of 1–5 mg solution (or 2.5–5 mg pellet) of prostaglandin F2 under sedation. Sustained contraction of uterus occurs within minutes for 7 minutes, followed by cyclic contractions for 3–4 hours. Bleeding starts and continues for 7–8 days.

Gossypol

- Only Male sterilization method
- Natural phenol, yellow coloured compound.
- Known to have anti-malarial, anti-cancer and male sterilizing properties
- It is derived from a Chinese cotton plant
- Adverse effects
  - Permanent sterilization
  - hypokalaemia

Terminal Methods of Sterilization

- Ideal for couples desiring no more children
- Female sterilization accounts for about 85% and male sterilization 10–15% of all sterilization in India
- Male sterilization in simpler, safer, faster and cheaper. No scalpel vasectomy is a new technique (safe, convenient and acceptable).

Advantages of Sterilization over Other Contraceptive Methods

- One-time method and does not requires sustained motivation of the user for its effectiveness
- Most effective protection against pregnancy

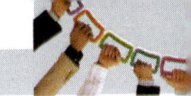

- Risk of complications is small if performed according to accepted medical standards
- Most cost-effective.

Male Sterilization or Vasectomy

- Minimum 1 cm of vas deferens is removed and ends are ligated
- Postoperative advice
- Acceptor is not immediately sterile after operation (Another method of contraception (condom) must be used until aspermia is established-usually until approx 20 ejaculations or 3 months whichever is earlier)[Q]
- Avoid taking bath for at least 24 hours after the operation
- Wear a T-bandage or scrotal support (langot) for 15 days and keep the site clean and dry
- Avoid cycling or lifting heavy weights for 15 days
- Complete bed rest is not needed
- Stitches are to be removed on 5th day after the operation.

Complications of vasectomy

- Operative pain, scrotal hematoma and local infection
- Sperm granules
- **Spontaneous recanalization:** (Incidence between 0% and 6%)
- Autoimmune response to sperm.
- **Psychological:** Diminution of sexual vigor, impotence, headache, fatigue,etc.
- Failure rate of vasectomy is generally low, 0.15 per 100 person-years.[Q]

46 **Good to Remember**

Essure: A method of permanent sterilization, where micro inserts are inserted into fallopian tube via a catheter that result in scarring and tubal blockage. It is 99% effective. Disadvantage is ectopic pregnancy.

Tubectomy

- Also known as 'Voluntary surgical contraception', 'Tubal ligation', and 'Minilap'
- Both the fallopian tubes are blocked by minilaparotomy or laparoscopy.
- In Minilaperotomy:
  - Under light sedation and local anesthesia, a small incision of 2–5 cm is made in the anesthetized area, just above the pubic hair line.
  - Uterus is raised and each tube is tied and cut or else closed with a clipor ring. Incision is closed with stitches and bandage is put.
  - More suitable than laparoscopy for immediate postpartum period
- Ideally, the operation should be performed within a week of the menstrual period on confirming the fertility and absence of pregnancy in the woman.

Latest Updates

Sterilization Guidelines (2013):
Terminal methods of sterilization are indicated for:
- Ever married male (<60 years) and female (22–49 years)
- Couple with at least one child more than 1 year of age
- No past history of sterilization of self/spouse
- Person being in sound mental health (postpsychiatric evaluation and certification).

Essure

- Essure is a permanent method for contraception
- A soft flexible insert is inserted via vaginal endoscope and "essure delivery system"
- The essure coils later will form adhesions and scarring inside the fallopian tube leading to permanent tubal occlusion and sterilization
- The female may be declared as sterile after confirmation by a TVU (transvaginal ultrasonography) or HSG (hysterosalpingography) usually after 6 weeks of inserting the essure.

Recent Advances in Family Planning Methods

Microbicides

Vaginally applied substances to reduce the transmission of HIV and other RTI/STIs

- Most microbicides under development Act in one or more of the following ways:
  - **Vaginal defense enhancers:** Boost body's natural defenses against infection.
  - **Surfactants:** Damage and disable disease pathogens to prevent them from causing infection.
  - **Entry and fusion inhibitors:** Bind to disease pathogens or to healthy cells before pathogens can invade them.
  - **Replication inhibitors:** Prevent viruses from replicating in cells that they have entered.

Protectaid

- New polyurethane foam sponge, packed with spermicide gel F-5®
- Manufacturer plans to apply for US FDA approval
- **Effectiveness:** 23 pregnancies per 100 users in one year as typically used. (JRME-2007)

Condom

- **Female condoms:**
  - FC2 female condoms
  - VA feminine female condom
- **Newer condoms:**
  - Polyurethane based
  - Styrene based plastic – Tactylon, Unique, Unisex
  - Invisible condoms/spray-on condom – ultra thin with gel formation
  - Molecular condoms
    - Smart drug delivery system
    - A biologically responsive liquid forms gel when in contact with human tissue at a specified temperature. The gel is pH sensitive and release chemicals and germicidal when in contact with semen in the vagina.

Other Contraceptive Methods

- **Drospirenone – newer OCP**
  - New progestin, available in India
  - Analogue of spironolactone and thus can increase potassium levels
  - It has antiovulatory and antimineralocorticoid activity
  - **Avoid/Caution:** Long term of NSAIDs, potassium sparing diuretics, Pott. Supplements, ACE inhibitors
  - **Trade name:** Yasmin, Tarana, Janya, Dronis
- **Progesterone only pills**
  - **Ezy pill:** 75 mcg levonorgestrel
  - **Organon, cerazette:** Progesterone only pill – 75 mcg desogestrel
- **Injectables:**
  - ***ANTRA:*** Recently launched Medroxyprogesterone acetate injectable
  - **Cyclofem:** Combined injectable – DMPA 25 mg + estradiol cypionate 5 mg
  - **Mesigyna:** Combined injectable: NET-EN 50 mg + estradiol valerate 5 mg
  - **LNG butanoate:** 5 mg 6 monthly LNG injections
  - **DMPA-SC:** Subcutaneous injection with prefilled uniject injection. Better hormonal balance and absorption.
- **Implants:**
  - **Norplant:** Levonorgestrel containing – for 5 years
  - **Implanon:** Single rod, etonogestrel containing, 3 years
  - **Norplant II:** LNG containing, 2 rods, 5 years
  - New implants under trial:
    - **Jadelle:** 75 mcg LNG
    - **Nestorone:** Elcometrine containing, for 2 years, maybe used in lactation.

EVALUATION OF CONTRACEPTIVE METHODS

Failure Rate of Contraception

The failure rate of contraception can be assessed using:

- Life table analysis
- Pearls index

Life Table Analysis

- It calculates the failure rate for each month of contraceptive use
- It is an ideal indicator, though practically not possible

Pearls Index

- It is defined as the failure rate of contraception per 100 women years of exposure
- Formula:

$$\text{Pearls index} = \frac{\textit{total accidental pregnancies}}{\textit{total women years of exposure}} \times 100$$

Taking practical aspects into consideration, the pearls index is calculated on monthly basis as:

$$\text{Pearls index} = \frac{\textit{total accidental pregnancies}}{\textit{total women months of exposure}} \times 100 \times 2 \textit{ (months in a year)}$$

Women months of exposure = Number of women using the contraception x months of exposure

Effectivity of Contraception

The effectivity of contraception is basically a public health indicator inversely corresponding to the pearl's index.

The effectivity of the contraception is:

- Condoms 50% effective
- IUD 95% effective
- OCP's ~99.9% effective

Table 13: Effectiveness of birth control measures

Methods of contraception	Failure Rate (per 100 women-years of exposure)
Condom	5–14
Female condom	5–21
Diaphragm or Dutch cap with spermicide	6–12
Today (vaginal sponge)	20–40 (Parous women) and 9–20 (Nullipara)
Lippes loop	3
Cu T-200	3
Cu T-380A	0.5–0.8
LNG 20 or Mirena (3rd generation IUD)	0.2
Progestasert (3rd generation IUD)	1.3–1.6
OCP	0.1–0.5
DMPA	0.3
NET–EN	0.4
Norplant	1–6
Combined Injectible Contraceptive-Cyclofem/Cyclo-Provera	0.2
Centchroman	1.8–2.8
Rhythm or safe period method	24
Coitus interruptus	18
No method	80

Sterilization Equivalency

The sterilization equivalency is as follows:

1 tubectomy = 1 sterilization unit

1 vasectomy = 1 sterilization unit

3 Equivalent IUD users* = 1 sterilization unit

9 equivalent OCP users$ = 1 sterilization unit

18 equivalent condom users# = 1sterilization unit

*equivalent IUD user is a user who has used CuT 380 at least for one year

$equivalent OCP user is a female who has consumed OCPs for atleast 11 months in a year

#equivalent condom user is a male who uses atleast 2 condoms in a year

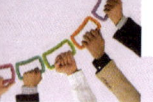

PUBLIC HEALTH ACTS AND GUIDELINES

COMPENSATION FOR COMPLICATIONS IN STERILIZATION

Table 14: Compensation limits for complications of sterilization

Coverage	Compensation Limits
Death following sterilization at hospital or within 7 days from date of discharge from hospital	***₹ 2 Lakh***
Death due to sterilization within 8–30 days of discharge from hospital	***₹ 50,000***
Failure of sterilization	***₹ 30,000***
Cost of treatment for medical complication of sterilization up to 60 days from date of discharge	As per actual expenditure incurred up to ₹ 25000
Indemnity Insurance per Doctor/Facility (not more than 4 cases a year)	***Up to ₹ 2 Lakh (Not per claim)***

NATIONAL POPULATION POLICY

- *National Population Policy, 1976* → Legal minimum age of marriage was increased from 15 to 18 years for females and from 18 to 21 years for males.
- *National Population Policy, 1977* → Small family norm without compulsion (Family Welfare Program) was implemented.
- National population policy 2000
  - Reach the replacement level for TFR = 2.1
  - Attain the NRR of 1
  - Address unmet needs for family planning
  - Promote small family norm
  - Free elementary school education to all children <14 years of age
  - Age of marriage for girls not less than 18, preferably more than 20 years
  - 100% registration of births and death
  - Reduce IMR < 30/1000 live births
  - Reduce MMR < 100 / 100,000 live births

MTP ACT 1971

MTP is permissible

- Up to 20 weeks gestation
- With the consent of the women. If the women is below 18 years or is mentally ill, then with consent of a guardian
- With the opinion of a registered medical practitioner, formed in good faith, under certain circumstances
- Opinion of single registered medical practitioner (RMP) for termination up to 12 weeks
- Opinion of two RMPs required for termination of pregnancy between 12 and 20 weeks.

Medical abortion: MTP using Mifepristone (RU 486) & Misoprostol approved for up to 7 weeks termination.

For termination up to 12 weeks:

A practitioner who has assisted a registered medical practitioner in performing 25 cases of MTP of which at least 5 were performed independently in a hospital established or maintained or a training institute approved for this purpose by the Government.

For termination up to 20 weeks (opinion of 2 RMPs required)

- A practitioner who holds a postgraduate degree or diploma in obstetrics and gynaecology
- A practitioner who has completed six months house job in obstetrics and gynaecology

- A practitioner who has at least one-year experience in practice of obstetrics and gynaecology at a hospital which has all facilities
- A practitioner registered in state medical register immediately before commencement of the Act, experience in practice of obstetrics and gynaecology for a period not less than three years.

MTP Indications

Medical Indications

To save life of mother but limited and scarcely justifiable except in:

- Cardiac disease (NYHA gr III/IV) with history of decompensation in previous pregnancies or in between pregnancies
- Chronic glomerulonephritis
- Malignant hypertension
- Intractable hyperemesis gravidarum
- Cervical and breast malignancies
- DM with retinopathy
- Epilepsy or psychiatric illness

Social/Humanitarian Indications

- This is almost sole indications to prevent grave injury to physical and mental health of pregnant woman
- Pregnancy is caused by rape both in case of major and minor girl and in mentally imbalanced women
- As a result of failure of contraception
- In 80% cases it is limited to parous women having unplanned pregnancy with low SE status.

Eugenic Indications

Provision of substantial risk of child being born with serious mental and physical abnormalities so as to be handicapped in life

- Structural (anencephaly), chromosomal (Downs syndrome) genetic (hemophilia) abnormalities in fetus
- Fetus likely to be deformed due to action of teratogenic drugs or radiation exposure in early pregnancy
- Rubella and viral infections in 1st trimester.

MTP Amendment Act 2002

- Term Lunatic was replaced by—Mentally ill
- MTP place to be approved by a district level committee chaired by CMO / DHO
  - MTP Place should have facility for blood transfusion, parenteral fluids
  - OT facility for laparotomy and/or major gynecological surgeries (for sites up to 20 weeks termination)
  - Backup facility for transportation
- Defaulters—rigorous punishment for 2–7 years
- Owner of the place also responsible if defaulter

Regulatory Body

District level MTP committee:

- Minimum 3 members, maximum 5 members.
- The chairman of the committee will be the chief medical and health officer of the district (also known as district medical officer or medical officer of health)
- One member of the local NGO and Panchayati Raj Institution of the district
- At least one female member.

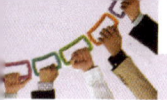

NEWER INITIATIVE FOR FAMILY PLANNING UNDER NHM (2017-2018)

Incentives for Sterilization

Incentives for acceptors of sterilization services

Conventional Tubectomy:

- High focus States/UT (All women) – ₹600 onetime payment.
- Non High focus States/UT - BPL + SC/ST women - ₹600 onetime payment
- Non BPL + Non SC/ST women – ₹250 onetime payment

Laparoscopic tubectomy- ₹145 onetime payment

Vasectomy – ₹1100 onetime payment (High Focus and Non Focus States/UT)

Motivator – ₹150 for tubectomy and ₹200 for vasectomy

IUD receptors – ₹75

Increments for government employees and ***Green card***- to individual acceptors of terminal method after 2 children.

Incentives for Family Planning Services

ASHA incentives are:

- Ensuring spacing at birth:
  - Services of ASHAs is to be utilized for counseling the newly married couples to ensure spacing of 2 years after marriage and couples with 1 child to have spacing of 3 years after the birth of 1st child.
- INR 500/- to ASHA for delaying first child birth by 2 years after marriage.
- INR 500/- to ASHA for ensuring spacing of 3 years after the birth of first child.
- INR 1000/- in case the couple opts for a permanent limiting method up to 2 children only.

Home Delivery of Contraceptive

- Applicable all over India from 17th December 2012.
- ASHA is to deliver contraceptives at doorstep of beneficiaries.
- ASHA is to charge a nominal amount from beneficiaries for her effort.
- (INR 1 for a pack of 3 condoms. INR 1 for a cycle of OCPs and INR 2 for a pack of one tablet of ECP.)

Newer IUD's under NHM

- Short term IUCD (5 years) and Cu IUCD 375 introduced under the national family planning program.
- A new method of IUCD insertion (Postpartum IUCD insertion) has been introduced by the government.
- Promotion of Postpartum family planning services at district hospitals by providing for placement of dedicated family planning counsellors and training of personnel.

Female Empowerment

Pregnancy Testing Kits (Nishchay–Home based pregnancy test kit) was launched under NRHM in 2008 across the country.

Available at sub centers and with ASHAs to facilitate early detection and decision making for the outcome of pregnancy.

Image-Based Questions

1. The symbol shown in figure is related to:

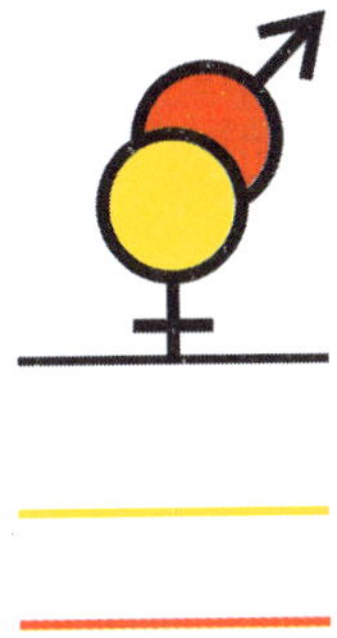

a. Jansankhya Sthirata Kosh
b. Gender equality
c. Population Services International
d. Indian Institute of Population Sciences

2. How can the efficacy of the contraceptive in figure be improved:

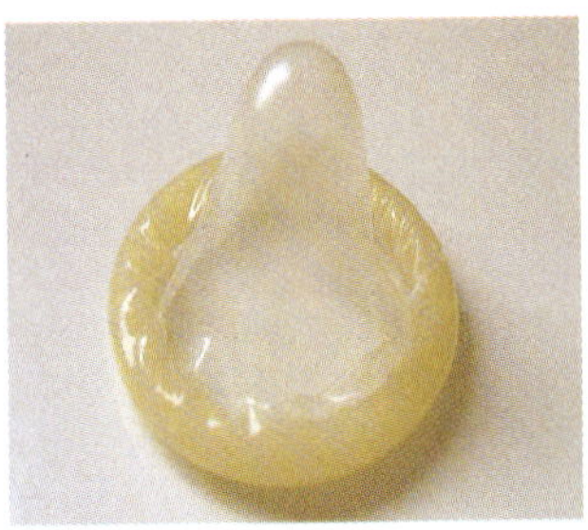

a. By using water based lubricant
b. By using oil based lubricant
c. By using spermicidal jelly
d. By making small hole near teat

3. Identify the contraceptive device shown in figure:

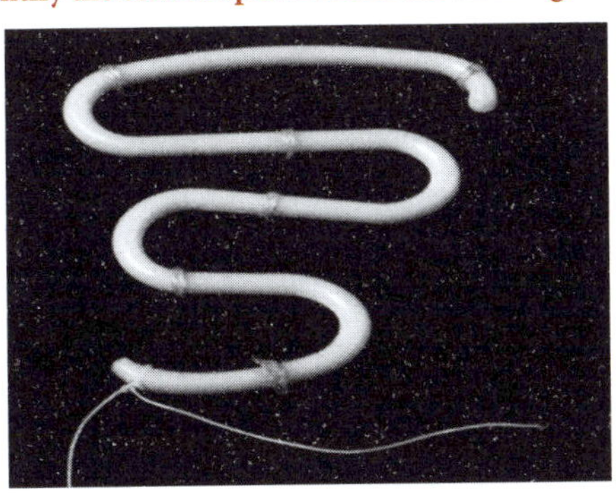

a. Cu-T 200
b. Lippes loop
c. Cu-T 380 A
d. Nova T

4. Identify the contraceptive in figure:

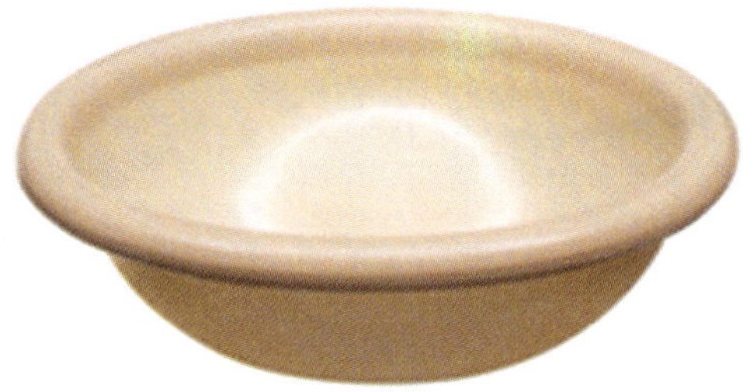

a. Diaphragm
b. Cervical cap
c. Vaginal sponge
d. Lippes loop

5. Identify the contraceptive in figure:

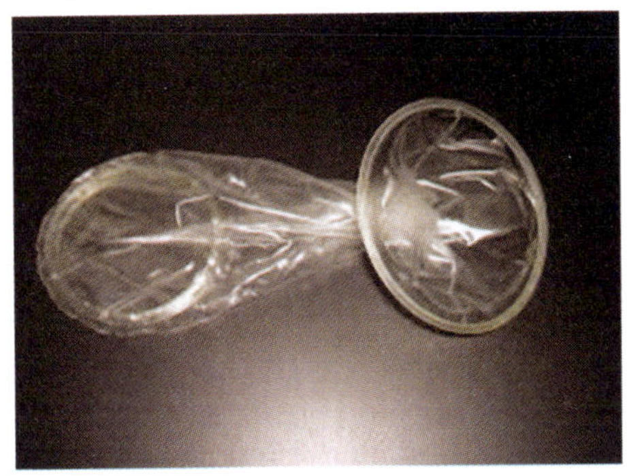

a. Male condom
b. Diaphragm
c. Female condom
d. Graffenberg ring

6. Identify the blister pack shown in figure:

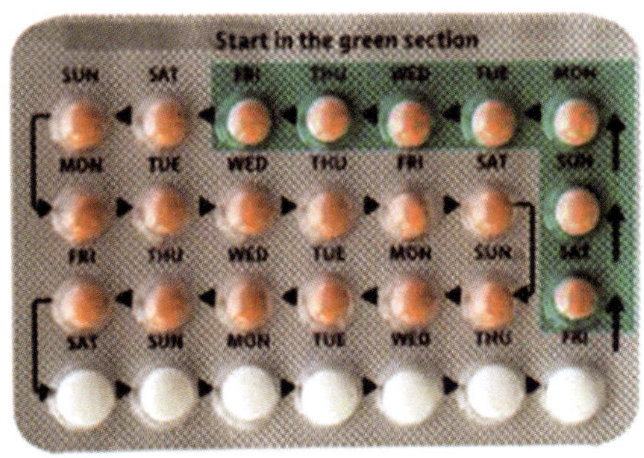

a. MDT PBL blister
b. Iron folic acid (IFA) tablets
c. Combined OCPs
d. Pediatric DOTS

7. Identify the contraceptive shown in figure:

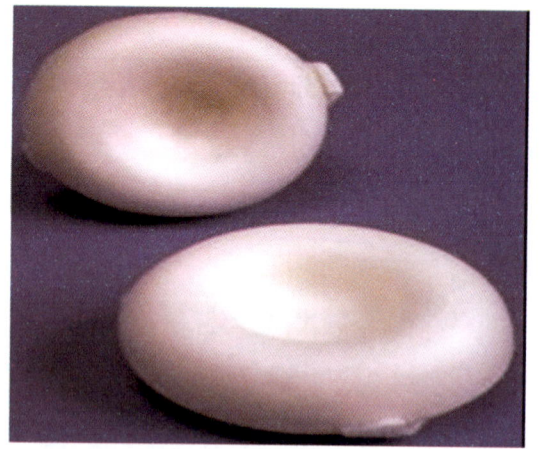

a. Dutch Cap
b. Cervical Cap
c. Diaphragm
d. Vaginal sponge

8. The diagram shown in figure represents:

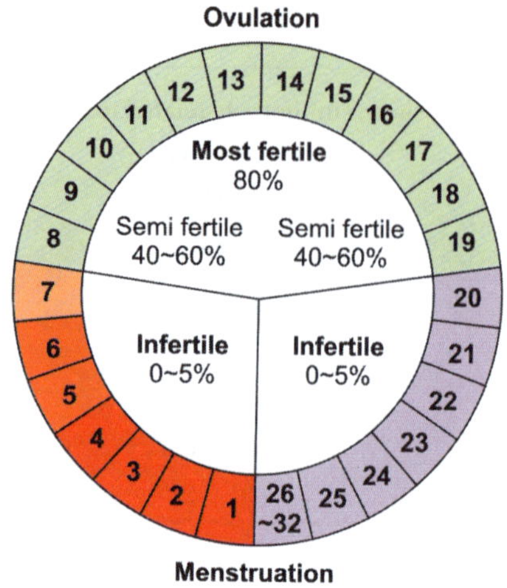

a. Ideal Tubectomy time estimation
b. BBT Method
c. Cervical mucus method
d. Rhythm method

Answers of Image-Based Questions

1. **Ans. (a) Jansankhya Sthirata Kosh**

2. **Ans. (c) By using spermicidal jelly**

3. **Ans. (b) Lippes loop**

4. **Ans. (a) Diaphragm**

5. **Ans. (c) Female condom**

6. **Ans. (c) Combined OCPs**

7. **Ans. (d) Vaginal sponge**

8. **Ans. (d) Rhythm method**

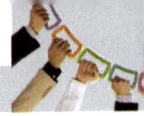

Multiple Choice Questions

1. **To achieve a net reproduction rate (NRR) of 1, the couple protection rate (CPR) should be:** ***(AIIMS May 2017)***
   a. 20% b. 30%
   c. 40% d. 60%
2. **100 women were surveyed for oral contraceptive pill usage for 24 months, out of which 10 became pregnant. Calculate the pearl index?** ***(Recent Question 2018)***
   a. 2.5 b. 5
   c. 10 d. 20
3. **True about Demographic cycle of India:** ***(PGI May 2017)***
   a. Entered into low stationary phase
   b. Dependency ratio <40%
   c. Year of Big divide-1921A.D
   d. Population pyramid has a broad base and a tapering top
   e. First regular census in India was carried in 1881
4. **Definition of pearl index is?** ***(Recent Question 2017)***
   a. Failure rate in 100 couple
   b. Failure rate in 1000 couple
   c. Failures per 100 women years of exposure
   d. Failures per 1000 women years of exposure
5. **Net reproduction rate is defined as:** ***(Recent Question 2017)***
   a. Number of live birth in the reproductive age group of a female
   b. Average number of children born to a married woman
   c. Average number of girls born to a woman assuming no mortality
   d. Number of girls born to a woman during her lifetime assuming mortality
6. **100 females used contraceptive for 1 year. Out of the females exposed, one female got pregnant due to contraceptive failure. How much is the accidental pregnancy rate?**
   a. 0.01 b. 1
   c. 1.5 d. 2.0
7. **If Net reproduction rate is desired to be 1, what should be the couple protection rate:** ***(Recent Question 2017)***
   a. 42 b. 60
   c. 70 d. 82
8. **Birth rate reduced and death rate reduced. Population is in which stage:** ***(Recent Question 2016)***
   a. 1 b. 2
   c. 4 d. 5
9. **Which is not a demographic indicator?**
   a. Social mobility b. Malnutrition
   c. Immigration d. Emigration
10. **Sex ratio in India is:**
    a. 940 b. 930
    c. 914 d. 924
11. **Perinatal mortality rate includes:**
    a. Still births + neonatal deaths per 1000 births
    b. Intrapartum deaths + neonatal deaths per 1000 births
    c. Intrapartum deaths + early neonatal deaths per 1000 live births
    d. Still births + early neonatal deaths per 1000 live births
12. **Birth and death registration should be done within:**
    a. 7 days b. 14 days
    c. 21 days d. 28 days
13. **For measuring premature death, life expectancy of the following country's people is used as a standard** ***(New Question 2015)***
    a. India b. China
    c. Japan d. USA

RCH

14. **Data regarding recent trends in Immunization in the community can be found by** ***(Recent Question 2016)***
    a. Census b. Sample Registration System
    c. Rural Household Survey d. DLHS
15. **According to 2006 government of India guidelines for sterilization all are true except**
    a. Should be married
    b. Female clients should be below the age of 45 years and above the age of 20 years
    c. The couple should have at least one child whose age is above one year unless the sterilization is medically indicated
    d. Clients or their spouses/partner must not have undergone sterilization in the past

MISCELLANEOUS

16. **Survey that yields data on recent trends of Immunization in community is** ***(Recent Question 2016)***
    a. Rural Health survey
    b. District level household survey
    c. Census data
    d. Sample registration system
17. **Birth and Death registration Act came into force on 1st April**
    a. 1968 b. 1969
    c. 1970 d. 1971
18. **Naranjo algorithms is used for:** ***(Recent Question 2016)***
    a. Environmental factors effecting drug
    b. Parameter based data evaluation
    c. Calculating probability of adverse drug reaction
    d. Demographic factor affecting drugs action

DEMOGAPHIC CYCLE, PROCESS, POPULATION GROWTH

19. **National Population Stabilisation Fund seeks to achieve population stabilization consistent with needs of sustainable economic growth, social development and environment protection by the year**
    a. 2045
    b. 2015
    c. 2040
    d. 2030

Ans.

1. d
2. b
3. c,d e
4. c
5. d
6. b
7. b
8. c
9. b
10. a
11. d
12. c
13. c
14. d
15. b
16. b
17. c
18. c
19. a

Most Recent Questions of 2019-18 are given at the end of MCQs

20. Growth rate is defined as *(Recent Question 2016)*
a. Difference between crude birth rate and crude death rate
b. Difference between general fertility rate and crude death rate
c. Difference between net reproduction rate and crude death rate
d. Difference between gross reproduction rate and crude death rate

21. Which of the following is true about the late expansion phase of demographic cycle?
a. High birth rate and high death rate
b. High birth rate and low death rate
c. Low birth rate and low death rate
d. Low birth rate and high death rate

22. Not true regarding second stage of demographic cycle is
a. Early expanding stage
b. Death rates decline
c. Birth rates decline
d. Population grows

23. India has entered the following stage of demographic cycle
a. Second stage
b. Third stage
c. Fourth stage
d. Fifth stage

24. Demographic gap attains its maximum limit in
a. Early stage 1
b. Late stage II
c. Late stage III
d. Early stage IV

25. Which of the following is a vital statistic in population
a. Birth rate b. Sex Ratio
c. Dependency Ratio d. Age composition

26. Which of the following state is considered as a Yard Stick of health in India *(Recent Question 2016)*
a. Gujarat b. Haryana
c. Kerala d. Tamil Nadu

27. Which is NOT a demographic indicator?
a. Social Mobility b. Mortality
c. Immigration d. Morbidity

28. True about late expanding phase of demography cycle:
a. Birth rate is lower than death rate
b. Death rate begins to decline, with the birth rate remains unchanged
c. Death rate declines still further, and the birth rate tends to fall
d. High birth rate and high death rate

29. Which year in history of demography of India is known as the year of big divide
a. 1881 b. 1921
c. 1947 d. 1978

30. In which stage of the demographic cycle in India currently? *(Recent Question 2015)*
a. High stationary
b. Late expanding
c. Early stationary
d. Low stationary

31. Movement in socio economic level is:
a. Social equality
b. Social mobility
c. Socio economic upliftment
d. Social mobilization

32. If the annual growth rate of a population is between 1.0- - 1.5, number of years required to double the population size: *(Recent Question 2015)*
a. 28–35 years b. 35–47 years
c. 47–70 years d. 70–39 years

33. The total percentage of women of reproductive age group falls within? *(Recent Question 2015)*
a. 22.2% b. 22.4%
c. 22.5% d. 22.6%

34. India is supporting almost % of world population
a. 12 b. 17
c. 20 d. 23

35. Percentage of urban population as per 2011 census
a. 32 b. 44
c. 56 d. 68

36. All the following are classified as urban areas except
a. Places having 5000 or more inhabitants
b. Density of not less than 1000 persons per square mile or 390 per sq. km
c. Safe water supply available for at least 80% population
d. At least three fourths of the adult male population employed in pursuits other than agriculture

37. The following indicator is not among the population statistics *(Recent Question 2014)*
a. Sex ratio
b. Population density
c. Growth rate
d. Dependency ratio

38. World population growth rate in 2010 was
a. 1.2 b. 1.5
c. 1.9 d. 2.1

39. Nishchay is a *(Recent Question 2014)*
a. Pregnancy test kit
b. STD test kit
c. Kit for rapid malaria diagnosis
d. Spot test for HIV

40. Population growth is rated to be 'explosive' if the annual growth rate exceeds: *(Recent Question 2014)*
a. 2.0% b. 1.5%
c. 1.0% d. 0.5

41. What is exponential growth:
a. Rapid growth of population that leads to misbalance in birth and death
b. Slow growth rate
c. Growth limited by limiting factors
d. None of the above

42. In a demographic cycle low stationary phase corresponds to which stage?:
a. First b. Second
c. Third d. Fourth

43. Demographic bonus is *(Recent Question 2014)*
a. Decrease in dependency ratio
b. Decrease in sex ratio
c. Increase in dependency ratio
d. Increase in sex ratio

44. WHO defines adolescent age between:
a. 10-19 years of age b. 10-14 years of age
c. 10-25 years of age d. 9-14 years of age

Ans.

20. a	21. c
22. c	23. b
24. b	25. a
26. c	27. d
28. c	29. b
30. b	31. b
32. c	33. a
34. b	35. a
36. c	37. c
38. a	39. a
40. a	41. a
42. d	43. a
44. a	

Most Recent Questions of 2019-18 are given at the end of MCQs

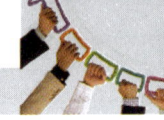

45. 'Explosive' growth rate occurs when annual rate of growth percent is *(Recent Question 2014)*
a. 0.5–1.0 b. 1–1.5
c. 1.5–2.0 d. >2.0

DEMOGRAPHIC RATES AND RATIOS

CBR – Crude Birth Rate

46. Crude birth rate in India is–
a. 80.3 b. 20.5
c. 30.1 d. 35

47. In a community of 5000 people, the crude birth rate is 30 per 1000 people. The number of pregnant females is:
a. 150 b. 165
c. 175 d. 200

48. True about crude birth rate is the following except:
a. Better measure of fertility than the GFR
b. Fertility indicator
c. Still born excluded
d. Not affected by the age distribution of the population

49. States, where crude birth rate is higher than the national level: *(Recent Question 2014)*
a. West Bengal b. Maharashtra
c. Rajasthan d. Madhya Pradesh
e. Himachal Pradesh

Total fertility rate (TFR)

50. Average number of children a woman would have if she were to pass through her reproductive years bearing children at the same rates as the women now in each age group is known as: *(Recent Question 2014)*
a. General fertility rate
b. Total fertility rate
c. Gross reproduction rate
d. Net reproduction rate

51. In demography, family size means
a. Total number of persons in a family
b. Total number of children in a family
c. Total number of women in the family
d. Total number of women in the reproductive age-group (15-45) in a family

52. The following fertility rate gives the approximate magnitude of the completed family size: *(Recent Question 2014)*
a. TFR
b. Total marital Fertility rate
c. General Fertility rate
d. General Marital Fertility rate

GFR – Gross Fertility Rate/ GMFR

53. Number of live births per 1000 women in the reproducti ve age group in a year is: *(Recent Question 2013)*
a. Total fertility rate
b. Gross Reproduction Rate
c. General Marital Fertility Rate
d. General Fertility Rate

54. Total live birth/women in reproductive age is
a. General fertility rate
b. Birth rate
c. General marital fertility rate
d. None

55. Gross Reproduction Rate is — *(Recent Question 2013)*
a. Number of girls born to a mother in her reproductive age
b. Number of boys born to a mother in her reproductive age
c. Number of total children born to a mother in her reproductive age
d. Number of lives births per 1000 women

56. Average number of girl child that a woman will give birth to assuming she experiences the current fertility rate throughout her reproductive span with no mortality is referred to as
a. General Fertility Rate b. Gross Reproduction Rate
c. Net Reproduction Rate d. Total Fertility Rate

57. Number of live birth per 1000 women in reproductive age group (15–45 year) in a year is
a. TFR
b. NRR
c. CBR
d. GFR

58. True about General fertility rate is
a. Indicator of complete family size
b. Measure of fertility
c. Not better than crude birth rate
d. All of the above

59. General fertility rate (GFR) is:
a. Number of live birth in women in the reproductive age-group 15-44 years
b. Number of live birth in unmarried women in the age group 15-44 years
c. Number of children a women would have if she were to pass through her reproductive years
d. Number of abortions, usually per 1000 women of child bearing age

NRR – NET REPRODUCTIVE RATE

60. What is net reproduction rate
a. No of children a newborn girl has in her life time
b. No of female children a newborn girl has in life time
c. No of male children a newborn girl has in her life time
d. No of female children a newborn girl has in her life time taking into account the mortality

61. NRR (Net Reproduction Rate) is defined as?
a. Average number of children a woman would bear during her reproductive life
b. Number of daughters that would be born to a woman if she survived to the age of 45
c. Number of daughters a woman would bear in her lifetime if she experiences prevailing age-specific fertility, 'assuming no mortality'
d. Number of daughters a woman would have in her lifetime if she experiences prevailing age-specific fertility and mortality rates

62. To attain the two-child norm, the net reproductive rate to be obtained is *(Recent Question 2013)*
a. 0.5 b. 1
c. 1.5 d. 2

63. Net reproductive rate of 1 can be achieved only when the couple protection rate exceeds *(Recent Question 2013)*
a. 40% b. 50%
c. 60% d. 70%

Ans.

45. d
46. b
47. b
48. a
49. c,d
50. b
51. b
52. a
53. d
54. a
55. a
56. b
57. d
58. b
59. a
60. d
61. d
62. b
63. c

Most Recent Questions of 2019-18 are given at the end of MCQs

64. **In 2011, % of eligible couples in the age group 15–44 years were effectively protected against contraception.**
a. 40 b. 50
c. 60 d. 70

65. **Number of eligible couples per 1000 population**
a. 100 - 120 b. 150 - 180
c. 200 - 240 d. 250 - 300

66. **For NRR to be 1, Couple Protection Rate should be…**
a. 20% b. 40%
c. 60% d. 80%

67. **Which of the following fertility rates include mortality in it:** *(Recent Question 2012)*
a. TFR b. GFR
c. NRR d. GRR

DEPENDENCY RATIO

68. **Dependency ratio numerator is:**
a. Less than 15 years and more than 65 years
b. Less than 85 years
c. 30–35 years
d. 25–65 years

69. **Calculate the Dependency ratio for a community, where 30% of the population is below 15 years of age and 10% of population is over 65 years of age:** *(Recent Question 2012)*
a. 20%
b. 66.6%
c. 3%
d. 40%

70. **Potential Support Ratio (PSR) refers to:**
a. Number of people aged 15 to 65 years per child below 15 years of age
b. Number of people aged 15 to 65 years per adult aged > 60 and young person aged < 15 years
c. Number of people aged 15 to 65 years per adult aged ≥ 65 years
d. Number of people aged 15 to 65 years per adult aged > 65 years and young person aged < 15 years

SEX RATIO

71. **What is the current sex ratio in India as per census 2011?**
a. 940 females per 1000 males
b. 986 females per 1000 males
c. 914 females per 1000 males
d. 942 females per 1000 males

72. **Sex ratio at birth in India in 2011 is** *(Recent Question 2012)*
a. 878 b. 927
c. 933 d. 940

73. **Sex ratio in India at birth is highest in**
a. Goa b. Kerala
c. Tamil Nadu d. Mizoram

LITERACY RATE

74. **A community has total population 10000. Children ranging 0-6 years are 2000. Literate persons among >7 years old are 4000. What is effective literacy rate –**
a. 20% b. 40%
c. 50% d. 60%

75. **In calculating effective literacy rate, the denominator is**
a. Total population
b. Mid-year population
c. Total population >12 years
d. Total population >7 years

76. **National effective literacy rate among females in 2011**
a. 56% b. 65%
c. 74% d. 82%

77. **Effective literacy rate is calculated from:**
a. Those above age of 7 years
b. Those who have completed 10 year schooling
c. Those who have completed 1 year schooling
d. Total population

POPULATION PYRAMID

78. **Age pyramid of India is:** *(Recent Question 2012)*
a. Broad base and narrow at apex
b. Broad from base to apex
c. Broad at apex and narrow at base
d. All

79. **The spindle shaped age pyramid denotes:**
a. Developing country b. Developed country
c. Underdeveloped d. Middle east country

80. **Which is/are true for Kerala in relation to India**
a. High literacy rate
b. High doctor population ratio
c. High growth rate
d. Older age of marriage
e. Higher life expectancy

CONCEPT AND SCOPE OF FAMILY PLANNING

81. **Unmet need for contraception in a 35 years female is for –**
a. Spacing birth b. Limiting birth
c. Improve maternal health d. Improve family health

82. **Family planning services were voluntary in India from**
a. 1956 b. 1977
c. 1992 d. 1997

83. **KAP studies in India were first used to study:** *(Recent Question 2012)*
a. HIV b. Malaria
c. Family planning d. Cancer cervix

84. **Setting up of condom vending machines at public places in high HIV prevalence areas is an example of**
a. Community Involvement
b. Socialisation
c. Social Marketing
d. Appropriate Technology

85. **Spacing methods used by family welfare programs are:**
a. IUCD b. OCP
c. Vasectomy d. Condom
e. Tubectomy

PEARL INDEX

86. **Contraceptive efficacy is best measured by:** *(Recent Question 2012)*
a. Pearl Index b. Couple protection rate
c. Net reproduction rate d. Life-table analysis

Ans.

64. a
65. b
66. c
67. c
68. a
69. b
70. c
71. a
72. d
73. b
74. c
75. d
76. b
77. a
78. a
79. b
80. a, b, d, e
81. b
82. b
83. c
84. c
85. a, b, d
86. d

Most Recent Questions of 2019-18 are given at the end of MCQs

87. The following method calculates failure rate of a contraceptive for each month of use
a. Life table analysis
b. Pearl index
c. Couple protection rate
d. Net reproduction rate

88. Total unmet need for family planning according to national family health survey-3 *(Recent Question 2013)*
a. 12.8% b. 14.6%
c. 21.1% d. 27.1%

89. Pearl index is expressed in
a. Per 100 women years
b. Per 10 women years
c. Per 1000 women years
d. Per 50 women years

90. Pearl index is referred as *(Recent Question 2012)*
a. Accidental pregnancies per 1000 women years of exposure
b. Accidental pregnancies per 100 women years of exposure
c. Accidental pregnancies per 10 women years of exposure
d. Accidental pregnancies per women years of exposure

91. Pearl index is
a. Failures per 1000 women years of exposure
b. Failures per 100 women years of exposure
c. Failures per 10 women years of exposure
d. Failures per women years of exposure

BARRIER METHOD OF CONTRACEPTION

92. Which of the following is the correct use of barrier creams?
a. For contraception
b. Protection from occupational dermatitis
c. As mosquito repellent
d. Protection from contagious diseases

93. Mechanism of action of Intra Uterine Device is:
a. Interferes with fertilization
b. Stops ovulation
c. Prevention of implantation
d. Acts as Spermicide

94. IUD 'Mirena' release Levonorgestrel for ....years
a. 3 b. 5
c. 7 d. 10

95. Which of the following is a third generation IUCD:
a. ML CuT 250 b. MIRENA
c. CuT 380 A d. Copper T 200

96. CuT 380 has a life span of: *(Recent Question 2012)*
a. 10 years b. 5 years
c. 2 years d. 7 years

97. Characteristics of an ideal IUCD candidate include all of the following except – *(Recent Question 2013)*
a. Has borne at least 2 children
b. Is willing to check IUD tail
c. Has a history of ectopic pregnancy
d. Has normal menstrual periods

98. Mechanism of action of Intra Uterine Device is all except: *(Recent Question 2013)*
a. Foreign body reaction
b. Thickening of cervical mucus
c. Unfavorable endometrium for implantation
d. Thinning of fallopian tube

99. Non medicated Intra Devices (IUDs) are called as
a. 3rd generation IUDs
b. 2nd generation IUDs
c. 1st generation IUDs
d. Multi – load devices

100. CuT 380A IUD should be replaced once in
a. 4 years b. 6 years
c. 8 years d. 10 years

HORMONAL CONTRACEPTIVE

101. Best contraceptive for a newly married healthy couple:
a. Barrier method
b. IUCD
c. Oral contraceptive pills
d. Natural methods

102. In case a women on OCP forgets taking pills on 3 successive days. What should she do
a. Take 2 pills each for the remaining cycle
b. Take 3 pills next day , then continue with 1 pill per day
c. Use a barriers method for rest of cycle
d. Continue with the next pill next day onward

103. Non-contraceptive benefits of combined oral contraceptive to a woman are all except: *(Recent Question 2013)*
a. Protection against PID
b. Protection against colorectal cancer
c. Protection against ovarian cancer
d. Protection against cervical cancer

104. Contraceptive option available to a 28-year-old breast-feeding mother with 6 week old baby, wishing to avoid next pregnancy are the following except
a. Implanon b. IUD 380 A
c. LNG IUD d. OCP

105. Which of the following is/are benefits of combined OCPs use *(Recent Question 2012)*
a. Hepatocellular adenoma
b. PID
c. Ovarian cysts
d. Fibrocystic disease of breast
e. Ectopic pregnancy

MINIPILL

106. Minipill is contraceptive of choices for
a. Elderly females b. Lactating females
c. Obese women d. Menstruating women

TERMINAL METHOD OF CONTRACEPTION

107. According female sterilization 2014 guidelines, eligibility criteria for female sterilization are all except
a. Age between 22–49 years
b. Should have at least 1 child
c. Unmarried woman
d. Partner is not sterilized

108. Postpartum sterilization as per Government of India guidelines should be performed between
a. 12 hours to 7 days of delivery
b. 24 hours to 7 days of delivery
c. 48 hours to 7 days of delivery
d. Within 7 days of delivery

Ans.
87. a
88. a
89. a
90. b
91. b
92. a
93. a
94. b
95. b
96. a
97. c
98. d
99. c
100. d
101. c
102. c
103. d
104. d
105. c, d
106. b
107. c
108. b

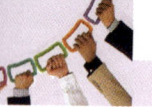

109. In a community health center, sterilization services are conducted every *(Recent Question 2012)*
a. Day
b. Week
c. Fortnight
d. Month

110. Failure rate of pomeroy's technique is
a. 0.1–0.5%
b. 0.5–1%
c. 1–2%
d. 5–10%

111. Most common method of sterilization practiced in India
a. Female sterilization
b. Male sterilization
c. Both equally common
d. None

EMERGENCY CONTRACEPTIVE

112. Yuzpe and Lancee regimen needs to be administered within a maximum of *(Recent Question 2012)*
a. 48 hours
b. 12 hours
c. 24 hours
d. 72 hours

113. Which of the following is used as an emergency contraceptive?
a. MALA-N
b. 0.75 mg Levonorgestrel
c. Copper T
d. All of the above

114. Drug of choice for Emergency contraception is?
a. Yuzpe and Lancee regimen (combined oral pill)
b. Levonorgestrel only pill
c. Danazol
d. High dose estrogen alone

115. IUCD can be inserted as emergency contraceptive up to:
a. 24 hours
b. 72 hours
c. 5 days
d. 7 days

MEDICAL TERMINATION OF PREGNANCY

116. The MTP Act does not allow termination of pregnancy after...... *(Recent Question 2013)*
a. 20 weeks
b. 24 weeks
c. 28 weeks
d. 30 weeks

117. MTP Act 1971, provides for termination of pregnancy till how many weeks of pregnancy-
a. 12 weeks
b. 16 weeks
c. 20 weeks
d. 24 weeks

SOURCES OF HEALTH INFORMATION

CENSUS

118. First census in India was done in *(Recent Question 2013)*
a. 1861
b. 1871
c. 1881
d. 1891

119. First disability census was done in the year
a. 1881
b. 1951
c. 1981
d. 2001

120. Birth and death registration act came into force on 1st April
a. 1968
b. 1969
c. 1970
d. 1971

121. True about Civil registration system in India: *(Recent Question 2013)*
a. Dual record system
b. Deficient
c. Head of institution or officer-in charge is responsible for registration
d. Birth and Death both are registered
e. Cause of death is recorded

REGISTRATION OF VITAL EVENTS

122. As per the Central Births and Deaths Registration Act, 1969, the time limit for registering birth and death is
a. 7 days
b. 14 days
c. 21 days
d. 30 days

SRS

123. In sample registration system, the investigator-supervisor conducts and independent survey every
a. 6 months
b. 1 year
c. 5 years
d. 10 years

124. Sample registration system done for both death and birth enumeration at *(Recent Question 2013)*
a. 6 months
b. 1 year
c. 5 years
d. 10 years

MISCELLANEOUS

125. National family health survey done in every.....years
a. 6 months
b. 1 year
c. 5 years
d. 10 years

126. NFHS has successfully completed:
a. 1 round
b. 2 round
c. 3 round
d. 4 round

127. For Net Reproduction rate to be 1, the couple protection rate should be:
a. 100%
b. 40%
c. 60%
d. 80%

128. 10 women got pregnant out of 100 women, mean interval was 2 years. Calculate pearl index.
a. 10
b. 2
c. 5
d. 4

Ans.
109. c
110. a
111. a
112. d
113. d
114. b
115. c
116. a
117. c
118. c
119. c
120. c
121. b, c, d, e
122. c
123. a
124. a
125. c
126. d
127. c
128. c

Most Recent Questions of 2019-18 are given at the end of MCQs

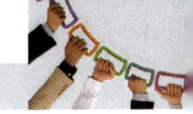

Most Recent Questions (2019-2018)

129. You went to a sub center as part of an audit. How many pregnant females should be registered with a health worker working there? *(AIIMS May 2018)*

a. 55
b. 100
c. 110
d. 200

130. A 30-year-old $G_2P_1A_1L_1$ female presents to PHC for contraception counseling. She is a known case of chronic hepatitis and has been on treatment for same. She also is a known case of diabetes (HbA1c 7.8%) on two oral hypoglycaemia agents. The contraception options for this female is/are *(PGI Nov 2018)*

a. Levonorgestrel IUD
b. Copper T before 5 days of unprotected intercourse
c. Progesterone only pills
d. Oral combined contraceptive pills
e. Barrier methods

131. All are true about vasectomy except: *(PGI May 2018)*

a. Non-scalpel vasectomy has less complication than conventional method of vasectomy
b. Unprotected intercourse is allowed only after two consecutive semen analyses show absence of spermatozoa
c. Failure rate is 1 in 300
d. Increased risk of testicular cancer
e. Antibodies to sperm may formed

132. In a town of 20,000 population, total 456 births were there in a year out of which 56 were dead born. The total deaths were 247 out of which 56 deaths were within first 28 days of life and another 34 had died after 28 days and before completing the first birthday. Calculate the infant mortality rate of the area. *(AIIMS May 2019)*

a. 225
b. 197
c. 392
d. 344

Ans.

129. a
130. a, c, e
131. b, c, d
132. a

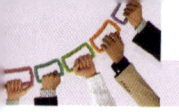

Answers with Explanations

1. Ans. (d) 60%

2. Ans. (b) 5

$$\textbf{Pearls index} = \frac{\text{Number of accidental pregnancies}}{\text{Total women years of exposure}} \times 100$$

Hence,

Total females exposed = 100 females for 24 months (2 years) = 200 women years

Accidental pregnancy = 10

Therefore,

$$PI = \frac{10}{200} \times 100 = 5$$

3. Ans. (c) Year of Big divide-1921A.D; (d) Population pyramid has a broad base and a tapering top; (e) First regular census in India was carried in 1881

4. Ans. (c) Failures per 100 women years of exposure

Ref: K. Park, 24th ed. p 544

5. Ans. (d) Number of girls born to a woman…

Ref: K. Park, 24th ed. p 523

6. Ans. (b) 1

Ref: K. Park, 24th ed. p 544

Pearls index – number of failures per 100 women years of exposure

$$\text{Failure rate} = \frac{\text{Total accidental pregnancy}}{\text{Total months of exposure}} \times 1200$$

Or

$$\text{Failure rate} = \frac{\text{Total accidental pregnancy}}{\text{Total women years of exposure}} \times 100$$

Hence as per the MCQ given

Accidental pregnancy = 1

Total women years = 100 females for one year = 100 women years (or 1200 months of exposure)

So, substituting in the formula:

$$\text{Failure rate} = \frac{1}{100} \times 100 = 1 \text{ per 100 women years of exposure}$$

47 **Good to Remember**

- The multiplicative factor 1200 is 100 years (with 12 months per year)
- The total months of exposure in denominator is calculated as (Total females exposed to contraception x number of months of exposure) – (the period not under exposure)*

*In case of pregnancy – it is 10 months per pregnancy to be subtracted

* In case of abortions – 4 months per abortions should be subtracted from the denominator

7. Ans. (b) 60

Ref: K. Park, 24th ed. p 527

8. Ans. (c) 4

Ref: K. Park, 24th ed. p 513

9. Ans. (b) Malnutrition rates

Ref: K. Park 24th ed. p 513

The demographic indicators are:

- Births
- Deaths
- Social mobility (change in the socioeconomic strata)
- Migrations
- Female literacy
- Age at marriage
- Duration of married life
- Spacing of children

10. Ans. (a) 940 (as per census 2011)

Ref: K. Park, 24th ed. p 517

- The sex ratio is the number of females per 1000 males.
- The female deficit syndrome is an adverse outcome of multiple social and economic adversities in a community. A low sex ratio indicates male child preference and further gender inequalities.

11. Ans. (d) Still births + early neonatal deaths per 1000 live births

Ref: K. Park, 24th ed. p 599

12. Ans. (c) 21 days

Ref: S Lal, Textbook of Community Medicine, 1st ed. p 350-51

13. Ans. (c) Japan

Ref: K. Park, 24th ed. p 18

RCH

14. Ans. (d) DLHS

Ref: https://data.gov.in/catalog/district-level-household-and-facility-survey-dlhs-4

The District Level Household and Facility Survey

- It is a nationwide survey, 4th round was conducted during 2012-13 (DLHS-4)
- It collected data on
    - Maternal care (Quality of antenatal and delivery care, % of women who received JSY benefits, % of women with any pregnancy/delivery/postdelivery complication,

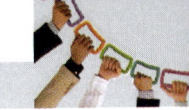

problem of vaginal discharge and menstrual related problems, % of pregnancy resulting in live birth, still birth, induced and spontaneous abortion)

- Immunization and childcare
- Contraception and fertility preferences
- Reproductive health including knowledge about HIV/ AIDS.
- Availability of health, education and other facilities in the village and accessibility and utilization, Human resources, infrastructure, and services available
- District wise data on population and household profile, % of households having electricity, improved source of drinking water, having access to improved toilet facility, use clean fuel for cooking
- Mean age of marriage for girls and boys
- Percentage of currently married women married below age 18 years and 21 years,
- Birth registration, personal habits, reported prevalence of morbidity, chronic illness during last one year, Anemia status by Hemoglobin level, blood sugar level and hypertension

DLHS-4. First time, a population-linked facility survey was conducted in all Community Health Centers (CHCs), District Hospitals and Sub Divisional Hospitals. All Sub-Health Centers and Primary Health Centers (PHCs) which serve the population of the selected PSUs were also covered.

15. Ans. (b) Female clients should be below the age of 45 years and above the age of 20 years

Ref: Standards for female and male sterilization services, Government of India, 2006

Sterilization	Services	Basic qualification requirement of provider
Female	Minilap services	Trained MBBS doctor
	Laparoscopic sterilization	DGO, MD (OandG), MS (Surgery) (trained in laparoscopic sterilization)
Male	Conventional vasectomy and No-scalpel vasectomy (NSV)	Trained MBBS doctor

Case Selection Criteria: (Self-declaration by client is used to compile information)

- Clients should be married (including ever-married).
- Age:
  - Female clients should be below 49 years age and above 22 years of age.
  - Male clients should be below 60 years of age
- Couple should have at least 1 child above 1year age unless sterilization is medically indicated.
- Clients or their spouses/partners must not have undergone sterilization in past (not applicable in case of failure of previous sterilization).
- Clients must be in a sound state of mind
- Mentally ill clients must be certified by a psychiatrist, and a statement be given by the legal guardian/spouse regarding the soundness of the client's state of mind.

Also Know......................

Timing of the Surgical Procedure

- Interval sterilization - performed within 7 days of the menstrual period
- Post-partum sterilization - done after 24 hours up to 7 days of delivery.
- Sterilization with MTP can be performed concurrently.
- Sterilization following spontaneous abortion can be performed if client fulfils the medical eligibility criteria.
- Laparoscopic tubal ligation should not be done concurrently with 2nd trimester abortion and in post-partum period.
- Male sterilization can be done at any convenient time on healthy clients.

Latest Updates

The consent of the spouse is not required for sterilization.

MISCELLANEOUS

16. Ans. (b) District level household survey

Ref: J Kishore, National Health Programs of India, 11th ed. p-20

17. Ans. (c) 1970

Ref: 24th ed. p 877

Central Births and Deaths Registration Act in 1969 (came into force on 1 April 1970) provides for *compulsory registration of births and deaths throughout the country.*[Q]

Also Know......................

- *Time limit for registering births and death* is within 21 days of occurrence, with local registrar.

18. Ans. (c) Calculating probability of adverse ...

Ref: www. nih.gov

DEMOGAPHIC CYCLE, PROCESS, POPULATION GROWTH

19. Ans. (a) 2045

(Ref: www.jsk.gov.in)

National Population Stabilization Fund: Objectives

- To provide or undertake activities aimed to achieve population stabilization, at a level consistent with the needs of sustainable economic growth, social development and environment protection, by 2045.
- To promote and support schemes, programs, projects and initiatives for meeting the unmet needs for contraception and reproductive and child health care.

- To promote and support innovative ideas in the Government, private and voluntary sector
- To facilitate the development of a vigorous people's movement in favor of the national effort for population stabilization.
- To provide a window for channelizing contributions from individuals, trade organizations and others within the country and outside, in furtherance of the national cause of population stabilization.
- No discrimination on the ground of religion, community, caste or class.

20. Ans. (a) Difference between crude birth rate and crude death rate

Ref: K. Park, 23rd ed. p 481

Annual growth rate[Q] = Crude Birth Rate – Crude Death Rate.

21. Ans. (c) Low birth rate and low death rate

Ref: K. Park, 23rd ed. p 479

Refer to Notes

22. Ans. (c) Birth rates decline

Ref: 24th ed. p 513

23. Ans. (b) Third stage

Ref: 24th ed. p 513

24. Ans. (b) Late stage II

Ref: K. Park 24th ed. p 513

Demographic gap is the difference between *Crude Birth rate and Crude Death rate.*

- *Demographic gap attains its maximum limit in the late stage II*[Q]
- Demographic gap starts to contract in early stage III.[Q]
- *Demographic gap is negative in stage V.*

25. Ans. (a) Birth rate

Ref: K. Park 24th ed. p 515

Vital statistics comprise → Birth, Death, Marriage, Divorce, Legal separation, Adaptation and Disease

26. Ans. (c) Kerala

Ref: K. Park 24th ed. p 23

27. Ans. (d) Morbidity

Ref: K. Park 24th ed. p 513

Demographic processes'[Q] continuously at work within a population determining size, composition and distribution.

- Fertility
- Mortality
- Marriage
- Migration
- *Social mobility* (Movement from one socioeconomic class to other.)

28. Ans. (c) Death rate declines still further, and the birth rate tends to fall.

Ref: K. Park, 24th ed. p 513

29. Ans. (b) 1921

Ref: park 24th ed. p 515

The year 1921 is called the ***"big divide"*** because absolute number of people added to the population in each decade thereafter has been on the rise since 1921

30. Ans. (b) Late expanding

Ref: K. Park, 24th ed. p 513

31. Ans. (b) Social mobility

Ref: S Lal, Textbook of community Medicine, 4th edition p-18

Social mobility is the phenomenon of movement of an individual (or family) from one socioeconomic class to another over a time period with attainment of literacy, better occupation and enhanced income.

32. Ans. (c) 47-70 years

Ref: K. Park, 24th ed. p 515

Population growth Phase	(Annual Growth Rate(AGR) = CBR-CDR)	Population Doubling Time
Stationary	No growth	
Slow growth	< 0.5	>139 years
Moderate growth	0.5 – 1	139- 70
Rapid growth	1- 1.5	70-47
Very rapid	1.5- 2	47-35
Explosive[Q] *or Population explosion*	2-2.5	35-28
	2.5-3	28-23
	3-3.5	23-20
	3.5-4	20-18

Explosive growth rate occurs when AGR exceeds 2%. (Maximum population doubling time is **35 years**)

33. Ans. (a) 22.2%

Ref: K. Park, 24th ed. p 555

34. Ans. (b) 17

Ref: K. Park, 24th ed. p 514

- *India is the 2nd most populous country in the world with a population of 1311 million (2016).*
- *India has 2.4 % of the world's land area and it supports 17.5% of world's population*

35. Ans. (a) 32

Ref: K. Park, 24th ed. p 518

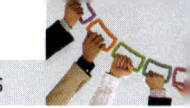

As per Census 2011

- *India's rural population is about 68%. and Urban population is 32%*
- *UP has the largest rural population (18.6%) and Maharashtra has the highest urban population (13.5%)*

36. Ans. (c) Safe water supply available for ...

Ref: K. Park, 24th ed. p 518

Urban Community Means a Place with

- Population > 5000
- Population density at least 390/km^2 OR 1000 per square mile
- At least 75% adult male population is engaged in non-agricultural occupation.

37. Ans. (c) Growth rate

Ref: K. Park, 24th ed. p 515

38. Ans. (a) 1.2

Ref: K. Park, 24th ed. p 515

World population growth rate stood at 1.2 % in 2015.

- It was at its peak 1.92% in 1970

39. Ans. (a) Pregnancy test kit

Ref: K. Park, 24th ed. p 548

Nishchay is a home based self-administered pregnancy test kit launched under NRHM in 2008.

- It is available free of cost at Sub Center and with ASHA to facilitate early detection of pregnancy and decision making

40. Ans. (a) 2.0%

Ref: K. Park, 24th ed. p 515

41. Ans. (a) Rapid growth of population that leads to misbalance in birth and death

Ref: Textbook of Public health and Community medicine, 1st edition, AFMC-WHO, p-892

Mathematical models commonly used for estimating inter-census and post census population estimates are:

- Arithmetic growth method: Assumes that there is an equal addition every year to the population during the inter census period and this addition is taken to be average increase per year.
- Geometric growth method: Assumes that population begets population at a constant rate (compound interest law)
- Exponential growth method: Assumes that there is an exponential growth.
- Component projection method is used for future population projections (future estimates)

42. Ans. (d) Fourth

Ref: K. Park, 24th ed. p 513

- **Low stationary phase** characterized by *low birth rate and low death rate* is the 4th stage in demographic cycle.

43. Ans. (a) Decrease in dependency ratio

Ref: K. Park, 24th ed. p 518

Demographic dividend (bonus) is rise in economic growth rate due to a rising share of working age people in a population.

- It usually occurs late in the demographic transition
- *It is characterized by fall in fertility rate and dependency ratio*[Q].

Demographic burden is increase in the total dependency ratio, mostly caused by increased old age dependency ratio.

44. Ans. (a) 10-19 years of age

Ref: S Lal, Textbook of community medicine, 4th edition p-167

Adolescence is the period between puberty and end of physiological maturation.

- **WHO** has defined adolescent as a *person in the age group 10–19 years*[Q] (10-13, 14-15 and 16–19 *year comprise early, mid and late adolescent respectively)*
- ***Youth*** *is defined as the age group 15-24 years and* ***Young people*** *as the age group 10-24 years*
- ***Juvenile***-boy or girl less than 18 years

Also Know......................

- Legal age for marriage and consent for sexual intercourse by girl is 18 years
- Legal age for marriage for boys is 21 year.
- Legal age for voting is 18 years and above for both gender
- Legal age for employment is more than 14 year
- SALE to Tobacco is prohibited to those < 18 year age and of Alcohol is prohibited to those < 25 year age

45. Ans. (d) >2.0

Ref: K. Park, 24th ed. p 515

DEMOGRAPHIC RATES AND RATIOS

46. Ans. (b) 20.5

Ref: K. Park, 24th ed. p 522

Crude birth rate (CBR) is the simplest indicator of fertility in the population[Q]

$$\text{Crude Birth Rate} = \frac{\text{Number of live births during the year}}{\text{Estimated mid -year population}} \times 1000$$

47. Ans. (b) 165

Ref: K. Park, 24th ed. p 522

Here, CBR (number of live births per 1000 midyear population in a given year) of the community is 30 per 1000

- Hence, number of live birth in the community in a year = 30/1000 × 5000 = 150
- Hence, total Number of pregnancies in a year = Number of live births + Number of pregnancy wastage (i.e. 10% of live birth) = 150 + 15 = 165

However number of detectable pregnancies at any point of time will be only 3/4th of total pregnancies (Since pregnancy is detectable usually after the first 3 months.)

48. Ans. (a) Better measure of fertility than the GFR

Ref: K. Park, 24th ed. p 522

Crude Birth Rate

- Denominator is estimated midyear population, no age or sex distribution comes into play
- It is an unsatisfactory measure of fertility because the total population is not exposed to child bearing.

GFR is a better measure of fertility than CBR

49. Ans. (c) Rajasthan; (d) Madhya Pradesh

Ref: K. Park, 24th ed. p 524

Also Know......................

India – Crude birth rate is = 21, TFR = 2.3

- **States with CBR higher than national level** are à Uttar Pradesh (27), Rajasthan (25), Bihar (25.9), Madhya Pradesh (25.7), Assam (22.4), Jharkhand (23.8) and Chhattisgarh (23.4)
- **States with TFR higher than national level** are - Uttar Pradesh (3.2), Rajasthan (2.8), Bihar (3.2) and Madhya Pradesh (2.8), Jharkhand (2.8) and Chhattisgarh (2.6)

50. Ans. (b) Total fertility rate

Ref: K. Park, 24th ed. p 523

Total Fertility Rate (TFR) *is the average number of children a woman would have if she were to pass through her reproductive years bearing children at the same rates as women now in each age group*[Q].

- TFR *gives approximate magnitude of* ***"completed family size"***.[Q]
- It is computed by summing age-specific fertility rates for all ages.

National Population Policy 2000- Medium term objective is to bring TFR to replacement levels by 2010

51. Ans. (b) Total number of children in a family

Ref: K. Park 24th ed. p 519

Family size is total number of children a woman has borne at a point in time and ***Completed Family size***[Q] is total number of children borne by a woman in her child bearing age (15-44 or 49)

52. Ans. (a) TFR

Ref: K. Park 24th ed. p 519

53. Ans. (d) General Fertility Rate

Ref: K. Park, 24th ed. p 522

General Fertility Rate (GFR) is the number of live births per 1000 women in the reproductive age-group (15–44 or 49 years) in a given year.

Also Know......................

- Current GFR of India is 77.6 (Rural-85.4, Urban -61.7).

54. Ans. (a) General fertility rate

Ref: K. Park, 24th ed. p 522

55. Ans. (a) Number of girls born to a mother in...

Ref: K. Park, 24th ed. p 523

Gross reproduction rate (GRR) is average number of girls to be born to a woman if she experiences the current fertility pattern throughout her reproductive span (15–44 or 49 years), assuming no mortality.

Also Know......................

- *GRR is thus equivalent to TFR for female children only*[Q]

56. Ans. (b) Gross Reproduction Rate

Ref: K. Park, 24th ed. p 523

57. Ans. (d) GFR

Ref: K. Park, 24th ed. p 522

58. Ans. (b) Measure of fertility

Ref: K. Park, 24th ed. p 522

GFR is a better measure of fertility than Crude Birth Rate, as denominator is restricted to women of child bearing age, rather than whole population.

- **Weakness** → Not all women in the reproductive age group are exposed to risk of childbirth.
- **TFR gives** *approximate magnitude of* ***"completed family size"***.[Q]

59. Ans. (a) Number of live birth in women in the reproductive age-group 15-44 years

Ref: K. Park 24th ed. p 522

NRR – NET REPRODUCTIVE RATE

60. Ans. (d) No of female children a newborn girl has in her life time taking into account the mortality

Ref: K. Park 24th ed. p 523

Net reproduction rate (NRR)[Q] *is the number of* ***daughters*** *a newborn girl will bear during her lifetime assuming fixed age -specific fertility and mortality rates.*

61. Ans. (d) Number of daughters a woman...

Ref: K. Park 24th ed. p 523

62. Ans. (b) 1

Ref: K. Park 24th ed. p 523

Also Know.......................

NRR = 1 is equivalent to **attaining** approximately the 2-child norm.
(**NRR > 1** → Population increases, NRR < **1** → Population decreases, NRR = **1** → Population is constant)

63. Ans. (c) 60%

Ref: K. Park 24th ed. p 527

Also Know.......................

- NRR = 1 can be achieved only if at least *60% of eligible couples are effectively practising family planning i.e. CPR = 60%.*[Q]
- National Health Policy, 1983 long term demographic goal was to achieve NRR = 1 by 2000. National Health Policy 2000 seeks to attain NRR = 1 by 2010[Q].

64. Ans. (a) 40

Ref: K. Park 24th ed. p 527

65. Ans. (b) 150–180

Ref: K. Park 24th ed. p 526

Eligible couple is a married couple wherein the wife is in the reproductive age group (15–45 year)

- There are about 150 to 180 eligible couples per 1000 population in India.
- About 20% of eligible couples are found in the age group 15–24 years
- On an average 2.5 million couples are joining the reproductive group every year.

66. Ans. (c) 60%

Ref: K. Park 24th ed. p 527

67. Ans. (c) NRR

Ref: K. Park 24th ed. p 523

DEPENDENCY RATIO

68. Ans. (a) Less than 15 years and more than…

Ref: K. Park 24th ed. p 518

Total Dependency Ratio (*Societal dependency ratio*[Q]) is the ratio of the combined age groups 0 -14 years and 65 years and above (considered dependent) to 15 - 64 year age group (economically productive age group)

- **TDR**=*Young age dependency ratio (0-14 year) + Old age dependency ratio (≥ 65 years)*
- Demerit → Elderly or young persons who are employed and working aged persons (>65 year) who are unemployed are not considered.

Trends of dependency ratio in India

Year	Total dependency	Young age dependency	Old age dependency
2005	61.1%	53.1%	8.02%
2016 (July)	53%	44.7%	8.4%

- There is a shift from young age dependency to old age dependency, as fertility declines and longevity increases.

69. Ans. (b) 66.6%

Ref: K. Park 24th ed. p 518

$$\text{Total dependency ratio} = \frac{\text{Persons less than 15 year + Persons more than or equal to 65 years}}{\text{Persons in age group 15-64 years}} \times 1000$$

$$= \frac{30\% + 10\%}{60\%} = 66.6\%$$

70. Ans. (c) Number of people aged 15 to 65 years per adult aged ≥ 65 years

Ref: Bernd Marin, M. Asghar Zaidi Mainstreaming Ageing: Indicators to Monitor Sustainable Policies, p-126

Potential Support Ratio (PSR) *Refers to the number of people of potential working age group (i.e. 15-64 years) for every person of dependent age group (i.e. ≥ 65 years)*

SEX RATIO

71. Ans. (a) 940 females per 1000 males

Ref: K. Park 24th ed. p 517

72. Ans. (d) 940

Ref: K. Park 24th ed. p 517

73. Ans. (b) Kerala

Ref: K. Park 24th ed. p 517

Also Know.......................

As per 2011 Estimates

- *Sex Ratio at Birth, India is* 906 (Rural =907, Urban=905)
- *Overall State wise Sex Ratio at Birth* is highest in Kerala (974) and lowest is in Haryana (866)
- *State-wise Sex Ratio at Birth* in rural areas is highest in Chhattisgarh (982) and lowest is in Punjab (863)
- *State-wise Sex Ratio at Birth* in urban areas is highest in Kerala (985) and lowest is in Haryana (859)

LITERACY RATE

74. Ans. (c) 50%

Ref: K. Park, 24th ed. p 519-20

Effective Literacy RateQ *is number of persons aged 7 year or more, who can read and write with understanding any language per 1000 population of persons 7 years of age and above.*

Crude Literacy Rate".Q is the Literacy rate calculated with the total population as denominator

Total persons *aged 7 year or more, = 10000–2000 = 8000*
Literate persons among > '7 years old are 4000.
Effective literacy rate = 4000/8000 × 100 = 50%

75. Ans. (d) Total population >7 years

Ref: K. Park, 24th ed. p 519-20

A person is deemed as literate if he/she can read and write with understanding in any language.

- Literacy rate calculated only for *population 7 years of age and above is "**Effective Literacy Rate**".*QQ
- Government of India has made education compulsory up to age 14 years.

Also Know......................

- Literacy rate of Indian population as per census 2011 is 74% *(Male 82% and Female 65.46%)*
- *Highest literacy rate*Q is in Kerala (93.9%). Mizoram (91.58%) and Lakshadweep (92.28 %)
- *Lowest literacy rate*Q is in Bihar (63.8%) and Arunachal Pradesh (66.9%)
- States with literacy rates below national average are Arunachal Pradesh, Andhra Pradesh, Bihar, Jammu and Kashmir, Uttar Pradesh, Rajasthan, M.P., Assam, Jharkhand, Chhattisgarh and Orissa.
- **International Literacy day is on 8th September:** UNESCO defines a "Literate person" as a one who can with understanding both read and write a short simple statement relevant to his everyday life.
- **National Literacy Mission** defines literacy as acquiring skills of reading, writing and arithmetic and ability to apply them to one's day-to-day life. Achievement of functional literacy implies:
- Becoming aware of the causes of deprivation and moving towards amelioration by participating in development process
- Acquiring skills to improve their economics status and general well-being
- Imbibing values of national integration, conservation of environment, women's equality, observance of small family norms, etc.

76. Ans. (b) 65%

Ref: K. Park 24th ed. p 520

National Literacy Mission (1998)

- Goal is to attain full literacy (i.e., a sustainable threshold level of 75 percent) by 2007.
- Mission seeks to impart functional literacy to all non-literate persons in 15–35 age group.
- It has been expanded to include people in the age group 9 to 14 years, in areas not covered by the non-formal education program, to ensure that the benefits of TLCs are made available to out-of-school children as well

Also Know......................

Sarva Shiksha Abhiyan (SSA)

- It is Government of India's flagship program for achievement of Universalization of Elementary Education (UEE) in a time bound manner.
- It seeks to provide quality Free and compulsory education including life skills to Children of 6–14 years age group.

77. Ans. (a) Those above age of 7 years

Ref: 24th ed. p 519

POPULATION PYRAMID

78. Ans. (a) Broad base and narrow at apex

Ref: K. Park 24th ed. p 517

*Age pyramid of India is typical of developing countries, with broad base and a tapering top*Q.

Age pyramid of India

Reflects:

- High fertility
- High dependency rate
- Growing proportion of elderly people
- High mortality in young age females

79. Ans. (b) Developed country

Ref: K. Park 24th ed. p 517

Population pyramid *is a graphical representation* (horizontal bar diagram) *of age (vertical axis) and sex distribution (horizontal axis- Male on right and Female on Left side) of a population*Q.

- *It shape reflects fertility pattern, height indicates life expectancy (Taller pyramid -Higher life expectancy) and symmetry indicates ideal sex ratio*Q

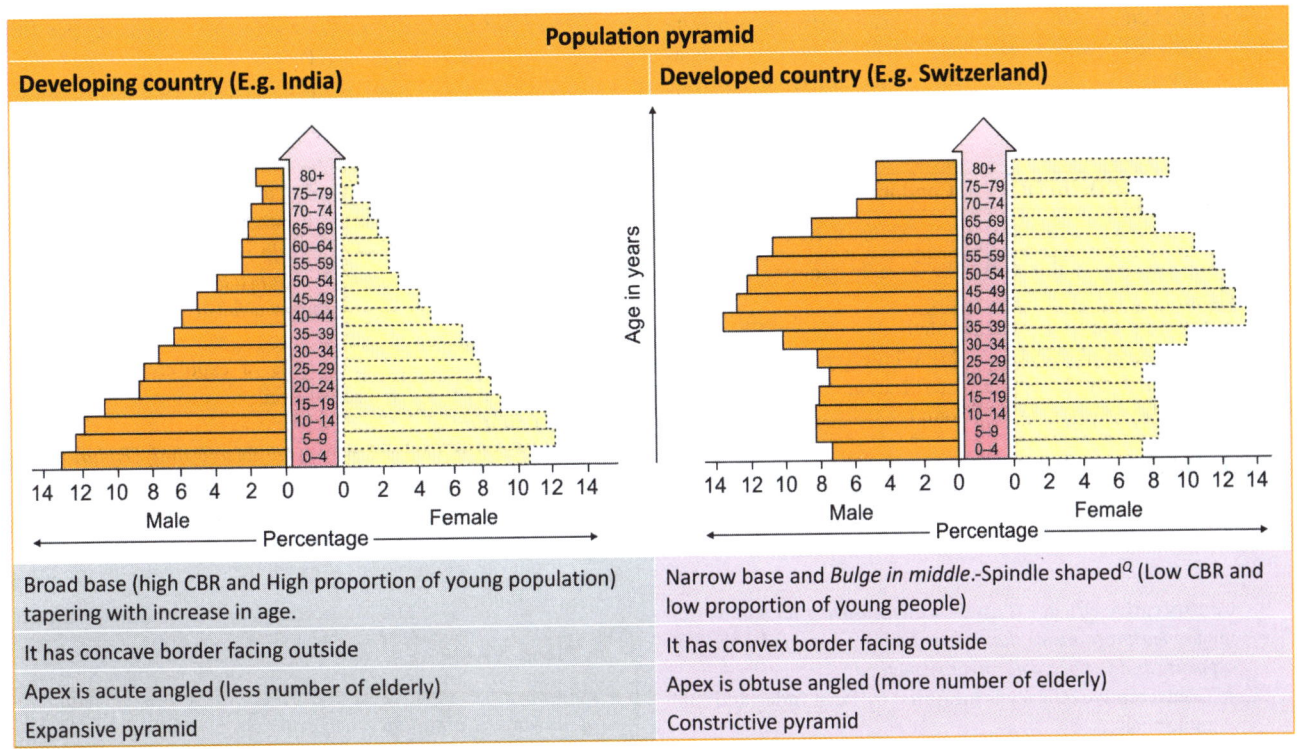

Population pyramid	
Developing country (E.g. India)	**Developed country (E.g. Switzerland)**
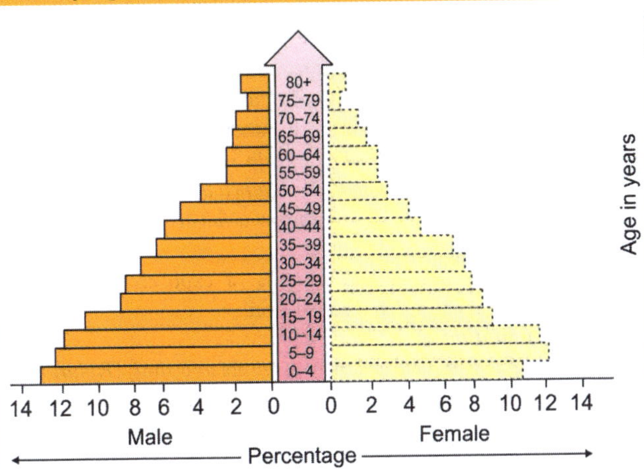	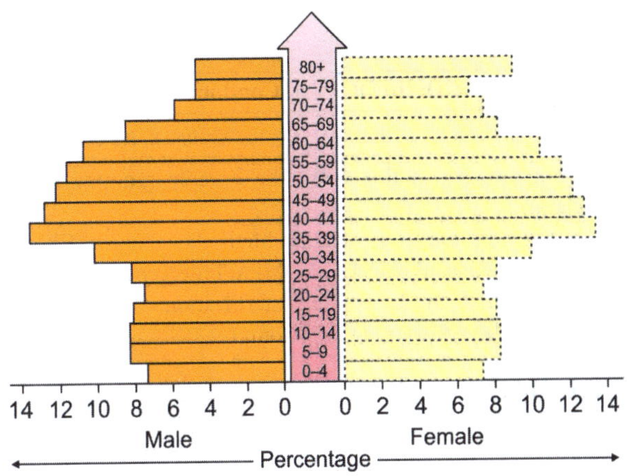
Broad base (high CBR and High proportion of young population) tapering with increase in age.	Narrow base and *Bulge in middle*.-Spindle shaped[Q] (Low CBR and low proportion of young people)
It has concave border facing outside	It has convex border facing outside
Apex is acute angled (less number of elderly)	Apex is obtuse angled (more number of elderly)
Expansive pyramid	Constrictive pyramid

80. Ans. (a) High literacy rate; (b) High doctor population ratio; (d) Older age of marriage; (e) Higher life expectancy

Ref: K. Park 24th ed. p 520

Ref multiple documents

CONCEPT AND SCOPE OF FAMILY PLANNING

81. Ans. (b) Limiting birth

Ref: K. Park 24th ed. p 545

Sexually active women who wish to avoid pregnancy but are not using any method of contraception (including use by their partner) are considered to have an **"Unmet need" for family planning**

- Applied to married women
- Unmet need for family planning is highest in women below 20 year age
- Among women below 20 year age unmet need is entirely for limiting birth
- Women 20–24 year age unmet need is mainly (about 75%) for spacing birth
- Women 30 year and above unmet need is mainly for limiting birth

82. Ans. (b) 1977

Ref: Community Medicine Recent Advances, Suryakanta, 3rd edition. P-629

India was the 1st country to launch family planning program in 1951.[Q]

In 1977, Family planning program was renamed "Family Welfare Program" with following features

- "Cafeteria" approach –All available contraceptive methods are offered to an individual, out of which one can choose according to his needs and wishes.
- Welfare approach
- Basket approach
- No compulsion for family planning.

83. Ans. (c) Family planning

Ref: K. Park 24th ed. p 545 http://www.jstor.org/pss/1964798

KAP (Knowledge Attitude Practices) study *have been part of studies on family planning since independence in India.*[Q]

- Concept of unmet need of family planning – (Gap between a women's reproductive intention and contraceptive behavior.) was 1st explored in 1960 post KAP surveys.
- ***KAP Gap*** *-refers to inconsistencies between a person's stated Knowledge and Attitude on one hand and their practice on other hand.*

84. Ans. (c) Social Marketing

Ref: High Impact Practices in Family Planning (HIP. Social marketing: leveraging the private sector to improve contraceptive access, choice, and use. Washington, DC: USAID; 2013

Social marketing approach in family planning programs makes contraceptive

- Accessible and Affordable
- It uses commercial marketing techniques to achieve specific behavioral goals.
- Social marketers combine product, price, place (distribution), and promotion— "4Ps" or the "marketing mix"—to maximize use of specific health products among targeted population groups.

- It seeks to improve access by tapping into networks of private providers and non-governmental sector outlets, such as pharmacies, shops, community-based distributors, private health care providers/outlets, kiosks, and community health workers.

85. Ans. (a) IUCD; (b) OCP; (d) Condom

Ref: K. Park 24th ed. p 528

Contraceptive methods may be broadly grouped into two classes

- **Spacing methods**–Barrier Methods (Physical/Chemical/ Combined), IUCD, OCP, DMPA, Emergency pill etc.
- **Terminal methods**–Male sterilization (Vasectomy) and Female sterilization (Tubectomy)

PEARL INDEX

86. Ans. (d) Life-table analysis

Ref: K. Park 24th ed. p 544

***Contraceptive efficacy** is assessed by measuring the number of unplanned pregnancies that occur during a specified period of exposure and use of a contraceptive method.*[Q]

- Contraceptive efficacy is measured by Pearl Index and Life table analysis

Life-Table Analysis: (Better)

- *It is better compared to Pearl Index*
- *It calculates a failure rate for each month of use.* A cumulative failure rate can compare methods for any specific length of exposure.
- Women who leave a study for any reason other than unintended pregnancy are removed from the analysis, contributing their exposure until the time of the exit.

87. Ans. (a) Life-table analysis

Ref: K. Park 24th ed. p 544

88. Ans. (a) 12.8%

Ref: K. Park 24th ed. p 545

- As per NFHS-3 Unmet need for family planning is 12.8% (For spacing—6.2% and for limiting—6.6%)
- Unmet need for family planning is highest in women below 20 years age—27.1% (Almost entirely for spacing)
- It is higher in rural, illiterate, poor socioeconomic status women

NFHS 4 report:

- Unmet need for family planning among currently married women ranges from a low of 3% among women age 45-49 to a high of 22% among women age 15-24
- Unmet need for family planning is 20% or more in Manipur, Nagaland, Sikkim, Arunachal Pradesh, Meghalaya, Bihar, Mizoram, and Daman & Diu. Unmet need is less than 10% in Andhra Pradesh, Punjab, Chandigarh, Telangana, West Bengal, Puducherry, and Haryana.

89. Ans. (a) Per 100 women years

Ref: K. Park 24th ed. p 544

Pearl index is the number of accidental pregnancy per 100 woman-years of exposure (HWY).[Q]

- ***Pearl Index*** $= \dfrac{\text{Total accidental pregnancies}}{\text{Total months of exposure}} \times 1200$
- Total accidental pregnancies include every known conception, irrespective of outcome (live births, still-births or abortions or not yet terminated).
- *1200 is the number of months in 100 years.*
- *Total month of exposure is obtained by deducting from period under review of 10 months for a full-term pregnancy and 4 months for an abortion.*[Q]
- A minimum of 600 months of exposure is considered necessary to reach a conclusion.
- ***Limitation-***
  - *It assumes a constant failure rate over time. (Failure rate of* most contraceptives decline with duration of use)
  - Pearl index is based on a specific exposure (usually 1 year) and hence it fails to accurately compare methods at various durations of exposure. (Overcome by ***life-table analysis.***)

Also Know........................

- *Contraceptive efficacy is measured in terms of number of unwanted pregnancy occurring in a specified period of exposure or use of contraceptive.*

90. Ans. (b) Accidental pregnancies per 100...

Ref: K. Park 24th ed. p 544

91. Ans. (b) Failures per 100 women years of...

Ref: K. Park 24th ed. p 544

BARRIER METHOD OF CONTRACEPTION

92. Ans. (a) For contraception

Ref: K. Park 24th ed. p 529

Barrier cream are "surface-active agents" that attach to spermatozoa and inhibit oxygen uptake and kill sperms (Spermicides). They are available as

- Foams: Foam tablets, foam aerosols
- Creams, jellies and pastes–squeezed from a tube
- Suppositories–inserted manually
- Soluble films–C-film inserted manually

93. Ans. (a) Interferes with fertilization

Ref: K. Park 24th ed. p 531

94. Ans. (b) 5 years

Ref: K. Park 24th ed. p 530

Source: Bayer HealthCare Pharmaceuticals Inc. 2008, Product Information Brochure.

Mirena is 3rd generation hormonal IUD.

It secretes 20 mcg/day of levonorgestrol (and hence called as LNG-20)

Mirena may be effective for 5–7 years (and some studies have reported effect lasting up to 10 years also), but the guidelines suggest mirena to be used for 5 years and later should be replaced.

Mirena contains 52 mg of levonorgestrel. Initially, levonorgestrel is released at a rate of approximately 20 µg/day. This rate decreases progressively to half that value after 5 years. Hence in the MCQ given, though multiple answers could be followed, best to mark would be option B (5 years)

Mirena is contraindicated when one or more of the following conditions exist:

- Pregnancy or suspicion of pregnancy.
- Congenital or acquired uterine anomaly including fibroids if they distort the uterine cavity.
- Acute pelvic inflammatory disease or a history of pelvic inflammatory disease unless there has been a subsequent intrauterine pregnancy.
- Postpartum endometritis or infected abortion in the past 3 months.
- Known or suspected uterine or cervical neoplasia or unresolved, abnormal Pap smear.
- Genital bleeding of unknown etiology.
- Untreated acute cervicitis or vaginitis, including bacterial vaginosis or other lower genital tract infections until infection is controlled.
- Acute liver disease or liver tumor (benign or malignant).
- Conditions associated with increased susceptibility to pelvic infections.
- A previously inserted IUD that has not been removed.
- Hypersensitivity to any component of this product.
- Known or suspected carcinoma of the breast.

95. Ans. (b) MIRENA

Ref: K. Park 24th ed. p 530

LNG -20 (Mirena) is a T shaped 3rd generation IUD.

- It releases 20 microgram of Levonorgestrel and has an effective life of 10 years.
- Pregnancy rate is low (0.2 per 100 women) and ectopic pregnancy is also less
- Associated with low menstrual blood loss and fewer days of bleeding

96. Ans. (a) 10 years

Ref: K. Park 24th ed. p 531

Copper and hormone-releasing IUCD devices *need periodic replacement.*

- ***Cu-T 380A*** is approved for use for 10 *years*^{Q}.
- ***Cu-T 200*** is approved for 4 *years*^{Q}
- **Nova T** is approved for 5 *years*^{Q}.
- ***Progesterone-releasing IUD*** must be replaced every *years*^{Q}.
- **Levonorgestrel IUD** can be used for 5-7 years^{Q}

Inert IUDs (Lippes Loop) may be left in place as long as required, if there are no side-effects

97. Ans. (c) Has a history of ectopic pregnancy

Ref: K. Park 24th ed. p 531

Ideal IUD candidate–Planned Parenthood Federation of America (PPFA) has described ideal IUD candidate as a woman:

- Who has borne at least one child (*IUD is not a method of first choice for nulliparous women*)
- Who has no history of pelvic disease
- Who has normal menstrual periods
- Who is willing to check the IUD tail
- Who has access to follow-up and treatment of potential problems, and
- Who is in a monogamous relationship (multiple partners → risk of PID) and possible infertility".

Contraindications to IUD

Absolute contraindications:

- Suspected pregnancy
- Pelvic inflammatory disease
- Vaginal bleeding of undiagnosed etiology
- Ca Cervix, uterus or pelvic adnexa
- Previous ectopic pregnancy

Relative contraindications:

- Anemia
- Menorrhagia
- History of PID since last pregnancy
- Purulent cervical discharge
- Distortions of the uterine cavity due to congenital malformations, fibroids
- Unmotivated person

98. Ans. (d) Thinning of fallopian tube

Ref: K. Park 24th ed. p 531

99. Ans. (c) 1st generation IUDs

Ref: K. Park 24th ed. p 530

Advantage of IUD -Refer to Notes

100. Ans. (d) 10 years

Ref: K. Park 24th ed. p 531

- Inert IUDs (Lippes Loop) may be left in place as long as required, if there are no side-effects.
- Copper devices and hormone-releasing IUD need periodic replacement- TCu-380A–10 years^{Q}, TCu-200–4 year, Nova T -5 year^{Q}, Progesterone IUD-every year^{Q}, Levonorgestrel IUD- 7 year.

HORMONAL CONTRACEPTIVE

101. Ans. (c) Oral contraceptive pills

Ref: K. Park 24th ed. p 534

Best contraceptive for a newly married couple is OCP *(Almost 100% effective in preventing pregnancy and removing anxiety about risk of unplanned pregnancy). It also has non contraceptive health benefits*

- **IUD** is not *preferred for nulliparous women because of higher incidence of expulsion, lower abdominal pain and pelvic infections*^{Q}
- **Barrier method and Natural methods** have a high failure rate and natural methods also need considerable period of abstinence.

102. Ans. (c) Use a barriers method for rest of cycle.

Ref; Mahajan and Gupta, Textbook of Community Medicine 4th ed p-613

If the client misses OCP for 3 successive days – Check for withdrawal bleeding

- ***Withdrawal bleeding present–Stop OCP*** and use condom for the rest of the cycle, if needed. Start a new pill course from 1st day of the beginning of the next cycle.
- **Withdrawal bleeding not started**
- Had intercourse–Take 2 doses of emergency contraceptive pills and after that continue to take the rest of the OCP (1 Tab daily) till the next menstrual cycle starts and use a condom for any further intercourse and start a new packet of OCP on the first day of the next cycle.
- No Intercourse–Stop OCP and use condoms (if any intercourse happens) till the next menstrual period begins and start a new packet of oral contraceptive pills on the first day of the next cycle.

103. Ans. (d) Protection against cervical cancer

Ref: K. Park 24th ed. p 536

Refer to Notes

104. Ans. (d) OCP

Ref: K. Park 24th ed. p 536

OCP in Lactating mother can

- Adversely affect the quantity and constituents of breast milk
- May result premature cessation of lactation

105. Ans. (c) Ovarian cysts; (d) Fibrocystic disease of breast

Ref: K. Park 24th ed. p 536

MINIPILL

106. Ans. (b) Lactating females

Ref: K. Park, 24th ed. p 535 24th ed. p Community Medicine Recent Advances, 3rd edition, p-641

Progestogen-only pill (POP)/"minipill" or "micropill"

- Contains only progestogen (Norethisterone and Levonorgestrel) in small dose given throughout the cycle
- Demerit is poor cycle control and an increased pregnancy rate.
- Indication
  - *Old women (age>35 year/ Smokers)*
  - *Young women with risk factors for neoplasia*
  - *Nursing woman*

TERMINAL METHOD OF CONTRACEPTION

107. Ans. (c) Unmarried woman

Ref –Guidelines for standards for female and male sterilization services, NHM, MOHFW, Govt. Of India

Sterilization Guidelines (2014)-Terminal methods of sterilization are indicated for

- Ever married male (<60 years) and female (22–49 years)
- Couple with at least one child more than 1 year of age,
- No past history of sterilization of self/spouse
- Person being in sound mental health (postpsychiatric evaluation and certification).

108. Ans. (b) 24 hours to 7 days of delivery

Ref: Standards for Female and Male Sterilization Services, Ministry of Health and Family Welfare, Government of India, October 2006

Timing for Surgical Sterilization Procedure

Procedure	Timing
Interval sterilization	Within 7 days of the menstrual period (in the follicular phase of the menstrual cycle)
Post-partum sterilization	Between 24 hours to 7 days of delivery
Sterilization with MTP	Concurrently
Sterilization following spontaneous abortion	Performed if the client fulfils the medical eligibility criteria

**Laparoscopic tubal ligation should not be done concurrently with second-trimester abortion and in the post-partum period*

109. Ans. (c) Fortnight

Ref: 24th ed. p 548

FDS–Fixed Day Static Services Approach–Sterilization services are to be provided at different health facilities within the public health system on fixed days to improve access.

Health Facility	Frequency
District hospital	Weekly
Sub district hospital	Weekly
CHC/Block PHC	Fortnightly
PHC	Monthly

110. Ans. (a) 0.1-0.5%

Ref: Berek and Novaks Gynaecology, 15th ed. p-287

Pomeroy's technique has a failure rate of 1-4 per 1000 cases

111. Ans. (a) Female sterilization

Ref: K. Park, 24th ed. p 542

Terminal methods of sterilization

- Ideal contraceptive procedure for couples desiring no more children.
- Currently female sterilizations account for about 85% and male sterilizations 10–15% of all sterilizations in India
- Male sterilization is simpler, safer, faster and cheaper. It can be performed at PHC by trained doctors under local anesthesia. **No scalpel vasectomy** is a new technique (safe, convenient and acceptable)

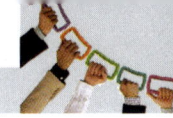

EMERGENCY CONTRACEPTIVE

112. Ans. (d) 72 hours

Ref: 24th ed. p 535

Yuzpe and Lancee ***regimen*** is indicated within 72 hours of unprotected intercourse.

113. Ans. (d) All of the above

Ref: 24th ed. p 535

Recommended Methods as per WHO (FACT SHEET RELAESED IN FEB 2016)-

- Emergency Contraception Pills (ECPs): WHO recommends either of the following drugs for emergency contraception, for use within 5 days (120 hours) of unprotected sexual intercourse: Effectiveness - 52–94%
  - Levonorgestrel single dose (1.5 mg) Or
  - Levonorgestrel taken in 2 doses (0.75 mg each, 12 hours apart) Or
  - Ulipristal acetate, single dose (30 mg).
- Yuzpe method
  Combined OCP (Each dose containing Estrogen (100–120 mg Ethinylestradiol) and Progestin (0.50–0.60 mg Levonorgestrel or 1.0–1.2 mg Norgestrel) is to be taken in two doses. 1st dose to be taken as soon as possible after unprotected intercourse *(preferably within 72 hours but as late as 120 hours, or 5 days) and the 2nd dose to be taken 12 hours later. If vomiting occurs within 2 hours of taking a dose, the dose should be repeated.*
- Copper-bearing Intrauterine Devices (IUDs)
  - To be inserted within 5 days of unprotected intercourse

Also Know......................

- Copper-bearing Intrauterine Devices (IUDs) is the most effective form of emergency contraception (Effectiveness 99%)

114. Ans. (b) Levonorgestrel only pill

Ref: National Health Program, J Kishore, 9th ed. p-131

- **i-pill** (0.75 mg of Levonorgestrel) is the only dedicated product for emergency contraception approved by Drug controller of India.
- **i-pill** *was introduced in National family welfare program in 2002.*[Q]

115. Ans. (c) 5 days

Ref: 24th ed. p 535

MEDICAL TERMINATION OF PREGNANCY

116. Ans. (a) 20 weeks

Ref: K. Park, 24th ed. p 540

Refer to theory

117. Ans. (c) 20 weeks

Ref: K. Park, 24th ed. p 540

SOURCES OF HEALTH INFORMATION

CENSUS

118. Ans. (c) 1881

Ref: K. Park, 24th ed. p 887

- It is carried out by most countries worldwide at regular intervals, usually of 10 years.
- *1st regular census in India was done in 1881*
- The last census was held in March 2011.
- Census enumerators are school teachers, government staff and local body employee trained in advance and paid honorarium

Also Know......................

Census 2011 – Tagline was 'Our census our future'

- Method used was ***de facto canvasser.***

119. Ans. (c) 1981

Ref: Drop-in-Article: Census of India 2011, p-8 Available athttp://censusindia.gov.in/Ad_Campaign/drop_in_articles/05-History_of_Census_in_India.pdf

Also Know......................

- Article 256 of the constitution of India mandates the Union Government to conduct census

120. Ans. (c) 1970

Ref: k Park, 24th ed p-877

The Central Births and Deaths Registration Act 1969 (Came into force on 1 April 1970)

121. Ans. (b) Deficient; (c) Head of institution or...; (d) Birth and Death both are registered; (e) Cause of death is recorded

Ref: S Lal, Textbook of community medicine, 4th ed. p-350-51

Civil Registration System in India

- It does *registration of births and deaths across the country and compiles vital statistics*
- Responsibility for reporting births and deaths
  - Public (e.g. Parents, Relatives) are to report events occurring in their households
  - Heads of institution or Officer in charge in case of hospitals, nursing homes etc.
- Responsibility for registration
  - **Urban area:** Municipal committee or corporation
  - **Rural:** Panchayat secretary (In its absence BDO/ Revenue official)

Time limit for registering births and death[Q] - Within 21 days of occurrence, with local registrar.

SRS is a dual record system

REGISTRATION OF VITAL EVENTS

122. Ans. (c) 21 days

Ref: S Lal, Textbook of community medicine, 1st ed. p-350-51

SRS

123. Ans. (a) 6 months

Ref: K. Park, 24th ed p878

124. Ans. (a) 6 months

Ref: K. Park, 24th ed. p 878

MISCELLANEOUS

125. Ans. (c) 5 years

Ref: Mahajan and Gupta, Textbook of Preventive and Social medicine, 4th ed. p 626

126. Ans. (d) 4 round

127. Ans. (c) 60%

The couple protection rate is 60%
The total fertility rate = 2.1
The net reproduction rate will be 1

128. Ans. (c) 5

$$\text{Pearl Index} = \frac{\text{Number of accidental pregnancies}}{\text{Total women years of exposure}} \times 100$$

$$= \frac{10}{2 \times 100} \times 100 = 5 \text{ per 100 women years}$$

129. Ans. (a) 55

Ref: K Park, 25ed 576 http://censusindia.gov.in/vital_statistics/SRS_Bulletins/Bylletins.html

The number of live births in an area is - Live births

$$= \frac{\text{Crude birth rate per 1000 population} \times \text{population}}{1000}$$

Assuming the birth rate for India as 20, the expected live births in the area (considering Subcentre population as 5000) would be:

$$= \frac{20 \times 5000}{1000} = 100$$

The number of pregnant females = Live births + pregnancy wastage (10% of live births)

= 100 + 10 = 110

as a rule, in any given month, approximately half of number of females estimated as per records should be registered with the health worker

So, in any month the ANM should have at least 55 pregnant females registered at the sub centre.

130. Ans. (a) Levonorgestrel IUD, (c) Progesterone only pills, (e) Barrier methods

Option	T/F	Comment
Levonorgestrel IUD	T	Yes correct.
Copper T before 5 days of unprotected intercourse	F	No this is highly unreliable and not a very good choice
Progesterone only pills	T	Yes possibly can be given
Oral combined contraceptive pills	F	No, OCPs is not indicated for metabolic disease and liver disease
Barrier methods	T	Yes possibly, can be given as another option along with some other definitive methods as injectable (antra) or IUD

131. Ans. (b) Unprotected intercourse is allowed only after two consecutive semen analyses show absence of spermatozoa, c. Failure rate is 1 in 300, d. Increased risk of testicular cancer

Option	T/F	Remarks
Non-scalpel vasectomy has less complication than conventional method ofvasectomy	T	Yes, NSV (non-scalpel vasectomy) is safe and convenient method. It does have lesser operative complications compared to the conventional technique
Unprotected intercourse is allowed only after two consecutive semen analyses show absence of spermatozoa	F	No, the male is said to be sterile after 30 ejaculation or after a period of 8-9 weeks
Failure rate is 1 in 300	F	No, the failure rate is 0.15 per 100 person years. The most common cause is mistaken identification of vas
Increased risk of testicular cancer	F	No, not correct. the complications are few as: ▪ Operative complications: pain/ infection ▪ Sperm granules – appear after 10-14 days, eventually subside ▪ Autoimmune response – antibodies to sperm may develop. Though these are harmless and carry no clinical relevance ▪ Psychological
Antibodies to sperm may formed	T	Yes correct.

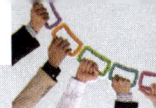

132. Ans. (a) **225**

Ref: Park 25th ed.; 622

The total population is 20,000
Total Births = 456
Still Births = 56
Neonatal deaths = 56
Post neonatal deaths (28 days – 1year) = 34

STEP 1

- Total Infant deaths = neonatal + post-neonatal deaths = 56 + 34 = 90
- Total Live births = Total births – still births = 456 – 56 = 400

STEP 2

$$\text{Infant mortality rate} = \frac{\text{Total Infant deaths in a year}}{\text{Total Live births in the same year}} \times 1000$$

$$\text{Infant mortality rate} = \frac{90}{400} \times 1000 = 225 \text{ per } 1000$$

NOTES

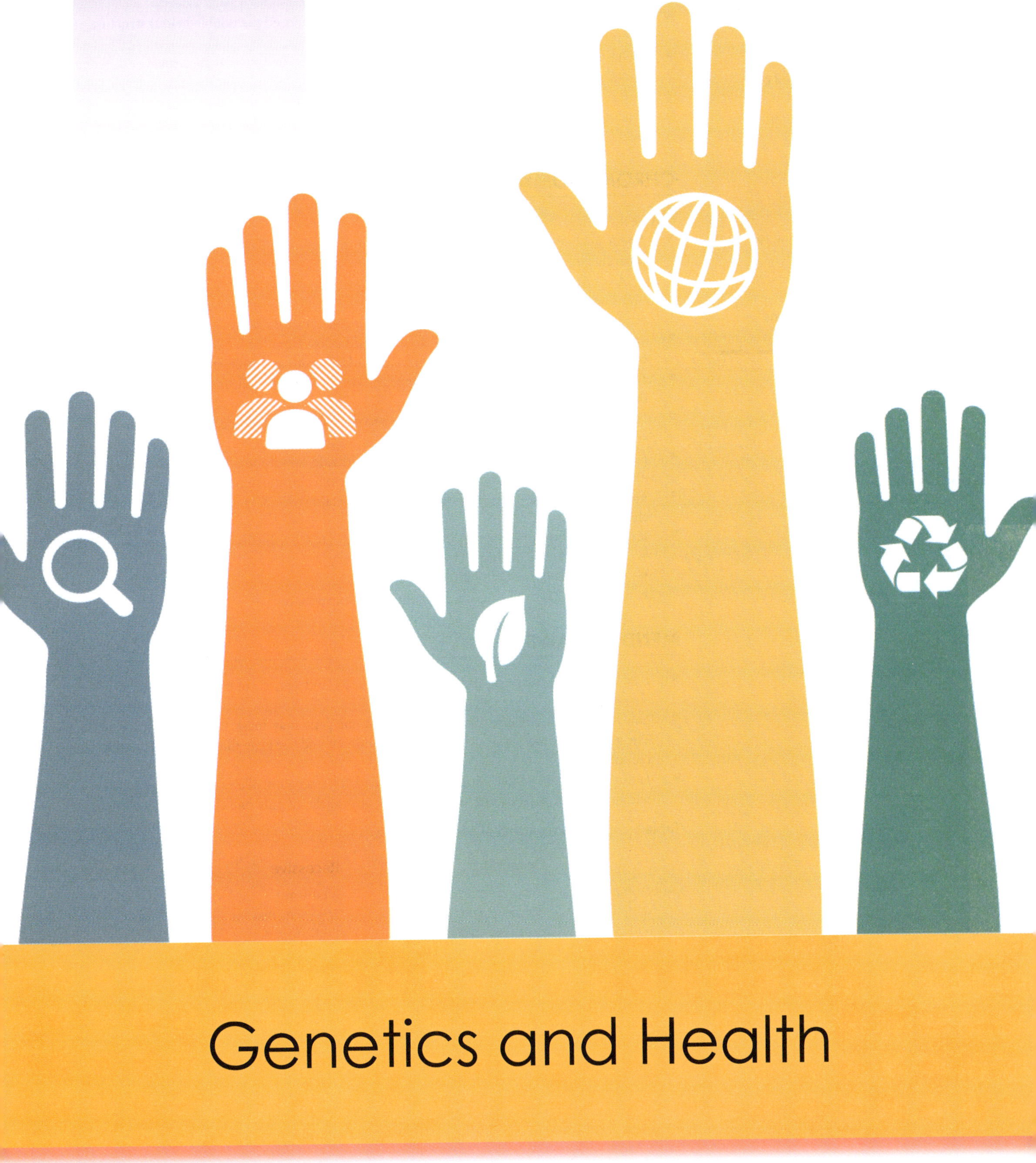

Genetics and Health

Chapter Outline

INTRODUCTION

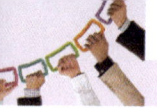

Genes are units of heredity information contained in chromosomes.

- The term "gene" was coined by Danish botanist, Johannsen.
- The human genome is estimated to have 30,000 genes[Q].
- Francis Crick, James Watson and Maurice Wilkins proposed the double helical structure of DNA[Q].
- Genes occur in pairs: Homozygous (pair of alike genes) or Heterozygous (pair of different genes).
- Polygenes or "multiple genes" are genes whose combined action affects a particular trait. Example, Color of skin, height and weight, life span, degree of resistance to disease, rate of heart beat, etc.

CHROMOSOMAL ABNORMALITIES

May be numerical or structural abnormalities.

- *Nondisjunction*: This is an error in the nuclear division. The pair of chromosomes does not separate and both are carried to one pole, resulting in an unequal number of chromosomes, i.e. 45 or 47. This numerical abnormality is called aneuploidy.
- *Translocation:* During nuclear division, if a portion of one chromosome breaks away and gets attached to another different chromosome, it is called translocation.
- *Deletion*: A part of chromosome is detached and is lost from the karyotype, resulting in loss of one or more genes. If the loss is severe, it leads to death and stillbirth.
- *Duplication*: Sometimes genes may appear twice in the same chromosome. This is called duplication.
- *Inversion*: A segment of the chromosome becomes inverted resulting in the alteration of the sequence of genes.
- *Isochromosomes*: Normally, the chromosomes divide longitudinally. But sometimes, they divide transversely, resulting in structurally abnormal chromosomes.
- *Mosaicism*: In the type, the somatic cells contain two or more genetically different chromosomes.
- *Incidence* of chromosomal abnormalities is 5.6 per 1000 live births.
  - 2 per 1000 live births represent sex aneuploidy.
  - 1.7 per 1000 live births autosomal aneuploidy.
  - 1.9 per 1000 live births chromosomal translocations

MENDEL'S LAWS

- *Law of Unit Characters:* All characters are units and genes control expression of these characters.
- *Law of Dominance:* Genes occur in pairs and one gene may mask the expression of other. The gene that expresses itself is said to be dominant and the gene that does not is said to be recessive.
- *Law of Segregation:* When germ cells are formed, it has a pair of alleles for any particular trait and each parent passes a randomly selected copy (allele) of only one of these to its offspring.

Table 1: Inheritance pattern of genetic diseases

	Dominant	Recessive
Autosomal	Achondroplasia Polyposis coli Brachydactyly Polycystic kidney Polydactyly Marfan's syndrome Retinoblastoma Huntington chorea Neurofibromatosis ABO blood group system Hyperlipoproteinemia Hereditary Spherocytosis	Albinism Tay-Sachs disease Cystic fibrosis Galactosemia Agammaglobulinemia (Swiss) Fibrocystic disease of pancreas Phenylketonuria Alkaptonuria Hemoglobinopathies Maple syrup urine disease Hirschsprung disease

Contd...

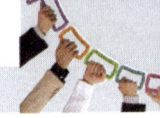

	Dominant	Recessive
Sex-linked	Familial hypophosphatemia Vitamin D resistant rickets	Hemophilia (A and B) Duchenne Muscular Dystrophy
		Hydrocephalus Retinitis pigmentosa Color blindness G6 PD Deficiency Agammaglobulinemia - (Bruton)

ABO Blood Group System

Table 2: ABO blood group

Genotype	Phenotype (blood group)	Frequency in Indian population
OO	O	40%
AA or AO	A	22%
BB or BO	B	33%
AB	AB	5% [*Rarest*]

- *Gene O* is recessive; RBC of a person whose blood group is O has no antigens.
- *Genes A and B* are codominant; when both are present, RBC carry antigen-A and antigen-B.

Blood group is helpful in case of paternity dispute and to determine if twins are identical or not.

- *RHESUS system* depends upon 3 genes C, D and E and their allele's c, d and e.
- Rh antigens are present only on the surface of red cells.
- Possible genotype in Rh system can be CDE, CDe, cDE, cdE, cDe and cde.
- Antigen D (the most potent) → "Rh +ve" means possessing D antigen and "Rh –ve" lacking it.
- In India → 93% of population are Rh +ve compared to 85% in of Northern Europe and North America.
- Rh system is important because of Erythroblastosis fetalis in newborn.

HARDY-WEINBERG LAW[Q]

"Relative frequencies of each gene allele tends to remain constant from generation to generation" in the absence of forces that change the gene frequencies.

Factors influencing gene frequency equilibrium in Hardy Weinberg law are:

- Mutation
- Natural selection (Survival of the fittest) proposed by Darwin
- Population Movements lead to intermixing of people and new genetic combinations.
- Assortative (Nonrandom) mating: Selective mating within subgroups disturbs genetic equilibrium.
- Public Health Measures by saving more lives, decrease selection rates and increase genetic burden.

Concept of "regression coefficient" in genetics was given by Francis Galton for estimating the degree of resemblance between relatives.

Penetrance is the extent to which a genetically determined condition is expressed in an individual. Lack of penetrance is one reason for skipped generations and unexpected pedigree patterns.

FOUNDER EFFECTS

- Differences in distribution of disease between populations can be explained by "founder effects".
  When a population expands from a few founding members, some contribute more and some less to the genetic make-up of subsequent generations.
- If one prolific founder carries a genetic abnormality, it can lead to a localized cluster of affected individuals.

79 *High Yield Points*

Duodenal and gastric ulcer are common in "O" group[Q] and stomach cancer in "A" group individuals.

55 *Must Remember*

Burden of genetic diseases in a community is determined by gene pool, breeding pattern and migration.

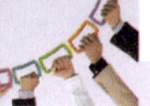

PREVENTION AND CONTROL OF GENETIC DISORDERS

Eugenics and Euthenics

- **Eugenics** is the science that aims to improve the genetic endowment of human population through breeding.
- The term 'Eugenics' was proposed by Sir Francis Galton.

Table 3: Types of eugenics their aims and limitations

Types	Aims	Measures	Limitations
Negative eugenics	Reduce frequency of hereditary disease and disability in community to as low as possible	Killing the weak and defective (Hitler in Germany), Sterilizing or debarring people suffering from serious hereditary diseases from producing children, Abortions	New cases of hereditary diseases will occur because of fresh mutations and partly because of marital alliances between hidden carriers (heterozygotes) of recessive defects
Positive eugenics	Improve genetic composition of population	Encouraging carriers of desirable genotypes to assume parenthood. (Very little application)	Majority of socially valuable traits (e.g. Intelligence) have a complex multifactorial determination, both genetic and environmental. We cannot determine which gene we transmit to our children

- **Euthenics** means environmental manipulation to give a suitable environment that will enable the genes to express themselves readily. The point of improving the human race using the advanced eugenic advancements will alone not suffice and mutual interaction with the environmental and hereditary factors may help for success in improved outcomes.

Genetic Counseling

Table 4: Prospective and retrospective genetic counseling

Prospective genetic counseling	Retrospective genetic counseling
Offered to individuals or couples who are at genetic risk	Offered to the couples, who report voluntarily after the birth of affected children
Counseling is provided before they develop symptoms or produce their first affected child.	Counseling about the probable risks associated with further pregnancies is given to couples
Diseases like thalassemia, sickle cell anemia and G6PD deficiency are prevented.	

- *Prevention of consanguineous marriages* (Marriage among blood relatives) to decrease the risk in offspring of traits controlled by recessive genes and polygenes. e.g. Albinism, Alkaptonuria, Phenylketonuria, etc.
- *Avoiding late marriages among women*- "Trisomy 21" is more frequent in children born to elderly mothers
- Avoiding *exposure* mutagens, such as X-rays, ionizing radiations and chemicals
- Immunization of reproductive age group females against rubella
- Immunization of Rh–ve mothers with anti-D globulin to prevent erythroblastosis fetalis
- Prenatal screening procedures may be carried out by ultrasonography, amniocentesis and chorionic villus sampling procedures.

Prenatal Diagnostics

Table 5: Prenatal diagnostic techniques and screening

Fetal age	Techniques	Tests	Genetic conditions diagnosed
10–11 weeks	Chorionic villus sampling	Chromosome analysis	**Chromosomal abnormalities**
		Biochemical assay	Metabolic disorders, Molecular defects
16 weeks	Amniocentesis	α-fetoprotein raised	Neural tube defects
		Chromosome analysis	**Chromosomal abnormalities**
		Biochemical assay	Metabolic disorders, Molecular defects
	Maternal serum screening (standard screening for "at risk" mothers)	Fetoprotein raised	**Neural tube defects**
		Quad test α-fetoprotein reduced Unconjugated estriol reduced hCG increased **Inhibin A increased**	**Down's syndrome**
18 weeks	**Ultrasound**		Structural abnormalities (heart, kidney, limbs, CVS)
2nd trimester	Fetoscopy		Structural abnormalities

- Indications for Prenatal diagnostic screening – Mother's age is >35 years, Previous child with mental abnormality/metabolic defect, parents with chromosomal translocation

Amniocentesis

Examination of a sample of amniotic fluid by amniocentesis is done as early as 14 weeks of pregnancy when abortion of the affected fetus is still possible. The diagnosis of chromosomal anomalies is done by culture and karyotyping of fetal cells from the amniotic fluid, and of metabolic defects by biochemical analysis of the fluid.

Indications for amniocentesis:

- Mother >35 years of age.
- Older child with Down's syndrome or other chromosomal anomalies.
- Parents known to have chromosomal translocation.
- Parents who have had a child with metabolic defect – detectable by amniocentesis.
- Detection of sex-linked genetic disease in couples with positive family history.

Treatment of Genetic Disorders

Table 6: Treatment of some genetic disorders

Diseases	Treatments
Phenylketonuria	Diet low in phenylalanine
Hemophilia	Factor VIII (antihemophilic globulin)
Spina bifida	Surgery
Galactosemia	Restriction of galactose
Lactase deficiency	Restriction of lactose
Agammaglobulinemia	Administration of gamma-globulin
Homocystinuria	Administration of pyridoxine
Maple syrup urine disease	Administration of thiamine
Hereditary spherocytosis	Splenectomy
Familial polyposis of colon	Colectomy
Adult polycystic kidney disease	Kidney transplantation
Gaucher's disease	Replacement of deficient enzyme α-glucosidase
Fam. Hypercholesterolemia	Diet low in Cholesterol
Cystic fibrosis	Pancreatic enzymes
Wilson's disease	Penicillamine
X-linked SCID	Bone marrow transplant

Population Screening for Genetic Diseases

Table 7: Some genetic population-screening services

Type of services	Conditions	Preventive or screening actions
Primary prevention	Rhesus hemolytic disease; Congenital rubella Congenital malformations	Postpartum use of Anti-D globulin Immunization of girls, Addition of folic acid to the maternal diet (may prevent neural tube defects), Control of maternal diabetes; Avoidance of mutagens and teratogens such as alcohol, certain drugs and possibly tobacco
Antenatal screening	Congenital malformations; Chromosomal abnormalities; Inherited disease	Ultrasound fetal anomaly scan, maternal serum alpha fetoprotein estimation; Noting maternal age and maternal serum factor levels Checking family history; Carrier screening for hemoglobinopathies, Tay-Sachs disease
Neonatal screening	Congenital malformations; Phenylketonuria, congenital hypothyroidism, sickle-cell disease	Examination of the newborn for early treatment (e.g., of congenital dislocation of the hip); Biochemical tests or early treatment

ADVANCES IN MOLECULAR GENETICS

GRAPH Int (Genome based Research and Population Health International) is an initiative to facilitate responsible and effective integration of genome-based knowledge/technology into public policies, program and services for improving health of populations.

- *Gene therapy* is introduction of a gene sequence into a cell using a virus (Retrovirus or Adenovirus) or by receptor targeting, to modify the cell's behavior in a clinically relevant fashion. E.g. Correcting a genetic mutation (cystic fibrosis), killing a cell (in cancer), etc.
- *Human genome project (1990):* It is an attempt to systematize the research on mapping and isolating human genes in order to create a single linear map of the human genome, with each coding gene defined and sequenced. Under James D Watson was an international, collaborative research aimed at complete mapping and understanding of human genome (Approximately 25,000 genes).
- *Human genome diversity project*: It aims to collect and preserve biologic samples (blood, cheek scrapings, saliva and hair roots) from hundreds of indigenous populations throughout the world on assumption that the indigenous populations are going to disappear to explore genetic diversity. The samples collected will be immortalized.
- *Dysgenics* is progressive evolutionary weakening or deterioration of a population of organisms relative to environment.

GENETIC EPIDEMIOLOGY

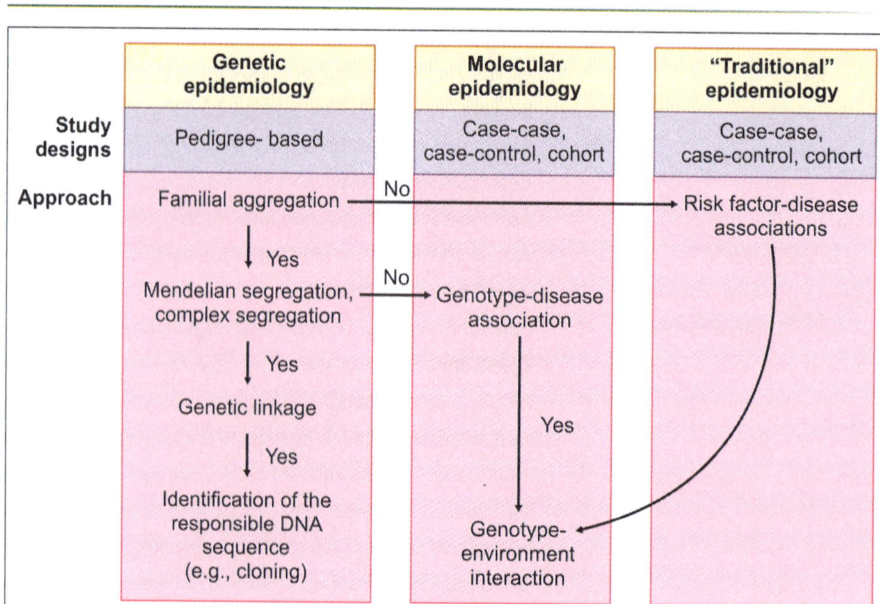

Types of Studies Based on Genetic Research Methods

- **Familial aggregation studies**: This is method to study if there is any genetic component to the disease, and what are the relative contributions of genes and environment?
- **Segregation studies**: What is the pattern of inheritance of the disease, (e.g. dominant or recessive) Linkage studies: On which part of which chromosome is the disease gene located?
- **Association studies**: Which allele of which gene is associated with the disease?

Pedigree Chart Symbols

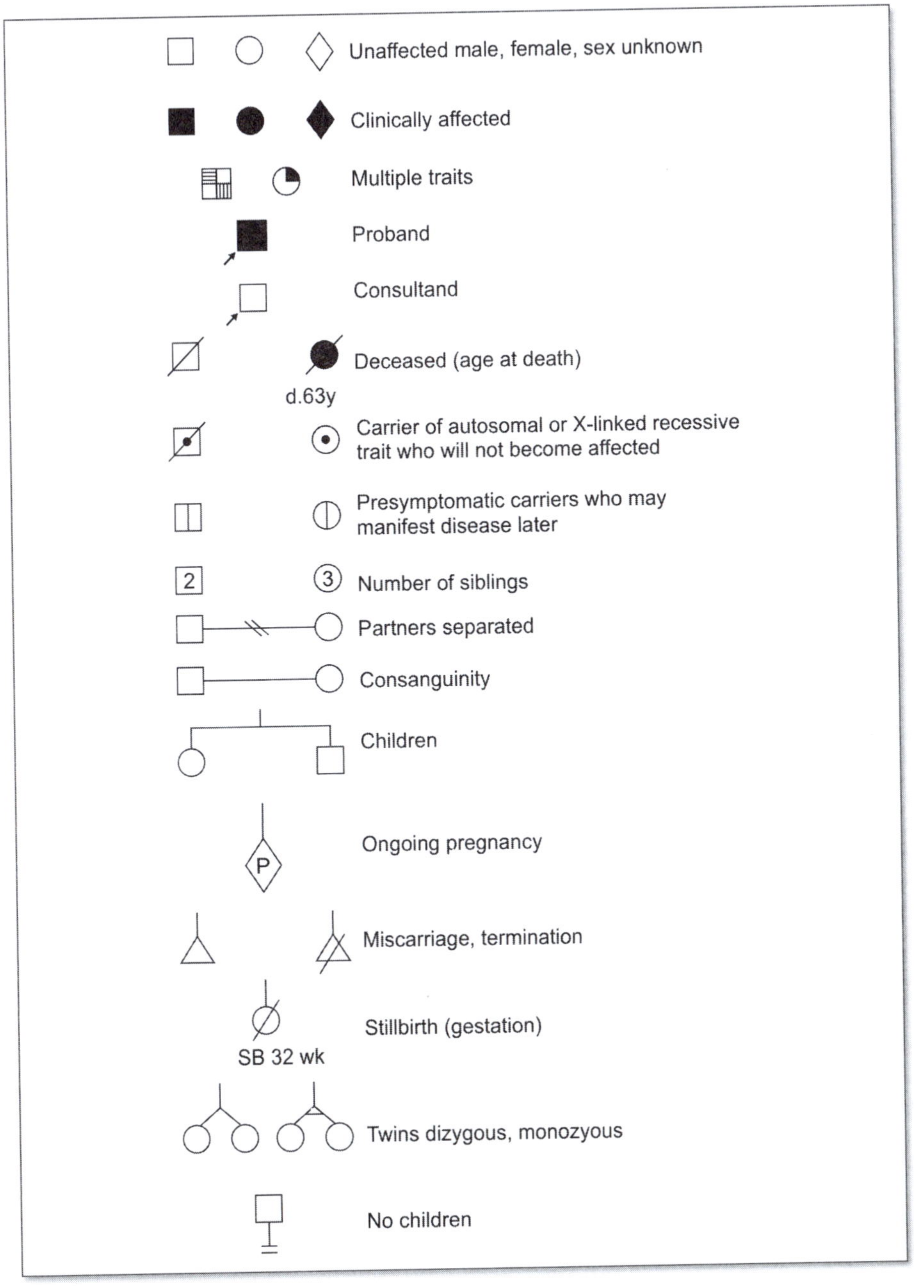

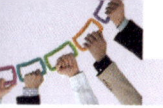

Multiple Choice Questions

1. **Which of the following methods prevent marriage between two heterozygous individuals for the same disorder:**
   a. Retrospective genetic counseling *(Recent Question 2017)*
   b. Prospective genetic counseling
   c. Legislation
   d. Mass health education
2. **X chromosome is classified under which group:**
   a. A b. C
   c. E d. G
3. **Peptic ulcer is associated with the following blood group:**
   a. O b. A
   c. B d. AB
4. **Hardy-Weinberg law deals with:** *(Recent Question 2017)*
   a. Molecular genetics
   b. Population genetics
   c. Human genome project
   d. Human genome diversity project
5. **Hardy Weinberg law is related to:** *(Recent Question 2017)*
   a. Gene therapy
   b. Human genome project
   c. Population genetics
   d. Eugenics
6. **All of the following affect the equilibrium in Hardy Weinberg law, except:**
   a. Small population
   b. Random mating
   c. Mutations
   d. Gene outflow
7. **Which is not a X linked disorder?** *(Recent Question 2016)*
   a. Wilson's disease b. Hemophilia
   c. Thalassemia d. G6PD deficiency
   e. ABO blood group system
8. **Effect of environment on genes is called:**
   a. Positive eugenics b. Negative eugenics
   c. Euthenics d. Enthenics
9. **Punnett Square is used for:** *(Recent Question 2016)*
   a. Statistical analysis
   b. Testing significance
   c. Random sampling
   d. Genotype determination in offspring
10. **Mentally retarded child with reasonable education and unskilled work without supervision:**
    a. Mild MR b. Moderate MR
    c. Severe MR d. Profound MR
11. **Most common drug abused in India is:**
    a. Cannabis indica b. Tobacco
    c. Heroine d. Amphetamine
12. **Mental age of a 6 year old child is 4 calculate IQ.**
    a. 150 b. 100
    c. 75 d. 66
13. **IQ of a child with mild mental retardation will be between:**
    a. 90–100 b. 71–90
    c. 50–70 d. 35–49
14. **IQ in profound mental retardation is:**
    a. 50–70 b. 35–50
    c. 20–35 d. <20
15. **IQ in severe mental retardation:** *(Recent Question 2016)*
    a. 50–70 b. 35–49
    c. 20–34 d. < 20
16. **Chronological age of 10 years and a mental age of 4 year, then the person is:**
    a. Idiot b. Imbecile
    c. Normal d. Genius
17. **If the mental age is 8 and chronological age is 10, the child is having:** *(Recent Question 2015)*
    a. No mental retardation
    b. Mild mental retardation
    c. Moderate mental retardation
    d. Severe mental retardation
18. **Which of the following regarding IQ is not true:**
    a. Idiot: IQ of 0–24 *(Recent Question 2014)*
    b. Imbecile: IQ of 25–49
    c. Moron: IQ of 50–69
    d. Borderline: IQ of 71–90
19. **WHO classifies mental retardation into four categories: mild, moderate, severe and profound. IQ range in moderate MR is:**
    a. 35-49 b. 20-34
    c. 50-69 d. 70-90
20. **An IQ = 51 is a case of:**
    a. Mild MR b. Moderate MR
    c. Severe MR d. Profound MR
21. **Average mental IQ according to Wechsler's scale is:**
    a. 70-79 b. 80-89
    c. 90-109 d. 110-119
22. **Mild mental retardation does not include IQ level(s):**
    a. 45 b. 55
    c. 65 d. 75
    e. 85
23. **IQ is calculated using the formula:**
    a. Mental age/chronological age × 100
    b. Mental age –chronological age × 100
    c. Chronological age/mental age × 100
    d. Chronological age – mental age × 100
24. **For mental retardation, IQ = 20-34 is:**
    a. Severe MR *(Recent Question 2013)*
    b. Profound MR
    c. Moderate MR
    d. Mild MR

Ans.

1. b
2. b
3. a
4. b
5. c
6. b
7. a, c, e
8. c
9. d
10. a
11. a
12. d
13. None
14. d
15. c
16. b
17. a
18. d
19. a
20. a
21. c
22. a, d, e
23. a
24. a

Most Recent Questions of 2019-18 are given at the end of MCQs

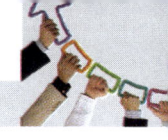

Most Recent Questions (2019–2018)

25. Which of the following is an incorrect match pair *(PGI Nov 2018)*

	Disease	Chromosome abnormality
a.	Patau Syndrome	Trisomy 18
b.	Edwards Syndrome	Trisomy 13
c.	Prader-Willi Syndrome	Deletion on Chromosome 15
d.	Downs syndrome	Trisomy 21
e.	Cri-du-chat Syndrome	Translocation on chromosome 9

26. Which of the following is/are true for down syndrome *(PGI Nov 2018)*

a. Higher risk in case the maternal age more than 35 years
b. Higher risk in case the paternal age more than 35 years
c. Most commonly due to translocation on chromosome 21
d. Cardiac defects and atresia of G tract are common complications
e. Translocation downs syndrome may be inherited

27. What is the study design used for consanguineous marriage and genetic abnormalities? *(JIPMER Nov 2018)*

a. Ecological study
b. Family pedigree study
c. Case control study
d. Twin study

Ans.

25. a, b, e
26. a, d, e
27. b

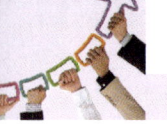

Answers with Explanations

1. Ans. (b) Prospective genetic counseling

Ref: K. Park, 24th ed. p 865

Genetic counseling is a process of communication and education that addresses concerns relating to the development and/or transmission of a hereditary disorder.

- Person seeking genetic counseling is known as "consultand"
- It is *non directive.* Consultand make their own decisions.
- The counsellor tries to provide the consultand with information that enables him/her to understand:
  - Medical diagnosis, prognosis and possible treatment
  - Mode of inheritance of the disorder and Risk of developing and/or transmitting it
  - Choices or options available for dealing with the risks
- Types of genetic counseling:
  - **Prospective:** It involves identification of heterozygous individuals for any particular defect (e.g. Sickle cell anemia, Thalassemia) by screening and counseling them on risk of having affected children if they marry another heterozygote for same gene.
  - **Retrospective:** It is genetic counseling when the hereditary disorder has already occurred within family. Methods suggested are contraception, pregnancy termination, sterilization

Also Know......................

Most genetic counseling at present is Retrospective

2. Ans. (b) C

Ref: K. Park, 24th ed. p 857

Autosomes are classified into 7 groups based on the length and morphological similarities:

- Group A - 1 to 3 pairs
- Group B - 4 and 5 pairs
- Group C - 6 to 12 pairs
- Group D - 13 to 15 pairs
- Group E - 16 to 18 pairs
- Group F - 19 and 20 pairs
- Group G - 21 and 22 pairs

X chromosome is included in Group C and Y chromosome in Group G

3. Ans. (a) O

Ref: K. Park, 24th ed. p 861

Blood Group Diseases

O - Duodenal ulcer, Gastric ulcer, Hemolytic diseases*
A - Stomach cancer, Pernicious anemia*, Carcinoma of uterine cervix*, Thrombosis.*

*** Suspected Association**

4. Ans. (b) Population genetics

Ref: K. Park, 24th ed. p 864

Population genetics is the study of genetic composition [gene pool] of the population and factors which operate to alter the "gene pool" and their long-term consequences that determine incidence of inherited traits.

- It is based on ***Hardy-Weinberg law*** given by Hardy (England) and Weinberg (Germany) in 1908.
- It states that the relative frequency of each gene allele tends to remain constant from generation to generation in absence of disturbing forces that change gene frequencies.

Also Know......................

- Hardy-Weinberg law assumes that human gene pool is static, infinitely large and random mating. Whereas in reality human population gene pool is never static

5. Ans. (c) Population genetics

Ref: K. Park, 24th ed. p 864

6. Ans. (b) Random mating

Ref: K. Park, 24th ed. p 864

Factors influencing gene frequency equilibrium in Hardy Weinberg law:

- Mutation
- Natural selection (*Survival of the fittest)* proposed by ***Darwin***. Harmful genes are eliminated from gene pool and genes favorable to an individual tend to be preserved and passed on to the offspring.
- Population Movements lead to intermixing of people and new genetic combinations.
- Assortative (Non Random) mating: Selective mating within subgroups based on religion, economic and educational status disturbs genetic equilibrium. [E.g. Doctors marry doctors or nurses; musicians marry musicians].
- Public Health Measures: by saving more lives, decrease selection rates and increase genetic burden.

7. Ans. (a) Wilson's disease (c) Thalassemia (e) ABO blood group system

Ref: K. Park, 24th ed. p 860

Refer to Annexure-16.1

Thalassemia is a disorder characterized by reduction in globin chain synthesis (α Thalassemia is due to gene deletion and β Thalassemia is due to point mutations)

8. Ans. (c) Euthenics

Ref: K. Park, 24th ed. p 865

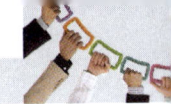

Euthenics

- Environmental manipulation to give a suitable environment that will enable the genes to express themselves readily.
- Improving human race involves mutual interaction of heredity and environmental factors.
- A mentally retarded (mild) child's exposure to environmental stimulation improves their IQ.

9. Ans. (d) Genotype determination in offspring

Ref: Internet

Punnet Square is a chart that predicts all possible gene combination in a cross breeding of parents with known genotype.
Named on English geneticist –Reginald Punnett.

10. Ans. (a) Mild MR

Ref: Jean-François Lemay, Anthony R Herbert et al. A rational approach to the child with mental retardation for the paediatrician. Paediatr Child Health. 2003 Jul-Aug; 8(6): 345–356.

Category of Mental Retardation	Prognosis
Mild	Often acquire social and vocational skills adequate for minimum self-support [May need supervision and assistance, especially when under stress]
Moderate	Acquire communication skills during early childhood years. May learn to travel independently to familiar places. In adult years are able to perform unskilled or semiskilled work under supervision
Severe	May learn to talk during the school years and can be trained in elementary self-care skills. In the adult years, they can perform simple tasks in closely supervised settings.

11. Ans. (a) Cannabis indica

Ref: K. Park, 24th ed. p 871

Drug abuse refers to self-administration of a drug for non-medical reasons, in quantities and frequencies which may impair an individual's ability to function effectively and which may result in social, physical or emotional harm.

- Alcohol is the only drug whose self-induced intoxication is socially acceptable.
- Cannabis is the most common drug abused today [Forms are Bhang, Charas, Ganja Marijuana]
- Heroin-Worst type of addiction

Dependence producing drug (ICD 10)- Alcohol, Opioids, Cannabinoids, Sedatives or hypnotics, Cocaine etc.

Also Know.......................

- ***Superman drugs*** → Amphetamines and cocaine- give a tremendous boost to self-confidence and energy while increasing endurance.
- ***Wrong drug*** → It has no legitimate use, but causes potential damages that are extremely high no matter how or when they are taken. To use these drugs is to abuse them e.g. Brown sugar.

12. Ans. (d) 66

Ref: K. Park, 24th ed. p 716

IQ = Mental Age/ Chronological age × 100 = 4/6 × 100 = 66.5

13. Ans. (c) 50-70

Ref: K. Park, 24th ed. p 618

14. Ans. (d) <20

Ref: K. Park, 23rd ed. p 582

WHO Classification of Mental Retardation[Q]

- Mild mental retardation – IQ – 50-70
- Moderate mental retardation- IQ – 35-49
- Severe mental retardation – IQ – 20-34
- Profound mental retardation – IQ - < 20

15. Ans. (c) 20 - 34

Ref: K. Park, 23rd ed. p 582

16. Ans. (b) Imbecile

Ref: K. Park, 23rd ed. p 679

IQ = (Mental Age/Chronological age) × 100

Levels of Intelligence	IQ Range
Idiot	0-24
Imbecile	25-49
Moron	50-69
Border Line	70-79
Low normal	80-89
Normal	90-109
Superior	110-119
Very Superior	120-139
Near Genius	140 and over

17. Ans. (a) No mental retardation

Ref: K. Park, 24th ed. p 618, 716

IQ = (Mental Age/ Chronological age) × 100 = 8/10 × 100 = 80.0

18. Ans. (d) Borderline: IQ of 71–90

Ref: K. Park, 24th ed. p 618

19. Ans. (a) 35-49

Ref: K. Park, 24th ed. p 618

20. Ans. (a) Mild MR

Ref: K. Park, 24th ed. p 716

21. Ans. (c) 90-109

Ref: www.assessment psychology.com

Wechsler Adult Intelligence Scale [3rd Edition, 1997]

Scale of Intelligence	IQ Levels
Very Superior	≥130
Superior	120–129
High Average	110–119
Average	90–109
Low Average	80–89
Borderline	70–79
Extremely Low	≤69

22. Ans. (a) 45; (d) 75; (e) 85

Ref: K. Park, 24th ed. p 618

23. Ans. (a) Mental age/chronological age × 100

Ref: K. Park, 24th ed. p 716

24. Ans. (a) Severe MR

Ref: K. Park, 24th ed. p 716

25. Ans. (a, b, e)

Syndrome	Chromosomal abnormality	"Karyotype"
Down syndrome	Trisomy 21 type	47, XX, + 21
	Translocation type	46, XX, 14, +t (14;21)
	Mosaic type	46, XX/47, XX, +21
Turner syndrome	Monosomy X	45,X
Klinefelter syndrome		46, XXY or XXXY or XY/XXY mosaic
Edwards' syndrome	Trisomy 18 type	47,XX/ + 18
	Mosaic type	46,XX/47, XX, + 18

Contd...

Syndrome	Chromosomal abnormality	"Karyotype"
Patau syndrome	Trisomy 13 type	47,XX/+13
	Translocation type	46,XX/–14, +t(14:13)
	Mosaic type	46,XX/47,XX/+13
Trisomy 9 Mosaicism syndrome	Trisomy 9	47,XY,+9
Cri-du-chat syndrome	Deletion	del (5 p 15)
Wolf–Hirschhorn syndrome	Deletion	del (4pl4)
Trisomy 8	Trisomy 8	
	Mosaic	
Prader–Willi and Angelman syndromes	Deletion	47, XX. + 8 46, XX/47, XX, + 8 Del 15 (11;13)

26. Ans. (a) Higher risk in case the maternal age more than 35 years, (d) Cardiac defects and atresia of G tract are common complications, (e) Translocation downs syndrome may be inherited

Ref: Park 25th pg 883

Downs syndrome:

Genetic variations of Down's syndrome:

- Trisomy 21 (> 95% of all Down's syndrome – most common form of Down's)
- Translocation 21 (rare)
- Mosaic 21 (very rare) – includes mosaic of trisomy 21 and abnormal translocations on chromosome 21

Risk factors:

- Higher maternal age > 35 years
- Parent is carrier of translocation 21 chromosome – unbalanced transmission of the translocation 21 chromosome may lead to inherited Down's Syndrome
- Previous child with down's syndrome

Complications with Down's

- Typical Down's facies – small round head, tilted eye slits, malformed ears
- Cardiac defects, GI atresia, obesity, immunological deficiencies, leukaemia, dementia

27. Ans. (b) Family pedigree study

A simple family pedigree analysis may show how genetic disorders are inherited in a family. They can use this to work out the probability that someone in a family will inherit a condition

Section

C

Public Health

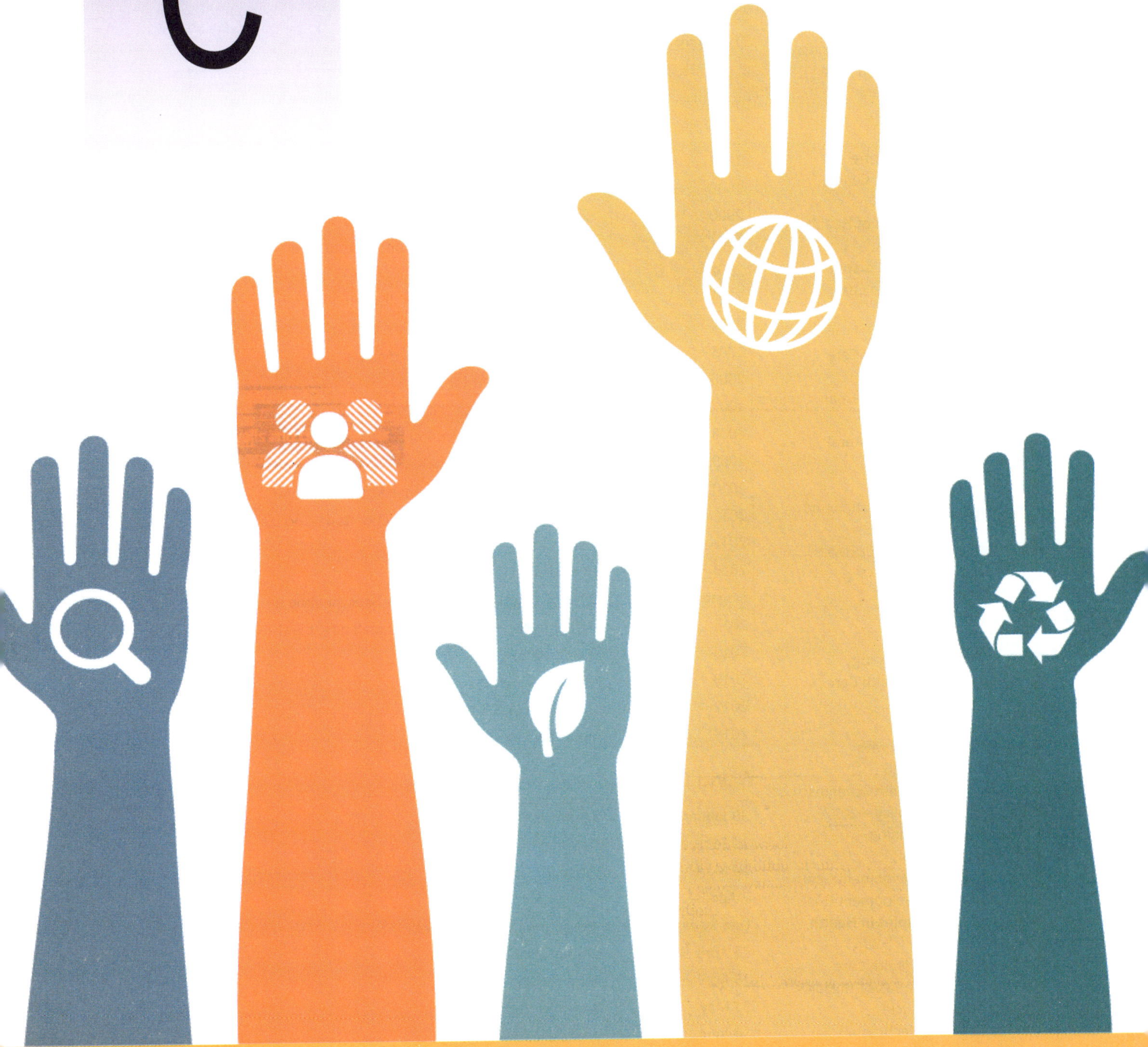

Health Planning and Health Care Management

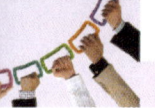

Chapter Outline

PRINCIPLES OF HEALTH CARE AND PLANNING

HEALTH CARE PLANNING

World Health Day

Themes—All in One

1995	Global polio eradication
1996	Healthy cities for better life
1997	Emerging infectious diseases
1998	Safe motherhood
1999	Active aging makes the difference
2000	Safe blood start with me
2001	Mental health: Stop Exclusion, Dare to care
2002	Move for Health
2003	Shape the future of Life: Healthy Environment for children
2004	Road safety
2005	Make every mother and child count
2006	Working together for health
2007	International health security
2008	Protecting health from the adverse effect of climate change
2009	Save lives, Make hospitals safe in emergencies
2010	Urbanization and health: make cities healthier
2011	Antimicrobial resistance: no action today, no cure tomorrow
2012	Good health adds life to years
2013	Hypertension
Slogans	BP-Take control; Healthy heart beat, healthy BP
2014	Vector borne disease Slogan: Small bite, big threat
2015	Food safety
2016	Diabetes : Beat the diabetes
2017	Depression, Let's talk
2018	Universal health coverage

World Days

30 January	World Leprosy Day
10 February	National Deworming Day
24 March	World TB Day
7 April	World Health Day
Last week of April	World Immunization Week
25 April	World Malaria Day
25 April 2016	Polio switch Day
31 May	World No Tobacco Day
14 June	World Blood Donor Day
28 July	World Hepatitis Day
28 September	World Rabies Day
24 October	World Polio Day
10 October	World Mental Health Day
1 December	World AIDS Day

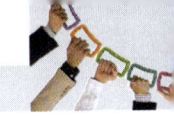

World Health Day 2019—Universal Health Coverage—Everyone, Everywhere

Slogan

- Inspire—Motivate—Guide
- All people to receive health care without financial hardships
- Access to good quality health care.
- **Inspire**—by highlighting policy-makers' power to transform the health of their nation, framing the challenge as exciting and ambitious, and inviting them to be part of the change.
- **Motivate**—by sharing examples of how countries are already progressing towards UHC and encourage others to find their own path.
- **Guide**—by providing tools for structured policy dialogue on how to advance UHC domestically or supporting such efforts in other countries (e.g. expanding service coverage, improving quality of services, reducing out-of-pocket payments).

EVOLUTION OF HEALTH CARE IN INDIA

Health related committees and recommendations have been summarized in the table below.

Table 1: Different committees and their recommendations for health care

Committee	Recommendation
Bhore Committee, 1946 *[Health Survey and Development Committee]*	▪ Comprehensive [Preventive, Promotive Curative] health care at PHC level. 1 PHC per 40000 population with 30 beds ▪ 3 months training in PSM- Social Physicians[Q] ▪ *3 Million Plan*[Q](Development of PHC in 2 stages: Short-term and Long-term)
Chopra Committee [1948]	▪ Integrating the several systems of medicine with allopathic system and evolution of an integrated system of medical education.
Balwant Rai Mehta Committee [1957]	▪ Recommended setting up of 3 Tier system of Panchayati Raj at village, block and district level
Mudaliar Committee, 1962 *[Health Survey and Planning Committee]*	▪ Strengthening of district hospital with specialist services ▪ Regional organizations in each state between headquarters and district ▪ Each PHC not to serve more than 40,000 population ▪ Improve the quality of health care provided by the PHC ▪ Integration of medical and health services ▪ *Constitution of an All India Health Service on pattern of IAS.*[Q]
Chadha Committee, 1963	▪ General health services to be responsible for vigilance operations [by monthly home visits] w.r.t. National Malaria Eradication Program ▪ 1 Basic Health Worker per 10,000 population. Duty of collection of vital statistics and family planning, in addition to malaria vigilance. ▪ Family Planning Health Assistants to supervise 3 or 4 basic health workers.
Mukherjee Committee, 1965	▪ Separate staff for family planning program and to delink the malaria activities from family planning.
Jain Committee, 1966	▪ 1 bed per 1000 population, 50 beds hospital at taluka level ▪ Health insurance for large population coverage
Jungalwalla Committee, 1967 *[Committee on Integration of Health Services]*	▪ Integration of health services with unified cadre and common seniority ▪ Recognition of extra qualifications ▪ Equal pay for equal work and special pay for specialized work ▪ No private practice and good service conditions.
Kartar Singh committee, 1973	▪ Male and Female Multipurpose Health Workers. ▪ 1 PHC for a population of 50,000 with 16 SC each for 3,000 to 3,500 population.
[Committee on Multipurpose Workers under Health and Family Planning]	▪ Each Subcenter [SC] to be staffed by a 1 male and 1 female health worker ▪ A male health supervisor to supervise the work of 3 to 4 male health workers and female health supervisor to supervise the work of 4 female health workers ▪ Lady health vision (LHV) to be designated as Female Health Supervisor
Shrivastav Committee, 1975 *'Group on Medical Education and Support Manpower'*	▪ Creation of bands of para-professional and semi-professional health workers from within the community (e.g., school teachers, postmasters) to provide simple, promotive, preventive and curative health services - ***Rural Health Scheme***[Q]

Contd...

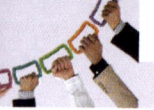

Committee	Recommendation
	▪ 2 cadres of health workers, MHW and HA (Health Assistant) between community level workers and medical officer at PHC ▪ Develop a 'Referral Services Complex' between PHC and higher level centers ▪ Medical and Health Education Commission on lines of the UGC. ▪ Concept of Village Health Guide ▪ ROME scheme [*Reorientation of medical education*]
Krishnan committee, 1983	▪ Revamping of Primary urban health services– Health posts in urban slums. ▪ Basic health and Family welfare services to be made available within 1–3 km of dwelling, with appropriate link to secondary and tertiary care centers
Bajaj Committee, 1986 *'Expert committee for Health Manpower Planning, Production and Management'.*	▪ Formulation of a national medical and health education policy ▪ Formulation of a national health manpower policy ▪ Establishment of health science universities. ▪ Vocationalization of education at 10 + 2 level with regards to health. ▪ Carry out realistic health manpower survey.

> 48 *Good to Remember*
>
> Primary health care is "essential health care made universally accessible to individuals and acceptable to them, through their full participation and at a cost the community and country can afford."[Q]
> - Primary health care is the key to the attainment of health for all by 2000 AD.[Q]
> - It came into existence in 1978, following an international conference at Alma-Ata (USSR).[Q]

LEVELS OF HEALTH CARE IN INDIA

Levels of Health Care – (3 Levels)

- **Primary care level**
  - 1st level of contact of individuals, family and community with the national health system[Q]
  - Primary health care is provided by Primary health center and Sub center.[Q]
- **Secondary (Intermediate) care level**
  - Provided in district hospitals and CHC[Q] which also serve as the First referral units [FRU]
  - Specialist services are available [Medicine, Surgery, Obs & Gyn, Pediatrics]
- **Tertiary care level**
  - More specialized and sophisticated care and attention of highly specialized health workers.

Provided by the regional or central level institutions, e.g., Medical College Hospitals, All India Institutes, Regional Hospitals, Specialized Hospitals and other Apex Institutions.[Q]

Primary Health Care

- It is the essential health care made universally accessible to all sectors of community.
- The **hallmarks of primary health care** are (4As)
  - Accessible
  - Available
  - Acceptable
  - Affordable
- The **principles of primary health care** are (TICE)
  - Community participation
  - Intersectoral coordination
  - Technology use
  - Equitable distribution
- The **Elements of Primary health care** (ELEMENTS)
  - E – education for health and disease prevention
  - L – locally endemic disease prevention
  - E – EPI – expanded program for immunization and prevention of vaccine preventable disease
  - M – maternal and child health care
  - E – essential drugs to be provided for secondary prevention
  - N – nutritional diseases to be prevented
  - T – treatment for common disease and accidents
  - S – safe water supply, hygiene and sanitation

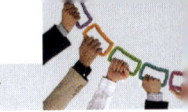

Subcenter

As per population norms, there shall be one Subcenter established for every 5000 population in plain areas and for every 3000 population in hilly/tribal/desert areas.

Type A Subcenter

- Located in remote, difficult, hilly or tribal area
- No/poor infrastructure to conduct delivery in the subcenter.
- Expected number of deliveries with birth rate 30 per month would be approximately 12 deliveries per month
- Poor referral services

Type B Subcenter (MCH Subcenter)

- Better facility and better connectivity of the subcenter
- Good case load of deliveries
- They provide reasonable RCH, MCH and neonatal care with outreach services
- They are expected to conduct more than 20 deliveries per month.

Table 2: Manpower for subcenters

Type of subcenter	Subcenter A		Subcenter B (MCH Subcenter)	
Staff	Essential	Desirable	Essential	Desirable
ANM/Health worker (Female)	1	+1	2	
Health worker (Male)	1		1	
Staff nurse (or ANM, if staff nurse is not available)				1**
Safai-Karamchari*	1 (Part-time)		1 (Full-time)	

*To be outsourced

**If number of deliveries at the Subcenter is 20 or more in a month

Primary Health Center

The 6th Five-year Plan (1983–88) proposed reorganization of PHCs on the basis of one PHC for every 30,000 rural populations in the plains and one PHC for every 20,000 population in hilly, tribal and desert areas for more effective coverage

Type A PHC → Delivery load less than 20/month

Type B PHC → Delivery load of 20 or more per month

Table 3: Proposed reorganization for primary health center

Staff	Type A		Type B	
	Essential	Desirable	Essential	Desirable
Medical officer-MBBS	1		1	1#
Medical officer-AYUSH		1*		1*
Accountant cum data operator	1		1	
Pharmacist	1		1	
Nurse-midwife (Staff-Nurse)	3	+1**	4	+1**
Health worker (Female)	1*		1*	
Health assistant (Male)	1		1	
Health assistant (Female)/Lady health visitor	1		1	
Health educator		1		1
Laboratory technician	1		1	
Cold chain and vaccine logistic assistant		1		1
Multi-skilled group D worker	2		2	
Sanitary worker cum watchman	1		1	+1
Total	13	18	14	21

* For subcenter area of PHC.

**To provide choices to the people wherever an AYUSH public facility is not available in the near vicinity. PHC are referral center for 6 Subcenter

#If the delivery case load is 30 or more per month. One of the two medical officers (MBBS) should be female.

High Yield Points

Health for all 2000 is an attainment of a level of health that will enable every individual to lead a socially and economically productive life.[Q]

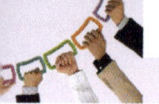

Community Health Center

- Has a staff of 46-52 personnel
- It is for a population of
  - Hilly/tribal/forest areas – 80,000 population
  - Plains – 120,000 population
- Beds strength in CHC – up to 30 beds
- Staffing pattern in CHC
  - Specialists
    - Medicine
    - Surgery
    - Obs and gyne
    - Pediatrics
    - Anesthesia
    - Ophthalmology (preferable)
    - Public health
  - Medical officer
    - Incharge
    - AYUSH
    - Dental
    - General duty MO
  - ANMs, staff nurses, laboratory technicians, radiographers, pharmacists, health workers and other staff

Norms under the IPHS (2016-2017 Update)

IPHS – Indian public health standards

Table 4: Desirable norms to staff of health centers and kits available

Health centers	Norm	Staff	Kits available
Subcenter (SC) (No. of SC In India 1,55,069 [2016])-100% Central Govt. Assistance #	▪ 1 for every 5000 population in plains[Q] and 3000 population in hilly, tribal and backward areas[Q]	Health worker male [MPW] and Health worker female. Volunteer worker (Optional) Total = 34	A, B and C
Primary Health Center (PHC)- Integrated curative and preventive health care (No. of PHC In India 25,354 [2016)-Maintained by State Govt.	▪ 1 for every 30000 population in plains[Q] and 20000 population in hilly, tribal and backward areas[Q] ▪ 6 bedded	Medical Officer: 1 Health assistant male-1 Health assistant female-1 Health educator-1 ANM, LDC, UDC, LT, Pharmacist, Staff nurse, Driver-1 each, *Class IV-4* **Total = 13-14/18-21***	D
Community Health Center (CHC) *Specialist care[Q] (No. of CHC in India 5510 [2016]) Maintained by State Govt.*	▪ *1 for a population of 80000 to 1,20,000[Q]* ▪ 30 bedded[Q]	Specialist doctors- 4 (Surgery, Medicine, Obs and Gyn, Pediatrics-1 each) Ophthalmic surgeon -1 Anesthetist -1, Public Health Manager-1 **Total = 46/52***	E, F G H, I, J, K, L, M, N, O and P

*Desirable as per IPHS (Revised 2012). ROME Scheme–3 PHC have been attached to each medical college#

Only salary of Male Health Worker is borne by state Govt.

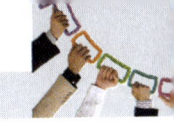

NORMS AND FUNCTIONS OF HEALTH CARE PROFESSIONALS

Norms for Health Personal

Table 5: National strategy for health for all (HFA) 2000

Health worker	Population covered[a]	Level[a]
AWW (ICDS)—4 months training	400–800 in plain, 300–800 in hill/tribal area	Village
ASHA (NRHM)—23 days training	1000	Village
Village Health Guide—200 hours training in 3 months	1000	Village
Trained Dai	1 in each village	Village
USHA [NUHM]	2500	Urban areas
MPW [Male/Female]	5000 [3000 hill/tribal]	SC
Health Assistant [Male/Female]	30000 [20000 hill/tribal]	PHC

Table 6: Suggested norms for health personnel

Category of personnel	Norms suggested
▪ Nurses	1 per 5,000 population
▪ Health worker female and male	1 per 5,000 population in plain area and 3,000 population in tribal and hilly areas
▪ Trained dai	One for each village
▪ Health assistant (male and female)	1 per 30,000 population in plain area and 20,000 population in tribal and hilly areas. Provides supportive supervision to 6 health workers (male/female)
▪ Pharmacists	1 per 10,000 population
▪ Laboratory technicians	1 per 10,000 population
▪ ASHA	1 per 1,000 population

Functions of Health Care Workers

Table 7: Job profile of health care workers staff

Staff	Job profile
Health worker female [HW (F)] (covers 350–500 families)	▪ Maternal and Child Health • **Antenatal care**—Ensure 4 ANC visits. Test for hemoglobin, urine • **Health education** to mother on family planning, nutrition, immunization, control of communicable disease and personal + environmental hygiene • **Natal care**—Conduct and supervise deliveries by dais. Refer complicated cases. • **Postnatal care**—Minimum 2 postnatal visits and render advice (IYCF = infant and young child feeding). • Assist MO and Health Assistant (Female) in antenatal/postnatal clinic at subcenter ▪ Family planning • Maintain and update eligible couple register, distribute contraceptives and establish female depot holders, health education on family planning, follow-up services and attend Mahila Mandal meetings ▪ MTP • Identify women who need MTP services and refer, to authorized center. ▪ Nutrition • Health education, distribute IFA, administer vitamin A to children, identify malnutrition in infants and young child and give treatment/advice/referral ▪ Immunization • TT in pregnant women, Vaccination of children as per immunization schedule, Injection safety ▪ DAI training • List dais, assist HA (F) in their training, utilize their services for family welfare ▪ Communicable disease • Notify abnormal rise in cases to MO, assist HW(M), educate/counsel/follow-up • Vital events—Record and Report to health authorities • Record keeping—Eligible couple register, register of pregnant women/infant/distribution of ORS, Condom • Treatment of minor ailments—First aid and ISM medicines, referral • Team activities—Coordinate with HA (F), ASHA, AWW, PRI. Attend staff meeting, Cleanliness at SC and disposal of medical waste

Contd...

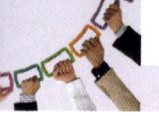

Staff	Job profile
Health worker male [HW (M)]	▪ Record keeping • Survey and maintain records (vital events, immunization, etc.), maps, vital event ▪ National Health Program • Malaria—Active surveillance (Fortnightly), collect thick/thin blood smear, radical treatment for positive cases • Identify and refer cases of Kala-azar, JE, Filariasis, Leprosy, TB (Collect sputum samples/Ensure treatment compliance), Blindness to MO (PHC) and provide health education. ▪ Immunization – administer vaccines ▪ RCH • Distribute contraceptives, ORS, Health education on family planning, Follow-up services to male family planning acceptors, Identify male leaders, educate on MTP • Report outbreak of diarrhea and home based management of diarrhea ▪ Environment sanitation • Chlorination of drinking water source, encourage use of latrines, stress on sanitation ▪ Communicable diseases—Identify and refer to MO, educate/counsel/follow-up of cases ▪ Nutrition • Health education, identify malnourished infants and young children and give treatment/advice/referral ▪ Treatment of minor ailments—First aid and ISM medicines, referral
Health assistant male [HA (M)]	▪ Malaria—Supervise work of HW (M), Check minimum 10% houses in a village, collect thick and thin smears from fever case. Administer radical treatment to positive cases. Supervise spraying of insecticides ▪ Communicable disease—Remain alert on outbreak of epidemics and take necessary control measures ▪ Leprosy and TB—Ensure regular and complete treatment and inform MO of defaulters to treatment. ▪ Environmental Sanitation—Help in construction of safe water source, Soakage pit, sanitary latrine, smokeless chulha ▪ Immunization—Conduct and supervise immunization of children 1–5 years ▪ Family planning—Guide HW (M) to establish male depot holders. Assist MO (PHC) in Family planning camps, provide information on MTP and follow-up of vasectomy/tubectomy case ▪ Nutrition—Ensure necessary treatment/advise/referral for malnutrition cases in infants and young children (0–5 years), IFA, vitamin A to beneficiaries ▪ Blindness control—Referral of all cases of cataract to MO (PHC)
Health assistant female	▪ Supervision and guidance • Enhancement of knowledge, skills, Planning and organizing activities of HW (F) • Visit each Subcenter at least once a week, supervisory home visits in area of HW (F). ▪ Coordinate her activities with HA (M), Dais, workers of other departments, Conduct regular staff meetings with health workers in coordination with the HA (M), Attend staff meetings at PHC, Block level, Participate as a member of the health team in mass camps and campaigns and assist MO (PHC) ▪ Check stores and procure supplies, equipment. Maintain subcenter ▪ Records and reports—Review reports of HW (F), consolidate and submit to MO (PHC). ▪ Kala-azar/Lymphatic filariasis/JE— • Check minimum 10% of the houses in a village, Ensure complete treatment, complete coverage during spray activities and search operation and Health education activities. ▪ MCH—Conduct weekly MCH clinics at each Subcenter conduct deliveries at PHC ▪ Family welfare and MTP—Conduct weekly family welfare clinics, Guide HW (F) in establishing female depot holders, spot checking eligible couple register. IUD services, assist MO (PHC) in family planning camps. ▪ Nutrition—Identify cases of malnutrition in children (0–5 years), give treatment/advice/refer. Ensure IFA, vitamin A distribution. Educate expectant mother on breastfeeding. ▪ Immunization—Supervise the immunization of all pregnant women and children (0–5) years. ▪ Acute respiratory infection—Ensure early diagnosis/treatment/referral ▪ School Health—Help medical officer in school health services. ▪ Treatment for minor ailments, first aid for accidents and attend referred cases by HW. ▪ Health education

Table 8: Population covered and levels of health workers

Health worker	Population covered[Q]	Level[Q]
AWW (ICDS)—4 months training	400–800 in plain, 300–800 in hill/ tribal area	Village
ASHA (NRHM)—23 days training	1000	Village
Village Health Guide—200 hours training in 3 months	1000	Village
Trained Dai	1 in each village	Village
USHA [NUHM]	2500	Urban areas
MPW [Male/Female]	5000 [3000 hill/tribal]	SC
Health Assistant [Male/Female]	30000 [20000 hill/tribal]	PHC

49 *Good to Remember*

Gram sevak is a village level multipurpose link worker. 1 Gram sevak serves 10 villages [5000–6000 population]. He probes into "felt-needs" of villagers and seeks to arouse in them interest in all round family/village development.

ASHA—is an "Accredited Social Health Activist"

Selection Criteria for ASHA

- ASHA must be primarily a woman resident of the village—'Married/Widow/Divorced/ Separated' and preferably in the age group of 25–45 years.
- ASHA should have effective communication skills, leadership qualities and be able to reach out to the community.
- She should be a literate woman with due preference in selection to those who are qualified up to 10 standard wherever they are interested and available in good numbers. This may be relaxed only if no suitable person with this qualification is available
- Adequate representation from disadvantaged population/marginalized groups should be ensured to serve such population/groups better.
- ASHA should have family and social support to enable her to find the time to carry out her tasks in the community on regular basis.

Unit for Selection of ASHA

ASHAs shall be selected only in slum areas of the cities/towns (as per schedule of GOI)

- One ASHA shall be selected as per the main Anganwadi Center exists in the city/towns
- In case of non-existence of the AWC in the cities/towns, ASHA shall be selected from slum areas having 200-300 households.
- Any slums having less than 100 households within 1 km will be tagged with nearby slum(s) for selection of ASHA.
- Another ASHA shall be selected if the slum having more than 300 households.

Functions of ASHA

Mobilize Community

- Depot holder for essential drugs and consumables
- Liaison with AWW, VHSC
- Counseling of females for safe delivery and MCH practices

Health activist and one stop portal of health services

ASHA Remuneration Norms

Note for reader: Please refer to the latest guidelines.

The payment norms maybe subject to change as per NRHM guidelines by the Ministry of health and family welfare and also may vary from state to state.

This source is from: http://www.pbnrhm.org/docs/asha/incentives_to_asha_2016_17.pdf Accessed on 18 may 2018

Table 9: Remuneration norms of ASHA as per NRHM guidelines

Service	Amount (in INR)
Immunization	
Polio program	100 per case
RNTCP	
New TB case	1000 per case
Category II	1500 per case
MDR or XDR case	5000 per case
NLEP	
Referral for PB leprosy	250 per case
Referral for MB leprosy	250+600 per case
NVBDCP	
Preparing PBF slides	15 per slide
Providing drugs as per NMDP	75 per case
Referral of Kala-azar case	300 per case
Lymphatic filariasis – MDT therapy	200 per day for maximum of 3 days, up to 50 houses or 250 persons
Lymphatic filariasis – listing of cases	200 one time
Referral of AES/JE cases to DH	300 per case
Family Planning	
Referral for PPIUCD	150 per case
Follow up of child after discharge from health facility	150 per case
Ensuring home visits for LBW babies or malnourished babies after treatment from SNCU	50 per case
Others	
Line listing of houses in village	100 one time
Maintaining village health register in village on monthly basis	100 one time
List of children due for immunization in village on monthly basis	100 one time
List of ANC beneficiaries in village on monthly basis	100 one time
List of eligible couples in village on monthly basis	100 one time

For the ASHA to be effective in providing HBNC and to enable reductions in neonatal mortality, the following support needs to be provided:

Payment: The ASHA is to be paid ₹250 for conducting home visits for the care of the newborn and postpartum mother. The schedule of payment is as follows:

- Six visits in the case of institutional delivery (Days 3, 7, 14, 21, 28 and 42), and
- Seven visits in the case of home delivery (Days 1, 3, 7, 14, 21, 28, and 42)

The amount is to be paid based on the completed home visit form and first examination of the newborn, forms, validated by the facilitator. The payments to the ASHA should be made on time and with dignity. The payments are made on the 45th day (using the state mechanism for JSY payment) subject to the following:

(i) Ensuring that birth weight is recorded in the maternal and child protection (MCP) card
(ii) Ensuring that the newborn is immunized with: BCG, first doses of OPV and DPT, and entered into the MCP card
(iii) Ensuring birth registration
(iv) Both mother and newborn are safe until the 42nd day of delivery

MANAGEMENT OF HEALTH CARE AND SYSTEMS IN INDIA

Principal unit of administration in India is District (Under a Collector). Within each district there are 6 types of administrative areas:

- Subdivisions [Most districts have 2 or more subdivisions, each in charge of an Assistant/Sub Collector]
- Tehsils (Talukas) [In charge of a Tehsildar. Usually comprises between 200 to 600 villages]
- Community Development Blocks [Unit of rural planning and development. It comprises about 100 villages (80,000 to 1,20,000 population). Incharge is BDO

- Municipalities and Corporations
- Villages
- Panchayat

Institutions of Local Self-government in Urban Areas

- Town area committees—(in areas with population between 5,000 and 10,000)
- Municipal Boards—(population between 10,000 to 2 lakh[Q])—headed by a Chairman/President, elected by members. for a term 3–5 years.
- Corporations—(with population above 2 lakh[Q])—headed by Mayors

Institutions of Local Self-government in Rural Areas

- Panchayati raj (3-Tier structure)
  - Panchayat—(Includes Gram Sabha, Gram Panchayat and Nyaya Panchayat)—at village level
  - Panchayat Samiti—at block level
  - Zila Parishad—at district level.

RoGI Kalyan Smiti (RKS)

- These are community level management for the public health facilities
- There is RKS for PHC's, CHC's to monitor and support for the day to day functioning of the health facility.
- The RKS may work in coordination with the existing health infrastructure to enhance and upgrade the facilities being provided therein

Village Health, Sanitation and Nutrition Committee (VHSNC)

- These are lower level community participation models for effective implementation of the national health programs at the consumer level.
- The panchayat, prominent members of the village, ASHA worker, Anganwadi worker are member of the committee, which shall work together to implement the health programs and benefits to the community.
- VHSN committee is responsible for timely payments to the users under health programs, other works as building of toilets, subsidy for solar systems, general cleanliness drives, celebrating national health days

56 *Must Remember*

Village Health Sanitation and Nutrition Committee (VHSNC):

- Formed at village level for 'local level community action'
- The committee has been formed to take collective actions on issues related to health and its social determinants at the village level under NRHM
- Thus the committee is envisaged to take leadership in providing a platform for improving health awareness and access of community for health services, address specific local needs and serve as a mechanism for community based planning and monitoring.

81 *High Yield Points*

Comprehensive health care:

- The term was first used by Bhore Committee in 1946.
- Comprehensive services mean provision of integrated preventive, curative and promotional health services from "womb to tomb" to every individual residing in a defined geographic area

Advantages:

- As close to the beneficiaries as possible
- Widest cooperation between the people, the service and the profession
- Available to all irrespective of their ability to pay [Specifically vulnerable and weaker sections]
- Create and maintain a healthy environment both in homes as well as working places.

Basic health services—[1965]

- Defined by UNICEF/ WHO as "a network of coordinated, peripheral and intermediate health units capable of performing effectively a selected group of functions essential to the health of an area and assuring availability of competent professional and auxiliary personnel to perform these functions."

Drawbacks:

- Lack of community participation
- Lack of intersectoral coordination
- Dissociation from the socio-economic aspects of health

INNOVATIVE PROGRAMS FOR HEALTH CARE - INDIA

Ayusman Bharat

- Ayushman bharat – "Healthy India" is an enthusiastic scheme for providing preventive and curative health care at primary secondary and tertiary levels to the community
- Elements are:
  - Comprehensive primary health care by Health and wellness centers
  - PM JAY - Prime Minister Jan Arogya Yojana – providing health protection cover to poor and vulnerable families
- The functions of the PM JAY scheme are being monitored, implemented by the NHA – national health authority, constituted under MoHFW
- **PM JAY (Pradhan Mantri Jan Arogya Yojana) benefits:**
  - Financial health protection to 10.74 crore poor, deprived rural families and identified occupational categories of urban workers' families as per the latest Socio-Economic Caste Census (SECC) data
  - Approx. 50 crore beneficiaries
  - Benefit cover of ₹500,000 per family per year (on a family floater basis)
  - For any primary, secondary tertiary level care for any disease and 1350 medical packages including surgery, medical and day care treatments, cost of medicines and diagnostics

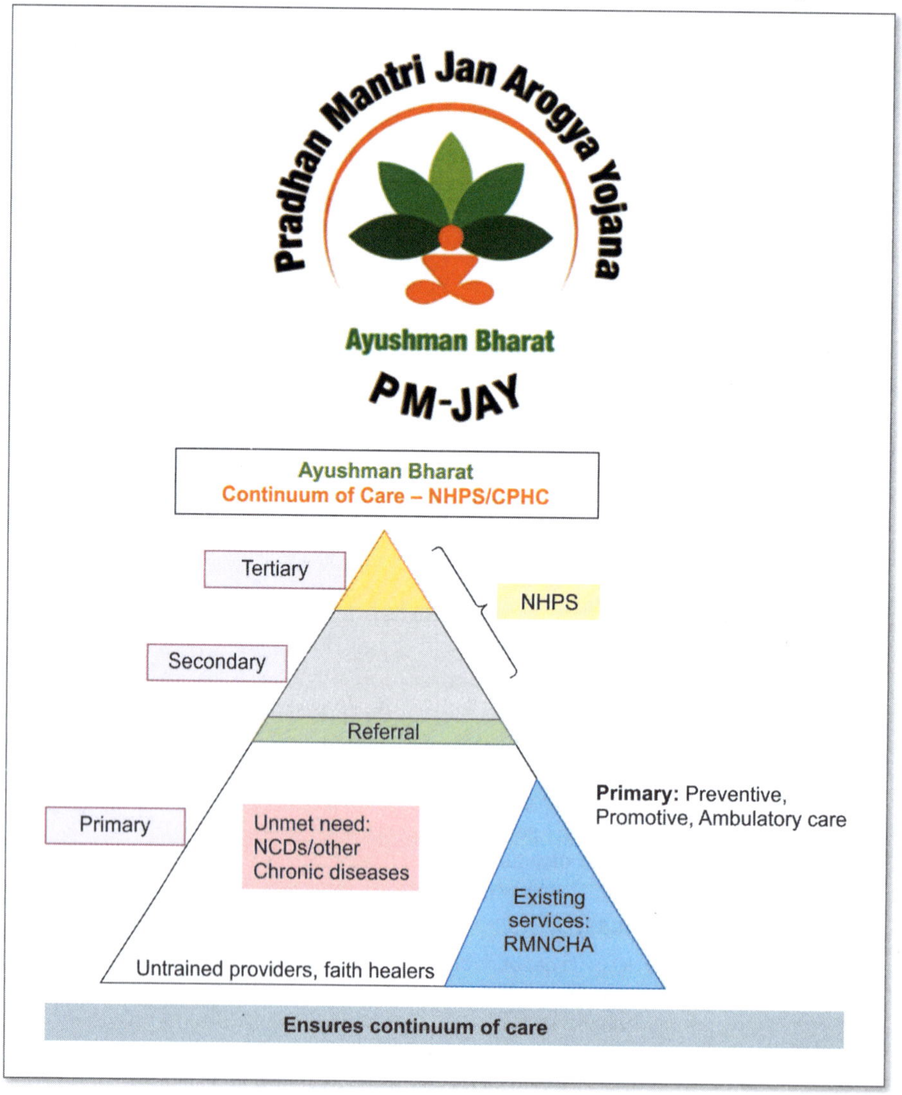

Fig. 1: Strategy of health care under CPHC – comprehensive primary health care

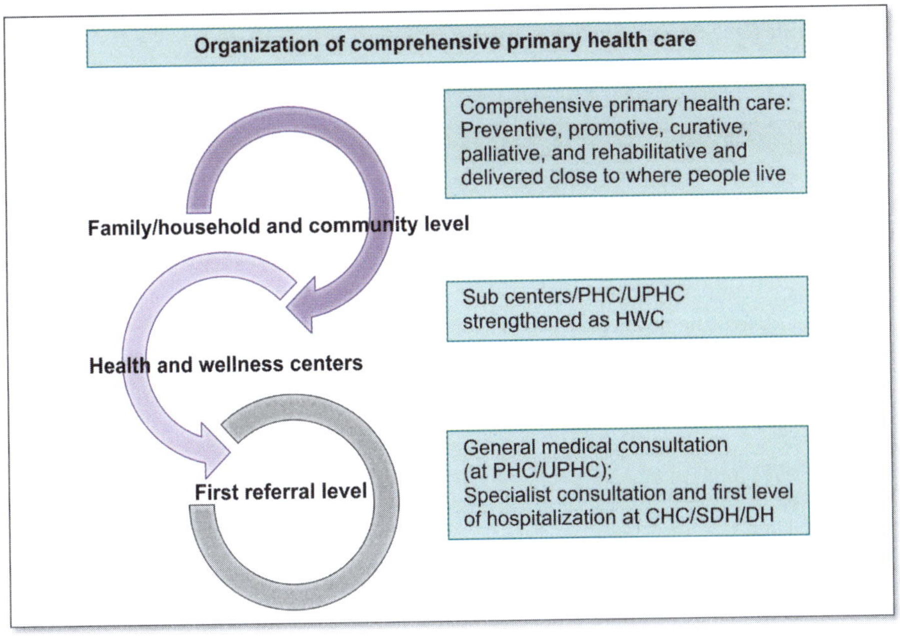

Fig. 2: Organization of health care under CPHC – comprehensive primary health care

Poshan Abhiyan

- POSHAN is acronym for PM's overarching scheme for holistic nutrition
- To improve nutritional outcome in females, pregnant women, lactating mothers, and children
- It is under the ministry of women and child development

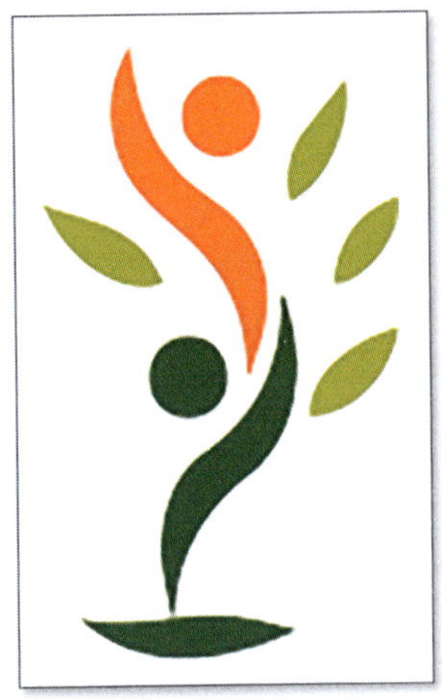

Fig. 3: Logo for Poshan abhiyan

NITI Ayog

- The National Institution for Transforming India, also called NITI Aayog, was formed via a resolution of the Union Cabinet on January 1, 2015.
- NITI Aayog is the premier policy 'Think Tank' of the Government of India, providing both directional and policy inputs.
- At the core of NITI Aayog's creation are two hubs –
  - Team India Hub and
  - The Knowledge and Innovation Hub.
- The Team India Hub leads the engagement of states with the Central government, while the Knowledge and Innovation Hub builds NITI's think-tank capabilities. These hubs reflect the two key tasks of the Aayog.
- NITI Aayog is also developing itself as a State of the Art Resource Centre, with the necessary resources, knowledge and skills, that will enable it to act with speed, promote research and innovation, provide strategic policy vision for the government, and deal with contingent issues.

Information Technology Innovations in Health Care

- Kilkari mobile app—it is an app for child development and growth monitoring
- M-cessation—for behavioral change and communication for quit smoking
- Health management and information system (HMIS)—for development of digital medical records
- Mother and child tracking system (MCTS)—for providing a unique ID to the mother and child as one unit
- ANM Online (ANMOL)—for providing digital access to the ANM's while at work in the field
- National health portal (NHP)—for providing access to the basic and essential statistics of the country—for use in research and policy framework.

Integrated Disease Surveillance Project (IDSP), 2009

Integrated disease surveillance project (IDSP)—for providing surveillance of epidemic prone diseases in a geographical area.

Syndromic Case Surveillance
It has six syndromes—cough, fever, acute flaccid paralysis (AFP), diarrhea, jaundice, unusual death.
Probable case surveillance
▪ Acute diarrheal disease (including acute gastroenteritis) ▪ Bacillary dysentery ▪ Viral hepatitis ▪ Enteric fever ▪ Malaria ▪ Dengue/dengue hemorrhagic fever/dengue shock syndrome (DHF/DSS) ▪ Chikungunya ▪ Acute Encephalitis syndrome ▪ Meningitis ▪ Measles ▪ Diphtheria ▪ Pertussis ▪ Chicken pox ▪ Fever of unknown origin (PUO) ▪ Acute respiratory infection (ARI)/Influenza like Illness (ILI) ▪ Pneumonia ▪ Leptospirosis ▪ Acute flaccid paralysis <15 years of age ▪ Dog bite ▪ Snake bite ▪ Any other state specific disease (Specify) ▪ Unusual syndromes not captured above (Specify clinical diagnosis)
Laboratory case surveillance
▪ Dengue/DHF/DSS ▪ Chikungunya ▪ Japanese encephalitis (JE) ▪ Meningococcal Meningitis ▪ Typhoid fever ▪ Diphtheria ▪ Cholera ▪ Shigella dysentery ▪ Viral hepatitis A ▪ Viral hepatitis E ▪ Leptospirosis ▪ Malaria • Plasmodium vivax (PV) • Plasmodium falciparum (PF)

Central Bureau of Health Information (CBHI)

CBHI is the National Nodal Institution for Health Intelligence in the country with broad objectives to:

- Maintain and disseminate the
  - National Health Profile (NHP)
  - Health Sector Policy Reform Options Database (HS-PROD)
  - Inventory and GIS Mapping of Govt. Health Facilities in India, etc.
- Review the Progress of Health Sector Millennium Development Goal (MDG) in India
- Annual Road Safety Profile of India
- Facilitate Capacity Building and Human Resource Development
- Need Based Operational Research for Efficient Health Information System (HIS) as well as use of Family of International Classification in India and South East Asia Region

50 *Good to Remember*

Swasthya slate—field-based system for providing lab tests in the field only using appropriate technology

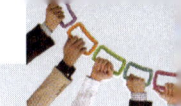

The Rights of Persons with Disabilities Bill—2016

The types of disabilities have been increased from existing 7 to 21 and the Central Government will have the power to add more types of disabilities. The 21 disabilities are given below:

- Blindness
- Low-vision
- Leprosy cured persons
- Hearing impairment (deaf and hard of hearing)
- Locomotor disbility
- Dwarfism
- Intellectual disability
- Mental illness
- Autism spectrum disorder
- Cerebral palsy
- Muscular dystrophy
- Chronic neurological conditions
- Specific learning disabilities
- Multiple sclerosis
- Speech and language disability
- Thalassemia
- Hemophilla
- Sickle cell disease
- Multiple disabilities including deaf blindness
- Acid attack victim
- Parkinson's disease

Other Public Health Schemes by GoI

Accessible India Campaign

Department of Empowerment of Persons with Disabilities (DEPwD) has launched Accessible India Campaign (Sugamya Bharat Abhiyan) as a nation-wide Campaign for achieving universal accessibility for Persons with Disabilities (PwDs)

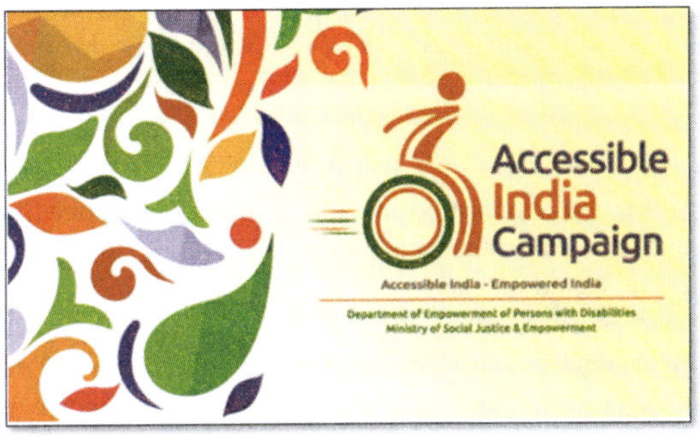

Fig. 4: Emblem of accessible India campaign

Rashtriya Vayoshri Yojana"

Ministry of social justice and empowerment, GOI

A Scheme for providing Physical Aids and Assisted-living Devices for Senior citizens belonging to BPL category.

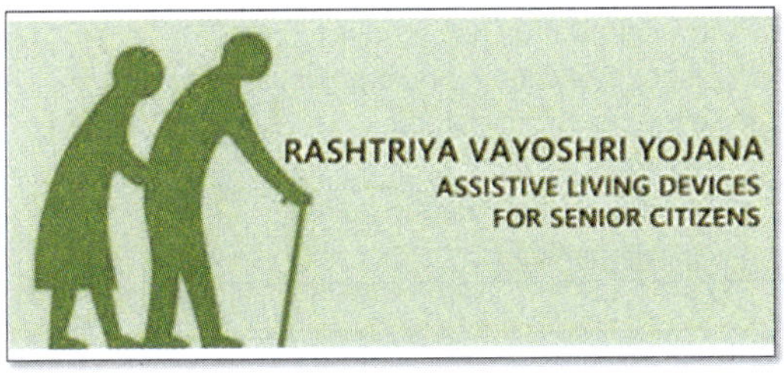

Fig. 5: Emblem of rashtriya vayoshri yojana

Juvenile Justice (Care and Protection of Children) Act, 2015

It replaced the Indian juvenile delinquency law, Juvenile Justice (Care and Protection of Children) Act, 2000, and allows for juveniles in conflict with Law in the age group of 16–18, involved in heinous offences, to be tried as adults. The Act came into force from January 15, 2016.

HMIS and MCH Scoring Indicators

HMIS – health management and information systems
MCH – maternal and child health
There has been a considerable development for data management for the MCH indicators. The NHM (national health mission) has built a scoring system for the MCH and other health care indicators.

It takes into account:

- Mortality indicators
- Fertility indicators
- Nutrition indicators
- Immunization
- Diarrhea
- Pneumonia
- Service delivery indicators

For all mortality, nutrition and fertility indicators:

- **Green:** Less than 20% of national average
- **Yellow:** Within 20% below or above the national average
- **Red:** More than 20% of the national average

All other indicators:

- **Green:** >20% of national average
- **Yellow:** Within 20% below and above the average
- **Red:** Less than 20% of the national average

82 High Yield Points

The Norway-India Partnership Initiative (NIPI) works within the National Rural Health Mission (NRHM) of India. NRHM aims to provide effective health care to the rural population, especially tribal groups including women and children, by improving access, enabling ownership and demand for services.

Child Death Review

Child death review (CDR) is a strategy to understand the geographical variation in causes of child deaths and thereby initiating specific child health interventions

- Reporting by ASHA (primary respondent) within 24 hours
- Family visit by ASHA and notification within 48 hours
- Followed by verbal autopsy and further investigation

Lactation Management Centers

The NHM has also added to the health care innovation by implementation of lactation management centers at various health facilities across the country.

Target

- Ensuring timely initiation of breastfeeding and promoting breastfeeding practices.
- Setting up of lactation management centers
  - Comprehensive lactation management centers (CLMCs) for donor human milk collection, storage, processing and dispensing for babies admitted in health facilities.
  - Lactation management units (LMUs) for collecting, storing and dispensing of mother's breast milk, expressed and stored for consumption by her own baby.
  - Lactation support Units (LSUs) for providing lactation support to mothers at all delivery points.

51 Good to Remember

NITI Aayog (National Institutions of Transforming India)—Replaced Planning Commission on 1st January 2015. Its functions are:

- To provide center and state with strategic and technical advice on a range of key elements of policy.
- To monitor and evaluate implementation of programs
- Technology upgradation and capacity building.

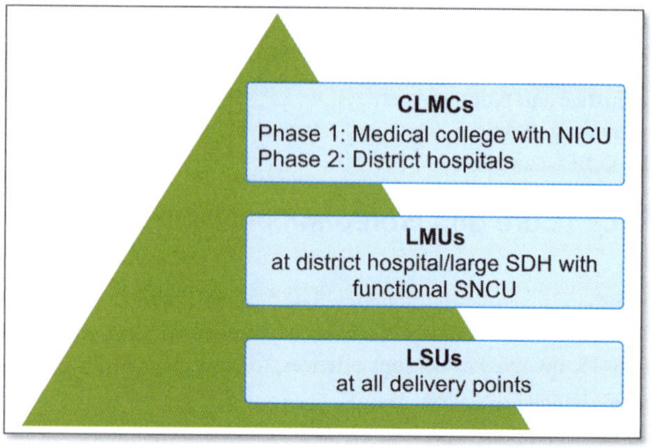

Fig. 6: Lactation management centers

Transplantation of Human Organ Act, 1994

Donor is any person, not less than 18 years who authorizes [parents in case of minor] for removal of any organ of his body before his death.

- A registered medical practitioner must certify that life or brainstem function have ceased before removal of body organs.
- *Penalty for illegal supply or advertisement or removal of human organ without authority*
  - A term of not less than 10 years + fine ₹20 Lakh- 1 Crore
  - In case of involvement of the doctor, penal erasure for 2 years for 1st act and for life for subsequent act.

Rashtriya Swasthya Bima Yojna (RSBY), 2007

National Health Insurance Scheme

- It was launched on 1st October, 2007
- Finance - Central government (75% of annual premium of ₹750 = ₹565/ family), State government (25% of annual premium)
- Beneficiary has to pay a onetime registration fee of ₹30.
- The beneficiary is any below poverty line (BPL) family, whose information is included in the district BPL list prepared by the State government.

Benefits

- The beneficiaries under RSBY are entitled to hospitalization coverage up to ₹30,000/- per annum on family floater basis, for most of the diseases that require hospitalization.
- The benefit will be available under the defined diseases in the package list.
- The government has framed indicative package rates for the hospitals for a large number of interventions. Pre-existing conditions are covered from day one and there is no age limit. The coverage extends to maximum five members of the family which includes the head of household, spouse and up to three dependents.
- Additionally, transport expenses of ₹100/- per hospitalization will also be paid to the beneficiary subject to a maximum of ₹1000/- per year per family.
- The beneficiaries need to pay only ₹30/- as registration fee for a year while Central and State Government pays the premium as per their sharing ratio to the insurer selected by the State Government on the basis of a competitive bidding.

At every state, the State Government sets up a State Nodal Agency (SNA) that is responsible for implementing, monitoring supervision and part-financing of the scheme by coordinating with Insurance Company, Hospital, District Authorities and other local stake holders.

Exclusions

Congenital external disease, conditions that do not need hospitalization, drug/alcohol induced illness, vaccination, suicide, AYUSH, sterilization and fertility related procedures, war.

Pradhan Mantri Jeevan Jyoti Bima Yojana (PMJJBY)

- PMJJBY scheme offers a life cover of ₹2 lakhs for a one year period (from 1st June-31st May)
- It is renewable every year.
- A premium of ₹330/annum/member is applicable.
- It offers cover for death due to any reason and is available to people in the age group of 18 to 50 years (life cover up to age 55) having a savings bank account who give their consent to join and enable auto-debit.
- The risk cover on the lives of the enrolled persons has commenced from 1st June 2015
- Participating Bank is the Master policy holder and have tied up with LIC and other Indian private Life Insurance companies
- The assurance on life of the member shall terminate on any of the following events and no benefit will be payable there under to individuals:
  - Who attain age of 55 years
  - Closure of account with the Bank or insufficiency of balance to keep the insurance in force
- A person can join PMJJBY with one Insurance company with one bank account only

57 **Must Remember**

Pradhan Mantri Swasthya Suraksha Yojana (PMSSY):

Objectives of correcting regional imbalances in the availability of affordable/reliable tertiary healthcare services and also to augment facilities for quality medical education in the country.

- Setting up of new AIIMS like institutions
- Upgradation of medical colleges

52 **Good to Remember**

Pradhan Mantri Suraksha Bima Yojana

- It is aimed at covering the uncovered population at a highly affordable premium of just ₹12 per year.
- The scheme will be available to people in the age group 18 to 70 years with a savings bank account who give their consent to join and enable autodebit on or before 31st May for the coverage period-1st June to 31st May on an annual renewal basis.
- Risk coverage available will be ₹2 lakh for accidental death and permanent total disability and ₹1 lakh for permanent partial disability, for a one year period stretching from 1st June to 31st May.

- One can exit the scheme at any point may re-join the scheme in future years by paying the annual premium and submitting a self-declaration of good health. However, it will not be possible to join beyond the age of 50 years.

National Rural Employment Guarantee Act, 2005

- 100 days of guaranteed wage employment per year for adult members of a rural household who volunteer to do unskilled manual work.
- Work is provided within 5 km radius of village or else with 10% extra wages.
- Willing person apply for registration to gram panchayat, which issues job card after verification
- Job card holder seeking work has to be employed by gram panchayat within 15 days of application or else daily unemployment allowance in cash has to be paid, borne by state government.
- At least one third of persons to whom work is allotted must be women.
- Nature of work is to be decided by the gram sabha
- Wages are as per Minimum Wages Act 1948 and disbursed weekly
- To ensure receipt of full amount to person concerned, labor amount is paid in bank or post office account.
- Help line is 1800110707 or in case of inconvenience it can be discussed at the gram sabha level.

Atal Pension Yojana

- It is for all citizens in the unorganized sector (who are not members of any statutory social security scheme and who are not income tax payers)
- Monthly pension would be available to subscriber and after him to his spouse After his death, the pension corpus accumulated at the age of 60 will be returned to the nominee.
- Subscribers would receive a fixed minimum pension ₹1000 per month or higher ₹5000 per month (Maximum) depending on their contribution.
- Subscriber joining at age 18 for 1000 pension has to pay a monthly contribution of ₹42 and for ₹5000 pension has to pay ₹210 /month. Contribution amount will vary with the pension amount desired and age of entry
- Central government will contribute 50% of total contribution or ₹1000 per annum whichever is lower for a period of 5 year from 2015-16 to 2019-2020, for those who join before 31st December 2015
- Minimum age of joining is 18 years and maximum age is 40 years.
- Minimum period of contribution by any subscriber would be 20 years.

Right to Information Act, 2005

- Extends to the whole of India except J&K.
- The provisions of this Act have come into force on 12 October, 2005
- The act provides for setting up:
    - Access to citizens of secure information under control of public authorities, in order to promote transparency and accountability in the working of every public authority
    - Constitution of a Central Information Commission and State Information Commissions.

Pradhan Mantri Gramin Digital Saskharta Abhiyan or DISHA (Digital Saksharta Abhiyaan)–to Improve Digital Literacy Mission

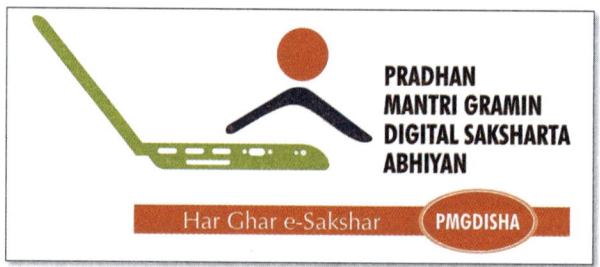

Fig. 7: Emblem of pradhan mantri gramin digital saksharta abhiyan

53 Good to Remember

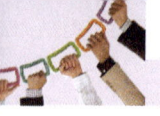

Some Schemes under GoI (Government of India)with similar name –

"Ujjawala"

- **Ujjawala** scheme:
    - Under ministry of women and child development
    - A Comprehensive Scheme for Prevention of trafficking and Rescue, Rehabilitation and Re-integration of Victims of Trafficking and Commercial Sexual Exploitation
- Pradhan Mantri **Ujjwala** Yojna:
    - Under ministry of petroleum & Natural Gas.
    - Providing safer fuels – LPG to BPL females
- **Ujala** Scheme: ***U**nnat **J**yoti by **A**ffordable **L**EDs for **A**ll*; "Prakash Path – Way to light"
    - Under Ministry of Power
    - 20W LED tube lights and BEE 5-star rated energy efficient fans are also distributed to the consumers.

"Indradhanush"

- Mission Indradhanush – by NHM for quality and better coverage of vaccines and strengthening of immunization program in India
- Indradhanush Scheme – by ESI corporation for colourful bedsheets for each day in week. This scheme represents the commitment for quality in health care

National Health Mission (NHM)

- It is an endeavor – mission to achieve the following targets to reflect:
- Equity
- Equality
- Effectivity
- Efficiency

Of the health system

- It was launched in India in 2005 as N(R)HM (rural), later combined with the NUMH (urban)
- It is an umbrella program, which encompasses all national health programs under one roof.

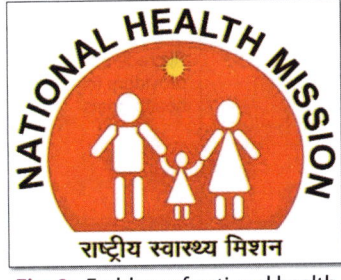

Fig. 8: Emblem of national health mission

83 *High Yield Points*

Targets

- Reduce MMR to 1/1000 live births
- Reduce IMR to 25/1000 live births
- Reduce TFR to 2.1
- Prevention and reduction of anemia in women aged 15–49 years
- Prevent and reduce mortality and morbidity from communicable, non-communicable; injuries and emerging diseases
- Reduce household out-of-pocket expenditure on total health care expenditure
- Reduce annual incidence and mortality from tuberculosis by half
- Reduce prevalence of leprosy to <1/10000 population and incidence to zero in all districts
- Annual Malaria Incidence to be <1/1000
- Less than 1 per cent microfilaria prevalence in all districts
- Kala-azar elimination by 2015, <1 case per 10000 population in all blocks.

NRHM

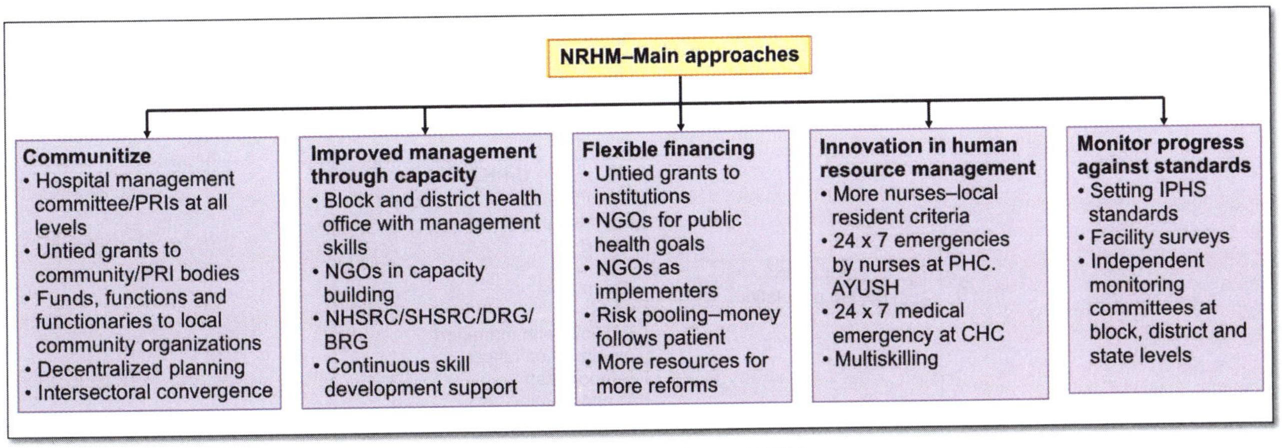

Fig. 9: Main approaches to NRHM

The organization structure is as follows (also refer to health care system in India in this chapter)

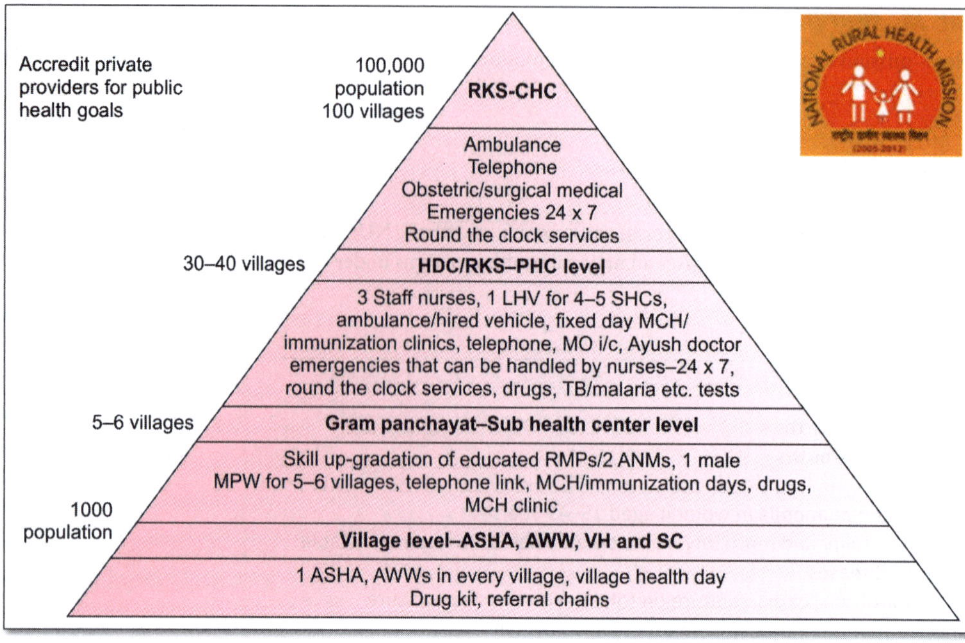

Fig. 10: Organization structure of NRHM

NUHM

The National Urban Health Mission (NUHM) as a sub-mission of National Health Mission (NHM) has been approved by the Cabinet on 1st May 2013.

NUHM is for the health care needs of the urban population with the focus on urban poor, by making available to them essential primary health care services and reducing their out of pocket expenses for treatment.

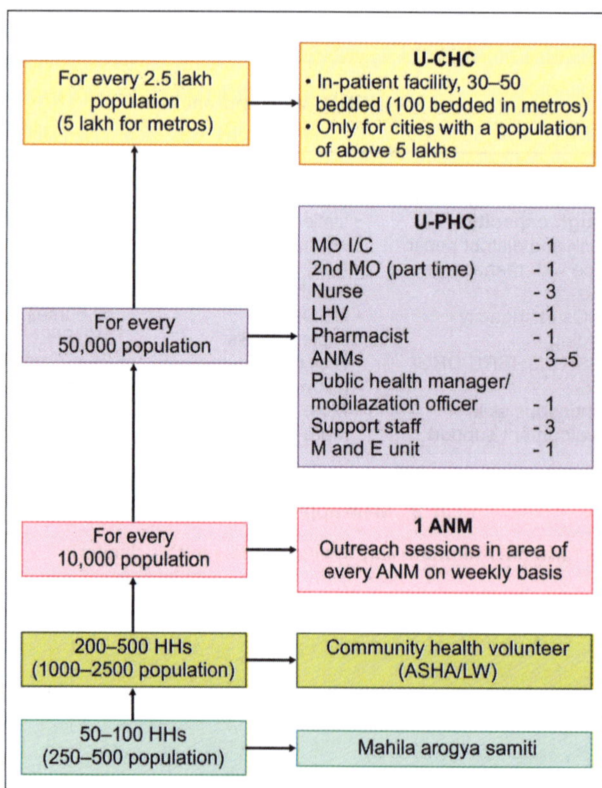

Fig. 11: Urban health care facilities

NATIONAL HEALTH POLICY 2017

Concise National Health Policy 2017

Table 10: Health status and program impact

Life expectancy and healthy life	Increase life expectancy at birth from 67.5 To 70 by 2025
	Establish regular tracking of disability adjusted life years (DALY) index as a measure of burden of disease and its trends by major categories by 2022.
	Reduce total fertility rate (TFR) to 2.1 at national and sub-national level by 2025
Mortality by age and/or cause	Reduce Under Five Mortality to 23 by 2025
	Reduce maternal mortality rate (MMR) from current levels to 100 by 2020
	Reduce infant mortality rate (IMR) to 28 by 2019
	Reduce neonatal mortality rate (NMR) to 16 and still birth rate to "Single digit" by 2025
Reduction of disease prevalence/incidence	Achieve global target of 2020 -Target of 90:90:90, for HIV/AIDS ▪ 90% of all people living with HIV know their HIV status ▪ 90% of all people diagnosed with HIV infection receive sustained antiretroviral therapy (ART) ▪ 90% of all people receiving ART have viral suppression.
	Achieve and maintain elimination status of Leprosy by 2018, Kala-azar by 2017 and Lymphatic Filariasis in endemic pockets by 2017.
	Achieve and maintain a cure rate of >85% in new sputum positive patients for TB and reduce incidence of new cases, to reach elimination status by 2025.
	Reduce prevalence of blindness to 0.25/1000 by 2025 and disease burden by one third from current levels.
	Reduce premature mortality from cardiovascular diseases, cancer, diabetes or chronic respiratory diseases by 25% by 2025.
Health systems performance	
Coverage of health services	Increase utilization of public health facilities by 50% from current levels by 2025
	ANC care coverage to be sustained above 90% and skilled attendance at birth above 90% by 2025
	More than 90% of the newborn are fully immunized by one year of age by 2025
	Meet need of family planning above 90% at national and sub-national level by 2025
	80% of known hypertensive and diabetics at household level maintain "controlled disease status" by 2025
Cross-sectoral goals related to health	Relative reduction in prevalence of current tobacco use by 15% by 2020 and 30% by 2025
	Reduction of 40% in prevalence of stunting of under-five children by 2025
	Access to safe water and sanitation to all by 2020 (Swachh Bharat Mission)
	Reduction of occupational injury by 50% from current level (334/Lakh agricultural workers) by 2020
	National/State level tracking of selected health behavior.
Health Systems Strengthening	
Health finance	Increase Govt. health expenditure from existing 1.15% of GDP to 2.5% of GDP by 2025.
	Increase State sector health spending to >8% of their budget by 2020
	Decrease proportion of households facing catastrophic health expenditure from the current levels by 25% by 2025.
Health infrastructure and human resource	Ensure availability of paramedics and doctors as per IPHS norm in high priority districts by 2020
	Increase community health volunteers to population ratio as per IPHS norm in high priority districts by 2025.
	Establish primary and secondary care facility as per norms in high priority districts by 2025

Contd...

Health management information	Ensure district-level electronic database of information on health system components by 2020
	Strengthen health surveillance system and establish registries for diseases of public health importance by 2020
	Establish federated integrated health information architecture, Health Information Exchanges and National Health Information Network by 2025

84 High Yield Points

Recent policies: (Update – January 2017)

1.	Swachh Bharat Abhiyan	Safe water and sanitation
2.	Yatri Suraksha Mission	Preventing deaths due to rail and road accidents
3.	Nirbhaya Nari	Action against gender violence
4.	Pradhan Mantri Surakshit Matritva Abhiyan	▪ Maternity benefits >26 weeks for all deliveries ▪ Safe antenatal care (ANC) and postnatal care (PNC)
5.	Ujjwala Scheme	Safe fuel for cooking for decreasing indoor air pollution

54 Good to Remember

Ayushman Bharat:

- Health and wellness center (HWC) – Subcenters to be upgraded to the HWCs which provide more comprehensive package of health care services including RMNCH+A, communicable, noncommunicable, ENT, dental, geriatric diseases and mental health care
- **National health protection scheme:** Providing blanket health insurance
- Increase GDP spending on health to 2.5%

GLOBAL HEALTH PLANNING–DEVELOPMENT GOALS

Millennium Development Goals (MDGs) 2000–2015

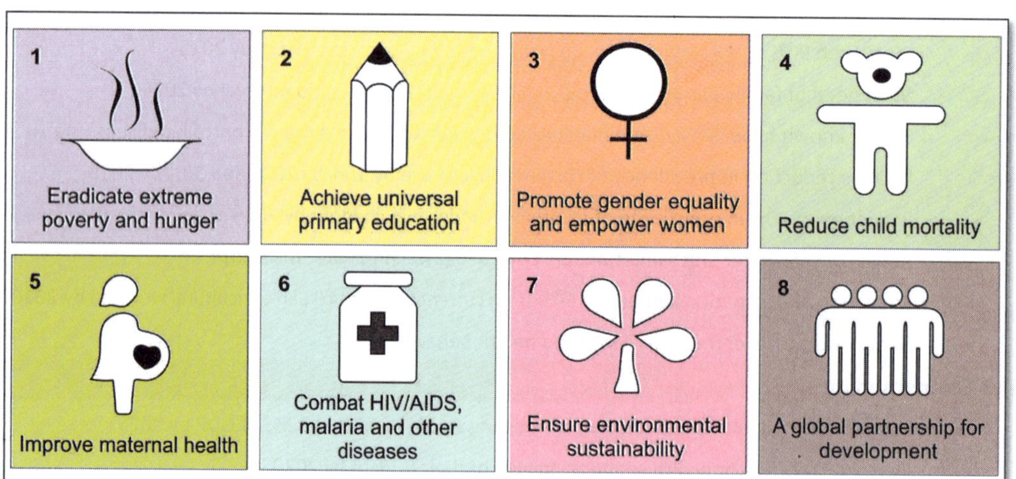

Fig. 12: Millennium development goals 2000–2015

Goals and Targets under MDG

Goal 1: Eradicate extreme poverty and hunger

Target 1A: Halve, between 1990 and 2015, the proportion of people living on less than $1.25 a day

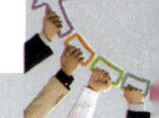

Target 1B: Achieve decent employment for women, men, and young people
Target 1C: Halve, between 1990 and 2015, the proportion of people who suffer from hunger

Goal 2: Achieve universal primary education
Target 2A: By 2015, all children can complete a full course of primary schooling, girls and boys

Goal 3: Promote gender equality and empower women
Target 3A: Eliminate gender disparity in primary and secondary education preferably by 2005, and at all levels by 2015

Goal 4: Reduce child mortality rates
Target 4A: Reduce by two-thirds, between 1990 and 2015, the under-five mortality rate
- Under-five mortality rate
- Infant (under 1) mortality rate
- Proportion of 1-year-old children immunized against measles

Goal 5: Improve maternal health

Goal 6: Combat HIV/AIDS, malaria, and other diseases
Target 6A: Have halted by 2015 and begun to reverse the spread of HIV/AIDS
Target 6B: Achieve, by 2010, universal access to treatment for HIV/AIDS for all those who need it
Target 6C: Have halted by 2015 and begun to reverse the incidence of malaria and other major diseases

Goal 7: Ensure environmental sustainability
Target 7A: Integrate the principles of sustainable development into country policies and programs; reverse loss of environmental resources
Target 7B: Reduce biodiversity loss, achieving, by 2010, a significant reduction in the rate of loss
Target 7C: Halve, by 2015, the proportion of the population without sustainable access to safe drinking water and basic sanitation

Goal 8: Develop a global partnership for development

Sustainable Development Goals (2015–2030)

Survive – thrive and transform health
Important points to remember:
- Reduce global maternal mortality to less than 70 per 100,000 live births
- Reduce newborn mortality to at least as low as 12 per 1,000 live births in every country
- Reduce under-five mortality to at least as low as 25 per 1,000 live births in every country
- End epidemics of HIV, tuberculosis, malaria, neglected tropical diseases and other communicable diseases
- Reduce by one third premature mortality from noncommunicable diseases and promote mental health and well-being.

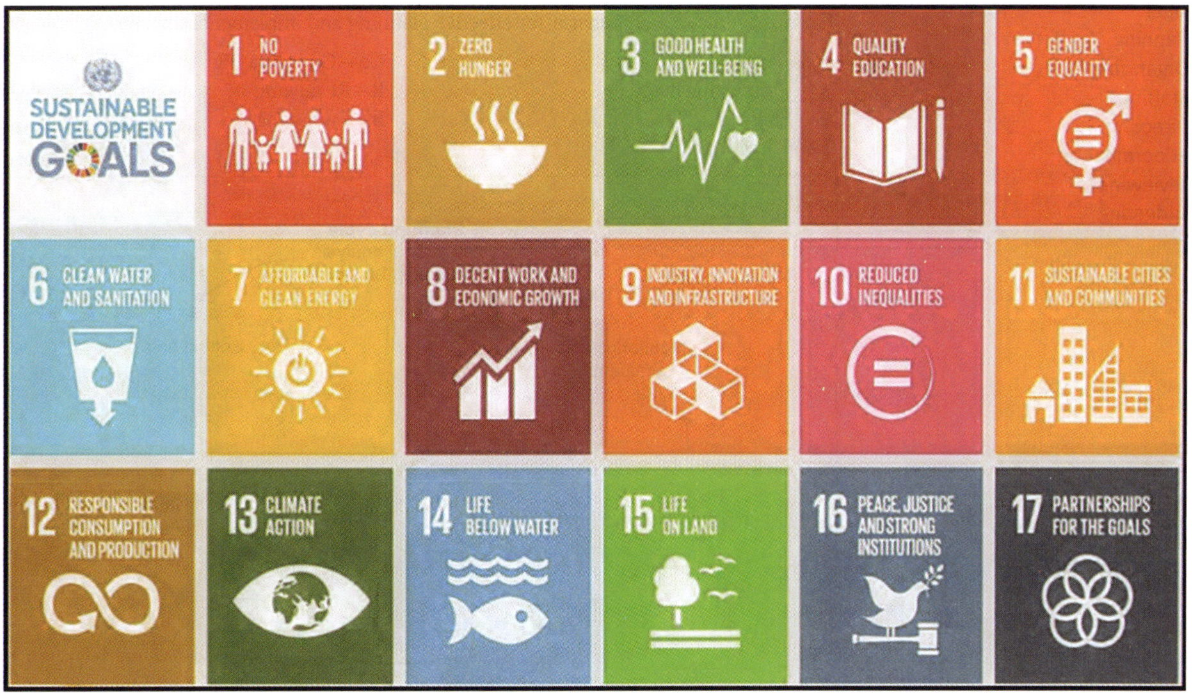
SUSTAINABLE DEVELOPMENT GOALS
1 NO POVERTY
2 ZERO HUNGER
3 GOOD HEALTH AND WELL-BEING
4 QUALITY EDUCATION
5 GENDER EQUALITY
6 CLEAN WATER AND SANITATION
7 AFFORDABLE AND CLEAN ENERGY
8 DECENT WORK AND ECONOMIC GROWTH
9 INDUSTRY, INNOVATION AND INFRASTRUCTURE
10 REDUCED INEQUALITIES
11 SUSTAINABLE CITIES AND COMMUNITIES
12 RESPONSIBLE CONSUMPTION AND PRODUCTION
13 CLIMATE ACTION
14 LIFE BELOW WATER
15 LIFE ON LAND
16 PEACE, JUSTICE AND STRONG INSTITUTIONS
17 PARTNERSHIPS FOR THE GOALS

Fig. 13: Sustainable development goals

85 *High Yield Points*

Management by Objectives (MBO): Objectives are set forth for different units and subunits, each of which prepares its own plan of action on a short-term basis. It helps in achieving the results more effectively and smoothly.

MANAGEMENT PRINCIPLES IN HEALTH CARE

MANAGEMENT IN HEALTH CARE

Management—Basic Principles

Management is purposeful and effective use of resources for fulfilling a predetermined objective. It involves 4 basic activities: Planning, organizing, communication and monitoring.

Goal: It is the ultimate desired state toward which objectives and resources are directed. Goals are not necessarily attainable (No constraint of time or resources).

Objective:
- It is the planned endpoint of all activities.
- It is very precise and either achieved or not achieved.

Target:
- It is related to a discrete activity.
- Targets are mid-term quantifiable milestones
- It is concerned with degree of achievement and factors involved.

Mission:
- It is a statement of purpose is supported by objectives. (Objective is more grounded and more attainable than the mission). It is time bound.

The Planning Cycle

Planning is a basic foundation for any process implementation and its management. The planning cycle is a process of analyzing a system, assessment, implementation and monitoring of the program cycle. It has various stages as:
- Analysis of health situation
- Establishment of objectives and goals
- Assessment of resources available
- Prioritization of activities
- Write up the formulated plan
- Programming and implementation
- Monitoring
- Evaluation

The main functions of manager for effective planning and implementation are:

P—Planning
O—Organizing
S— Staffing
D—Directing
Co—Coordinating
R—Reviewing
B—Budgeting

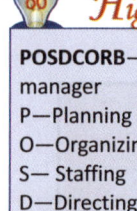

86 *High Yield Points*

POSDCORB—Functions of a manager
P—Planning
O—Organizing
S— Staffing
D—Directing
CO—Coordinating
R—Reviewing
B—Budgeting

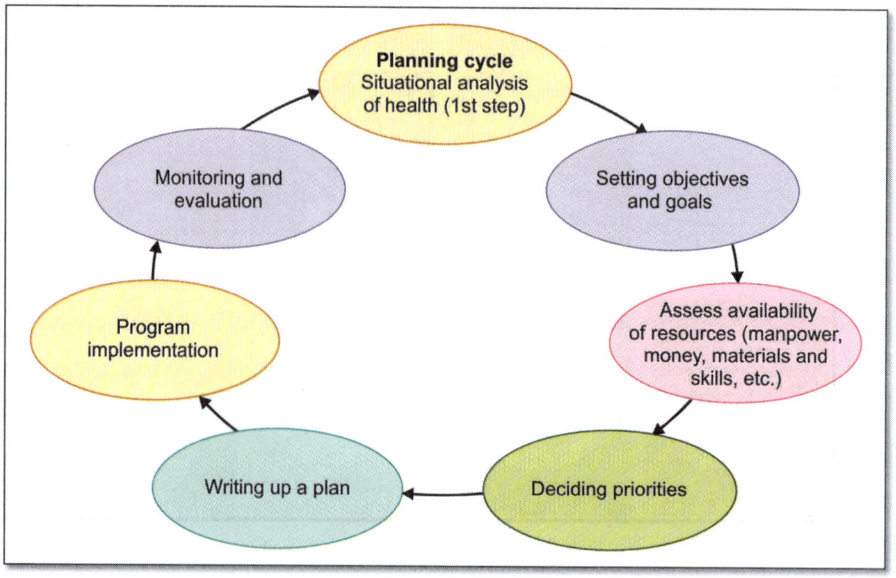

Fig. 14: Planning cycle of health care

Management Techniques

Input Output Analysis

How much of each "Input" is needed to produce a unit amount of each "Output".

Cost-benefit Analysis: Economic benefits of any program are compared with cost of that program.
Drawback: Benefits in health field as a result of a particular program cannot always be expressed in monetary means.

Cost-effective Analysis: Here, benefit is expressed in terms of results achieved, e.g. number of lives saved and number of days free from disease.

Network Analysis

Branch deals with proper planning, drafting, testing, implementation and execution of a series of activities oriented towards a common goal. It is a graphic plan of all events to be completed in order to reach an end objective.

Critical path method:

- It is a "deterministic model" strategic quantitative method for network analysis.
- ***Keyword*** – event time management
- Takes into account most time taking activity and allows to analyze activity as per time consumed.
- It helps asses for the most time taking event (or the critical event) which should be started first in order to finish the complex task in shortest time.
- Usually done along with the PERT technique

Example: Helps asses the time for each activity, so as to plan the initiation time for same and save on time as resource

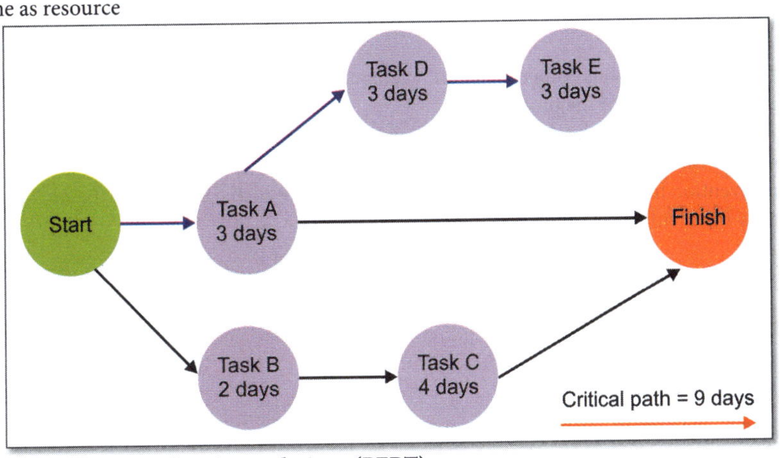

Program evaluation and review technique (PERT):

- It is a "probabilistic model" management technique whereby the sequence of smaller events is strategically planned to avoid loss
- It is an arrow and line diagram representing which event will follow another event.
- ***Keyword*** –event sequencing
- It is a management technique which makes possible more detailed planning and more comprehensive supervision.

Example – PERT for starting a clinic /laboratory service in an urban township

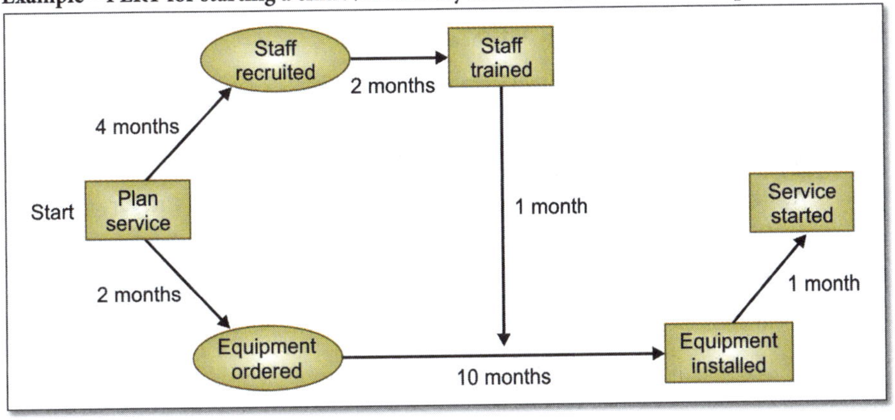

Work Sampling

- Systematic observation and recording of activities of one or more individuals carried out at random levels
- Provides quantitative measurement of various activities
- **Use:**
  - Determination of manpower needs
  - Assessment of performance of jobs by worker

55 Good to Remember

Cost accounting: It provides data on cost structure of any program. It has 3 important purpose: Cost control, Planning and allocation of resources and Pricing of cost reimbursement.

Budgeting Techniques

Planning Programming and Budgeting System (PPBS)

[Developed by Rand Corporation of USA]

- It calls for grouping of activities into programs related to each objective, so as to help decision makers to allocate resources efficiently.
- Activities are grouped into programs related to each objective, to utilize available resources most effectively.
- It emphasizes on clearly defined objectives and a well-established information system.
- Researches for alternative programs based on cost benefit implications and future cost implications.
- **Limitation:** Long planning period often more than 1 year.

56 Good to Remember

Six sigma level—this is benchmark level for quality assurance and the number of defects/errors committed.

Evaluation Techniques

Monitoring: Continuous supervision of the events or activities to assess/evaluate a program or series of events.

Surveillance: Continuous supervision of events to achieve the desired end result or the quantifiable end result of the program.

Evaluation is measure of the degree to which predetermined objectives and targets are fulfilled.

Incremental cost effectiveness ratio (ICER)

If an intervention found to be more effective but is also more costly. So to make the final decision, ICER may be calculated.

$$\text{ICER} = \frac{\text{Cost of A} - \text{Cost of B}}{\text{Effectiveness of A} - \text{Effectiveness of B}}$$

87 High Yield Points

Pareto's law forms the basis for inventory control

Inventory Management

Methods for stock management are:

- FIFO—first in first out
- GIGO—garbage in, garbage out
- EFFO—expiry first, first out

Methods for procurement and inventory management are:

- **ABC analysis** – based on the cost. "A-B-C" tagging is done to the products based on the scale of least expensive to most expensive item (or based on consumption of resources in terms of manpower or money resources)
- **VED analysis** – based on the need (requirement) of the product, where
  - V = vital
  - E = Essential but not vital
  - D = Desirable

Example matrix for ABC/VED analysis in health care

Table 11: Combination of these two categories like a matrix combining ABC and VED categories

	V	E	D	
A	AV defibrillator	AE X-ray machine	AD air curtains	Category I
B	BV ventillator	BE electric cautery	BD Bp instrument	Category II
C	CV SpO_2 machine	CE patient trolley	CD thermometer	Category III

*This matrix is more relevant in the hospitals

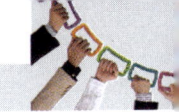

Usually
- "A" group items would consume more resources and are in few numbers
- "C" group items would consume less resources and are in large numbers
- So, "AV product" purchase is selected by the top management and requires higher management level approval or decision.
- "CD product" takes the other extreme end of the spectrum, which is desirable and non-expensive, and the procurement process may be delegated to a different (or lower) management level.

Organizational Management

Indoctrination is introducing a new employee to a job/organization in a way that, he takes pride in his new job and association with the organization.

Types of Organization

- **Line:** No subordinate is under more than one superior and scalar principle and principle of unity of command are strictly adhered.
- **Matrix:** An employee is accountable and takes orders from 2 different superiors at the same time
- **Functional:** Worker is accountable to 2 or more executives for a given specific and specialized function.

Swot Analysis

Strengths (S), Weaknesses (W), Opportunities (O) and Threats (T)
- S (strengths) and W (weakness) are permanent phenomena that exist within the organization or community
- T (threats) are temporary, often fleeting, phenomena that exist in the external environment.

Example:

SWOT analysis – RNTCP	
Strengths: • Strong political and administrative commitment • Secured medium to long term financing • Wide network of Tus and quality assured DMCs across the country • Decentralized DOTs (~ 0.43 million DOT centers) • Consistently achieving global targets for past few years • TBHIV & DOT plus services introduced-Nation vide scale up by 2012 • Wide participation of NGOs, PPs, corporate, professional bodies and other Government departments • Engaged CS partners viz. Union, WV, CBCI to enhance reach & empower TB cases/communities	**Weaknesses:** • Unorganized private sector • Weak general health systems in some states • Shortage of key managerial staff (one person handling multiple portfolio)
Opportunities: • Universal access • Airborne infection control guidelines developed • Newer diagnostic under RNTCP in collaboration with find - Pan sensitive TB - LED microscopy, GeneXpert - M/XDR TB diagnosis - LPA, liquid culture, capillia test, GeneXpert	**Threats:** • HR turnover • Sustainability of finances • Irrational use of 1st & 2nd line drugs due to market forces

Medical Audit

It is evaluation of the quality of medical care or performance by analysis of medical records.
Broad objectives of medical audit are as follows:
- Improve quality of care
- A clear definition of responsibilities
- Stimulation of research and developments
- Improved safety
- Providing a basis for providing care.

57 **Good to Remember**

- **Incremental budgeting**—Previous year's budget is used as a base for preparing next year's budget. Only the increment is to be justified.
- **Zero base budgeting**—Starting from a zero base of no funds for a program, every rupee is sanctioned, even for ongoing program.

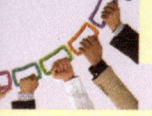

Image-Based Questions

1. The symbol shown in figure is related to?

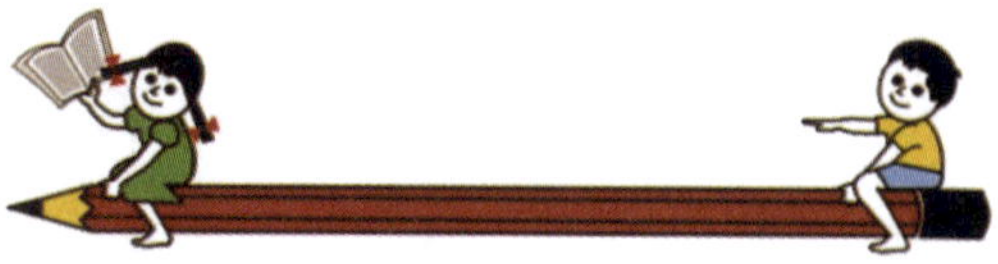

a. National Literacy Mission
b. Sarva Siksha Abhiyan
c. ICDS
d. ICPS

2. The symbol shown in figure is related to?

a. National Human Rights Commission
b. Sarva Siksha Abhiyan
c. National Literacy Mission
d. International Yoga Day

3. The symbol shown in figure is related to?

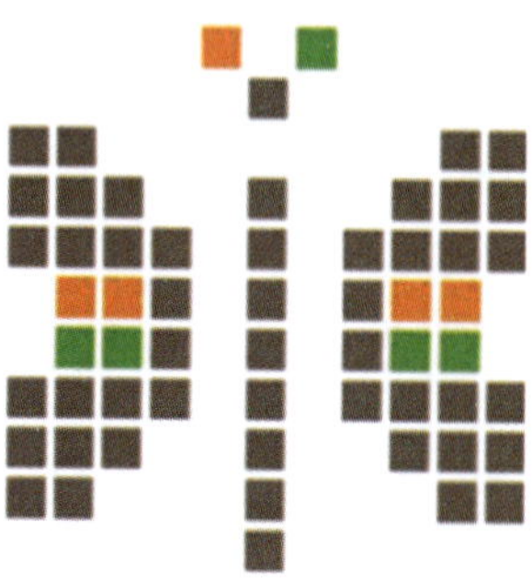

a. NUHM
b. Smart city
c. NHAI
d. Swachh Bharat

4. The figure shown in figure depicts India's campaign against?

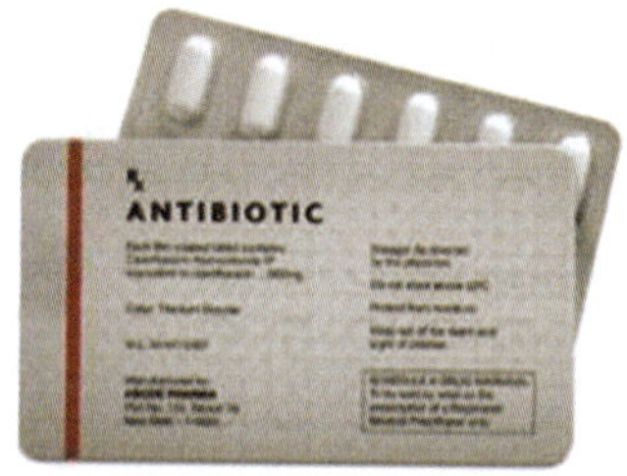

a. Misuse of antibiotics
b. Counterfeit medicines
c. Drug resistance
d. Drug price control

5. Identify the act depicted by the symbol in figure?

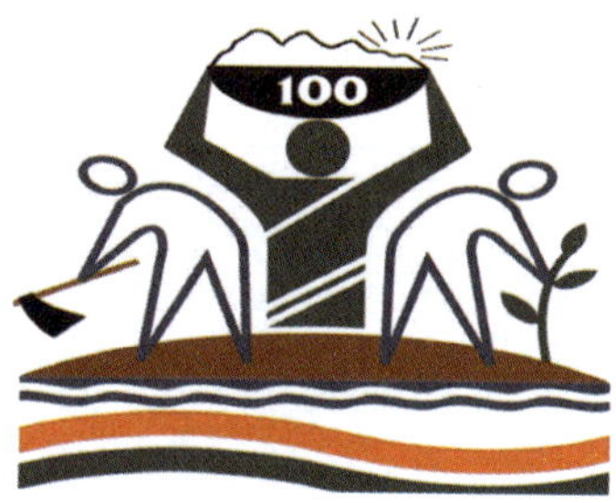

a. Workmen's Compensation Act, 1973
b. Employee State Insurance Act, 1948
c. Child Labor Act, 1986
d. NREGA Act, 2005

6. Identify the program represented by symbol in figure?

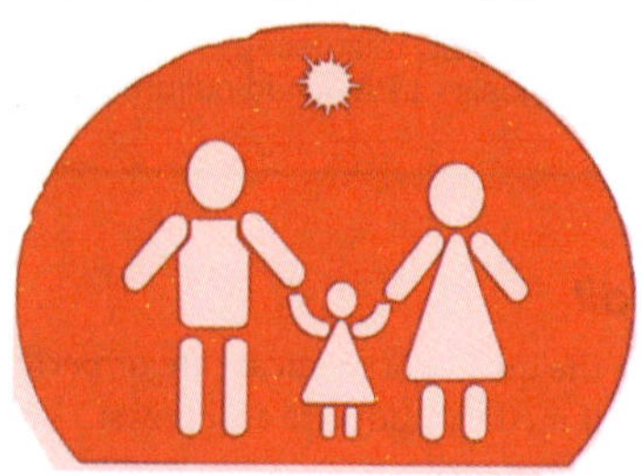

a. RNTCP
b. NLEP
c. NHM
d. NACP

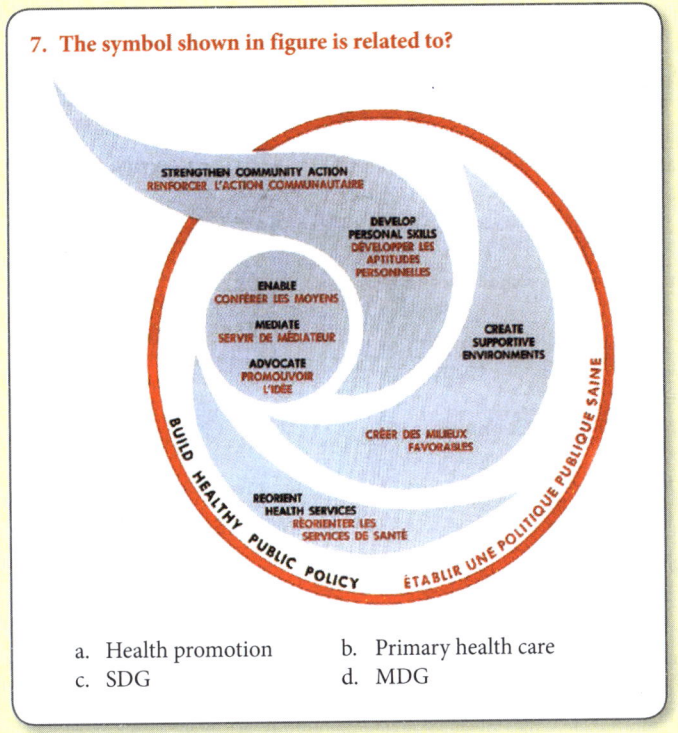

7. The symbol shown in figure is related to?

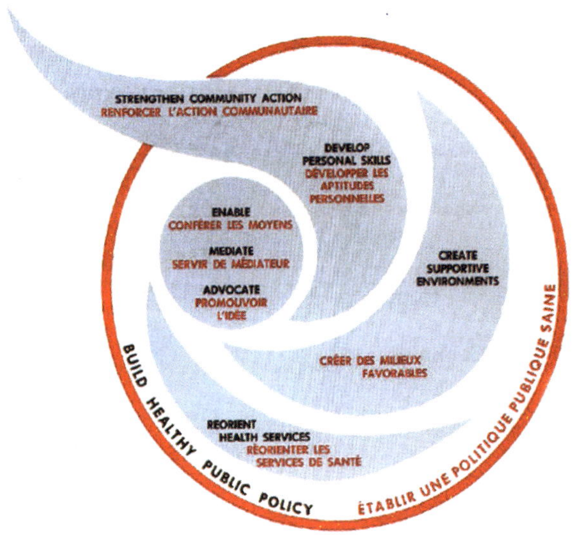

a. Health promotion
b. Primary health care
c. SDG
d. MDG

Answers of Image-Based Questions

1. **Ans. (b)** **Sarva Siksha Abhiyan**
2. **Ans. (c)** **National Literacy Mission**
3. **Ans. (b)** **Smart city**
4. **Ans. (a)** **Misuse of antibiotics**
5. **Ans. (d)** **NREGA Act 2005**
6. **Ans. (c)** **NHM**
7. **Ans. (a)** **Ottawa charter for health promotion**

The Ottawa Charter for Health Promotion is the name of an international agreement signed at the First International Conference on Health Promotion, organized by the World Health Organization (WHO) and held in Ottawa, Canada, in November 1986

Five action areas for health promotion were identified in the charter:
- Building healthy public policy
- Creating supportive environments
- Strengthening community action
- Developing personal skills
- Re-orienting health care services toward prevention of illness and promotion of health

58 *Good to Remember*

8th Global Conference on Health Promotion – Helsinki, 2013

The main theme of the conference was "Health in All Policies" (HiAP) and its focus was on implementation, the "how-to". It was structured around six themes.
- The conference aims to:
  - **Intersectoral action**: Facilitate the exchange of experiences and lessons learnt and give guidance on effective mechanisms for promoting intersectoral action;
  - **Health in all Policies (HiAP)**: Review approaches to address barriers and build capacity for implementing Health in All Policies;
  - **Social determinants of health**: Identify opportunities to implement the recommendations of the Commission on Social Determinants of Health through Health in All Policies;
  - **Investing in HiAP**: Establish and review economic, developmental and social case for investing in HiAP
  - **Primary health care**: Address the contribution of health promotion in the renewal and reform of primary health care
  - **Review**: Review progress, impact and achievements of health promotion since the Ottawa Conference.

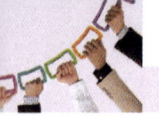

Multiple Choice Questions

1. **In a subcenter population, the CBR is 20, what should be the rate of ANC registration.** *(AIIMS Nov 2017)*
   a. 120 b. 80
   c. 60 d. 100
2. **True about population coverage of primary health center:** *(PGI May 2017)*
   a. 20000 in plain area b. 30000 in plain area
   c. 10000 in tribal area d. 20000 in tribal area
   e. 30000 in tribal area
3. **Which is correct about Kartar Singh Committee:** *(Recent Question 2017)*
   a. No private practice
   b. Multi-purpose worker scheme
   c. ROME scheme
   d. Equal pay for equal work
4. **ASHA covers how much population in a plain?**
   a. 1000 b. 2000
   c. 1500 d. 2500
5. **1 male health worker, 1 female health worker should be present at each PHC. This is given by which committee?** *(Recent Question 2017)*
   a. Jungalwalla Committee
   b. Kartar Singh Committee
   c. Bhore Committee
   d. Mudaliar Committee
6. **As per norms pharmacist and lab technician are suggested per how much population?**
   a. 5000
   b. 10,000
   c. 15,000
   d. 20,000
7. **Number of visits to be carried out by ASHA in a home delivery:** *(Recent Question 2016)*
   a. 3 b. 4
   c. 6 d. 7
8. **Observation under nursing care for 24 hours in an hospital is defined as:**
   a. Outpatient
   b. Inpatient
   c. Urgent care patient
   d. Observation status patient

BOOKS AND TITLES

9. **"Secret of national health is to be found in the homes of people" was stated by:**
   a. Indira Gandhi
   b. Abraham Lincoln
   c. Joseph Bhore
   d. Florence Nightingale

MODERN MEDICINE AND MEDICAL REVOLUTION

10. **Personal services rendered by doctors to patients in hospital, nursing home and at home is:** *(Recent Question 2016)*
    a. Health care b. Medical care
    c. Domiciliary care d. Nursing care
11. **AYUSH Ministry was set up in 2014, for education and research in:** *(Recent Question 2015)*
    a. Ayurveda, Yoga and Naturopathy
    b. Unani and Siddha
    c. Homeopathy
    d. All

MISCELLANEOUS

12. **"Right to life" is under which article of our constitution:**
    a. 11 b. 21
    c. 23 d. 25
13. **Nursing care in a hospital for a duration more than 24 hours is defined as:** *(Recent Question 2015)*
    a. Outpatient care b. Emergency care
    c. Inpatient care d. Observation status patient

NRHM

14. **All of the following are true about ASHA except:**
    a. She is trained for a period of 21 days
    b. Works with the Village Health and Sanitation Committee
    c. Act as depot holder for IFA, ORS
    d. She is in the age group 25–45 years
15. **Duty of ASHA worker include?**
    a. Escort pregnant women to hospital for delivery
    b. Screen village population for NCD
    c. Administer immunoglobulin to all eligible children
    d. Optimum coverage of all government program under supervision of ANM
16. **ASHA is not the depot holder for:**
    a. IFA b. OPV
    c. Contraceptive d. ORS
17. **USHA (Urban Social Health Activist) covers a population of:** *(Recent Question 2015)*
    a. 5000–10000 b. 1000–2500
    c. 4000–5000 d. 2500–5000
18. **All of the following are criteria for selection of ASHA, except:**
    a. Resident of village
    b. Women in the age group 25–45 years
    c. Education minimum 8th class
    d. In tribal areas one ASHA per 1000 population

Ans.

1.	c
2.	b, d
3.	b
4.	a
5.	b
6.	b
7.	d
8.	d
9.	d
10.	b
11.	d
12.	b
13.	d
14.	a
15.	a
16.	b
17.	b
18.	d

Most Recent Questions of 2019-18 are given at the end of MCQs

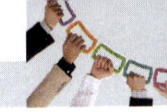

19. **ASHA is located at**
    a. Subcenter b. PHC
    c. CHC d. Village
20. **ASHA worker works for .... Population**
    a. 3000 b. 1000
    c. 5000 d. 400
21. **NRHM was started in:** *(Recent Question 2015)*
    a. 2005 b. 2006
    c. 2007 d. 2009
22. **ASHA gets remuneration on all, expect:**
    a. Institutional delivery
    b. Zero dose of OPV and BCG
    c. Recording birth weight
    d. Birth registration
23. **ASHA covers how much population in a plain?**
    a. 1000 b. 2000
    c. 1500 d. 2500
24. **In rural plane area, 1 ASHA is employed for how many people?** *(Recent Question 2015)*
    a. 500 b. 1000
    c. 3000 d. 5000
25. **True about ASHA is:**
    a. Male
    b. Resident of village
    c. 35–55 years age
    d. Literate up to class five
26. **Selection criteria for ASHA are all, except:** *(Recent Question 2015)*
    a. Woman
    b. Resident of village
    c. Education up to class five
    d. Literate
27. **Function of ASHA comprise:**
    a. Mobilization for institutional deliveries
    b. Conduction of Home delivery
    c. Give Immunization at birth
    d. Provide DEC for filarial treatment
28. **ASHA is recruited under:** *(Recent Question 2015)*
    a. NRHM
    b. National urban health mission
    c. ICDS
    d. Village health system
29. **ASHA full form is:**
    a. Accredited Social Health Activist
    b. A social health agent
    c. A specific health agent
    d. Advanced scientific health agent
30. **Which of the following is the 'Impact indicator' for evaluation of ASHA performance?**
    a. Number of meetings attended
    b. Number of institutional deliveries
    c. Reduction in infant mortality
    d. Hours of training
31. **All are included in National Rural Health Mission (NRHM), except:** *(Recent Question 2014)*
    a. Strengthening of JSY (Janani Suraksha Yojana)
    b. Formation of family health and social welfare societies
    c. State and district health mission
    d. Recruitment and training of ASHA

RCH

32. **Drug-kit B is given at:** *(Recent Question 2014)*
    a. PHC b. Subcenter
    c. CHC d. FRU level

NATIONAL HEALTH POLICY & NATIONAL POPULATION POLICY

33. **National Health Policy true are all, except,** *(Kol 2009)*
    a. Eradicate polio-2005
    b. Eliminate leprosy-2005
    c. Eliminate lymphatic filariasis-2010
    d. Achieve zero level growth of HIV-2007

MISCELLANEOUS

34. **Central Drugs Standard Control Organization Zonal Offices are located at all of the following places, except:**
    a. Mumbai b. Chennai
    c. Kolkata d. Jaipur
35. **PERT is:**
    a. The longest path of the network
    b. An arrow diagram which represents the logical sequence in which events must take place
    c. Helps decision makers to allocate resources so that they are used in the most effective way
    d. Systematic observation and recording of activities of one or more individuals carried out at random or predetermined intervals
36. **The longest path of the network is given by:**
    a. PERT b. CPM
    c. Work sampling d. Model
37. **A program where everything starts from "scratch:**
    a. Simple budgeting system
    b. Custom budgeting system
    c. Zero budget approach
    d. Critical path method
38. **Rural health scheme was formed based on the recommendation of** *(Recent Question 2014)*
    a. Shrivastava Committee
    b. Bhore Committee
    c. Mudaliar Committee
    d. Mukherjee Committee
39. **The concept of social physicians was given by**
    a. Shrivastava Committee
    b. Bhore Committee
    c. Mudaliarcommittee
    d. Mukherjee Committee
40. **The concept of PHC was given by:** *(Recent Question 2014)*
    a. Shrivastava Committee
    b. Bhore Committee
    c. Mudaliar Committee
    d. Mukherjee Committee
41. **"Critical path" in network analysis is:**
    a. Most expensive path in a network
    b. Congested path in a network
    c. Shortest path in a networ
    d. Longest path in a network

Ans.

19.	d
20.	b
21.	a
22.	b
23.	a
24.	b
25.	b
26.	c
27.	a
28.	a
29.	a
30.	c
31.	b
32.	b
33.	c
34.	d
35.	b
36.	b
37.	c
38.	a
39.	b
40.	b
41.	d

Most Recent Questions of 2019-18 are given at the end of MCQs

42. Systemic observation and recording of activities of one/ more individuals carried out at predetermined/random intervals is: *(Recent Question 2015)*
a. Decision making
b. System analysis
c. Network analysis
d. Work sampling

43. In health management, cost benefit analysis in an example of:
a. Critical path method
b. Program evaluation and review technique
c. Management by objectives
d. Total quality management

44. Analysis done for expenditure of a large proportion for small number of items and vice versa is:
a. ABC b. SDE
c. VED d. PSN

45. PERT technique is used in following:
a. Network analysis
b. Cost effective analysis
c. Input output analysis
d. System analysis

46. Planned end point of all activities is:
a. Objective b. Target
c. Goal d. Policy

47. A method which compares benefits of a program without taking into account for the cost of the program is called: *(Recent Question 2015)*
a. Cost benefits analysis
b. Cost effective analysis
c. Cost accounting
d. Input-output analysis

48. Which one of the following is a quantitative method of health management?
a. Cost effectiveness analysis
b. Human Resource Management
c. Communication management
d. Supportive supervision and leadership

49. Planning cycle includes: *(Recent Question 2015)*
a. Analysis of situation
b. Evaluation
c. Resource assessment
d. All

50. Set of statement for monitoring progress towards goal is referred as: *(Recent Question 2014)*
a. Target b. Objective
c. Program d. Procedure

51. Multipurpose Worker scheme in India was introduced following the recommendation of: *(Recent Question 2014)*
a. Shrivastava Committee
b. Bhore Committee
c. Kartar Singh Committee
d. Mudaliar Committee

52. Universal health coverage of India was recently approved by which health committee?
a. Medical education health group
b. MPW in health and family planning
c. High level expert group
d. Health survey and development committee

53. MPW Scheme in India was introduced following the recommendation of: *(Recent Question 2014)*
a. Srivastava Committee
b. Bhore Committee
c. Kartar Singh Committee
d. Mudaliar Committee

54. Bajaj Committee, true is:
a. Constituted in 1946
b. Recommended formation of PHC
c. Recommended health manpower policy
d. None

55. Rural health scheme was introduced by:
a. Bhore Committee
b. Mukherjee Committee
c. Srivastava Committee
d. Mudaliar Committee

56. A 3-year graduate MBBS program was suggested by:
a. Sundar Committee
b. Srivastava Committee
c. Expert level committee on universal health coverage
d. Krishnan Committee

57. As per NHP 2002, which of the following is to be eliminated by 2015
a. Malaria b. Leprosy
c. Filariasis d. Yaws

58. Male health worker, 1 female health worker should be present at each PHC. This is given by which committee?
a. Jungalwalla Committee
b. Kartar singh Committee
c. Bhore Committee
d. Mudaliar Committee

59. 3 tier rural health infrastructure was proposed by:
a. Bhore Committee b. Mukherjee Committee
c. Chadha Committee d. Bajaj Committee

60. VED Analysis is a term in management that stands for:
a. Vital essential desirable
b. Valuable essential desirable
c. Vital essential discrete
d. Valuable easily available discrete

61. ABC and VED analysis in management applies to:
a. Inventory management
b. Personal management
c. Emergency services management
d. Human resource management

PRIMARY HEALTH CARE/HEALTH FOR ALL

62. The Alma-Ata conference defines *(Recent Question 2013)*
a. Primary prevention b. Quality of life
c. Positive health d. Primary health care

63. Alma-Alta declaration came in the year:
a. 1948 b. 1978
c. 1952 d. 1921

64. The following is not an element of primary health care
a. Maternal and child healthcare, including family planning
b. Immunization against infectious diseases
c. Prevention and control of endemic diseases
d. Appropriate treatment of rare diseases and injuries

Ans.

42. d
43. d
44. a
45. a
46. a
47. b
48. a
49. d
50. a
51. c
52. c
53. c
54. c
55. c
56. c
57. c
58. b
59. a
60. a
61. a
62. d
63. b
64. d

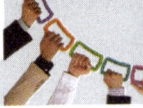

65. Elements of primary health care include all of the following, except: *(Recent Question 2013)*
a. Adequate supply of safe water and basic sanitation
b. Preventive and control of local endemic disease
c. Providing employment to every youth
d. Immunization against major infectious disease

66. Elements of primary health care include all of the following, except:
a. Adequate supply of safe water and basic sanitation
b. Providing essential drugs
c. Sound referral system
d. Health education

67. All of the following are pillars of primary health care except: *(Recent Question 2013)*
a. Equitable distribution
b. Community participation
c. Health education
d. Intersectoral coordination

68. Principles of Primary Health Care includes all, except:
a. Intersectoral coordination
b. Appropriate technology
c. Mainly coordinated by doctors
d. Community participation

69. All are principles of Primary Health Care except:
a. Intersectoral Coordination
b. Community Participation
c. Appropriate Technology
d. Decentralized Approach

70. Primary Health care concept was promoted and brought forward by: *(Recent Question 2013)*
a. Bhore Committee
b. Alma-Ata Declaration
c. Shrivastava Committee
d. National Health Policy

71. Which of the following is not an essential component of primary health care? *(Recent Question 2013)*
a. Provision of Essential Drugs
b. Cost effectiveness
c. Immunization against major infectious diseases
d. Health education

72. Which of the following is the current trend in Health Care?
a. Qualitative enquiry
b. Community participation
c. Equitable distribution
d. Primary health care

73. Which of the following best reflects the highest level of community participation.
a. Planning of intervention by community
b. Intervention based on assessment of community needs
c. Provision of resources by community
d. Community supports and cooperates with workers

MILLENIUM DEVELOPMENT GOALS

74. The following is not a health related Millennium development goal 2000 *(Recent Question 2013)*
a. Eradicate extreme poverty and hunger
b. Increase doctor-population ratio
c. Reduce child mortality
d. Combat HIV/AIDS, malaria and other diseases

75. 1st goal in Millennium development goals
a. Reduce poverty and extreme hunger
b. Improve maternal health
c. Reduce child mortality
d. Develop a global partnership for development

76. True regarding the launch of Millennium Development Goals is *(Recent Question 2013)*
a. Launched by WHO in 1998
b. Launched by UN in 2000
c. Launched by UN in 1998
d. Launched by WHO in 2000

77. Millennium Development Goal, targets to reduce maternal mortality rate by: *(Recent Question 2013)*
a. 0.25 b. 0.50
c. 0.75 d. 1.00

78. Number of health related goals in millennium development goals?
a. 1 b. 2
c. 3 d. 4

79. According to MDG child mortality has to be reduced by:
a. 1/3 b. 1/2
c. 2/3 d. 1/4

80. Millennium developmental goals pertaining to HIV/AIDS:
a. 6 b. 3
c. 8 d. 1

LEVELS OF HEALTH CARE

81. The national health plan recommended one PHC for how many people in hilly and tribal areas:
a. 5000 b. 10000
c. 20000 d. 30000

82. The level of care that is closest to the people is: *(Recent Question 2013)*
a. Primary health care
b. Secondary health care
c. Tertiary health care
d. All the above

83. One health worker (male) is expected to cover a population of ___ in plain areas.
a. 1000 b. 2000
c. 3000 d. 5000

84. What is the suggested population norm for Health Assistant in a tribal area?
a. 1 per 50,000 b. 1 per 30,000
c. 1 per 20,000 d. 1 per 5000

85. Female Health Worker covers a population of: *(Recent Question 2013)*
a. 100 population
b. 1000 population
c. 5000 population
d. 30000 population

86. Multipurpose Health Worker works for a population of:
a. 1000
b. 3000
c. 100
d. 5000

87. Functions of a Female Health Worker include:
a. Visit 4 Subcenters/month
b. Collection of blood sample
c. Conduct 50% delivery
d. Chlorination of water

Ans.

65.	c
66.	c
67.	c
68.	c
69.	d
70.	b
71.	b
72.	b
73.	a
74.	b
75.	a
76.	b
77.	c
78.	c
79.	c
80.	a
81.	c
82.	a
83.	d
84.	c
85.	c
86.	d
87.	c

Most Recent Questions of 2019-18 are given at the end of MCQs

88. A subcenter in a hilly area caters to population of:
a. 1000
b. 2000
c. 3000
d. 5000

89. A trained Dai caters to a population of
a. 1000
b. 2000
c. 3000
d. 4000

90. Which of the following is not a work of female MHW?
a. Malaria surveillance
b. Distribution of condoms
c. Immunization
d. DOTS activities

91. Which of the following is true about Female Health Worker?
a. Acts at PHC level
b. Covers population of 5000
c. Chlorinates well at regular intervals
d. Make at least 3 post natal visits for each delivery

92. Staff at PHC includes: *(Recent Question 2013)*
a. Pharmacist
b. Clerk
c. Radiologist
d. Laboratory technician
e. Pediatrician

93. How many beds are there in PHC for indoor patients?
a. 2 b. 3
c. 6 d. 9

94. Job functions of Health Assistant males are:
a. ORS distribution
b. Collect Smear from any fever case
c. Collection of sputum smear from having person prolonged cough
d. Immunization
e. Check minimum of 10% house in a village

95. Community Health Center caters a population of:
a. 10,000 to 20,000 b. 30,000 to 50,000
c. 50,000 to 80,000 d. 80,000 to 1,20,000

96. Minimum number of beds in Community Health Center is:
a. 4-6 b. 15
c. 30 d. 100

97. Population covered by community health center:
a. 5000 b. 30000
c. 50000 d. 80000-120000

98. True about Anganwadi worker are all, except:
a. Mostly female *(Recent Question 2013)*
b. Training for 4 months
c. Under ICDS scheme
d. Covers a population of 2000

99. False regarding Anganwadi worker –
a. Training for 4 months
b. Under ICDS scheme
c. Gets ₹1500 per month
d. Full-time worker

100. Objectives of IPHS for PHC comprise all except
a. Ensure availability of accident and emergency care
b. Provide Primary Health Care
c. Provision of quality health care
d. Provide services responsive to community needs

101. Number of Female Health Worker proposed at Subcenter as per revised IPHS guidelines 2012 is:
a. 3 b. 1
c. 2 d. None

102. As per revised IPHS guidelines, an Ophthalmologist is proposed for: *(Recent Question 2013)*
a. Every 3 CHC
b. Every 5 CHC
c. Each CHC
d. Every 2 CHC

103. Which of the following statements about Rashtriya Swasthya Bima Yojana is true?
a. Cashless benefit on presenting smartcard and fingerprints
b. Valid for up to 4 family members
c. Can be used in 1 district
d. Treatment only in government hospitals

104. Rashtriya Swasthya Bima Yojana, all are true, except:
a. Applicable for BPL only
b. Entitled for 30000 rupees
c. Pay and reimbursement follows
d. Is a type of employment scheme

105. Rashtriya Swasthya Bima Yojana is:
a. Government run insurance scheme for its employees
b. Government run insurance scheme for all citizens
c. Government run insurance scheme for poor
d. Private insurance company run scheme for all poor

106. True about Rashtriya Swasthya Bima Yojana is:
a. Applies to BPL families only
b. Annual cover is rupees 30000/- per family member
c. 75% premium is borne by family
d. Implemented all over India

107. In IDSP, lab report of disease sent as "L form" is:
a. Syndromic diagnosis b. Confirmed
c. Presumptive d. Active surveillance

108. In IDSP India, which of the following type of diagnosis is done by PHC Medical Officer?
a. Syndromic b. Probable case
c. Confirmed d. Laboratory

109. Which of the following disease is not under surveillance in integrated disease surveillance project (P-FORM):
a. Snake bite *(Recent Question 2013)*
b. Acute respiratory tract infections
c. Tuberculosis
d. Leptospirosis

110. Disease NOT covered under integrated disease surveillance project (IDSP) is: *(Recent Question 2013)*
a. Meningococcal disease
b. Tuberculosis
c. Herpes zoster
d. Cholera

Ans.

88. c
89. a
90. a
91. b
92. a,b,d
93. c
94. b,d,e
95. d
96. c
97. d
98. d
99. d
100. a
101. c
102. a
103. a
104. d
105. c
106. a
107. b
108. b
109. a
110. c

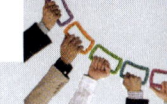

111. **Type of surveillance included in IDSP for non-communicable disease is:** *(Recent Question 2013)*
   a. Sentinel surveillance
   b. Regular surveillance
   c. Periodic regular survey
   d. Additional state priority

112. **Mega city is with population of**
   a. 1 L – 5 Lakh
   b. 5 Lakh – 1 million
   c. >1 million – 4.5 million
   d. >4.5 million

113. **Under IDSP, the surveillance reporting is done every**
   a. Daily
   b. Weekly
   c. Fortnightly
   d. Monthly

Most Recent Questions (2019–2018)

114. **Under National Health Mission which committee makes plan for village health?** *(AIIMS May 2018)*
   a. Panchayat health committee (PHC)
   b. Village health planning and management committee (VHPMC)
   c. Village health sanitation and nutrition committee (VHSNC)
   d. Rogi kalyan samiti

115. **Regarding public health surveillance, which of the following is/are true is:** *(PGI May 2018)*
   a. Done to evaluate the disease load in the society
   b. Identify risk factors associated with health conditions
   c. It can be both active and passive
   d. It helps in framing new health programme
   e. Only done for rare disease

116. **Single disease programme known as** *(JIPMER Nov 2018)*
   a. Horizontal
   b. Vertical
   c. Interventional
   d. Integrated

117. **PHC's are available for providing community based health care services. The quality assurance and resource management is done by** *(JIPMER Nov 2018)*
   a. WHO external monitoring committee
   b. NGO's involvement
   c. IPHS
   d. NABH

118. **AIIMS New Delhi was established by which health agency...** *(JIPMER Nov 2018)*
   a. WHO
   b. UNICEF
   c. SIDA
   d. The Colombo plan

119. **Regarding functions of ASHA, all are true except?** *(AIIMS May 2019)*
   a. Malaria Slide preparation
   b. Facilitate Immunization
   c. Accompany pregnant females to hospital
   d. Spread awareness about contraception

120. **Which of the following comes under concurrent list:** *(Recent Question 2019)*
   a. International immigration for quarantine
   b. Prevention of communicable diseases
   c. Mines and oilfield workers rules
   d. Establishment and maintenance of drug standards

Ans.

111. c
112. c
113. c
114. c
115. a, b, c, d
116. b
117. c
118. d
119. a
120. b

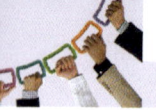

Answers with Explanations

1. Ans. (c) 60

If the subcenter population is 5000 and CBR is 20.

The number of live births is = (CBR / 1000) * population = (20/1000) *5000 = 100

The number of pregnant females = Live births + 10% (of LB) (pregnancy wastage factor)

So, the pregnant females in a year would be = 100 + 10 = 110 At any given time, the Sub center should have minimum at least 50% of the ANC registrations. Hence the sub Centre in the MCQ given would have at least 55-60 registrations at any given time.

2. Ans. (b) 30000 in plain area; (d) 20000 in tribal area

3. Ans. (b) Multi-purpose worker scheme

Ref: K. Park, 24th ed. p 912

4. Ans. (a) 1000

Ref: K. Park, 24th ed. p 470

5. Ans. (b) Kartar singh Committee

Ref: K. Park, 24th ed. p 912

6. Ans. (b) 10,000

Ref: K. Park, 24th ed. p 938

7. Ans. (d) 7

Ref: K. Park, 24th ed. p 480

8. Ans. (d) Observation status patient

Ref: http://www.ncpssm.org/Portals/0/pdf/hospital-observation.pdf

BOOKS AND TITLES

9. Ans. (d) Florence Nightingale

Ref: Sir Edward Tyas Cook, The Life of Florence Nightingale, Volume 1

MODERN MEDICINE AND MEDICAL REVOLUTION

10. Ans. (b) Medical care

Ref: Reasoning

11. Ans. (d) All

Ref: www.ayush.gov.in

AYUSH stands for **A**yurveda, **Y**oga and Naturopathy, **U**nani, **S**iddha and **H**omeopathy[Q].

Also Know......................

Ministry of AYUSH was formed on 9th Nov 2014

MISCELLANEOUS

12. Ans. (b) 21

(Ref: Voice of Research, Vol. 2 Issue 2, September 2013, p-61-66

Article 21 secures two rights:

- **Right to life** (including right to livelihood and work)
- **Right to personal liberty**

13. Ans. (d) Observation status patient

Ref: The World Health Report 2000 – Health systems: improving performance https://www.ncbi.nlm.nih.gov

Inpatient care: Admission to a health-care facility and discharge after one or more days.

Outpatient care: A person who goes to a health-care facility for a consultation, and who leaves the facility within three hours of the start of consultation. An outpatient is not formally admitted to the facility.

Ambulatory care: Medical and paramedical services delivered to patients, formally admitted for diagnosis, treatment or other types of health care with the intention of discharging the patient the same day.

Long-term care: Care is concerned with maintaining or improving the ability of patient with disabilities to function as independently as possible for as long as possible; it also encompasses social and environmental needs. It is broader than the medical model that dominates acute care.

NRHM

14. Ans. (a) She is trained for a period of 21 days

Ref: K. Park, 24th ed. p 470, Press Information Bureau GOI, MOHFW, 16-May, 2013

Training of ASHA

- The induction training of ASHA is for 23 days in 5 episodes *spread over 1 year.*[Q]
- After 6 months of her functioning in the village, she is sensitized on HIV/AIDS, STI, RTI, prevention and referrals.
- She is also trained on newborn care.
- The Central Government bears the cost of training, incentives and medical kits.

15. Ans. (a) Escort pregnant women to hospital for delivery

Ref: K. Park, 24th ed. p 936

16. Ans. (b) OPV

Ref: K. Park, 24th ed. p 936

17. Ans. (b) 1000-2500

Ref: K. Park, 24th ed. p 466

18. Ans. (d) In tribal areas one ASHA per 1000 population

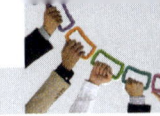

19. Ans. (d) Village

Ref: K. Park, 24th ed. p 470

ASHA or Accredited Social Health Activist is a link person between community and health care services.

- Norm → 1 ASHA for 1000 population. [Tribal, hilly and desert areas 1 ASHA per habitation].

Also Know......................

- Other village level worker → Anganwadi worker, Village Health guide, Trained dai

20. Ans. (b) 1000

Ref: K. Park, 24th ed. p 470

21. Ans. (a) 2005

Ref: K. Park, 24th ed. p 469

National Rural Health Mission (NRHM) was launched on 12th April 2005, for a period of 7 years (2005-2012).[Q]

Refer to Notes for Details

22. Ans. (b) Zero dose of OPV and BCG

Ref: K. Park, 23rd ed. p 450, DK Taneja, Health Policies and Programs in India,13th ed. p-89; 24th ed. p 89

- ASHA gets an incentive for institutional delivery under JSY (not for zero dose OPV).

Role and Responsibilities of ASHA

Also Know......................

- ASHA working on a 1000 population gets about ₹3000/ month approx. as performance based incentives.

23. Ans. (a) 1000

Ref: K. Park, 24th ed. p 36

24. Ans. (b) 1000

Ref: K. Park, 24th ed. p 936

25. Ans. (b) Resident of village

Ref: K. Park, 24th ed. p 936

26. Ans. (c) Education up to class five

Ref: K. Park, 24th ed. p 936

27. Ans. (a) Mobilization for institutional deliveries

Ref: K. Park, 24th ed. p 936

28. Ans. (a) NRHM

Ref: K. Park, 24th ed. p 469

29. Ans. (a) Accredited Social Health Activist

Ref: K. Park, 24th ed. p 469

30. Ans. (c) Reduction in infant mortality

Ref: K. Park, 24th ed. p 469

31. Ans. (b) Formation of family health and...

Ref: K. Park, 24th ed. p 469

RCH

32. Ans. (b) Subcenter

Ref: MoHFW, IPHS 2012 Guidelines

Level of health care	Drug/Equipment kit supplied
Sub Center	Drug kit A and B, Midwifery kit and Sub-center equipment kit
PHC	PHC equipment kit, Essential Obstetric Care kit*
CHC/FRU	Equipment kit E to P

**Category C districts*

NATIONAL HEALTH POLICY & NATIONAL POPULATION POLICY

33. Ans. (c) Eliminate lymphatic filariasis-2010

Ref: K. Park, 25th ed. p 936

MISCELLANEOUS

34. Ans. (d) Jaipur

Ref: www.cdsco.nic.in, Central Drugs Standard Control Organization, DGHS, Ministry of Health and Family Welfare

Also Know......................

Human blood is covered under the definition of 'Drug' under Sec. 3((b) of Drugs and Cosmetics Act 1940)

- Blood Banks are regulated under the Drugs and Cosmetics Act and rules.

CDSCO: Central Drug Standard Control Organization [Headed by Drugs Controller General (Indi(a)]

- It has 4 Zonal offices at Mumbai, Ghaziabad, Kolkata, Chennai, 3 sub zonal and 7 port offices

Main Functions

- Control of quality of drugs imported into the country
- Coordination of activities of state/UT drug control authorities.
- Approval of new drugs proposed to be imported or manufactured in the country
- Lay down standards and regulatory measures
- Act as Central License Approving Authority (CLA(a) in respect of whole human blood and blood products, I.V. Fluids, Vaccines, Sera and r –DNA.

- Regulate the quality of cosmetics manufactured and marketed in the country.

Also Know.......................

- Testing Human Blood for HIV and Hepatitis C is a mandatory requirement before transfusion.

35. Ans. (b) An arrow diagram which represents...

Ref: K. Park, 24th ed. p 909

Network analysis[Q] is a graphic plan of all events and activities that need to be completed in order to reach an end objective. It has 2 components–**PERT and CPM**

Program Evaluation and Review Technique (PERT)

- An Arrow Diagram[Q] of logical sequence of events that must take place is made along with calculation of time needed for each activity to be completed
- Critical activities are identified.
- It minimizes any delay or crises in implementation of the plan and can calculate time taken for any project
- Potential problems are identified
- It aids in planning, scheduling and monitoring of any project
- It leads to preparation of continuous, timely progress reports

Also Know.......................

- Arrow Diagram is the *Essence of PERT.*

36. Ans. (b) CPM

Ref: K. Park, 24th ed. p 909

37. Ans. (c) Zero budget approach

Ref: Textbook of Community Medicine 3rd Edition, B Rao Thirunavalli p 729

Zero Base Budgeting

- It was used for the 1st time in USA in 1962 by former President of America, Jimmy Carter.
- It starts from "scratch." Previous year's budget is not used as a base for preparing this year's budget.
- It does not assume that all the activities of the previous year must be continued
- Zero is taken as a base and likely future activities are decided according to the present situations.
- It requires every manager to justify the entire budget in detail from 'scratch'

Advantages of ZBB

- It helps to identify waste and useless activities.
- It helps to identify efficient alternative approaches.
- It facilitates better communication between various levels of management.

Disadvantage of ZBB

- A lot of discussion, review and paper work is involved

38. Ans. (a) Shrivastava Committee

Ref: K. Park, 24th ed. p 912

39. Ans. (b) Bhore Committee

Ref: K. Park, 24th ed. p 910-11

40. Ans. (b) Bhore Committee

Ref: K. Park, 24th ed. p 910-11

41. Ans. (d) Longest path in a network

Ref: K. Park, 24th ed. p 909

42. Ans. (d) Work sampling

Ref: K. Park, 24th ed. p 909

Work Sampling

- *It is systematic observation and recording of various activities of one or more people, at different intervals (predetermined or random).*
- ***Major parameters analyzed are***→*Type of activity performed and time spent to perform specific jobs.*
- It has been done on doctors, nurses, pharmacists and laboratory technicians.
- It permits judgments to the appropriateness of current staff, job description and training.
- Helps in standardizing methods of performing jobs and determining manpower needs in any organization.

43. Ans. (d) Total quality management

Ref: K. Park, 24th ed. p 908

44. Ans. (a) ABC

Ref: Post Graduate Certificate Course on Health system and management. Module 5 Chapter 3, p 8

ABC inventory control method is based on the principle that a small portion of items consume bulk of the budget.

Whereas a relatively large number of items may consume a small part of the budget

Also Know.......................

Other Inventory Control Measures

- **ABC analysis** [Always Better Control]
- **VED** [Vital Essential and Desirable]
- **HML** [Based on cost of individual item as High Medium and Low]
- **SDE** system [Based on ease of availability of items Scarce, Difficult and Easy]
- **GOLF** [Based on source of supply Govt., Ordinary , Local and Foreign]
- **FSN** [Rate of issue from stores Fast moving (F), Slow moving (S) and Nonmoving]
- SOS [Based on Seasonal (S) and Off-seasonal (OS) availability]

45. Ans. (a) Network analysis

Ref: K. Park, 24th ed. p 909

46. Ans. (a) Objective

Ref: K. Park, 24th ed. p 905

Objective [Q] *is the planned end point of all activities directly concerned with a specific problem. It is* precise and may or may not be achieved.

Also Know.......................

Target is the degree of achievement *of a discrete activity and* factors involved. E.g. *number of blood films collected, tubectomy/vasectomy performed etc.*

47. Ans. (b) Cost effective analysis

Ref: K. Park, 24th ed. p 908

Cost effective analysis [CEA]- Here benefits of the program are expressed in terms of results achieved (e.g., number of lives saved) are compared to cost of the program.

$$\text{CEA} = \frac{\text{Cost incurred}}{\text{Number of lives saved}}$$

48. Ans. (a) Cost effectiveness analysis

Ref: K. Park, 24th ed. p 908

Quantitative Management Techniques Comprise

- Cost effective analysis
- Cost benefit analysis
- Cost accounting
- System analysis
- Work sampling
- Input output Analysis
- Network analysis [PERT and CPM]
- Planning-Programming-Budgeting System
- Zero budgeting.
- Model

49. Ans. (d) All

Ref: K. Park, 24th ed. p 906

Steps in Planning

Plan formulation (Defining problem, Setting goals/objective) → Execution → Monitoring and Evaluation

50. Ans. (a) Target

Ref: K. Park, 24th ed. p 905

51. Ans. (c) Kartar Singh Committee

Ref: K. Park, 24th ed. p 912

52. Ans. (c) High level expert group

Ref: K. Park, 24th ed. p 914

Latest Updates

Universal Health Coverage (UHC) means "Equitable access of all Indian citizens across the country, regardless of income, social status, gender, caste or religion to affordable accountable, appropriate and quality assured health services (Promotive, Preventive, Curative and Rehabilitative) as well as services addressing wider determinants of health"

- Government is to act as a guarantor and enabler for the health services.
- Healthcare services to all citizens UHC is to be made available via the public sector and contracted-in private facilities (including NGOs and nonprofits).
- Universal Health Coverage was approved by the High Level Expert Group.

Also Know.......................

Core areas of HLEG recommendations to augment and strengthen capacity of India's health system to fulfill vision of UHC

- Health Financing and Financial Protection
- Health Service Norms
- Human Resources for Health (HRH)
- Community Participation and Citizen Engagement
- Access to Medicines, Vaccines and Technology
- Management and Institutional Reforms

53. Ans. (c) Kartar Singh Committee

Ref: K. Park, 24th ed. p 912

54. Ans. (c) Recommended health manpower...

Ref: J Kishore, National Health Program, 9th ed. p 46; 12th ed. p 55

55. Ans. (c) Srivastava Committee

Ref: K. Park, 24th ed. p 912

56. Ans. (c) Expert level committee on universal health coverage

Ref: High Level Expert Group Report on Universal Health Coverage for India, p 148;http://planningcommission.nic.in/reports/genrep/rep_uhc0812.pdf

HLEG endorsed a 'Bachelor of Rural Health Care' (BRHC) course with a 3-year curriculum

- It is not a mini-MBBS course.
- District Health Knowledge Institutes would offer BRHC degree (linked to State Health Sciences Universities)
- BRHC students should be taught in local settings where they live and work
- Focus to be on essential skills package to ensure a high quality of competence in preventive, promotive and rehabilitative services essential for rural populations. The pedagogy should be focused on primary health care.
- BRHC faculty should be from existing teaching institutions or retired teachers or specialists from public health and social sciences.

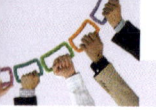

- It would be mandated by legislation that a graduate of BRHC will be licensed to serve only in specific notified areas in the government health system

57. Ans. (c) Filariasis

Ref: K. Park, 24th ed. p. 910

58. Ans. (b) Kartar Singh Committee

Ref: K. Park, 24th ed. p 912

59. Ans. (a) Bhore Committee

Ref: K. Park, 24th ed. p 910

60. Ans. (a) Vital Essential Desirable

Ref: Principles of Hospital Administration and Planning, BM Sakharkar, 2nd ed. p 262

VED Analysis [Vital Essential Desirable]: It is a Inventory Management Technique based on critical value and shortage cost of an item. It is a subjective analysis.

Type of Item	Quality
Vital	Shortage cannot be tolerated
Essential	Shortage can be tolerated for a short period
Desirable	Shortage does not adversely affect, but may be using more resources. Need to be strictly Scrutinized

	V	E	D		ITEM	Cost
A	AV	AE	AD	Category 1	10	70%
B	BV	BE	BD	Category 2	20	20%
C	CV	CE	CD	Category 3	70	10%

Category 1: Need Close Monitoring and Control
Category 2: Moderate Control.
Category 3: No Need For Control

61. Ans. (a) Inventory management

Ref: Principles of Hospital Administration and Planning, BM Sakharkar, 2nd ed. p 262

ABC Analysis (ABC = Always Better Control)

Type of Item	Quality	Management
A (Small in number, but consume large amount of resources)	About 10 % of items consume 70 % of resources	Tight control and Rigid estimate of requirements Strict and close watch Low safety stocks Managed by top level management
B (Intermediate)	About 20% of items consume 20% of resources	Moderate control Purchase based on rigid requirements Reasonably strict watch and control Moderate safety stocks Managed by middle level management
C (Larger in number, but consume lesser amount of resources)	About 70% of items consume 10% of resources	Ordinary control measures Purchase based on usage estimates High safety stocks

Contd...

PRIMARY HEALTH CARE/HEALTH FOR ALL

62. Ans. (d) Primary health care

Ref: K. Park, 24th ed. p 929

Primary Health Care approach came into existence in 1978, following an international conference at Alma-Ata

- Primary health care is "essential health care made universally accessible to individuals and acceptable to them, through their full participation and at a cost the community and country can afford."Q
- In India, primary health care is provided by complex of Primary Health Centers and Subcenters.

Also Know......................

- Primary health care is the key to the attainment of Health for All by 2000 AD.Q

63. Ans. (b) 1978

Ref: K. Park, 24th ed. p 929

64. Ans. (d) Appropriate treatment of rare diseases and injuries

Ref: K. Park, 23rd ed. p 891; 24th ed. p 928

Elements of Primary Health Care Include:Q

- Education concerning prevailing health problems and the methods of preventing and controlling them.
- Locally endemic diseases prevention and control
- Essential drugs provision
- Maternal and child health care, including family planning.
- EPI Immunization against major infectious diseases.
- Nutrition and Promotion of food supply
- Treatment of common diseases and injuries
- Safe water and basic sanitation

65. Ans. (c) Providing employment to every youth

Ref: K. Park, 24th ed. p 928

66. Ans. (c) Sound referral system

Ref: K. Park, 24th ed. p 928

67. Ans. (c) Health education

Ref: K. Park, 24th ed. p 928-29

Principles/Pillars of Primary Health Care

- Equitable distribution
- Community participation
- Intersectoral coordination
- Appropriate technology

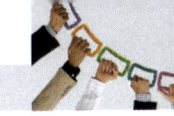

68. Ans. (c) Mainly coordinated by doctors

Ref: K. Park, 24th ed. p 928-29

69. Ans. (d) Decentralized approach

Ref: K. Park, 24th ed. p 928-29

70. Ans. (b) Alma-Ata Declaration

Ref: K. Park, 24th ed. p 929

71. Ans. (b) Cost effectiveness

Ref: K. Park, 24th ed. p 928

72. Ans. (b) Community Participation

Ref: K. Park, 24th ed. p 929

Primary health care is health by the people, placing people's health in people's hands.[Q]

- Primary health care is to be achieved by Community participation

73. Ans. (a) Planning of intervention by community

Ref: Guidebook for planning education in emergency and reconstruction, IIEP, Community participation chapter 32, p-12. UNESCO

Highest level of community participation is where communities initiate and share all aspects of decision making process.[Q]

Levels of Community Involvement

Manipulation	▪ Communities do not understand the issues with which they are confronted ▪ Communities are not given any feedback on actions taken ▪ Problem analysis is not shared with community
Decoration	▪ Communities are not involved with root of the problem and their participation is incidental ▪ External providers use community members to support their cause in a indirect manner
Tokenism	▪ Communities appear to have been given a voice, but in reality have little or no choice about subject matter. ▪ Communities have little or no opportunity to formulate their own opinion
Communities are assigned but informed	▪ Communities are given complete, accurate information about their actions and understand why their participation is needed. ▪ They know who made the decisions concerning their involvement and why ▪ They have a meaningful role to play in the development of a project ▪ They volunteer for a project after having been given all the necessary information
Communities are consulted and informed	▪ Projects are run and designed by external agencies, but communities understand the process and their opinions are treated seriously
Communities participate in project implementation	▪ Decisions are initiated externally ▪ Communities have high degree of responsibility and are involved in the production and design aspects of projects
	▪ Communities contribute their opinions before final projects are implemented
Communities initiate and direct decisions	▪ External agencies do not interfere or direct community run projects.
Communities initiate, plan, direct and implement decisions	▪ Community develops decisions and projects ▪ Actions are implemented by the community.

MILLENIUM DEVELOPMENT GOALS

74. Ans. (b) Increase doctor-population ratio

Ref: K. Park, 24th ed. p 505

75. Ans. (a) Reduce poverty and extreme hunger

Ref: K. Park, 24th ed. p 505

76. Ans. (b) Launched by UN in 2000

Ref: K. Park, 24th ed. p 505, 930

77. Ans. (c) 0.75

Ref: K. Park, 24th ed. p 505

78. Ans. (c) 3

Ref: K. Park, 24th ed. p 930

MDG →3 of the 8 goals, 8 of the 18 targets and 18 of the 48 indicators are health related. [Q]

79. Ans. (c) 2/3

Ref: K. Park, 24th ed. p 505

80. Ans. (a) 6

Ref: K. Park, 24th ed. p 505

LEVELS OF HEALTH CARE

81. Ans. (c) 20000

Ref: K. Park, 24th ed. p 911

82. Ans. (a) Primary health care

Ref: K Park, 24th ed. p 940

Primary Level of Health Care

1. It is the 1st level of contact of beneficiaries with the health system.
2. It is close to the beneficiaries and tuned to local needs
3. Problems are mostly simple in nature

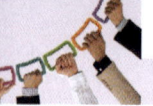

4. Provides "essential" health care: More stress on Preventive and Promotive services.
5. Institutions and personnel providing these services outnumber the secondary level.

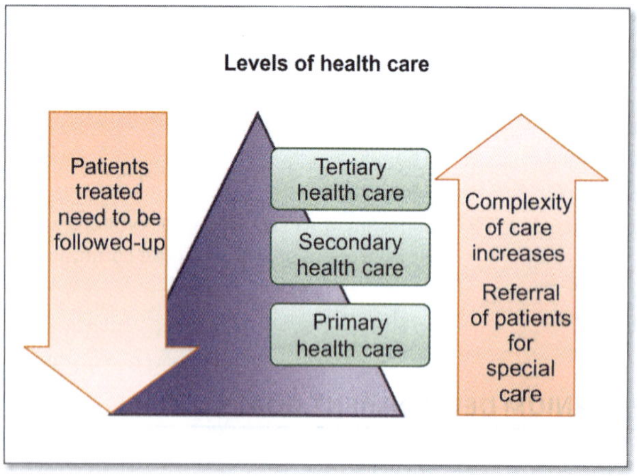

83. Ans. (d) 5000

Ref: K. Park, 24th ed. p 937

84. Ans. (c) 1 per 20,000

Ref: K. Park, 24th ed. p 941

85. Ans. (c) 5000 population

Ref: K. Park, 24th ed. p 937, 940

86. Ans. (d) 5000 population

Ref: K. Park, 24th ed. p 937, 940

87. Ans. (c) Conduct 50% delivery

Ref: K. Park, 24th ed. p 948

88. Ans. (c) 3000

Ref: K. Park, 24th ed. p 937

89. Ans. (a) 1000

Ref: K. Park, 24th ed. p 937

- National target → To train one local dai in each village. Average population of 1000.

90. Ans. (a) Malaria surveillance

Ref: K. Park, 24th ed. p 948

91. Ans. (b) Covers population of 5000

Ref: K. Park, 24th ed. p 940

92. Ans. (a) Pharmacist; (b) Clerk; (d) Laboratory technician

Ref: K. Park, 24th ed. p 944

93. Ans. (c) 6

Ref: K. Park, 24th ed. p 941

94. Ans. (b) Collect Smear from any fever case; (d) Immunization; (e) Check minimum of 10% house in a village

Ref: K. Park, 24th ed. p 952

95. Ans. (d) 80000-1,20,000

Ref: K. Park, 24th ed. p 944

Each CHC covers a population of 80,000 to 1.20 lakh (one in each community development block)

- It has 30 beds[Q]
- It has specialists in surgery, medicine, obstetrics and gynecology and pediatrics[Q]
- It has X-ray and laboratory facilities. [Q]
- Community health officer [new non-medical post at each CHC] is for strengthening preventive and promotive aspects of health care. Some states have opted for a second medical officer.
- Specialists at CHC may refer a patient directly to State level hospital or Medical College Hospital, as may be necessary, without the patient having to go first to the sub-divisional or District Hospital.

96. Ans. (c) 30

Ref: K. Park, 24th ed. p 944

97. Ans. (d) 80000-1,20,000

Ref: K. Park, 24th ed. p-944

98. Ans. (d) Covers a population of 2000

Ref: K. Park, 24th ed. p- 936

ICDS (Integrated Child Development Services) Scheme

- 1 Anganwadi worker for 1000 population.
- About 100 Anganwadi worker in each ICDS Project.
- Anganwadi worker is a part-time worker selected from the community
- Trained for 4 months in various aspects of health, nutrition, and child development
- She gets an honorarium of ₹1500 per month for services rendered (i.e. Health check-up, immunization, supplementary nutrition, health education, non-formal pre-school education and referral services.

99. Ans. (d) Full-time worker

Ref: K. Park, 24th ed. p- 936

100. Ans. (a) Ensure availability of accident and emergency care

Ref: K. Park, 24th ed. p- 941

Objective of IPHS for PHC is
- To provide quality health care
- To provide care responsive and sensitive to community needs
- To provide comprehensive Primary Health Care

101. Ans. (c) 2

Ref: K. Park, 24th ed. p- 940

102. Ans. (a) Every 5 CHC

Ref: Indian Public Health Standards (IPHS) Guidelines for Community Health Centers

103. Ans. (a) Cashless benefit on presenting smartcard and fingerprints

Ref: RSBY Document, Government of India, J Kishore, National Health Programs, 11th ed, p- 87

104. Ans. (d) Is a type of employment scheme

Ref: RSBY Document, Government of India, J Kishore, National Health Programs, 11th ed, p- 33-37

105. Ans. (c) Government run insurance scheme for poor

Ref: RSBY Document, Government of India, J Kishore, National Health Programs, 11th ed, p- 33-37

106. Ans. (a) Applies to BPL families only

Ref: RSBY Document, Government of India, J Kishore, National Health Programs, 11th ed, p- 33-37

107. Ans. (b) Confirmed

Ref: K. Park, 24th ed. p 498

IDSP – Data is collected on "S", "P" and "L" forms on weekly basis

L Form – Confirmed Diagnosis (Clinical diagnosis by Medical officer and or Lab confirmation)

P Form – Presumptive diagnosis (Diagnosis based on history and clinical examination by medical officer)

S Form – Syndromic diagnosis (Diagnosis based on clinical pattern by paramedical personnel)

108. Ans. (b) Probable case

Ref: K. Park, 24th ed. p 498

Type of Surveillance	Basis of diagnosis	Who does it
Syndromic	Clinical pattern	Paramedical personnel and members of community
Probable case	Typical history and clinical examination	Medical Officer of PHC/CHC
Confirmed	Clinical diagnosis by a medical officer and positive laboratory identification	Medical officer Laboratory

109. Ans. (a) Snake bite

Ref: K. Park, 24th ed. p 498

Diseases under Surveillance in IDSP

Syndromic Surveillance

- Fever with or without localizing signs- Malaria, Typhoid, JE, Dengue, Measles
- Cough > 2 week – TB
- Acute Flaccid Paralysis- Polio
- Diarrhea – Cholera
- Jaundice- Hepatitis, Leptospirosis, Dengue, Malaria, Yellow Fever
- Unusual syndrome – Anthrax, Plague, Emerging epidemics

Regular Surveillance

- Vector Borne disease – Malaria
- Water Borne disease - Acute diarrheal disease (Choler(a), Typhoid
- Respiratory disease – TB
- Vaccine Preventable disease – Measles
- Disease under eradication – Polio
- Others – Road Traffic Accidents
- Other International Commitment – Plague
- Unusual clinical syndromes leading to death /hospitalization – Meningitis/ Respiratory distress, Hemorrhagic fever, Other diagnosed conditions

Sentinel Surveillance

- STD/ Blood borne- HIV, Hepatitis B and C
- Others – Water quality monitoring, Outdoor air quality monitoring (Large Urban Centers)

Regular Periodic Survey-

- NCD risk factor, Anthropometry, Physical activity, Blood pressure, Tobacco, Nutrition etc.

Additional state priorities

110. Ans. (c) Herpes zoster

Ref: K. Park, 24th ed. p 498

111. Ans. (c) Periodic regular survey

Ref: K. Park, 24th ed. p 498

112. Ans. (c) >1 million – 4.5 million

Town/ city = 1 lakh–5 lakh

Medium city = > 5 lac to 1 million

Mega city = >1 million – 4.5 million

Metro city = >4.5 million

113. Ans. (c) Fortnightly

IDSP – a newly launched program in 2009.

Contains Syndromic case surveillance – done by health workers: It has six syndromes – cough, fever, AFP, diarrhoea, jaundice, unusual death

Probable case surveillance – by medical officers; with 22 Epidemic prone diseases

Laboratory surveillance – by laboratories

114. Ans. (c) Village health sanitation and nutrition committee (VHSNC)

Ref: K park, 25th ed., Pg. 481 and Health Policies and programme in India, DK Taneja, 12th ed., Pg. 82

The village health and sanitation committee

Composition of VHSC:

- Chairperson – ward member of the village
- Gram panchayat members from village
- ASHA, anganwadi worker, ANM

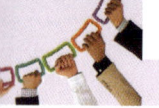

- Self-help group members
- Secretary - primary school teacher association
- Village representative from community-based organization

Functions

- To discuss the problems of the community and the health and nutrition care providers and suggest mechanism to solve it
- To create awareness in the village about available health services and their health entitlements
- To develop a Village Health Plan based on an assessment of the situation and priorities of the community
- To oversee the work of the AWW, ASHA and be involved in the management of local subcentre
- To discuss the bimonthly village report submitted by ANM

Discuss the cause of death – Death Audit and registration of the death with panchayat

115. Ans. (a) Done to evaluate the disease load in the society, (b) Identify risk factors associated with health conditions, (c) It can be both active and passive, (d) It helps in framing new health programme

Option	T/F	Remarks
Done to evaluate the disease load in the society	T	Yes, health surveillance may be taken as a mode to assess the case load in the community. it is a direct morbidity indicator
Identify risk factors associated with health conditions	T	Yes, health surveillance may help to ascertain the case load and also assess for the promotive risk factors
It can be both active and passive	T	Yes correct
It helps in framing new health programme	T	Yes, correct
Only done for rare disease	F	Not, it is done for any health related problem which may be of public health importance

116. Ans. (b) Vertical

Vertical programmes have three components: intervention strategy, monitoring and evaluation, and intervention delivery. The first two are inherently vertical in nature. The intervention strategy sets out in detail how best to handle the health problem at hand. The monitoring and evaluation component follows the impact of the intervention strategy at population level and is essential to improve it continuously

Usually health care systems (or health care programs) are horizontal system, offering promotive, curative and preventive health care for variety of prevailing health conditions.

Vertical systems (or programs) in health care imply for the specific health conditions, where the workforce, resources are targets are for specific disease or agent or intervention

117. Ans. (c) IPHS

- IPHS are a set of uniform standards envisaged to improve the quality of health care delivery in the country.
- The Indian Public Health Standards (IPHS) for Sub-centres, Primary Health Centres (PHCs), Community Health Centres (CHCs), Sub-District and District Hospitals were published in January/February, 2007 and have been used as the reference point for public health care infrastructure planning and upgradation in the States and UTs.

118. Ans. (d) Colombo plan

With the recommendation by Bhore Committee, an establishment of a national medical centre which would concentrate on meeting the need for highly qualified manpower to look after the nation's expanding health care activities was planned. A generous grant from New Zealand under the Colombo Plan made it possible to lay the foundation stone of All India Institute of Medical Sciences (AIIMS) in 1952. The AIIMS was finally created in 1956, as an autonomous institution through an Act of Parliament, to serve as a nucleus for nurturing excellence in all aspect of health care.

119. Ans. (a) Malaria Slide preparation

Ref: Park 25th ed. Pg 487

Options	T/F	Comment
Slide preparation	F	No, it is done by the Health worker (MPW) male
Facilitate Immunization	T	ASHA worker is the key functionary to facilitate for immunization sessions and liaison of vaccinators (ANM / MPW-female) with general community
Mobilize cases to hospital	T	Yes, correct
Spread awareness about sterilization	T	Yes, correct
Home delivery of contraceptives	T	Yes, correct

120. Ans. (b) Prevention of communicable diseases

The powers of the state and the Central government is scheduled under the 'seventh schedule' of the Indian Constitution. The seventh schedule has three lists – Union, state and concurrent list: The union list has a range of subjects under which the Parliament may make laws. This includes defence, foreign affairs, railways, banking, among others.

The state list lists subjects under which the legislature of a state may make laws. Public order, police, public health and sanitation; hospitals and dispensaries, betting and gambling are some of the subjects that come under the state.

The concurrent list includes subjects that give powers to both the Centre and state governments. Subjects like Education including technical education, medical education and universities, population control and family planning, criminal law, prevention of cruelty to animals, protection of wildlife and animals, forests etc. However, given that there can be conflict when it comes to laws passed by Parliament and state legislatures on the same subject, the Constitution provides for a central law to override a state law.

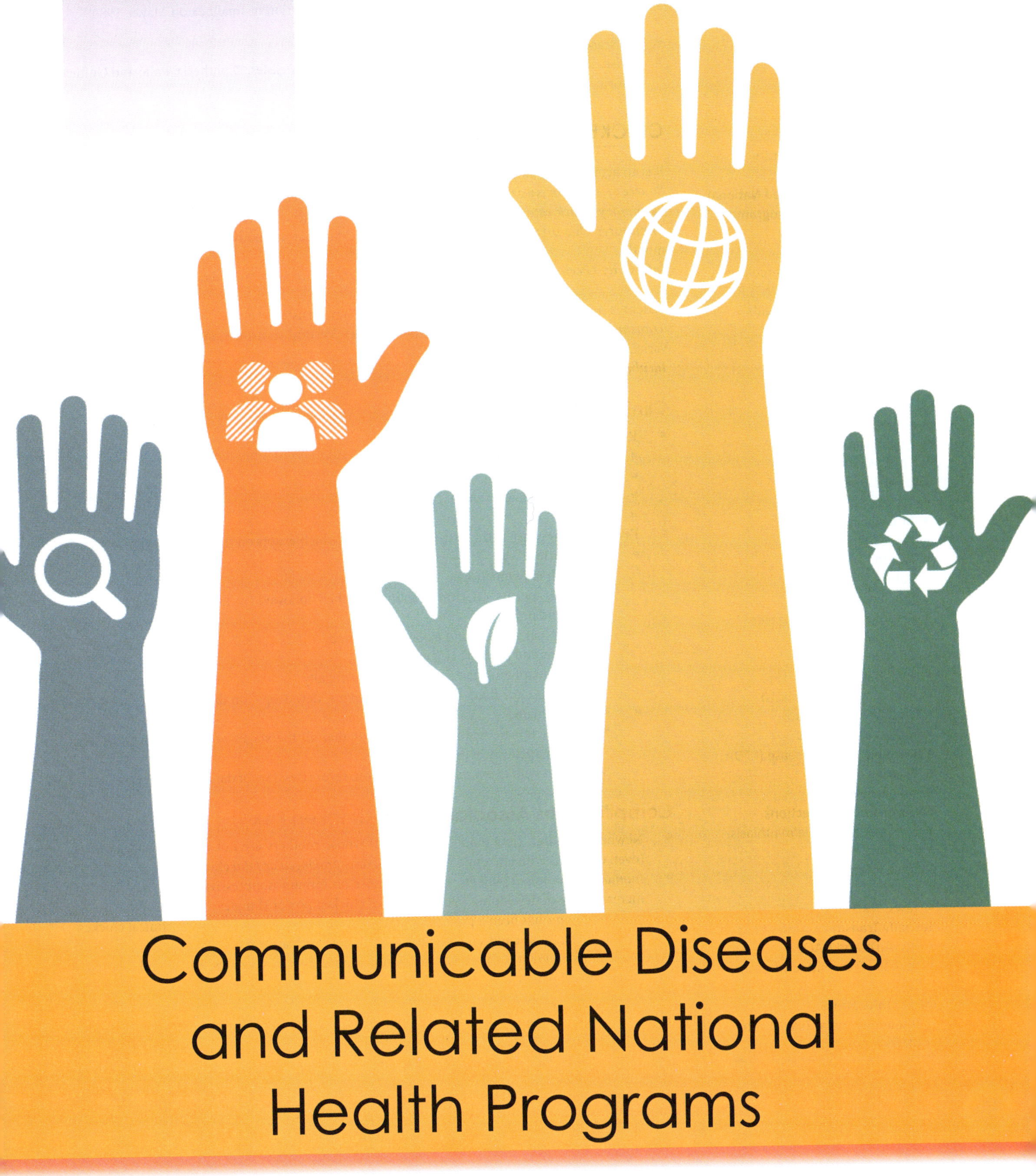

Communicable Diseases and Related National Health Programs

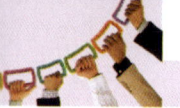

Chapter Outline

AIRBORNE INFECTIONS

SMALLPOX

World Health Organization (WHO) declared global eradication of smallpox on May 8, 1980[Q]

- India was declared smallpox-free[Q] in April 1977
- Disease eradicated globally till date is—Smallpox.[Q]
- Diseases targeted for global eradication[Q] in future are Measles, Diphtheria, Polio and Guinea worm

CHICKEN POX (VARICELLA)

It is an acute infectious disease caused by Varicella-zoster virus [Human (alpha) herpes virus 3]
Source of infection is a case of chicken pox (oropharyngeal secretions and lesions of skin/mucosa).
Secondary attack rate = 90% in household contacts (Highly communicable)
Immunity: One attack gives durable immunity. Maternal antibody protect infant in 1st few months.
Infectivity (Period of communicability) is 1–2 days before and 4 to 5 days after appearance of rash.
Patient is noninfectious once the lesions (Vesicles) have crusted
Transmission: Droplet infection and droplet nuclei. Vertical transmission leading to congenital varicella.
Incubation period: 14 to 16 days

Clinical Features

- **Pre-eruptive stage:**
  - Sudden onset of mild to moderate fever
  - Back pain
  - Shivering and
  - Malaise
- **Eruptive stage:** Rash is the first sign in children which erupts on the day the fever starts.
  - **Distribution:**
    - Rash is symmetrical
    - First appears on trunk (abundant) then followed by face, arms and legs (less abundant)
    - Mucosal surfaces and axilla are involved
    - Palms and soles are not involved
    - Density of eruption diminishes centrifugally
    - Rash is clear fluid vesicle and look like a "dew drops" on the skin
  - **Pleomorphism:**
    - Characteristic feature of the rash is that all the stages of the rash may be seen simultaneously at one time
    - Fever: with every new crop eruption, fever rises. (Secondary rise of fever).

Complications Associated with Chicken Pox

- Newborn children (less than 1 month old) whose mothers are not immune and patients (even children) with leukemia may suffer *severe, prolonged or fatal* chicken pox
- *Immunocompromised patients*, including those on immunosuppressive drugs, may have an increased risk of developing a severe form of chicken pox or shingles
- *Reye's Syndrome* has been a potentially serious complication associated with clinical chicken pox involving those children who have been treated with aspirin
- *Varicella pneumonia* is the most common complications in neonates, adults and immune-compromised patients
- Maternal varicella during pregnancy may cause *fetal wastage and birth defects* such as:
  - Cutaneous scars
  - Atrophied limbs
  - Microcephaly

- Low birthweight
- Cataract
- Microphthalmia
- Chorioretinitis
- Deafness
- Cerebrocortical atrophy

- Varicella zoster virus is major association with acute retinal necrosis and progressive outer retinal necrosis among AIDS patients.

Laboratory Diagnosis

Laboratory diagnosis has been done for confirmation

- Detecting VZV DNA using polymerase chain reaction (PCR) or isolating VZV in cell culture from vesicular fluids, crusts, saliva, CSF or other specimens. (most sensitive tests)
- Less sensitive methods are:
  - Direct immunofluorescence
  - Detection of VZV- specific serum IgM antibody
- Serological screening of serum for IgG antibodies to assess immunity or susceptibility to infection in unvaccinated persons like health workers.

Prevention

- **Varicella zoster immunoglobulin (VZIG):**
  - In exposed susceptible persons especially in immunocompromised patients should be given within 72 hours of exposure
  - It has no therapeutic value in established disease
  - Schedule: IM injection in a dose of 12.5 units/kg body weight up to maximum of 625 units, with repeat dose in 3 weeks, if high-risk patient remains exposed.
  - It binds with varicella vaccine, so the 2 should not be given concomitantly.
- **Vaccine:**
  - A vaccine to protect children against chicken pox was first licensed in March 1995.
  - It is a live attenuated varicella vaccine recommended for 12–18 months children who have not had chicken pox.
- **Monovalent vaccine:**
  - Two-dose schedule of 0.5 mL each by subcutaneous route with an interval of either 6 weeks or 3 months for children (12 months to 12 years of age inclusion), and 4 or 6 weeks for adolescents and adults.
- **Combination vaccines (MMRV):**
  - Administered to 9 months to 12 years of children
  - Two-dose schedule with an interval of 4 weeks
  - It is preferred that 2nd dose be administered 6 weeks to 3 months after first dose or at 4–6 years of age.
- Duration of immunity probably 10 years.
- Vaccine can be considered in clinically stable HIV patient CD4+T cell levels ≥15% including those receiving highly active ART.
- **Vaccine is contradicted in:**
  - Pregnancy
  - Immune-compromised patient
  - Person allergic to neomycin
- Salicylates should be avoided for 6 weeks following vaccination to prevent Reye's syndrome.

MEASLES (RUBEOLA)

Measles is an acute infectious disease caused by RNA paramyxovirus

- **Infective material:** Secretions from the nose, throat and respiratory tract in case of measles
- Epidemics occur when the proportion of susceptible children reaches about 40%
- Epidemics are common in India during winter and early spring (January to April)
- Incidence is equal in both sexes
- Highly infectious in prodromal phase and during eruption of rash. Infectivity decreases after appearance of rash.[Q]

88 High Yield Points

- OKA Strain is used for varicella
- CDC recommendation: Children 12 months through 12 years of age should get 2 doses of chicken pox vaccine

59 Good to Remember

Chicken pox and herpes zoster are different host responses to same etiological agent. A fall in CMI (Cell-Mediated Immunity) leads to reactivation of virus in 10–30% cases resulting in herpes zoster

89 High Yield Points

- Infection in pregnant women (<20 week of gestation) leads to Congenital Varicella Syndrome (in 0.4–2.0% children)
- Seasonal (winter and spring in temperate/tropical country) and Periodic outbreaks (once in 2–5 years) occur

58 Must Remember

- Only one antigenic type of measles virus exist.
- Infection confers lifelong immunity.[Q]

59 Must Remember

Measles is responsible for around 2% of under-5 mortality in India.

- *Transmission:* Droplet infection and Droplet nuclei
- SAR of Measles = 80%
  - Incubation period: Vaccine induced is 7 day and10/14* day for natural infection (Exposure to onset of Fever/Rash*)
  - Measles vaccine can provide postexposure prophylaxis, if given within 3 days of exposure
  - Prevention: Vaccination (1st dose of vaccine gives 95% protection) at 9 completed month and 16–24 month (2 Dose)
  - Period of communicability is 4 days before and 4 days after appearance of the rash
  - Control measures:
- Isolation for 7 days after onset of rash
- Immunization of contacts within 2 days of exposure or at the start of an epidemic.

90 High Yield Points

Sometimes measles and chicken pox may occur together, so the most remarkable finding is that the first infection may diminish the severity of the rash of the second infection.

Clinical Features

Prodromal phase: Fever, coryza, nasal discharge, cough, redness of eyes, lacrimation and Photophobia. Koplik's spots are pathognomionc of measles.

60 Good to Remember

Measles may be prevented by early use of immunoglobulin in the incubation period.
Dose: 0.25 mL per kg of body weight – best within 3-4 days of exposure

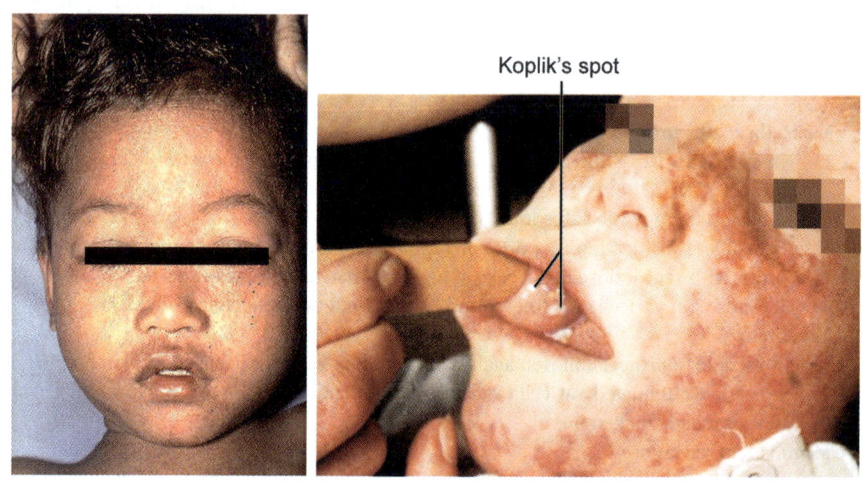

Fig. 1: Koplik's spot

60 Must Remember

In 2010, China held the largest supplementary immunization activity (SIA), vaccinating >130 million children and India started implementation of a 2 dose vaccination strategy.

- **Eruptive phase:** Dusky red, maculopapular rash (erupt behind ears and spread rapidly). Rash fade in order of appearance. A brown discoloration may persist for 2 months or more.

91 High Yield Points

Second dose of measles vaccine added to the routine immunization schedule in countries that have achieved ≥80% coverage of the first dose of the vaccine at the national level for 3 consecutive years, as determined by WHO/UNICEF estimates.

Complications of Measles

- **Most common complication:** Diarrhea, pneumonia and other respiratory complications and otitis media
- Measles leads to acute Vitamin A deficiency (Keratomalacia, corneal scar and blindness)
- **Serious complication:** Febrile convulsion, Encephalitis and SSPE (Dawsons disease)
- SSPE is a rare complication that develops after many years of initial measles infection (1 in 3 Lakh)

Diagnosis

Diagnosis of measles is done clinically by Koplik's spot and maculopapular rash.

Prevention

- **Vaccination**
  - Live attenuated vaccine
  - Each dose of 0.5 mL contains ≥1,000 viral infective units of the vaccine strains
  - Vaccine contains sorbitol and hydrolyzed gelatin as stabilizers and small amount of neomycin

- After reconstitution, vaccine must be kept in dark due to sensitive to sunlight at 2–8°C and used within 4 hours
- Vaccine should be administered as close to the age of 9 months
- In case of measles outbreak, it can be given at 6 months of age and second dose as close to 9 months with 4 weeks interval
- It is administered generally subcutaneously but can be effective if given intramuscularly
- Immunity develops after 11–12 days of vaccination with 99% protection with first dose
- Combined vaccine like MMR, measles and rubella (MR) and measles, mumps, rubella and varicella (MMRV) are also effective

- **Immunoglobulin**
  - Measles may be prevented by administering immunoglobulin early in the incubation period
  - Dose recommended by WHO is 0.25 mL/kg of body weight
  - Should be given within 3-4 days of exposure, then passively immunized the person by giving live vaccine 8–12 weeks later.

Measles Elimination and Eradication

16 March – world measles immunization day.

Measles is eradicable disease. It is amenable for eradication because of the following reasons:

- It is a disease of human beings only.
- There is no animal reservoir.
- There is neither subclinical state nor carrier state.
- Potent, live, vaccine is available
- Single dose administration.
  - The only two limitations for the eradication are:
  - 95 percent of infant population must be immunized
  - Immunization must be a continuous ongoing program.

WHO measles elimination plan:

As the initial strategy to eliminate measles, WHO proposed a 3 phase strategy:

- **Catch up** – This is a nationwide campaign to vaccinate all children between the ages of 9 months and 14 years regardless of measles history or vaccination status
- **Keep up** – This is the routine vaccination schedule in which the aim is to vaccinate at least 95% of children in each successive birth cohort
- **Follow up** – It is conducted every 2-4 years after the catch-up phase. All children born after the catch-up phase are vaccinated.

Later, the targets proposed as milestones towards the goal of eradication of measles include:

- More than 95% coverage with first dose of measles vaccine.
- Reduce annual measles incidence to less than 5 cases per million population and maintain at that level.
- Reduce measles mortality by 95 percent or more compared to 2000 estimates.

2012-20 Global Measles and Rubella Strategic Plan

- Achieve and maintain high levels of population immunity-2 doses of Measles Vaccine.
- Establish effective surveillance
- Outbreak preparedness for rapid response and case management
- Communicate and engage to build public confidence in, and demand for vaccination
- Conduct research and development to support operations and improve vaccination and diagnostic tools.

MUMPS

- It is an acute infection caused by RNA virus classified as genus Rubella virus of the family paramyxoviridae.
- This virus has a predilection for glandular and nervous tissues.

Epidemiological Determinants

Agent Factors

- The causative agent is Myxovirus parotiditis is a RNA virus of myxovirus family
- Both clinical and subclinical cases are source of infection, but subclinical cases are more responsible
- Virus is isolated from the saliva or the swabs taken from the surface of Stenson's duct
- Period of communicability is usually *4–6 days before the onset* of symptoms and *1 week thereafter.*
- This disease has estimated 85% secondary attack rate.

Host Factors

- Mumps is the most frequent cause of parotitis in 5–9 years age group children
- Disease tends to be more severe in adults as compared to children
- One attack gives lifelong immunity.

Environmental Factors

- It is an endemic disease
- It has peak incidence in winter and spring.

Mode of Transmission

- Mainly by droplet infection and after contact with an infected person.

Incubation Period

- Varies from 2–4 weeks, usually 14–18 days.

Clinical Features

- Pain and swelling in either one or both parotid glands
- Child complains of 'ear ache' on the affected side prior to the onset of swelling
- Pain and stiffness on opening of mouth before the onset of swelling
- Mumps may also affect testes, pancreas, CNS, ovaries, prostate, etc.
- Severe cases, there may be fever and headache last for 3–5 days.

92 ***High Yield Points***

Laboratory Confirmed Mumps

- Positive mumps IgM antibody without mumps immunization in previous 6 weeks; or
- Seroconversion with 4-fold or greater rise in mumps IgG titer; or
- Isolation of mumps virus from saliva, urine or CSF.

Complications

- Orchitis (Commonly unilateral and M/C extra-salivary gland manifestation)
- Ovaritis
- Pancreatitis (*Mumps is the leading cause of pancreatitis in children)*
- Meningoencephalitis
- Thyroiditis
- Neuritis
- Hepatitis
- Myocarditis
- Oophoritis (Mostly unilateral)
- Infection in first trimester of pregnancy can cause spontaneous abortion.
- Sensorineural deafness (Mumps is one of the main infectious cause).

Prevention

Vaccination

- Live attenuated vaccine.
- Mumps vaccine strains include:
  - Jeryl-Lynn (Commonly used and have lowest incidence of postvaccine aseptic meningitis)
  - RIT 4385
  - Leningrad-3
  - L-Zagreb
  - Urabe strains

61 ***Must Remember***

Vaccine strains used on limited scale include:

- Hoshino
- Torii
- NKM-46

- WHO recommended Rubini vaccine strain should not be used in National Immunization Programme because of it low effectiveness.
- A single dose of 0.5 mL IM recommended for routine immunization for children over 1 year of age, either alone or in combination vaccine (MMR, MMRV)
- The second dose is recommended for children at 4–6 years of age, i.e. before starting the school.

RUBELLA (GERMAN MEASLES)

- It is an acute childhood infection.
- Disease follows the cyclic trend of epidemic, in nonimmunized populations, every 6 to 8 years.

Epidemiological Determinants

Agent Factors

- It is caused by an RNA virus of the togavirus family.
- Only 1 antigenic type of virus exists.
- Clinical or subclinical case of rubella is the source of infection.
- Period of communicability is probably 1 week before symptoms to 1 week after rash appears.

Host Factors

- It mainly affects 3–10 years of age group children.
- One attack results in lifelong immunity.

Environmental Factors

- It has a seasonal pattern, i.e. in temperate zones during the late winter and spring, with epidemic every 4–9 years.

Transmission

- Transmits directly from person to person by droplets from nose and throat, and droplet nuclei (aerosols).
- The virus can cross the placenta (vertical transmission).

Incubation Period

- 2–3 weeks; average 18 days.

Clinical Features

- **Prodromal:** Coryza; Sore throat; Low grade fever
- **Lymphadenopathy:**
  - Enlargement of postauricular and posterior cervical lymph nodes
  - Enlargement of glands
- **Rash:**
  - It is the first indication of disease in children.
  - It appears first on face, usually within 24 hours of the onset of prodromal symptoms.
  - It is minute, discrete, pinkish and macular rash.
  - Rash spreads rapidly to the trunk and extremities, by which time it is not apparent on face.
  - It disappears on third day.
  - Rash is absent in subclinical cases, so it is not pathognomonic sign.

Complications

Congenital Rubella

- *Congenital rubella syndrome (CRS)* refers to infants born with defects secondary to intrauterine infection or who manifest symptoms or signs of intrauterine infection sometime after birth.

61 Good to Remember

History

- In 1941, Norman Gregg, an ophthalmologist reported an epidemic of congenital cataracts associated with other congenital defects in children born to mothers who had rubella during pregnancy.
- 1962, the virus was isolated.
- 1967, an attenuated vaccine was developed.

62 Must Remember

Source of infection: large number of subclinical cases

Period of communicability: Rubella is less communicable than measles due to absence of cough.

93 High Yield Points

- **Other defects are:**
  - Glaucoma
  - Retinopathy
  - Microcephalus
  - Cerebral palsy
- Intrauterine growth retardation
- Hepatosplenomegaly
- Mental and motor retardation

63 Must Remember

Rate of infection and organ damage to fetus is highest in 1st trimester of pregnancy. Those infected after 20 weeks suffer no major abnormalities[Q]

- It is a chronic infection.
- The classical triad of congenital defects are:
  - Deafness
  - Cardiac malformations
  - Cataracts
- Nearly 85% of abnormalities occur in fetus if the infection occurs in first trimester of pregnancy as compared to second trimester
- Birth defects are uncommon, if maternal infection occurs after 20 weeks of gestation.
- At birth, virus is easily detected in pharyngeal secretions, multiple organs, CSF, urine and rectal swabs.
- Presence of IgM or IgG (for 6 months) indicates presence of congenital infection.
- Viral excretion may last for 12–18 months after birth.

Diagnosis

- Virus isolation
- **Serology:**
  - Hemagglutination inhibition (HI) test
  - ELISA tests
  - Demonstration of rise in antibody titer between 2 serum samples taken 10 days apart or rubella specific IgM in single sample, accurately confirms the recent infection.

> 94 *High Yield Points*
>
> **Rubella Vaccination Strategy**
> - 1st priority- women of child-bearing age (15–34 or 39 years of age)
> - 2nd priority- Interrupt transmission by vaccinating all children 1–14 years age
> - 3rd priority- Routine immunization of all children <1 year (using combined MR or MMR vaccine)

Prevention

Rubella Vaccine

- RA 27/3 vaccine is live attenuated vaccine administered in a single dose of 0.5 mL subcutaneously.
- The recipients of vaccine should be advised not to become pregnant over the next 3 years.
- Also available in combined vaccine with measles and mumps (MMR).

	1st trimester	2nd trimester	3rd trimester	At delivery
Disease showing vertical trans-mission	Rubella, Varicella	Parvovirus	Syphilis, Toxoplasma, Hepatitis B, CMV,	HIV, Hepatitis C, Herpes

PERTUSSIS

- The Chinese call it a "Hundred Day Cough".

Epidemiological Determinants

Agent Factors

- B. pertussis is the causative agent.
- In 5% cases, B. parapertussis is responsible.
- B. pertussis infects only man.
- The source of infection is a case of pertussis.
- Nasopharyngeal secretions, bronchial secretions and objects contaminated with secretions are the infective materials.
- Infective period ranges from a week after exposure to about 3 weeks after the onset of paroxysmal stage.
- 90% of secondary attack rate in unimmunized household contacts.

Host Factors

- It is a disease of *infants and pre-school children.*
- The highest incidence is found below the age of 5 years.
- Infants below 6 months have the highest mortality.
- Incidence and fatality is more among female as compared to male children.

Environmental Factors

- Occurs throughout the year but more cases during winter and spring months

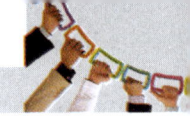

Transmission

- Droplet infection and direct contact

Incubation Period

- Usually 7-14 days, but not more than 3 weeks

Clinical Features

- **Catarrhal stage**
  - Last for 10 days
  - Insidious onset
  - Lacrimation
  - Sneezing and coryza
  - Anorexia
  - Malaise
  - Hacking night cough that becomes diurnal
- **Paroxysmal stage**
  - Lasting for 2–4 weeks
  - Bursts of rapid, consecutive coughs followed by a deep, high pitched inspiration (whoop)
  - Followed by vomiting
  - Cyanosis and apnea
- Convalescent stage
  - Last for 1–2 weeks

Complications

- Bronchitis
- Bronchopneumonia
- Bronchiectasis
- Subconjunctival hemorrhages
- Epistaxis
- Hemoptysis
- Punctuate cerebral hemorrhages

Laboratory Diagnosis

- Bacteriological examination of nose and throat secretions obtained by swab.

Treatment

- Erythromycin, 30-50 mg/kg of body weight in 4 divided doses for 10 days is the drug of choice.

DIPHTHERIA

- It is an acute infectious disease having 4 major clinical types: anterior, nasal, faucial and laryngeal.
- It is a rare disease in developed countries due to routine immunization but occasionally seen among nonimmunized children.
- In India, it is an endemic disease.
- Case fatality rate of about 2.61 (GOI {2014}, National Health Profile 2013, DGHS)

Epidemiological Determinants

Agent Factors

- Diphtheria is caused by toxigenic strains of *Corynebacterium diphtheria*.
- 4 types of diphtheria bacilli are: *gravis* (***more severe infection***), *mitis, belfanti* and *intermedius*, all pathogenic to man.

- Case or carrier may be the source of infection.
- Immunization does not prevent carrier state.
- Nasopharyngeal secretions, discharges from the skin lesions, contaminated fomites and possibly infected dust.
- Period of infectivity is from 14 days to 28 days before the onset of the disease.

Host Factors

1. It particularly affects children aged 1–5 years.
2. Both the sexes equally affected.

Environmental Factors

- Cases occur in all seasons, but winter month is favorable.

Mode of Transmission

- By droplet infection
- Cutaneous lesions of infected person
- Objects contaminated by nasopharyngeal secretions of infected person.

Incubation Period

- 2–6 days

Clinical Features

Pharyngotonsillar Diphtheria

- Sore throat
- Difficulty in swallowing
- Low grade fever
- Formation of a greyish or yellowish membrane (***false membrane***) commonly over the tonsils, pharynx or larynx (or at the site of implantation), with well-defined edges and the membrane cannot be wiped away.
- "*Bull-necked*" appearance- marked edema of the submandibular area and anterior portion of the neck, along with lymphadenopathy.

Laryngotracheal Diphtheria

- Fever
- Hoarseness
- Croupy cough
- Dyspnea due to obstruction caused by membrane

Nasal Diphtheria

- Mildest form
- Localized to septum or turbinates of one side of the nose

Cutaneous Diphtheria

- Common in tropical areas
- It appears as a secondary infection
- The lesion presented as ulcer, may be surrounded by erythema and covered with a membrane

Complications

- Toxin is absorbed and results in distant toxic damage, particularly:
- Parenchymatous degeneration
- Fatty infiltration
- Necrosis of heat muscles, liver, kidneys and adrenals
- Nerve damage results in paralysis of soft palate, eye muscles or extremities.

Treatment

Cases

- Diphtheria antitoxin should be given IM or IV immediately after a preliminary test dose of 0.2 mL S/C to detect sensitization to horse serum.
- For mild disease- 20,000–40,000 units
- For moderate disease- 40,000–60,000 units
- For severe disease- 80,000–100,000 units
- In addition to antitoxin, every case should be treated with penicillin or erythromycin for 5–6 days

Carriers

- Oral erythromycin for 10 days is the most effective drug treatment

DPT Vaccine

- Pertussis component in combined vaccine enhances the potency of diphtheria toxoid.
- WHO recommends that only adjuvant DPT preparations be utilized in immunization programme
- Store at the temperature of ***2-8°C***.
- As early as 6 weeks is the optimum age for administration of this vaccine.
- 3 primary doses of 0.5 mL given at the interval of 4 weeks, with booster injection at one and a half year to 2 years, followed by another booster (DT only) at the age of 5–6 years.
- Vaccine should be injected deep intramuscular on upper and outer quadrant of the gluteal region or lateral aspect of thigh in children below 1 year of age.

Schick test is an intradermal test that gives information about:

- Presence of antitoxin and the immunity status
- State of hypersensitivity to diphtheria toxin or other proteins of diphtheria cells

Procedure: 0.2 mL (1/50 MLD) of Schick test toxin is injected intradermally into skin of forearm and as "control" same amount of inactivated and diluted toxin is injected intradermally into the opposite arm.

- ***Negative reaction:*** (Child is immune to diphtheria and no need for immunization). No reaction of any kind observed on either arm. (Serum antitoxin level >0.03 units/mL)
- ***Positive reaction:***(Child is susceptible to diphtheria and needs immunization).
- **Test arm**: Erythema >10 mm diameter within 24-48 hrs, reaching its maximum by 4th-7th day.

  Control arm shows no change.
- ***Pseudopositive reaction:*** (Child is immune and hypersensitive and no need for immunization). A transient erythema <10 mm in both arms by day 2, maximum by day 3 and fades by day 4.
- ***Combined reaction:*** (Person is susceptible, hypersensitive and needs immunization (vaccinated with caution)). Control arm shows a pseudopositive reaction and the test arm a true positive reaction.
- Schick test has largely been replaced by measurement of serum antitoxin level by the hemagglutination test.

INFLUENZA

- It is an acute respiratory tract infection caused by influenza virus, of which there are 3 types- A, B and C.
- The unique features of influenza epidemics are the suddenness with which they arise, and the speed and ease with which they spread.
- At present 3 types of influenza viruses are circulating in the world: ***A (H1N1), A (H3N2) and B*** viruses.
- Influenza A (H1N1) virus of swine origin emerged in Mexico in 2009 and given name pandemic influenza A (H1N1) 2009 virus.

64 **Must Remember**

Diphtheria immunization

- **Combined or mixed vaccines:**
  - DPT (diphtheria-pertussis-tetanus vaccine)
  - DTPw (diphtheria, tetanus, whole cell pertussis)
  - DTPa (diphtheria, tetanus, acellular pertussis)
  - DT (diphtheria-tetanus toxoid)
  - dT (diphtheria-tetanus, adult type)
- **Single vaccines**
  - FT (formal-toxoid)
  - APT (alum-precipitated toxoid)
  - PTAP (purified toxoid aluminium phosphate)
  - PTAH (purified toxoid aluminium hydroxide)
  - TAF (toxoid-antitoxin floccules)
- **Antisera:**
  - Diphtheria antitoxin

95 **High Yield Points**

Positive Schick test and Negative Tuberculin Test – indicate need for vaccination.

65 **Must Remember**

All known pandemics were caused by influenza A strains.

- It may occur in pandemics every 10-40 years due to major antigenic changes, as occurred in:
  - 1918, Spanish influenza
  - 1957, Asian influenza
  - 1968, Hong Kong influenza
- In between pandemics, epidemics tend to occur at intervals of 2–3 years in case of influenza A and 3–6 years in the case of influenza B.

Epidemiological Determinants

Agent Factors

- Influenza viruses are classified within the family Orthomyxoviridae.
- Three antigenically distinct viral subtypes namely influenza type A, type B and type C.
- No cross immunity between 3 subtypes.
- Influenza A and B viruses are responsible for epidemics throughout the world.
- Influenza A virus has two distinct surface antigens namely:
  - *Haemagglutinin (H)*
  - *Neuraminidase (N)*
- Humans are generally infected by subtypes of H1, H2 or H3 and N1 or N2.
- The influenza A virus is unique because it is frequently subject to antigenic variation, both major change or sudden complete change called as **shift** and minor change or change is gradual over a period of time called as **drift.**
- **Antigenic shift** occurs due to result from genetic recombination of human with animal or avian virus; cause major epidemics or pandemics and **antigenic drift** involves point mutation in the gene.
- Type B virus exhibit lesser degree of antigenic changes and is not divided into subtypes.
- Type C virus appears to be antigenically stable.
- Major reservoir of influenza virus exists in animals and birds e.g. swine, horses, dogs, cats, domestic poultry, wild birds, etc.
- *Source of infection* is a case or subclinical case and respiratory secretions from them.
- Period of infectivity is from 1–2 days before and 1–2 days after onset of symptoms.

Host Factors

- Influenza affects all ages and both sexes
- Human mobility is an important factor in the spread of infection
- Antibodies against HA and NA are important in immunity to influenza.

Environmental Factors

- **Season**
  - Northern hemisphere- in winter months
  - Southern hemisphere- in winter or rainy season
  - Tropical area- virus circulates throughout the year with 1 or 2 peaks during rainy season
- **Overcrowding**

Transmission

- Directly from person to person by droplet infection or droplet nuclei.

Incubation Period

- 18–72 hours

96 High Yield Points

HIV infected persons can be safely vaccinated against influenza. Vaccination is less effective when CD4 counts are less than 100/mcL

Clinical Features

- Fever for 1–5 days
- Chills
- Aches
- Pains
- Coughing
- Generalized weakness.

Complications

- Acute sinusitis
- Otitis media
- Purulent bronchitis
- Pneumonia (most dreaded complication)
- Reye syndrome

- Hepatic failure
- Encephalopathy

Laboratory Diagnosis

- **Virus isolation:**
  - Nasopharyngeal secretions are the best specimens
  - Indirect fluorescent antibody technique and egg inoculation technique are used
- **Serology:**
  - Hemagglutination inhibition (HI)
  - ELISA (more sensitive)

Prevention

- Good ventilation of public buildings
- Avoidance of crowded places
- Encouraging suffers to cover their faces with a handkerchief when coughing and sneezing
- To stay at home at the first sign of influenza
- Immunization
- Thorough cooking to more than 70°C, of poultry products

Vaccines

- **Killed vaccines**
  - The recommended vaccine strains for vaccine production are grown in the allantoic cavity of developing chick embryos, harvested, purified, killed by formalin or beta-propiolactone, and standardized according to the hemagglutinin content.
  - One dose of vaccine contains approximately 15 micrograms of HA.
  - A single subcutaneous or intramuscular inoculation (0.5 mL for adults and children over 3 years and 0.25 mL for children from 6 months to 36 months of age) is usually given
  - 2 doses of vaccine are recommended, separated by an interval of 3-4 weeks if person below 9 years is not immunized.
  - The immunity lasts for only 6–12 months, so revaccination on an annual basis is recommended.
- **Live attenuated vaccines**
  - A trivalent, live attenuated influenza vaccine administered as a single dose intranasal spray is as effective as inactivated vaccine.
  - It is approved for use in healthy individuals between age of 2 and 49 years but there is always a risk of transmission of live attenuated vaccine virus to immunocompromised individuals.

Immunity

- Vaccine does not give 100% protection against disease.
- Vaccine only becomes effective after 14 days, so persons get infected shortly before (1-3 days) and shortly after immunization can still get the disease.

Influenza Updates 2018

Categorization of Cases for Containment of Outbreaks

Category A

- Mild fever cough/sore throat
  Recommendation
- Do not require oseltamivir
- Monitored for 24-48 hrs by physician
- No testing required for H1N1

Category B

Include Category A symptoms +

- High grade fever + severe sore throat

66 **Must Remember**

Mass vaccination to prevent influenza epidemic is not recommended

62 **Good to Remember**

WHO recommends to immunize following groups according to their priority:

- Health care workers (to prevent nosocomial transmission)
- Pregnant women
- Individuals aged more than 6 months with one or more several chronic medical conditions.
- Healthy young adults between 15–49 years
- Healthy children
- Healthy adults between age 49–65 years
- Healthy adults aged more than 65 years

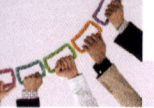

- High risk factor group
    - Age <5 years or >65 years
    - Pregnant female
    - Chronic underlying condition as cancer, HIV/AIDS
    - Patients on long term immunosuppressive therapy

Recommendation:
- Home isolation + oseltamivir
- No tests are required for category B (i) and B (ii)

Category C

Includes Category A, Category B AND
- Breathlessness, chest pain, hypotension, haemoptysis, cyanosis
- Children: Irritability and refusal to feed
- Worsening of any underlying chronic condition

Recommendation:
- Immediate hospitalization and treatment

Phases for Influenza Pandemic

Phase 1-3: predominantly animal infections, very few human infections
Phase 4: sustained human to human transmission. Effective response to preventive measures can avert an impending epidemic
Phase 5 – widespread human disease but restricted to one WHO region
Phase 6: declared pandemic – widespread human infection – cross two WHO regions
Post peak – possibility of recurrent infections
Post pandemic – disease activity at seasonal levels

Management Guidelines for Influenza 2018

Pandemic influenza A (H1N1) is currently susceptible to the neuraminidase inhibitors (NAIs) oseltamivir and zanamivir but resistant to the M2 inhibitors amantidine or rimantidine. Standard antiviral treatment regimens:

- **Oseltamivir**
    - It is a neuraminidase inhibitor
    - It is taken orally activated by hepatic esterase.
    - Dose is 75 mg twice daily for 5 days as treatment.
    - 75 mg once daily as prevention.
    - Modified in renal patients.

Table 1: Antiviral treatment for infants under 1 year of age

Age	Dosage
>3 months – 12 months	3 mg/kg, twice daily for 5 days
>1 month – 3 months	2.5 mg/kg, twice daily for 5 days
0 – 1 month	2 mg/kg, twice daily for 5 days

Table 2: Older children dosage according to weight

Weight	Dosage
15 kg or less	30 mg twice a day for 5 days
15-23 kg	45 mg twice a day for 5 days
24-40 kg	60 mg twice a day for 5 days
>40 kg	75 mg twice a day for 5 days

- **Zanamivir**

The recommended dose for treatment of adults and children from age of 5 years is 2 inhalations (2 × 5 mg) twice daily for 5 days

Severe, non-responding cases:

In patients who have persistent severe illness despite oseltamivir treatment, there are few licensed alternative antiviral treatments. In these situations, consider intravenous administration of alternative antiviral drugs such as zanamivir, peramivir, and ribavirin. The use of such treatments should be done only with following cautions:

- Ribavirin should not be administered as monotherapy
- Ribavirin should not be administered to pregnant women
- Zanamivir formulated as a powder -for inhalation should not be delivered via nebulization due to the presence of lactose, which may compromise ventilator function

Chemoprophylaxis

Oseltamivir is the drug of choice for suspected, probable or confirmed cases.

It should be given till 10 days of after last exposure.

Table 3: Dosage of oseltamivir according to age and weight of patient

Weight	Dosage
15 kg or less	30 mg OD
15–23 kg	45 mg OD
24–40 kg	60 mg OD
>40 kg	75 mg OD
For infants	
Age	**Dosage**
<3 months	Not recommended unless situation is critical
3–5 months	20 mg OD
6–11 months	25 mg OD

Vaccines

Killed (Inactivated) Vaccines

- The recommended vaccine strains for vaccine production are grown in the allantoic cavity of developing chick embryos, harvested, purified, killed by formalin or beta-propiolactone, and standardized according to the hemagglutinin content.
- One dose of vaccine contains approximately 15 micrograms of HA.
- A single subcutaneous or intramuscular inoculation (0.5 mL for adults and children over 3 years and 0.25 mL for children from 6 months to 36 months of age) is usually given
- 2 doses of vaccine are recommended, separated by an interval of 3–4 weeks if person below 9 years is not immunized.
- The immunity lasts for only 6–12 months, so revaccination on an annual basis is recommended.

Flu – Inactivated Vaccine

- **Egg based quadrivalent vaccines** for use in the 2019 southern hemisphere influenza season contain the following:
  - An A/Michigan/45/2015 (H1N1) pdm09-like virus;
  - A/Switzerland/8060/2017 (H3N2)-like virus
  - B/Colorado/06/2017-like virus (B/Victoria/2/87 lineage)
  - B/Phuket/3073/2013-like virus (B/Yamagata/16/88 lineage).
- **Egg based trivalent vaccines** for use in the 2019 southern hemisphere influenza season contain the following:
  - A/Michigan/45/2015 (H1N1) pdm09-like virus;
  - A/Switzerland/8060/2017 (H3N2)-like virus; and
  - B/Colorado/06/2017-like virus (B/Victoria/2/87 lineage).
- **Non Egg Based Vaccine:**
  - A/Singapore/INFIMH-16-0019/2016-like virus (H3N2 component) along with other vaccine components

Route: Single dose intramuscular injection – upper arm

Flu Live Attenuated Vaccine (Flu-LAV)– via nasal spray

Flu-LAV contraindications

- Immunocompromised patients
- Pregnant women
- Individuals who have taken an influenza antiviral medication within the previous 48 hours
- Adults aged ≥50 years

Note: Vaccines are associated with higher risk of Guillain Barre syndrome

Indications

The influenza vaccine is recommended only for the category of 'high-risk children'.
This category contains the following:

- Chronic cardiac, pulmonary (excluding asthma)
- Hematologic and Renal (including nephrotic syndrome) condition,
- Chronic liver diseases
- Congenital or acquired immunodeficiency (including HIV infection)
- Children on long term salicylates therapy

WHO suggests the following groups for vaccination according to their order of priority:

- Pregnant women
- Individuals aged more than 6 months with one of the several chronic medical conditions;
- Healthy young adults between age 15–49 years
- Healthy children
- Healthy adults between age 49–65 years
- Healthy adults aged more than 65 years

Recent Advance

Baloxavir marboxil is a novel **oral selective inhibitor of influenza cap-dependent endonuclease** that blocks influenza proliferation by inhibiting the initiation of mRNA synthesis.

Baloxavir was associated with more rapid declines in infectious viral load than placebo or oseltamivir.

Dose-

- For 40 to <80 kg- 40 mg PO single dose
- For 80 kg and more- 80 mg PO single dose

FDA approved (24/10/18) baloxavir for the treatment of acute uncomplicated influenza (flu) in patients 12 years of age and older who have been symptomatic for no more than 48 hours.

ACUTE RESPIRATORY INFECTIONS

- Acute respiratory infections (ARI) may cause inflammation of the respiratory tract anywhere from nose to alveoli.
- It can be upper ARI or lower ARI
- ARI responsible for about 30–50% of visits to health facilities and about 20–40% of admissions to hospitals globally
- It is the leading cause of disabilities including deafness as sequelae of otitis media
- Streptococcus pneumonia is the major cause of illness and death in children as well as in adults followed by H. influenzae type B (Hib).

Epidemiological Determinants

Agent Factors

Table 4: Agents causing acute respiratory infections

Agents	Age group most frequently affected	Characteristics clinical features
Bacteria		
B. pertussis	Infants and young children	Paroxysmal cough
C. diphtheriae	Children	Nasal/tonsillar/pharyngeal membranous exudate ± severe toxaemia

Contd...

Agents	Age group most frequently affected	Characteristics clinical features
H. influenza	Adults	Acute exacerbations of chronic bronchitis pneumonia
	Children	Acute epiglottitis (type B)
Klebsiella pneumonia	Adults	Lobar pneumonia± lung abscess
Legionella pneumonia	Adults	Pneumonia
Staphylococcus pyogenes	All ages	Lobar and bronchopneumonia (esp. secondary to influenza) ± lung abscess
Streptococcus pneumonia	All ages	Pneumonia (lobar or multilobular) acute exacerbations of chronic bronchitis
Streptococcus pyogenes	All ages	Acute pharyngitis and tonsillitis
Virus		
Adenoviruses – endemic types (1,2,5)	Young adults	Lower respiratory
-epidemic types (3,4,7)	Older children and young adults	Febrile pharyngitis and influenza like illness
Enteroviruses (ECHO and coxsakie)	All ages	Variable respiratory
Influenza A and B	All ages and Children	Fever, aching, malaise, variable respiratory and occasional primary pneumonia and secondary bacterial pneumonia in elderly
Influenza type C	Rare	Mild upper respiratory
Measles	Young children	Variable respiratory with characteristic rash
Parainfluenza 1;2;3	Young children; infants	Croup; bronchiolitis and pneumonia
Respiratory syncytial virus	Infants and young children	Severe bronchiolitis and pneumonia
Rhinoviruses and coronavirus	All ages	Common cold
Other agents		
Chlamydia type B (Psittacosis)	Adults exposed to infected birds	Influenza like illness and atypical pneumonia
Coxiella burnetti (Q fever)	Adults exposed to sheep and cattle	Atypical pneumonia
Mycoplasma pneumonia	School children and young adults	Febrile bronchitis and atypical pneumonia

Host Factors

- Young infants
- Malnourished children
- Under 3 years of age boys are more affected often and more severe

Risk Factors

- Overcrowding
- Poor nutrition
- Low birthweight
- Indoor smoke pollution
- Urban communities

> 63 **Good to Remember**
>
> Any pneumonia in a young infant <2-month age is either very severe pneumonia or severe pneumonia

Transmission

- Direct to direct person transmission by airborne route

Table 5: Classification of illness in child aged 2 months to 5 years

Very severe pneumonia	Severe pneumonia
▪ **Signs** • Not able to drink • Convulsions • Abnormally sleepy or difficult to wake • Stridor in calm child, or • Severe malnutrition	▪ **Signs** • Chest in drawing (most important) • Fast respiratory breathing • Nasal flaring • Grunting • Cyanosis

Contd...

▪ **Treatment** • Refer urgently to hospital • Give first dose of an antibiotic • Treat fever, if present • Treat wheezing, if present • If cerebral malaria possible, give an antimalarial	▪ **Treatment** • Refer urgently to hospital • Give first dose of an antibiotic • Treat fever, if present • Treat wheezing
Pneumonia	**No pneumonia**
▪ **Signs** • Fast breathing • No chest in drawing	▪ **Signs** • Cough and cold • Difficulty in breathing
▪ **Treatment** • Advice mother to give home care • Give antibiotic • Treat fever and wheezing • Advice mother to return with child after 2 days for reassessment • After 2 days ◆ If worse, refer urgently ◆ If same, change antibiotic or refer ◆ If improving, finish 5 days of antibiotic	▪ **Treatment** • If cough for more than 30 days, refer for assessment • Assess and treat ear problem or sore throat or fever or wheezing or other problems, if present • Advice mother to give home care.

Table 6: Classifying illness of young infant (less than 2 months)

Very severe pneumonia	Severe pneumonia
▪ **Signs** • Stopped feeding well • Convulsions • Abnormally sleepy or difficult to wake • Stridor in calm child • Wheezing, or • Fever or low body temperature	▪ **Signs** • Severe chest indrawing, fast breathing (60/min or more)
▪ **Treatment** • Refer urgently to hospital • Keep young infant warm • Give first dose of an antibiotic	▪ **Treatment** • Refer urgently to hospital. • Keep young infant warm. Give first dose of antibiotic
No pneumonia (Cough or cold)	
▪ **Signs** • No severe chest indrawing and no fast breathing	▪ **Treatment** • Advice mother to keep young infant warm, breast feed frequently and clear nose if interferes with feeding • Return quickly if: breathing becomes difficult, becomes fast, feeding becomes problem and infant becomes sicker

Treatment

- Children aged 2 months up to 5 years
- **Pneumonia:** Cotrimoxazole is the drug of choice.

Table 7: Dosage in child as per their age and weight

Age/weight	Pediatric tablet: sulfamethoxazole 100 mg and Trimethoprim 20 mg	Pediatric syrup: each spoon (5 mL): sulfamethoxazole 200 mg and trimethoprim 40 mg
<2 months (wt. 3–5 kg)	One tablet twice a day	Half spoon (2.5 mL) twice a day
2–12 months (wt. 6–9 kg)	Two tablets twice a day	One spoon twice a day
1–5 years (wt. 10–19 kg)	Three tablets twice a day	One and a half spoon twice a day

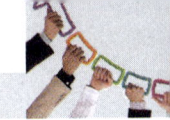

Severe Pneumonia

Table 8: Dosage of antibiotics in case of severe pneumonia

Antibiotics	Dose	Interval	Mode
A. First 48 hours			
Benzyl penicillin, or	50,000 IU/kg/dose	6 hourly	IM
Ampicillin, or	50 mg/kg/dose	6 hourly	IM
Chloramphenicol	25 mg/kg/dose	6 hourly	IM
B. 1. If condition improves, then for the next 3 days give			
Procaine penicillin, or	50,000 IU/kg	Once	IM
Ampicillin, or	50 mg/kg/dose	6 hourly	Oral
Chloramphenicol	25 mg/kg/dose	6 hourly	Oral
B. 2. If no improvement, then for next 48 hours			
Change antibiotic			

Very Severe Disease

- Chloramphenicol IM is the drug of choice
- Treat for 48 hours, if condition improves switch over to oral chloramphenicol and give for 10 days
- If condition worsens or does not improve after 48 hours, switch to IM injections of cloxacillin and gentamycin.

Table 9: Pneumonia in young infants under 2 months of age

Antibiotic	Dose	Frequency	
		Age <7 days	Age 7 days to 2 months
Inj. Benzyl Penicillin, or	50,000 IU/kg/dose	12 hourly	6 hourly
Inj. Ampicillin, and	50 mg/kg/dose	12 hourly	8 hourly
Inj. Gentamycin	2.5 mg/kg/dose	12 hourly	8 hourly

Immunization

- Measles vaccine:
- HIB vaccine
  - Schedule: 6, 10, 14 weeks of age along with DPT followed by booster dose between 12 and 18 months.
  - Administered IM
- **Pneumococcal pneumonia vaccine**
  - **PPV23**
    - Polysaccharide nonconjugate vaccine containing 23 serotypes
    - Recommended for adults and children over 2 years of age
    - A dose of 0.5 mL of PPV23 contains 25 micrograms of purified capsular polysaccharide
    - A single primary dose is administered as IM dose preferably in deltoid muscle or as subcutaneous dose.
  - **PCV**
    - Two conjugate vaccines are available: PCV 10 and PCV 13.
    - WHO recommends 2 schedule:
      - **3P+0 schedule:** Vaccination initiated as early as 6 weeks of age with interval between doses 4 and 8 weeks with dose given at 6, 10, 14 weeks or 2, 4, and 6 months.
      - **2P+1 schedule:** 2 primary doses are given during infancy as early as 6 weeks of age at an interval preferably of 8 weeks or more for young infants, and 4-8 weeks or more between primary doses for infants ≥7 months of age. One booster should be given between 9 and 15 months of age.

Integrated Global Action Plan for Prevention and Control of Pneumonia and Diarrhea

Latest Updates

Goals set for 2025 in under 5 children is to reduce the following:
- Pneumonia mortality less than 3 per 1,000 live births
- Diarrhea mortality less than 1 per 1,000 live births
- Severe pneumonia and diarrhea incidence by 75% compared to 2010 levels
- Stunting by 40% compared to 2010 levels

Latest Updates

Coverage targets set to attain above goals are:

By the end of 2025	90% full dose coverage of each relevant vaccine (80% coverage in every district)
	90% access to appropriate pneumonia and diarrhea case management (80% coverage in every district)
	Virtual elimination of pediatric HIV
	At least 50% coverage of exclusive breastfeeding in infants 0–6 months
By end of 2030	Universal access to basic drinking water, adequate sanitation*, hand–washing facility (water + soap) and clean and safe energy technologies in health care facilities and homes

*By 2040 in homes

64 Good to Remember

IHR of WHO covers 7 diseases: ***Cholera, Plague, Yellow fever, Polio, Human influenza, SARS, Small pox***

SEVERE ACUTE RESPIRATORY SYNDROME (SARS)

- It is a communicable viral disease.
- It is a notifiable disease under IHR (2005).

Incubation Period

- Estimated to be 2–7 days commonly 3–5 days

Transmission

- Direct or indirect contact of mucous membranes of eyes, nose or mouth with respiratory droplets or fomites
- Aerosol generating procedures (endotracheal intubation, bronchoscopy, nebulization treatments) in hospitals
- Natural reservoir appears to be horseshoe bat.

97 High Yield Points

Case definition of SARS
- A history of fever, or documented fever and
- One or more symptoms of lower respiratory tract illness (cough, difficulty in breathing, shortness of breath) and
- Radiological evidence of lung infiltrates consistent with pneumonia or acute respiratory distress syndrome (ARDS) or autopsy findings consistent with pneumonia or ARDS without an identifiable cause and
- No alternative diagnosis fully explaining the illness.

Diagnostic Tests Required for Lab Confirmation

- ***Conventional reverse transcriptase PCR (RT-PCR)*** and real time reverse transcriptase PCR (real time RT-PCR) assay detecting viral RNA present in:
  - At least 2 different clinical specimens (nasopharyngeal or stool specimen) or
  - The same clinical specimen collected on 2 or more occasions during the course of illness (e.g. sequential nasopharyngeal aspirates) or
  - A new extract from the original clinical sample tested positive by 2 different assays or repeat RT-PCR or real time RT-PCR on each occasion of testing or
  - Virus culture form any clinical specimen
- ***ELISA and immunofluorescent assay (IFA)***
  - Negative antibody test on serum collected during the acute phase of illness, followed by positive antibody test on convalescent phase serum, tested simultaneously, or
  - A 4-fold or greater rise in antibody titer against SARS-CoV between an acute phase serum specimen and a convalescent phase serum specimen (paired sera), tested simultaneously.

Complications

- Viral pneumonia
- Pulmonary decompensation

Management

The CDC recommends that patients suspected of or confirmed as having SARS receive the same treatment that would be administered if they had any serious, community-acquired pneumonia.

Recent approach to management of SARS

- SARS cocktail management
  - Antiviral drugs: ribavirin
  - Corticosteroids
- Other drugs may be used
  - Lopinavir/ritonavir
  - Interferons
  - **Monoclonal antibody:** A high-affinity human monoclonal antibody (huMab) to the SARS-CoV S protein, known as 80 R, has potent neutralizing activity *in vitro* and *in vivo*. This antibody was shown to neutralize SARS-CoV and inhibit syncytia formation between cells expressing the S protein and those expressing the SARS-CoV receptor ACE2.

> 65 Good to Remember
>
> **SARS**
>
> - Severe acute respiratory syndrome (SARS) is a viral respiratory illness that was recognized as a global threat in March 2003, after first appearing in Southern China in November 2002.

TUBERCULOSIS AND REVISED NATIONAL TUBERCULOSIS CONTROL PROGRAMME (RNTCP)

Topics discussed under this section are as follows:

Tuberculosis

- Epidemiology and introduction to TB
  - TB epidemiology
- Epidemiological determinants
  - Agent, host environment factors
- Diagnosis of TB

RNTCP

- Background
  - National strategic plan for elimination of TB
  - Approach TB
  - Strategy TB
  - New terminologies
- Guidelines for Diagnosis of TB
  - Adult - pulmonary TB
  - Pediatric Pulmonary TB
  - Guidelines for EPTB (extrapulmonary TB)
  - Guidelines for DRTB (drug resistant TB)
  - Summary of guidelines for Diagnosis of TB under RNTCP
- Guidelines for Treatment of Tuberculosis under RNTCP
  - DOTS (directly observed treatment short course)
  - FL- DSTB (First line regime for Drug sensitive tuberculosis)
    - Regime for DS-TB
    - Treatment for DS-TB - adults
    - Treatment plan for DSTB – Pediatric population
  - Guidelines for H -mono drug resistance
  - Guidelines for RR TB/MDR-TB
  - Follow up guidelines for MDR TB
  - Guidelines for MDR TB in pregnancy
  - Guidelines for XDR TB
  - Newer TB drugs Bedaquiline
  - Newer TB drugs Delamanid
  - Summary of treatment regimes

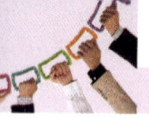

66 **Good to Remember**

END TB Targets:
90% case detection rate
90% cure rate

67 **Good to Remember**

- Over 95% of TB deaths occurred in low- and middle-income countries.
- TB is a leading killer of HIV-positive people: In 2015, 1 in 3 HIV deaths was due to TB.
- Natural course (without proper treatment) -People with active TB can infect 10–15 other people over the course of a year. Without proper treatment,45% of HIV-negative people with TB and nearly all HIV- positive people with TB will die.
- People infected with HIV are 20 to 30 times more likely to develop active TB
- Tobacco use greatly increases the risk of TB disease and death. More than 20% of TB cases worldwide are attributable to smoking.

67 **Must Remember**

Tuberculosis is considered barometer of social welfare.[Q]

- Chemoprophylaxis of TB
- RTNCP Organogram
- TB and global health
- Summary – what's new in RNTCP -India 2019

TUBERCULOSIS

Epidemiology and Introduction to TB

- It is a specific infectious disease primarily affects lungs and causes pulmonary tuberculosis.
- It can also affect intestine, meninges, bones and joints, lymph glands, skin and other tissues of the body.
- It also affects animals like cattle; which is known as Bovine tuberculosis, which may sometime transmitted to man
- Patient with infectious pulmonary tuberculosis can infect 10–15 persons per year
- It is a social disease with medical aspects, so it is also described as a barometer of social welfare.
- WHO has launched global plan for **Stop TB Strategy (2006-2015),** with the objective of reducing incidence of TB.
- In developing countries, every 1% of annual risk of infection is said to correspond to 50 new cases of smear positive pulmonary TB, per year for 100,000 general population.
- TB is the first opportunistic infection occurring in young people suffering from HIV.

TB Epidemiology (Burden of TB in India 2017)

Incidence of tuberculosis	204/100,000 population
Incidence of MDR TB	10/100,000 population
Mortality in Tuberculosis	32/100,000 population
TB case fatality ratio (mortality/incidence)	0.16/100,000 population
Among the new TB cases	
▪ % with known HIV status	64%
▪ % pulmonary TB	85%
▪ % bacteriologically confirmed among pulmonary	60%
Anti TB Drug resistance survey (2016)	
▪ MDR TB	6.19% of all TB patients
▪ New TB patients	2.8%
▪ Previously treated patients	11.6%
▪ Mono drug resistance	28%
▪ INH resistance in new TB cases	11%
▪ INH resistance in previously treated TB cases	25%

Epidemiological Determinants

Agent Factors

- The causative agent is *Mycobacterium tuberculosis* which is a facultative intracellular parasite.
- Indian tubercle bacillus is less virulent than European bacillus
- Atypical mycobacteria are isolated from man, which are saprophytic and diseases caused by them resembles pulmonary TB and chronic cervical lymphadenitis:
  - *Photochromogens (e.g. M. kansasii)*
  - *Scotochromogens (e.g. M. scrofulaceum)*
  - *Nonphotochromogens (e.g M. intercellulare)*
  - *Rapid growers (e.g. M. fortuitum)*
- **Source of infection:**
  - ***Human source***: The most common source of infection is the human case whose sputum is positive for tubercle bacilli and who has either received no treatment or has not been treated fully.
  - ***Bovine source***: Usually infected milk.
- Patients are infective as long as they remain untreated.
- Effective antimicrobial treatment reduces infectivity by 90% within 48 hours.

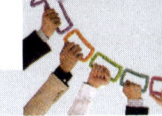

Host Factors

- Tuberculosis affects all ages but more prevalent in adults (15–54 years) than in children.
- Disease is more prevalent in males
- It is not hereditary disease
- Malnutrition is the most common risk factor
- No inherited immunity against TB.

Transmission

- Transmitted mainly by droplet infection and droplet nuclei generated by sputum positive patients with pulmonary TB.
- TB is not transmitted by fomites, such as dishes and other articles used by the patients.

Incubation Period

- It may be weeks, months or years.

Diagnosis of Tuberculosis

- **Sputum microscopy**
  - 2 sputum samples are taken; 1 sample on the spot and other sample an early morning sample brings by patient.
  - Sputum smear microscopy for tubercle bacilli is positive when there are at least 10,000 organisms present per mL of sputum.
  - Slide reporting

Number of bacilli	Oil immersion fields	Result reported
None	AFB per 100 oil immersion fields	0
1–9	AFB per 100 oil immersion fields	Scanty (or number AFB seen)
10–99	AFB per 100 oil immersion fields	+ (1+)
1–10	AFB per oil immersion field	++ (2+)
>10	AFB per oil immersion field	+++ (3+)

- **Fluorescence microscopy**
  - Mainly used in industrialized countries
  - Performed with ***auramine stain***
  - Advantage- speed of examination.
  - Field view is 5–10 times bigger.
  - Scanning of one length of smear will require only 1–2 minutes.
- **Light-emitting diode fluorescence microscopy (LEDs)**
  - Less expensive than fluorescence microscopy
  - Diagnostic accuracy of LED microscopy was found to be comparable to that of conventional microscopy and superior to that of Ziehl-Nelsen microscopy.
- **Radiography**
  - Chest X-rays are useful for diagnosis of smear negative pulmonary TB and TB in children
  - Valuable tools for diagnosis of pleural and pericardial effusion, especially in early stages of the disease when clinical signs are minimal
  - Essential in the diagnosis of military TB.
- **Sputum culture**
  - It can be performed on:
    - Conventional egg based solid medium: ***Lowenstein-Jensen medium***
    - Agar based ones- ***Middle brook 7H10 or 7H11***
    - Liquid media- ***Kirchner's or Middle brook 7H9 broth***
  - **Disadvantage:** Slow growth of mycobacterium which necessitates a mean incubation period of at least 4 weeks and the drug susceptibility tests to antituberculosis drugs require additional 4 weeks.
- **Microcolony detection on solid media**
  - Middle brook 7H11 agar medium is used
  - In less than 7 days, microcolonies of M. tuberculosis can be detected

98 *High Yield Points*

Drug susceptibility testing is done to find out drug resistant TB

It could be of two types:

- Culture (drug sensitivity and testing) technique
- Molecular susceptibility tests

- Method is less expensive and requires half the time needed for conventional culture.
- It is labor intensive.
- Method better alternative for culturing tubercle bacilli.

- **Radiometric BACTEC 460 TB method**
  - C labeled palmitic acid in 7H12 medium is used.
  - System detects the presence of mycobacteria based on their metabolism.
  - When C labeled substrate present in the medium is metabolized, CO_2 is produced and measured by the BACTEC system instrument and reported in terms of growth index (GI) value.
  - Identification is done using specific inhibitor, paranitro-a-acetylamino-b-hydroxypropiophenone.
  - Drug susceptibility can also be performed.
- **MGIT 960 mycobacteria detection system**
  - It is an automated system for the growth and detection of mycobacteria with a capacity to incubate and continuously monitor 960 mycobacteria growth indicator tube (MGIT) every 60 minutes for increase in fluorescence.
  - Growth detection is based on the AFB metabolic O_2 utilization and subsequent intensification of an O_2 quenched fluorescent dye contained in a tube of modified MGIT.
- **MB/BaCT system**
  - Nonradiometric continuous monitoring system with a computerized database management.
  - System is based on colorimetric detection of CO_2.
- **Detection and identification of mycobacteria directly from clinical samples**
  - **Genotypic methods**
    - **Polymerase chain reaction**
      - Allows sequences of DNA present in only a few copies of mycobacteria to be amplified in vitro.
      - If specific sequence is selected for bacteria, then 10-1000 organisms can be readily identified.
      - The most common target used in PCR is IS6110.
      - It is a rapid test.
    - **Transcription-mediated amplification (TMA) and nucleic acid amplification (NAA)**
      - It identifies the presence of genetic information unique to bacteria complex directly from preprocessed clinical specimens
      - NAA technique uses chemical to produce nucleic acid, so that within few hours these test can distinguish between *M. tuberculosis* complex and non-tuberculous mycobateria in an AFB positive specimen.
    - **Cartridge-based nucleic acid amplification test**
      - The second generation NAAT-based TB diagnostics with very high sensitivity and the current gold standard for TB diagnosis
      - It can early provide information on drug susceptibility to rifampicin, thus allowing the early initiation of standardized 2nd line TB treatment.
    - **GeneXpert MTB/RIF**
      - It detects DNA sequence specific for bacteria and rifampicin resistance by PCR.
      - It is based on the Cepheid GeneXpert system, a platform for rapid and simple to use NAAT.
      - The process identifies all the clinically relevant rifampicin resistance inducing mutations in the RNA polymerase beta (rpoB) gene in the mycobacterium in a real time format using fluorescent probes called molecular beacons.
      - Results are obtained from unprocessed sputum samples in 90 mins.
- **Phenotypic methods**

  FAST plaque TB: it is original phage based test for detection of M.TB directly from sputum samples

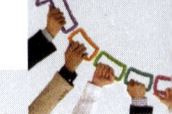

Other tests:

- Serological TB detection –
  - Advantage: Is rapid and has 'high' negative predictive value
  - Disadvantage: Low sensitivity in smear negative patients, HIV cases and in high infection rate areas
- TB STAT-PAK–immunochromatographic test based on the detection of antibodies
- Insta test TB–in-vitro assay for detection of the antibodies in active TB disease
- IGRAs–Interferon gamma release assay
  - These are tests for diagnosing TB infection and not TB disease. They do not help differentiate latent tuberculosis infection (LTBI) from tuberculosis disease
  - FDA/CDC approved IGRA are: QuantiFERON-TB Gold In-Tube test (QFT-GIT) and T-SPOT TB test
  - The IGRA test is 'not' valid for diagnosis of TB in India, as it simply detects infection rather than disease
- Tuberculin Test: To detect previous or present B infection
  - In India PPT RT-23 with tween 80 is used
  - Criteria for declaring positive tuberculin test:
  - ≥5 mm
    - HIV positive
    - Recent contacts with active TB
    - Fibrotic changes on CXR with prior TB
    - Organ transplants and other immunosuppressive patients
  - ≥10 mm
    - Recent immigrants from high TB prevalence countries
    - HIV negative drug abusers
    - Mycobacteriology laboratory personnel
    - Residents and employees of high risk occupation groups – nursing homes, health care facilities, correctional homes, hospice centers.
    - Medical conditions which increase TB risk – gastrectomy, DM, silicosis, advanced kidney disease, chronic blood disorders, leukemia, cancers
    - Children age <4 years
  - ≥15 mm – for persons with no risk factors

Two Step Tuberculin Testing

It is done for health personnel or specific groups who are routinely tested. In some people who were previously infected, the tuberculin test may be negative (as the immune system wanes off). This initial test done, may now boost the immune system to react to the tuberculin test, if given in future. So, a subsequent test may be misinterpreted as a new infection, but is due to the immune modulation by the previous test.

Therefore, a two-step tuberculin test is recommended for people who are to be tested often and periodically:

- First test is read within 48-72 hrs
  - If positive – person is tuberculin test positive
  - If negative – do second test after 3 weeks
- Second test is done after 3 weeks and result read after 48-72 hrs
  - If 2nd positive - person infected
  - If 2nd negative – person uninfected

REVISED NATIONAL TUBERCULOSIS CONTROL PROGRAMME (RNTCP)

Background

Goal: To decrease the mortality and morbidity due to tuberculosis and cut down the chain of transmission of infection until TB ceases to be a public health problem.

Objectives: To achieve and maintain:

- 90% Cure rate for treatment in tuberculosis[Q]
- 90% Case detection in the community
- Eliminate TB by 2025

99 *High Yield Points*

Molecular susceptibility tests:

As the resistance would arise from genetic mutations, the mutations themselves may be detected using molecular diagnostics.

- **GeneXpert** – Detect M.TB and associated rifampicin sensitivity directly from the sputum samples
- **Line probe assay**: Tests that use PCR and reverse hybridization methods for the rapid detection of mutations associated with drug resistance. Line probe assays are designed to identify *M. tuberculosis* complex and simultaneously detect mutations associated with drug resistance. One of the disadvantages with these assays is that they have an open-tube format, which can lead to cross contamination and an increased risk of false positive results.

100 *High Yield Points*

- Number of specimen required for diagnosis is 2 (1 spot and the other early morning specimen)
- Any person with cough of more than 2 weeks, 2 sputum samples are taken (Spot and Morning) and Sputum smear examination is done by direct microscopy (method of choice)
- On sputum smear microscopy → If 1 out of the 2 sputum sample is positive, it is termed as smear positive pulmonary TB[Q]

Latest Updates

- **NIKSHAY**- is a case based web enabled TB surveillance system *(launched in May 2012)*
- As per GOI notification 7th May 2012- TB is a *Notifiable disease* (mandatory for all health care providers)

History of RNTCP

Table 10: National tuberculosis program and revised national tuberculosis program

	NTP (1962)	RNTCP (1992)
Emphasis	Early diagnosis and Treatment	Break the chain of Transmission
Operational	Not defined targets	Cure rate >85%, Case finding >70%
Strategy	SCC supervised and conventional	DOTS Uninterrupted drug supply
Diagnosis	More emphasis on X-rays	Emphasis on sputum smear microscopy

The global plan targets are:

- To Reach 90% of all people with TB
- To Reach 90% of all 'KEY POPULATIONS" (vulnerable, underserved at risk population)
- To Achieve 90% treatment

Global End TB strategy global milestones and targets:

Indicators	Milestones		Targets	
	2020	2025	*SDG* 2030	*End TB* 2035
Reduction in number of TB deaths compared with 2015 (%)	35%	75%	**90%**	**95%**
Reduction in TB incidence rate compared with 2015 (%)	20% (<85/100 000)	50% (<55/100 000)	**80% (<20/100 000)**	**90% (<10/100 000)**
TB-affected families facing catastrophic expenditures due to TB (%)	Zero	Zero	**Zero**	**Zero**

Eliminate TB mission 2020 is an enthusiastic close target achievement strategy by the ministry of health and family welfare. The government of India also provided the complete support and announced targets for Ending TB by 2025, much ahead of the global SDG targets of 2030.

National Strategic Plan for Tuberculosis Elimination (2017–2025)

Vision: TB-Free India with zero deaths, disease and poverty due to tuberculosis
Goal: To achieve a rapid decline in burden of TB, morbidity and mortality while working towards elimination of TB in India by 2025.

Objectives

- To achieve 90% notification rate for all cases
- To achieve 90% success rate for all new and 85% for re-treatment case
- To significantly improve the successful outcome of treatment for DRTB cases
- To achieve decreased morbidity and mortality for HIV-associated TB cases
- To improve the outcome of TB care in the private sectors.

Approach RNTCP – INDIA 2019

Find a TB cases with an emphasis on reaching every TB patient in the private sector
Treat a TB cases with high quality anti TB drugs
Prevent the emergence of TB in susceptible populations and stop catastrophic expenditure due to TB
Build and strengthen supportive systems including enabling policies, empowered institutions and human resources with enhanced capacities

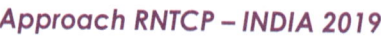

Must Remember

Intensive phase–Each blister pack has 1 day dose
Continuation phase–Each blister has 1 week's medication

Anti-Tubercular Drug Contraindications

- Pregnancy- Streptomycin
- Child <6 year- Ethambutol
- HIV – Thioacetazone

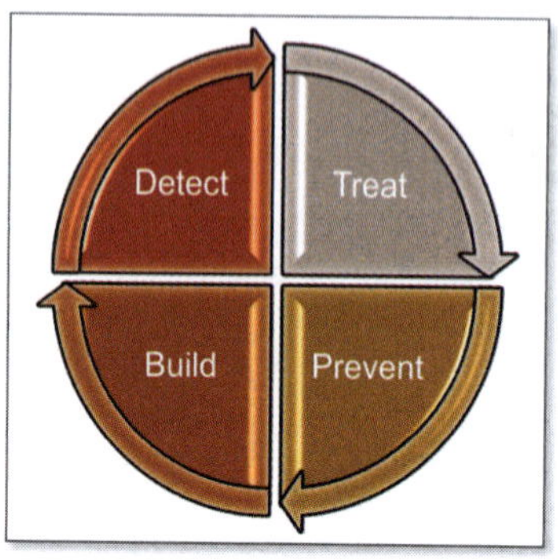

Strategies under RNTCP – India 2019 for:

- Early diagnosis and prompt treatment with high quality anti TB drugs
- Active case search for presumptive TB cases by house to house survey
- Mandatory TB notification for diagnosing of TB and treatment for TB – ***NIKSHAY notification system***
- Starting of ***NIKSHAY Poshan Yojna*** – for nutritional support for TB patients by Government of India (GoI)
- Incentive-based system for treatment compliance:
  - **Private provider ₹1000/–**
  - **Patients – ₹500/- pm**
  - **Tribal patient – ₹750/–**
  - Incentive for Treatment support
    - New Case: ₹1000/- at completion of treatment
    - Previously Treated Case: ₹1500/- at completion of treatment
    - Drug Resistant Case: ₹2000/- at completion of intensive phase, ₹3000/- at completion of treatment
  - Incentive for Informant: INR 500 for notification of TB case to any health facility

New Terminologies–under RNTCP 2018-2019

- TB suspect is now changed to – presumptive TB case
- Sputum positive TB and sputum negative TB is changed to bacteriologically confirmed and clinically confirmed case
- CBNAAT is the diagnostic test for children and HIV population

Latest Updates

- *Confirmed TB case*- Biological specimen is positive by smear microscopy, culture or CBNAAT.
- *Clinically diagnosed TB case* - Does not fulfill the criteria for bacteriological confirmed TB but has been diagnosed with active TB by a clinician and decided to be given full course of TB treatment.

Presumptive Pulmonary TB Case[Q]

- Any person with cough for 2 weeks, or more
- An individual having fever or night sweats or appreciable weight loss of 2 weeks or more.
- Contacts of a smear positive TB patients having cough of any duration
- Suspected/confirmed extrapulmonary TB having cough of any duration
- HIV positive patient having cough of any duration

Extrapulmonary TB

Tuberculosis of organs other than lungs such as pleura, lymph nodes, intestine, genitourinary tract, joint and bones, meninges of the brain, etc.

Guidelines for Diagnosis of Tuberculosis—2018–2019

2019 present Categorization for tuberculosis

- Available categories are category I, IV and V
- CAT III Removed in 2010
- CAT II Removed in 2018

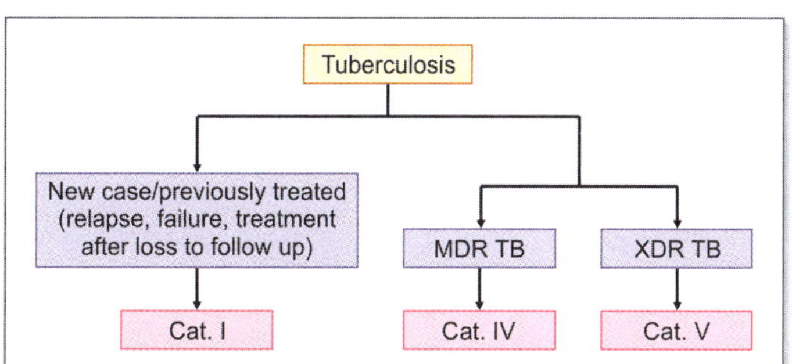

69 Must Remember

GLOBAL END TB targets – 90-90-90
90% case detection
90% of all key populations
90% of treatment success
Drug resistant Types:
Mono drug resistance:
Resistance to first line single drug only
MDR (Multidrug) resistance:
Resistance to Rifampicin and Isoniazid
Poly Drug Resistance:
Resistant to more than one first-line anti-TB drug, other than both H and R
XDR TB (extensively drug resistance TB):
MDR + Additional resistance to a fluoroquinolone (Ofx, Lfx, or Mfx) and a second-line injectable anti TB drug (Km, Am or Cm)

68 Good to Remember

Sputum smears are stained for AFB with "Ziehl-Neelsen" stain. 25% Sulphuric acid is the decolorizer and 0.1% Loefflers Methylene Blue is the counter stain

70 Must Remember

As per the New diagnostic algorithm all pulmonary TB suspects should have 2 sputum samples (Spot and morning) examined for AFB

101 High Yield Points

If a patient has both smear-positive pulmonary TB and extrapulmonary TB, the patient is classified as having pulmonary TB and site of extrapulmonary TB is recorded.

69 Good to Remember

Serological tests for TB detection have been banned in India

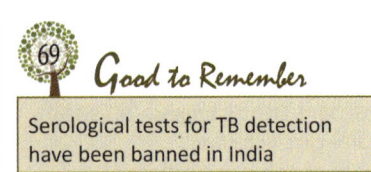

Diagnosis of Pulmonary Tuberculosis–Adults

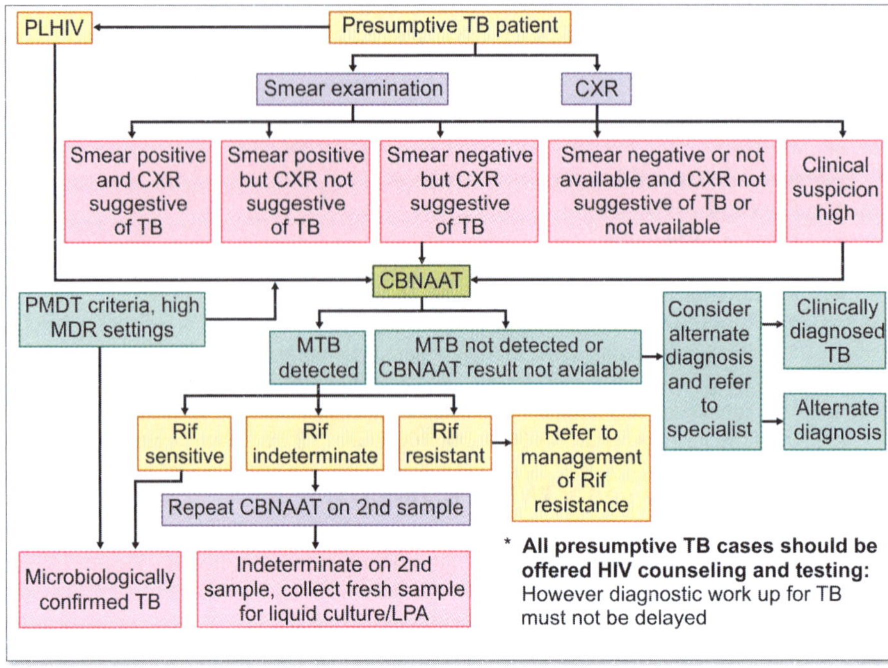

Fig. 2: Diagnostic algorithm for pulmonary

Diagnosis of Pediatric Pulmonary TB

- Childhood TB is usually due to failure of TB control in adults
- Most common age of childhood TB is 1–4 years
- CBNAAT is the preferred investigation of choice

Diagnostic algorithm for Pediatric Pulmonary TB

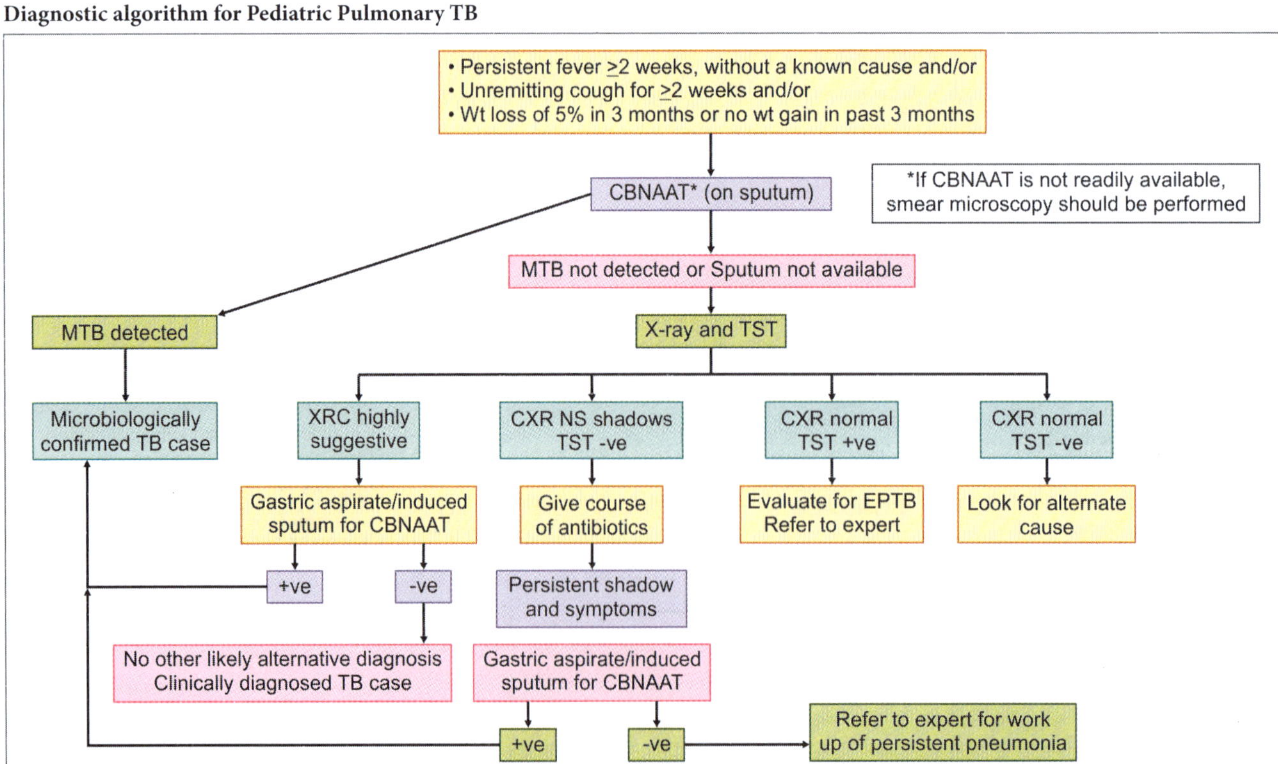

Diagnostic Algorithm for Extrapulmonary TB

- Usually are sputum negative
- Maybe associated with HIV infections

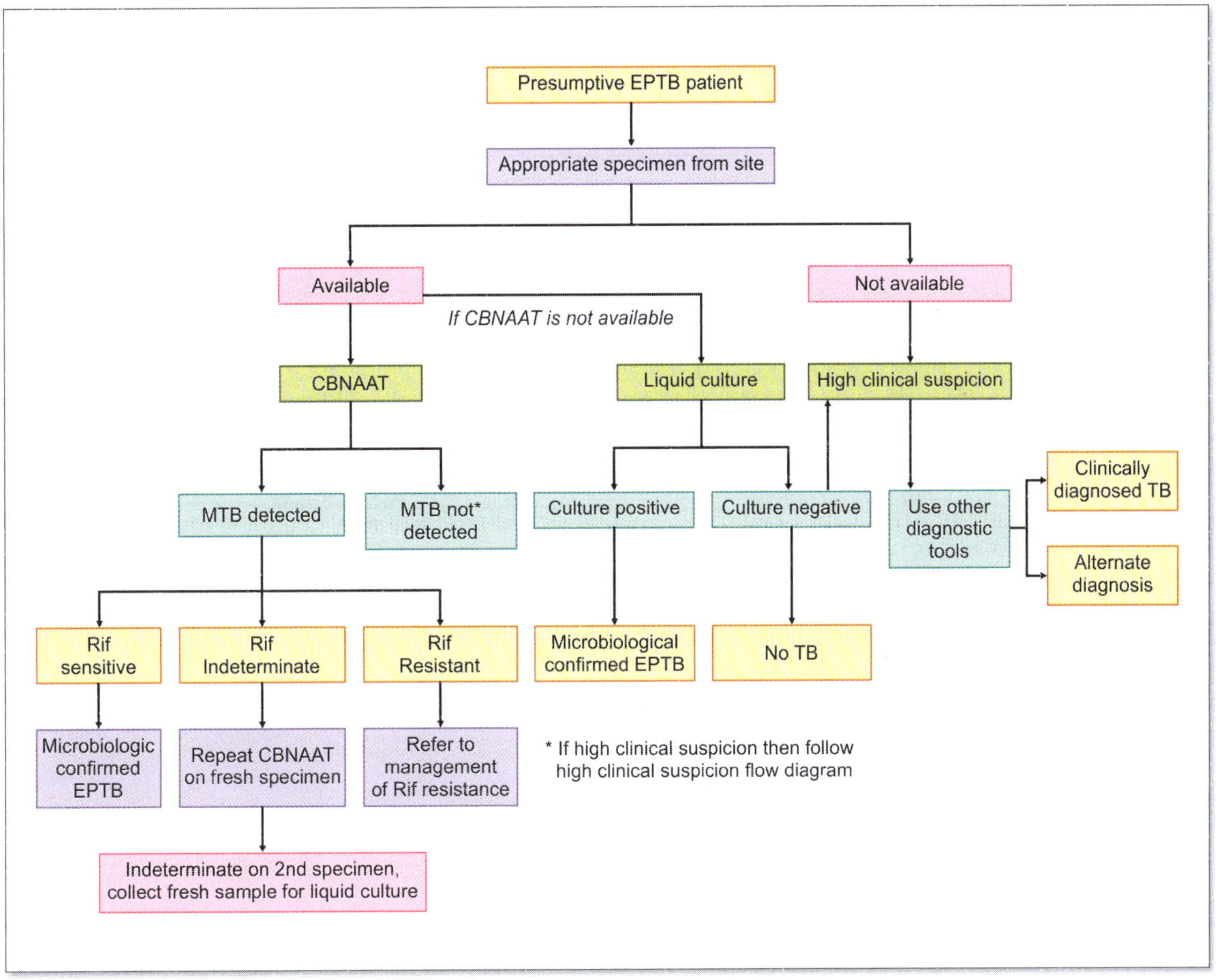

Diagnostic Algorithm for Drug-resistant TB

It is defined as *M. tuberculosis* resistant to isoniazid and rifampicin with or without resistance to other drugs at a RNTCP-certified culture and DST Laboratory

MDR-TB suspect is identified based on pre-decided suspect criteria in district and investigated further to diagnose MDR-TB.

Criteria A:

- All failures of new TB cases
- Smear +ve previously treated cases who remain smear +ve at 4th month onward
- All pulmonary TB cases who are contacts of known MDR TB case

Criteria B: *In addition to Criteria A*

- All smear +ve previously treated pulmonary TB cases at diagnosis
- Any smear +ve follow-up results in new or previously treated cases

Criteria C: *In addition to Criteria B*

- All smear -ve previously treated pulmonary TB cases at diagnosis.
- HIV TB coinfected cases at diagnosis.

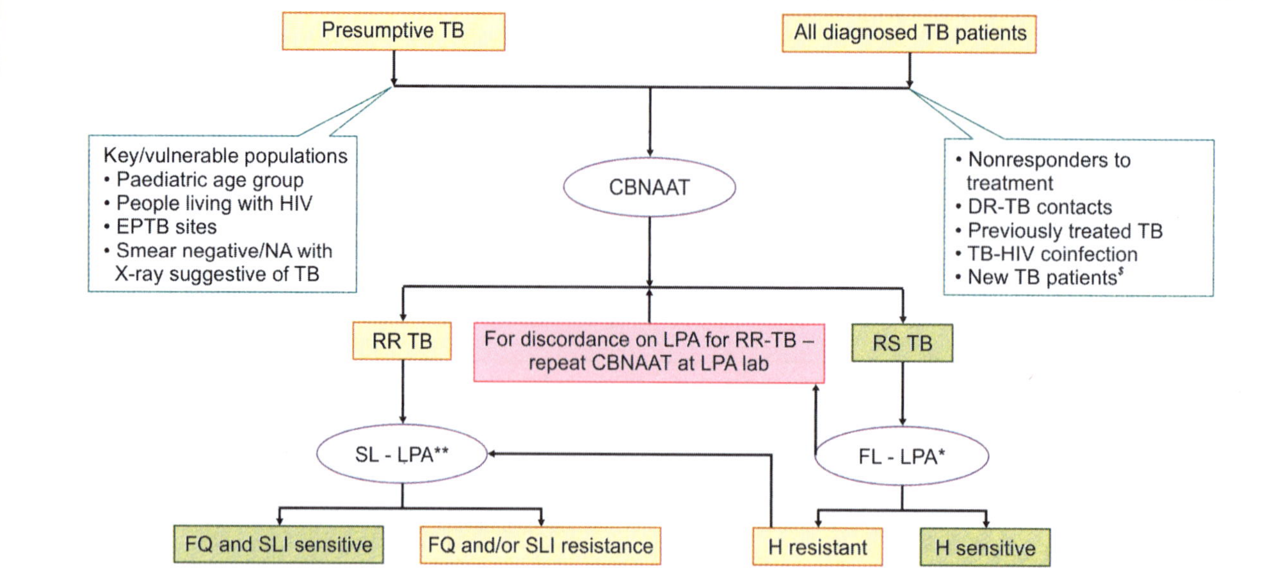

*Offer molecular testing for H mono/poly resistance to TB patients prioritized by risk as per the available lab capacity
**LC DST (Mfx 2.0, Km, Cm, Lzd) will be done only for patients with any resistance of baseline SL-LPA. DST to Z, Cfz, Bdq & Dlm would be considered for policy in future, whenever available, standardized & WHO endorsed.
$States to advance in phased manner as per PMDT scale up plan for universal DST based on lab capacity and policy on use of diagnostics.

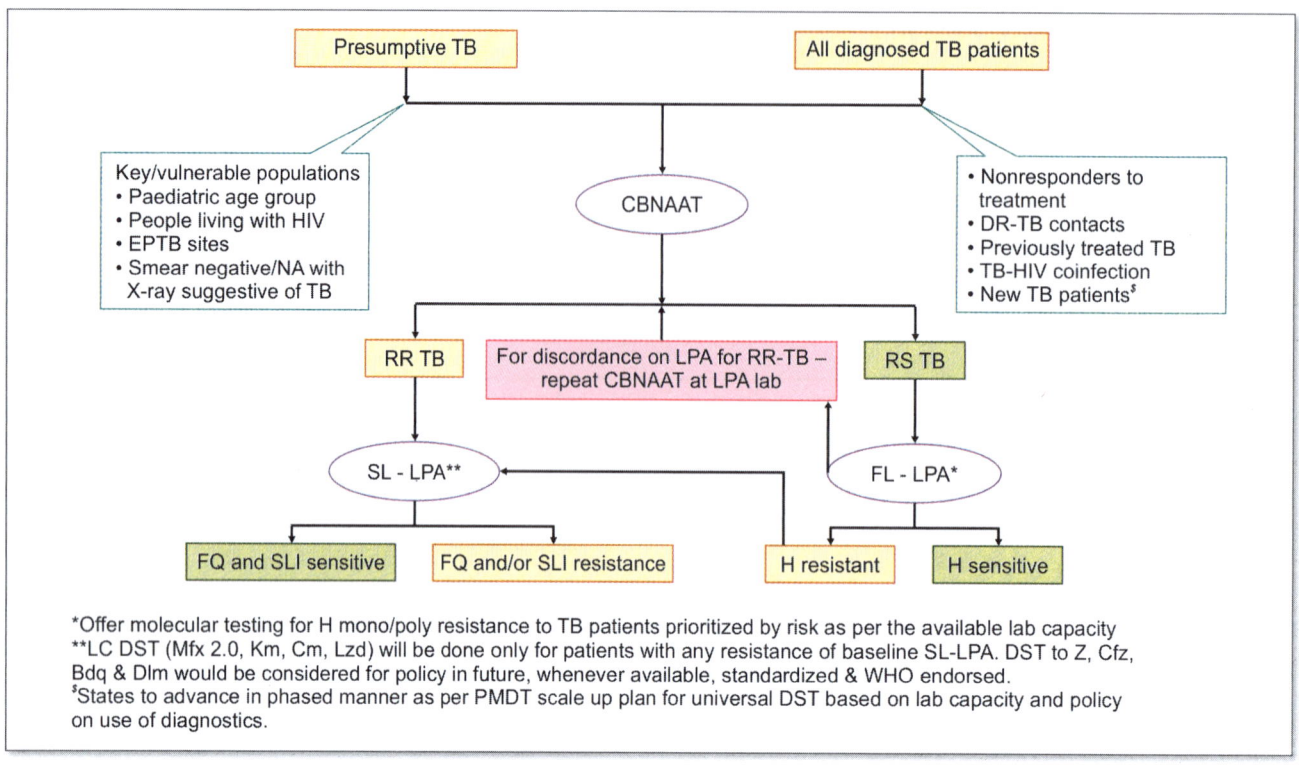

Abbreviations: RR TB, rifampicin resistant tuberculosis; RS TB, rifampicin sensitive tuberculosis; FL LPA, first line – line probe assay, SL LPA, second line – line probe assay; FQ, fluoroquinolone; SLI, second line injectable; H, isoniazid

Summary for Diagnostic Protocols

For drug sensitive TB:
- Smear microscopy
- Smear negative, with any CXR abnormality - CB NAAT
- Direct Upfront CBNAAT – Children, PLHIV and Extrapulmonary
- Cytology, Histopathology, Radio-imaging are used for supporting extrapulmonary TB diagnosis.
- A diagnosis of clinical TB to be made by specialist in case of CBNAAT not available and high clinical suspicion of TB. All efforts to undertake microbiologically confirmation in the diagnosis

Drug resistant TB
- All high risk populations, vulnerable populations to be tested for rifampicin sensitivity using CBNAAT
- All Rifampicin Sensitive TB patients tested for INH Drug Susceptibility
- All Rifampicin Sensitive, INH Resistant TB patients to be tested for second line drug susceptibility- SL LPA
- All Rifampicin Resistant TB patients to be tested for second line drug susceptibility- SL LPA

Treatment for TB under RNTCP (2019)

Directly Observed Treatment Short Course (DOTS)

It is the standardized treatment protocol for management of tuberculosis under RNTCP. DOTS is governed by the principle of "directly observed" treatment system to ensure proper doses and adherence to complete treatment. It has five components as:
- Political and administrative commitment (Continued financial assistance, human resources and administrative support)
- Good quality diagnosis, primarily by sputum smear microscopy[Q] at designated RNTCP microscopy centers (1 every 1 lakh population[Q]).
- Uninterrupted supply of quality drugs (In blister combipacks in patient wise drug boxes for adults and weight band drug boxes for pediatric cases for the entire course of treatment)

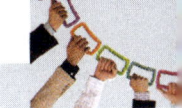

- Directly observed treatment (DOT) (An observer (MPW or trained community volunteer - e.g. Teacher, Anganwadi worker, dais, ex patients and social workers etc. other than family member) watches and supports the patient in taking drugs. It ensures treatment adherence, with the right drugs in right doses and at the right intervals.)
- Systematic monitoring and accountability

Abbreviations used in treatment regimens:

H (INH) - Isoniazid	R - Rifampicin
Z - Pyrazinamide	E - Ethambutol
Cm - capreomycin	PAS - para-aminosalicylic acid
Mfx - moxifloxacin	H^h-dose - high-dose Isoniazid
Lfx - Levofloxacin	Cfz - Clofazimine
Lzd - linezolid	Amx/clv - amoxicillin and clavulanic acid
Km - Kanamycin	Eto - Ethionamide
Pto = Prothionamide	

First Line Regimen for Drug Sensitive TB

- The drugs are given daily
- The dose of drugs are according to body weight
- Fixed Dose Combination (FDC) tablets are used
- Loose Drugs would be needed as substitutions in case of adverse drug reaction or with co-morbid conditions.
- No need for extension of IP
- CP may be extended by 12-24 weeks in certain forms of TB like CNS TB, Skeletal TB, Disseminated TB etc. based on clinical decision of the treating physician.
- Extension beyond 12 weeks should only be on recommendation of experts of the concerned field.
- No separate regimen for Re treatment cases.

Regime for First line – Drug sensitive TB:

Type of TB Case	Treatment regimen in IP	Treatment regimen in CP
New/Previously Treated	(2) HRZE	(4) HRE

Note:

- All previously treated cases also need to be initiated on standard first line regimen (2 HRZE+4 HRE)
- CB NAAT at baseline to rule our Rifampicin resistance.
- FL-LPA to be offered to all Previously treated patients at baseline itself to know INH susceptibility status.
- No need to wait for the FL-LPA results to start on First line regimen.
- Cases without specimens can be directly initiated on First-line regime (need to be followed up clinically/radiologically to identify any non-response).
- Honorarium for treatment supporters same as New patient.

Treatment Plan for Drug Sensitive TB–Adults

Weight category	Tablets as FDC – (Fixed dose combination)	
	Intensive phase	Continuation phase
	HRZE	HRE
	75/150/400/275 (mg/tablet)	75/150/275 (mg/tablet)
25–39 kg	2	2
40–54 kg	3	3
55–69 kg	4	4
≥70	5	5

Note:

- *Adults weighing <25 kg will be given loose drugs as per body weight.*
- *Tab pyridoxine for Alcoholics, Malnourished persons, Pregnant and lactating women, Patients with chronic renal failure, diabetes, HIV infection*

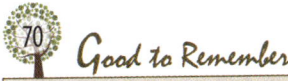

70 *Good to Remember*

National anti-TB drug resistance survey 2016.

The results are reported as follows:

MDR TB: 6.19% of all TB patients
New TB patients – 2.8%
Previously treated patients – 11.6%

Mono-drug resistance (any drug) among all TB Patients – 28%

INH resistance in
New TB cases – 11%
Previously treated TB cases – 25%

Treatment Plan for Drug Sensitive TB – Pediatric Cases

Weight category	Number of tablets (dispersible FDCs)			
	Intensive phase		Continuation phase	
	HRZ	E	HR	E
	50/75/150	100	50/75	100
4-7 kg	1	1	1	1
8-11 kg	2	2	2	2
12-15 kg	3	3	3	3
16-24 kg	4	4	4	4
25-29 kg	3 + 1A*	3	3 + 1A*	3
30-39 kg	2 + 2A*	2	2 + 2A*	2

*A = Adult FDC (HRZE = 75/150/400/275; HRE = 75/150/275 mg/tablet)

71 Good to Remember

Shorter MDR Regime: New regime for RR-TB/MDR TB
Intensive phase: 4–6 Km; Mfx; pto; cfz; H (high dose); E
Continuation phase: 5 Mfx; Cfz; Z; E

Treatment for H-Mono Drug Resistance

R susceptible; H resistant TB & DST of SEZ not known -
6 months of Levofloxacin, Rifampicin, Ethambutol, Pyrazinamide

- No separate Intensive phase and continuation phase
- Base line SL LPA to be offered for all patients with H resistance. No need to wait for the results of SL LPA to initiate treatment. If additional resistance to FQ found- replace Lfx with High dose Moxifloxacin.
- Follow up smear to be done monthly from the end of third month. Culture at the end of 3rd month and at end of treatment, then at 12,18,24 months flowing treatment.
- Treatment duration may be extended up to 9 months based on smear, culture and clinical progress.

Treatment Plan for MDR-TB/RR TB (Multidrug Resistance TB/Rifampicin Resistant TB)

Regimen Class	Resistance Pattern	Intensive Phase	Continuation Phase	Total duration
Shorter MDR-TB Regimen	RR/MDR TB	(4-6) Mfx^h Km* Eto Cfz Z H^h E	(5) Mfx^h Cfz Z E	9-11 months
Conventional MDR-TB Regimen	MDR TB	(6-9) Lfx Km Eto Cs Z E	(18) Lfx Eto Cs E	24-27 months

102 High Yield Points

MDR/RR-TB treatment (both shorter MDR and conventional MDR regime) is available at District DR TB centers MDR/ RR TB, XDR TB other mixed pattern resistant TB cases are managed at the nodal DR-TB centers

Follow-up Protocol for Drug Resistance TB

- Follow up is done by Sputum/culture monthly in IP and culture every 3 months in CP
- IP is extended, if culture is positive in IP
- DST is repeated, if culture is positive at end of IP and extended IP or any time during CP
- **Weight:** Monthly
- **Chest X-Ray** at end of IP, end of treatment and whenever clinically Indicated
- **Physician evaluation** including adverse drug reaction monitoring every month for six months, then every three months for two years
- **S. Creatinine** monthly for first 3 months, then every 3 months during the injectable phase

- **Thyroid Function Test** during pre-treatment evaluation and whenever indicated

For additional drug resistance:—

- **ECG**: Once a month in IP whenever Moxifloxacin is used
- **Complete Blood Count with Platelets Count:** Weekly in first month, then monthly to rule out bone marrow suppression and anaemia as a side effect of Linezolid
- **Kidney Function Test**- monthly creatinine and addition of monthly serum electrolytes to the monthly creatinine during the period that Inj. Capreomycin is being administered
- **Liver Function Tests**: monthly in IP and 3 monthly during CP

Pregnancy with MDR TB

- All MDR TB suspects and patients of child bearing age should be tested for pregnancy as part of pre-treatment evaluation and also while on the treatment.
- Family planning methods: OCP's are avoided during the treatment. Barrier methods, IUD's are recommended.
- Management protocol for MDR TB and pregnancy:

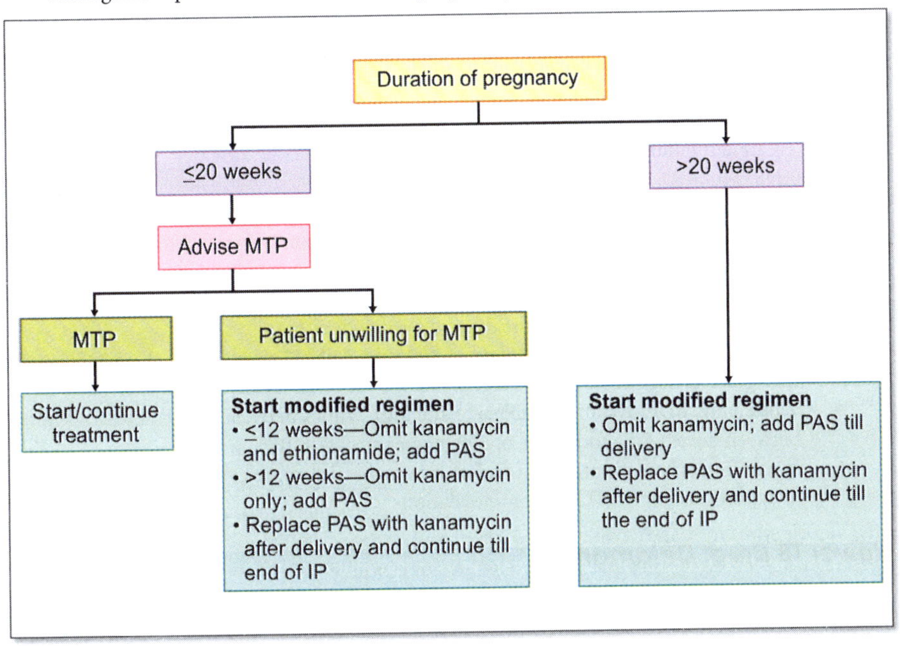

72 *Good to Remember*

Conventional MDR DOTS – plus regime:
RNTCP Regimen for MDR-TB: 6 (9) Km Lvx Eto Cs Z E/ 18 Lvx Eto Cs E
(Reserve/substitute drugs: PAS, Mfx, Cm)
Total duration. 24–27 months

XDR TB Case

An MDR TB case whose recovered *M. tuberculosis* isolate is resistant to

- At least Isoniazid and Rifampicin,
- A fluoroquinolone (Ofloxacin, Levofloxacin or Moxifloxacin) and
- A second-line injectable anti TB drug (Kanamycin, Amikacin or Capreomycin at a RNTCP-certified Culture and DST Laboratory.

MDR-TB patient diagnosed as XDR-TB is labelled an outcome of "Switched to regimen for XDR-TB". The XDR case is managed as per the Drug sensitivity testing (DST) report.

The Standard management recommendation of XDR TB case with Optimisation of background Regime drugs:

- **Intensive phase**:
  - 6-12 months – Cm, PAS, Mfx, High dose-H, Cfz, Lzd, Amx/Clv
- **Continuation phase**:
  - 18 months - PAS, Mfx, High dose-H, Cfz, Lzd, AMx/Clv

Newer TB Drug: Bedaquiline

- It is a new class of drug diarylquinoline and targets ATP synthase
- It is bactericidal and causes high volume of tissue distribution

- It is metabolized in liver and has extended half-life
- Patient selection criteria:
  - Age ≥18 years with MDR/ RR or XDR TB,
  - Female -nonpregnant, using nonhormonal contraceptives throughout treatment or postmenopausal for past 2 years.
- Contraindication:
  - Cardiac arrhythmia
  - A marked prolongation of QT/QTc interval, e.g. repeated demonstration of QTc interval >450 ms.
  - A history of additional risk factors for Torsade de Pointes, e.g. heart failure, hypokalemia, family history of long QT syndrome;
  - Has evidence of chorioretinitis, optic neuritis, or uveitis at screening which precludes long term linezolid (Lzd) therapy;
- The following patients are eligible for Bedaquiline
  - MDR TB with resistance to all FQs
  - MDR TB with resistance to all SLIs
  - All FQ and All SLI resistant
  - All FQ and any SLI resistant
  - Any FQ and all SLI resistant
  - Any FQ and Any SLI resistant
  - Treatment failure of Cat IV –MDR
  - XDR-TB
  - Treatment failure for XDR TB
  - MDR/RR-TB patients with extensive pulmonary lesions, advanced disease and others deemed at higher baseline risk for poor outcomes
- Dosage:
  - It is given orally usually with meal, swallowed with water
  - Week 0–2: BDQ 400 mg (4 tablets of 100 mg) daily (7 days per week) + Optimized Background Regime (OBR)
  - Week 3–24: BDQ 200 mg (2 tablets of 100 mg) 3 times per week (with at least 48 hours between doses) for a total dose of 600 mg per week + OBR
  - Week 25 (start of month 7) to end of treatment: Continue other second-line anti-TB drugs only as per RNTCP recommendations

> 103 *High Yield Points*
>
> **Bedaquiline (BDQ)**
> - ATP synthase inhibitor with extended half-life of 5.5 months after stopping BDQ.
> - Pregnancy and cardiac arrhythmias are specific contraindications for BDQ

Newer TB Drug: Delamanid

- First approved drug in the class of nitro-dihydro-imidazo-oxazoles for the treatment of MDR-TB.
- Bactericidal with Half-life of 36 hours.
- Dlm may have a protective role in preventing the emergence of additional drug resistance.
- Special caution
  - HIV+ (in consultation with ART centers)
  - Risk factors as: 65 yrs +, patients with diabetes, hepatic or severe renal impairment, those with serum albumin <2.8 g/dL or those who use alcohol or substances.
- Exclusion Criteria:
  - Children under 6 years.
  - Pregnant & breastfeeding women.
  - Patients with repeated demonstration of a QT interval >500 ms, history of torsades de pointes or cardiac ventricular arrhythmias
  - Hypersensitivity to the active substance or to any of the excipients
- Dose: Week 0–24: Delamanid 100 mg (two tablets of 50 mg) orally twice a day + OBR.

Summary – Treatment Regimens

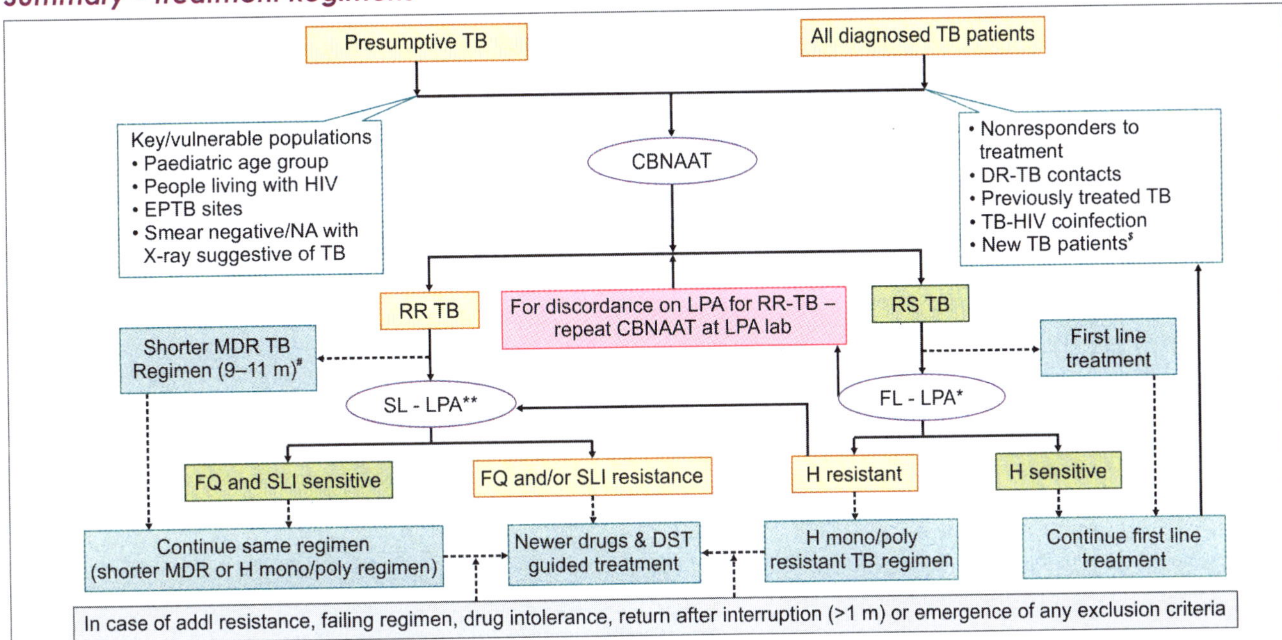

#Conventional MDR TB regimen [24 m] for pregnant women or for EP TB patients those who are not eligible for shorter regiment.
*Offer molecular testing and treatment for H mono/poly resistance to TB patients prioritized by risk as per the available lab capacity
**LC DST (Mfx 2.0, Km, Cm, Lzd) will be done only for patients with any resistance on baseline SL-LPA. DST to Z, Cfz, Bdq & Dlm would be considered for policy in future, whenever available, standardized & WHO endorsed.
$States to advance in phased manner as per PMDT scale up plan for universal DST based on lab capacity and policy on use of diagnostics.

Chemoprophylaxis of TB

TB preventive Therapy:
INH is given as 10 mg/kg daily for 6 months. The indications for TB preventive therapy are:

- All asymptomatic contacts (<6 years) for a sputum positive case.
- All HIV positive cases who had a known exposure or are TST (tuberculin skin test) positive but no active disease
- All TST (tuberculin sensitivity test) positive children on immunosuppressive therapy
- A child born to mother diagnosed with TB in pregnancy (and congenital TB is ruled out followed by BCG vaccination)

RNTCP Organogram

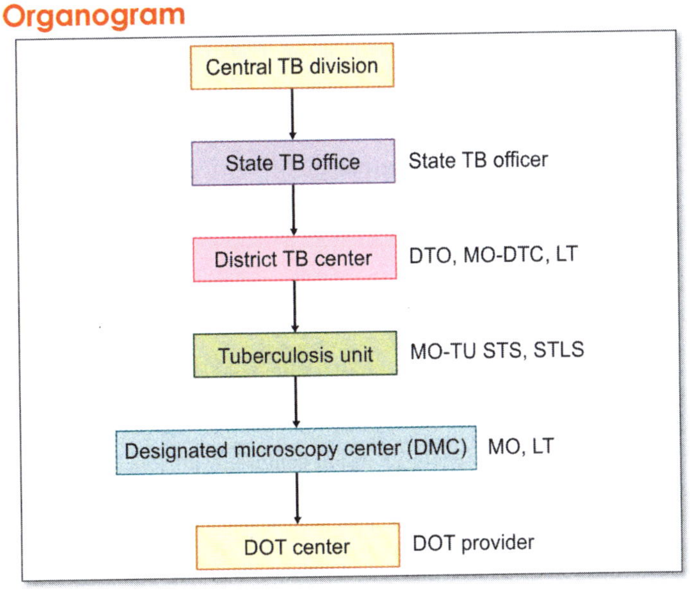

IRL – Intermediate reference laboratory
MO – Medical officer
LT – Lab technician
STS – Senior Treatment supervisor
STLS – Senior TB laboratory supervisor
DTO – District TB officer
STO - State TB Officer
DMC – Designated microscopy center

Availability of Diagnostic Services in RNTCP Laboratory Network

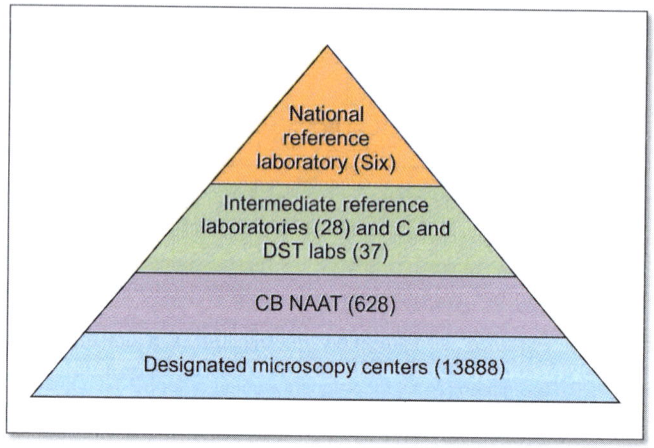

Availability of Regimes at TB Centers

Treatment regimen	Availability
▪ First Line Regimen	At all DOTS centers, PHC, CHC
▪ MDR/RR-TB • Shorter MDR-TB Regimen • Conventional MDR- TB Regimen	At District DR-TB centers
▪ H Mono/Poly Drug-Resistant TB	
▪ MDR/RR-TB with additional resistance to any/all FQ or SLI	At National Nodal DR-TB centers
▪ XDR-TB	
▪ Mixed pattern resistant TB • With H mono + FQ/SLI/Lzd resistance • With MDR/RR-TB + FQ/SLI ± Lzd resistance • Other patients who need careful regimen designing • Non tuberculous mycobacterium (NTM)	

Tuberculosis and Global Health

The End TB Strategy (2016–2035)

Vision: A world free of TB. Zero deaths, disease and suffering due to TB.
Goal: End the Global epidemic of TB
Indicators

- 95% reduction by 2035 in number of TB deaths compared with 2015.
- 90% reduction (<10/100000) by 2035 in TB incidence rate compared with 2015.
- Zero TB-affected families facing catastrophic costs due to TB by 2035.

	Reduction in number of TB deaths compared with 2015	Reduction in TB incidence rate compared with 2015	Reduction in TB-affected families facing catastrophic costs compared with 2015
By 2020	35%	**20%** (<85/100000)	Zero
By 2025	75%	**50%** (<55/100000)	Zero
By 2020 (SDG)	90%	**80%** (<20/100000)	Zero
Target 2035	95%	**90%** (<10/100000)	Zero

The High Burden Country (HBC) List by WHO

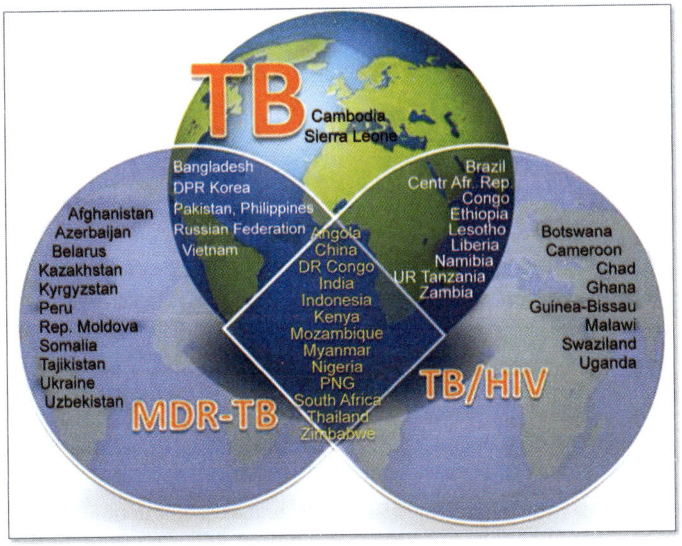

Fig. 3: The three HBC lists of 30 countries each that will be used by WHO 2016–2020

73 *Good to Remember*

Global 90-90-90 Targets

- Reach 90% of all people with TB and place all of them on appropriate therapy—first line, second line or preventative TB therapy.
- Reach at least 90% of the key at risk population (most vulnerable and underserved)
- Achieve at least 90% treatment success for all people diagnosed with TB through affordable treatment services along with adherence and social support.

The 30 TB HBCs (those in all 3 lists in bold) are: **Angola**, Bangladesh, Brazil, Cambodia, **China**, Congo, Central African Republic, DPR Korea, **DR Congo, Ethiopia, India, Indonesia, Kenya**, Lesotho, Liberia, **Mozambique, Myanmar**, Namibia, **Nigeria**, Pakistan, **Papua New Guinea**, Philippines, Russian Federation, Sierra Leone, **South Africa, Thailand**, the United Republic of Tanzania, Vietnam, Zambia and **Zimbabwe**.

Summary - What's New in RNTCP-2019 (India)

Recent Initiatives by RNTCP (at State Level)

- **99DOTS – compliance system**
  - This is a low-cost approach for monitoring and improving TB medication adherence and compliance.
  - Using 99DOTS, each anti-TB blister pack is wrapped in a custom envelope, which includes hidden phone numbers that are visible only when doses are dispensed.
  - After taking daily medication, patients make a Toll-free call to the hidden phone number and confirming to the compliance for medications.
- **Nikshay Poshan Yojana** to All TB patients (Financial Support to Patients @Rs.500/-month) as Direct Benefit Transfer
- **Incentives to Private Providers**: Government of Kerala has taken policy decision to give ₹1000 to the private treating facility who notifies and follow up the patient till end and declare outcome.
- **TB notification:** Real time updating and notification in NIKSHAY software
- **Clinical Review:** All TB patients on ATT should undergo clinical review by Medical Officer PHC/CHC once a fortnight.
- **Honorarium to Treatment Supporters**
  - First line regimen/H monopoly TB: ₹1000/- at completion of treatment
  - Drug Resistant TB case: ₹2000/- at completion of intensive phase, ₹3000/- at completion of treatment

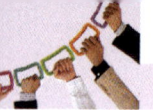

Time Line for Major Recommendations for RNTCP

END TB BY 2025	2018
Category II abolished	2018
Withdrawal of Kanamycin from H mono/poly DR TB Regimen	2018
Non declaration of TB made punishable	2018
Nutritional support for TB patients (500/month)	2018
Incentive for private doctors 1000 per patient at completion of treatment	2018
Daily regimen introduction	2016
Newer definition and diagnostic algorithm for TB (pulmonary, extrapulmonary, Pediatric TB and HIV-TB	2016
Introduction of Bedaquiline for DR-TB patients	2016
Introduction of Delamanid for DR-TB patient	2016
Ban on serological test for TB diagnosis	2012
TB declared as a Notifiable disease	2012
Category III of RNTCP abolished	2010
Introduction of CBNAAT/Gene expert for TB diagnosis	2010

MENINGOCOCCAL MENINGITIS

- Caused by *N. meningitidis.*
- There are 12 serogroups of N. meningitidis that have been identified, 6 of which (A, B, C, W, X and Y) can cause epidemics
- Serotypes Groups A and C and to a lesser extent Group B are capable of causing major epidemics
- Meningitis belt- zone between 5 and 15 degree N of the equator in tropical Africa
- *Source of infection:* Clinical cases (a negligible source) and Carriers (Most important source).

Epidemiology

During epidemics, carrier rate may be 70–80%

- *Period of communicability* is until meningococci is no longer present in discharges from nose and throat. Cases rapidly lose their infectiousness within 24 hours of specific treatment
- All ages are susceptible (Younger > older groups).
- Immunity is acquired by subclinical infection (mostly), clinical disease or vaccination. Infants derive passive immunity from the mother.
- CFR of typical untreated cases = 80 %. With early diagnosis and treatment, CFR declines to < 10%
- Outbreaks occur more frequently in dry and cold months of the year.Q
- Overcrowding is an important predisposing factor. The incidence is also greater in the low socioeconomic groups.
- *Mode of transmission:* Droplet infection. (Portal of entry is nasopharynx)
- *N.* Meningitides infects only humans, and there is no known animal reservoir.
- *Incubation period:* 3 to 4 days (range 2-10 days)

Diagnosis

Initial screening by rapid diagnostic tests, clinical evaluations

Confirmatory test: growing the bacteria from specimens of spinal fluid or blood, by agglutination tests or by polymerase chain reaction (PCR)

Treatment

In low resource settings, Ceftriaxone is the drug of choice. Other drugs which maybe used for treatment are penicillin, ampicillin, chloramphenicol.

Prevention

Vaccine

Vaccines are serogroup specific and have varying degrees of protection. Three types of vaccines are available:

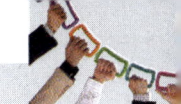

- Polysaccharide vaccine-
  - Bivalent (A and C), Trivalent (A, C, Y, W135) or Quadrivalent (Group A, C, Y, W135) are available
  - Contain 50 microgram of polysaccharide of each individual strain
  - This vaccine is given only after > 2 years of age and does NOT provide herd immunity.
  - It is protective for 3 years
- Conjugate vaccine
  - It is used in routine immunizations and is available as
    - Monovalent (A or C)
    - Quadrivalent (A, C, Y, W135)
    - Combined vaccine (Hib/MenC)
  - They confer longer-lasting immunity (5 years and more), prevent carriage and induce herd immunity.
  - They can be used as soon as of one year of age
- Protein based vaccine – Newley developed, still to be implemented for wide use

Chemoprophylaxis

Antibiotic prophylaxis for close contacts, when given promptly, decreases the risk of transmission.
Close contact, households: Most cases occur within 72 hours, hence it is important to provide prophylaxis within 24 hours to close contacts. In Indian settings, the chemoprophylaxis for close contacts is recommended in non-epidemic situations.
Meningococcal epidemic: Mass chemoprophylaxis may be administered.

Table 11: Drugs used for primary prevention of meningococcal meningitis

	First drug of choice	Alternate
Treatment of cases	Ceftriaxone	Other alternates: penicillin, ampicillin, chloramphenicol
Chemoprophylaxis	Ciprofloxacin* (500 mg, single dose) *Not given to children	Ceftriaxone

*In low resource setting, ciprofloxacin is the drug of choice and ceftriaxone is an alternate

FOODBORNE INFECTIONS

DIARRHEA

Oral Rehydration Therapy

Table 12: Guidelines for ORT in first four hours

Age (used if weight is not known)	<4–months	4–11 months	1–2 years	2–4 years	5–14 years	>15 years
Weight (kg)	Under 5	5–7.9	8–10.9	11–15.9	16–29.9	>30
ORS (mL)	200–400	400–600	600–800	800–1200	1200–2200	2200–4000

Table 13: Composition of reduced osmolarity who ORS

Ingredient	Quantity	Osmolar concentration	(mmol/L)
Sodium chloride	2.6 g /L	Sodium	75
Trisodium Citrate (makes ORS stable and reduces stool output	2.9 g/L	Potassium	20
Potassium chloride	1.5 g/L	Chloride	65
Glucose (anhydrous)	13.5 g/L	Citrate	10
Potable water	1 L	Glucose (Anhydrous)	75
Total weight	20.5 g	Total	245

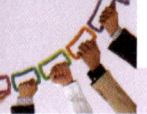

Appropriate use of technology
- India was the 1st country to launch Reduced osmolarity WHO ORS- June 2004.

Super ORS

- Special ORS containing complex sugars. It may be food- based (Rice-based) or be starch-free (Glycine/alanine based or Glucose polymer based).

Advantages of Super ORS
- Provides rehydration
- Reduces the stool output, frequency of stools and duration of diarrhea
- Provide calories (180 kcal/L and contribute toward weight gain. Especially useful for malnourished.
- With gradual release of glucose, prevents secondary disaccharide intolerance.

Limitation
- Short shelf-life (<10 hours), need to be freshly prepared 2–3 times a day

ReSoMal

- ReSoMal (Rehydration Solution for Severely Malnourished) is recommended for the treatment of dehydration in severely malnourished children.

Composition

WHO ORS packet + 2 L water + 50 g sucrose + 40 mL electrolyte/ mineral solution (or 45 mL of KCl solution (100 g KCl in 1 litre of water), Mg^{++}, Zn^{++}, Cu^{++})

GLOBAL ACTION PLAN FOR PNEUMONIA AND DIARRHEA (GAPPD)

Targets

By the end of 2025: 90% full-dose coverage of each relevant vaccine (with 80% coverage in every district); 90% access to appropriate pneumonia and diarrhea case management (with 80% coverage in every district); at least 50% coverage of exclusive breastfeeding during the first 6 months of life; virtual elimination of pediatric HIV.

By the end of 2030: Universal access to basic drinking-water in health care facilities and homes; universal access to adequate sanitation in health care facilities by 2030 and in homes by 2040; universal access to hand-washing facilities (water and soap) in health care facilities and homes; universal access to clean and safe energy technologies in health care facilities and homes.

CHOLERA

Epidemiology

- Caused by V cholera O1 (classical or El tor) and O139
- Most common: El tor biotype and O139
- Features of cholera epidemics
  - Sudden rise and fall of the epidemic curve
  - Tail of the epidemic curve is due to ongoing transmission between carriers and contacts
  - Cholera does occur and is hidden among carries during inter-epidemic periods

Agent Factors

- Classified into two groups
  - Vibrio cholera O group 1 (or cholera O1): common vibrio in India and south Asia. Contain two biotypes
    - Classical
    - El Tor
  - Each biotype is further divided into
    - Ogawa
    - Inaba
    - Hikojima

- Note:
  - Non O group 1 strains: further classified into
    - Epidemic strains
    - Non epidemic strains

El Tor has special features differentiating from other vibrio as it:

- Agglutinates chicken and sheep erythrocytes
- Is resistant to Polymyxin B and to classical phage IV
- Gives positive reaction (non-consistent) to Vogues – Proskauer test
- Survives in adverse conditions
- Causes higher number of milder cases with more number of carrier states
- Vibrio characteristics
  - Highest attack rate in children
  - Destroyed by acidity of pH <5
  - Incubation period: few hours up to 5 days
- **Infective material:** Stool and vomitus of case/carrier
- **Period of infectivity:**
  - Case: 8-10 days
  - Incubatory carrier: 1-5 days
  - Contact carrier: 10 days
  - Convalescent carrier: 2-3 weeks
  - Chronic carrier: Months – Years
- **Reservoir of infection:** Humans are only reservoir
- Cholera case:
  - For every case of cholera, there are 50-100 subclinical cases
- Carrier of cholera
  - Preclinical/incubatory carrier
  - Convalescent carrier
  - Contact/healthy carrier
  - Chronic carrier

74 Good to Remember

In India, almost all cases of cholera belong to El Tor biotype, Ogawa serotype.

104 High Yield Points

- ~75% of people infected with cholera do NOT develop symptoms, although the bacteria are present in the stools for 7-14 days

Pathogenesis

- Vibrio secrete mucinase and enters gut mucosa
- Secretes adherence factor and adheres to the intestinal epithelium
- Produces toxin
  - Light (L) toxin: Combines with gangliosides in cell membrane and binds the vibrio to the cell
  - Heavy (H) toxin: Activates the adenyl cyclase and cAMP, which further secretes fluid in to the intestinal lumen and produces diarrhea

Clinical Features

It has three stages:

- Stage of evacuation: Profuse, painless diarrhea (rice water stools)
- Stage of collapse: intense diarrhea and signs of dehydration
- Stage of recovery

Diagnosis

Lab diagnosis of cholera

- Stool collection and transportation
  - Use McCartney bottles for transport of stool
  - Transport (holding) media – Venkatraman Ramakrishna (VR) media
  - Best to use is sterile rubber catheter
  - Rectal swabs transported in alkaline peptone water or Cary Blair media
- Culture methods
  - Enrichment: Inoculation onto peptone water tellurite (PWT) media
  - Sub culture: Bile salt agar media (BSA, pH 8.6)
  - Gm -ve rods
  - Hanging drop preparation: Show scintillating movements. Mixing with polyvalent antisera stops motility
  - Dark field illumination: Shooting stars in dark sky
- Serological tests: To differentiate the sub types of cholera

Management of Cholera

- **Isolation** –2–3 Negative stool culture reports
- Concurrent and terminal disinfection is required in hospital. Stool and vomits to be disinfected with cresol (always use a disinfectant with Rideal Walker (RW) coefficient of 10 or more)
- Fluid rehydration is the mainstay of treatment
- Antibiotics as per the culture report. A brief WHO guideline for choosing antibiotic is as follows:

Guidelines for cholera Treatment with Antibiotics

Organization	Recommendation	First-line drug choice	Alternate drug choices	Drug choices for special population
World health organization	Antibiotic treatment for cholera patients with severe dehydration only	Doxycycline	Tetracycline	Erythromycin is recommended drug for children
Pan American health organization	Antibiotic treatment for cholera patients with moderate or severe dehydration	Doxycycline	Ciprofloxacin azithromycin	Erythromycin or azithromycin recommended as first-line drugs for pregnant women and children ciprofloxacin and doxycycline recommended as second-line drugs for children
International center for diarrheal disease research, Bangladesh	Antibiotic treatment for cholera patients with some or severe dehydration	Doxycycline	Ciprofloxacin azithromycin	Erythromycin recommended as first-line drug for children and pregnant women
Medicins sans frontieres	Antibiotic treatment for severely dehydrated patients only	Doxycycline	Erythromycin cotrimoxazole chloramphenicol furazolidone	

Control for Cholera

- Chemoprophylaxis of cholera
  - DOC – Tetracycline
    - Adults 500 mg BD × 3 days
    - Children (4-13 years) 125 mg BD × 3 days
    - Children (0-3 years) 50 mg BD × 3 days
  - Doxycycline @ 300 mg single dose oral drug
- Immunization
  - Parenteral Vaccine : heat killed, phenol preserved vaccine.
    - 0.5 ml contains 3000 million killed organisms
    - Primary immunization 2 doses 0.5mL, deep i/m, with interval 4-6 weeks
    - Immunity developed after 15 days till 5-6 months. Protective value is 50%
    - Not useful in outbreaks. If used, should be given 1 month before impending outbreak
  - Oral Vaccine
    - Dukoral (WC-rBS – whole cell recombinant cholera toxin B subunit)
      - Heat killed whole cell of cholera O1 serotype + B subunit
      - 3ml single dose vials with bicarbonate buffer (protect the vaccine from being destroyed by gastric acidity)
      - How to use
        - Vaccine + buffer to be mixed in 150 ml of water and consumed orally
        - Adults: 2 doses, ≥7 days apart but <6 weeks

- Children 3 doses, ≥7 days apart but <6 weeks
- To be restarted if the second dose is delayed by >6 weeks
- Avoid food/water at least 1 hour before and after vaccine
- Protection after 1 weeks of the last dose
- Not licensed for use in children <2 years

- Sanchol and mORCVAX
  - Bivalent oral cholera vaccine based on serogroups O139 and O1
  - Do not contain the cholera toxin B subunit, do not require gastric buffer
  - 2 doses, 14 days apart for children >1 year
- Euvichol – recently approved vaccine
- Live attenuated CVD 103 HgR vaccine – abolished, no longer used

- Prevention and control of cholera:
  - Constructing a strict 'sanitation barrier' is the BEST way to control cholera outbreak
  - Mass chemoprophylaxis is NEVER advised in control of cholera outbreak, as to prevent a single case of cholera, 10,000 individuals must be provided chemoprophylaxis

75 Good to Remember

- Drug of choice for cholera - doxycycline
- Mass vaccination for cholera or mass chemoprophylaxis for cholera
- Is not recommended

TYPHOID

- Typhoid fever is endemic in India

Epidemiology

Agent factors

- S. typhi has three main antigens:
  - Somatic 'O' antigen – specific for group
  - Flagellar 'H' antigen – specific for type
  - Capsular 'Vi' antigen – virulence of organism
- Gram -ve, flagellated, actively motile
- Reservoir of infection: Man is the only known reservoir of infection
- Carrier:
  - Convalescent carrier – excrete bacilli for 6-8 weeks
  - Chronic carrier: Persons who excrete bacilli for more than a year
  - Fecal carrier more common than urinary carriers. However, chronic carrier state is usually associated with some urinary tract abnormality
- Source of infection:
  - Primary source – faeces or urine
  - Secondary source: Contaminated water, food, fingers, fomites
- Incubation period: 10-14 days

Host/Environment Factors

- Maximum incidence of cases 5-19 years
- Males >females
- Antibody to 'O' (somatic) antigen is higher in infected individuals
- Antibody to 'H' (flagellar) antigen is higher in immunized individuals
- Cell mediated immunity pays a major role in pathogenesis of typhoid
- Peak incidence July – September
- The typhoid bacilli may survive in food/vegetables/soil for up to a month or even more
- Mode of transmission – Feco-oral route

Clinical Features

Early phase:

- Fever/malaise/Leukopenia
- Pea soup diarrhea
- Blood/stool/urine culture positive for Salmonella typhi

Late phase (after 7-10 days):

- Splenomegaly/abdominal distension/tenderness
- Rose spots – popular rash on trunk – appear during 2nd week of disease
- Case fatality rate: 1-4%

Complications

- Relapse
- Haemorrhage (from intestinal ulcers)
- Perforation

Diagnosis

- Blood culture -- gold standard
- Serology:
  - Widal felix test
    - O antibodies appear on day 6-8
    - H antibodies appear on day 10-12
    - It may be negative in 30% of cases
  - Rapid serological test –
    - IDL tubex test
    - Typhi Dot – detects both IgM and IgG antibody

Plan for Investigations

■ 1st week of illness	Blood for culture
■ 2nd week of illness	Blood for Widal, leucopoenia
■ 3rd week of illness	Blood for repeat Widal (and/or) Stool/urine for culture

Control of Typhoid

- Early diagnosis, treatment and notification
  - Isolation is recommended for at least 3 negative stool culture reports
- Treatment for uncomplicated typhoid
  - Fully sensitive
    - Fluoroquinolone @ 15 mg/kg 5-7 days
  - Multi drug resistance but quinolone sensitive
    - Fluoroquinolone @ 15 mg/kg 5-7 days 'or'
    - Cefixime @ 15 mg/kg 2 weeks
  - Quinolone resistance
    - Azithromycin @ 10 mg/kg 7 days 'or'
    - Cefixime @ 15 mg/kg 2 weeks
- Disinfection:
  - Stool and urine 5% cresol × 2 hours
  - Clothes and linen 2% chlorine and steam sterilized
- Control of carrier states
  - Identify carries
    - Serology or culture is done to identify carriers
    - Vi antibodies are present in 80% of all carriers
  - Treatment for typhoid carrier state
    - Ampicillin or amoxicillin @4-6 g/day
    - AND Probenecid @2 g/day
- Sanitation control
- Immunization
  - **Vi polysaccharide vaccine**
    - Not for age <2 years
    - Subcutaneous or intramuscular injection
    - Single dose – protection starts after 7 days, revaccination required after 3 years
    - Contraindications – hypersensitivity
  - **Ty21 a vaccine**
    - Oral enteric coated capsules, Ty2 strain of S. typhi
    - 3 dose regime – day 1,3,5 – protection starts after 7 days, revaccination required after 3 years
    - Licensed for use ≥5 years
    - Precautions:

105 High Yield Points

- Treatment for typhoid carrier state
  - Ampicillin or amoxicillin @4-6 g/day
  - AND Probenecid@2 g/day

- Stop antibiotics, proguanil – 3 days before and 3 days after vaccine
- May-not be effective in acute diarrheal condition
- Not recommended for active HIV disease (CD4 <200), immunosuppressed states

HEPATITIS

Table 14: Types of hepatitis their incubation period

Types of hepatitis	Incubation period	Modes of transmission
A	10–50 days	Feco-oral, Sexual (Homosexuals)
B	30–180 days	Parenteral, Perinatal, Sexual and Other routes: (horizontal transmission)
C	2 week –6 month	Parenteral Perinatal
D	2 week –12 week	Parenteral, Perinatal
E	3 week-8 weeks	Feco-oral, Parenteral, Perinatal
G	–	Suspected association with blood transfusion

Hepatits B

Hepatitis B is transmitted through body fluids including blood and through sex where exchange of body fluids takes place. The routes of transmission can be categorized as follows

- **Parenteral or percutaneous:** Through infected blood, blood products, syringes, transfusion apparatus, etc.
- **Vertical or perinatal spread:** Mother to infant transmission can occur when the mother is a chronic carrier or suffers from acute infection during the first trimester of pregnancy. The infection can also occur during passage through the birth canal or during the post-natal period due to close contact.
- **Permucosal spread:** Blood, saliva, vaginal fluids and semen are infective.

Table 15: Markers of hepatitis B infection

Markers	Interpretation
Surface antigen *(Australia antigen/ HbsAg)*	*1st to be detected*[Q]*, Signals infection (acute or chronic) or carrier.*[Q]
"e" antigen (HBeAg)	*Signals virus replication and that the patient is highly infectious.*[Q]
Core antibody (anti- HBc)	IgM signals *New infection*[Q], IgG anti HBc Ag signals *Old infection*[Q]
"e" antibody (anti- HBe)	Good prognostic feature. *Signals low infectivity.*
Surface antibody (anti-HBs)	Signals *recovery from HBV infection, development of immunity and cured*[Q]

Hepatitis C

- Clinical presentation is mild/asymptomatic
- More than >50% cases develop chronic hepatitis and subsequently cirrhosis of liver or liver cancer (in about >20 years) more common in men compared to women and in alcoholics.
- Major route of transmission -Transfusion of contaminated blood or blood products.
- High risk groups→ IV drug users (50% cases).
- *Incubation period* is 6–7weeks.
- Diagnosis → anti-HCV blood test kits. Confirmation is by Recombinant Immuno Blot Assay (**RIBA**)
- Testing donated blood for HCV reduces transfusion associated risk from 10% to 1%. It is mandatory in India for all blood banks from July 1, 1997.
- Treatment → Interferon and is effective.

106 High Yield Points

Transplacental transmission is also seen in HIV, Varicella, Rubella, Syphilis, Chagas disease, Toxoplasmosis, CMV, E. coli, P. falciparum, Group B Streptococci, Herpes Simplex Virus (I and II)

Prevention of Hepatitis

Vaccination for Hepatitis A

- Formaldehyde inactivated vaccines:
  - For age more than 1 year
  - Two-dose schedule with interval of 6–18 months

Live attenuated vaccine: Single and subcutaneous dose

Human immunoglobulin:

- IgG to be given within 2 weeks of exposure:
- Dose @ 0.02 mL/kg – effective for 1-2 months
- Dose @ 0.06 mL/kg – effective for 3-5 months

Prevention of Hepatits B

Hep B Diagnosis

Table 16: Common serologic patterns in hepatitis B virus infection and their interpretation

HBsAg	Anti-HBs	Anti-HBs	HBeAg	Anti-HBe	Interpretation
+	–	IgM	+	–	Acute hepatitis B
+	–	IgG	+	–	Chronic hepatitis B with active viral replication
+	–	IgG	–	+	Chronic hepatitis B with low viral replication
+	+	IgG	+ or –	+ or –	Chronic hepatitis B with heterotypic anti-HBs (about 10% of cases)
–	–	IgM	+ or –	–	Acute hepatitis B
–	+	IgG	–	+ or –	Recovery from hepatitis B (immunity)
–	+	–	–	–	Vaccination (Immunity)
–	–	IgG	–	–	False positive, less commonly, infection in remote past

Vaccine

Recombinant monovalent combination or fixed combination with other vaccines as DPT, polio dose –

- 20 mcg at 0 dose, 1 month and 6 months given as IM injection
- Note – 20 mcg Hep B = 1 mL of Hep B vaccine

Interruption of vaccine at any age, may be continued (no need to restart whole schedule because of interruption)

- High risk individuals:
- High risk sexual behavior
- IV drug users
- Frequent blood transfusion
- Organ transplant recipients
- Health care workers, international travellers to HBV endemic countries

Contraindication: Allergy (pregnancy, lactation, TB, underweight – are NOT contraindications)

Hep B Immunoglobulin

- For acute exposure to HBsAg positive blood
- Given within 6 hours not later than 48 hours.

Post-Exposure Prophylaxis

- Administer HBIG 0.05 mL/kg BW – 2 doses one month apart
- Check for antibody to HBsAg (surface antigen)
  - If positive, no further action required
  - If negative, Hep B vaccination to be started immediately (Hep B 1.0 mL IM at 0,1,6 months)

Hepatitis C

Treatment modality with direct acting antivirals (DAA)

Table 17: Classes of DDAs

The four classes of DAAs	Very roughly what the DAAs do
NS3/4A protease inhibitors (PIs)	NS3/4A protease inhibitors work by blocking a viral enzyme (protease) that enables the Hep C virus to survive and replicate in host cells
Nucleoside and nucleotide NS5B polymerase inhibitors	They directly target the Hep C virus to stop it from making copies of itself in the liver. They attach themselves onto the genetic information, called RNA, to block the virus from multiplying
NS5A inhibitors	They block a virus protein, NS5A, that HCV needs to reproduce and for various stages of infection
Non-nucleoside NS5B polymerase inhibitors	They work to stop HCV from reproducing by inserting themselves into the virus so that other pieces of the Hep C virus cannot attach to it.

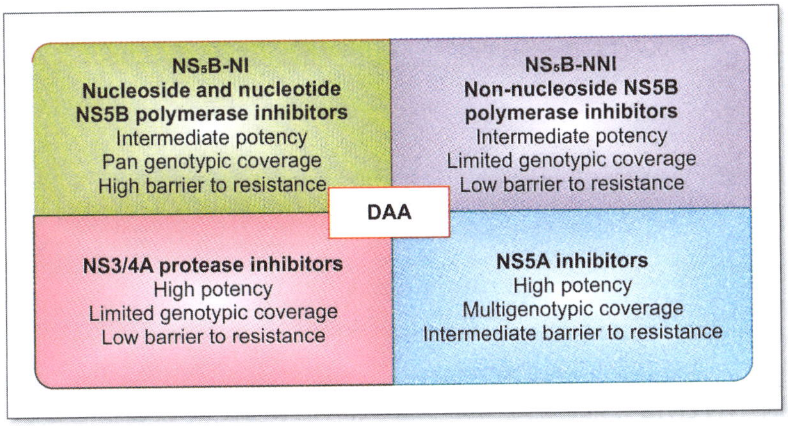

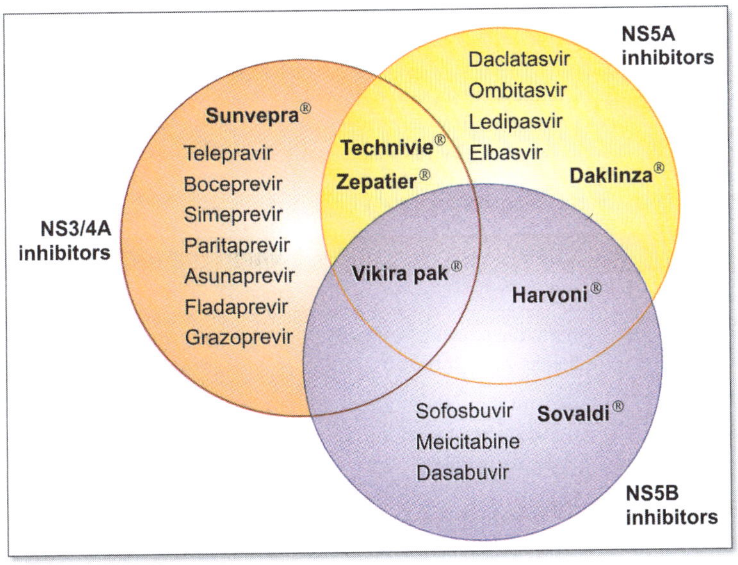

Fig. 4: Direct-acting antiviral agents for Hepatitis C
(®*Trade names are registered under International Pharmacopoeia*)

Hepatitis E

- Found worldwide
- Various genotypes
  - Genotype 1: Developing countries and may lead to community level outbreaks
  - Genotype 3: Developed countries, no outbreaks

Table 18: Comparison of various types of hepatitis

	HAV	HBV	Hep C	Hep E
Transmission	Feco-oral	Parenteral route, perinatal, sexual route	Parenteral route Blood transfusion, syringes, organ donations	Waterborne
IP	10–50 days	30–180 days	2 weeks to 6 months	3–8 weeks
Clinical spectrum	In apparent: 80-90% Icteric: 5-20% Complete recovery >98%	Insidious onset with chronicity in 5-10% of cases	80% asymptomatic, fatigue, jaundice, dark urine, grey color feces	▪ Common in young ▪ Chances of having serious or fulminant hepatitis is more in pregnancy ▪ More common in immunocom-promised individuals
Diagnosis	▪ HAV detection from stool sample ▪ Anti-HAV IgM anti-body after 2 weeks of increase in liver enzymes	HBs Ag and HBe Ag (refer to table given below)	▪ Recombinant Immuno Blot Assay (RIBA) ▪ Antibody to HCV persisting for more than 6 months	Anti-HEV IgM and IgG antibody rtPCR to detect HEV particles
Prevention	Formaldehyde inactivated vaccine - age >12 yrs ▪ 2 dose, with interval of 6–12 months Live-attenuated vaccine	▪ Recombinant Hep B Vaccine ▪ HBIG	▪ Screening for HCV in high risk groups ▪ Primary prevention strategies ▪ *Direct Antiviral Agents* (DAA) –	HEV vaccine (still under trials and not available

POLIOMYLITIS

Causative agent has 3 serotypes—P1, P2 and P3.

- P1 virus is most common cause of outbreaks of paralytic polio or polio epidemic. It can survive for long period in the external environment (4 months in water, 6 months in feces)
- P3 virus is most common cause of Vaccine Associated Paralytic Polio, followed by P2 and P1.
- P2 virus is most antigenic. Type 2 virus was eradicated from the world in1999.

Table 19: Comparison between VDPV and VAPP

	VDPV	VAPP
Most common	P2	P3
Frequency	Rare, only 24 cVDPV cases across 21 countries	1 in 2.7 million doses, usually by single dose of OPV
Why?	De-mutation, Re-mutation in the vaccine virus of the OPV "Vaccine problem"	Aberrant change in the vaccine virus leading to paralysis. "Low RI coverage leading to proliferation of virus"
Epidemic potential	Yes	No

VDPV—vaccine derived polio virus
cVDPV—circulating VDPV
VAPP—vaccine-associated paralytic polio

Table 20: Types of polio vaccines

	Oral polio vaccine (OPV)	Inactivated polio vaccine (IPV)
Contains	Mixture of live, weakened poliovirus strains ▪ *Trivalent OPV:* All 3 poliovirus types ▪ *Bivalent OPV:* Types 1 and 3 ▪ *Monovalent OPV:* Any 1 individual type	Mixture of inactivated, killed strains of all three poliovirus types
How it works	Body produces antibodies in the blood and gut in response to the weakened virus. Helps stop transmission by limiting the virus' ability to replicate in the gut and spread to infect others	Body produces antibodies in the blood in response to the inactivated virus. Protects the individual, but the virus may still replicate in the gut and could spread to infect others.
Administration	Easy, oral administration can be conducted by volunteers and is part of many countries' routine immunization program. Used extensively in immunization campaigns to root out poliovirus. Costs less than US$0.15 per dose.	Vaccine injection is administered primarily through routine immunization program by trained health workers. Higher cost, starting at US$1 per dose for low-income countries
Use	Extremely effective in protecting children from WPV and cVDPV. Nearly every country has used OPV to stop wild poliovirus transmission because it prevents person-to-person spread of the virus, protecting both the individual and the community	Extremely effective in protecting children from polio disease due to WPV and cVDPV, but cannot stop spread of virus in a community
cVDPV risk	Can cause cVDPV in under-immunized population, through very rare	Cannot cause cVDPV

National Polio Surveillance Programme (NPSP)

Selected Polio case definitions:

- **Suspected case:** Any case of acute-onset flaccid paralysis (AFP), including Guillain-Barré syndrome, in a person under 15 years of age for any reason other than severe trauma, or paralytic illness in a person of any age in which polio is suspected. The classification "suspected case" is temporary. It should be reclassified as "probable" or "discarded" within 48 hours of notification.
- **Probable case:** A case in which AFP is found, and no other cause for the paralysis can be identified immediately. The classification of "probable case" is also temporary; within 10 weeks of onset of the case should be reclassified as "confirmed", "compatible", "vaccine-associated" or "discarded."
    - **Confirmed case:** A case with acute paralytic illness, with or without residual paralysis, and isolation of wild poliovirus from the stools of either the case or its contacts.
    - **Polio-compatible case:** A case in which one adequate stool specimen was not collected from a probable case within 2 weeks of the onset of paralysis, and there is either an acute paralytic illness with polio-compatible residual paralysis at 60 days, or death takes place within 60 days, or the case is lost to follow-up.
    - **Vaccine-associated paralytic poliomyelitis case:** A case with acute paralytic illness in which vaccine-like poliovirus is isolated from stool samples, and the virus is believed to be the cause of the disease. There are two possible types of vaccine-associated paralytic poliomyelitis (VAPP): Recipient and contact. A case classified as a recipient is a person who has onset of AFP 4 to 40 days after receiving OPV and has neurologic

76 *Good to Remember*

Vaccines for polio:-There are two types of vaccines available for prevention against polio – One is a killed vaccine and is injected (Salk vaccine) and the other is a live vaccine which is given orally (Sabin vaccine).

107 *High Yield Points*

- India was declared polio-free on 27th March 2014 (Last case was reported in Howrah in Jan 2011).
- Polio is now endemic in only 3 countries: Afghanistan, Pakistan Nigeria (2016)
- 4 of the six WHO regions with 80% of global population (America, West Pacific, Europe and South East Asia) have been certified Polio Free in 2014

sequelae compatible with polio 60 days after the paralysis began. A case is classified as a contact VAAP when a person who has residual paralysis 60 days after the onset of AFP had contact 4 to 40 days before the paralysis began with a person who received OPV somewhere between 4 and 85 days before the contact's paralysis began.

- **Discarded (Not poliomyelitis) case:** A case with acute paralytic illness for which one adequate stool specimen was obtained within 2 weeks after onset of paralysis and was negative for poliovirus.

71 **Must Remember**

Major cause of VDPV outbreaks is type 2 polio virus component in OPV. Wild polio virus 2 last case was in 1999

Polio Eradication and End Game Strategic Plan, 2013–2018

Goal is polio free world by 2018, by eradication of all types of polio (Wild and Vaccine derived).

Objectives:

- Detect and interrupt all poliovirus transmission
- Strengthen immunization system and withdraw oral polio Vaccine
- Containment and certification.
- Legacy planning- mainstreaming polio functions into on-going national health program at different levels

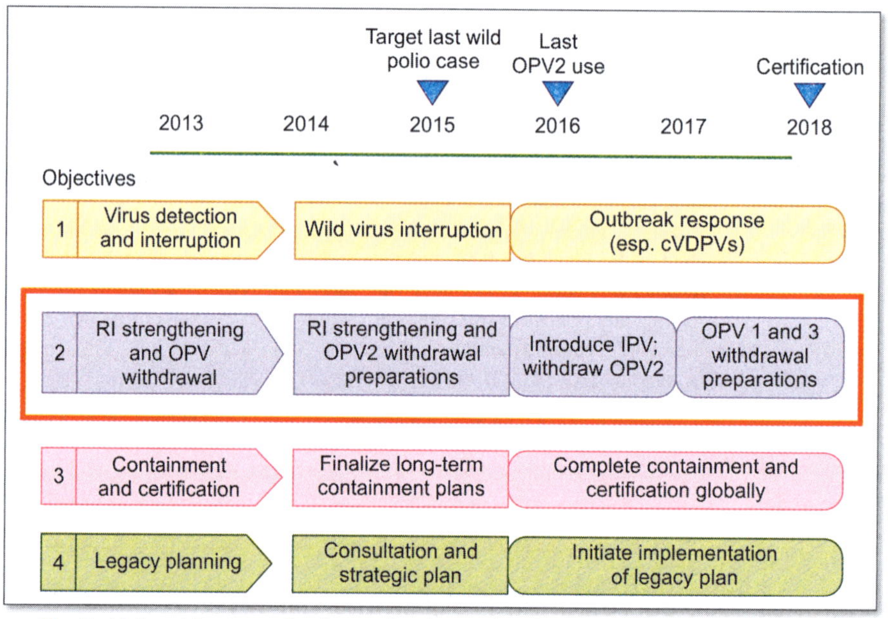

Fig. 5: Major objectives of polio eradication and endgame strategic plan 2013–2018

108 **High Yield Points**

The Switch

It is synchronised cessation of tOPV between 18th April and 1st May 2016, replacing tOPV with bOPV containing only type 1 and type 3 polio viruses and withdrawing type 2 from all immunization activities around the world.

Strategies for Polio Eradication in India –(4 Pillars)

- Routine immunization
- Conduct National Immunization Days (Intensive Pulse Polio Immunization)
- AFP Surveillance
- Mopping Up

Epidemiological Basis for Poliomyelitis Eradication

- Man is the only host
- A long-term carrier state is not known to occur
- Half-life of excreted virus in sewage is about 48 hours, and spread can only occur during this period
- OPV is easy to administer, cheap and ideally suited for poliomyelitis eradication
- Pulse Polio Program interrupts transmission of wild polio virus by displacing it from intestine.

72 **Must Remember**

Surveillance system should be sensitive enough to detect at least one AFP case for every 100,000 under 15 children even in absence of polio.

Introduction of IPV

- Endgame strategy, IPV was introduced in Dec 2015 in India, 3rd dose of OPV was coupled within intramuscular IPV at 14 weeks of age.

- ***Fractional IPV***: Introduced in April 2016, now introduced in routine immunization
    - Two fractional doses of IPV (1/5 of the full dose), given intradermal at 6 and14 weeks provide higher seroconversion rates than a single full dose (intramuscular) given at 14weeks.
    - 2 fractional doses should be separated by a minimum interval of 4 weeks.
    - One fractional dose of IPV may be suitable for outbreak response.

Acute Flaccid Paralysis (AFP) Surveillance

- Active case finding and passive reporting of AFP in children (≤15 year)
- Stool collection (2 samples, 24 hour apart) and transport to lab (Reverse cold chain 4-8° C) ideally within 14 days of onset of paralysis, but can be collected till 2 months
- Isolation of wild poliovirus and mapping
- Mop up operation if wild polio virus is detected.
- ***Environmental surveillance***- Testing sewage or other environmental samples for the presence of poliovirus. (4 sites in India)

FOOD POISONING

Table 21: Incubation period different food poisoning

Incubation	Organisms	Common food
0.5 – 6 hrs	*S. aureus* toxins (Preformed)	Meat and dairy products Reheated rice
1 – 6 hrs	*Bacillus cereus emetic* from preformed toxins	Emetic toxin Heart stable 1 -6 hrs Enterotoxin – heat labile cholera toxin
10-12 hrs	Clostridium perfringens toxin (Preformed)	Reheated meat foods
8 hrs – 2d	Ays *Vibrio parahemolyticus*	Shellfish
18-36 hrs	*Salmonella*	Poultry eggs
22- >48 hrs	*C. botulinum* toxin (botulism)	Canned food
1-5 days	EHEC (VTEC) 0157 H7	Meat hamburger unpasteurized milk
2- 11 days	Campylobacter	Poultry, unpasteurized milk
4-7 days	Yersenia enterocolitica	Raw or under cooked Pork

ZOONOTIC DISEASES

Diseases which are naturally transmitted between vertebrate animals and human

TYPES OF ZOONOSIS

- **Based on reservoir hosts**
    - Anthropo-zoonosis–from animals to humans
    - Zoo-anthroponosis–from humans to animals
    - Amphixenosis–infection transmitted in either direction
- **Based on type of life cycle and infecting organism**
    - Direct zoonosis–by direct contact
        - Example: Rabies, trichinosis, brucellosis
    - Cyclo zoonosis: More than one vertebrate host species are involved and **NO invertebrate host is** involved to complete the life cycle
        - Example: Taeniasis, echinococcosis
    - Meta zoonosis: Transmitted biologically by invertebrate hosts
        - Example: Vector borne diseases, plague, schistosomiasis

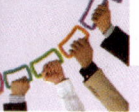

- Sapro zoonosis: include both vertebrate host and non animal developmental site (as soil, food, plants)
    - Example: Mycoses, larva migrans

BRUCELLOSIS

- Also known as undulant fever, Malta fever or Mediterranean fever
- Endemic in areas where – domestic animals, cattle farms, horses, pigs, goats, sheep are in large numbers
- National and international center for Brucellosis: WHO Brucella reference center, Veterinary research institute, Izatnagar. Uttar Pradesh, India

Epidemiology

- Gram negative, Non motile, non-sporing, intracellular coccoballius.
- Four species are responsible for brucellosis:
    - B. miltensis — Most virulent and invasive species
    - B. abortus — Less virulent, primarily disease in cattle
    - B. suis — Intermediate virulence
    - B. canis — Majorly affects dogs
- Reservoir: Domestic animals
- Source of infection: Infected animals may excrete Brucella in urine, faeces, milk, placenta, vaginal discharges
- Mode of transmission — Mostly from animal to man
    - Contact infection
    - Food borne infection
    - Air borne infection
- Incubation period: 1-3 weeks (maybe as long as 6 months or even more)

Clinical Picture

- Swinging pyrexia, rigors
- Monoarticular Arthralgia – involving large joints as hip, knee, shoulder, ankle
- Hepatosplenomegaly

Brucellosis Control

- Control of brucellosis in animals by mass surveys
- Vaccine for B. abortus strain 19 for young animals
- Hygiene and sanitation
    - Clean sanitary environment for animals
    - Sanitary disposal of or urine and feces
    - Safe handling of placenta, animal discharges
    - Avoid contact with suspected animals
- Early diagnosis and treatment
    - DOC - tetracycline dose: 500 mg every 6 hours for 3 weeks
    - Severe brucellosis: i/m streptomycin 1 g daily in addition to tetracycline
- Milk pasteurization

LEPTOSPIROSIS

- Weils disease is a manifestation of leptospirosis
- High prevalence in warm countries with outbreaks during rainfall

Epidemiology

- *L. interrogans* are the pathogenic strains, these are thin motile spirochetes.
- Reservoir: Wild, domestic animals

- Rodents are most common reservoir – *Rattus norvegicus, Mus musculus*
- Domestic animals: Cattle, sheep, goats

- Source of infection:
  - Direct contact or environment contaminated with excreta, urine of infected animals
  - Leptospira may survive in soil for months. They can optimally at average depth of 50 cms and optimum temperature of 22°C.
- Mode of transmission:
  - Direct contact
  - Indirect contact – contact of broken skin with soil, water, vegetation contaminated with Leptospira
  - Droplet infection – inhalation while milking of cows
- Incubation period: 4-20 days
- Mostly males are affected, m/c age: 20-45 years

Clinical Picture

- Anicteric leptospirosis
  - Milder form
  - Pulmonary manifestations are primary concern
- Icteric leptospirosis
  - More severe form
  - Jaundice, fever, myalgia, hypotension, circulatory failure
- Pregnancy: fetal complications, abortions

Diagnosis

- Blood smear – Dark field examination
- IgM ELISA – Sensitive test for diagnosis.
- Urine culture possible after 2 weeks of infection
- Rapid test: Leptodipstick test

Management and Control

- DOC – Penicillin, 6 mill units daily i/v
- Alternate drugs: Tetracycline, amoxycillin, ampicillin

HYDATID DISEASE

- Pathogen: Echinococcus (Metacystode stage)
- Found in many food animal rearing communities and countries (especially with sheep rearing)
- It is considered as an occupational disease in certain groups

Epidemiology

- Echinococcus are intestinal, canine tapeworms with four valid species:
  - E. granulosus
    - Most common distribution
    - Most common cause for unilocular echinococcosis
  - E. multilocularis
    - Causes the alveolar echinococcosis
  - E. oligarthus: Found in central and South America
  - E. Vogeli: Found in central and South America, cause polycystic hydatidosis
- Life cycle: Dog – sheep life cycle. Man is an intermediate, accidental host
- Mode of transmission:
  - By ingestion of eggs of echinococcus with food, unwashed vegetables
  - Handling dogs, infected animals
  - Man-man transmission is not known
- Incubation period: months to years

Clinical Features

- Hydatidosis has insidious onset – usually taking several years after exposure.
- Most common location of the cyst – liver right lobe (70%) followed by other organs as lung, brain, kidney or even bones
- Cyst is filled with watery fluid and contain tapeworm heads, hence rupture of cysts may lead to dissemination and metastasis of hydatid cysts to other locations
- Most symptoms are due to space occupying lesions

Diagnosis

- Clinical and X-rays are the mainstay for diagnosis
- ELISA – high sensitivity
- Casoni's test – may be used, but has low specificity

Management

- Surgical Removal of Cyst:
  PAIR (Puncture, Aspiration, Injection, Re aspiration) is an option for surgical removal of the cyst.
  Indications for PAIR. Patients with:
  - Non-echoic lesion ≥5 cm in diameter
  - Cysts with daughter cysts, and/or with detachment of membranes
  - Multiple cysts if accessible to puncture
  - Infected cysts

  Also
  - Pregnant women
  - Children >3 years old
  - Patients who fail to respond to chemotherapy alone
  - Patients in whom surgery is contraindicated
  - Patient who refuse surgery
  - Patients who relapse after surgery
  - Non-cooperative patients and inaccessible or risky location of the cyst in the liver
  - Cyst in spine, brain and/or heart
  - Inactive or calcified lesion
  - Cysts communicating with the biliary tree
  - Cysts open into the abdominal cavity, bronchi and urinary tract
- Hygiene and sanitation

RABIES

Causative organism for rabies is Lyssavirus type 1, a neurotropic virus belonging to the family of Rhabdoviruses. The incubation period is usually between 2 and 8 weeks.

Table 22: Classification of exposure to suspect or confirmed rabid animal bite

Categories	Types of contacts	Types of exposure	Recommended postexposure prophylaxis
I	Touching or feeding of animals Licks on intact skin	None	▪ None, if reliable case history is available
II	Nibbling of uncovered skin Minor scratches or abrasions without bleeding	Minor	▪ Wound management ▪ Anti-rabies vaccine
III	Single or multiple transdermal bites or scratches, licks on broken skin Contamination of mucous membrane with saliva (i.e. licks)	Severe	▪ Wound management ▪ Rabies immunoglobulin ▪ Anti-rabies vaccine

- **Bite by wild animals:** Bite by all wild animals should be treated as category III exposure
- **Bite by rodents:** It should be noted that bites by domestic rats, mice, squirrel, hare and rabbits seldom require treatment
- **Bat rabies:** Bat rabies has not been conclusively proved in India and hence exposure to bats does not warrant treatment

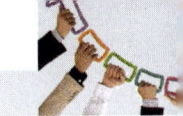

- Pregnancy, lactation, infancy, old age and concurrent illness are no contraindications for rabies postexposure prophylaxis in the event of an exposure
- **HIV:** Even immunocompromised patients with category II exposures should receive rabies immunoglobulin in addition to a full post-exposure vaccination. Preferably, if the facilities are available, antirabies antibody estimation should be done 10 days after the completion of course of vaccination.
- Anti-rabies sera should always be brought to room temperature (20–25° C) before use
- Reconstituted vaccines must be stored at 2–8° C and discarded after 6–8 hours.

Wound Management

Do's		
Physical	Wash with running tap water	Mechanical removal of virus from the wound
Chemical	Wash the wound with soap and water Apply disinfectant	Inactivation of the virus
Biological	Infiltrate immunoglobulins in the depth and around the wound in category III exposures	Neutralization of the virus
Don'ts		
▪ Touch the wound with bare hand ▪ Apply irritants like chillies, oil, herbs, chalk, betel leaves, etc.		

Management of Rabid Animal Bite

- Local treatment
  - Cleaning/flushing the wound with soap and water (preferably under running tap water) for 15 min. Irrigation with catheter in case of punctured wound
    - **Chemical treatment:** Virucidal agents, alcohol and tincture iodine
  - Wound should never be sutured immediately (if necessary, it should be done after 24–48 hour, applying minimum stitches and undercover of Anti Rabies Serum locally)
- Rabies vaccination
- Antirabies serum in severe exposure (class III)
- Antibiotic and tetanus toxoid, if indicated

Note: (Stop treatment if animal remains healthy throughout an observation period of 10 days, or if animal is killed and found to be negative for rabies by appropriate laboratory techniques)

Good to Remember

- Avoid sutures (loose, if required)
- No cauterization 85%
- TT, Antibiotics as per case

Rabies Immunoglobulin (RIG)

- Equine RIG—40 IU per kg
- Human RIG—Better—20 IU per kg

The RIG is administered as 70% in and around the wound site and remaining 30% IM

(**Note:** The data is controversial and different sources provide different opinion. However, for exam purpose, we can remember that most of the immunoglobulins are administered in and around wound, while remaining as IM injection at a distant site).

Special Considerations

- The only contraindication to PrEP is severe reaction to rabies vaccine (which is very rare)
- There is NO contraindication to postexposure prophylaxis as rabies is fatal disease
- Pregnancy, malnutrition, HIV, immunocompromised, infants, children – do NOT form any contraindications to this vaccine
- Individuals on "chloroquine treatment" for malaria or any other purpose will require intramuscular injections rather than intradermal injection (due to reduced response of vaccine)

Skin Test Before ERIG

- Inject 0.1 mL ERIG diluted 1:10 in physiological saline intradermally into the flexor surface of the forearm to raise a bleb of about 3-4 mm diameter.

- Inject an equal amount of normal saline as a negative control on the flexor surface of the other forearm
- After 15 minutes an increase in diameter to >10 mm of induration surrounded by flare is taken as positive skin test, provided the reaction on the saline test was negative
- An increase or abrupt fall in blood pressure, syncope, hurried breathing, palpitations and any other systemic manifestations should be taken as positive test

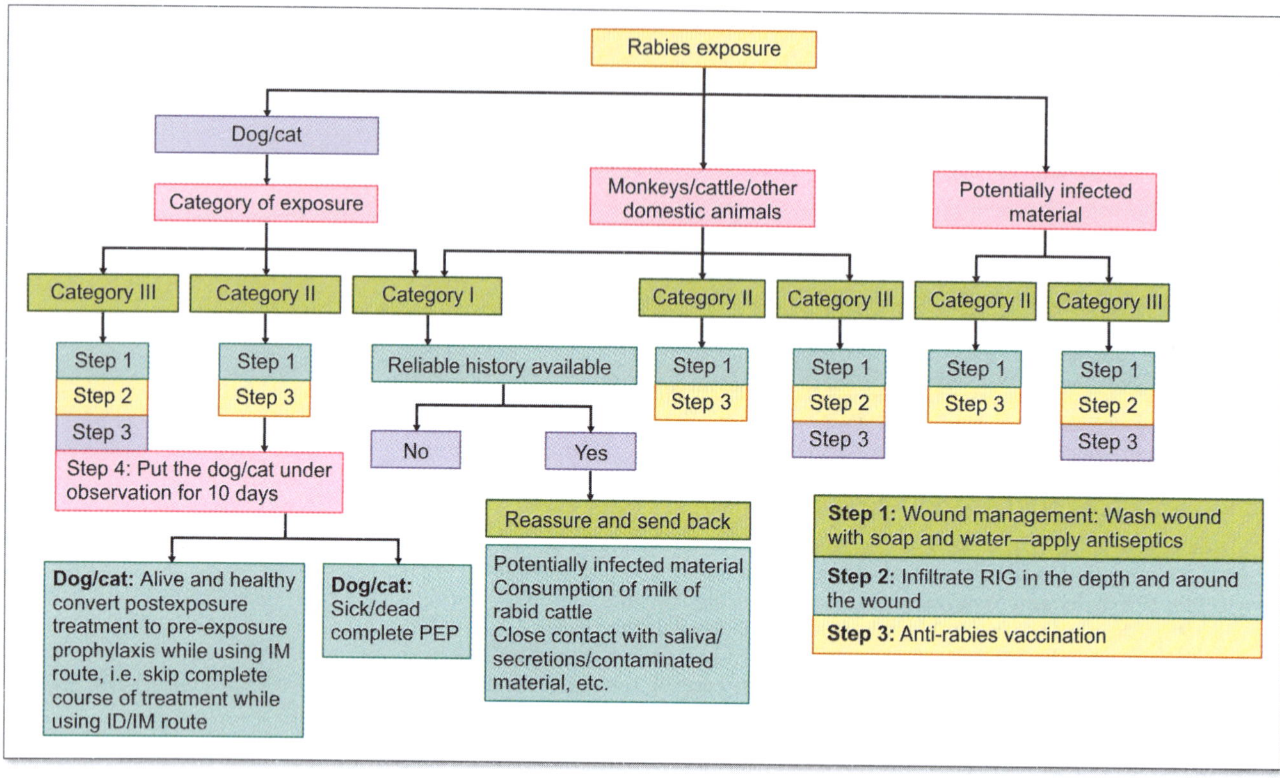

Fig. 6: Flow of rabies exposure

78 Good to Remember

The following vaccines have been approved by DCGI currently for use by intradermal route :
PVRV: Verorab, Aventis Pasteur (Sanofi Pasteur) India Pvt. Ltd.
PCECV: Rabipur, Chiron Behring Vaccines Pvt. Ltd.
PVRV: Pasteur Institute of India
PVRV: Abhayrab, Human Biologicals Institute.

79 Good to Remember

Re-Exposure guidelines:
Vaccine is NOT given if previously immunized within 3 months
RIG is NOT given if previous dose was given within 1 year
Re-vaccination is required if the VNA levels are below 0.5 IU/mL

Anti-Rabies Vaccine

The different types of antirabies vaccines are as follows:

- **Nerve tissue vaccines:** Semple's vaccine, etc.
- **Avian embryo vaccine:** Chick or duck embryo vaccines
- **Primary cell culture vaccines:** Human diploid cell vaccine.

April 2018 – WHO position paper on rabies immunization:
The current WHO recommendations are:

Categorization of wounds:
Category I – Touching or feeding animals with licks on intact skin
Category II – Nibbling of uncovered skin, minor scratch or abrasions without bleeding
Category III – Single or multiple bites or scratches, contamination of mucous membrane.

Management

Wound wash:

- At least 15 mins with soap and generous water. Iodine based or virucidal agents may be applied on wound
- Wounds which require suture – should have loose sutures
- RIG for category III wounds

Postexposure Prophylaxis–Recommended Schedules

	Category 1	Category 2	Category 3
No previous immunization	Wound wash No PEP required	Wound wash ▪ ID - 2 site – 0,3,7days ▪ IM – 1 site – 0,3,7,28 days ▪ IM 2 site day 0 + 1 site IM 7,21 days RIG is NOT indicated	Wound wash ▪ ID - 2 site – 0,3,7 days ▪ IM – 1 site – 0,3,7,28 days ▪ IM 2 site day 0 + 1 site IM 7,21 days RIG is recommended
Previously immunized individuals of all ages (*Vaccine is NOT given if PEP received within <3 months previously)	Wound wash No PEP required	Wound Wash + vaccine* ▪ ID – 1 site 0,3 days ▪ ID – 4 site day 0 ▪ IM – 1 site 0,3 days RIG is NOT indicated	Wound Wash + vaccine* ▪ ID – 1 site 0,3 days ▪ ID – 4 site day 0 ▪ IM – 1 site day 0,3 days RIG is NOT indicated

Summary of Schedules

- ONE week; 2 site; ID regime; *Institut pasteur du cambodge* regime; 2-2-2-0-0
- Two week; 1 site; IM regime; 4 dose; ESSEN regime; 1-1-1-1-0
- Three week; IM regime; 5 dose; ZAGREB regime; 2-0-1-0-1
- Four Week; ID regime; 8 dose; Thai Redcross regime; 2-2-2-0-2

Note:

- All dates of doses are 0,3,7,14,28 days
- All Intradermal (ID) doses are 0.1 ml/dose; Intramuscular (IM) Dose is 0.5 - 1.0 mL/dose

India MoHFW recommendations:

Previous WHO-recommended rabies vaccine schedules for IM administration remain acceptable, but in comparison the ID schedules offer advantages through savings in costs, doses and time. The national health system in India recommends ID – *Updated Thai Red cross regime.*

- If the doses are delayed, they should be resumed, not restarted.
- In case of complete vaccination <3 months, repeat vaccine is not required.
- In case of time lapse is >3 months, repeat vaccine maybe administered as required.
- RIG (Rabies immunogloblin) is not required to be repeated till 1 year of age.
- RIG - IM injection at a distant site is NO longer recommended
- NO contraindication for ID or IM vaccine with chloroquine or hydroxychloroquine
- Vaccine may be given to PREGNANT females

Exposure in HIV

- HIV individuals receiving ART (CD4 >200 for age >5 years) - can receive Rabies vaccine .
- HIV - immunocompromised patients - VACCINE (cat II, III + RIG in all cases)
  Day 0,7,21 - ID or IM vaccination

Pre-exposure Prophylaxis

To high risk occupation individuals

- 2 site ID on day 0, 7 days
- 1 site IM on day 0,7 days

Revaccination is recommended if the Vaccine induced neutralizing antibody (VNA levels) are lower than <0.5 IU/mL

VECTOR-BORNE DISEASES

ARTHROPOD-BORNE DISEASES

Mosquito	Malaria, Filaria, Japanese encephalitis, Dengue, West Nile fever, Yellow fever, dengue haemorrhagic fever
Housefly	Typhoid and Paratyphoid fever, Diarrhea, Dysentery, Cholera, Amebiasis, Helminthic infestations, Poliomyelitis, Conjunctivitis, Trachoma, Anthrax and Yaws

Contd...

High Yield Points

Postexposure prophylaxis is indicated in[Q] (Mnemonic: HMV Ring Tone)

- Hepatitis B and HIV (ART)
- Measles (Within 2 days of exposure)
- Varicella (Varicella Zoster Immunoglobulin within 72 hours of exposure)
- Rabies
- Tetanus

Sandfly	Kala-azar, Oriental sore, Sandfly fever, Oraya fever
Tsetse fly	Sleeping sickness
Louse	Epidemic typhus, Relapsing fever, Trench fever, Pediculosis
Rat flea	Bubonic plague, Endemic typhus, Chiggerosis, Hymenolepis diminuta
Blackfly	Onchocerciasis
Reduviid bug	Chagas disease
Hard tick	Tick typhus (Rocky Mountain spotted fever), Viral encephalitis (Russian spring-summer encephalitis), Viral fevers (Colorado tick fever), Viral hemorrhagic fever, (e.g., Kyasanur forest disease), Tularemia, Tick paralysis, human babesiosis
Soft tick	Q fever, Relapsing fever
Trombiculid mite	Scrub typhus, Rickettsial-pox
Itch-mite	Scabies
Cyclops	Guinea-worm disease, Fish tapeworm (D. latus)
Cockroaches	Enteric pathogens

MALARIA

- Man is the *intermediate host*[Q] (Asexual cycle) and
- Mosquito the *definitive host*[Q] (Sexual cycle)
- Malaria is a seasonal (Maximum prevalence between July to Nov in Monsoon rains).
- Extrinsic Incubation period is 10–20 days, depending upon conditions of atmospheric temperature and humidity.

> **110 High Yield Points**
> - Anopheles culicifacies is major vector in rural/semi urban areas[Q]
> - Anopheles stephensi in urban areas[Q].
> - Anopheles fluviatilis–forest areas and foothills

Mode of Transmission

Vector borne: (Most common[Q]) Bite of infected female anopheles mosquito.

Direct: Accidental injections of blood or plasma (Parasites remain infective for at least 14 days in blood bottles stored at - 4°C).

Congenital: Rare

- Newborn infants have resistance to infection with *P. falciparum.*
- Pregnancy increases the risk of malaria in women. Febrile herpes is common in all malaria patients.

Diagnosis and Treatment of Malaria

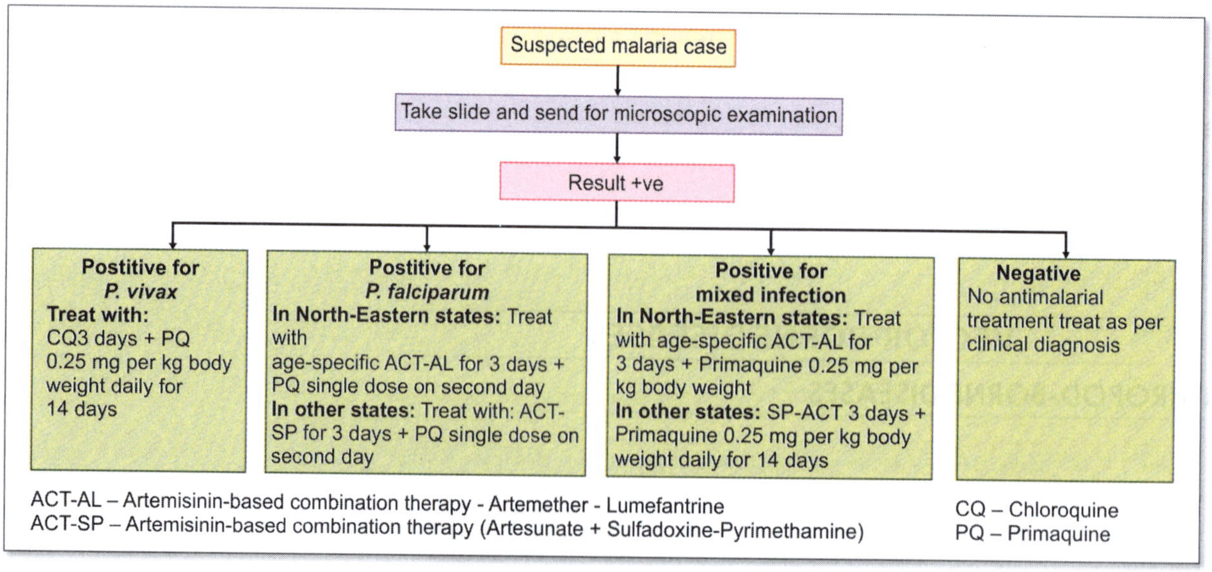

Fig. 7: Suspected malaria cases treatment and diagnosis

Malaria Diagnosis and Treatment Guideline

Treatment of uncomplicated malaria

- No more presumptive treatment[Q].
- All fever cases suspected to be malaria must be investigated by microscopy or RDT.
- **P. vivax cases** → Chloroquine: 10 mg/kg on day 1 and 2 and 5 mg/kg on day 3. + Primaquine* 0.25 mg/ kg body weight daily for 14 days. (**contraindicated in pregnancy, G6PD deficiency).*
- ***P. falciparum* cases** → Artemisinin based combination therapy (ACT-SP)** + Primaquine: 0.75 mg/kg body weight on day 2 (**Artesunate 4 mg/kg body weight daily for 3 days + Sulfadoxine 25 mg/kg body weight) and Pyrimethamine 1.25 mg/kg on day 1)
- **Mixed infection (*P. falciparum* + *P. vivax*)**– ACT SP×3days + Primaquine 0.25 mg/kg bodyweight daily for 14 days.

Table 23: Dosage chart for treatment of vivax malaria

Age	Day 1		Day 2		Day 3		Day 4 to 14
	CQ (150 mg base)	PQ (2.5 mg)	CQ (150 mg base)	PQ (2.5 mg)	CQ (150 mg base)	PQ (2.5 mg)	PQ (2.5 mg)
Less than 1 year	1/2	0	1/2	0	1/4	0	0
1–4 years	1	1	1	1	1/2	1	1
5–8 years	2	2	2	2	1	2	1
9–14 years	3	4	3	4	1 1/2	4	4
15 years or more*	4	6	4	6	2	6	6
Pregnancy	4	0	4	0	2	0	0

* CQ 250 mg tablet is having 150 mg base

Table 24: Dosage chart for treatment of falciparum malaria with ACT-SP

Age group (Years)	1 st day		2nd day		3rd day
	AS	SP	AS	PQ	AS
0–1* pink blister	1 (25 mg)	1 (250 + 12.5 mg)	1 (25 mg)	Nil	1 25 (mg)
1–4 yellow blister	1 (50 mg)	1 (500 + 25 mg each)	1 (50 mg)	1 (7.5 mg base)	1 (50 mg)
5–8 green blister	1 (100 mg)	1 (750 + 37.5 mg each)	1 (100 mg)	2 (7.5 mg base)	1 (100 mg)
9–14 red blister	1 (150 mg)	2 (500 + 25 mg each)	1 (150 mg)	4 (7.5 mg base)	1 (150 mg)
15 and above white blister	1 (200 mg)	2 (750 + 37.5 mg each)	1 (200 mg)	6 (7.5 mg base each)	1 (200 mg)

* SP is not to be prescribed for children <5 months of age and should be treated with alternate ACT
* ACT-AL is not to be prescribed for children weighing less than 5 kg.

High Yield Points

In North Eastern states

- *P. falciparum* cases- ACT-AL (Coformulated tablet of Artemether (20 mg) + Lumefantrine (120 mg) as per age specific schedule) + Primaquine: 0.75 mg/kg body weight on day 2.
- Mixed infection (*P. falciparum* + *P. vivax*)– ACT-AL × 3 days +Primaquine 0.25 mg/kg body weight daily for 14 days.

Table 25: Recommended regimen by weight and age group the packing size for different age groups base on Kg body weight

Co-formulate tablet ACT-AL	5–14 kg (>5 months to <3 years)	15–24 kg (>3 to 8 years)	25–34 kg (>9 to 14 years)	>34 kg (>14 years)
Total dose of ACT-AL	20 mg/120 mg twice daily for 3 days	40 mg/240 mg twice daily for 3 days	60 mg 360 mg twice daily for 3 days	80 mg/480 mg twice daily for 3 day
Pack size				
No. of tablets in the packing	6	12	18	24
Give	1 tablet twice daily for 3 days	2 tablets twice daily for 3 days	3 tablets twice daily for 3 days	4 tablets twice daily for 3 days
Color of the pack	Yellow	Green	Red	White

General recommendations for starting anti-malaria treatment:
- Do not give empty stomach
- First doe should be observed dose
- Dose should be repeated if vomit occurs within 15 minutes of taking the tablets. Open a new blister pack and discard what is remaining in the previous blister pack. (in case of repeat vomit, consider severe malaria and shifting the patient to higher referral center and management according to severe malaria)
- Always explain danger signs

Management of Malaria

Malaria in Pregnancy

P. falciparum cases → 1st Trimester: Quinine, 2nd and 3rd Trimester: ACT
P. vivax cases → Chloroquine

Resistant Cases

- Resistance is suspected if full treatment, shows no response in 72 hour.
- Treatment- Oral Quinine + Tetracycline/Doxycycline

Severe Malaria

Characterized by one or more features:
- Impaired consciousness/coma
- Repeated generalized convulsions
- Renal failure
- Jaundice
- Severe anemia
- Pulmonary edema
- Hypoglycemia
- Metabolic syndrome
- Circulatory collapse/shock/abnormal bleeding and disseminated intravascular coagulation.

Treatment for Severe Malaria

- Artesunate: 2.4 mg/kg IV or IM on admission, then at 12 h and 24 h and then once a day or
- Artemether: 3.2 mg/kg body weight IM on admission and then 1.6 mg/kg per day or
- Arteether: 150 mg IM daily for 3 days in adults only or
- Quinine: 20 mg/kg body weight on admission (IV or IM) followed by maintenance dose of 10 mg/kg body weight 8 hourly.

Treatment Failure

Early treatment failure: Development of danger signs or severe malaria on day 1, 2, 3 in presence of parasitemia
Late clinical failure: Development of danger signs or severe malaria in presence of parasitemia between day 4 and day 28
Late parasitological failure: Presence of parasitemia on any day between day 7 and day 28

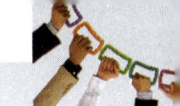

Chemoprophylaxis

(To be Complemented with Personal Protection and Other Methods)

- **Indication:** Selective groups (Military and Para-military forces, labour forces, travelers from nonendemic area for long stay in high *P. falciparum* endemic areas.
- **Short-term chemoprophylaxis (up to 6 weeks)**
  - All drugs to be taken strictly on time and continued for 4 weeks after the last possible exposure to infection.
  - **Doxycycline:** 100 mg OD for adults and 1.5 mg/kg OD for children started 2 days before travel.
  - Not recommended for pregnant women and children <8 years. Dose in children >8 year is to be based on bodyweight.
  - **Chloroquine:** 300 mg (base) once weekly or 100 mg (base) OD for 6 days a week. Initiated a week before arrival.
  - **Mefloquine:** 250 mg weekly. Initiated 2–3 weeks before arrival
- **Chemophrophylaxis for longer stay (>6 weeks)**
  - **Mefloquine:** 250 mg weekly for adults, administered 2 weeks before, during and 4 weeks after exposure.
  - Chloroquine (300 mg weekly/100 mg OD) + Proguanil (100 mg OD) – (Screening for retinal changes to be done 6 months after 5 year (weekly regimen) and 3 year (daily regimen)

> **112 High Yield Points**
>
> ***Complications of P. falciparum malaria*** are cerebral malaria, acute renal failure, liver damage, gastro-intestinal symptoms, dehydration, collapse, anaemia, black-water fever etc.
> ***Complications of P. vivax, P. ovale and P. malariae*** infections are anaemia, splenomegaly, enlargement of liver, herpes, renal complications etc.

National Vector Borne Disease Control Program (NVBDCP)

(NVBDCP) Evolution and Timeline at a Glance

- **1953 National Malaria Control Program**
- **1958 National Malaria Eradication Program**
- **1977 Modified Plan of Operations**
- **1997 Enhanced Malaria Control Project**
- **2002 National Vector Borne Disease Control Program**
- **2005 Rapid diagnostic tests (RDT) introduced and integrated as part of NRHM**

Strategy to Combat Malaria

- Disease management and early diagnosis:
  - Peripheral blood Smears—Microscopic examination
  - National Malaria Drug Policy update (2014–2017)
- Integrated vector management
  - Anti-larval measures
  - Larvicides: Paris green, temefos
    - Source reduction: drainage, flushing, irrigation
  - Anti-adult measures
    - Residual spray
    - DDT
    - Malathion
    - Fenthion
  - Space application: Pyrethrum spray—fogging
  - Individual protection
  - Use of bed nets
  - Protective clothing
  - Mosquito repellents

Behavior change, communication, use of legislation and other social support system.

> **113 High Yield Points**
>
> - **Urban Malaria Scheme (1971) :** As in early 1970s resurgence of malaria, most of malaria vector was from urban areas.
> - Install civil byelaws for mosquito-genic situations
> - Set up of malaria clinics at all peripheral health centers for fever survey and malaria microscopy slide examination
> - Strengthen drug distribution centers and fever treatment depots

Organization

State level: State program officer – state vector borne control society
Zonal level: Senior divisional officer
District level: District health officer, Assistant malaria Officer, Malaria inspector

Table 26: Classification of states/UTS based on API as primary criteria

Categories of states/UTs	Definition
Category 0: Prevention of re-establishment phase	States/UTs with zero indigenous cases of malaria.
Category 1: Elimination phase	States/UTs (15) including their districts reporting an API of less than 1 case per 1,000 population at risk.
Category 2: Pre-elimination phase	States/UTs (11) with an API of less than 1 case per 1,000 population at risk, but some of their districts are reporting an API of 1 case per 1000 population at risk or above.
Category 3: Intensified control phase	States/UTs (10) with an API of 1 case per 1,000 population at risk or above.

Indicators under NVBDCP

- **The main indices are:**
  - **Infant parasite rate:** Sensitive indicator, for assessment of the program in annual basis
  - **Slide positivity rate:** Useful for predicting an impending outbreak
  - **Annual parasitic incidence:** Is an indicator for **malaria prevalence** in the area.

$$API = \frac{\text{Confirmed case during one year (by PBF/RDT-wherever approved)}}{\text{Population under surveillance}} \times 1000$$

    Useful indicator for assessment of impact of the program and to formulate the prevention strategy for a particular area

  - **Annual blood examination rate** –is an indicator for fever prevalence in an area.

$$ABER = \frac{\text{Number of slides examined}}{\text{Population under surveillance}} \times 100$$

    Useful indicator for assessment of the operational activity of the program in the area. It indicates the level of utilization of the malaria preventive services in the area reflecting the functionality of the program

Entomological Indices

- **Human blood index:** Proportion of freshly fed female anopheles mosquito whose stomach contains human blood
- **Mosquito density:** Number of mosquitoes per person per hour. (Usually expressed as per man hours)

NVBDCP Update–2017

Strategic Action Plan for Malaria Control in India, 2007-2012 (NVBDCP)

The strategies for *prevention and control of malaria and its transmission* are:

- Surveillance and case management
- Case detection (passive and active)
- Early diagnosis and complete treatment
- Sentinel surveillance.

Integrated Vector Management

- Indoor residual spray (IRS)
- Insecticide treated bed nets (ITNs) and long lasting insecticidal nets (LLINs)
- Antilarval measures including source reduction.

Epidemic Preparedness and Early Response

Supportive Interventions

- Capacity building
- Behavioral change communication

80 Good to Remember

Children aged 2 – 10 years are examined for enlargement of spleen and areas are classified according to endemicity as indicated by the spleen rate:

Below 10%	–	Nonendemic
10 – 25%	–	Hypoendemic
25 – 40%	–	Endemic
>40%	–	Hyperendemic

114 High Yield Points

- **Spleen rate*** - though an old indicator from the pre-eradication malariometric indicator – is still the sensitive indicator for evaluation of the malaria program
- **ABER**- is the operational indicator
- **Slide positivity rate** is a useful indicator for assessment of an impendoing outbreak or onset of malaria season in an area.
- **API** is the principal impact indicator along with falciparum and vivax incidence rates
- **Anti-malaria month** – June every year
- ***Chloroquine*** is contraindicated as presumptive treatment

115 High Yield Points

- **Treatment of choice for *P. vivax*** – Chloroquine + primaquine
- **Treatment of choice for *P. falciparum*** – Artesunate combination therapy (+ Primaquine as single dose)

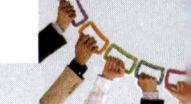

- Intersectoral collaboration
- Monitoring and Evaluation
- Operational research and applied field research.

National Framework for Malaria Elimination in India (2016–2030)

Vision
- Eliminate malaria nationally and contribute to improved health, quality of life and alleviation of poverty.

Goals
- Eliminate malaria (zero indigenous cases) throughout country by 2030
- Maintain malaria–free status in areas where malaria transmission has been interrupted and prevent reintroduction of malaria.

Objectives
- Eliminate malaria from all 26 low (Category 1) and moderate (Category 2) transmission states/union territories (UTs) by 2022
- Reduce the incidence of malaria to less than 1 case per 1000 population per year in all states and UTs and their districts by 2024
- Interrupt indigenous transmission of malaria throughout the country by 2027
- Prevent the establishment of local transmission of malaria in areas where it has been eliminated and maintain national malaria-free status by 2030 and beyond.

Table 27: The goals, milestones and targets for the Global Technical strategy for malaria 2016–2030

Goals	Milestones		Targets
	2020	2025	2013
▪ Reduce malaria mortality rates globally compared with 2015	At least 40%	At least 75%	At least 90%
▪ Reduce malaria case incidence globally compared with 2015	At least 40%	At least 75%	At least 90%
▪ Eliminate malaria from countries in which malaria was transmitted in 205	At least 10 countries	At least 20 countries	At least 35 countries
▪ Prevent re-establishment of malaria in all countries that are malaria-free	Re-establishment prevented	Re-establishment prevented	Re-establishment prevented

Malaria Vaccine Implementation Program (MVIP) – Trade Name 'Mosquirix'

- Positive opinion by 'European medicines agency' 2015
- RTS, S/AS01 (RTS, S) shows partial protection against malaria
- It is a pre-erythrocytic stage hybrid recombinant protein vaccine, based on the RTS, S recombinant antigen.
- It comprises the hybrid polypeptide RTS in which regions of the P. falciparum circum-sporozoite protein known to induce humoral (R region) and cellular immune (T region) responses are covalently bound to the hepatitis B surface antigen (S).
- This recombinant fusion protein (RTS) is expressed in *Saccharomyces cerevisiae* together with free hepatitis B surface antigen (S), to form RTS, S virus-like particles.
- The formulation comprises 25 µg of RTS, S (pharmaceutical powder form) with the AS01E adjuvant system (suspension).

81 Good to Remember

- *Aedes aegypti* – is a nervous and discordant feeder – needs more than one feed to complete its gonotropic cycle, hence may cause many cases clustered in an area or region.

82 Good to Remember

Symptoms usually last for 2–7 days, after an incubation period of 4–10 days after the bite from an infected mosquito.

DENGUE

Vector - Female Aedes aegypti and Aedes albopictus (Lesser extent) mosquito
Aedes Aegypti

- Diseases transmitted – Dengue, Chikungunya, Yellow fever and Zika infection.
- Lives in urban habitats and breeds in man-made containers.
- It is a day-time feeder, peak biting hours being 2 hours after sunrise and 2 hours before sunset
- Usually endophilic and causes a painful bite
- Once the mosquito is infective, it remains so for the rest of its life.
- Aedes albopictus – aggressive and concordant feeder – does not require a second blood meal
- Best temperature = 16-20°C, with 60–80% humidity

4 distinct, but closely related serotypes of the virus cause dengue (***DEN-1, DEN- 2, DEN-3 and DEN-4).*** Recovery from infection by one serotype provides lifelong immunity against that particular serotype.

Cross-immunity to the other serotypes after recovery is only partial and temporary.

Subsequent infections by other serotypes increase the risk of developing severe dengue.

Clinical Features

Dengue should be suspected when a high fever (40°C/104°F) is accompanied by two of the following symptoms:

- Severe headache
- Pain behind the eyes
- Muscle and joint pains
- Nausea
- Vomiting
- Swollen glands or rash.

Classical Dengue or "Break-bone Fever"

This is an acute viral infection, caused by 4 serotypes (1, 2, 3 and 4) of dengue virus.

- Reservoir of infection is man and mosquito.
- Transmission cycle is "Man-mosquito-Man".
- All ages and both sexes are susceptible to dengue fever.
- Children usually have a milder disease than adults.[Q]
- Incubation period is of 3 to 10 days (commonly 5–6 days).

Dengue Hemorrhagic Fever

- Febrile illness:
  4–6 days, high grade fever
- Maculopapular rash – Rubelliform type
- Lab: High hematocrit and moderate to severe thrombocytopenia
- Positive tourniquet test
- Test is positive if more than 10 petechiae/2.5 × 2.5 cm (or one sq. Inch) area

Critical Phase

- Approx. 3-7 days - Around the time of defervescence – temperature is 27.5-38°C
- Significant plasma leakage for 24–48 hours
- Progressive leukopenia and rapid decline in platelet count is associated
- Pleural effusion, ascites, gallbladder edema and liver engorgement
- Usually lasts for 24–48 hours

Recovery Phase

- Follows the critical phase
- Gradual re-absorption of the fluid and return from the critical phase
- The rash starts to fade. Typically known as 'isles of white in the sea of red'
- Excessive or aggressive fluid resuscitation may result in pulmonary edema or CCF
- Severe dengue:

- Plasma leakage leading to shock
- Severe bleeding
- Sever organ impairment

Warning Signs of Severe Dengue

Occur 3–7 days after 1st symptoms in conjunction with a decrease in temperature (below 38°C/100°F) and include:

- Severe abdominal pain
- Persistent vomiting
- Rapid breathing
- Bleeding gums
- Fatigue
- Restlessness and
- Blood in vomit.

The next 24–48 hours of the critical stage can be lethal; proper medical care is needed to avoid complications and risk of death.

Course of Disease—Dengue

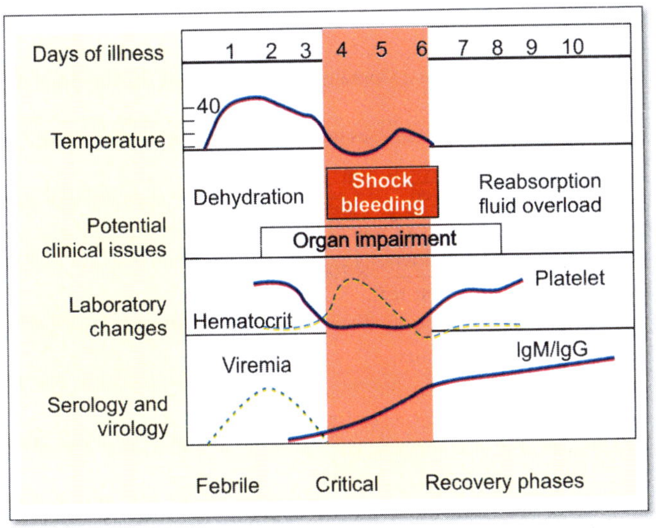

Fig. 8: Course of dengue illness

Center for disease control and prevention. Clinician's case management card. Available at http://www.cdc.gov/Dengue/resources/Dengue% 20 Case% 20 Management card 125085 12 × 6 Zcard Dengue.pdf

Guidelines for Treatment of Dengue Syndrome

- *Management of Dengue fever*: Patient able to tolerate oral fluids and passes urine once in 6 hours, no warning signs and stable hematocrit-
- Encourage fluid intake, paracetamol 6 hourly for high fever, no other NSAID, advice regarding warning signs- (no clinical improvement, severe abdominal pain, persistent vomiting, cold and clammy extremities, bleeding, not passing urine for more than 6 hours etc). Daily monitoring needed.
- *Management of DHF (Febrile phase)*: Paracetamol to keep temp below 39° C, copious amount of fluid to the extent of tolerance, close monitoring for initial signs of shock, serial hematocrit determinations daily from third day onwards.
- IV crystalloids, blood transfusion (if internal bleeding suspected)

Prevention and Control

WHO Dengue Prevention Control Strategy 2012–2020

- Reduce Dengue mortality by 50% by2020*
- Reduce Dengue Morbidity by 25% by 2020*

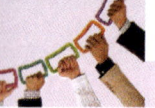

- Estimate real burden of disease by 2015*
- Baseline year2010

Treatment: There is no specific treatment for dengue fever.

Dengue Vaccine

Vaccination: 1st dengue vaccine, **Dengvaxia (CYD- TDV)**, was registered in several countries for use in individuals 9–45 years of age living in endemic areas.

Preventing mosquitoes from accessing egg-laying habitats by environmental management and modification;

- Disposing of solid waste properly and removing artificial man-made habitats
- Covering, emptying and cleaning of domestic water storage containers on a weekly basis
- Applying appropriate insecticides to water storage outdoor containers
- Personal household protection (window screens, long-sleeved clothes, insecticide treated materials, coils and vaporizers)
- Community participation and mobilization for sustained vector control
- Insecticides as space spray during outbreaks is one of the emergency vector-control measures.

Vector Surveillance

Larval Surveillance

For larval surveys, the basic sampling unit is the house or premise, which is systematically searched for water holding containers. Containers are examined for the presence of mosquito larvae and pupae. The indices used are:

- House Index (HI) : percentage of houses infected with larvae and/or pupae

$$HI = \frac{\text{Number of houses infected}}{\text{Number of houses survived}} \times 100$$

- Container index (CI): Percentage of water holding containers infected with larvae or pupae.

$$CI = \frac{\text{Number of positive containers}}{\text{Number of containers inspected}} \times 100$$

- Breteau index (BI): Number of positive containers per 100 houses inspected

$$BI = \frac{\text{Number of positive containers}}{\text{Number of houses inspected}} \times 100$$

- Pupae index (PI): Number of pupae per 100 houses

$$PI = \frac{\text{Number of pupae}}{\text{Number of houses inspected}} \times 100$$

Adult Mosquito Surveillance

- Mosquito Landing Counts per man hour
- Oviposition traps:
  - Ovitraps are devices used to detect the presence of Aegypti where the population density is low and larval surveys are largely unproductive (when the Breteau index is less than 5) as well as normal conditions.
  - The ovitrap is used for *Ae aegypti* surveillance in urban areas to evaluate the impact of adulticidal space spraying on adult female population

Vector Management

Involves management of the vector Aedes aegypti mosquito at the larval or adult level and personal protection measures.

Chemical Control

- Larvicide: Temephos (50EC) – 1 ppm (i.e. 1 mg/L of Water)
- Adulticide: for control of adult mosquitos are:
  - Pyrethrum spray: used in concentration of 0.1% - 0.2% @ 30-60 ml/1000 cu. ft. Commercial formulation of 2% pyrethrum extract is diluted with kerosene in the ratio of one part of 2% pyrethrum extract with 19 parts of kerosene (volume/volume). Thus, one liter of 2% pyrethrum extract is diluted by kerosene into 20 liters to make 0.1% pyrethrum formulation (ready-to-spray formulation).

- Malathion or Ultra low volume (ULV) Fogging: in ULV, the insecticide is sprayed with small droplets of 'volume median diameter' (VMD) of 40-80 microns. As no diluent is used, this technique is more effective than thermal fogging and does not generate visible fog

Biological Control: The Larval Control can be Done Using

- Larvivorous fish – *Gambusia affinis, Betta splendens, Trichogaster trichopterus* and *Poecilia reticulate (Guppy fish)*
- Endotoxin producing bacteria: *Bacillus thuringiensis serotype H-14*

LYMPHATIC FILARIASIS (LF)

Caused by three nematodes
- *W. bancrofti*
- *B. malayi*
- *B. timori*

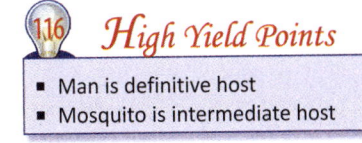

High Yield Points
- Man is definitive host
- Mosquito is intermediate host

Epidemiology

LF in India:
MDA is being implemented in India since 2004
LF is public health problem in 8 states
- Uttar Pradesh
- Andhra Pradesh
- West Bengal
- Maharashtra
- Bihar
- Jharkhand
- Odisha
- Telangana

Agent Factors

- W. bancrofti
  - Vector – *Culex fatigans* mosquito
  - Sweeping curves, no terminal nuclei present at the caudal end
  - Maximum density in blood – 10 pm – 2 am
- B. malayi
  - Vector - *Mansonia* mosquito
  - Crinkled secondary curves, with two terminal nuclei present at the caudal end
  - Maximum density in blood – 10 pm – 2 am

Life Cycle

- Mosquito cycle begins when Mf are picked up by vector mosquito
- The stages in vector are:

Exsheathing	Within 1-2 hours of ingestion
First stage larva	Penetrate the stomach wall of mosquito in 6-12 hours and migrate to thoracic muscles. It grows into 'sausage' shape
Second stage larva	Larva moults and increases in length
Third stage larva	Larva migrates to the proboscis and is the infective stage of larva.

- Extrinsic incubation period (duration of the mosquito cycle) is 10-14 days under optimal humidity and temperature
- Reservoir of infection: humans (predominantly in India) and animals

Host and Environmental Factors

- All age groups may be affected, with male preponderance due to higher exposure to outdoor environments.
- Optimum temperature: 22-38°C and Humidity 70%
- Inadequate sewage disposal, bad town planning, bad drainage predispose to LF outbreaks or hyper-endemicity

83 Good to Remember

- Main vector in India are:
  - C. quinquefasciatus (C. fatigans) Bancroftian filariasis
  - Mansonia annulifers, M. uniformis Burgian filariasis

- Main vector in India are:
  - C. quinquefasciatus (C. fatigans) — Bancroftian filariasis
  - Mansonia annulifers, M. uniformis — Burgian filariasis

Clinical Features

- Lymphatic filariasis parasite in Lymphatic system
  - Asymptomatic amicrofilaraemia – in some endemic areas, the Mf is not detectable in blood, though the person is infected and is symptomatic
  - Asymptomatic filaraemia – these are important sources of infection. The person is asymptomatic and shows evidence of filaraemia
  - Stage of acute manifestation: filarial fever, lymphangitis, lymphadenitis, lymphoedema, Epididymo-orchitis
  - Stage of chronic obstructive lesions: usually develops after 10-15 years of onset of infection. Characterised by
    - Fibrosis and obstruction of lymph vessels causing permanent damage
  - Bancroftian filariasis:
    - Hydrocele, elephantiasis, chyluria (rare)
  - Burgian filariasis
    - Rare genitalia involvement
- Occult filariasis
  - Absence of classical symptoms of filariasis and Mf are not found in blood
  - Hyper-responsiveness of immune system derived from the Mf
  - Tropical pulmonary eosinophilia

Management

- Uncomplicated acute dermato-lymphangioadenitis (ADLA)
  - Analgesics
  - Antibiotics
    - Amoxycilin 1.5 g in 3 divided doses for 8 days [OR]
    - Oral erythromycin 1gm TDS × 8 days
  - Wound/limb care
  - anti-filarial medicine is not given
- For Severe ADLA
  - i/v Penicillin G 5million units TDS [OR]
  - i/m procaine benzyl penicillin 5 million units given 2 times/day until fever subsides [OR]
  - Penicillin Allergy – i/v erythromycin 1 g × 3 times/day
  - Analgesic, antipyretics

Filarial Survey

- 5-7% of the population should be surveyed
- Mass Blood Survey – night blood survey
  - Thick film
  - Membrane filter concentration (MFC) method
    - Most sensitive technique, but very low density Mf carriers will not be detected
  - DEC provocation test:
    - The Mf are induced to appear in blood in daytime
    - DEC 100 mg is given orally and blood film examined after 1 hour
- Clinical survey
  - Presence of clinical manifestation in the population under survey
- Serological survey
  - Detection of antibodies ad antigens in the blood or urine
- Xenodiagnoses
  - Use of mosquitos for detection of very low level microfilaria in the blood
- Entomological survey
  - General mosquito collection

Monitoring and Evaluation Indicators

- Microfilaria rate: %age of persons showing Mf in blood
- Filarial endemicity rate: proportion of population showing either Mf in blood or symptoms of filariasis or both
- Microfilarial density: Number of microfilaria/unit volume of blood (20 mm^3)
- Average infestation rate: It is the number of Mf per positive slide being made from a unit of blood (20 mm^3). It indicates the prevalence of microfilaria in the population

Control Measures

Chemotherapy

- DEC (Di-Ethyl-Carbamazine)
  - Dose: 6 mg/kg body weight per day orally for 12 days (total 72 mg/Kg DEC)
  - Adverse reactions
    - By the drug – vomiting, dizziness
    - By allergic reactions due to destruction of Mf – fever, local inflammation around the dead worms
- Preventive chemotherapy – prophylaxis:
  - Single dose 2 drug regime
    - Albendazole 400 mg stat + Ivermectin (150-200 mcg/kg) [OR]
    - Albendazole 400 mg stat + DEC 6 mg/kg
  - Conducted for 4-6 years consecutively
- Selective treatment is given in selected cases from low endemic area
- DEC medicated salt
  - A type of mass treatment, common salt is medicated with 1-4 g/kg DEC
- Ivermectin
  - Semisynthetic macrolide antibiotic
  - Dose: 150-200 mcg/kg body weight

Vector Control

- Antilarval methods
  - Larvicidal oils
  - Pyrosene oils – pyrethrum based oils
  - Organophosphate larvicides – Temephos, fenthion
  - De-weeding and removal of aquatic plants
- Anti-adult measures
  - Fogging methods – pyrethrum prays
- Personal protection

WHO's Global Programme to Eliminate Lymphatic Filariasis (GPELF)

- Target to stop transmission is to achieve:
  - Prevalence <1% in community – to interrupt transmission
  - ≥5 annual rounds of MDA (Mass Drug administration)
  - ≥65% coverage in each round
- MDA with 2 drug regime
  - DEC + albendazole [OR] Ivermectin + albendazole
  - Single dose annually for 4-6 years

Aim: To eliminate lymphatic filariasis (LF) by 2020.

LF elimination level: The number of filarial cases <1% and children born are free from circulating antigenemia.

The WHO's strategy is based on 2 key components:

- Stopping the spread of infection by large-scale annual treatment of all eligible people in an area where infection is present
- Alleviating suffering caused by lymphatic filariasis through increased morbidity management and disability prevention activities.

117 *High Yield Points*

- **2018 update:** (started from endemic districts in Maharashtra)
- Triple drug therapy (TDT) for filariasis to eliminate filariasis by 2020
- **TDT:** Ivermectin + Diethyl carbamazine citrate (DEC) + albendazole

LF Mass Drug Administration

- The Mass drug administration (MDA) is done AFTER conducting the survey. The survey is done in 4 sentinel sites and 4 random sites collecting total 4,000 slides
- The MDA is done with DEC + albendazole - with at least >80% coverage for 5–6 years continuously
- Large-scale treatment involves a single dose of 2 medicines given annually to an entire at-risk population in the following ways:
  - Diethylcarbamazine citrate (DEC) (6mg/kg) and Albendazole (400 mg)
    Or
  - Albendazole (400 mg) with Ivermectin (150-200 mcg/kg)

KALA-AZAR (LEISHMANIASIS)

Endemic in Bihar (31 district), West Bengal (11 district) and UP and Jharkhand (4 district each)

- **Causative agent:**
  - Kala-azar (Visceral) → *L. donovani,*
  - Cutaneous (oriental sore) → L. tropica
  - Mucocutaneous → L. braziliensis.
- Life cycle in Kala-azar is completed in 2 hosts:
  - A vertebrate (amastigote form “leishmania bodies”)
  - An insect (flagellated promastigote)
- All age groups are affected. Peak age is 5 to 9 years
  - More common in Males (2 times).

Vectors

- Sandfly (Kalaazar-*Phlebotomous argentipes*, Cutaneous leishmaniasis - P. papatasi and P. sergenti.)
- Sandfly breed in cracks/crevices in soil, buildings, tree holes, caves, etc. Overcrowding, ill-ventilation and accumulation of organic matter facilitate transmission
- It is a hairy insect, it hops and cannot fly – though it has wings !
- Insecticide of choice–DDT (1-2 g/m^2 up to 6feet)

Epidemiology and Mode of Transmission

- Bite of female sand-fly (nocturnal and highly anthrophilic).
- Contamination of bite wound (Insect is crushed during feeding)
- Blood transfusion
- Incubation period in man – 1 to 4 months Reservoir → Indian Kala-azar (Non zoonotic)-Man is the sole reservoir.
- Associated with occupation like farming, forestry, mining and fishing. Disease occurs more often in rural areas (strikes the poorest) and in plains.
- Prevalence is high during and after rains.
- Recovery from kala -azar and oriental sore gives a lasting immunity.

Diagnosis

- **rk39**: Rapid dipstick test is the method of choice for diagnosis of kalaazar.
- ***Caution***: Not to be used in Kalaazar relapse, reinfection and HIV coinfection
- Demonstration of parasite LD bodies in aspirates of spleen, liver, bone marrow, lymph nodes or skin is only way to confirm Visceral Leishmaniasis or Cutaneous Leishmaniasis conclusively.
- ***Aldehyde test of Napier*** (non specific) -good for surveillance. [Q]
- ***Leishmanin (Montenegro) test:*** It is of value in distinguishing immune from non-immune subjects.
- ***Haematological test***: Leucopenia, anaemia, reversed albumin-globulin ratio, increased IgG. and WBC: RBC ratio (1:1500 to 1:2000 (normal 1:750)) and ESR

Treatment

- Drug of choice is injection Lysosomal Amphotericin B
- Oral drug given under the program is miltefosine 50-10 mg BD for 4 weeks
- Alternate drugs are – paramomycin, ketoconazole, itraconazole, sitamaquine

Treatment Guidelines for Kala-Azar-2017

- Single dose IV inj. Liposomal Amphotericin B ***(LAMB)*** for all age groups- dose 10 mg/kg body weight.
- Cap. Miltefosine 10 mg (pediatric) and 50 mg (adults) in the age group 2–65 years. C/I in pregnant and lactating women. Dose is 2.5 mg/kg once daily for children 2-11 years for 28 days and 50 mg Twice daily for age >12 years and wt >25 kg for 28 days.
- Amphotericin B deoxycholate IV inj at dose 1mg/kg body weight on alternate days for 15 days.
- Combination of Paramomycin inj IM and Miltefosine for 10 days.
- HIV coinfected patients: LAMB 40 mg/kg bw as total dose of 3–5 mg/kg bw daily or intermittently for 10days
- PKDL: Drug of Choice is Miltefosine 100 mg/day for 12 weeks. Alternatively, Amphotericin B deoxycholate inj 1mg/kg bodyweight over 4 month (60–80 doses)

JAPANESE ENCEPHALITIS

- Mosquito-borne encephalitis
- Group B arbovirus (Flavivirus)
- Mosquito bite → initial viral replication in local and regional lymph nodes → viral invasion of the CNS via blood

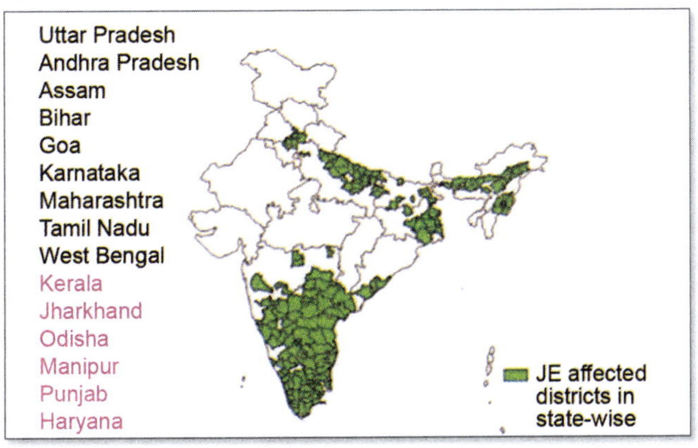

Fig. 9: Japanese encephalitis endemic area in India

JE Life Cycle

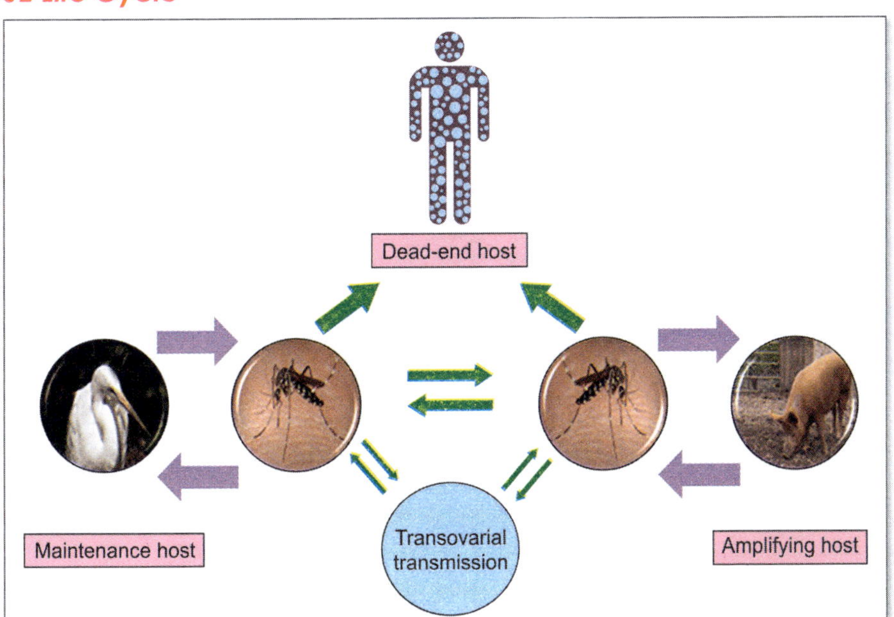

Fig. 10: Life cycle of Japanese encephalitis

118 High Yield Points

Man is an incidental dead end host

84 Good to Remember

Ardied birds: long legged birds comprising of herons and egrets.

- Pig → mosquito → pig
- Ardied bird → mosquito → ardied bird
- Pig – Amplifying host
- Ardied birds – maintenance host
- **Mosquito:** Predominantly – C. tritaeniorhynchus, C. vishnui are implicated as vector for JE

Clinical Features

- Prodromal stage: 1-6 days – lethargy, fever and GI complaints
- Acute encephalitic stage: fever is high, focal CNS signs, convulsions, raised ICP, speech, gait, hemi/quadriplagia, altered sensorium
- Late and sequel stage: inflammation subsides, CNS signs tend to regress, l
- Case fatality – approx. 20-40%

Causes of AES (Acute Encephalitis Syndrome)

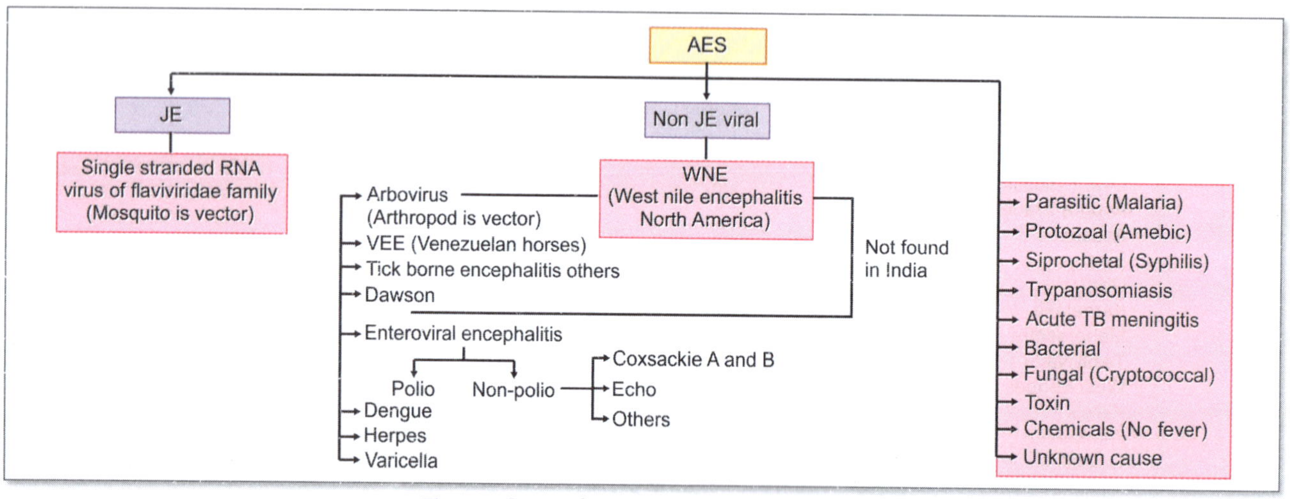

Fig. 11: Cause of acute encephalitis syndrome

Diagnosis

IgM ELISA

Management of AES at Community Level

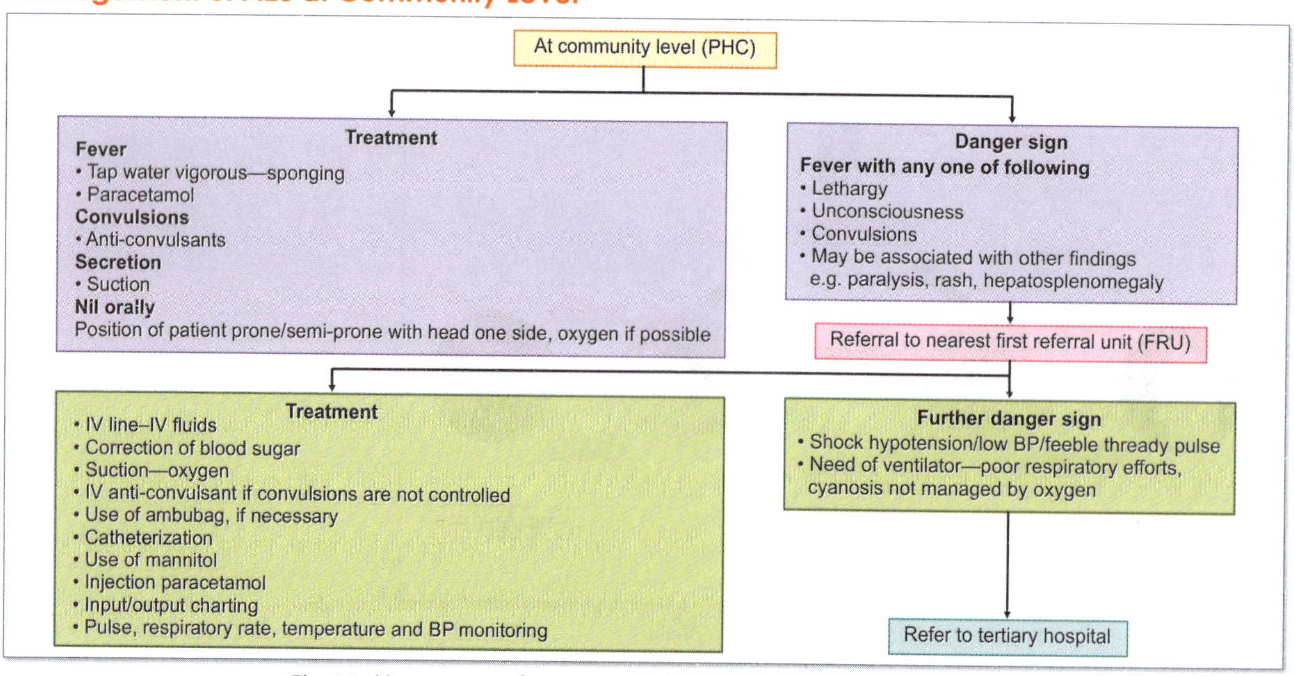

Fig. 12: Management of acute encephalitis syndrome at community level

Prevention

JE Vaccination

- Mouse brain derived – purified killed strain
  - Beijing
  - Nakayama strain
- Cell culture-derived inactivated vaccine Beijing P3 strain
- Cell culture derived live, attenuated SA -14-14-2 strain of JE Virus

In Universal immunization program, the cell culture, live attenuated vaccine is used schedule at 9 months and 16–24 months

RICKETTSIAL DISEASES

Table 28: Diseases caused by rickettsia

	Diseases	Rickettsia agents	Insect vector	Mammalian reservoir
Typhus Group	Epidemic typhus	*R prowazekii*	Louse	Humans
	Endemic (murine) typhus	*R typhi*	Flea	Rodents
	Scrub typhus	*R tsutsugamushi*	Mite	Rodents
Spotted Fever Group	Indian tick typhus	*R conorii*	Hard tick	Rodents, dogs
	Rocky Mountain Spotted Fever	*R rickettsii*	Hard tick	Rodents, dogs
	Rickettsial pox	*R akari*	Mite	Mice
Others	Q fever	*C. burnettii*	Nil	Cattle, Sheep, Goats
	Trench fever	*R. quintana*	Louse	Humans
	Relapsing fever	*B. recurrentis*	Louse	

KYASANUR FOREST DISEASE (KFD)

- Is an arbovirus disease caused by Group B toga viruses (flavi viruses)
- Incubation period = 3–8 day
- Case Fatality Rate = 5–10%
- Vector → Hard ticks (Hemaphysalis spinigera and Hemaphysalis turtura in India).
- Transmitted to man by bite of infective ticks (especially nymphal stages).
- Man is an incidental or dead end host. There is no evidence of man to man transmission
- Main reservoir – Rats, squirrels
- Amplifying host – Monkey and cattles
- Majority of cases are between 20–40 years, males >females
- Mostly in people dependent on forests for livelihood.

Control of Ticks

- Insecticide spray (Carbaryl, Fenthion or Propoxur- 2.24 kg/Hectare) in 'hot spot' (50 m around the spot of monkey death) besides endemic foci.
- Restriction of cattle movement in forest
- Vaccination of at risk population
- Personal protection: Adequate clothing, insect repellent (Dimethyl phthalate (DMP, DEET))

Must Remember

Soft tick also transmits KFD.

Good to Remember

KFD is a 'Biosafety level 4'pathogen.

PLAGUE

Agent: Caused by by Yersinia pestis

- Gram positive, nonmotile, coccobacillus
- Bipolar staining with Wayson stain
- Produce both endotoxin and exotoxin

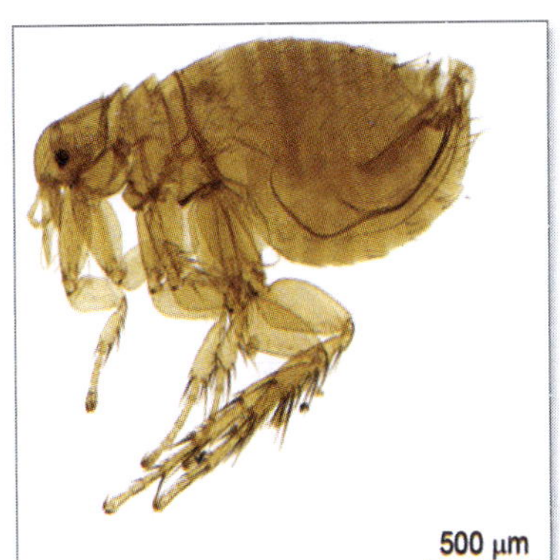

Fig. 13: *Xenopsylla cheopis* (Rat flea)

119 High Yield Points

Plague is a zoonoses, with epidemic potential. Plague is presently a WHO notifiable disease

120 High Yield Points

Reservoir

Rodents: In india: wild rodent – tatera indica is the main reservoir of infection

74 Must Remember

Plague season: September to May, disease decreases with summer

Vector: Xenopsylla cheopis (both sexes)

121 High Yield Points

Incubation Period

Septicemic plague – 2–7 days
Bubonic plague – 2–7 Days
Pneumonic plague – 1–3 days

122 High Yield Points

- In case of outbreak situation, primary dose @ 3 mL for adult is given
- Immunity is developed 5–7 days after vaccination
- Booster dose for high risk individuals – at 6 monthly interval

The principal vector for transmission of plague is a blocked flea or chocked flea. The Fleas show a propagative mode of transmission (allowing replication of the plague bacilli in terms of number)

Flea Index

- Total flea index – Average number of fleas per rat
- Cheopis index – Average number of cheopis per rat. If it is more than one – indicates explosiveness of the plague disease
- Burrow index – Average number of free living fleas per species per rodent burrow.

Clinical Features

- Bubonic plague
  - Most common type
  - Rat flea bite on lower limbs → inoculation of the bacilli → intercepted by the local lymphatics
  - Fever, chills, painful lymphadenitis
  - Cannot spread from person to person
- Pneumonic plague
  - Usually rare <1%
  - It is usually a complication of bubonic septicemic plague
  - It is infectious and spread from person to person
- Septicemic plague
  - Primary septicemic plague is rare

Diagnosis

- **Staining:** Demonstration of bipolar staining on Giemsa or Wayson stain
- **Culture:** For isolation of the bacilli. The transport media used is Cary Blair media
- **Serology:** For Antibody detection

Prevention and Management

- Isolation – recommended wherever possible. It is essential in pneumonic plague
- Treatment
  - Streptomycin 30 mg/kg BW, BD × 7–10 days
  - Tetracycline 30-40 mg/kg BW OD × 7–10 days
- Vector control
  - 10% DDT
  - 3% BHC
  - Alternate: 2% carbaryl, 5% malathion
- Vaccination
  - It is effective usually, if carried out 1 week before anticipated plague outbreak
  - It is essentially for 'primary prevention' rather than secondary prevention or control of human plague cases.
- Vaccine
  - Stain: Sokhey modified Haffkine vaccine
  - Day 0: 0.5 mL s/c at day 0
  - Day 14: 1.0 mL s/c at day 7–14
- Chemoprophylaxis
  - DOC – tetracycline @ 500 mg 6 hourly × 5 days

YELLOW FEVER

It is a zoonotic disease caused by arbovirus
Endemic areas: Tropical Latin America and Africa
Yellow fever is exotic for Indian subcontinent

Epidemiology

- Caused by *flavivirus fibricus*
- Reservoir: Monkeys, and other wild animals

- Period of communicability:
  - Man is infective for 3-4 days of illness
  - Mosquitos are also infective after completing the incubation period of 8-10 days. Once infective the mosquito shall remain so all its life
- One attack gives life long immunity
- Host factors
  - Infants born to immune mothers have antibodies up to 6 months of life
- Environment factors:
  - Humidity >60% and temperature 24-36°C is optimum for the mosquito transmission cycle of the virus
- Modes of transmission:
  - Sylvatic (or jungle) yellow fever
    - Monkey → mosquito → human
  - Intermediate yellow fever
    - Monkey 'and/or' humans → mosquito → humans
  - Urban yellow fever
    - Human → mosquito → human
- Incubation period –3-6 days

Prevention and Control of Yellow Fever

- Vaccination
  - 17D vaccine is available
    - Storage +5 to –30°C, preferably below 0°C
    - Reconstituted vaccine should be kept on ice, away from light and discarded if not used with half an hour
    - 0.5 ml subcutaneous at insertion of deltoid
    - Immunity starts after 7 days and lasts for almost a life time
    - All travellers passing through the endemic zones for yellow fever must have a valid vaccination certificate
- Vector control
  - Aedes aegypti index (AAI)
    - It is the number of Aedes mosquito found with 400 mts of an area
    - The AAI is kept as <1 (or zero) for all international connections airports, sea ports

Elimination of Yellow Fever Epidemic (EYE) Strategy

It was developed by the WHO, UNICEF and GAVI to contain the threat for yellow fever in the world.

- Protect at risk population – by affordable vaccine
- Prevent spread of disease – by international health regulations and notification of disease
- Contains the outbreaks rapidly – with intersectoral coordination, political commitment and research

SOIL TRANSMITTED INFECTIONS

SOIL TRANSMITTED HELMINTHIASIS

These refer to a group of infections caused by:

- Intestinal round worms (*ascariasis*)
- Hook worms (*Ancylostoma duodenale, Necator americanus*)
- Whipworms (*trichuris trichura*)

Mode of Transmission

- By eggs that are passed through the feces of infected persons
- The eggs are released in the soil, where they mature and infect the host

Ascariasis

Agent Factors

- Cosmopolitan distribution. Most common soil transmitted helminthic infection
- Ascariasis lumbricoides lives in lumen of small intestine

Must Remember

- Hookworm eggs hatch in the soil to release larvae that mature into a form that can actively penetrate into the skin
- There is no person to person transmission
- There is no transmission from fresh feces as eggs require several weeks to mature and become infective
- Worms do not multiply in the host and hence, re-infection can only occur through the contact with infective eggs in soil

High Yield Points

- Clay soil is most suitable for ascariasis
- Moist porous soil is most suitable for hookworms

124 High Yield Points

Chandler's index is used to identify the importance of Hookworm infestation as a public health problem in a community. It is calculated based on average number of Hookworm eggs/gram of stool.

- <200: Not a significant public health problem
- 200-250: Potential danger
- 250-300: minor public health problem
- >300: Major public health problem

125 High Yield Points

- Heavy infection is >50,000 roundworm eggs per gram of stool

76 Must Remember

- Hookworms – cause significant public health problems pertaining to child health.
- Cause significant morbidity as low birth weight, stillbirths, growth retardation

- Female 20-35 cms; male 12-30 cms
- Sexes are separate. Females lay approx. 2.5 lac eggs per day!
- Eggs become mature and infective in 2-3 weeks
- Reservoir: Man is the only reservoir

Incubation period: 18 days to several weeks

Symptoms

- Intestinal symptoms: diarrhea, abdominal pain
- General – malaise, weakness
- Larva migration:
- Pulmonary system: asthma, fever, skin rash, cough, eosinophilia
- GI – volvulus, intussusception, Intestinal obstruction

Hookworms

Agent Factors

- Lives in small intestine, mainly jejunum
- Males: 8-11 mm; females 10-31 mm
- Eggs per day:
- *Ancylostoma duodenale:* 10,000 – 30,000 eggs
- *Necator americanus* – 5000 – 10,000 eggs
- The eggs hatch to larvae with 5-7 days (best condition is moist porous soil) and are infective
- Once inside the host, they migrate via the lymphatics and blood to the lungs, into the alveoli, coughed up and are swallowed again to reach the intestines where they become sexually mature

Reservoir: Man is the only most important reservoir known

Incubation period:

- *Ancylostoma duodenale:* 5 weeks – 9 months (unpredictable)
- *Necator americanus* – 5-8 weeks

Symptoms

- Chronic blood loss and iron deficiency anemia
- Loss of blood plasms into intestine leading to hypoalbuminemia

Whipworms

Agent Factors

- Live in large intestine
- Male: 30-45 mm; female 30-35 mm
- Life cycle
- The female lays 200-10,000 eggs per day, and is excreted in feces
- Eggs mature (embryonization) takes place in 21 days in the soil
- The eggs are ingested and reach the intestine where they hatch into larvae in the villi of the small intestine
- Later the larva re-emerges and attaches to mucosa of the colon and grows into adult

Incubation period: 60–90 days

Symptoms

Majority of infections only cause mild symptoms as nausea, distension, flatulence, epigastric pain.

Prevention and Management of STH

Primary prevention: Sanitation, health education

Secondary prevention:

- Albendazole (>2 years @ 400 mg as single dose)
- Mebendazole (@ 100 mg BD × 3 days, >2 years)
- Levamisole (@ 2.5 mg/kg bw, single dose)
- Pyrentral (@ 10 mg/kg bw)

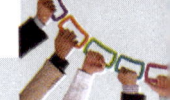

National Deworming Day

NDD is observed on 10th February and 10th august every year for mass drug administration.
Age covered: 1-19 years of age, given drug through schools or anganwadis
The recommended dosage is as follows

- **For children of 2 years and above**: 1 tablet Albendazole (400 mg) or 1 tablet Mebendazole (500 mg)
- **For children of age 1 – 2 years** - ½ tablet of Albendazole (400 mg) or 1 tablet of Mebendazole (500 mg)

Appropriate administration of tablets to children between the ages of 1 and 3 years is important. The tablet should be broken and crushed between 2 spoons, then safe water added to help administer the drug. The older children should chew the tablet and if required should consume some water.

TETANUS

Epidemiology

- It is due to the exotoxin of the Clostridium tetani.

Agent Factors

- Gm positive, anaerobic, drum stick appearance, spore forming organism
- Spores are resistant to: boiling, autoclaving, phenol, cresol
- Spores are best destroyed by:
    - Steam under pressure at 120°C for 20 mins
    - Gamma radiation
- The organism is sensitive to heat and cannot survive in the presence of oxygen
- *C. tetani* has two toxins:
    - Tetanolysin – not much is known for this toxin
    - Tetanospasmin – most potent toxin known
- **Reservoir:** Soil and dust
- Infants may get disease due to septic conditions while performing delivery
- **Mode of transmission:** Contamination of wounds by tetanus spores. Not transmitted from person to person
- **Incubation period:** 6-10 days (may be prolonged to months)

Pathogenesis

- *C. tetani* enters the body through the wound and in anaerobic conditions, the spores will germinate.
- The toxins are produced which act via the central nervous system including peripheral motor end plates, spinal cord, and brain, and in the sympathetic nervous system
- The tetanus toxin blocks the inhibitor impulses by inhibiting the release of the neurotransmitters
- This leads to un-opposed muscle contraction, spams, seizures and other sequel

Tetanus Complications

- Laryngospasm
- Fractures
- Pulmonary embolism
- Aspiration pneumonia
- Nosocomial infections

Types of Tetanus

- Traumatic tetanus – major and most common type
- Puerperal tetanus – following abortion (more commonly) or normal labour
- Otogenic tetanus (cephalic tetanus) – from the foreign body in ear or head injury.
- Tetanus neonatorum – tetanus in neonatal period.
    - Also known as 8th day disease
    - Most common cause is infection of the umbilical stump after birth

Prevention and Control of Tetanus

Active Immunization

- To vaccinate entire community and ensure an antitoxin level of more than 0.01 IU/ml throughout life
- Types
  - Combined vaccine – DPT, pentavalent vaccine
    - 3 doses of pentavalent vaccine at 6,10,14 weeks followed by
    - 1st booster of DPT vaccine at 18 months age
    - 2nd booster (DPT) at 5-6 years of age
    - 3rd booster (TT) at 10 years of age
  - Monovalent vaccine – purified tetanus toxoid (adsorbed) vaccine
    - 2 doses (0.5ml) intramuscular at interval of 2 months

Passive Immunization

- Human tetanus immunoglobulin
  - Dose 250 IU for all ages – protection for 30 days.
- Horse Anti Tetanus Serum (ATS)
  - 1500 IU subcutaneous after sensitivity testing
  - Higher chances of hypersensitivity reactions
  - **Precaution:** The following MUST always be kept in hand BEFORE administering the ATS – to manage any generalised anaphylactoid reaction
    - Always adrenaline solution 1:1000 for i.m. injection in dose of 0.5-1 ml AND
    - Injection hydrocortisone 100 mg for i.v. injection

Antibiotics

- Indicated in non-immune persons, sustained injury with definitive exposure.
- Used for 'immediate' prophylaxis against tetanus – but is NOT active against the spores
- 1.2 mega units of Benzathine penicillin

Prevention of Maternal and Neonatal Tetanus

- Safe, clean delivery
- Disposable delivery kits to be used
- Maintain the essential 7 cleans
  - Clean surface
  - Clean hands
  - Clean cord
  - Clean cut
  - Clean tie
  - Clean water
  - Clean towel
- Essential obstetric package to immunize all pregnant females with TT (2018 update –Td – tetanus diphtheria vaccine to replace the previous TT vaccines)
  - Previous unimmunized female: 2 doses of TT vaccine - first dose as soon as possible and second dose at least after 4 weeks, but at least 3 weeks before delivery
  - Previous immunized female: Single booster dose during 1st – 2nd trimester of pregnancy

Prevention of Traumatic Tetanus

Patient category		Wound category	
		Clean, non penetrating wound	Any other wound
Category A	Has complete course of TT vaccine or booster dose within 5years	Nothing required	Nothing required
Category B	Has complete course of TT vaccine or booster dose more than 5 years ago but within 10 years	TT 1 dose	TT 1 dose
Category C	Has complete course of TT vaccine or booster dose more than 10 years ago	TT 1 dose	TT 1 dose + human TIG
Category D	Unknown status	TT complete course	TT complete course + Human TIG

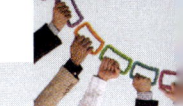

SURFACE INFECTIONS

LEPROSY

- Caused by *M. leprae* (acid fast)
- Occur in clumps, affinity for Schwann and RES cells
- A case is source of infection
- Nose is major portal of exit
- Has high infectivity and low pathogenicity
- **Transmission:** Droplet and contact method
- **Incubation period** – Ranging from 3-5 years or more

Classification

Indian Madrid: Intermediate, tuberculoid, borderline, lepromatous, polyneuritic

Lepromin test detects cell-mediated immunity. It simply measures the individual susceptibility or resistance. It does not indicate past or present infection. Lepromin positivity is associated with resistance to leprosy infection. After intrademal injection of 0.1 mL of lepromin antigen, two types of reactions can be seen.

These are referred to as the early (Fernandez), which is read at 48 hours and the late (Mitsuda) reaction, which is read at 21 days.

The early reaction comprises of redness and induration and is regarded as positive if the area of redness is greater than 10 mm at 48 hours. The late reaction consists of a papule or nodule, which is first measured after 2 weeks, and then at weekly intervals.

Diagnosis of Leprosy

- **Clinical examination:** This is the main stay for diagnosis (and classification) of leprosy
  - Loss of sensation – for heat, cold or light touch
  - Palpation of nerves – for thickening or tenderness in ulnar nerve, greater auricular nerve, lateral popliteal nerve
  - Hypopigmented patches
- **Bacteriological examination:** To have the bacteriological assessment, various methods may be used to 'extract' the bacilli as:
  - Skin smears – was earlier used for diagnosing multibacillary leprosy
  - Nasal smears/blows
    - Prepared from early morning nasal blows
    - Maybe used to assess the infectivity potential for leprosy cases
  - Nasal scrapings (obsolete measure) – usually not done

  Further, the bacilli may be used to find the following indices:
  - **Bacteriological index**

    This index denotes change in the number of leprosy bacilli present in the tissues. Smears are made from at least 7 sites, including a nasal smear, both earlobes and 4 skin lesions. Each smear is graded separately. If there are no bacilli, a score of '0' is given while if bacilli are found in some fields (mean <1 bacilli per field), it is scored as '1'; If bacilli are found in all fields it is scored as '2' and if many bacilli are found in all fields it is scored as '3'. All scores of all smears are added and a mean calculated. If the index is <2, it is paucibacillary leprosy and if it is >2 it is classified as multibacillary leprosy.

0	No bacilli	in 100 oil immersion fields
1+	1-10 bacilli	in 100 oil immersion fields
2+	1-10 bacilli	in 10 oil immersion fields
3+	1-10 bacilli	in each oil immersion field
4+	10-100 bacilli	in each oil immersion field
5+	100-1000 bacilli	in each oil immersion field
6+	More than 1000 bacilli	in each oil immersion field

126 *High Yield Points*

Triad of symptoms:
- Hypopigmented patches
- Loss of cutaneous sensation
- Thickened nerves

Latest Updates

(Latest data – 2014 report)
ANCDR: 0.9
PR: 0.67 Per 10,000 populations

The Bacteriological index is calculated as = $\frac{\textit{Adding the indx from each site examined}}{\textit{Total number of sites examined}}$

- **Morphological index**

  This index is the percentage of solid rods among 200 organisms counted in a smear stained for demonstrating M. *leprae*. Solid rods represent the viable bacilli. This index changes more rapidly than the bacteriological Index. If it shows a rise after an initial decline, it could indicate either inadequate drug intake or development of drug resistance.

  Solid fragmented granular (SFG) percentage: Calculating the percentage of solid bacilli, fragmented bacilli and granular bacilli separately gives a slightly more sensitive indicator for understanding of the patient's response to the treatment

- **Foot pad culture**
  - Foot pad culture is 10 times more sensitive than slit smears
  - Disadvantage: more time consuming -6-9 months for providing the results
- **Histamine test**
  - Detecting early stage of peripheral nerve damage
  - Injecting 0.1 ml of 1:1000 solution of histamine phosphate in to the hypopigmented patches – the normal wheal- flare response (lewis triple response) is abolished
- **Biopsy**
  - More accurate method of diagnosis
- **Immunological tests**

Tests for Detecting Cell Mediated Immunity

- Lepromin test:
  - Injecting intradermally 0.1 ml of lepromin into the inner aspect of forearm of individual.
  - The reaction is read at 48 hours and 21 days
  - Two types of reactions can be present:
    - Early reaction (Fernandez reaction) – an inflammatory response develops in 24-48 hrs
      - **Reading:** Positive early reaction: If the red area >10 mm at the end of 48 hrs
      - **Pathology:** Delayed hypersensitivity reaction due to the 'soluble' components of leprosy bacilli
      - **Interpretation:** If positive, the person is previously sensitized by exposure to and infection by the leprosy bacilli
    - **Late reaction (Mitsuda reaction):** Reaction is apparent in 7-10 days till 3-4 weeks. The reaction is noted on 21st day.
      - **Reading:** Positive test – If the nodule size >5 mm in diameter at end of 21 days
      - **Pathology:** Induced by the bacillary component of the leprosy antigen. It indicates cell mediated immunity
  - **Use of the test:** It is "NOT" a diagnostic test – due to high false positive and false negative cases. The usefulness is in evaluating the
    - Cell mediated immunity in leprosy patients
    - Confirm the classification of leprosy based on clinical and bacteriological grounds
    - Estimating the prognosis of disease
      - Tuberculoid leprosy has strongly positive result, while
      - Lepromatous leprosy has almost lepromin negative test result
- Lymphocyte transformation test (LTT) and leucocyte migration inhibition test (LMIT)
  - These are in vitro tests
  - May be used to detect a proportion of subclinical cases from suspected cases of leprosy

Tests for Humoral Response to M. *Leprae*

- FLA-ABS test (Fluroscent leprosy antibody absorption test) –
  - Most commonly and widely used for detecting clinical, subclinical cases
  - 92% sensitive and almost 99.99% specific
- Monoclonal antibodies: expensive test and not useful as mass screening
- ELISA based on the 'phenolic glycolipid (PGL) antigen'

National Leprosy Eradication Program (NLEP)

Diagnosis of Leprosy

Diagnosis of leprosy under NLEP is based only on the presence of the characteristic lesions (supplemented by thickened peripheral nerve). Skin smears are not taken to reach a diagnosis.

Classification of Leprosy

- ***Paucibacillary leprosy:*** 1–5 Skin lesion (Bacteriological Index <2, Includes TT, BT of Ridley Jopling Classification)
- ***Multibacillary leprosy:*** More than 5 Skin lesion (Bacteriological Index ≥2, Includes LL, BL, BB of Ridley Jopling Classification)

Rationale for MDT in Leprosy

- MDT in leprosy is very useful because of the following reasons:
  - To interrupt transmission of the infection in the community as rapidly as possible using a combination of bactericidal drugs
  - It provides an opportunity for cure
  - It helps to prevent drug resistance
  - A shorter course of therapy ensures a better compliance
  - There is reduced work load on the health-care delivery system.

WHO Guidelines Development Group Recommendation 2018

As per the revision 2018 for Diagnosis, treatment and prevention of Leprosy – WHO 2018, the new recommendations by the GDG (guidelines development Group – WHO 2018) are:

- Revision in the treatment for leprosy PB and MB cases

Table 29: Recommended treatment regimens

Age group	Drug	Dosage and frequency	Duration	
			MB	PB
Adult	Rifampicin	600 mg once a month	12 months	6 months
	Clofaziminie	300 mg once a months and 50 mg daily		
	Dapsone	100 mg daily		
Children (10–14 years)	Rifampicin	450 mg once a month	12 months	6 months
	Clofazimine	150 mg once a month, 50 mg daily		
	Dapsone	50 mg daily		
Children <10 years old or <40 kg	Dapsone	10–mg/kg once month	12 months	6 months
	Rifampicin	6 mg/kg once a months and 1 mg/kg daily		
	Clofazimine	2 mg/kg daily		

Note: The treatment for children with body weight below 40 kg requires single formuiation medications since no MDT combination blister packs are available. For children between 20 and 40 kg, it would be possible to follow the instructions of the Operational Manual, Global Leprosy Strategy 2016–2020 on how to partly use (MB-Child) blister packs for treatment (60).

- Recommendation for drug resistant leprosy

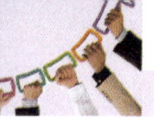

Table 30: Recommended regimens for drug-resistant leprosy

Resistance type	Treatment	
	First 6 months (daily)	Next 18 months (daily)
Rifampicin resistance	Ofloxacin 400 mg* + minocycline 100 mg + clofazimine 50 mg	Ofloxacin 400 mg* OR minocycline 100 mg + clofazimine 50 mg
	Ofloxacin 400 mg* + minocycline 500 mg + clofazimine 50 mg	Ofloxacin 400 mg* + clofazimine 50 mg
Rifampicin and ofloxacin resistance	Clarithromycin 500 mg + minocycline 100 mg + clofazimine 50 mg	Clarithromycin 500 mg OR minocycline 100 mg + clofazimine 50 mg

**Ofloxacin 400 mg can be replaced by levofloxacin 500 mg OR moxifloxacin 400 mg*

- Recommendation for prevention of leprosy by chemoprophylaxis
  The GDG recommends the use of SDR as preventive treatment for contacts of leprosy patients (adults and children 2 years of age and above), after excluding leprosy and TB disease, and in the absence of other contraindications

Table 31: Rifampicin dose for single-dose rifampicin (SDR)

Age/weight	Rifampicin single dose
15 years and above	600 mg
10–14 years	450 mg
Children 6–9 years (weight ≥20 kg)	300 mg
Children <20 kg (≥2 years)	10–15 mg/kg

- Prevention of leprosy by immune-prophylaxis (vaccination)
  - BCG at birth is effective at reducing the risk of leprosy; therefore, its use should be maintained at least in all leprosy high-burden countries or settings (good quality of evidence).
  - BCG at birth appears to potentiate the protective effect of SDR in contacts from 57% to 80% (low quality of evidence).

***Note:** The WHO – 2018 updates have been incorporated in the NLEP-India and various activities for manpower training, resource selection, quality control, monitoring mechanisms are currently being strategically planned to expedite the implementation of the above said recommendations in India.

Drug Side Effects and Adverse Drug Reactions

Table 32: Common side effects of dapsone, their signs and symptoms

	Common side effects	Signs and symptoms	What to do if side effects occur
Minor	Anemia	Paleness inside the lower eyelids, tongue and fingernails, Tiredness, edema of feet and breathlessness	Give anti-worm treatment and iron and folic acid tables folic acid tablets continue dapsone
	Abdominal symptoms	Abdominal pain, nausea and vomiting with high doses	Symptomatic treatment reassure the patient give drugs with food
Serious	Severe skin complication (Exfoliate dermatitis) Sulphone hypersensitivity hemolytic anemia	Extensive scaling, itching, ulcers in the month and eyes, jaundice and reduced urine output Itchy skin rash	Stop dapsone Refer to hospital immediately. Never restart
	Liver damage (hepatitis)	Jaundice (Yellow color of skin, eyeballs and urine) Loss of appetite and vomiting	Stop dapsone. Refer to hospital Restart after the jaundice subsides
	Kidney damage (Nephritis)	Edema of face and feet Reduced urine output	Stop dapsone. Refer to hospital

Table 33: Common side effects of rifampicin their signs and symptoms

	Side effect	Signs and symptoms	What to do if side effects occur
Minor adverse effects	▪ Red discoloration of body fluids	▪ Reddish coloration of urine, saliva and sweat	▪ Reassure the patient and continue treatment
	▪ Flu-like illness	▪ Fever, malaise and body ache	▪ Symptomatic treatment
	▪ Abdominal symptoms	▪ Abdominal pain, nausea and vomiting	▪ Symptomatic treatment ▪ Reassure the patient ▪ Give drug with food
Serious adverse effects	▪ Hepatitis (liver damage)	▪ Jaundice (yellow color of skin, eyeballs and urine). Loss of appetite and vomiting	▪ Stop Rifampicin refer to hospital. Restart after the jaundice subsides
	▪ Allergy	▪ Skin rash or shock, purpura renal failure	▪ Stop Rifampicin

Table 34: Common side effects of clofazamine

Side effects	Signs and symptoms	What to do if side effects occur
Skin pigmentation (Not significant)	Brownish-red discoloration of skin, urine and body fluids	▪ Reassure the patient, it disappears after completion of treatment
Acute abdominal symptoms	Abdominal pain, nausea and vomiting on high doses	▪ Symptomatic treatment ▪ Reassure the patient ▪ Give drug with food ▪ If intractable stop clofazimine
Ichthyosis (diminished sweating)	Dryness and scaling of the skin, itching	▪ Apply oil the skin ▪ Reassure the patient
Eye	Conjunctival dryness	▪ Moistening eye drops/frequent washing of eyes

Note:
- Dapsone may cause hemolysis of red blood cells
- People with glucose-6-phosphatase dehydrogenase deficiency are more susceptible to hemolysis. It is usually mild and symptomless.
- Methemoglobinemia may also occur due to dapsone therapy.
- Lips and nails may develop blue hue that may disappear spontaneously or on reducing the dose but is NOT an indication to interrupt therapy.
- Stop both dapsone and rifampicin in case of hepatic/renal symptoms and clofazimine in severe gastritis.

Core Indicators of NLEP

- Number of new cases detected per year
- Rate of new cases with grade two disability/100,000 population** (Recently added indicator)
- Treatment completion
- Cure rate
- Child cases among new cases
- Elimination of leprosy as public health problem was achieved globally in 2000 and India (at national level) in Dec 2005
  - In India 34 states/UT have achieved leprosy elimination level

Must Remember

Lepra Reactions

Type 1: Reversal:
- Delayed hypersensitivity
- Skin lesions become red, painful. New lesions appear

Type II reactions [Erythema nodosum reaction (ENL)]
- Antigen-antibody reaction
- Red painful skin, subcutaneous nodules appear
- Affecting multiorgan

DOC for reactions: Corticosteroids + Clofazimine in ENL

- Chhattisgarh and Dadra and Nagar Haveli have a prevalence of 2–5 per10,000.
- Total of 1.25 lac new cases in 2014-15 in India, ANCDR of 9.73 per lac population.

- Global prevalence of disease has dropped to 0.29 per 10 000 in 2015.
- 14 countries accounted for 95% of all cases in 2015, India contributing to around 60% of cases.
- Proportion of MB cases was 60.2%
- Females comprised 36.9% of cases and children 9.49% of cases. About 4% cases had grade II deformity
- The age-old stigma associated with the disease remains an obstacle to self-reporting and early treatment.
- Leprosy prevalence rate more than 1 per 10,000 is considered a public health problem.[Q]

127 *High Yield Points*

For disability assessment: organs noted are: Hand, Feet, Eye.

Surveys for Leprosy

- **Contact survey:** Prevalence is less than1per1000
- **Group survey:** Prevalence is more than or equal to 1 per 1000
- **Mass survey:** Prevalence is more than or equal to10 per 1000.

Leprosy control units are established in endemic zones with a prevalence rate of 5 per 1,000 and above and cover a rural population of 4–5 lakhs. There is a central leprosy clinic at the headquarters.

SET centers under NLEP stands for survey, education and training and these are the main functions of these centers. These are established in endemic zones where prevalence rate is <5 per 1,000.

For **tertiary prevention and locomotor rehabilitation** of patients: MCR – microcellular rubber footwear is special footwear for leprosy patients

78 *Must Remember*

Targets of the New Global Strategy to be met by 2020 are

- Zero disabilities among new pediatric patients.
- A grade-2 disability rate of less than 1 per 1 million people.
- Zero countries with legislation allowing discrimination on basis of leprosy.

Global Leprosy Strategy 2016–2020

It is based around 3 core pillars:

"Pillar I: Strengthen government ownership, coordination and partnership	▪ Ensuring political commitment and adequate resources for leprosy programmes. ▪ Contributing to universal health coverage with a special focus on children, women and underserved populations including migrants and displaced people. ▪ Promoting partnerships with state and nonstate actors and promote intersectoral collaboration and partnerships at the international level and within countries. ▪ Facilitating and conducting basic and operational research. ▪ Strengthening surveillance and health information systems (including GIS)
Pillar II: Stop leprosy and its complications	▪ Strengthening patient and community awareness of leprosy. ▪ Promoting early case detection through active case-finding (such as campaigns) in areas of higher endemicity and contact management. ▪ Ensuring prompt start of and adherence to treatment, including working toward improved treatment regimens. ▪ Improving prevention and management of disabilities. ▪ Strengthening surveillance for antimicrobial resistance including laboratory network.
	▪ Promoting innovative approaches for training, referrals and sustaining expertise in leprosy ▪ Promoting interventions for the prevention of infection and disease.
Pillar III: Stop discrimination and promote inclusion	▪ Promoting societal inclusion by addressing all forms of discrimination and stigma. ▪ Empowering persons affected by leprosy and strengthening their capacity to participate actively in leprosy services. ▪ Involving communities in action for improvement of leprosy services. ▪ Promoting coalition-building among persons affected by leprosy and encouraging the integration of these coalitions and or their members with other community-based organizations. ▪ Promoting access to social and financial support services, for example to facilitate income generation for persons affected by leprosy and their families. ▪ Supporting community-based rehabilitation for people with leprosy-related disabilities. ▪ Working toward abolishing discriminatory laws and promoting policies facilitating inclusion of persons affected by leprosy.

Major initiative under NLEP 2017-2018

- Focus on new case detection - main indicator for program monitoring
- Treatment completion rate as operational indicator

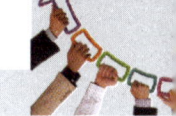

- Emphasis on Disability Prevention and Medical Rehabilitation (DPMR)
  - Dressing materials, ulcer kits, supportive medicine
  - Providing micro-cellular rubber footwear
  - Incentive to leprosy patients from BPL families
  - Incentive to health facility as INR 5000 for reconstructive surgery conducted
- ASHA incentives
  - INR 250 – confirmed diagnosis
  - On treatment completion – PB leprosy case INR 400, MB case INR 600
- Intensive IEC (information, education and communication) – awareness campaigns

Sparsh

Rolled on 30 January 2017 for increasing awareness and address the issue of leprosy stigma in the society.

'Sapna' is a concept designed and developed keeping in mind a common girl living in community, who will help to spread awareness in the community, through key IEC messages

Who can be 'Sapna'
A local school going girl who is willing to be 'Sapna' from the same locality preferably.

There can be any number of Sapna in a village

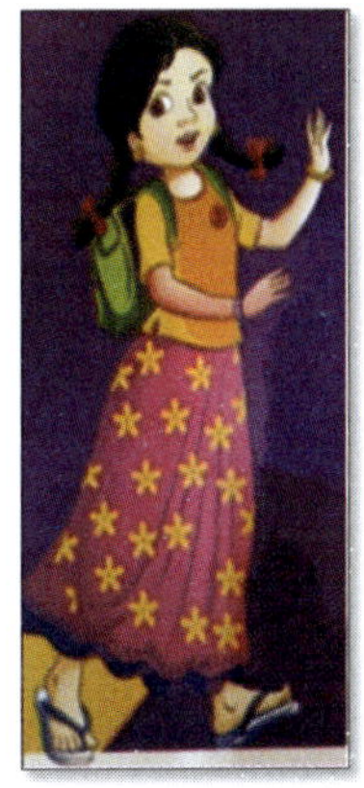

Fig. 14: 'SAPNA', the Mascot

TRACHOMA

- Chronic infectious disease of conjunctiva and cornea – by chlamydia trachomatis.
- Responsible for 0.1% of the visual impairment and blindness in India

Epidemiology

Agent factors:
- C. trachomatis (serotypes A, B, C). Chlamydia serotypes D-K – are implicated for sexually transmitted infections
- Other pathogenic microorganisms *may contribute* to disease pathology
  - Morax-axenfeld — Most innocuous
  - Koch-weeks bacillus — Most widespread
  - Gonococcus — Most dangerous
- Reservoir: Children with active disease
- Source of infection: Persons with active disease. After complete cicatrisation the person is non infectious
- Communicability: Has low infectivity
- Incubation period: 5-12 days

Host/Environmental factors:
- Most commonly in children 2–5 years
- Equal gender involvement in younger age groups
- In adults: females >males
- m/c during April-May and July-sept
- It is a familial disease, with many members of a family being infected at a point of time

Diagnosis

At least two out of four criteria should be present:
1. Follicles in the upper tarsal conjunctiva
2. Limbal follicles, Herbert's pits
3. Typical conjunctival scarring (trichiasis, entropion)
4. Vascular pannus, most marked in the superior limbus

Trachoma Control

- **Chemotherapy**
  - DOC – 1% tetracyclines ophthalmic ointment
  - Alternate – erythromycin ointment

- **Mass treatment**
  - Mass (blanket) treatment may be done to control outbreaks in community
  - Prevalence >5% of moderate/severe trachoma is indication for mass treatment
  - DOC – 1% tetracycline ointment given as:
- Twice daily, 5 days every month for 6 months
- Once daily, 10 days every month for 6 months
- Surgery
  - Surgical correction of lid deformities – entropion, trichiasis

WHO's Global Campaign to Eliminate Trachoma

S-A-F-E strategy:

- S- Surgery for deformed eyelids (trichiasis and entropion)
- Antibiotic treatment: Periodic mass treatment with Azithromycin
- F- Face washing
- E- Environmental improvements

Table 35: Key findings of the national trachoma rapid assessment survey 2014–17

Districts included in survey Households visited	17 districts 39,910
Total population examined and coverage 1–9 years 10+ years	 8,807 9,225
Burden of active trachoma infection (TF + TI) in population aged 1–9 years	104 (1.2%)
Trachomatous trichiasis (TT) in population aged 10+ years	19 (2.1/1000)
Uncelean faces in population aged 1–9 years	1,463 (16.6%)
Water source unavailable within 30-minute walking distance from households	2,651 (67.8%)
Absent functional latrine among visited households	2,090 (53.5%)

YAWS

- It is a chronic contagious non -venereal disease[Q] caused by *T. pertenue*[Q].
- Confined to the belt between Tropic of Capricorn and Tropic of Cancer.
- It is a disease of childhood and adolescence[Q]
- Treponemal infection (yaws, pinta and endemic syphilis) cannot be differentiated serologically[Q]
- No case reported in India since 2004. It was endemic among tribals in India.
- *Reservoir of infection* → Man
- *Source of infection* → skin lesions and exudates from early lesions.
- *Communicability* → Variable may extend over several years
- Prevalence is high in males.
- It is a crippling disease ***(Late yaws)*** → Lesions of sole and palms are called "*crab yaws*", lesions of soft palate, hard palate and nose are called "*Gangosa*". Swelling by the side of the nose due to osteo-periostitis of the superior maxillary bone is called "*Goundu*".
- Transmitted nonvenerally by → Direct contact, fomites, vector (flies and insects feeding on the lesion).
- Incubation period - 3 to 5 weeks

New strategy involves single dose treatment with Azithromycin with following approach-

- ***Total Community Treatment (TCT)*** → Treatment of entire endemic community
- ***Total Targeted Treatment (TTT)*** → Treatment of all active clinical cases and their contacts.

86 Good to Remember

Yaws provides partial immunity to venereal syphilis.[Q]

Latest Updates

YAWS – Year 2020 is the target set by WHO for Yaws eradication globally.

Treatment

- Azithromycin (oral) or Benzathine penicillin G (Inj) single dose is treatment of choice.
- Simultaneous treatment of all clinical cases and their contacts in the community interrupts transmission.

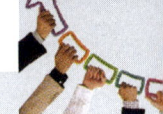

- WHO has recommended 3 treatment policies:
  - ***Total mass treatment***: hyperendemic areas (>10% prevalence of clinically active yaws).
  - ***Juvenile mass treatment***: mesoendemic communities (5–10% prevalence), treatment is given to all cases, all children under 15 years of age and other obvious contacts of infectious cases.
  - ***Selective mass treatment:*** In hypoendemic or areas of low prevalence (<5%) treatment is confined to cases, their household and other obvious contacts of infectious cases.

Table 36: Differentiating features in syphillis, yaws and pinta

	Venereal syphilis	Yaws	Endemic syphilis	Pinta
Mode of transmission	Sexual, Trans-placental	Skin to skin	Household contact, mouth to mouth or via shared drinking/ eating utensils	Skin to skin
Age of acquisition	Adulthood	Early childhood	Early childhood	Early childhood

SEXUALLY TRANSMITTED INFECTIONS

HIV/AIDS AND NACO (NATIONAL AIDS CONTROL ORGANISATION)

Human Immunodeficiency Virus

- **Lentivirus** (Slowly replicating retrovirus) that causes the acquired immunodeficiency syndrome (AIDS), also known as slim's disease
- Heat labile, inactivated by alcohol, Sodium Hypochlorite solution
- Resistant to UV and ionizing radiation
- Reservoir is a case
- Source is blood, fluids, tear, semen, CSF
- HIV-1—most common type, more virulent
- HIV-2—less frequent, less virulent
- HIV-1 three subgroups
  - M (major)
  - O (outlier)
  - N (neither M nor O)
- Group M (subtypes A to K)
  - Subtype B—most common in US, Europe
  - Subtype E—most common in Thailand, Bangkok, Vietnam
  - Subtype C (fastest-spreading type worldwide) --- most common in India, Ethiopia, and Southern Africa.
- Most common cause of AIDS in India--- HIV-1 group-M, Subtype-C.

128 High Yield Points

(Remember HIV 1 MC (most common)
Most common route of HIV transmission is Sexual -89.7% cases (Heterosexual-88.2%)

HIV Epidemiology

HIV/AIDS as disease has high DALY (disability adjusted life years) and is a part of MDG (millennium development goal) # 6 - combat HIV/AIDS, malaria and other diseases

India 2017

- 2.1 million people living with HIV
- 0.29% HIV prevalence among ANC clinic attendees (considered as proxy for general population)
- 1.6% HIV among the female sex workers
- 6.3% HIV among the i/v drug abusers [ranging from 3% (Nagaland) - 12% (Manipur)]
- 3% HIV among transgender

Source: UNAIDS 2017

87 Good to Remember

- Women comprise about half of all people living with HIV worldwide ***(India -39%).***
- India - 83% of HIV infections occur in the age group ***15-49 year.***
- Andhra Paradesh and Telangana>Bihar>Gujarat and Uttar Pradesh account for 47% of total new HIV infections in adults.

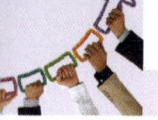

High Risk Categories in India

Table 37: HIV Prevalence in adult Population in India

Groups	Criteria	States/UT
I: High Prevalence States	HIV infection >5% in high-risk group and ≥1% in antenatal women	Maharashtra, Tamil Nadu, Karnataka, Andhra Pradesh, Manipur, and Nagaland
II: Moderate Prevalence States	HIV infection >5% high risk groups but <1% in antenatal women	Gujarat, Goa, and Puducherry
III: Low Prevalence States	HIV infection <5% in high risk groups and <1% in antenatal women	Remaining states

Table 38: NACO District categorization based on HIV burden and HIV as public health problem

Types of Epidemic	Definition	Surveillance
Generalized (HIV is established in general population)	HIV prevalence>1% in the pregnant women in antenatal care (Taken as proxy of general population)	Focus on monitoring HIV infection and risk behavior in general population.
Concentrated (HIV is not established in general population)	HIV prevalence >5% in any of the sub-population at higher risk of infection (e.g. Drug injectors, Sex workers, Men who have sex with men) but <1% in pregnant women (Taken as proxy of general population)	Focus is on monitoring infection in high risk (HR) groups and behavioural links between members of HR groups and the general population. Surveillance systems also monitor the general population, especially young people, for high-risk sexual behaviour and trends in STI

Table 39: NACO district categorization based on prevalence of HIV in ANC females and high risk groups (HRG)

District categorization	Prevalence in antenatal women (Last 3 year)	Prevalence in high risk groups
A	>1%	—
B	<1%	>5% (Any HRG)
C	<1%	<5% (All HRG with known hot spots/STD clinic)
D	<1%	<5% (All HRG /STD clinic, No known hot spot*)

*Hot spots—Aggregation of migrants, truckers, factory workers

Table 40: Mode of transmission

Transmission	Efficiency	%age total
Blood transfusion	90–95%	5%
Perinatal	20–40%	10%
Sexual	0.1–10%	75 – 80%
IDU	0.7%	10%
Needle stick	0.3%	<1%

Clinical Features

129 *High Yield Points*

Initial infection
- Asymptomatic Carrier
- ARC (AIDS related complex)
  - Weight loss>10%, persistent fever, chronic diarrhea
  - G. LAP, candidiasis, opportunistic Infections

AIDS
- End stage
- Opportunistic infections

WHO Staging

Stage 1: Asymptomatic, LAP
Stage 2: Moderate w/l (<10%), mild surface infections and chronic diarrhea
Stage 3: Severe w/l (>10%), chronic diarrhea, persistent fever, moderate to severe infections involving deep tissue or organs.
Stage 4: HIV wasting syndrome, Pneumocystis carinii pneumonia, candidiasis, malignancy

Relation of CD4 Count with the Opportunistic Infections

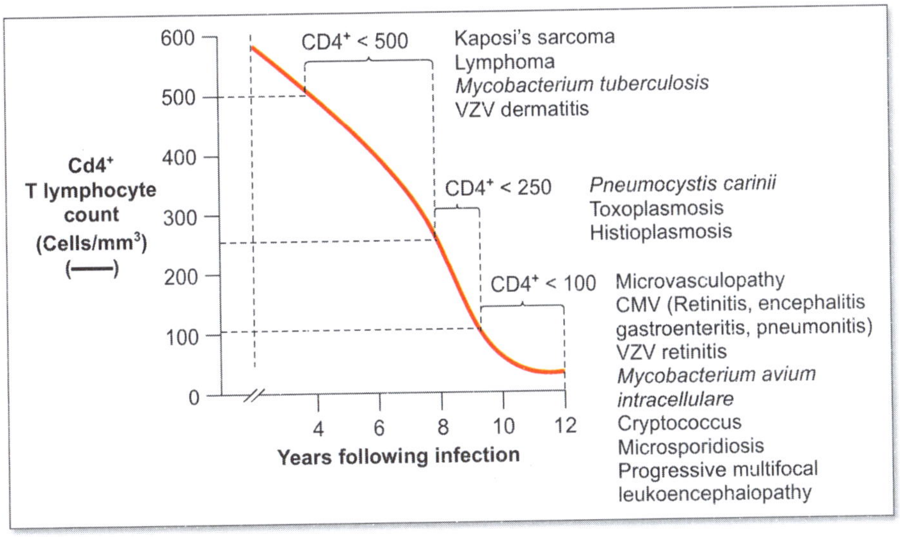

The Center for Disease Control and Prevention (CDC) USA "AIDS defining illness" are

- Bacterial infections, multiple or recurrent*
- Candidiasis of bronchi, trachea or lungs
- Candidiasis of esophagus†
- Cervical cancer, invasive©§
- Coccidioidomycosis, disseminated or extrapulmonary
- Cryptosporidiosis, chronic intestinal (>1 month's duration)
- Cytomegalovirus disease (other than liver, spleen, or nodes), onset at age >1 month
- Cytomegalovirus retinitis (with loss of vision)†
- Encephalopathy, HIV related
- Herpes simplex: Chronic ulcers (>1 month's duration) or bronchitis, pneumonitis, or esophagitis (onset at age >1 month)
- Histoplasmosis, disseminated or extrapulmonary
- Isosporiasis, chronic intestinal (>1 month's duration)
- Kaposi sarcoma†
- Lymphoid interstitial pneumonia or pulmonary lymphoid hyperplasia complex*†
- Lymphoma, Burkitt (or equivalent term)
- Lymphoma, primary, or brain
- *Mycobacterium avium complex or mycobacterium kansaii, disseminated or extrapulmonary*†
- *Mycobacterium tuberculosis* of any site, pulmonary,†§ disseminated,† or extrapulmonary†
- *Mycobacterium*, other species or unidentified species, disseminated† or extrapulmonary†
- *Pneumocystis jirovecii* pneumonia†
- Pneumonia, recurrent†§
- Progressive multifocal leukoencephalopathy
- Salmonella of brain, onset at age >1 month†
- Wasting syndrome attributed to HIV

*Only for children age <13 years
†Condition that might be diagnosed presumptively.
§Only among adults and adolescents aged >13 years.

AIDS Case Definition/WHO Case Definvition

- Major and minor signs our 12 years of age as per WHO

Table 41: Major and minor cases of HIV as per HIV

Major	Minor
Unexplained chronic diarrhea for >1 month Loss of >1 0% body weight Prolonged fever for >1 month	Persistent cough for >1 month Generalized pruritic dermatitis History of Herpes zoster Oropharyngeal candidiasis Chronic progressive or disseminated HSV infection Generalized lymphadenopathy AIDS illness—Kaposi's sarcoma, cryptococcal meningitis cervical carcinoma and primary lymphoma of brain

- For children (age <12 years) 2 Major + 2 Minor signs

Table 42: Major and minor signs under 12 years of age as per WHO

Major Signs	Minor Signs
▪ Weight loss >10% of body weight, or abnormal slow growth ▪ Chronic diarrhea >1 month ▪ Persistent fever >1 month	▪ General lymph node enlargement ▪ Oropharyngeal candidiasis ▪ Recurrent common infections ▪ Persistent cough ▪ Generalized rash

130 *High Yield Points*

Viral load estimation is the best parameter for assessment of response to treatment in PLHIV (People living with HIV)

Expanded WHO Case Definition

HIV serological test positive with one of the following conditions

- Unexplained chronic diarrhea for >1 month, Loss of >10% body weight (BW); prolonged fever for >1 month
- Cryptococcal meningitis
- Pulmonary or extrapulmonary tuberculosis.
- Kaposi's sarcoma
- Neurological impairment sufficient to prevent independent daily activity.
- Candidiasis of the esophagus.
- Recurrent episodes of life-threatening pneumonia with or without etiological confirmation.
- Invasive cervical cancer.

Note: Most common opportunistic infection tuberculosis.

Advanced HIV Disease

- Age >5 years, CD4 <200
- Age >5 years, Any CD4, stage III or Stage IV
- Age <5 years, any CD4, any stage, HIV +

131 *High Yield Points*

HIV-related most common infections

Table 43: HIV-related infections most frequently encountered in India

Bacterial	Viral	Fungal	Parasitic	Other illnesses
Tuberculosis	Herpes simplex virus infection	Candidiasis	Cryptosporidiosis	AIDS dementia complex
Bacterial respiratory infection	Oral hairy leukoplakia	Cyptococcosis	Microsporidiosis	Invasive cervical cancer
	Varicella zoster virus disease	Pneumocystis jiroveci *Pneoumonia*	Isosporiasis	Non-hodgkin lymphoma
Salmonella infection	Cytomegalovirus disease	Penicilliosis	Giardiasis stongyloides	
	Human papilloma virus infections		Toxoplasmosis	

Pulmonary TB is one of the most common opportunistic infections in HIV

Diagnosis of HIV-Infections

Screening Test

- Elisa, Rapid and Spot test: E,R,S – are at ICTC centers
- Under the NACP, the most commonly employed rapid tests are based on the principle of enzyme immunoassay, immunochromatography (lateral flow), immunoconcentration/dot-blot assays (vertical flow) and particle agglutination
- All samples reactive in the first test should further undergo confirmatory 2nd/3rd tests based on different principles/antigens using the same serum/plasma sample as that in the 1st test

Laboratory Criteria

The diagnosis of HIV is done at the **Integrated Counseling and Testing Centers (ICTC)** and the reference laboratories

- ELISA
  - Most sensitive test – screening
- Western blot
  - Detecting antibody to specific viral core protein (p24 Ag)
  - Most specific – diagnostic test
- CD 4 Lymphocyte count (normal is >950 CD4/micro Liter)
  - Most widely used predictor of HIV progression
  - High risk of opportunistic infections/malignancy at CD4 <200
- CD4 percentage
  - Better than absolute CD4 count
  - CD4 percentage <14% indicates high risk for infections/malignancy
- Viral HIV loads
  - Measures the amount of actively replicating HIV.
  - Correlates to HIV disease progression and response to ART
  - P24 Antigen
    - Indicates acute HIV replication

133 High Yield Points

- Most sensitive **(=best screening method)**----- ELISA
- Most specific **(=confirmatory)**---- WESTERN BLOT (positive if antibodies exist against 2 out of 3 HIV-proteins, i.e. p24; gp 41; gp120/60)

Viral load estimation (level of HIV in body) is measured by number of copies of HIV-1 per milliliter of blood plasma (copies/mL).

It is an important marker for prognosis and response of treatment by the patient

132 High Yield Points

- For blood safety: Any one positive: Labeled as HIV and blood discarded
- Symptomatic patient: Any Two positive: Labeled as HIV
- In case of asymptomatic patient: all three have to be positive

79 Must Remember

- For HIV screening in pregnant females: Opt out screening
- For HIV screening in blood banks: Unlinked anonymous testing of the sample

80 Must Remember

- **Window period** is the period between HIV infection and appearance of HIV antibodies. During this period the person is infectious (high concentration of virus in blood), but tests negative.
- HIV antibodies appear between 2 to 12 weeks in the blood stream. [Q]

Antiretroviral Therapy

The primary goal of the treatment is to lower viral load below 50 copies/mL within 6 months of treatment.

- It includes major three classes of drugs
  - Nucleoside analogs—Didanosine, zidovudine, zalcitabine, stavudine and lamivudine.
  - Protease inhibitors—Saquinavir, ritonavir, indinavir and nelfinavir.
  - Nonnucleoside reverse transcriptase inhibitors (NNRTIs): Nevirapine, delavirdine, and efavirenz.

Table 44: Drugs approved by FDA for use in HIV

Nucleoside Reverse Transcriptase Inhibitors (NRTIs)	
Mechanism: Block reverse transcriptase, an enzyme HIV needs to make copies of itself.	Abacavir (Abacavir sulfate, ABC)
	Emtricitabine (FTC)
	Lamivudine (3TC)
	Tenofovir disoproxil fumarate (tenofovir DF, TDF)
	Zidovudine (azidothymidine, AZT, ZDV)

Contd...

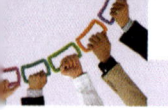

Nonnucleoside Reverse Transcriptase Inhibitors (NNRTIs)	
Mechanism: NNRTIs bind to and later alter reverse transcriptase, an enzyme HIV needs to make copies of itself.	Efavirenz (EFV) Etravirine (ETR) Nevirapine (Extended-release nevirapine, NVP) Rilpivirine (Rilpivirine hydrochloride, RPV)
Protease Inhibitors (PIs)	
Mechanism: PIs block HIV protease, an enzyme HIV needs to make copies of itself.	Atazanavir (atazanavir sulfate, ATV) Darunavir (darunavir ethanolate, DRV) Fosamprenavir (fosamprenavir calcium, FOS-APV, FPV) Ritonavir (RTV) *Although ritonavir is a PI, it is generally used as a pharmacokinetic enhancer as recommended in the *Guidelines for the Use of Antiretroviral Agents in Adults and Adolescents Living with HIV* and the *Guidelines for the Use of Antiretroviral Agents in Pediatric HIV Infection*. Saquinavir (saquinavir mesylate, SQV) Tipranavir (TPV)
Fusion Inhibitors	
Mechanism: Fusion inhibitors block HIV from entering the CD4 cells of the immune system.	Enfuvirtide (T-20)
CCR5 Antagonists	
Mechanism: CCR5 antagonists block CCR5 co-receptors on the surface of certain immune cells that HIV needs to enter the cells.	Maraviroc (MVC)
Integrase Inhibitors	
Mechanism: Integrase inhibitors block HIV integrase, an enzyme HIV needs to make copies of itself.	Dolutegravir (DTG, dolutegravir sodium) Raltegravir (Raltegravir potassium, RAL)
Post-attachment Inhibitors	
Mechanism: Post attachment inhibitors block CD4 receptors on the surface of certain immune cells that HIV needs to enter the cells.	Ibalizumab (Hu5A8, IBA, Ibalizumab-uiyk, TMB-355, TNX-355)
Pharmacokinetic Enhancers	
Mechanism: Pharmacokinetic enhancers are used in HIV treatment to increase the effectiveness of an HIV medicine included in an HIV regimen.	Cobicistat (COBI)
Source: ▪ FDA ▪ National institute of allergy and infectious disease ▪ National library of medicine *Aidsinfo.nih.gov, Accessed on date: 2018-05-18*	

National AIDS Control Program (NACP)

2016 WHO Revised Treatment Guidelines – Salient Features

- Initiation of anti-retroviral treatment (ART) in all adults and adolescent cases regardless of CD4 counts or WHO clinical staging
- Priority to severe/advanced HIV cases with CD4 count ≤ 350 cells/mm^3.
- Start ART irrespective of CD4 count in all HIV +ve persons with Active TB ***(Treatment of TB should be started first followed by ART within first 8 weeks)***, Hepatitis B coinfection with severe chronic liver disease, serodiscordant couples, pregnant and breast feeding women.

- All children <10 years regardless of WHO clinical staging and CD4 cell counts, should be started on ART.
- Infants diagnosed in the first year of life should be started on ART.
- *Children 1–10 years, conditional recommendations.*
  - As a priority ART should be started in all children <2 years or children <5 years with WHO clinical stage 3 or 4 or CD4 counts ≤750/mm^3 or CD4% <25%.
  - Children more than 5 years of age with WHO stage 3 or 4 or CD4 <350/mm^3 should be initiated on ART
- New preferred first line ART regimen for adults, pregnant and breastfeeding women, Children ≥3 year age.
- Phase out Stavudine (d4T) in first line ART regimen for adults and adolescent
- Use viral load testing as preferred approach for monitoring ART success and diagnose treatment failure in addition to clinical and CD4 monitoring
- Community based HIV testing and counseling.

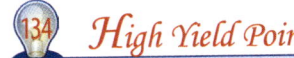

134 *High Yield Points*

Treat all PLHIV Regardless of the CD4 Count, Clinical Stage, Age or Population

2018 NACO Updates

- NACO has adopted the UNAIDS 90-90-90 target

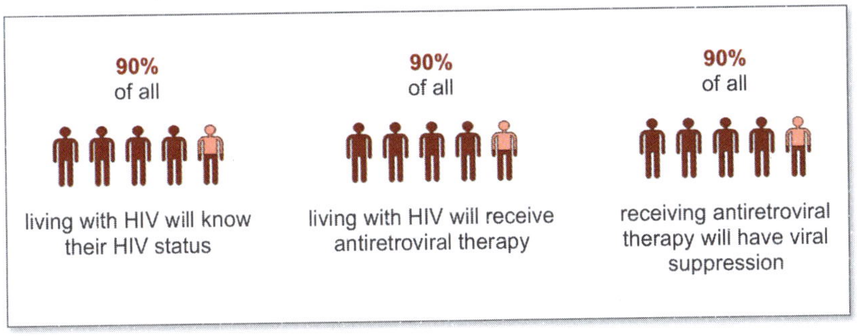

HIV Diagnosis under NACO Guidelines

- **HIV diagnosis:** It is based on use of THREE DIFFERENT ANTIGEN principles (assay 1, 2 and 3)
  - Diagnosis for clinically symptomatic individual

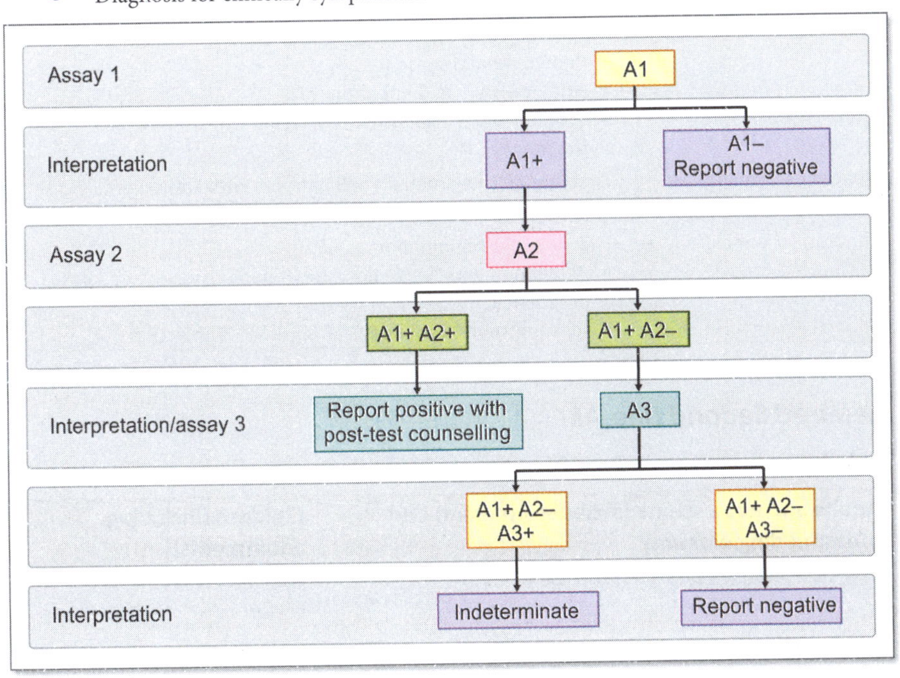

- Diagnostic algorithm for Asymptomatic individual

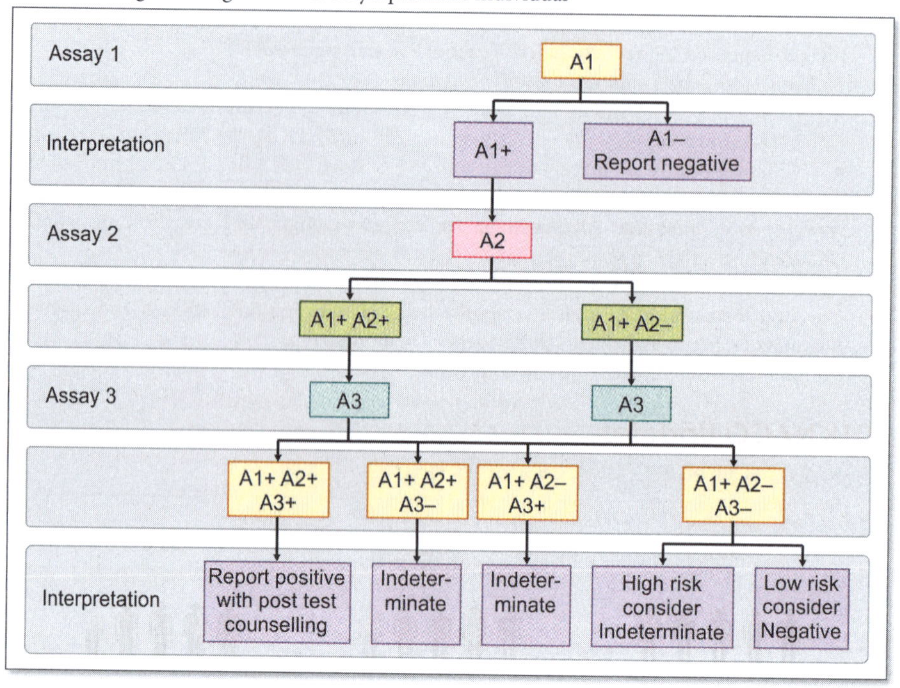

- Diagnosis of HIV infection in infants and children aged less than 18 months of age: DNA PCR test age >6 weeks but <18 months

▪ TREAT ALL people living with HIV (PLHIV)

ART Regimens under NACO Guidelines

Preferred 1st Line ART (2016)

Table 45: Preferred first line ART 2016 as per NACP

ART Regimen	Recommended For
Tenofovir + Lamivudine + Efavirenz	First line ART Regimen for: All ARV naive patients **except those** with ▪ Known renal disease (or) ▪ HIV-2 or HIV-1 & 2 infection (or) ▪ Women with single dose Nevirapine exposure in past pregnancy
Abacavir + Lamivudine + Efavirenz	First line ART Regimen for: All patients with known renal disease
Tenofovir + Lamivudine + Lopinavir/ritonavir	First line ART regimen for: ▪ All women with single dose Nevirapine exposure in a past pregnancy; ▪ All confirmed HIV-2 or HIV- 1 & HIV-2 co-Infection

▪ Drug resistance or 2nd and 3rd line ART

Preferred Second Line ART

Table 46: Preferred second line ART as per NACP

Adults and adolescents (includes pregnant and breastfeeding women)	Children (including adolescents)
2 NRTIs + Ritonavir boosted Protease Inhibitor (PI)	Boosted PI (LPV/r is the preferred) + 2 NRTIs

Third Line ART

New drugs (Integrase inhibitors and second generation NNRTIs and PIs) with minimal risk of cross resistance to previously used regimens. In children benefits and risks need to be balanced.

135 *High Yield Points*

Routine cotrimoxazole prophylaxis should be administered to all HIV "+"ve people with active TB regardless of CD4 cell count.

ART in Pregnant Females

Target Population	Drug Regimen	Remark
Pregnant and breastfeeding Women with HIV (ART Naive/"Not-already" receiving ART)	TDF + 3TC + EFV	FDC of TDF (300 mg) + 3TC (300 mg) + EFV (600 mg)- To be given 2 hours after low-fat or fat-free dinner
Pregnant and breastfeeding Women with HIV already receiving ART	The same ART regimen has to be continued	E.g. If they are already on AZT+3TC+NVP/EFV, continue the same regimen
ART regimen for pregnant women having prior exposure to NNRTI for PPTCT	TDF + 3TC and LPV/r	FDC of TDF (300 mg) + 3TC (300 mg) -- 1-tab OD and
FDC of LPV (200 mg)/r (50 mg) - 2-tab BD		

Antiretroviral Prophylaxis in HIV Exposed Infants

Syrup NVP has to be given for 6 weeks and these children have to be linked to the EID (early infant diagnosis) program

Infants Birth Weight	NVP daily dose (in mg)	NVP daily dose (in ml) (10 mg Nevirapine in 1 ml suspension)	Duration
Infants with birth weight <2000 g	2 mg/kg once daily	0.2 mL/kg once daily	Up to minimum of 6 weeks duration regardless of exclusively breast fed or exclusively replacement fed
Birth weight 2000–2500 g	10 mg once daily	1 mL once daily	
Birth weight >2500 g	15 mg once daily	1.5 mL once daily	Extended to 12 weeks, if the duration of ART of the mother is less than 24 weeks and she is breast feeding

ART in Children

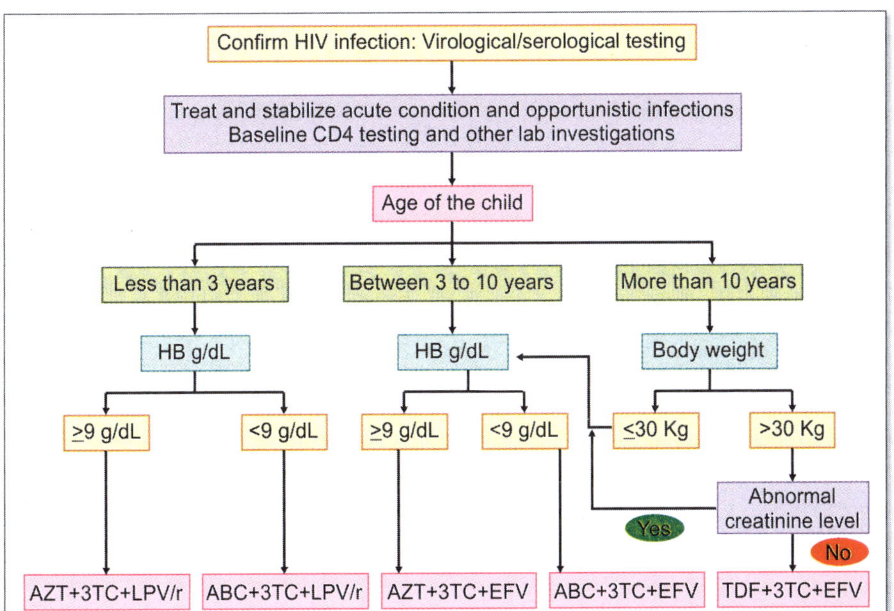

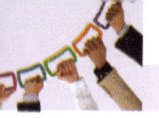

Postexposure Prophylaxis (PEP)

Dosages of drugs for PEP for Adults	Recommendations for PEP	Duration
Tenofovir (300) + Lamivudine (300)- One tablet once daily	One tablet immediately within 2 hours of accidental exposure either at day or night time	Next day one tablet once a day, continue for 4 weeks
Lopinavir (200) + Ritonavir (50)-Two FDC tablets twice daily	Two tablets immediately within 2 hours of accidental exposure either at day or night time	Next day two tablets twice daily, continue for 4 weeks
If Lopinavir/ritonavir is not available or cannot be used, Tenofovir (300) + Lamivudine (300) + Efavirenz (600) may be given 2 hours after dinner before going to bed daily for four weeks		

CPT (Cotrimoxazole Preventive Therapy) Prophylaxis

Prophylaxis	Recommendations
Commencing primary CPT	Co-trimoxazole prophylaxis has to be initiated in PLHIV with CD4 count <350/cmm or with WHO clinical stage 3 and 4 conditions
Commencing secondary CPT	For all patients who have completed successful treatment for PCP until CD4 is ≥350 cells/cmm (at least on two occasions, done 6 months apart)
Timing the initiation of Co-trimoxazole in relation to initiating ART	▪ Start co-trimoxazole prophylaxis first ▪ Start ART after start of co-trimoxazole or as soon as CPT is tolerated and patient has completed the "preparedness phase" of counselling
Dosage of Co-trimoxazole in adults and adolescents	One double-strength tablet or two single-strength tablets once daily–total daily dose of 960 mg (800 mg SMZ + 160 mg TMP)
Monitoring	No specific laboratory monitoring is required in patients receiving co-trimoxazole
Discontinuation of Co-trimoxazole prophylaxis	When CD4 count ≥350/cmm on two different occasions 6 months apart with an ascending trend and devoid of any WHO clinical stage 3 and 4 condition

88 Good to Remember

Though breastfeeding 'increases' the chances of HIV transmission, but the risks outweigh the benefits from the breastfeeding and hence is recommended in Indian setting.

Pediatric HIV Guidelines

Table 47: Risk of transmission of mother to child

Timing of HIV infection	% of children at risk
During pregnancy	5–10
During labor and delivery	10–15%
During breast feeding	5–2%
Overall risk without breastfeeding	15–25%
Overall risk with breastfeeding to 6 months	20–35%
Overall risk with breast feeding to 10 to 24 months	30–45%

Table 48: Breastfeeding guidelines

Situations	Until first 6 months	Beyond 6 months
Situation 1 Mother on ART for her own health	EBF¥ Mother on ART ensures safer breast feeding	Continue breast feeding till 12 months*

Contd...

Situations	Until first 6 months	Beyond 6 months
Situation 2 Mother and infant on ARV prophylaxis for PPTCT	EVF¥ Mother on triple ARV prophylaxis during breastfeeding will make breastfeeding safer	Introduce complementary feeding from 6 months onward**
Situation 3 No access to ARV during breastfeeding	EBF¥ (Unless conditions suitable for RF@)	Introduce complementary feeding from 6 months onwards. ▪ If nutritionally adequate and safe diet ensured, stop BF gradually ▪ If not feasible, continue BF until safe diet ensured.$
Situation 4 Infant detected HIV infected, and initiated on ART	EBF¥	Introduce complementary feeding from 6 months onward continue breast feeding up to two years or beyond. Stop breast feeding gradually as per mother's choices

**If child found to be HIV negative through EID, continue breastfeeding till 12 months. If found to be HIV positive through EID, continue breastfeeding till 2 years.*
***All children more than 6 months of age should be started on complementary feeding as per usual practice.*
¥EBF means that infants are given only breast milk and nothing else – no other milk, food, drinks and water.
The infant receives only breast milk and no other liquids, or solids; with the exception of drops or syrups consisting of vitamins, mineral supplements or medicines.
$Do not stop breastfeeding abruptly. Stop breastfeeding gradually according to comfort level of mother and infant.
@In situations where women opt for replacement feeding or where breastfeeding is not possible (maternal death or sickness), two options are available:
1. Locally available animal milk (unmodified)
2. Commercial infant feeding formula (as per the nutritional guidelines)

Immunization for Children Living with HIV (CLHIV)

HIV-exposed /infected children should be immunized according to the following schedule:

- Live vaccines should be avoided in all severely immune compromised infants (CD4%<25% or WHO stage 3 and 4).
- Vitamin A supplementation should be as per the national immunization schedule.
- In all other cases of children with HIV on treatment, the NIS (national immunization schedule) should be followed

Table 49: Immunization protocol for Child exposed to HIV

Age	Immunization protocol
At birth	BCG, OPV-0, Hep B Birth Dose
6 weeks	OPV-1, RVV-1, Pentavalent-1, fIPV-1#
10 weeks	OPV-2,RVV-2,Pentavalent-2
14 weeks	OPV-3, RVV-3, Pentavalent-3, fIPV-2#
9 months	MCV-1/MR-1, Vit A*, JE-1$
15 months	MCV-2/MR2
16-24 months	DPT-B1/DaPT-B2, OPV-B, JE-2$, Vit A*
5-6 years	DPT-B2/ DaPT-B2
10 years	TT/Td
16 years	TT/Td

*Vitamin A is given 6 monthly till 5 years
$JE vaccine in selected JE endemic states/districts
#schedule may vary from state to state

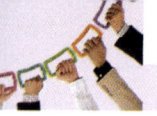

136 *High Yield Points*

Early Infant Diagnosis (EID) program, virological tests, i.e. HIV-1 DNA PCR by Dried Blood Spot (DBS) and on Whole Blood Sample (WBS) are being done for infants and children below 18 months of age.

89 *Good to Remember*

CDC recommends opt-out testing to be provided to all pregnant women.

Early Infant Diagnosis

The exposed infants and children should be followed up at ICTCs at 6, 10, 14 weeks of age and then at 6, 9, 12 and 18 months of age. If they test positive by DBS-DNA PCR test done at ICTC, they should be referred to ART center for confirmation of the diagnosis by WBS-DNA PCR

HIV Counseling and Testing

Opt-in testing → (Client initiated counseling and testing- Direct walk in clients) → Client visits ICTC on their own. He/She is counseled for HIV and then "Opts in" or agrees to be tested for HIV.

Opt-out testing (Provider initiated counseling and testing) → A clinician offers HIV counseling and testing services to patients who present at a health facility with symptoms suggestive of HIV infection.

With opt-out testing, women can specifically ask not to be tested and sign a form refusing HIV testing.

HIV Vaccines

Promising results are from: Ankara vaccine, rAAV vaccine

- **Recombinant subunit vaccines** stimulate antibodies to HIV by mimicking proteins on the surface of HIV. A range of HIV proteins has been produced as potential vaccines for HIV
- **Peptide vaccine:** A vaccine containing the V3 sequences from several strains of HIV has been used in animals and produced antibodies able to neutralize several laboratory-adapted virus strains. Peptide vaccines have been tested in HIV-positive patients, with some antibody and cellular immune responses against HIV
- **DNA vaccine:** After injection, the host's cells effectively make the vaccine themselves by expressing the HIV genes
- **Recombinant vector vaccines** are most often used for vaccines that attempt to stimulate cellular immunity, as the vaccine acts more literally like an infection than vaccines which simply contain proteins or DNA. These are made by incorporating fragments of HIV into the shells of viruses that can infect cells but cause no or few symptoms, such as the canarypox viruses or adenoviruses. Example: Ankara vaccine
- **Replicons** have the same physical properties as viruses and viral vectors, including the ability to enter cells of specific kinds, but they have the advantage of not reproducing after entering the human cell, so there is little or no immune response to the carrier virus. The replicon systems for HIV vaccines are based on Venezuelan equine encephalitis (VEE), Semliki forest virus (SFV), and adenoassociated virus (AAV). All three have shown some success in animal studies.

Live vaccines and inactivated have not been able to provide successful prevention from AIDS, rather showed a risk for development of HIV in later times.

Targeted Interventions

These are preventive interventions for HRG in a defined geographic area.

Objective

- To reduce the transmission of HIV amongst the most vulnerable segment of population.[Q]

Targeted interventions covers

Core Population[Q] →

- Sex workers and their clients
- Men who have sex with men (MSM)
- Transgender population and
- Injectable Drug Users (IDU)

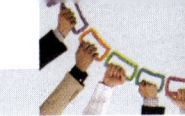

Bridge Population →

- Truck drivers
- Street children
- Prison inmates and
- Migrant workers

Services to be Provided

- Diagnosis and treatment of Sexually Transmitted Infections (STIs)
- Condom promotion via social marketing scheme
- Behavior change communication
- Creating an enabling environment (community involvement and participation)
- Linkage to integrated counseling and testing centers
- Linkage with care and support services for HIV positive HRGs
- Community organisation and ownership.

Specific Interventions for IDUs

- Distribution of clean needles/syringes
- Abscess prevention and management
- Opioid substitution therapy
- Linkage with detoxification/rehabilitation services.

Specific Intervention for MSM and Transgenders

- Provision of lubricating materials

NACP IV (2012–2017)

Objectives

- *Zero HIV*
- Reduce new infection by 50% (Baseline 2007)
- Provide comprehensive care and support to all PLHA and Treatment services for all those who require it.

Strategies

- Intensifying and consolidating prevention services with focus on HRG and Vulnerable population
- Increased access and promoting comprehensive care and support and treatment
- Expansion of IEC services with focus on BCC and demand generation
- Capacity building at all levels
- Strengthening strategic information management system.

HIV Testing Policy

- Voluntary with pre-and post-test counseling
- No individual can be forced to undergo a testing for HIV
- HIV testing cannot be imposed as a precondition for employment or providing health care
- Disclosure of HIV status to spouse depends on person's willingness. He is encouraged to share with spouse/family

Testing Strategy: (In Different Settings)

- ***Mandatory*** → In blood banks for transfusion safety
- ***Unlinked and anonymous*** → Epidemiological survey, HIV sentinel surveillance
- ***Voluntary and confidential*** → Confirmatory testing for subclinical/ clinical case and voluntary testing.
- ***Need based*** → for research – to maintain ethical standards

The investigation for assessment of response to treatment and effect of ART therapy is: Viral load estimation using rtPCR technique

90 Good to Remember

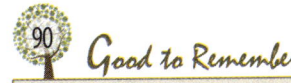

"3 BY 5 TARGET" – Historical Approach

- Provide antiretroviral treatment (ART) to 3 million people living with HIV/AIDS in developing countries by 2005.
- Ultimate goal was universal access to treatment for HIV/AIDS to all those who need it.
- "3 by 5" strategy, WHO strategic framework for scaling up ART had 5 pillars-
  - Global leadership, strong partnership and advocacy.
  - Urgent, sustained country support
  - Simplified, standardized tools to deliver ART
  - Effective reliable supply of medicines and diagnostics
  - Rapidly identifying and reapplying new knowledge and successes.

137 High Yield Points

90–90–90 - Treatment Target

It seeks to achieve by 2020

- 90% of all people living with HIV will know their HIV status
- 90% of all people with diagnosed HIV infection will receive sustained ART
- 90% of all people receiving ART will have viral suppression.

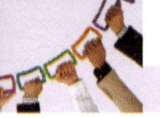

81 **Must Remember**

NACO Projects 2014-2020

The **Condom Social Marketing Program** (CSMP): aims to promote safer sex.

Project Sunrise: Responsible for the expansion of HIV interventions in north eastern states with a focus on key affected populations, particularly people who inject drugs.

Project NIRANTAR: This three-year project began in 2014 and focuses on building the capacity of civil society organizations working with key affected populations in the states of Chhattisgarh, Madhya Pradesh and Odisha. Its main aim is to improve access to HIV prevention, care and treatment services, including social protection schemes, in an enabling environment.

Link Worker Scheme: It involves highly motivated and trained community members, responsible for establishing links between the community on one hand and information, commodities and services on the other.

National Strategic Plan for HIV/AIDS - 2017-2024

Goal: To achieve

- Zero new infections
- Zero AIDS related deaths
- Zero discrimination

Objectives: This NSP proposes six objectives towards fulfilling its vision of an AIDS free India. These are:

- Objective 1: Reduce 80% new infections by 2024 (Baseline 2010)
- Objective 2: Ensure 95% of estimated PLHIV know their status by 2024
- Objective 3: Ensure 95% PLHIV have ART initiation and retention by 2024, for
- Sustained viral suppression
- Objective 4: Eliminate mother-to-child transmission of HIV and Syphilis by 2020
- Objective 5: Eliminate HIV/AIDS related stigma and discrimination by 2020
- Objective 6: Facilitate sustainable NACP service delivery by 2024

Broad strategies

Test & Treat policy relates to - PTT (prevent → test → treat)

Prevent	Test	Treat
▪ Increased coverage for improved prevention, testing and care linkages ▪ Systematic evidence generation to reach 'at risk' population ▪ Retain KP with adequate and adequate and appropriate services	▪ Geo-prioritise differential approach ▪ Use graded approach to increase HIV testing ▪ Pilot and scale up newer modalities of testing (e.g. CBT, self testing, etc.) ▪ Active use of IEC to increase demand for HIV testing	▪ Accelerate uptake of ART ▪ Improve ART retention by engaging community/NGOs/ private sector. ▪ Ensure supportive environment for achieving universal access to ART ▪ Address co-morbidities of HIV infection to lower mortality and morbidity

Glossary:

KP = knowledge and practice; CBT = community based testing; IEC = information education, communication; ART – anti retroviral treatment; NGO = non-government organisation.

Indicators for EMTCT (Elimination of Mother to Child Transmission) for HIV and Syphilis by 2020

Impact indicators [at least last one year data]

- Case rate of new paediatric HIV infections due to Mother-to-Child-Transmission (MTCT) of HIV of <50 cases per 100 000 live births and
- <50 cases of congenital Syphilis per 100,000 live births
- HIV transmission rate of <5% in breastfeeding population or <2% in non-breastfeeding population

Process indicators [at least last two-year data]
- Antenatal care (ANC) coverage (of at least one visit) of >95%
- Coverage of pregnant women who know their HIV status of >95%
- Antiretroviral (ARV) coverage of HIV positive pregnant women of >95%
- Treatment of Syphilis – sero-positive women of >95%

SEXUALLY TRANSMITTED DISEASES (STD)

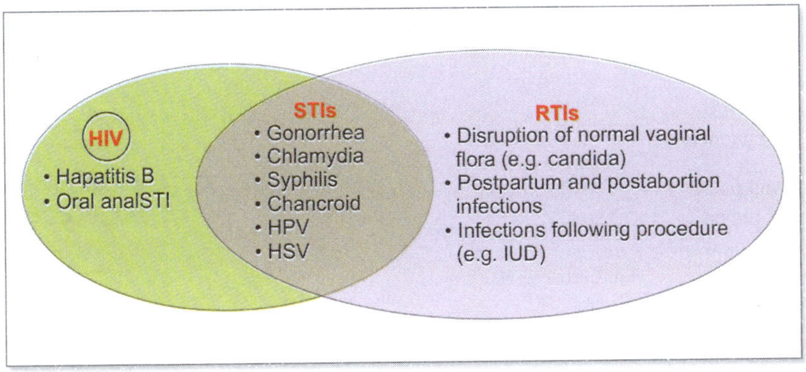

Fig. 15: Spectrum of RTI/STI

- 5 "Classical" STD/venereal diseases: Syphilis, Gonorrhea, Chancroid, LGV and Donovanosis.
- Syndromic approach in RTI/STI management: Diagnosis is based on identification of syndromes (a combination of symptoms and signs). It ensures correct and complete treatment against all common organisms responsible for a particular syndrome. It also includes client education and counseling.

Suraksha Clinics

These clinics have been set up which provide sexual and reproductive health services. These clinics also provide counseling from trained councilors and RTI/STI treatment kits
The kits provided are color coded for different syndromic manifestations as follows:

suraksha clinic
Sexual and Reproductive Health Services

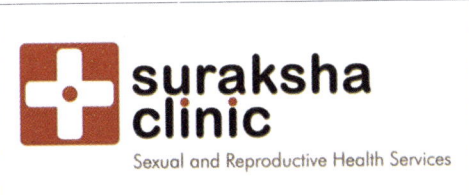

Fig. 16: Emblem of suraksha clinic

Table 50: Color coded kits for different syndromic manifestation in Suraksha clinics

Name of kit	Color	Syndrome	Symptomatology	Pharmacotherapy	Partner management	
Kit 1	Grey	Urethral discharge	▪ Urethral discharge (pus or mucopurulent) ▪ Pain or burning while passing urine ▪ Increased frequency of urination ▪ Systemic symptoms like malaise, fever	Tab Azithromycin 1 g – OD Stat + Tab Cefixime 400 mg OD Stat	Treat all recent partners	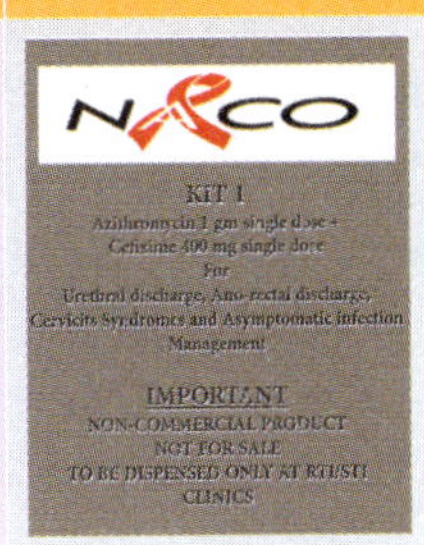

Contd...

Name of kit	Color	Syndrome	Symptomatology	Pharmacotherapy	Partner management	
Kit 1	Grey	Cervical discharge	▪ Nature and type of discharge (quantity, color and odor) ▪ Burning while passing uine, increased frequency ▪ Genital complaints by sexual partners ▪ Low backache *(Take menstrual history to rule out pregnancy)*	Tab Azithromycin 1 g – OD Stat + Tab Cefixime 400 mg OD Stat	Treat partners when symptomatic	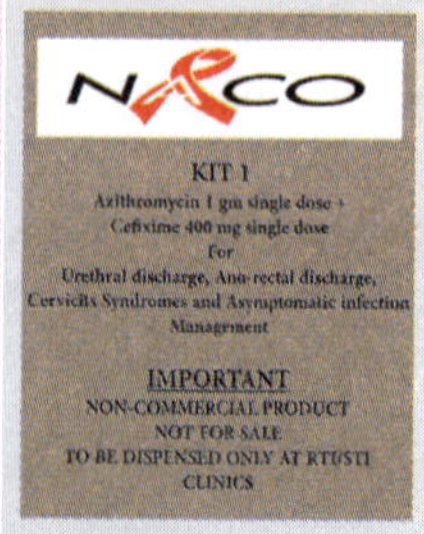
Kit 1	Grey	Painful scrotal swelling	▪ Swelling and pain in the scrotal region ▪ Pain or burning while passing urine ▪ Systemic symptoms like malaise, fever ▪ History of urethral discharge	Tab Azithromycin 1 g – OD Stat + Tab Cefixime 400 mg OD Stat	Treat all recent partners	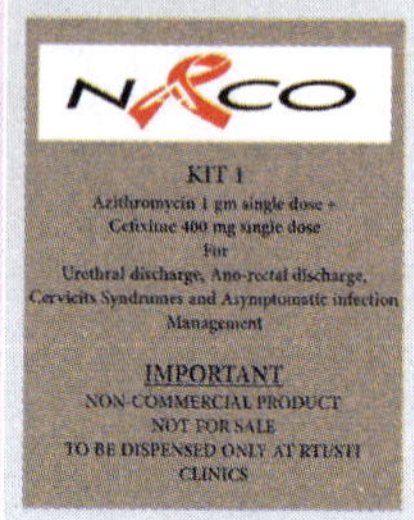
Kit 2	Green	Vaginal discharge	▪ Nature and type of discharge (quantity, color and odor) ▪ Burning while passing urine, increased frequency ▪ Genital complaints by sexual partners ▪ Low backache *(Take menstrual history to rule out pregnancy)*	Tab Secnidazole 2 g – OD Stat + Cap. Fluconazole 150 mg OD Stat	Treat partners when symptomatic	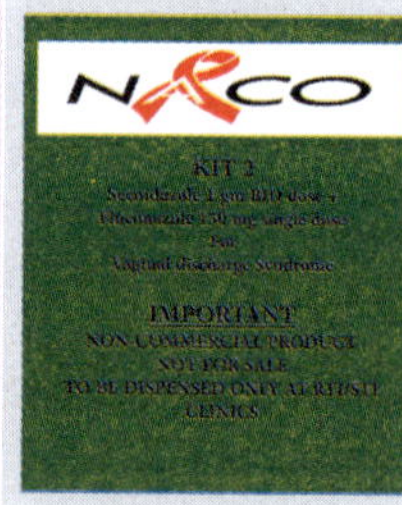
Kit 3	White	Genital ulcer non-herpetic	▪ Genital ulcer, single or multiple, painful or painless ▪ Burning sensation in the genital area ▪ Enlarged lymph nodes	Inj. Benzathine penicillin (2.4 MU)-1 vial Tab. Azithromycin (1 g)-single dose	Treat all sexual partners for past 3 months	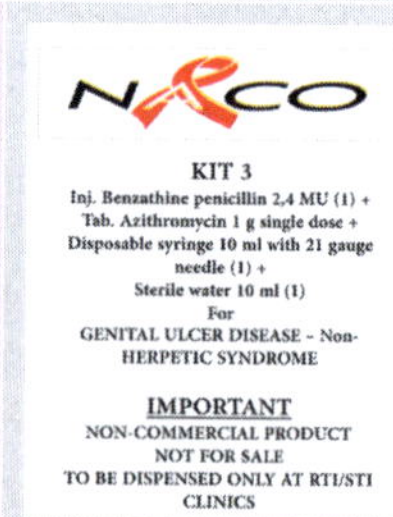
Kit 4	Blue			If allergic to Inj. penicillin: Doxycycline 100 mg (Bid for 15 days) Azithromycin 1 g (Single dose)		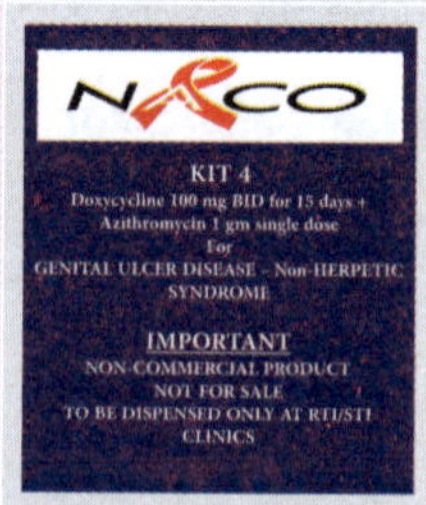

Contd...

Name of kit	Color	Syndrome	Symptomatology	Pharmacotherapy	Partner management	
Kit 5	Red	Genital ulcer-herpetic	▪ Genital ulcer or vesicles, single or multiple, painful, recurrent ▪ Burning sensation in the genital area	Tab. Acyclovir 400 mg TDS for 7 days	No partner treatment	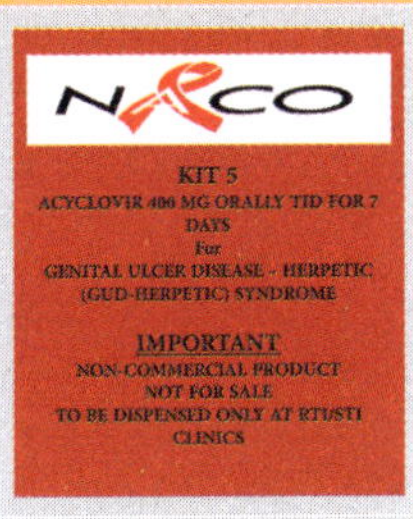
Kit 6	Yellow	Lower abdominal pain (LAP)	▪ Lower abdominal pain ▪ Fever ▪ Vaginal discharge ▪ Menstrual irregularities like heavy, irregular vaginal bleeding ▪ Dysmenorrhoea dysparenunia, dysuria, tenesmus ▪ Lower backache ▪ Cervical motion tenderness	Tab. Cefixime 400 mg OD stat + Tab. Metronidazole 400 mg BD × 14 days + Doxycycline 100 mg BD × 14 days	Treat male partners with Kit 1	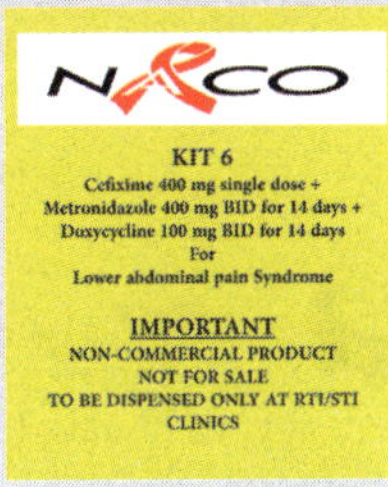
Kit 7	Black	Inguinal Bubo (IB)	▪ Swelling in inguinal region which may be painful ▪ Preceding history of genital ulcer or discharge ▪ Systemic symptoms like malaise, fever, etc	Tab. Azithromycin 1 g OD Stat + Tab. Doxycycline 100 mg BD for 21 days	Treat all sexual partners for past 3 weeks	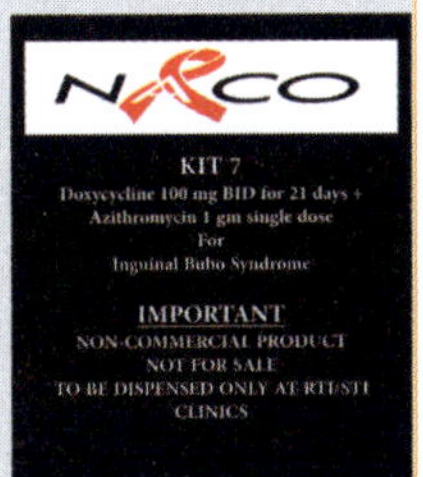

Other important considerations for management of RTI/STI

- Educate and counsel client and sexual partner(s) regarding STI/RTI, safer sex practices and importance of taking complete treatment
- Treat partners
- Advise sexual abstinence or condom use during the course of treatment
- Provide condoms, educate about correct and consistent use
- Refer all patients to ICTC
- Follow-up after 7 days for all STI, 3, 7, and 14 day for LAP and 7, 14, and 21 day for IB
- If symptoms persist, assess whether it is due to re-infection and advise prompt referral
- Consider immunization against Hepatitis B.

NEWER INFECTIONS

DISEASE X

The World Health Organization (WHO) has released a list of diseases that could cause an International health risk and Disease X is on the list.

Watch List | Diseases threatening a public health emergency*

- Crimean-Congo hemorrhagic fever (CCHF)
- Ebola virus disease and Marburg virus disease
- Lassa fever
- Middle East respiratory syndrome coronavirus (MERS-CoV)

91 *Good to Remember*

- **Disease X** could be sparked by a zoonotic disease—and then spreads to become an epidemic or pandemic in the same way **H1N1 Swine flu** virus did in 2009.
- Zoonotic infections that have wreaked havoc in the past include HIV, which is believed to have jumped from chimpanzees to humans through the eating of bushmeat and has killed 35 million people since the early 1980s.
- **Ebola** is also a zoonosis. As the ecosystem and human habitats change, there is always the risk of disease jumping from animals to humans.
- And same has happened with the **Nipah virus** (NiV) in Kerala, India (2018)

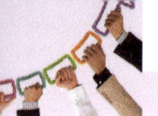

- Severe acute respiratory syndrome (SARS)
- Nipah and henipaviral diseases
- Rift Valley fever (RVF)
- Zika virus disease
- Disease X

"Diseases that currently have no cure and pose a threat to public health internationally."

Disease X could emerge as:

- An accident
- An act of terror
- Changing habits and habitats

EBOLA VIRUS

- **Causative agent:** Ebola virus (Filoviridae family) comprises 5 distinct species – Zaire, Reston, Sudan, Tai and Bundibugyo.
- Recent epidemic started in Dec 2013 in Guinea and spread to South Africa. A total of 7,192 cases with 3,286 deaths reported till 28/09/2014.
- **Case fatality rate:** Up to 70%.
- **Incubation period:** 2–21 days (Noninfectious during this period) Asymptomatic cases are also noninfectious
- **Modes of transmission-**
  - Direct contact with blood, organ, body secretion/fluids of infected animals or symptomatic person.
  - Exposure to objects (needles) contaminated with infected secretions.
  - Not transmitted through air, water or food or by sexual transmission

82 **Must Remember**

Ebola virus disease (Ebola Hemorrhagic Fever) -1st time reported in Zaire and Sudan in 1976 (Since then it has appeared periodically)

Clinical Presentation

- Sudden onset of fever, intense weakness, muscle pain, headache, sore throat, vomiting, diarrhea, rash, impaired, kidney and liver functions and in some cases both internal and external bleeding.

Treatment

- No specific treatment or Vaccine is available. Intensive supportive care is recommended to reduce mortality.
- Infection control measures need to be observed.

SWINE FLU (INFLUENZA A H1N1)

- Outbreak started in Mexico on 18th March, 2009.
- 1st pandemic since 1968.
- WHO has heightened the pandemic level to Phase 5 implying widespread human infection
- ***Transmission:*** By droplet infection and fomites
- ***Incubation period:*** 1-7 days
- ***Period of communicability:*** 1 day before to 7 days after the onset of symptoms.
- Children may spread the virus for a longer period.
- ***Clinical features:*** Fever, Upper Respiratory symptoms (cough and sore throat). Headache, body ache, fatigue diarrhea and vomiting.
- Individuals at extremes of age and with preexisting medical conditions are at higher risk of complications
- ***Complications:*** Sinusitis, otitis media, croup, pneumonia, bronchiolitis, status asthamaticus, myocarditis, pericarditis, myositis, rhabdomyolysis, encephalitis, seizures, toxic shock syndrome and secondary bacterial pneumonia with or without sepsis.
- *Confirmation of influenza A(H1N1)* in nasopharyngeal swab, throat swab, nasal swab, wash or aspirate, and tracheal aspirate (for intubated patients) is done using
- Real time RT PCR or
- Di Isolation of the virus in culture or
- Di Four-fold rise in virus specific neutralizing antibodies.
- *Oseltamivir* is the drug both for prophylaxis and treatment.
- Close Contacts of suspected, probable and confirmed cases are advised voluntary home quarantine for at least 7 days after the last contact with the case.
- *Monitoring* of fever should be done for at least 7 days.

83 **Must Remember**

In India, facilities for isolation of influenza virus are available at:

- Govt. of India, Influenza Center, Pasteur Institute, Coonoor, South India, Haffkine Institute, Mumbai,
- School of Tropical Medicine, Kolkata
- AIIMS, New Delhi
- Vallabhbhai Patel Chest Institute, Delhi,
- AFMC, Poona

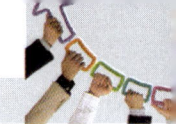

MIDDLE EAST RESPIRATORY SYNDROME (MERS)

- It Originated in Saudi Arabia in 2012
- Causative agent – corona virus(C).
- Incubation period: 2–14days
- Transmission: Droplet
- CFR: 30%
- No treatment available at present

ZIKA VIRUS

- **Causative agent:** Flavivirus (known to circulate in Africa, the Americas, Asia and the Pacific)
- First identified in Uganda in1947
- First large outbreak of disease was reported from island of Yap in 2007. Currently 22 countries and territories in Americas have reported local transmission of Zika virus.
- **Reservoir:** Unknown
- **Incubation period:** Not clear, likely to be few days.
- **Vector:** Aedes mosquitoes.
    - Also, vertical transmission is a possibility.
- **Symptom:** Mild fever, maculopapular skin rash (exanthema), conjunctivitis, muscle and joint pain, malaise, headache. Symptoms last for about 2–7 days. Only one in four infected people develop symptoms of disease. Clustering of cases of microcephaly (Vertical transmission).
- No specific treatment or vaccine currently available.
- Best form of prevention is protection against mosquito bites, safe sex
- *Diagnosis* –RT PCR (polymerase chain reaction) and virus isolation from blood samples
- NCDC, Delhi and NIV, Pune have the capacity to provide lab diagnosis.

WHO "Zika Strategic Response Framework"

- Define and prioritize research into Zika virus disease
- Enhance surveillance of Zika virus and potential complications.
- Strengthen capacity in risk communication to engage communities to better understand risks associated with Zika virus.
- Strengthen the capacity of laboratories to detect the virus.

NIPAH VIRUS

Outbreak in India

On May 19, 2018, three deaths due to Nipah virus infection were reported in Kozhikode District, Kerala State, India. The three deaths occurred in a family cluster and a fourth death was subsequently reported in a health care worker who was involved in treatment of the family in the local hospital.

Laboratory testing of throat swabs, urine and blood samples collected from four suspected patients have been conducted by the National Institute of Virology in Pune; three of the four reported deaths were confirmed positive for Nipah virus (NiV) by real-time polymerase chain reaction (RT-PCR) and IgM Elisa for NiV.

The field investigation team found bats living in the abandoned water well on the premises of a new house where the family had plans to move after renovation. One bat was caught and sent to the National Institute of Virology, Pune for laboratory testing.

In the current outbreak, acute respiratory distress syndrome and encephalitis have been observed.

This is the first NiV outbreak reported in Kerala State and third NiV outbreak known to have occurred in India, with the most recent outbreak reported in 2007.

> 84 **Must Remember**
>
> Nipah virus is classified internationally as a biosecurity level (BSL) 4 agent. BSL 2 facilities are sufficient if the virus can be first inactivated during specimen collection

NIV Features

Agent factors:

- Nipah virus infection, also known as Nipah virus encephalitis, was first isolated and described in 1999. The name, Nipah, is derived from the village in Malaysia where the person from whom the virus was first isolated succumbed to the disease
- The organism which causes Nipah virus encephalitis is an RNA virus of the family Paramyxoviridae, genus *Henipavirus*, and is closely related to Hendra virus.

Reservoir:

- Zoonotic disease
- Large fruit bats (genus *Pteropus)* (flying foxes) are the natural reservoirs of NiV

Mode of transmission:

- Three basic modes have been understood till now:
  - Pig to human
  - Bat to human
  - Human to human
- Consumption of infected fruits (with bites from bats)
- NiV is highly contagious among pigs and is spread by infected droplets. Pigs acquire NiV and act as an intermediate and possibly amplifying host after contact with infected bats or their secretions
- Human to human transmission can occur among close contacts and family members
- High risk of transmission of the virus from infected patients to health care workers through contact with infected secretions, excretions, blood or tissues.

Incubation period: 5–18 days

Symptoms

- Infection with Nipah virus is associated with encephalitis.
- 3–14 days of fever and headache, followed by drowsiness, disorientation and mental confusion. These signs and symptoms can progress to coma within 24–48 hours. Some patients have a respiratory illness during the early part of their infections, and half of the patients showing severe neurological signs showed also pulmonary signs.
- Long-term sequelae following Nipah virus infection have been noted, including persistent convulsions and personality changes.
- Latent infections with subsequent reactivation of Nipah virus and death have also been reported months and even years after exposure.
- High fatality rate—40–75%

Diagnosis

- Laboratory diagnosis of a patient with a clinical history of NiV can be made during the acute and convalescent phases of the disease by using a combination of tests.
- Virus isolation attempts and real time polymerase chain reaction (RT-PCR) from throat and nasal swabs, cerebrospinal fluid, urine, and blood should be performed in the early stages of disease.
- Antibody detection by ELISA (IgG and IgM) can be used later on.
- In fatal cases, immunohistochemistry on tissues collected during autopsy maybe the only way to confirm a diagnosis.

Prevention

- No specific treatment available
- Ribavirin has been shown to be effective, but the data is nonconclusive and uncertain
- Standard protocol for prevention of nosocomial infections.

92 Good to Remember

- NiV disease has been known to occur in pigs, and hence exposure to pigs is to be avoided for primary prevention strategies.
- NiV in pigs is known to cause respiratory and nervous system disorders as porcine respiratory and encephalitic syndrome (PRES), and barking pig syndrome (BPS)

Latest Updates

- Passive immunization using a human monoclonal antibody targeting the Nipah G glycoprotein has been evaluated in the postexposure therapy in the ferret model and found to be of benefit.
- A subunit vaccine, using the Hendra G protein, produces cross-protective antibodies against HENV and NIPV has been recently used in Australia to protect horses against Hendra virus. This vaccine offers great potential for henipavirus protection in humans as well.
- ALVAC Canarypox vectored Nipah F and G vaccine is also a potential vaccine

Image-Based Questions

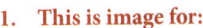

1. **This is image for:**

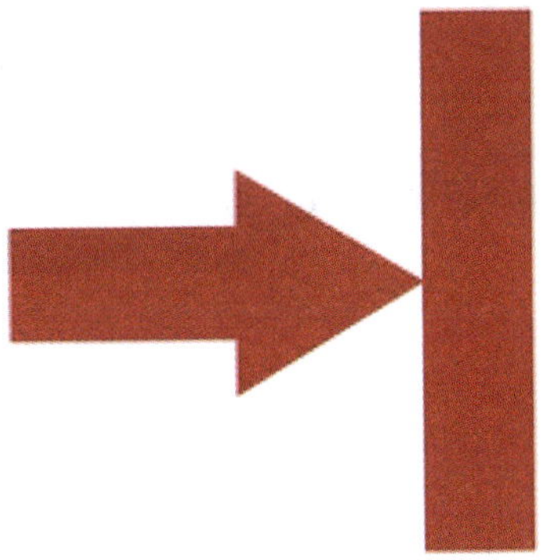

a. End Polio
b. End Leprosy
c. End TB
d. End Yaws

2. **Identify the lesion in the figure below:**

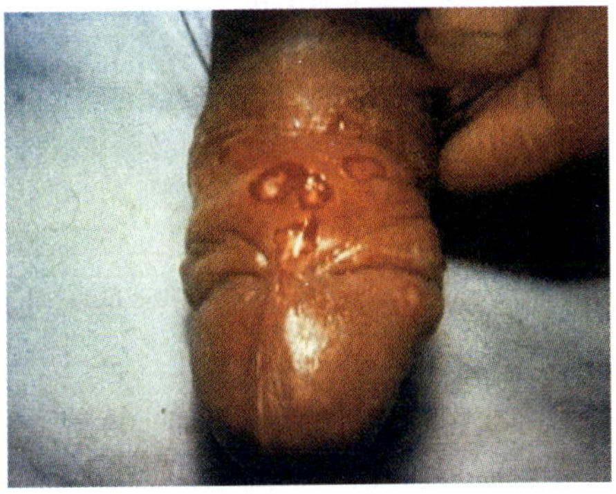

a. Herpes
b. Chancroid
c. Yaws
d. Neurofibromatosis

3. **Identify organism given in the figure below:**

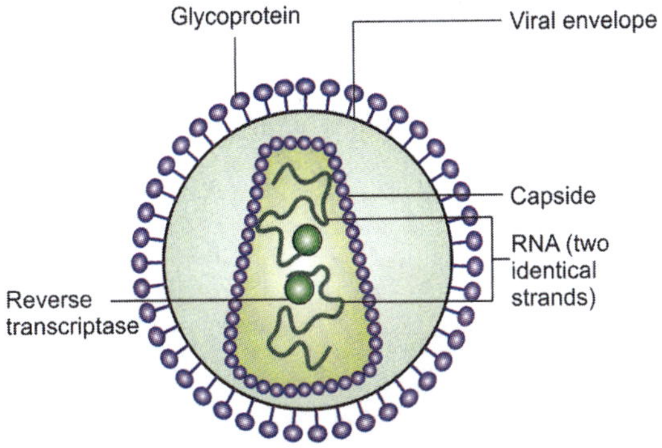

a. Influenza virus
b. Rabies virus
c. HIV virus
d. Ebola virus

4. **Identify the organism in the figure below:**

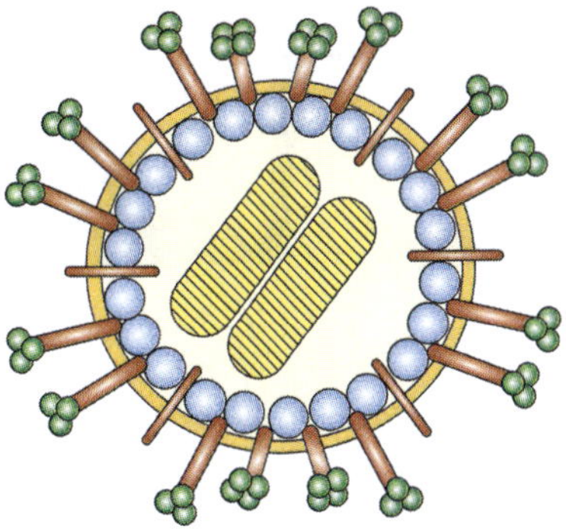

a. HIV virus
b. Influenza virus
c. Rabies virus
d. Ebola virus

5. **Identify the symbol as shown in the figure below:**

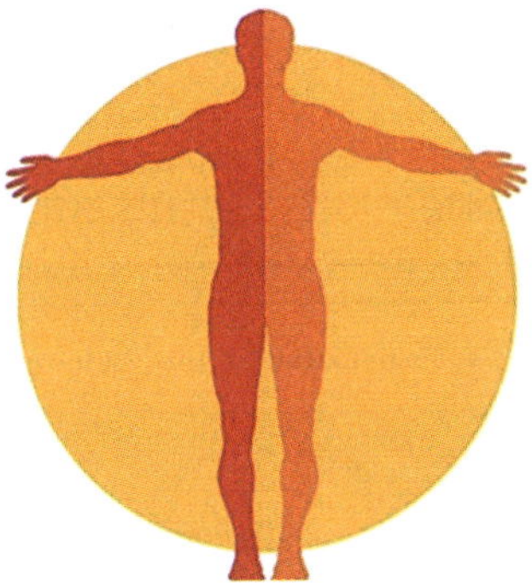

a. RNTCP
b. NPCB
c. NIDDCP
d. RBSK

6. **Identify the program depicted by the symbol in the figure below:**

a. RNTCP
b. NLEP
c. NVBDCP
d. NACP

7. Identify the most probable diagnosis of the condition shown in the figure below:

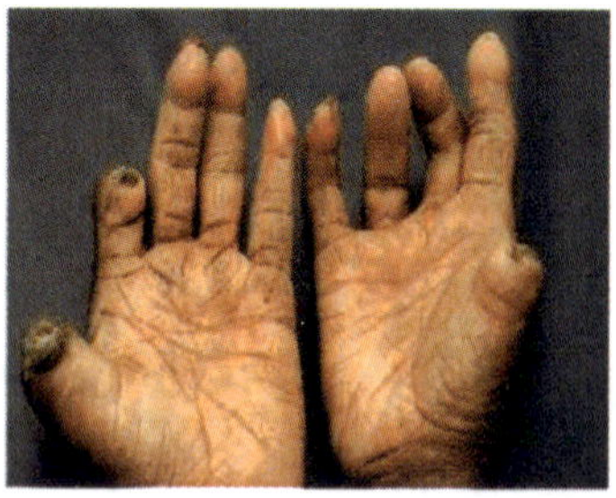

a. Leprosy b. Syphilis
c. Yaws d. Peripheral neuropathy

8. Identify the symbol shown in the figure below:

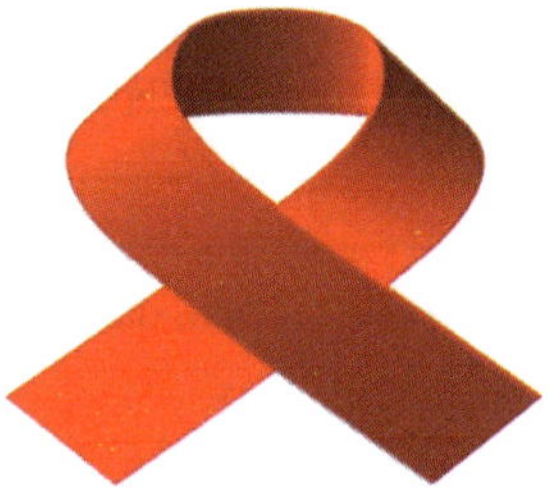

a. RTI/STI b. Blood bank
c. Haemophilia d. HIV/AIDS

9. Identify the scientist in the figure below:

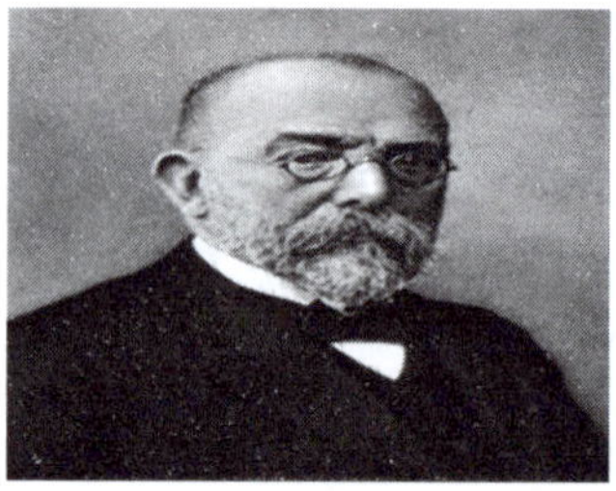

a. Robert Koch b. Laveran
c. Paul Muller d. Ronald Ross

10. Identify the condition shown in the figure below and give the most probable diagnosis among the given options:

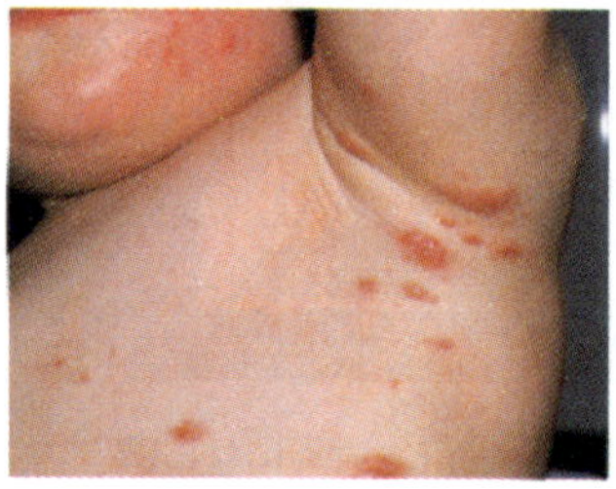

a. Chicken pox b. Measles
c. Smallpox d. Scabies

11. Identify the condition shown in the figure below & give the most probable diagnosis among the given options:

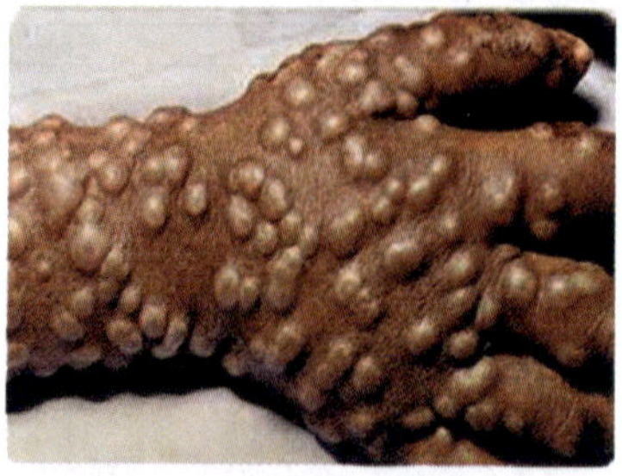

a. Chicken pox b. Measles
c. Small pox d. Scabies

12. Identify the condition shown in the figure below & give the most probable diagnosis among the given options:

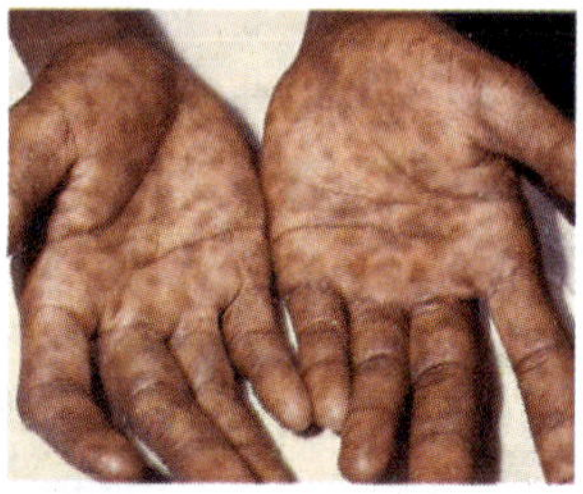

a. Chicken pox b. Syphilis
c. Smallpox d. Scabies

13. Identify the most probable diagnosis from the X ray given in the figure below:

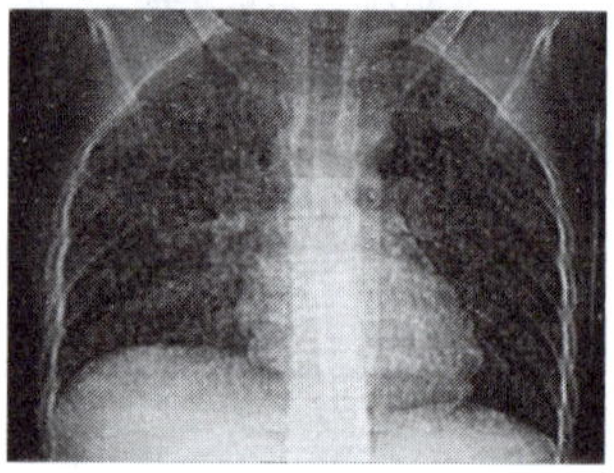

a. Pneumonia b. Plueral effusion
c. Collapse d. Milliary tuberculosis

14. Identify the symbol shown in the figure below:

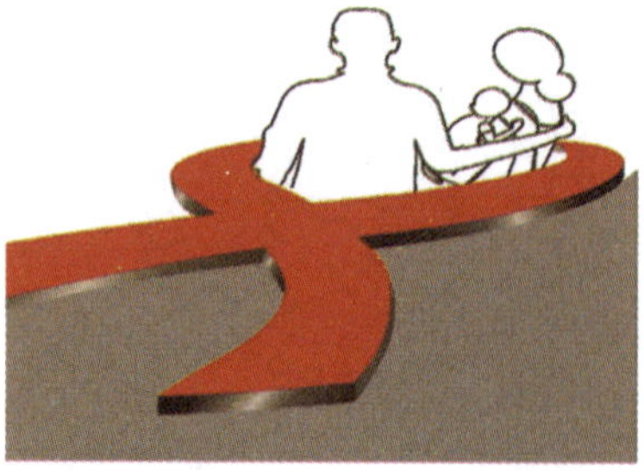

a. RMNCH+A b. Blood transfusion
c. PPTCT d. NACO

15. Identify the disease depicted in the figure below:

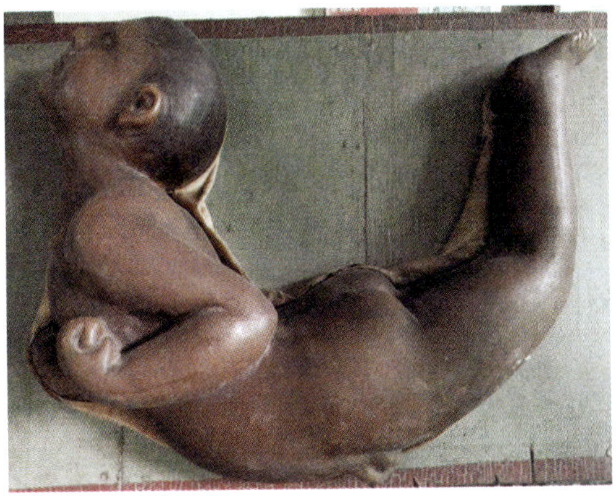

a. Tetanus
b. Cholera
c. Typhoid
d. Rabies

16. Identify the image and relate to the National program

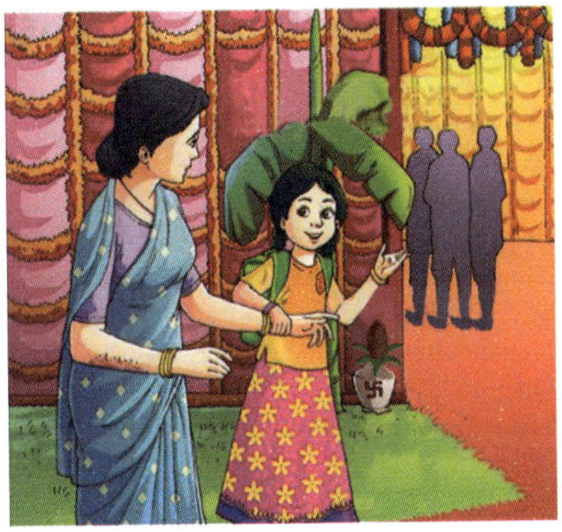

a. National Leprosy eradication program
b. Filariasis control program
c. Prevention of child abuse
d. Prevention of female Foeticide

17. The Kit shown in the figure below is available at:

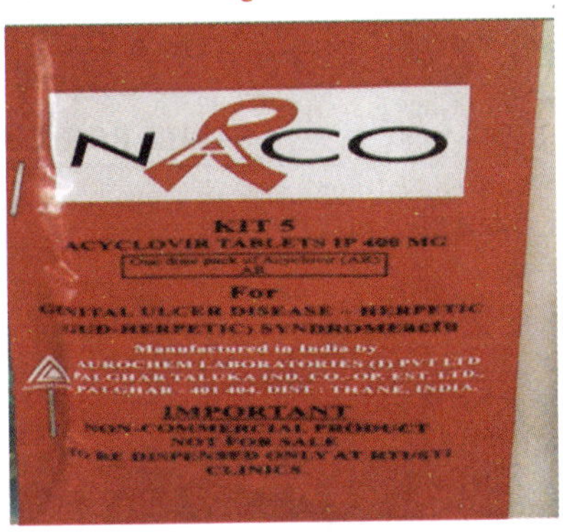

a. Suraksha Clinic
b. ART center
c. Asthma clinic
d. Geriatric clinic

Answers of Image-Based Questions

1. **Ans. (c)** **END TB**
2. **Ans. (b)** **Chancroid**
3. **Ans. (c)** **HIV virus**
4. **Ans. (b)** **Influenza virus**
5. **Ans. (a)** **RNTCP**
6. **Ans. (b)** **NLEP**
7. **Ans. (a)** **Leprosy**
8. **Ans. (d)** **HIV/AIDS**
9. **Ans. (a)** **Robert Koch**
10. **Ans. (d)** **Scabies**
11. **Ans. (c)** **Small pox**
12. **Ans. (b)** **Syphilis**
13. **Ans. (d)** **Milliary tuberculosis**
14. **Ans. (c)** **PPTCT**
15. **Ans. (a)** **Tetanus**
16. **Ans. (a)** **National Leprosy eradication program**
17. **Ans. (a)** **Suraksha clinic**

Multiple Choice Questions

1. **Annual case detection rate of leprosy is:** *(AIIMS Nov 2017)*
   a. 10.17/10,000 b. 10.17/100,000
   c. 0.64/100,000 d. 0.64/10,000
2. **A patient was sputum negative for TB, but chest X-Ray was suggestive for TB. Which is the next step according to RNTCP** *(AIIMS May 2017)*
   a. Liquid culture b. CB - NAAT
   c. Line probe assay d. None of the above
3. **Web based program for monitoring TB is:** *(Recent Question 2018)*
   a. Nikshay b. Nischay
   c. Nikusth d. e-DOTS
4. **Kala-azar is found in all endemic areas except.** *(Recent Question 2018)*
   a. West Bengal b. UP
   c. Bihar d. Assam
5. **Period of communicability of measles is:** *(PGI May 2017)*
   a. 3 days before and 10 days after appearance of rashes
   b. 3 weeks after appearance of rashes
   c. 1 week before appearance of rashes
   d. 4 days before and 5 days after appearance of rashes
   e. Up to 3months after appearance of rashes
6. **Which of the following is/are true about Revised National Tuberculosis Control Program (RNTCP):** *(PGI May 2017)*
   a. T.B is mandatory to notify
   b. Suspicious TB patients are screened through 2 sputum smear examinations
   c. MDR-TB is not included in RNTCP
   d. Case finding is active
   e. Covered the whole country since March 2006
7. **Which of the following is true about postexposure prophylaxis in rabies:** *(PGI May 2017)*
   a. Category I- Both vaccine and immunoglobulin are given
   b. Immunoglobulin not required if prior immunization and immunoglobulin is received within 1 year
   c. Local wound cleaning is done in all cases of dog wound
   d. Category I- requires vaccination only
   e. Vaccine is stopped if within 3 days of bite, dog dies
8. **Black RTI kit is used in:** *(Recent Question 2017)*
   a. Urogenital infection b. Genital ulcer
   c. Scrotum swelling d. Inguinal bubo
9. **What is the recommended dose for human rabies immunoglobulin (Ig) in 4 month old child?**
   a. 20 IU/kg b. 30 IU/kg
   c. 40 IU/kg d. 50 IU/kg
10. **What is the color of RTI/STI kit number 6?**
    a. Grey b. Yellow
    c. Red d. Black
11. **Under RNTCP, a designated microscopy lab covers how much population in plains:**
    a. 5000 b. 20,000-30,000
    c. 1 lakh d. 1 lakh to 5 lakh
12. **Incubation period for cholera:** *(Recent Question 2017)*
    a. 1–7 days b. Few hours to 5 days
    c. 2 weeks d. 4 weeks
13. **Measles is infective for how many days before the onset of rash:**
    a. on same b. 1 days
    c. 4 days d. 10 days
14. **Portal of entry in measles is:**
    a. Respiratory b. Oral route
    c. Through skin d. Fecal
15. **'NIKSHAY' software lunched by Central Government is used for tracking of:**
    a. High risk newborns
    b. High risk pregnancies
    c. Malaria
    d. Tuberculosis
16. **A patient was sputum negative for TB, but chest Xray was suggestive for TB. Which is the next step according to RNTCP:**
    a. Liquid culture b. CB - NAAT
    c. Line probe assay d. None of the above

SMALL POX/CHICKEN POX

17. **The last case of small pox was reported in India is**
    a. May 1975 b. May 1980
    c. July 1985 d. September 1990
18. **Immunity conferred by an attack of small pox is:**
    a. 10 yr b. 15yr
    c. 20 yr d. Life long
19. **Which of the following disease maybe associated sequel of measles**
    a. Herpes zoster b. Mumps
    c. Herpes simplex d. Micronutrient deficiency
20. **Regarding varicella which of the following is FALSE**
    a. Scabs are most infective
    b. Palms and soles are sparingly affected
    c. Rashes are symmetrical centripetal and like dew drop
    d. We may see pleomorphism in the rash
21. **Which of the following is not a complication of chicken pox?**
    a. Pneumonia
    b. Reye's syndrome
    c. Encephalitis
    d. Pancreatitis
22. **A class 2 child develops fever and vesicular rash on abdomen during school time. As a school medical officer, what is the next best step**
    a. Send the child to the nearest hospital
    b. Isolation of the boy
    c. Send the boy home in emergency
    d. Call the parents and report the emergency
23. **Chicken pox causes severe infection in:**
    a. Infant b. Children
    c. Adolescent d. Adults

Ans.

1.	b
2.	b
3.	a
4.	d
5.	d
6.	a, b, e
7.	b, c
8.	d
9.	a
10.	b
11.	c
12.	b
13.	c
14.	a
15.	d
16.	b
17.	a
18.	d
19.	a
20.	a
21.	d
22.	b
23.	d

Most Recent Questions of 2019-18 are given at the end of MCQs

24. The varicella vaccine is:
- a. Killed OKA strain
- b. Live attenuated OKA strain
- c. Killed VZ. strain
- d. Oral varicella vaccine

25. Chicken pox is infective:
- a. 2 days before and 2 days after rash appearance
- b. 2 days before and 5 days after rash appearance
- c. 4 days before and 4 days after rash appearance
- d. 4 days before and 5 days after rash appearance

26. All of the following are true about chicken pox, except:
- a. Superficial rash
- b. Secondary attack rate is 90%
- c. Causative agent is herpes simplex-3
- d. Only one stage of rash is seen

27. Varicella zoster immunization is given to all, except
- a. Contacts with Varicella Zoster
- b. To the newborn and pregnant female who was exposed 6 weeks before delivery
- c. All HIV positive patients
- d. Patients with varicella zoster

28. WHO declared global eradication of small pox on:
- a. 26th October 1977
- b. 5th July 1975
- c. 17th May 1975
- d. 8th May 1980

29. Small pox was eradicated in the year:
- a. 1975
- b. 1980
- c. 1981
- d. 1984

30. Secondary attack rate of chicken pox is:
- a. 60 b. 50
- c. 90 d. 40

31. Chicken pox vaccine is: *(Recent Question 2017)*
- a. Live vaccine
- b. Killed vaccine
- c. Conjugated vaccine
- d. Toxoid vaccine

32. Small pox eradication was not due to:
- a. Highly effective vaccine
- b. Cross-immunity with animal pox virus
- c. Subclinical infection do not transmit the disease
- d. Life long immunity

33. Not true about varicella infection
- a. Only single stage of lesion is present at a time
- b. Secondary attack rate is 90%
- c. Lesions occurs in flexors
- d. Reactivation occur in 10-30%

MEASLES

34. Which one of the following is most complication of measles infection in children?
- a. Otitis media b. Bronchopneumonia
- c. Encephalitis d. Diarrhea

35. In an area not covered by measles immunization, the attack rate of measles is
- a. 70% b. 80%
- c. 90% d. 100%

36. Measles is caused by:
- a. DNA paramyxovirus
- b. Human herpes virus 3
- c. Orthomyxo virus
- d. Toga virus

37. Measles epidemic can occur when proportion of susceptible children is about:
- a. 10% b. 20%
- c. 40% d. 60%

38. Case fatality rate of measles in India is:
- a. 1% b. 4%
- c. 7% d. 12%

39. Most common age of infection for measles:
- a. <6 months b. 6 months-3 yrs
- c. >5 yrs d. >10 yrs

40. Epidemics of measles are common in India in:
- a. October to April
- b. January to July
- c. July to December
- d. Throughout the year

41. Koplik's spot - which is not true?
- a. Appear 1–2 days before rash
- b. Appear opposite 1st & 2nd upper molar
- c. Small bluish white spots
- d. Occur in other exanthematous fever also

42. Which of the following is not a complication of measles?
- a. Diarrhea b. Pneumonia
- c. SSPE d. Pancreatitis

43. Vitamin deficiency common in severe measles is
- a. Vitamin K
- b. Vitamin D
- c. Vitamin A
- d. Vitamin C

44. Measles vaccine can be given at 6-8 months of age:
- a. In malnourished children
- b. If measles outbreak
- c. If child is unlikely to return at 9 months of age
- d. All of the above

45. Measles vaccination is effective if given within days of exposure to susceptible contacts:
- a. 1 day
- b. 3 days
- c. 7 days
- d. 10 days

46. For eradication of measles, immunization coverage should be at least:
- a. 60%
- b. 85%
- c. 95%
- d. 100%

47. Which of the following is the 'Least common' complications for measles? *(Recent Question 2017)*
- a. Diarrhea b. Pneumonia
- c. Otitis media d. SSPE

48. Most common cause of death due to measles is:
- a. Otitis media
- b. Diarrhea
- c. Measles encephalitis
- d. Pneumonia

Ans.

24. b
25. b
26. d
27. d
28. d
29. b
30. c
31. a
32. b
33. a
34. d
35. c
36. b
37. a
38. c
39. b
40. a
41. d
42. d
43. c
44. d
45. b
46. c
47. d
48. d

Most Recent Questions of 2019-18 are given at the end of MCQs

49. Isolation period, false is: *(Recent Question 2017)*
a. Chicken pox – 6 days after onset of rash
b. Herpes zoster- 6 days after onset of rash
c. Measles – up to 3 days after onset of rash
d. German measles – 7 days after onset of rash

50. The incubation period of Measles is:
a. 3 days
b. 10 days
c. 21 days
d. 30 days

51. Post-exposure Measles vaccine must be administered within how many day(s) of exposure:
a. 3 day
b. 7 days
c. 1 days
d. 10 days

52. Second attack rate is minimum in:
a. TB
b. Diphtheria
c. Measles
d. Whooping cough

53. Catch-up, keep-up and follow-up is the WHO's elimination strategy for:
a. Measles
b. Polio
c. Leprosy
d. Rubella

54. Supplementary immunization service for measles immunization comprise? *(Recent Question 2017)*
a. Keep up with >95% immunized
b. Catch up
c. Follow up
d. All of the above

55. Frequency of SSPE after measles attack is:
a. 1: 10000
b. 1: 100000
c. 1: 30000
d. 1: 300000

56. True statement regarding Measles are all, except:
a. Common in summer
b. Incubation period is 10-14 days
c. Infectivity decreases after the appearance of rash
d. Measles vaccine is live attenuated

57. True regarding the appearance of measles rash is:
a. Rash appears 1–2 days after appearance of Koplik spot
b. Rash appear 1–2 days before appearance of Koplik spot
c. Along with Koplik spot
d. None of the above

58. Measles vaccination campaign between 9-14 years age for elimination is: *(Recent Question 2017)*
a. Keep up
b. Fellow up
c. Mop up
d. Catch up

59. To eradicate measles the percentage of infant population to be vaccinated is at least ______%
a. 70
b. 80
c. 85
d. 95

60. Most serious complication of measles is:
a. Koplik spots
b. Parotitis
c. Meningoencephalitis
d. Nephritis

MUMPS AND RUBELLA

61. All of the following statements are true about Congenital Rubella <u>except:</u>
a. It is diagnosed when the infant has IgM antibodies at birth
b. It is diagnosed when IgG antibodies persist for more than 6 months
c. Most common congenital defects are deafness, cardiac malformations and cataract
d. Infections after 16 weeks of gestation result in major congenital defects

62. All are features of rubella <u>except</u>
a. Source of infection is a case
b. No subclinical case
c. No carrier state for postnatally acquired rubella
d. Infants with congenital rubella excrete virus

63. Complication of rubella is all <u>except</u>
a. Arthralgia
b. Thrombocytic purpura
c. Myocarditis
d. Congenital malformation

64. The most widely used diagnostic test for rubella is
a. Elisa
b. RIA
c. HaI Test
d. Virus isolation

65. Classical triad of congenital rubella syndrome includes all <u>except:</u>
a. PDA
b. Deafness
c. Microcephalus
d. Cataract

66. After which week of gestation, rubella does <u>not</u> cause major abnormalities of fetus
a. 8th
b. 12th
c. 16th
d. 20th

67. All are features of RA 27/3 rubella vaccine <u>except:</u>
a. Produced in human diploid fibroblast
b. Produces high antibody titre
c. Does not prevent subclinical infection with wild virus
d. Immunity is life-long.

68. Recommended vaccination strategy for rubella is to vaccinate which age group on priority during rubella outbreak
a. Women 15-39 yrs (non pregnant)
b. Infants
c. Women 15-39 yrs (pregnant)
d. Adolescent girls 10-19 years

69. Causative agent for mumps is:
a. Arbovirus
b. Rhabdovirus
c. Flavivirus
d. Myxo virus

70. Incidence of mumps is highest among:
a. 0-5 yrs
b. 5-15 yrs
c. 15-95 yrs
d. >25 yrs

71. Incubation period for mumps is:
a. 4-7 Days
b. 1-2 weeks
c. 2-4 weeks
d. >4 weeks

72. Incubation period of Mumps is:
a. 7 days
b. 10 days
c. 14 days
d. 18 days

INFLUENZA

73. The type of influenza causing pandemics:
a. A
b. B
c. C
d. Any of the above

Ans.
49. d
50. b
51. a
52. a
53. a
54. b
55. d
56. a
57. a
58. d
59. d
60. c
61. d
62. b
63. c
64. c
65. c
66. c
67. c
68. a
69. d
70. b
71. c
72. d
73. a

74. **Major epidemics of influenza A occurs at interval of:**
a. 2–3 yrs b. 3–5 yrs
c. 4–7 yrs d. 10–15 yrs

75. **All are features of influenza epidemics except:**
a. Affects majorly young girls 10–19 years
b. Increase incidence of respiratory infections
c. Sickness absenteeism from schools
d. Increase hospitalization of cases

76. **Rapid spread of influenza occurs because of all except:**
a. Short Incubation Period
b. Large no. of sub-clinical cases
c. Presence of cross immunity
d. Short duration of immunity
e. High proportion of susceptible population

77. **Which of the following is not true about influenza virus?**
a. Influenza virus A is subject to frequent antigenic variation
b. Antigenic drift is a gradual antigenic change over a period of time
c. Antigenic shift is due to genetic recombination of virus
d. Major epidemics are due to antigenic drift

78. **All of the following is true about influenza except:**
a. Antigenic drift is due to point mutation
b. Influenza C virus is antigenically stable
c. Recent epidemics are caused by HI N I type
d. Infant & person>65 yrs are low risk groups

79. **The most serious complication of influenza is:**
a. Myocarditis b. Pneumonia
c. Encephalitis d. Pancreatitis

80. **Which of the following influenza vaccine can be given as nasal drugs?**
a. Killed vaccine
b. Live attenuated vaccine
c. Split virus vaccine
d. Neuraminidase specific vaccine
e. Recombinant vaccine

81. **All of the following are used in treatment of Influenza B, except:**
a. Oseltamivir
b. Zanamivir
c. Peramivir
d. Ribavirin

82. **Incubation period less than 5 days is:** ***(Recent Question 2015)***
a. Influenza
b. Salmonella typhi
c. Vibrio parahemolyticus
d. Yersinia
e. Swine flu

83. **Major reason for H5N1 not to become a global pandemic is:**
a. Route of transmission is not respiratory
b. Man to man transmission is rare
c. Does not cause serious disease among humans
d. Restricted to few countries only

84. **Following statement is true about Influenza:**
a. Source of infection: is a case
b. Period of infectivity is 5 days before to 5 days after onset of symptoms
c. Subclinical case is not seen
d. All of the above

85. **As per WHO a confirmed case of Swine Flu (H1N1) is a person with acute febrile respiratory illness and lab confirmation by all the following tests, except:**
a. Real time PCR
b. ELISA
c. 4 fold rise in virus specific neutralising antibodies
d. Virus culture

86. **Drug used in treatment/prophylaxis of influenza is:**
a. Acyclovir b. Rimantidine
c. Oseltamivir d. Amantidine

87. **Incubation period of Swine flu:** ***(Recent Question 2016)***
a. 1-3 days b. 2-3 weeks
c. 10-15 days d. 5 weeks

88. **Which of the following lead to an outbreak of Influenza in China in 2013?**
a. H1N1 b. H3N2
c. H2N2 d. H7N9
e. H5N1

89. **Pig in H1N1 influenza acts as:**
a. Carrier b. Amplifying host
c. Intermediary host d. Vector

DIPHTHERIA

90. **Fatality rates for diphtheria in untreated cases is**
a. <0.5%
b. 2-3%
c. 10%
d. 70%

91. **The most common source of infection for diphtheria is:**
a. Clinical case
b. Subclinical case
c. Chronic Carrier
d. Incubatory Carriers

92. **The major clinical types of diphtheria include all except:**
a. Anterior nasal b. Conjunctival
c. Faucial d. Laryngeal

93. **All are true of carrier state in diphtheria except:**
a. Incidence 0.1-5% in community
b. Immunization prevents carrier state
c. Chronic carrier persists for a year
d. Nasal carriers are particularly dangerous

94. **Infective period of diphtheria is:**
a. From 1 wk after exposure to 3 months
b. 14–28 days from onset of the disease
c. 4–6 days before onset of symptoms and a week there after
d. None of the above

95. **Diphtheria is commonest in age group:**
a. <1 yrs b. 1–5 yrs
c. 1–15 yrs d. 10–15 yrs

96. **To prevent epidemic spread of diphtheria herd immunity should be at least:**
a. 50% b. 70%
c. 80% d. 90%

97. **More commonly immunity to diphtheria is acquired through:**
a. Maternal Ab
b. Immunization with DPT
c. Inapparent infection
d. Acquiring the disease

Ans.

74. a
75. a
76. c, d
77. d
78. d
79. b
80. b
81. d
82. a, c, d, e
83. b
84. a
85. b
86. c
87. a
88. d
89. c
90. c
91. c
92. b
93. b
94. b
95. b
96. b
97. c

Most Recent Questions of 2019-18 are given at the end of MCQs

98. Incubation period of diphtheria is:
a. 1–2 days b. 2–6 days
c. 6–10 days d. 10–14 days

99. Which of the following is not true about diphtheria?
a. Grayish black membrane on posterior pharynx or tonsil
b. Membrane can be removed easily
c. Minimal mucosal erythema surrounding the membrane
d. Cutaneous diphtheria is common in tropics

100. Isolation of all suspected diphtheria cases is done till:
a. Symptoms subside
b. 2 consecutive swabs are -ve
c. Schick test is -ve
d. Ab titre decrease

101. The drug of choice for treatment of diphtheria carrier is:
a. Sulphadiazine b. Erythromycin
c. Rifampicin d. Tetracycline

102. Management of non-immunized close contacts of diphtheria include:
a. Erythromycin b. Diphtheria antitoxin
c. Immunization d. All of the above

103. Severe reaction to DPT includes all except:
a. Progressive hepatitis
b. Convulsions
c. Anaphylactic reaction
d. Persistent screaming episode

104. Incubation period of Diphtheria and Salmonella is:
a. 1-2 days and 20-40 days b. 2-6 days and 7-21 days
c. 2-6 days and 10-14 days d. 1-2 days and 10-14 days

105. Management of non immunized diphtheria contacts include all, except: *(Recent Question 2016)*
a. Prophylactic penicillin
b. Single dose of Toxoid
c. Daily throat examination
d. Daily throat swab culture
e. Weekly throat swabs examination

106. Reduction in cases of Diphtheria, reported in recent surveillance reports is due to:
a. Immunization
b. Chemoprophylaxis
c. Health Education
d. Improvement in standard of living

107. A herd immunity of over..........% is considered necessary to prevent epidemic spread of diphtheria:
a. 50% b. 55%
c. 60% d. 70%

PERTUSSIS

108. Which is not true regarding B. pertussis?
a. The source of infection is only a case of pertussis
b. Chronic carriers are main source of infection
c. Chronic carriers are not known to occur
d. Subclinical infection is not known to occur

109. Which of the following is not true regarding Pertussis?
a. Most infections during paroxysmal stage
b. Affects infants & preschool children
c. Highest mortality in infants <6 months
d. Recovery is followed by immunity pertussis

110. A 5-year-old sister of a neonate is suffering from pertussis, which has been documented by isolation and culture of the organism. Most appropriate statement regarding this clinical situation is:
a. If mother has received pertussis vaccine, the neonate is protected
b. Hyperimmune globulins indicated for the neonate
c. Erythromycin prophylaxis is indicated in the neonate
d. DPT vaccine is recommended for the elder child before birth of a child

111. True about Pertussis is/are:
a. Incubation period is 7-14 days
b. Main source of infection is chronic carriers
c. All ages are affected
d. Secondary attack rate in unimmunized persons is 90%
e. More common in Summer

112. True about epidemiology of pertussis is?
a. Incubation period of 7-14 days
b. Chronic carriers are source of infection
c. All age groups are equally susceptible
d. Secondary attach rate is 40% in unimmunized children

MENINGOCOCCAL MENINGITIS

113. All are true regarding meningococcal meningitis except:
a. Cases are important source of infection
b. Case Fatality rate in treated cases is <10%
c. Group A & C causes epidemic
d. Predominant in children

114. Most common serotype of Meningococcus responsible for epidemics worldwide is: *(Recent Question 2016)*
a. A b. C
c. Y d. W-135

115. All of the following statements with reference to meningococcal meningitis are correct, except:
a. Fatality in untreated cases is 60%
b. Disease spreads mainly by droplet infection
c. Treatment of cases has no significant effect in epidemiological pattern of disease
d. Mass chemoprophylaxis causes immediate drop in incidence rate of cases

116. Vaccine for meningococcal meningitis should be routinely given to: *(Recent Question 2016)*
a. Laboratory workers
b. Young adolescents
c. 4-8 years old children
d. Elderly population

117. WHO criteria for high endemicity of meningococcal disease include:
a. 0.1%
b. 0.01%
c. 0.001%
d. 1.0%

118. Meningococcal vaccine available is:
a. ACW135Y
b. ABCW135
c. CYW135B
d. ABCY

Ans.

98. b
99. b
100. b
101. b
102. d
103. a
104. c
105. b, d
106. a
107. d
108. b
109. a
110. c
111. a, d
112. a
113. a
114. a
115. b
116. b
117. b
118. a

Most Recent Questions of 2019-18 are given at the end of MCQs

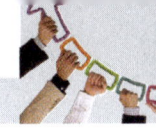

TUBERCULOSIS

119. Tuberculin test is a cheap and easily available test. In which of the following situations there is high failure in interpretation of result? ***(Recent Question 2016)***
a. Environmental mycobacterium infections are less
b. High prevalence of immunized people
c. High prevalence of disease
d. Lesser number of HIV positive cases

120. WHO defines Multi-drug resistant (MDR) Tuberculosis strain as one that is:
a. At least resistant to INH
b. At least resistant to Rifampicin
c. Resistant to INH and Rifampicin with or without resistant to other anti TB drugs
d. Resistant to Streptomycin only

121. Duration of treatment of MDRTB cases:
a. 8-12 months
b. 12-18 months
c. 18-24 months
d. 24-27 months

122. Extremely drug resistance Tuberculosis is defined as:
a. Resistance to isoniazid and rifampicin
b. Resistance to a fluoroquinolone
c. Resistance to amikacin
d. All the above

123. TB Research Center is located at: ***(Recent Question 2016)***
a. Chennai
b. New Delhi
c. Bangalore
d. Ahmedabad

124. True statement with regards to TB in a diabetic is:
a. Severity of TB increases
b. Incidence of TB increases
c. Course of TB disease changes
d. All of the above

125. Targets of WHO 'Stop TB strategy' are all, except:
a. 70% of people with sputum positive TB will be diagnosed by 2005
b. To cure 100% of sputum positive TB cases
c. Reducing prevalence to 150/100000/year by 2015
d. To reduce global incidence of TB less than or equal to 1 case per million per year by 2050

126. A patient with sputum positive pulmonary TB who has taken anti-TB drugs for <4 weeks is classified as: ***(Recent Question 2016)***
a. Relapse case
b. Default case
c. Treatment failure case
d. New case

127. A person presented with persistent cough for about 2 months along with low grade fever. His sputum smear examination was positive for AFB in the first examination; but negative in the second examination. The chest X-ray were consistent with pulmonary tuberculosis. The disease will be classified as:
a. Sputum negative pulmonary TB
b. Sputum positive pulmonary TB
c. To be reviewed after 2 weeks of antibiotic therapy
d. Repeat sputum microscopy after 1 month

128. Practical index of tuberculosis case load in the community is:
a. Incidence rate
b. Prevalence rate
c. Tuberculosis conversion index
d. Secondary attack rate

129. Percentage of individuals who show a positive reaction to a standard tuberculin test is the:
a. Prevalence of infection
b. Prevalence of disease
c. Incidence of infection
d. Tuberculin conversion index

130. In tuberculosis, the following rate reveals the impact of control measures: ***(Recent Question 2016)***
a. Prevalence of infection
b. Tuberculin conversion index
c. Case rate
d. Incidence of new cases

131. Epidemic marker of TB:
a. Sputum AFB positivity rate
b. Tuberculin test positivity rate
c. Chest X-ray positivity rate
d. None of the above

132. In RNTCP, one tubercular unit covers how much population:
a. 1,00,000
b. 5,00,000
c. 2,00,000
d. 1000

133. Cure rate to be achieved in RNTCP:
a. 70%
b. 85%
c. 60%
d. 95%

134. As per WHO, investigation for latent TB infection is not done in: ***(Recent Question 2014)***
a. Patients on dialysis
b. Silicosis
c. Patient on TNF inhibitors
d. Chronic alcoholics

135. The most appropriate test to assess the prevalence of tuberculosis infection in a community is:
a. Mass miniature Radiography
b. Sputum examination
c. Tuberculin test
d. Clinical examination

136. Incidence of TB in a community measured by:
a. Sputum smear positivity
b. Positive Tuberculin test
c. Sputum culture
d. Mantoux test positive

137. Contacts of sputum positive TB patient who should be given preventive chemotherapy: ***(Recent Question 2016)***
a. Pregnant women
b. Old people
c. Children above 6 years
d. Children below 6 years

138. Naranjo algorithm is used for:
a. Environmental factors effecting drug
b. Parameter based data evaluation
c. Calculating probability of adverse drug reaction
d. Demographic factor affecting drugs action

139. One of the following is known as Tuberculin conversion index:
a. Incidence of infection
b. Prevalence of infection
c. Incidence of disease
d. Prevalence of disease

140. Number of (+) for tubercle bacilli if count in AFB sample is >10 per oil immersion fields:
a. +
b. ++
c. +++
d. Scanty

141. Mycobacterium tuberculosis infection in humans is most common because of: ***(Recent Question 2016)***
a. Contact
b. Inhalation
c. Infiltration
d. Inoculation

Ans.
119. b
120. c
121. d
122. d
123. a
124. d
125. b
126. d
127. b
128. b
129. a
130. b
131. a
132. c
133. b
134. d
135. c
136. a
137. d
138. c
139. a
140. c
141. b

Most Recent Questions of 2019-18 are given at the end of MCQs

142. Xpert MTB/RIF test is used to detect:
a. For assessing resistance to isoniazid
b. For assessing multi drug resistant TB
c. For assessing Rifampicin resistance
d. Monitoring drug response in MDR TB
e. Diagnosis of TB

143. TB multidrug regimen is given to:
a. Prevent resistance b. Broad spectrum
c. Prevent side effects d. None

144. One TB infected person can infect how many people in one year:
a. 20 b. 30 *(Recent Question 2016)*
c. 10 d. 5

145. Tuberculin positive means:
a. Immunodeficient patient
b. Resistance to tuberculin protein
c. Patient is infected with mycobacterium
d. Patient is suffering from disease

146. Antitubercular drug which cause Optic neuritis is:
a. Ethambutol b. Rifampicin
c. Isoniazid d. Pyrizinamide

147. Treatment of choice for sputum positive pulmonary TB detected in the 1st trimester of pregnancy is:
a. Defer treatment till 1st trimester
b. Start category I immediately.
c. Start category II immediately
d. Start category III immediately

148. Mc Keown's theory on decline in the incidence of infectious disease like TB is better understood in terms of:
a. Increased awareness and knowledge
b. Medical advancement
c. Behavioural modification
d. Social and economic factors

149. The population of a community on the 1st of June was recorded as 1,65,000. Total no. of new cases of Tuberculosis, recorded from 1st January to 31st June were 22. Total Registered cases of tuberculosis in the community were recorded as 220. What is the incidence of TB in this community:
a. 133 per 100,000 b. 1.33 per 100,000
c. 220 per 100,000 d. 100 per 100,000

150. Which of the following is not false about annual risk of TB?
a. ARI of 1% = 75 cases new cases
b. Current ARI in India is 4.7
c. It represents new cases of TB
d. It is assessed by Tuberculin conversion in previously non-vaccinated children.

151. In which of the following patient, bedaquiline may not be administered:
a. 35-year-old, with XDR TB
b. 20-year-old, with XDR TB resistant to any FQ and any SLI
c. 16-year-old with XDR TB resistant to all FQ and any SLI
d. 58-year-old with treatment failure of XDR TB

INTESTINAL INFECTION

Poliomyelitis

152. Most out breaks of polio are due to:
a. Type I virus b. Type II virus
c. Type III virus d. All of the above

153. Which of the following is not true about polio
a. Man is the only reservoir
b. Subclinical infections occur and are the main role in spread
c. Females more commonly affected
d. Most vulnerable age is 6 months to 3yrs
e. IP - 7–14 days
f. Feco-oral spread

154. For every case of polio the estimated No. of subclinical cases is
a. 10 b. 50
c. 500 d. 1000

155. Vaccine associated paralytic polio is due to which virus in OPV:
a. Type I b. Type 2
c. Type 3 d. All

156. Incubation period of Vaccine associated paralytic poliomyelitis is: *(Recent Question 2016)*
a. 1-2 hours b. 1-3 days
c. 7-10 years d. 4-30 days

157. Which of the following statements about Polio is true:
a. Type 1 virus is the most antigenic
b. Type 2 virus causes most epidemics
c. Type 1 is most easily eradicable
d. Type 3 is responsible for VAPP

158. Which of the following serotypes of Polio virus is most commonly associated with vaccine associated paralytic poliomyelitis?
a. Serotype 1 b. Serotype 2
c. Serotype 3 d. Serotype 1 and 2

159. Incidence of Vaccine Associated Paralytic Poliomyelitis is:
a. 1 per 100000 birth cohort
b. 1 per 1000000 birth cohort
c. 4 per 100000 birth cohort
d. 4 per 1000000 birth cohort

160. Follow-up of a case of AFP to check for residual paralysis is done at
a. 30 days b. 45 days
c. 60 days d. 90 days

161. Find the false statement regarding polio:
a. Line listing is done to check for duplication
b. Line listing is done to identify high risk pockets
c. Mopping up is done in low risk districts
d. Mopping up is done where wild polio virus is suspected

162. All the following are true regarding pulse polio immunization, except: *(Recent Question 2015)*
a. Simultaneous mass administration of OPV on a single day to all children 0-5 years of age
b. Occurs as two rounds about 4-6 weeks apart during low transmission season of polio
c. The dose do not replace the doses received during routine immunization services
d. There should be minimum 4 weeks interval between PPI and scheduled OPV doses

163. The 107 block plan is related to the control/eradication on the following disease:
a. Plaque
b. Polio
c. Malaria
d. STD

Ans.
142. c, e
143. a
144. c
145. c
146. a
147. b
148. d
149. b
150. d
151. c
152. a
153. c
154. d
155. c
156. d
157. d
158. c
159. d
160. c
161. c
162. d
163. b

Most Recent Questions of 2019-18 are given at the end of MCQs

164. Which of the following is not a type of vaccine derived polio virus? *(Recent Question 2014)*
a. cVDPV b. i VDPV
c. aVDPV d. mVDPV

165. Polio virus is shed maximum in stool up to:
a. 6 weeks b. 8 weeks
c. 10 weeks d. 12 weeks

166. Wild poliomyelitis is still endemic in:
a. Sri Lanka b. Pakistan
c. India d. Afghanistan
e. Nigeria

167. True about complete eradication of poliomyelitis from India is:
a. From 2012 onwards, no vaccine associated polio case has been detected
b. Last polio case in India was reported in 13 January 2011
c. Mostly IPV is used currently
d. India is the only country which is not able to eliminate it completely

168. Regarding poliovirus responsible for poliomyelitis all are true, except: *(Recent Question 2015)*
a. Type 3 is most common is India
b. Type 1 is most common in India
c. Type 1 is responsible for most epidemics
d. Type 2 is eradicated worldwide

HEPATITIS

169. The 1st antibody to appear against Hepatitis B is
a. Anti HBs b. Anti HBe
c. Anti HBc d. Anti HBm

170. Marker for infectivity of serum in Hepatitis B is:
a. HBs Ag b. Anti HBc
c. HBe Ag d. Anti HBC

171. The persistent (Chronic) carrier state in hepatitis B is defined as HBs Ag present in Blood more than:
a. 2 months b. 6 months
c. 4 months d. 9 months

172. Which of the following is not a component of WHO 5 C's approach
a. Consent b. Communitisation
c. Counseling d. Confidentiality
e. Correct test results f. Connections

173. Which of the following is correct for control and management of hepatitis?
a. Treatment for hepatitis B is started when the HBV DNA is >2000 IU/mL
b. the assessment of cirrhosis is done when AST-to-platelet ration index of more than 10
c. HBV is a monovalent recombinant vaccine
d. Complete vaccination provides lifelong immunity for more than 95%

174. Correct statements about hepatitis E:
a. Water borne
b. Chronic carrier 5-15%
c. Fulminant infection in pregnancy
d. RT-PCR is the investigation of choice

175. Which of the following viral markers signify ongoing viral replication in Hepatitis-B infection?
a. Anti-HBs b. Anti-HBc
c. HBe Ag d. HBs Ag

176. Transplacental transmission is not seen in:
a. Hepatitis A
b. Hepatitis B
c. HIV
d. Varicella

177. Both HBsAg and HBeAg are positive in:
a. Acute infectious hepatitis B
b. Chronic hepatitis B
c. Recovery phase of Hepatitis B
d. Individuals vaccinated with Hepatitis B

178. A nurse was diagnosed to have HBeAg and HBsAg in serum. Most likely she is having:
a. Chronic hepatitis B
b. HBV + HBE coinfection
c. Active and infectious Hepatitis B disease
d. Recovery from Hepatitis B

179. Most important in diagnosing Acute Hepatitis B infection is: *(Recent Question 2015)*
a. IgG Anti HBc
b. IgM Anti HBc
c. Anti HBs
d. HbsAg

180. A person positive for HBsAg, Anti HBc IgG,HBeAg, Anti HBe antibody can be diagnosed as having:
a. Acute Hepatitis B infection
b. Recovered Hepatitis B infection
c. Chronic Hepatitis B infection with high infectivity
d. Vaccination

181. 1955 Hepatitis outbreak in Delhi was:
a. A b. B
c. C d. E

182. A mother is HBsAg positive at 32 weeks of pregnancy. What should be given to the newborn to prevent neonatal infection?
a. Hepatitis B vaccine + Immunoglobulin
b. Immunoglobulin only
c. Hepatitis B vaccine only
d. Immunoglobulin followed by vaccine 1 month later

183. Acute Hepatitis B marker(s) is/are:
a. HBsAg b. Anti-HBs
c. Anti-HBc d. HBeAg
e. Anti HBe

184. Isolation period of Hepatitis A:
a. 1 weeks b. 2 weeks
c. 3 weeks d. 4 weeks

ACUTE DIARRHEAL DISEASE

185. Total osmolarity of WHO reduced osmolarity ORS (in mmol/litre) is: *(Recent Question 2015)*
a. 245 b. 275
c. 300 d. 345

186. ORS once prepared should be used within....
a. 1 hour b. 6 hours
c. 12 hours d. 24 hours

187. Role of sodium citrate in ORS is all, except:
a. To correct dehydration
b. To correct acidosis
c. To increase absorption of glucose
d. To correct electrolyte imbalance

Ans.
164. d
165. d
166. b, d
167. b
168. a
169. c
170. c
171. b
172. b
173. c
174. a,c
175. c
176. a
177. a
178. c
179. b
180. c
181. d
182. a
183. a,c, d
184. c
185. a
186. d
187. c

Most Recent Questions of 2019-18 are given at the end of MCQs

188. Persistent diarrhea in infants:
a. 7 days
b. 14 days
c. 21 days
d. 1 month

189. ORS contains 75 mmol/litre of:
a. Sodium
b. Potassium
c. Glucose
d. Chloride

190. Ratio of Sodium: Glucose in WHO reduced Osmolarity ORS is: *(Recent Question 2015)*
a. 1:4
b. 1:3
c. 1:2
d. 1:1

191. Dehydration in a child with diarrhea, thirst present, tears absent is:
a. Mild
b. Moderate
c. Severe
d. None

192. A 12 kg child with diarrhea, fluid to be replaced in first 4 hours:
a. 0–400 mL
b. 400–800 mL
c. 800–1200 mL
d. 1200–1600 mL

193. ORS amount required in first 4 hours in a 1-year-old child with dehydration is:
a. 200–400 mL
b. 400–600 mL
c. 600–800 mL
d. 800–1200 mL

194. New WHO ORS osmolarity is:
a. 270
b. 245
c. 290
d. 310

195. ORS should be discarded after:
a. 54 hours
b. 6 hours
c. 12 hours
d. 24 hours

196. Concentration of sodium in mMol/L in low osmolar ORS is: *(Recent Question 2015)*
a. 45
b. 75
c. 90
d. 60

CHOLERA

197. Mechanism of action of Cholera toxin is through:
a. Gangliosides
b. Adenyl cyclase
c. Gangliosides + adenyl cyclase
d. Exotoxin

198. Chemoprophylaxis is indicated in all of the following, except: *(Recent Question 2014)*
a. Cholera
b. Meningococcal meningitis
c. Plague
d. Typhoid

199. Chemoprophylaxis is not required in:
a. Conjunctivitis
b. Meningitis
c. Measles
d. Plague

200. True of 8th Pandemic of Cholera:
a. Startedin Bangladesh
b. Originated in 2012
c. Due to O139 Strain
d. Low attack rate
e. Low proportion of adults in endemic regions

201. A village effected with epidemic of cholera, what is the 1st step which should be taken in village to decrease the death to cholera: *(Recent Question 2015)*
a. Safe water supply and sanitation
b. Cholera vaccination to all individuals
c. Primary chemoprophylaxis
d. Treat everyone in the village with tetracycline

202. Incubation period for cholera:
a. 1 – 7 days
b. Few hours to 5 days
c. 2 weeks
d. 4 weeks

203. Disinfection of stool to prevent contamination of cholera epidemic is: *(Recent Question 2015)*
a. Cresol
b. Bleaching powder
c. Phenol
d. Sodium hypochlorite

204. Drug of choice for cholera chemoprophylaxis is:
a. Erythromycin
b. Ampicillin
c. Ciprofloxacin
d. Tetracycline

205. Incubation period of which disease is less than 7 days:
a. Cholera
b. Measles
c. Leishmaniasis
d. Mumps

TYPHOID

206. Reservoir of Enteric fever is: *(Recent Question 2014)*
a. Birds
b. Cattle
c. Man
d. Cow

207. Incubation period of typhoid is:
a. 1-2 days
b. 10-14 days
c. 1 month
d. 4-6 hours

FOOD POISONING

208. Shortest incubation period in food poisoning is seen with:
a. C. botulinum
b. Bacillus
c. E. coli
d. Staph aureus

AMEBIASIS/ASCARIASIS/ HOOKWORM INFECTION/ DRACUNCULIASIS

209. Chandler's Index is used for which of the following:
a. Hookworms
b. Round worms
c. Guinea worms
d. Sand fly

210. Chandler index of 350 indicates:
a. Hookworm infection is not of much significance
b. Hookworm infection regarded as potential danger
c. Hookworm infection – a minor public health problem
d. Hookworm infection–an important public health problem

211. Hookworm infection is considered as a major health problem, if the chandler's index is:
a. >300
b. >200
c. >100
d. >50

212. Chandler's Index is used for:
a. Ankylostoma Duodenale
b. Ascariasis Lumbricoides
c. Strongyloides
d. Trichuris trichiura

Ans.
188. b
189. a,c
190. d
191. b
192. c
193. b
194. b
195. d
196. b
197. b
198. d
199. c
200. c, e
201. a
202. b
203. a
204. d
205. a
206. c
207. b
208. d
209. a
210. b
211. a
212. a

213. **Chandler's Index is:**
a. No. of eggs of hookworm in 100 gram soil
b. No of eggs of hookworm in 1 gram soil
c. No of eggs of hookworm in 1gram stool
d. Percentage of stool specimens positive for hookworms

214. **Use of Chandler Index for hookworm include all, except:**
a. Assessment of endemicity
b. Monitoring individual treatment
c. Monitoring mass treatment of community
d. Comparison of worm load in different populations

215. **WHO considerations regarding dracunculiasis eradication, all are true, except:**
a. Drinking piped water and installation of hand pumps
b. DDT spray
c. Health education and awareness of public
d. Control of Cyclops

RABIES

216. **A classical case of Rabies is characterized by all except**
a. Variable incubation period
b. Short period of illness
c. Encephalomyelitis always present
d. Fatal only some cases

217. **A rabies free area has been defined as one where no case of indigenously acquired rabies has occurred for**
a. 1 year
b. 2 years
c. 3 years
d. 5 years

218. **All are true of Rabies virus except**
a. Bullet shaped virus
b. RNA virus
c. Has four serotypes
d. All serotypes cause rabies

219. **The virus recovered from naturally occurring cases is called**
a. Natural virus
b. Street virus
c. Fixed virus
d. Free virus

220. **All of the following are characteristic features of fixed virus except**
a. Long incubation period
b. Reproducible incubation period
c. Does not form Negri bodies
d. Does not multiply in extra-neural tissues

221. **The virus used in preparation of anti-rabies vaccine is**
a. Street virus
b. Fixed virus
c. Both of these
d. None of these

222. **In India, urban rabies is maintained by**
a. 1
b. 2
c. 3
d. 4

223. **In India, urban rabies is maintained by**
a. Dogs
b. Cats
c. Rats
d. Mongoose

224. **In India, all the following animals are reported to transmit rabies except**
a. Dogs
b. Jackal
c. Fox
d. Vampire bats

225. **All are features of Rabies in man except**
a. Dead end infection
b. Aerosol transmission is quite common
c. Common age group 1–24 years
d. All animals are susceptible to rabies

226. **The incubation in period rabies in man depends on**
a. Site of bite
b. Severity of bite
c. Number of wounds
d. All of the above

227. **The incubation period of rabies in man depends on**
a. Site of bite
b. Severity of bite
c. Number of wounds
d. All of the above

228. **Specific treatment for rabies is**
a. Anti rabies vaccine
b. Anti rabies serum
c. FTS Antibody
d. None of the above

229. **The rabies vaccine not given to person with sensitivity to egg protein is**
a. Adult sheep brain vaccine
b. Suckling mouse brain vaccine
c. Duck embryo vaccine (DEV)
d. Cell culture vaccine

230. **Advantages of cell culture vaccine includes**
a. More potency
b. Less side effects
c. Fewer injections of lower volume
d. All of the above

231. **The action of soap in washing bile wound by a rabid dog is**
a. Removal of dirt
b. Kills virus
c. Prevents virus from getting attached to nerve endings
d. Relieves pain

232. **The unique feature in rabies vaccine compared to other vaccines is that:**
a. Immunity is absolute
b. It is effective even after nerve infection
c. Can be given after exposure to infection
d. Booster doses are not necessary

233. **All the following are considered as Class I wounds for rabies management except**
a. Lick on healthy skin
b. Consumption of unboiled milk suspected animal
c. Small Bite on thigh
d. Scratches without oozing of blood

234. **Bites on all the following are considered as Class III except:**
a. Head
b. Face
c. Fingers
d. Toes

235. **Bites from wild animals are classified as**
a. Class I
b. Class II
c. Class III
d. Any of the above

236. **Immunoglobulin is particularly useful in case**
a. Where incubation period is short
b. Of wild animal bite
c. With severe exposure
d. All of the above

237. **Recommended dose of human rabies immunoglobulin (HRIG) is**
a. 10 IU/Kg
b. 20 IU/Kg
c. 30 IU/Kg
d. 40 IU/Kg

Ans.
213. c
214. b
215. b
216. d
217. b
218. d
219. b
220. a
221. b
222. a
223. a
224. b
225. b
226. b
227. d
228. d
229. c
230. d
231. b
232. c
233. c
234. d
235. c
236. d
237. b

Most Recent Questions of 2019-18 are given at the end of MCQs

238. Oral rabies vaccine has been introduced. For immunization of

a. Humans b. Dogs
c. Foxes d. Horses

239. A 10-year-old child with history of unprovoked Dog bite comes to you. Appropriate action would be:

a. Withhold vaccine and observe dog for 10 days
b. Administer cell culture derived vaccine
c. No further action is required
d. Kill the dog and send brain for biopsy

240. For the prevention of human rabies, immediate flushing and washing the wound(s) in animal bite cases, with plenty of soap and water, under running tab should be carried out for how much time? *(Recent Question 2015)*

a. 2 minutes b. 1 minutes
c. 15 minutes d. 5 minutes

241. Which of the following is a rabies free country?

a. Sri Lanka b. Bangladesh
c. Russia d. Australia

242. Speed of rabies virus in nerve is:

a. 3 mm/day
b. 3 mm/hour
c. 5 mm/day
d. 5 mm/hour

243. Pre exposure prophylaxis for Rabies is given on:

a. Days 0, 3, 7, 14, 28, 90
b. Days 0, 3, 7, 28, 90
c. Days 0, 3
d. Days 0, 7

244. Intermediate host of Rabies is:

a. Man b. Dog
c. Cow d. Rat

245. What is the recommended dose for Human Rabies Immunoglobulin (Ig) in a 4 month old child?

a. 20 IU/kg b. 30 IU/kg
c. 40 IU/kg d. 50 IU/kg

246. Characteristics features of Rabies include all, except:

a. Can manifest as ascending paralysis
b. Hematogenous spread to brain
c. Can be transmitted by bites other than dogs also
d. In invariably fatal

247. The intradermal plan according to Institut pasteur du cambodge schedule for day 0,3,7,14,28 is:

a. 2-2-2-0-0 b. 2-2-2-0-2
c. 1-1-1-1-0 d. 8-0-4-0-1

248. Number of doses of Rabies HDCV vaccine required for pre-exposure prophylaxis: *(Recent Question 2015)*

a. 5 b. 2
c. 3 d. 1

249. Which virus is used to produce rabies vaccine:

a. Wild b. Street
c. Fixed d. Live attenuated

SURFACE INFECTION

Trachoma

250. Drug of choice for mass treatment of Trachoma is:

a. Ciprofloxacin b. Tetracycline
c. Penicillin G d. Chloramphenicol

251. Single drug treatment recommended for trachoma control in India is:

a. Azithromycin b. Tetracycline
c. Erythromycin d. Penicillin

252. Trachoma screening is done on which of the following age-groups:

a. <5 years b. 5–10 years
c. 5–15 years d. 1–9 years

TETANUS

253. Spores of Clostridium tetani are sterilized by

a. Boiling b. Cresol- 15%
c. Autoclaving at 110°C d. None of the above

254. The reservoir of infection in tetanus is

a. Active case
b. Chronic carrier
c. Convalescent
d. None of the above

255. The elimination for Maternal and neonatal tetanus is defined as

a. <1 case per 100,000 population
b. <10 case per 100,000 population
c. <1 case per 1000 live births
d. <1 case per 100,000 Live births in an area

256. Neonatal tetanus most often manifests at

a. Birth b. 48 hours
c. 7th day d. 14th day

257. Purified tetanus toxoid should be stored at a temperature of

a. (-) 20 degree C b. 0 degree C
c. 4 degree C d. Room temperature

258. The prophylactic does of human tetanus immunoglobulin is

a. 250 IU b. 1000 IU
c. 2000 IU d. 4000 IU

259. Tetanus toxin acts on all of the following areas of nervous system except:

a. Brain
b. Spinal cord
c. Parasympathetic system
d. Sympathetic system

260. A person has received complete immunization against tetanus 10 years ago, now he presents with a clean wound without any lacerations from an injury sustained 3 hours ago. He should now be given:

a. Full course of tetanus toxoid
b. Single dose of tetanus toxoid
c. Human tetanus globulin
d. Human tetanus globulin and single dose of toxoid

261. As per RMNCH/NHM guidelines, the state is called as Neonatal Eliminated state, if the neonatal tetanus rate in state is

a. >10 per 1000 b. >1 per 1000
c. <1 per 10,000 d. <0.1 per 1000

262. True about tetanus is all, except:

a. Tetanus protection 5 years if previously immunized
b. Herd immunity present
c. Cant be eradicated
d. Eliminantion is less than 0.1 case per 1000 births

Ans.

238. c
239. b
240. c
241. d
242. b
243. d
244. b
245. a
246. b
247. a
248. b
249. c
250. b
251. b
252. d
253. d
254. d
255. c
256. c
257. c
258. a
259. c
260. b
261. d
262. b

Most Recent Questions of 2019-18 are given at the end of MCQs

263. All of the following are true statement regarding clostridium tetani, except:
a. The main reservoir is soil and intestine of animal and human
b. Herd immunity is not of much value
c. Seen commonly in winter and dry season
d. The main mode of transmission is through trauma and contaminated wound

LEPROSY

264. Leprosy is considered as a public health problem if the prevalence is more than.
a. 1 per 1000 b. 5 per 1000
c. 10 per 1000 d. 10 per lakh population

265. Following are true of M. leprae except:
a. Grows slowly in artificial media
b. Intracellular bacteria
c. Acid fast bacilli
d. Affinity to Schwann cells

266. Leprosy is transmitted by
a. Droplet infection
b. Contact transmission
c. Via breast milk
d. All of the above

267. Target for cure rate for multibacillary leprosy under programme implementation plan for 12th plan period:
a. >85% b. >80%
c. >75% d. >95%

268. In India, prevalence of leprosy per 10000 cases in 2012
a. 0.42 b. 0.68
c. 0.89 d. 1.20

269. Under NLEP, the following social workers are involved in bringing out suspected leprosy cases from their villages:
a. ASHA
b. Anganwadi workers
c. Multipurpose workers
d. Village health guide

270. In a patient of leprosy, 4 split skin smears were taken. 2 samples had 10 bacilli out of 100 oil immersion fields and 2 samples had >1000 bacilli on average in each fields. The Bacteriological index will be: *(Recent Question 2015)*
a. 4.5 b. 3.5
c. 5.5 d. 6.5

271. The target of NLEP was to reduce case load to:
a. 1 per 1000 population b. 1 per 10000 population
c. 1 per 100000 population d. 1 per million population

272. True regarding leprosy:
a. Clofazimine included in treatment regimen
b. Any positive smear 1+ is MBL
c. Grenz zone is lepromatous spectrum
d. All deformity cases are MBL
e. MBL recommended treatment is for 12 months duration

273. Lepromin test is used for all of the following, except:
a. Classify the lesions of leprosy patients
b. Determine the prognosis of disease
c. Assess the resistance of individuals to leprosy
d. Diagnosis of leprosy

274. Multibacillary is a spectrum of disease seen in:
a. Leprosy b. TB
c. Tetanus d. Trachoma

275. Elimination of leprosy is defined as prevalence:
a. <1 per 1000 b. <1 per 10000
c. <1 per 100000 d. <1 per 100

276. Prevalence of leprosy in India per 10000 is:
a. >1 b. 0.88
c. 0.71 d. 0.69

277. Erythema nodosum is seen in treatment of which type of leprosy: *(Recent Question 2015)*
a. Borderline leprosy b. Lepromatous leprosy
c. Tuberculoid leprosy d. None of the above

278. Which of the following about Lepromin test is not true?
a. It is negative in most children in first six month
b. It is a diagnostic test
c. It is an important aid to classify type of leprosy
d. BCG vaccination may convert Lepra reaction from negative to positive

279. Leprosy involves all, except: *(Recent Question 2015)*
a. Uterus b. Ovary
c. Nerve d. Eye

280. Mass chemoprophylaxis is endemic area is recommended for all of the following, except:
a. Yaws b. Leprosy
c. Trachoma d. Filaria

SEXUALLY TRANSMITED DISEASE (STD)

281. Colour of Kit 3 for STD under AIDS control program is:
a. Red b. Blue
c. White d. Green

282. A sexually active, long distance truck driver's wife comes with vaginal discharge. Under syndromic approach, which drug should be given: *(Recent Question 2015)*
a. Metronidazole, Azithromycin, Fluconazole
b. Metronidazole
c. Azithromycin
d. Metronidazole and fluconazole

283. Case detection in STD's is done by all except:
a. Screening b. Contact tracing
c. Cluster testing d. Notification

284. Mass chemoprophylaxis to the whole population is not recommended in:
a. Lymphatic filariasis b. Worm infestation
c. Scabies d. Vit A administration

AIDS

285. In case of accidental exposure, the postexposure HIV prophylaxis should be started immediately best within:
a. 2 hours b. 4 hours
c. 24 hours d. 72 hours

286. Most effective intervention to prevent vertical transmission of HIV is: *(Recent Question 2015)*
a. HAART
b. Zidovudine
c. Nevirapine
d. Elective CS

Ans.
263. c
264. a
265. a
266. d
267. d
268. b
269. a
270. b
271. b
272. a,c,e
273. d
274. a
275. b
276. d
277. b
278. b
279. a
280. b
281. c
282. d
283. d
284. c
285. a
286. a

Most Recent Questions of 2019-18 are given at the end of MCQs

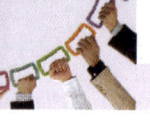

287. **Which states are qualified as high prevalence states in the context of HIV/AIDS?**
   a. When prevalence in high risk groups is more than 5%, and less than 1% in antenatal women
   b. When prevalence in high risk groups in more than 5%, and 1% or more in antenatal women
   c. When prevalence in high risk groups is less than 5%, and more than 1% in antenatal women
   d. None of these
288. **If the prevalence of HIV is >5% in one subpopulation and <1% in pregnant women it is called:**
   a. Generalized HIV epidemic
   b. Concentrated HIV epidemic
   c. High level HIV epidemic
   d. Low level HIV epidemic
289. **WHO defines HIV as generalized epidemic when the prevalence is:** *(Recent Question 2015)*
   a. >5% in a sub-population
   b. <5% in a sub-population
   c. <1% in pregnant women
   d. >1% in pregnant women
290. **All the following are components of national AIDS control and prevention policy 2002, except:**
   a. Blood safety program
   b. Avahan program
   c. Link worker scheme
   d. Targeted intervention among high risk groups
291. **Treatment 2.0 is a new approach for the treatment of:**
   a. HIV b. Tuberculosis
   c. Leprosy d. Obesity
292. **The services of Suraksha clinic are related to:**
   a. Acute diarrheal diseases b. Acute respiratory infections
   c. STD/RTI d. Family planning
293. **The following sub-population is considered as highest risk group of AIDS:** *(Recent Question 2015)*
   a. Homosexual men
   b. STD patients
   c. Population in conflict areas
   d. Clients of sex workers
294. **Antiretroviral prophylaxis decrease the chance of transmission of HIV to fetus during pregnancy by:**
   a. 35% b. 45%
   c. 50% d. 65%
295. **HIV virus was discovered in the year:**
   a. 1981 b. 1983
   c. 1986 d. 1996
296. **Risk of mother to child HIV transmission in pregnant women at the time of delivery, and after delivery in non breast feeding woman is:** *(Recent Question 2014)*
   a. 5-10% b. 10-15%
   c. 15-30% d. More than 50%
297. **HIV postexposure prophylaxis should be started in:**
   a. 2 hours b. 24 hours
   c. 48 hours d. 72 Hours
298. **HIV transmission mother to child can be stopped by all, except:**
   a. Cesarean section
   b. Vitamin A supplementation
   c. Stopping breast feeding
   d. Zidovudine mother antenatal and newborn after delivery
299. **Most common subtype HIV in India is:**
   a. HIV A
   b. HIV B
   c. HIV C
   d. None of above
300. **Criteria included in AIDS surveillance definition include:**
   a. Extrapulmonary TB b. Cryptococcosis
   c. Candidiasis d. All of above
301. **HIV sentinel surveillance is used to identify/ calculate:**
   a. High risk population
   b. Prevalence of HIV
   c. Trend finding among populations
   d. All of the above

MISCELLANEOUS

302. **Mode of spread of Ebola virus:** *(Recent Question 2014)*
   a. Aerogenous b. Body fluids
   c. Water-borne d. Insect bite
303. **All are true about SARS, except:**
   a. Incubation period is 3-5 days
   b. Effective vaccine with 82% protective efficacy
   c. Ribavirin is used for treatment
   d. Mortality rate is around 14%
304. **Rat is associated with:** *(Recent Question 2014)*
   a. Measles b. Leptospirosis
   c. Tetanus d. Influenza
305. **Drug of choice for Scabies in Pregnancy is:**
   a. Ivermectin b. Crotaminaton
   c. Benzyl benzoate d. Permethrin
306. **Most common subtype of Shigella in India is:**
   a. Shigella boydii b. Shigella sonnei
   c. Shigella dysenteriae d. Shigella flexneri
307. **Outbreaks of leptospirosis are usually expected after:**
   a. Earthquakes b. Floods
   c. Mud slides d. Avalanche
308. **Not true about Ebola virus is:** *(Recent Question 2014)*
   a. Caused by ss negative strand RNA virus
   b. Bats most likely reservoir
   c. Incubation period is less than 48 hours
   d. Sexual transmission possible
   e. Oseltamivir is quite effective in treatment

RNTCP

309. **According to WHO definition Tuberculosis control is achieved when TB positivity in age group 0 – 14 yrs is less then**
   a. 20% b. 10%
   c. 50% d. 1%
310. **Prevalence of disease in tuberculosis can be confirmed by:**
   a. Mass miniature radiograph
   b. Sputum microscopy
   c. Sputum culture d. Tuberculin test
311. **Trends of the TB problem in a community including impact of control measures is reflected by:**
   a. Prevalence of suspect cases
   b. Proportional mortality ratio
   c. Incidence of new cases
   d. All of the above

Ans.

287. b
288. b
289. d
290. b
291. a
292. c
293. a
294. c
295. b
296. c
297. a
298. b
299. c
300. d
301. d
302. b
303. b
304. b
305. d
306. d
307. b
308. c, e
309. d
310. b
311. c

312. After BCG vaccination individual become Mantoux positive after
a. 2 wks b. 5 wks
c. 8 wks d. 6 months

313. According to WHO, multidrug resistance strains is one that is at least resistant to:
a. Rifampicin and pyrazinamide
b. INH & thiacetazone
c. INH & ethambutol
d. INH & Rifampicin

314. Which of the following statements is true about BCG vaccination?
a. Distilled water is used as a diluent for BCG vaccine
b. The site for injection should be cleaned thoroughly with spirit
c. Mantoux test becomes positive after, 48 hours of vaccination
d. WHO recommends Danish 1331 strain for vaccine production

315. A patient with sputum positive pulmonary tuberculosis is on ATT for the last 5 months, but the patient is still positive for AFB in the sputum. This case refers to:
a. New case b. Failure case
c. Relapse case d. Drug defaulter

316. DOTS Supervisor under RNTCP cannot be:
a. Social Worker b. Father
c. Teacher d. Health Worker

317. Which of the following is a pitfall of DOTS?
a. High cure rate b. Prevents failure and MDR
c. Destigmatization d. High cost

318. Objective of RNTCP is to achieve cure rate of:
a. 70% b. 80%
c. 85% d. 100%

319. Drug not given under continuation phase of category I patient under RNTCP is:
a. Rifampicin b. Isoniazid
c. Ethambutol d. Pyrazinamide

320. National Strategic Plan for TB control (2012-2017) includes all, except:
a. Finding TB HIV +VE cases
b. Reduction in default case rate to <10% for new case and <5% for reinfection cases
c. Wages to ASHA on treatment completion
d. Benefit to patient treated in private hospital

321. Boxes given for sputum collection to a suspected TB case are labeled as: *(Recent Question 2014)*
a. a, b b. 1, 2
c. Y, Z d. A, B

322. A patient was diagnosed to have TB by a private practitioner. The case has to be informed to DTO within:
a. 1 day b. 7 days
c. 30 days d. 1 years

323. An 18-year-old HIV positive girl has been diagnosed to be suffering from sputum smear negative pulmonary tuberculosis. She had previously diagnosed with TB 5 years back and had complete course. The treatment regimen recommended under DOTS for her is:
a. 2 $(HRZE)_3$ + 4 $(HR)_3$
b. 2 $(HRZES)_3$ + 1 $(HRZE)_3$ + 5 $(HRE)_3$
c. 2 (HRZE) + 4 (HRE)
d. 2 (HRZE) + 6 (HRE)

324. 'NIKSHAY' software lunched by Central Government is used for tracking of:
a. High risk newborns b. Malaria
c. Tuberculosis d. High risk pregnancies

325. What is the category and color of the drug box for sputum smear positive cases who are 'treated after default' under the RNTCP?
a. Category 2, Yellow b. Category 1, Red
c. Category 2, Blue d. Category 1, Green

326. XDR – TB definition include resistance to:
a. Rifampicin b. Any one Fluoroquinolone
c. INH d. Kanamycin
e. Ethionamide

327. Under RNCTP diagnosis, TB bacilli take up AFB stain faster showing 'Beaded appearance' due to presence of:
a. Palmitic acid b. Wax D
c. Cord factor d. Mycolic acid

328. What is new change in Revised National Tuberculosis Control Programme (RNTCP):
a. DOTS based therapy
b. Diagnosis by Sputum smear miscroscopy
c. Non DOTS based therapy
d. Early diagnosis and treatment

329. Dose of Rifampicin in each FDC tablets for Adult patient with Tuberculosis is:
a. 150 mg b. 300 mg
c. 450 mg d. 600 mg

330. RNTCP diagnosis of TB is as follows:
a. 1 Sample out of 2 positive b. 2 Sample out of 3 positive
c. 3 Sample out 3 positive d. None

331. As per recent revision in RNTCP, Category II treatment comprises:
a. 2 HRZE + 4 HRE b. 4 HRZE + 2 HRE
c. 2 HRZES + 4 HRZE d. 4 HRZES + 2 HRZE

332. WHO was instrumental in foundation of which of the following program in India: *(Recent Question 2014)*
a. RNTCP
b. National Leprosy Eradication Program
c. Janani Suraksha Yojana
d. National old age pension plan

333. All are new revision to RNTCP except:
a. Same regime for Category I and II
b. Bedaquiline is drug of choice for Rifampicin resistant TB
c. In first line regime, the IP is not extended if sputum is positive at end of IP
d. Mono drug resistance with INH is treated with 6 months of Lfx R Z E

334. DOTS criteria for TB is positive if: *(Recent Question 2014)*
a. 1 out of 2 sputum positive
b. 2 out of 3 sputum positive
c. Chest X-ray positive
d. Mantoux positive

335. Why a TB patient is recommend a regimen of 4 drugs on 1st visit?
a. To avoid emergence of resistance
b. To avoid side effects
c. To cure disease early
d. None of the above

Ans.

312. c
313. d
314. d
315. b
316. b
317. d
318. c
319. d
320. b
321. a
322. c
323. c
324. c
325. c
326. a, b, c, d
327. d
328. c
329. a
330. a
331. a
332. a
333. b
334. a
335. a

Most Recent Questions of 2019-18 are given at the end of MCQs

336. RNTCP case finding is: *(Recent Question 2014)*
a. Active b. Passive
c. Both d. None

337. Features of RNTCP A/E:
a. Active case findings is not done
b. Included in NRHM in 2005
c. Teachers act as DOTS agent
d. Microscopy center is established/1 lakh population
e. Achievement of at least 70% cure rate

NACP

338. Postexposure prophylaxis for HIV is:
a. Lamivudine + Ritonavir for 4 weeks
b. Zidovudine + Lamivudine for 4 weeks
c. Zidovudine + Lamivudine + Indinavir for 4 weeks
d. Lamivudine + Tenofovir for 4 weeks

339. Behavioral surveillance survey is done if:
a. TB b. AIDS
c. Malaria d. Filaria

340. WHO recommendations for initiating anti-retroviral treatment (ART) in HIV +ve individuals is:
a. CD4 cells less than 250 cells/mm³
b. CD4 cells less than 200 cells/mm³
c. CD4 cells less than or equal to 350 cells/mm³
d. None of above

341. National Pediatrics AIDS Initiative was launched in:
a. 05 September 2005 b. 30 November 2006
c. 02 October 2008 d. 02 November 2010

342. Link worker scheme comes under which National health program:
a. RNTCP b. NACP
c. NLEP d. ICDS

343. Sentinel surveillance for HIV under National AIDS control program is used for all,except:
a. Estimation of total infection in community
b. Estimation of total cases in hospitals
c. Estimation of trend of the disease
d. Classifications of districts

344. Which of the following RTI/ STI color coded kits wrongly matched? *(Recent Question 2014)*
a. Kit 1 – Grey
b. Kit 2 – Green
c. Kit 3 – White
d. Kit 4 – Red

345. According to Suraksha Clinic National AIDS Control Program, a women coming with lower abdominal pain, the color code of kit in treatment is:
a. White
b. Yellow
c. Green
d. Grey

NATIONAL HEALTH POLICY & NATIONAL POPULATION POLICY

346. India aims to eliminate the following diseases except:
a. Leprosy b. Kala azar
c. Filariasis d. Dengue

NLEP

347. In case of multibacillary leprosy target cure rate under PIP for 12th Five-Year Plan:
a. >75% b. >80%
c. >85% d. >90%

348. Adequate treatment in case of Paucibacillary Leprosy is considered as if the patient has received the 6 monthly doses of combined therapy within:
a. 6 months b. 9 months
c. 12 months d. 15 months

349. Which of the following anti leprotic drugs is not given in blister packs of NLEP?
a. Dapsone b. Rifampicin
c. Clofazimine d. Minocycline

350. Multibacillary leprosy follow-up duration:
a. 12-18 months b. 2 years
c. 5 years d. 10 years

351. Treatment of paucibacillary leprosy drugs used are:
a. Dapsone
b. Dapsone, rifampicin
c. Rifampicin, Clofazimine
d. Dapsone, Rifampicin, Clafazimine

352. National Leprosy Eradication Program started in:
a. 1949 b. 1955
c. 1973 d. 1983

353. Two years duration in terms of leprosy is with regard to:
a. Treatment of paucibacillary leprosy
b. Treatment of multibacillary leprosy
c. Post-treatment surveillance of paucibacillary leprosy
d. Post-treatment surveillance of multibacillary leprosy

NATIONAL POLIO ERADICATION PROGRAMME

354. Target group for pulse polio immunization is:
a. 0-1 years b. 0-3 years
c. 0-5 years d. 0-10 years

355. In the listing of cases of acute flaccid paralysis is done for all of the following reasons except *(Recent Question 2014)*
a. To check for duplication
b. To document high risk groups
c. To confirm year of onset of illness
d. To identify high risk population

356. Acute flaccid paralysis surveillance, evaluation for residual paralysis is done at: *(Recent Question 2014)*
a. 6 weeks
b. 6 months
c. 60 days
d. 90 days

357. In Acute Flaccid paralysis, examination for residual paralysis should be done after:
a. 30 days
b. 60 days
c. 90 days
d. 120 days

358. Pulse polio immunisation covers:
a. 0–5 years children
b. 0–1 years children
c. 1–5 years children
d. 0–2 years children

Ans.
336. c
337. e
338. d
339. b
340. d
341. b
342. b
343. b
344. d
345. b
346. d
347. d
348. b
349. d
350. c
351. d
352. d
353. c
354. c
355. d
356. c
357. b
358. a

ARTHROPOD-BORNE DISEASE

359. All are true about dengue hemorrhagic fever, except:
a. Lamivudine is drug of choice
b. More than 20 petechiae/2.5 sq cm is positive tourniquet test
c. Transmitted by Aedes
d. Causative agent belongs to flaviviridae group

360. "Saddle back" fever is known as:
a. Brucellosis
b. Dengue fever
c. Malaria fever
d. Typhoid fever

361. Malaria recrudescence is: *(Recent Question 2014)*
a. Resistant to treatment
b. Relapse of infection
c. Relapse in Vivax and Ovale
d. Reappearance of sexual stage parasitemia after treatment

362. Cycle that is seen in RBC's in malaria
a. Sexual
b. Sporogony
c. Exogenous
d. Endogenous

363. Extrinsic incubation period of Plasmodium is:
a. 7-10 days
b. 10-20 days
c. 20-25 days
d. 21-30 days

364. Which is not true for dengue fever?
a. Aedes aegypti is the principal of vector
b. Break bone fever is characteristic
c. Serotype 4 is more dangerous than other serotypes
d. Tourniquet test is positive

MALARIA

365. In a patient of malaria, if fever has periodicity of 72 hours causative agent is: *(Recent Question 2014)*
a. P. falciparum
b. P. vivax
c. P. ovale
d. P. malariae

366. In area with API >2, if the insecticides are refractory to DDT:
a. Regular spray with 1 round of malathion
b. Regular spray with 3 rounds of malathion
c. Regular spray with 1 round of pyrethroids
d. Regular spray with 2 rounds of pyrethroids

367. Under national vector borne disease control program (NVBDCP), integrated vector management (IVM) is done by using identical vector control methods to control:
a. Malaria and leishmaniasis in rural area
b. Malaria and filarial in urban area
c. Malaria and dengue in rural area
d. Malaria and chikungunya in urban areas

368. Under Modified plan of operation, the criteria for indoor residual spray (IRS) are prioritized. All of the following are true, except:
a. Areas with >5 API where ABER is 10% or more
b. Areas reporting >5% SPR, if ABER is <10%
c. If Pf proportion is <50%
d. API <5 or SPR <5% in case of drug resistant foci, project areas with population migration and aggregation

369. Behavior change communication (BCC) is a systematic process that motivates individuals and communities to change their inappropriate or unhealthy behavior or to continue a healthy behavior. BCC is a key supportive strategy for: *(Recent Question 2013)*
a. Coronary heart disease prevention
b. Malaria prevention
c. STD prevention
d. Accident prevention

370. The following rate measures endemicity of malaria in the community:
a. Infant parasite rate
b. Annual parasite incidence
c. Annual blood examination rate
d. Spleen rate

371. Operational efficacy of malaria in a community is indicated by:
a. Slide positivity rate
b. Infant parasite rate
c. Annual parasite incidence
d. Annual blood examination rate

372. Find the false statement regarding malaria chemoprophylaxis for short term:
a. Doxycycline daily, stated the day before arrival
b. Chloroquine weekly, 1 week before arrival
c. Mefloquine weekly, 2-3 weeks before arrival
d. Artesunate weekly, 1 day before arrival

373. The following is an anti-larval measure in malaria vector control measure:
a. Indoor residual sprays
b. Space application
c. Individual protection
d. Source reduction

374. All the following are true regarding anopheles fluviatilis except: *(Recent Question 2013)*
a. Main vector in urban and industrial areas
b. Propagate malaria at lower densities (efficient vector)
c. Highly anthrophilic (high preference for human blood)
d. Breed in moving water

375. As per new WHO 2013 malaria treatment guidelines and drug policy 2013. True regarding falciparum malaria is:
a. No ACT in falciparum malaria
b. Presumptive treatment with chloroquine should be given
c. Primaquine is contraindicated in infants and pregnant women
d. No primaquine in falciparum malaria

376. The following is/are true regarding malaria surveillance and management
a. Active case detection in rural area by multipurpose workers during fortnightly house visits
b. Passive case detection at sub-centers by rapid diagnostic tests
c. Passive case detection at PHCs by examination of blood smears
d. All the above

377. Treatment of uncomplicated falciparum malaria in pregnancy: *(Recent Question 2013)*
a. Chloroquine
b. Artemisinin
c. Mefloquine
d. Doxycycline

378. Prophalaxis for malaria not used:
a. Doxycycline
b. Artesunate
c. Chloroquine
d. Mefloquine

Ans.
359. a
360. b
361. d
362. d
363. b
364. c
365. d
366. b
367. c
368. c
369. b
370. d
371. d
372. d
373. d
374. a
375. c
376. d
377. b
378. b

Most Recent Questions of 2019-18 are given at the end of MCQs

379. Chemoprophylaxis of malaria can be done by all, except:
a. Chloroquine b. Mefloquine
c. Proguanil d. Primaquine

380. Incubation period of Plasmodium vivax is:
a. 5-7 days b. 7-10 days
c. 10-14 days d. 15-30 days

381. Cyclopropagative cycle is seen in:
a. Malaria b. Filarial
c. Yellow fever d. Plague

382. True abut malaria in India is/are:
a. 1.5 million cases annually
b. Quinine is drug of choice in severe malaria in pregnancy
c. Anopheles culicifacies is vector in urban malaria
d. Plasmodium ovale is not seen in India
e. Falciparum malaria is most common type.

383. All of the following factors contribute to resurgence of malaria, except:
a. Drug Resistance in host
b. Drug Resistance in parasite
c. Vector resistance to DDT
d. Antigenic variations in parasite

384. Anti malaria month is: *(Recent Question 2013)*
a. April b. May
c. June d. September

LYMPHATIC FILARIASIS

385. The rate which measures the mosquito positive for stage III larvae is
a. Infection rate b. Infectivity rate
c. Endemicity rate d. Mosquito density rate

386. The currently given regimen for Bancroftian filariasis is
a. DEC - 6 mg/ kg/day × 21 days
b. DEC - 6 mg/kg/day × 12 days
c. DEC - 100 mg/day × 21 days
d. DEC - 100 mg/day × 12 days

387. Diethylcarbamazine is very effective in killing
a. Microfilaria
b. Adult filarial worms
c. Infective stage larva
d. All of these

388. Filariasis does not cause explosive epidemic because
a. Parasite does not multiply in vector
b. Larvae do not multiply in host.
c. Long life cycle
d. All of the above

389. To eliminate lymphatic filariasis, Government of India launched annual mass drug administration (MDA) in which co-administration of the following drugs has been upscaled to cover population at risk:
a. DEC + Albendazole
b. DEC + Mebendazole
c. DEC + Ivermectin
d. DEC + Dapsone

390. Mass drug therapy is used in:
a. Cholera
b. Typhoid
c. Filaria
d. Diphtheria

391. All of the following are helpful for elimination of filariasis, except:
a. Microfilariae do not multiply in vectors
b. They multiply in humans
c. Larvae are deposited on skin surface where they cannot survive
d. Mass drug administration

YELLOW FEVER

392. The causative organism of yellow fever belongs to the family of
a. Alpha virus b. Flavivirus
c. Reovirus d. Poxvirus

393. Jungle yellow fever is primarily a disease of
a. Man b. Dogs
c. Foxes d. Monkeys

394. All are features of yellow fever except
a. Sub clinical cases present
b. Fatality rate >90%
c. One attack gives life-long immunity
d. Hepatic and renal involvement in severe cases

395. Classical vector of yellow fever is
a. Aedes b. Culex
c. Anopheles d. All of the above

396. Incubation period of yellow fever is
a. 1–2 days b. 3–10 days
c. 10–20 days d. 20–25 days

397. The index measuring percentage of houses in an area showing actual bleeding of A. aegypti larvae is
a. Aedes aegypti index b. Yellow fever index
c. Container index d. Breteau index

398. The index measuring number of positive containers for 100 houses is
a. Ae. aegypti index
b. House index
c. Container index
d. Breteau index

399. Which is correct regarding administration of 17D vaccine
a. 0.5 mL Intramuscular dose
b. 1 mL Intramuscular dose
c. 0.5 mL subcutaneous dose
d. 1 mL subcutaneous dose

400. Following yellow vaccine, immunity begins within
a. 1–2 days
b. 10–12 days
c. 2–3 weeks
d. 4 weeks

401. The main reason why yellow fever does <u>not</u> exist in India is
a. High vaccination coverage
b. Vector is absent
c. Environmental conditions nor suitable
d. None of the above

402. Mass immunization is used for: *(Recent Question 2013)*
a. Cholera
b. Dengue fever
c. Yellow fever
d. KFD

Ans.
379. d
380. c
381. a
382. a, b, e
383. a
384. c
385. b
386. b
387. a
388. d
389. a
390. c
391. c
392. b
393. d
394. b
395. a
396. b
397. a
398. d
399. c
400. b
401. d
402. c

Most Recent Questions of 2019-18 are given at the end of MCQs

403. **All of the following statements about Yellow fever are true, except:**
  a. One attack confers lifelong immunity
  b. India is a "Receptive area"
  c. Causative agent is Flavivirus Fibricus
  d. Validity of certificate of vaccination begins 10 days after vaccination and extends till 5 years
404. **Yellow fever vaccination starts protection after how many days of injection:** *(Recent Question 2013)*
  a. 5 days b. 10 days
  c. 15 days d. 20 days
405. **Which is not true about yellow fever?**
  a. Exotic
  b. Incubation period 2-6 days
  c. Validity of vaccine 6 years
  d. Live attenuated 17D strain vaccine
406. **Yellow fever certificate of vaccination is valid for:**
  a. 1-year b. 10 years
  c. 35 years d. Lifelong
407. **To prevent yellow fever Aedes aegypti index should be less than....**
  a. 0.5% b. 1%
  c. 2% d. 5%
408. **Yellow fever certificate of vaccination is valid for:**
  a. 6 years, starting from 6 days after vaccination
  b. 10 years, starting from 10 days after vaccination
  c. 10 years, starting from 6 days after vaccination
  d. Lifelong, starting from 10 days after vaccination

JAPANESE ENCEPHALITIS

409. **All of the following are true regarding Japanese encephalitis vaccine, except:** *(Recent Question 2013)*
  a. Boaster does are given after 1 year and repeated every 3 years
  b. Not given for infants less than 6 months age
  c. Two primary doses given to children aged 1-3 years age
  d. In endemic areas, vaccination is given to cover children 1-9 years age
410. **JE virus life cycle is nature run between:**
  a. Pigs- Mosquito
  b. Cattle- Birds
  c. Pigs – Human
  d. Bird – Pigs
411. **Amplifier for Japanese encephalitis:**
  a. Horse b. Dogs
  c. Pigs d. Monkey
412. **Japanese encephalitis is transmitted by:**
  a. Culex b. Aedes
  c. Mansonia d. Anopheles
413. **Which is not transmitted by Aedes aegypti?**
  a. Yellow fever
  b. Dengue
  c. Japanese encephalitis
  d. Filariasis
414. **False regarding Japanese encephalitis is:**
  a. Occurs in children more than adults
  b. Mosquito bite always results in disease
  c. Apparent and nonapparent cases ratio is 1: 1000
  d. Epidemic is defined as occurrence of 2-3 cases in a village

KFD AND CHIKUNGUNYA FEVER

415. **All the following arbovirus belong to Group B flavivirus except:**
  a. Dengue b. JE
  c. KFD d. Chikungunya
416. **All are true of extra human hosts for JE virus except:**
  a. Pigs are major hosts
  b. Cattle & buffaloes are mosquito attractants
  c. Infected pigs manifest disease
  d. Some species of birds are involved
417. **The most important breeding place for Culex tritaeniorhynchus is**
  a. Overhead ranks b. Rice fields
  c. Shallow ditches d. Artificial water collections
418. **All the following regarding Japanese Encephalitis vaccine in India, are true except:**
  a. Live attenuated vaccine
  b. Single dose, booster not needed
  c. Dose – 0.5mL, subcutaneous
  d. It is given in 2 doses at least 3 months apart in upper left arm
419. **In which state in India is Kyasanur Forest disease prevalent?**
  a. Kerala b. Tamil Nadu
  c. Karnataka d. AP
420. **The vector for KFD is**
  a. Aedes aegypti b. Haemaphysalis
  c. Culex d. Xenopsylla
421. **The tick population involved in transmission of KFD is mostly maintained by**
  a. Monkey b. Cattle
  c. Ardeid birds d. Fox
422. **Chikungunya is transmitted by:** *(Recent Question 2013)*
  a. Aedes b. Culex
  c. Mansonoides d. Anopheles
423. **True about Arboviruses is:**
  a. Yellow fever is endemic in India
  b. Dengue has only one serotype
  c. KFD was first identified in West Bengal
  d. Chikungunya is transmitted by Aedes aegypti
424. **Arboviral infections include:**
  a. Chikungunya fever b. West Nile fever
  c. JE d. Sandfly fever
  e. Malaria

PLAGUE

425. **In India, the main reservoir of plague transmission is**
  a. *Rattus rattus*
  b. *Bandicota bengalensis*
  c. *Tatera indica*
  d. *Mus booduga*
426. **Index which is an indicator of potential explosiveness of plague outbreak:** *(Recent Question 2013)*
  a. Total flea index b. X. cheopis index
  c. Specific % of fleas d. Burrow index
427. **Plague is transmitted by:**
  a. Hard tick b. Soft tick
  c. Rat flea d. Louse

Ans.

403. d
404. b
405. c
406. d
407. b
408. d
409. d
410. a
411. c
412. a
413. c
414. b
415. d
416. c
417. b
418. b
419. c
420. b
421. c
422. a
423. d
424. a, b, c, d
425. c
426. b
427. c

Most Recent Questions of 2019-18 are given at the end of MCQs

428. Maximum explosiveness of plague is determined by:
a. Total flea index
b. Cheopis index
c. Borrow index
d. Specific percentage of fleas

429. Severity of spreading of plague detected by:
a. Burrow's index b. Cheopis index
c. Specific flea index d. Total flea index

430. Most important and potential agent that can be used in bioterrorism is: *(Recent Question 2013)*
a. Plague
b. Small pox
c. TB
d. Clostridium botulinum

RICKETTSIAL DISEASES

431. The antibiotics of choice for specific treatment of Rickettsial infection is:
a. Tetracycline b. Penicillin
c. Erythromycin d. Ampicillin

432. At present, vaccine is available against which Rickettsial infection
a. Scrub typhus b. Murine typhus
c. Indian tick typhus d. Q fever

433. Epidemic typhus is caused by
a. R. prowazeki b. R. typhi
c. R. tsutsugamushi d. R. conorii

434. The Rickettsial infection in which there is no skin lesion is
a. Epidemic typhus b. Indian tick typhus
c. Q Fever d. Scrub typhus

435. The most widespread Rickettsial infection is
a. Epidemic typhus b. Indian tick typhus
c. Murine typhus d. Scrub typhus

436. All are features of Scrub typhus except:
a. Resembles epidemic typhus clinically
b. Not reported in India
c. Strongly positive with Proteus OXK
d. Mite is reservoir of infection

437. All are true statements regarding Q fever except
a. Present in Punjab and Rajasthan
b. Caused by Coxiella burnetii
c. Tick borne infection
d. No rashes

438. Rash starting peripherally is a feature of:
a. Epidemic typhus
b. Endemic typhus
c. Scrub typhus
d. Q fever

439. Following is NOT caused by virus:
a. Rocky Mountain Spotted Fever
b. KFD
c. Dengue
d. Yellow fever

440. Epidemic typhus cause and vector is:
a. Rickettsia prowazekii and Louse
b. R. typhi and Mite
c. R. conori and Tick
d. R. akari and Mite

441. Scrub typhus is caused by:
a. R. typhi b. R. Akari
c. R. prowazekii d. R. tsutsugamushi

442. Transmission of Epidemic Typhus occurs by:
a. Bite of louse
b. Ingestion of infective material
c. Crushing of louse on body
d. All of the above

443. Vagabond disease transmitted by:
a. Louse b. Mite
c. Tick d. Black fly

444. Scrub typhus is transmitted by:
a. Flea b. Mite
c. Tick d. Mosquito

445. Endemic typhus is transmitted by:
a. Louse b. Flea
c. Mite d. Tick

446. Epidemic typhus is transmitted by:
a. Louse b. Soft tick
c. Hard tick d. Rat flea

447. Not spread by Louse is: *(Recent Question 2014)*
a. Epidemic Typhus b. Q fever
c. Relapsing fever d. Trench fever

448. All are true about Scrub Typhus, except:
a. Mite is a vector
b. Adult mite feeds on vertebral host
c. Caused by R. tsutsugamushi
d. Tetracycline is treatment

NVBDCP

449. Drug of choice for mass therapy under the Filaria control program is:
a. Albendazole b. DEC
c. Ivermectin d. Mebendazole
e. Praziquantel

450. Larvicide used under Urban Malaria scheme is
a. DDT b. Abate
c. Parathion d. Malathion

451. Malaria target for 2012-2017 is:
a. API <1 per 1000 b. API <0.5 per 1000
c. API <10 per 1000 d. API <15 per 1000

452. All of the following are true regarding Strategic Plan for Malaria Control 2012-17, except:
a. API <1 per 1000
b. 50% mortality reduction by 2017
c. Annual incidence <10 per 1000
d. Complete treatment to at least 80% patients

453. A patient was admitted with fever and microscopy of blood smear was positive for P. Falciparum. Treatment recommended as per the revised drug policy 2013 is:
a. 50 mg Artesunate × 3 day + Sulfadoxine and Pyrimethamine (500 mg and 25 mg) single dose + Primaquine × 14 days
b. 200 mg Artesunate + Sulfadoxine and Pyrimethamine (750 mg and 37.5 mg) daily for 3 days
c. 4 mg/kg daily Artesunate × 3 day + Sulfadoxine and Pyrimethamine (25 mg/1.25 mg/kg) single dose + Primaquine 0.75 mg /kg single dose
d. 4 mg/kg Artesunate if patient were pregnant and in 2nd trimester

Ans.
428. b
429. b
430. a
431. a
432. d
433. a
434. c
435. d
436. b
437. c
438. c
439. a
440. a
441. d
442. c
443. a
444. b
445. b
446. a
447. b
448. b
449. a, b, c
450. b
451. a
452. c
453. c

454. Diseases under National Vector Borne Disease Control Program are: *(Recent Question 2013)*
a. Malaria, Filariasis, KFD
b. Malaria, Filariasis, Epidemic Typhus
c. Malaria, Dengue, Kala-azar
d. Malaria, Chikungunya, KFD

455. Which of these is not an element of the Roll Back Malaria Project?
a. Early detection of malaria illness
b. Rapid treatment of those who are ill
c. Provision of Impregnated bed nets
d. Strengthening of health sector and intersectoral activities

456. A pregnant woman in third trimester having fever was diagnosed as a case of Falciparum malaria. Under the National Health Program, which drug is recommended?
a. ACT only
b. ACT with a single dose of Primaquine on day 2
c. Chloroquine
d. Quinine only

457. As per the revised 2013 Malaria Drug Policy 2013, true statement is: *(Recent Question 2013)*
a. Presumptive treatment with Chloroquine is given
b. ACT is not given in Falciparum malaria
c. Primaquine is contraindicated in infants and pregnant women
d. Primaquine is not given in Falciparum malaria

458. Dose of chloroquine when used for chemoprophylaxis of Malaria is:
a. 300 mg twice/week b. 600 mg once/week
c. 600 mg/week d. 300 mg once/week

459. Treatment of severe Falciparum malaria is:
a. Chloroquine b. Mefloquine
c. Quinine d. Primaquine

460. In a town of population of 100,000 the number of slides examined is 5000. Out of these, 100 slides were positive for malaria. The API is: *(Recent Question 2015)*
a. 2 b. 5
c. 1 d. 0.5

461. In Roll Back Malaria Program, which of the following is not a component:
a. Training for health care workers
b. Using insecticide-treated bed nets
c. Developing newer insecticides
d. Strengthening health system

462. NVBDCP does not include:
a. Zika virus disease b. Filariasis
c. Kala-azar d. Chikungunya fever

463. Urban malaria scheme is based on: *(Recent Question 2014)*
a. API levels
b. Anti-adult measures
c. Anti-larval measures
d. Drug based treatment

464. Burden of malaria is best established by:
a. Mosquito rate b. API
c. Parasite rate d. SPR

ARI

465. Average number of ARI attacks per child per year is:
a. 1–3 **b. 3–5**
c. 8–10 d. >10

466. Bronchopneumonia secondary to influenza is usually caused by:
a. Streptococcus pyogenes b. Staphylococcus pyogenes
c. Klebsiella pneumonia d. Legionella pneumonia

467. Indications for admission in a one year old child who is suffering from ARI is:
a. Chest in drawing b Respiratory rate >40
c. Cough d. Fever above 100F

468. A mother in a village has brought her 1 month baby with a complaint of fever to the PHC. You find that the baby's respiratory rate is 69/minute. The baby is irritable but able to feed; the baby does not have chest indrawing or stridor. There is no history of convulsions. According to the RCH program, the baby's illness is classified as:
a. Very severe disease b. No pneumonia: cough or cold
c. Severe pneumonia d. Pneumonia

469. A 1-year-old child is brought with symptoms suggesting pneumonia. One examination chest indrawing is present. No other severe abnormality found from history and examination. The child is classified to have
a. Very severe pneumonia *(Recent Question 2015)*
b. Severe pneumonia
c. Pneumonia
d. Cough and cold

470. A 1-month-old infant presenting with cough and sneezing, respiratory rate 40 per minute, and there is no chest in drawing. The management is:
a. Urgent referral to hospital
b. IV antibiotics
c. Frequent breastfeeding
d. Oral antibiotic syrup

471. An 11-month-old child brought to PHC with respiratory rate 58 per minute and cough, there is no chest in drawing. Next step of management: *(Recent Question 2013)*
a. Reassurance to parent b. Urgent referral to hospital
c. Antibiotic with home care
d. Nasal saline drop

472. A 10-month-old child is brought to a PHC with history of cough and cold. On examination, he has respiratory rate of 48 per minute and there is absence of chest indrawing. His weight is 5 kg. He is probably suffering from
a. No pneumonia b. Pneumonia
c. Severe pneumonia d. Very severe pneumonia

473. Not evaluated in Clinical evaluation pneumonia at PHC
a. Respiratory rate b. Inability to feed
c. Oxygen saturation d. Chest in drawing

474. Most important feature to diagnose severe pneumonia:
a. Cyanosis b. Chest indrawing
c. Nasal flaring d. Fast breathing

475. According to IMNCI, fast breathing in 5 months child is defined as *(Recent Question 2013)*
a. >30/min b. >40/min
c. >50/min d. >60/min

OTHER INFECTIONS

476. The most virulent and invasive species of Brucella is
a. B. melitensis b. B. abortus
c. B. suis d. B. canis

Ans.

454. c
455. a
456. a
457. c
458. d
459. c
460. c
461. c
462. a
463. c
464. b
465. b
466. b
467. a
468. d
469. b
470. c
471. c
472. d
473. c
474. b
475. c
476. a

Most Recent Questions of 2019-18 are given at the end of MCQs

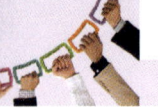

477. High risk groups for brucellosis include
a. Farmers b. Shepherds
c. Butchers d. All of the above

478. The most common mode of transmission of Brucellosis is through
a. Contact infection b. Food borne infection
c. Air borne infection d. Vectors

479. The antibiotic of choice, in uncomplicated case of Brucellosis is?
a. Tetracycline b. Streptomycin
c. Penicillin d. Ampicillin

480. Human live vaccine is available against which species of Brucella?
a. B. mefitensis b. B. abortus
c. B. suis d. B. canis

481. Trachoma is transmitted by following routes except
a. Direct contact
b. Venereal transmission
c. Vector borne transmission
d. Corneal transplantation

482. Human cysticerosis is caused by
a. T solium
b. T Saginata
c. Both the above
d. None of the above

483. Definitive host for T. saginata is
a. Man
b. Cattle
c. Pig
d. None of the above

484. 1nterrnediate host for T. solium is
a. Man b. Cattle
c. Pig d. None of the above

485. The definitive host for Echinococcus is
a. Man b. Dog
c. Sheep d. Cattle

486. The intermediate host for E. granulosis is
a. Man b. Sheep
c. Cattle d. All of the above

487. ln India highest prevalence of Hydatid disease are reported in
a. Kerala &. Karnataka b. AP &. Tamil Nadu
c. Rajasthan &. Gujara d. Bihar &. W. Bengal

488. The most prevalent from. of Leishmaniasis in India is _____ Leishmaniasis
a. Visceral
b. Cutaneous
c. Mucocutaneous
d. Post kala azar

489. The proven vector of Leishmaniasis in India is
a. P. argentipes
b. P. papatasi
c. P. sergentii
d. None of the above

490. Post kalaazar dermal Leishmaniasis is caused by
a. L. donovani
b. L. brazilensis
c. L. tropica
d. None of the above

491. The insecticide which is most efficient in the control of kalaazar is
a. DDT
b. Malathion
c. Fenitrothion
d. BHC

492. The most dangerous type of flea involved in Plague transmission is
a. Blocked flea
b. Partially blocked flea
c. Flea which just had blood meal
d. Flea not fed on blood meal

493. The drug of choice for Chemoprophylaxis of plague is
a. Erythromycin
b. Streptomycin
c. Tetracycline
d. Penicillin

494. The most common manifestation of Salmonellosis is
a. Gastroenteritis
b. Pyelonephritis
c. Arthritis
d. Meningitis

495. Most peripheral unit of microscopic center of TB is:
a. District microscopy center
b. Tuberculosis unit
c. Peripheral DOTS center
d. Designated microscopy center

496. New RNTCP software online TB monitoring is:
a. Nirbhya
b. e-DOT
c. Nikshay
d. Nischay

497. Prevalence of Kala-azar is not seen in:
a. UP
b. Bihar
c. Assam
d. West Bengal

498. Annual new case detection rate of leprosy as on 31st March, 2016 is:
a. 0.66/10,000 population b. 9.7/1,00,000 population
c. 0.66/1,00,000 population d. 9.7/10, population

499. World Rabies day is:
a. 29 April
b. 7 April
c. 30 January
d. 28 September

500. Which is true for MDA (Mass Drug Administration)
a. MDA is done with DEC and Ivermectin in India
b. Transmission assessment survey is done in under 5 children
c. MDA is done after a filariasis survey in all age groups
d. The MDA coverage should be more than 50% in the endemic zones

501. Random blinding, rechecking is for:
a. NHM
b. RNTCP
c. NACP
d. NPSP – national polio surveillance program

Ans.

477. d
478. a
479. a
480. b
481. d
482. a
483. a
484. c
485. d
486. d
487. b
488. b
489. a
490. a
491. a
492. b
493. c
494. a
495. d
496. c
497. c
498. b
499. c
500. c
501. b

Most Recent Questions of 2019-18 are given at the end of MCQs

502. **Regarding ZIKA virus all are correct except:**
   a. The sample should be refrigerated (2-8 deg) and sent within 48 hrs
   b. A BSL-2 containment level lab is required to process the suspect samples
   c. RT-PCR is diagnostic for zika disease
   d. Viral isolation is the gold standard

503. **The standard dose for human tetanus hyperimmunoglobulin is:**
   a. 100 IU b. 150 IU
   c. 200 IU d. 500 IU

504. **The dose for Sulphadoxine in 15 year old boy for Pl. Falciparum infection is:**
   a. 500 mg
   b. 750 mg
   c. 1500 mg
   d. 2500 mg

505. **The Theme for 2019 World TB day is:**
   a. It's time
   b. Universal Health coverage
   c. Everyone, Everywhere
   d. 90-90-90 target

Most Recent Questions (2019-2018)

506. **The below pictures indicated the life cycle of:** *(AIIMS Nov 2018)*

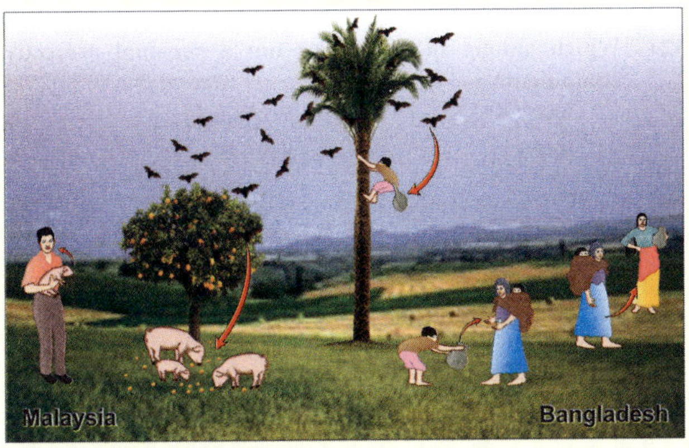

   a. Japanese encephalitis
   b. Influenza
   c. Nipah virus
   d. Chandipura virus

507. **Period of isolation for measles is from:** *(AIIMS Nov 2018)*
   a. Onset of catarrhal symptoms to 3 days after rash
   b. Onset of catarrhal symptoms to 14 days after rash
   c. Onset of rash to 7 days after
   d. Onset of rash to 14 days after

508. **Which of the following drugs are entry inhibitors for HIV** *(PGI Nov 2018)*
   a. Ibalizumab
   b. Maraviroc
   c. Raltegravir
   d. Enfuviritide
   e. Darunavir

509. **True statement regarding varicella zoster in pregnancy** *(PGI Nov 2018)*
   a. Congenital anomalies is more when 1st trimester infection
   b. Highest chances of anomalies are with 2nd trimester infection
   c. Max chances of transmission when 4 days before to 3 days after Pregnancy
   d. Higher chances of herpes zoster in infancy
   e. Higher chances of microcephaly in infants born to VZV exposed mothers

510. **Which of the following is correct for Hep B vaccination to pregnant females** *(PGI Nov 2018)*
   a. Dose is 10-20 mcg at 0,1,6 months during pregnancy
   b. In case of accidental exposure to Hepatitis B infected blood in a pregnant female, the HBIG is given in dose of 0.05 ml/kg within 6 hours of accidental exposure
   c. To prevent effectively prevent the perinatal transmission of HBV infection, the birth dose Hep B vaccine should be given within 7 days of birth
   d. Both Hep B Vaccine and HBIG is contraindicated in pregnancy
   e. HBIG (Hep B Immunoglobulin) may be given while HepB vaccine is contraindicated in pregnancy

511. **GeneXprt** *(PGI Nov 2018)*
   a. Detects DNA sequence by PCR
   b. Investigation for detection of HIV infection
   c. Investigation for detection of TB infection and rifampicin resistance
   d. Results obtained within 48 hours
   e. Based on assessment of growth index and O_2 utilization in a specialized media

512. **Mass chemoprophylaxis is done for** *(PGI Nov 2018)*
   a. Soil transmitted helminthiasis
   b. Lymphatic filariasis c. Trachoma
   d. Meningococcal infection e. Cholera

513. **Kit 1 syndromic approach, the drug(s) used is/are** *(PGI Nov 2018)*
   a. Doxycycline b. Azithromycin
   c. Cefixime d. Cefuroxime
   e. Metronidazole

514. **Which of the following are criteria for SIRS - systemic inflammatory response syndrome** *(PGI Nov 2018)*
   a. Fever >38°C b. TLC >9000 /μL
   c. Tachycardia >90 bpm d. PaO_2 <80
   e. $PaCO_2$ <32 mmHg

515. **After accidental needle stick exposure from a known Hep B positive case to a surgeon, the most probable risk of transmission is:** *(JIPMER Nov 2018)*
   a. 50% b. 10%
   c. 5% d. 0.3%

Ans.

502. d
503. d
504. c
505. a
506. c
507. a
508. b, d
509. a, d, e
510. a, b
511. a, c
512. a, b, c, d
513. b, c
514. a, c, e
515. b

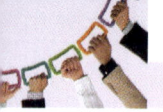

516. State which of the following statements is true: *(AIIMS May 2019)*
a. Surveillance only till 5 years of age
b. Sample collected for suspected AFP even after 15 years
c. At least one case of non-polio AFP should be detected annually per 100000 population
d. Stool specimen should reach the laboratory within 72 hours
e. At least 80% should have follow up after 60 days from the last stool sample

517. This insect transmits all of the following diseases except *(AIIMS May 2019)*

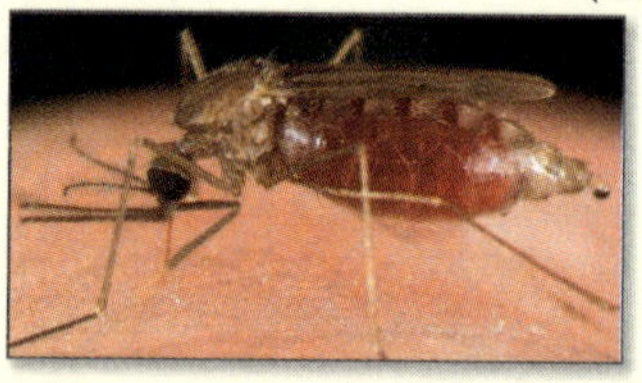

a. KFD
b. Kala Azar
c. babesiosis
d. Chandipura encephalitis
e. Oriental sore

518. What is the sequence for removal of the personal protective equipment? *(Sequential arrangement type; AIIMS May 2019)*
a. Facemask
b. Gloves
c. Eyewear
d. Apron

519. Which of the following disease with bird, arthropod and human chain: *(Recent Question 2019)*
a. Japanese encephalitis
b. Plague
c. Malaria
d. Onchocerciasis

520. Drug of choice for Diphtheria carriers is: *(Recent Question 2019)*
a. Penicillin
b. Erythromycin
c. Amoxycillin
d. Tetracycline

521. Which of the following not an epidemiological indicator for malaria: *(Recent Question 2019)*
a. Annual blood examination rate
b. Annual parasite incidence
c. Annual parasite index
d. Annual falciparum incidence

522. Dose of diphtheria antitoxin is: *(Recent Question 2019)*
a. 1000-5000 IU
b. 20000-1000000 IU
c. 1000-2000 IU
d. None

523. Which among the following not a personal protective equipment? *(Recent Question 2019)*
a. Goggles
b. Face shield
c. Gloves
d. Lab coat

Ans.

516. c, d
517. a
518. d, b, c, a
519. a
520. b
521. c
522. b
523. b

Answers with Explanations

1. Ans. (b) 10.17/100,000

Ref: Annual report, NLEP 2016-2017

- The ANCDR for leprosy is 10.17/100,000 population.
- Total 88166 cases were recorded giving prevalence rate of 0.66 per 10,000 population
- Grade II disability rate of 3.94 per million population
- Child case rate of 8.7%
- 34 states and UTs achieved elimination out of 36 States/ UTs. One State (Chhattisgarh) and one U.T. (Dadra & Nagar Haveli) are yet to achieve elimination.
- Five more states/UTs wherein elimination was achieved earlier, namely Odisha, Bihar, Chandigarh, Goa and Lakshadweep have reported with PR>1/10,000 population, as on 31st March 2017.

2. Ans. (b) CB - NAAT

Ref. Technical and Operational Guidelines for TB Control in India – 2016

3. Ans. (a) Nikshay

4. Ans. (d) Assam

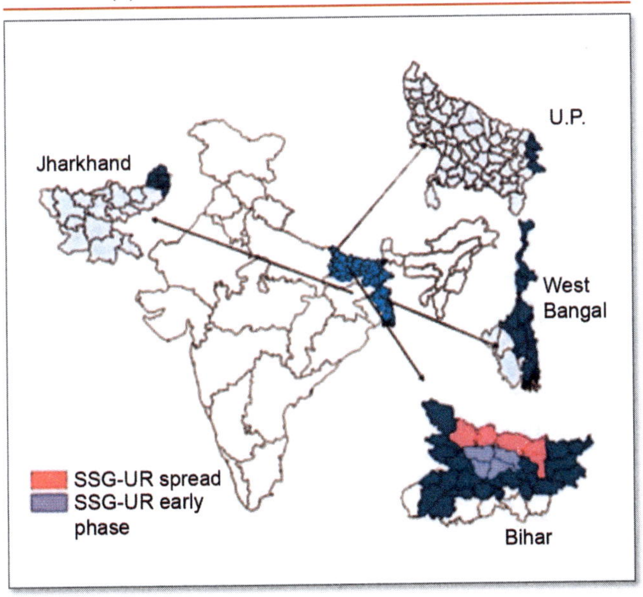

- Leishmania donovani is the only parasite causing this disease
- Post Kala-azar Dermal Leishmaniasis (PKDL) is a condition when Leishmania donovani invades skin cells, resides and develops there and manifests as dermal leisions. Some of the kala-azar cases manifests PKDL after a few years of treatment
- Endemic in eastern States of India namely Bihar, Jharkhand, Uttar Pradesh and West Bengal

Kala Azar Transmission

- Sandfly of genus Phlebotomus argentipes are the only known vectors of kala-azar in India
- Indian Kala-azar has a unique epidemiological feature of being Anthroponotic; human is the only known reservoir of infection
- Female snadflies pick up parasite (Amastigote or LD bodies) while feeding on an infected human host.
- Parasite undergo morphological change to become flagellate (Promastigote or Leptomonad), development and multiplication in the gut of sand-flies and move to mouthparts
- Healthy human hosts get infection when an infective sandfly vector bites them

Drugs used for Kala Azar (all are approved under the program)

- Sodium stibo gluconate IM/IV 20 mg/kg/day X 30 days
- Miltefosine 100 mg daily x 4 weeks
- Amphotericin B 1 mg/kg b.w. IV infusion daily or alternate day for 15-20 infusions
- Liposomal Amphotericin B

5. Ans. (d) 4 days before and 5 days after appearance of rashes

6. Ans. (a) T.B is mandatory to notify; (b) Suspicious TB patients are screened; (c) Covered the whole country since March 2006

7. Ans. (b) Immunoglobulin not required if prior immunization and immunoglobulin is received within 1 year; (c) Local wound cleaning is done in all cases of dog wound

8. Ans. (d) Inguinal bubo

Ref: K. Park, 24th ed. p 352

9. Ans. (a) 20 IU/kg

Ref: K. Park, 24th ed p 297

10. Ans. (b) Yellow

Ref: K. Park, 23rd ed. p 438, Operational Guidelines for STI/RTI, GOI.

11. Ans. (c) 1 lakh

Ref: K. Park, 24th ed. p 446

12. Ans. (b) Few hours to 5 days

Ref: K. Park, 24th ed. p 245

13. Ans. (c) 4 days

Ref: K. Park, 24th ed. p 181-183

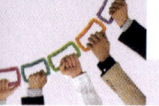

14. Ans. (a) Respiratory

Ref: K. Park, 24th ed. p 157

15. Ans. (d) Tuberculosis

Ref: K. Park, 24th ed. p 448

16. Ans. (b) CB - NAAT

Ref: Technical and Operational Guidelines for TB Control in India – 2016

SMALL POX/ CHICKEN POX

17. Ans. (a) May 1975

Small pox – timeline to eradication

Last known case of small pox	24 may 1975
India declared free from small pox	5th July 1975
Eradication confirmed in	April 1977
Global eradication	May 1980

18. Ans. (d) Life long

19. Ans. (a) Herpes zoster

20. Ans. (a) Scabs are most infective

21. Ans. (d) Pancreatitis

22. Ans. (b) Isolation of the boy

This is peculiar to chicken pox type rash. Creating panic and emergency will not be a good solution. Isolation of the child and appropriate counselling of the parents/guardians is the best next step.

23. Ans. (d) Adults

24. Ans. (d) Live attenuated OKA strain

25. Ans. (b) 2 days before and 5 days after rash appearance

Ref: K. Park, 24th ed. p 154

Chicken Pox (Varicella)

- Infectivity (Period of communicability) is 1–2 days before and 4 to 5 days after appearance of rash.
- Patient is non infectious once the lesions(Vesicles) have crusted

26. Ans. (d) Only one stage of rash is seen

Ref: K. Park, 24th ed.p-154

Chicken pox is an acute infectious disease caused by Varicella -Zoster virus (*Human (alpha) herpes virus 3*)

Clinical Features

- Vesicular rash (Superficial, Unilocular, Dew-drop like vesicles with surrounding inflammation)
- Rash is pleomorphic (different stage of rash seen at a time) and is accompanied by fever and malaise.
- Rash is symmetrical and centripetal in distribution (seen in axilla, flexor surfaces). Palm and sole are spared[Q]
- Secondary attack rate = 90% in household contacts (Highly communicable)

27. Ans. (d) Patients with varicella zoster

Ref: K. Park, 24th ed p-156

Recommendation for Varicella Zoster Immunization

- Children 12-18 months age who didn't had chicken pox
- HIV positive children/adult with CD_4 T level >15%

Contraindicated to those allergic to Neomycin

28. Ans. (d) 8th May 1980

Ref: K. Park, 24th ed. p 153

29. Ans. (b) 1980

Ref: K. Park, 24th ed. p 153

30. Ans. (c) 90

Ref: K. Park, 24th ed. p 154

31. Ans. (a) Live vaccine

Ref: K. Park, 24th ed. p 155

32. Ans. (b) Cross-immunity with animal pox virus

Epidemiological factors that led to eradication of smallpox:

- No known animal reservoir
- No long-term carrier of the virus
- Immunity post recovery from disease was life-long
- Detection of cases was simple (characteristic rash on visible parts of the body).
- Persons with subclinical infection did not transmit the disease
- Highly effective, easily administered and heat stable vaccine. Protection conferred was long-term
- International cooperation

33. Ans. (a) Only single stage of lesion is present at a time

Ref: K. Park, 24th ed. p 155

- Rash is pleomorphic (different stage of lesion present at a time)
- *Rash is symmetrical and centripetal in distribution (seen in axilla, flexor surfaces). Palm and sole are spared* [Q]
- *A fall in CMI (Cell Mediated Immunity) leads to reactivation of virus in 10-30%* cases resulting in *herpes zoster*[Q]
- Occurs mostly in children <10 years of age. Disease is severe in normal adults
- **Secondary attack rate** = 90%

MEASLES

34. Ans. (d) Diarrhea

35. Ans. (c) 90%

36. Ans. (b) Human herpes virus 3

Human herpes virus

Type	Synonym	Pathophysiology
HHV 1	HSV 1	Oral and Herptic whitlow and/or genital herpes (predominantly orofacial), as well as other herpes simplex infections
HHV 2	HSV 2	Oral, genital ulcers
HHV 3	VZV	Chicken pox and varicella
HHV 4	EBV	EBV associated lymphoproliferative diseases, Infectious mononucleosis, lymphomas
HHV 5	CMV	Infectious mononucleosis like illness
HHV 6	Roseola virus	Sixth disease – roseola infantum
HHV 7		Encephalopathy, myocarditis, hepatitis, mononucleosis like illness
HHV 8	Kaposi sarcoma associated virus	Kaposi sarcoma, primary effusion lymphoma

37. Ans. (a) 10%

38. Ans. (c) 7%

39. Ans. (b) 6 months-3yrs

40. Ans. (a) October to April

41. Ans. (d) Occur in other exanthematous fever also

42. Ans. (d) Pancreatitis

43. Ans. (c) Vitamin A

44. Ans. (d) All of the above

45. Ans. (b) 3 days

46. Ans. (c) 95%

47. Ans. (d) SSPE

Ref: K. Park, 24th ed. p 158

Complications of Measles

- *Most common complication*^Q-Diarrhea, Pneumonia and other respiratory complications and Otitis media
- Acute Vitamin A deficiency (Keratomalacia, Corneal scar and blindness)
- Serious complication – Febrile convulsion, Encephalitis and SSPE (Dawsons disease)
- *SSPE is a rare complication, that develops after many years of initial measles infection*^Q *(1 in 3 Lakh)*

48. Ans. (d) Pneumonia

Ref: https://www.cdc.gov/vaccines/pubs/pinkbook/meas.html#complications

- Post measles there is increased susceptibility to infections and nutritional/metabolic disorders
- Pulmonary conditions (secondary bacterial infections) contribute to >90% of measles related mortality in developing countries.
- Growth retardation, diarrhea, weight loss, cancrum oris, pyogenic infection, candidiasis and reactivation of pulmonary tuberculosis, etc. is common following an episode of measles.
- As many as one out of every 20 children with measles gets pneumonia, the most common cause of death from measles in young children.
- About one child out of every 1,000 who get measles will develop encephalitis (swelling of the brain) that can lead to convulsions and can leave the child deaf or with intellectual disability.
- For every 1,000 children who get measles, one or two will die from it.

Common complications following measles:

- Diarrhea 8%
- Otitis media 7%
- Pneumonia 6%
- Encephalitis 0.1%
- Seizures 0.6–0.7%
- Death 0.2%

93 *Good to Remember*

- Most common life threatening complication of measles is pneumonia.
- The most common complication arising from measles is diarrhea.

49. Ans. (d) German measles – 7 days after onset of rash

Ref: K. Park, 24th ed. p 160

Rubella (German measles)

- *Period of communicability*: 1 week before to 1 week after appearance of rash. Maximum at eruption of rash
- Duration of isolation is none (23rd edition, Park. p-120)

50. Ans. (b) 10 days

Ref: K. Park, 24th ed. p 157

Measles

- *Incubation period*→Vaccine induced is 7 day and10/14* day for natural infection (Exposure to onset of Fever/Rash*)

51. Ans. (a) 3 day

Ref: K. Park, 24th ed. p 157

To be effective measles vaccine in postexposure prophylaxis must be given within 3 days of exposure.

52. Ans. (a) TB

Ref: Infectious Disease Epidemiology Kenrad E. Nelson, Carolyn Williams, p-538

53. Ans. (a) Measles

Ref: K. Park, 24th ed. p 181

WHO's measles elimination strategy→*3 part vaccination strategy*

- ***Catch-up***→ One-time vaccination of all children 9 month -14 years age.(Irrespective of disease or vaccination status)
- ***Keep-up***→ Routine vaccination. Aim is to vaccinate >95% of each successive-birth cohort.
- ***Follow up***→Vaccination done every 2 -4 years targeting all children born after the catch-up campaign

54. Ans. (b) Catch up

Ref: K. Park, 24th ed. p 181

Supplementary immunization service mean immunisation offered in addition to Routine immunization. In case of measles it comprises "Catch up"

Targets for Global Measles Eradication

- Raise the routine immunization coverage with 1st dose of MCV (Measles Containing Vaccine) to ≥90% and ≥80% in every district or administrative unit
- Reduce and maintain annual measles incidence to <5 cases per million
- Reduce measles mortality by ≥95% compared with that in year 2000 (Baseline)

55. Ans. (d) 1: 300000

Ref: K. Park, 24th ed. p 158

SSPE (Sub-acute Sclerosing Pan Encephalitis)

- It is a *rare neurological complication, that develops after many years of initial measles infection*[Q]
- *It is a serious complication with 10-20% fatality rate. Death usually occurs within 1-3 day.*
- It presents as progressive mental deterioration leading to paralysis, involuntary movements, muscular rigidity and coma (may be due to persistence of the virus in the brain)
- Diagnosis is by the demonstration of high levels of measles complement fixing antibodies in CSF and serum.

Frequency of SSPE is 1:300000 cases of natural measles

56. Ans. (a) Common in summer

Ref: K. Park, 24th ed. p 157

57. Ans. (a) Rash appears 1-2 days after appearance of Koplik spot

Ref: Charles D. Bluestone, Pediatric Otolaryngology, Volume 2, p 1236

Koplik spots appear on the buccal mucosa opposite the 1st & 2nd upper molars in prodromal stage 24-48 hour before the appearance of rash

Small (pin head size) bluish white spots on a red base

58. Ans. (d) Catch up

Ref: K. Park, 24th ed. p 181

59. Ans. (d) 95

Ref: K. Park, 24th ed. p 159

Eradication of measles; requires

- *Immunization coverage of at least 96% in children under 1 year of age*[Q]
- Prevent cumulation of immunity gap or build up of susceptible.

60. Ans. (c) Mengioencephalitis

Ref: K. Park, 24th ed. p 158

MUMPS AND RUBELLA

61. Ans. (d) Infections after 16 weeks of gestation result in major congenital defects

Comment: No, the first trimester is the most dangerous time for congenital rubella syndrome as at that time the organs are developing.

62. Ans. (b) No subclinical case

Comment: Most common source of infection – clinical or subclinical case of rubella. rubella has a significant number of subclinical cases

63. Ans. (c) Myocarditis

64. Ans. (c) HaI Test

Comment: The hemagglutination inhibition (HaI) test is the most commonly accepted investigation for rapid diagnosis of rubella detection of IgG is an evidence of immunity towards rubella

ELISA test is better test than HaI as serum pre-treatment is not required.

65. Ans. (c) Microcephalus

66. Ans. (c) 16th

67. Ans. (c) Does not prevent subclinical infection with wild virus

Comment:

RA 27/3 produced in the human fibroblasts produces an immune response which closely parallels the natural infection immune response. It majorly also prevents the subclinical superinfections

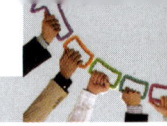

RA27/3 single dose 0.5 ml Subcutaneous

68. Ans. (a) Women 15-39 yrs (non pregnant)

69. Ans. (d) Myxo virus

70. Ans. (b) 5-15 yrs

Mumps Epidemiology:

- Most common age: 5-9 years
- Severe in adults
- One attack life-long immunity
- <6 months – babies are immune due to presence of maternal antibodies
- IP – 14 - 18 days
- Transmission: Droplet infection, direct contact

71. Ans. (c) 2-4 weeks

IP is 2-4 weeks (average 14-18 days)

72. Ans. (d) 18 days

Ref: K. Park, 24th ed. p 162

MUMPS

- Incubation period – 2 to 4 weeks (Average 14-18 days).

INFLUENZA

73. Ans. (a) A

74. Ans. (a) 2–3 yrs

75. Ans. (a) Affects majorly young girls 10–19 years

No, influenza affects all age groups and gender. Infact the attack rate is lower among the adults. however, there is higher mortality among the risk groups as:

- Age >65 years
- Comorbid conditions as stroke, diabetes, hypertension, chronic kidney disease or any other respiratory disease.
- Age <18 months
- Pregnancy

76. Ans. (c) Presence of cross immunity; (d) Short duration of immunity

Ref: Park 25th ed. p 167

Short Incubation Period	T	Yes, it has short IP of 18-72 hours
Large no. of sub-clinical cases	T	Yes, a large number of subclinical infections occur which play a major role in spread of infection
Presence of cross immunity	F	No, Not correct. The three types of influenza virus are antigenically distinct and induce no cross protection
Short duration of immunity	F	No, not correct. The antibodies in influenza starts to rise 7 days after attack and reach maximum by 14-20 days. After 10-12 months, the antibody titre reaches back to pre-infection levels
High proportion of susceptible population	T	Yes, correct. Influenza can attack any age group and any gender. However, higher fatality rate is observed in seniors (age >65 years), children (age <18 months) and persons with comorbidities.

Contd...

- Transmission – direct infection, droplet
- The portal of entry – respiratory tract
- IP – 18-72 hours
- Immunity:
  - Resistance to initiation of infection – antibody to HA
  - Resistance of severity of infection - antibody to NA
  - Resistance of transmission infection- antibody to NA

77. Ans. (d) Major epidemics are due to antigenic drift

Antigenic shift is a result of genetic recombination of the human with the animal viral genome, which may be responsible for major epidemics

78. Ans. (d) Infant & person > 65 yrs are low risk groups

79. Ans. (b) Pneumonia

80. Ans. (b) Live attenuated vaccine

81. Ans. (d) Ribavirin

Ref: K. Park, 24th ed. p 166

Treatment of Influenza

	Therapy	Chemoprophylaxis
Influenza A	Zanamivir or Oseltamivir + Rimantidine	Zanamivir (If contraindicated then Rimantidine)
Influenza B	Oseltamivir OR Zanamivir	Oseltamivir OR Zanamivir

- Dose → Oseltamivir (Tamiflu) 75mg* BD x 5 day for therapy and 75mg OD for prophylaxis (up to 10 days past last exposure).
- Zanamivir (Adults and child >5 year) – administered by inhaler (2 x 5 mg) – BD for therapy and OD for prophylaxis.

Duration of prophylaxis → depends on clinical setting.

Peramivir is also a neuraminidase inhibitor like Oseltamivir OR Zanamivir and is a licensed alternative antiviral in treatment of Influenza A and B

Also Know......................

- **Treatment of pandemic Influeza A** (H1N1)– In patients with persistent severe illness despite treatment on Oseltamivir: i.v. Zanamivir or Peramivir or Ribavirin is a licensed alternative.

82. Ans. (a) Influenza; (c) Vibrio parahemolyticus; (d) Yersinia; (e) Swine flu

Ref: K. Park, 24th ed. p 164, 166, 245, 312

83. Ans. (b) Man to man transmission is rare

Ref: K. Park, 24th ed. p 166

H5N1 is a strain of avian influenza that has potential to become a pandemic.

- Fortunately, the virus has not adopted itself to a strain contagious to humans (No man to man transmission)

84. Ans. (a) Source of infection: is a case

Ref: K. Park, 24th ed. p-164

Influenza

- *Source of infection*: Case or subclinical case.
- *Period of infectivity*: 1-2 days before and after onset of symptoms.

85. Ans. (b) ELISA

Ref: K. Park, 23rd ed. p 156

Confirmation of influenza A(H1N1) is done using

- Real time RT PCR or
- Isolation of the virus in culture or
- Four-fold rise in virus specific neutralizing antibodies.

86. Ans. (c) Oseltamivir

Ref: K. Park, 24th ed. p 164

Oseltamivir is the drug of choice for treatment and prophylaxis against influenza

87. Ans. (a) 1-3 days

Ref: K. Park, 24th ed. p 166

88. Ans. (d) H7N9

Ref: Centers for Disease Control and Prevention. February 12, 2014. http://www.cdc.gov/flu/avianflu/h7n9-virus.htm

Human infections with avian influenza A (H7N9) virus was first reported in China in 2013.

- Cause - Exposure to infected poultry or contaminated environments (Bird Market)
- No person-to-person transmission, Mode of transmission –Respiratory
- CFR = 33%,
- Treatment –Oseltamivir, Zanamivir

89. Ans. (c) Intermediary host

Ref: World Health Organisation. http://www.who.int/influenza/human_animal_interface/swine_influenza/en/

Pigs are the most important reservoir for influenza A viruses, acting as an intermediary host for both interspecies transmission and genetic reassortment. This is due to the high susceptibility of pigs to human and avian influenza viruses, the mixing of which can produce viruses with increased pandemic potential in different hosts, and coinfection with both avian and human influenza viruses has been observed in pigs.

DIPHTHERIA

90. Ans. (c) 10%

Ref: K. Park, 25th ed. p 172–176, www.cbhidghs.nic.in (CBHI profile 2018)

Diphtheria is a public health problem, which affects majority of the younger children, with following epidemiological features:

- Case fatality rate ~ 10% in untreated children (slightly higher in children <5 years)
- Case fatality in India is 2-3% (with treatment and with DPT vaccination in place)
- Carriers are common in diphtheria (95:5 – carrier: case ratio)
- Nasal Carriers are more important than throat carriers
- Incidence of carrier in community – 0.1-5%
- Infective material – nasopharyngeal secretions
- Period of infectivity – 14-28 days from onset of disease
- Case is labelled as no -infective – 2 cultures (24 hrs apart, from nose and throat) are reported negative

91. Ans. (c) Chronic Carrier

Most important source of infection is – chronic carriers (nasal carriers are more dangerous than throat carriers)

92. Ans. (b) Conjunctival

93. Ans. (b) Immunization prevents carrier state

94. Ans. (b) 14–28 days from onset of the disease

95. Ans. (b) 1–5 yrs

In developed countries, with widespread immunization coverage, the age group of children affected is slightly raised and affects maximally, the school going children

96. Ans. (b) 70%

97. Ans. (c) Inapparent infection

98. Ans. (b) 2–6 days

99. Ans. (b) Membrane can be removed easily

No, the attempt to remove the membrane may result in bleeding.

100. Ans. (b) 2 consecutive swabs are -ve

Isolation is done till:
- At least 14 days
- 2 consecutive culture swabs (24 hrs apart from nose and throat) are negative

101. Ans. (b) Erythromycin

Ref: K. Park, 25th ed. p 174

Management protocol for Suspected diphtheria cases:
- **Mild pharyngeal** or laryngeal disease 20,000 – 40,000 Units diphtheria antitoxin IM/IV
- **Moderate pharyngeal** or laryngeal disease 40,000 – 60,000 Units diphtheria antitoxin IM/IV
- **Severe pharyngeal** or laryngeal disease 80,000 – 100,000 Units diphtheria antitoxin IM/IV

  +
- Penicillin or erythromycin for 5-6 days
- **Management of Diphtheria Carriers**: 10 days oral erythromycin

Management for Close Contacts of Diphtheria

Primary immunization	Action to be taken	Follow up
Within previous 2 years	No further action	Placed under medical surveillance and examined daily for signs of diphtheria for at least 7 days following exposure
More than previous 2 years	Booster dose of Td or diphtheria toxoid	
Non immunized/ unknown status	Prophylactic penicillin/ erythromycin + Active immunization for Diphtheria + 1000-2000 Units of diphtheria antitoxin	

102. Ans. (d) All of the above

103. Ans. (a) Progressive hepatitis

The reactions of the DPT vaccine are:
- Uncontrollable crying (most common, considered as vaccine side effect rather than adverse vaccine reaction)
- Local pain and swelling 10%–20% (most common adverse reaction)
- Fever 2–6%
- Severe complication are rare – mostly due to pertussis component:
  - Encephalopathy
  - Prolonged convulsions
  - Infantile spasms
  - Reye's syndrome (rare)

104. Ans. (c) 2-6 days and 10-14 days

Ref: K. Park, 24th ed. p 164

105. Ans. (b) Single dose of Toxoid (d) Daily throat swab culture

Ref: K. Park, 24th ed. p 171

Management of Contacts in Diphtheria

Primary immunization/ Booster	Course of action
Within 2 years	Nothing
More than 2 years before	Booster of Diphtheria Toxoid
Non immunized close contacts	Prophylactic Penicillin or Erythromycin. Diphtheria antitoxin (1000-2000 units) and Full course of vaccine against Diphtheria Daily medical surveillance for minimum 1 week after exposure Weekly bacteriological surveillance (Throat swab) for several weeks

106. Ans. (a) Immunization

Ref: K. Park, 24th ed. p-170

107. Ans. (d) 70%

Ref: K. Park, 24th ed. p 170-71

Immunity in Diphtheria
- Maternal antibodies (immune mothers) protect infants in the first few weeks or months of life.
- Inapparent infection also contributes to immunity in developing countries
- A herd immunity of more than 70% is necessary to prevent epidemic spread, (it may be as high as 90%)

PERTUSSIS

108. Ans. (b) Chronic carriers are main source of infection

Ref: K. Park, 25th ed. p 176–178

Pertussis Epidemiology:
- Most common due to *B. Pertussis* (*B.parapertussis* – rarely)
- Source of infection: humans – a known case of pertussis
- No evidence of subclinical infections or carrier state of pertussis
- Infective material – nasopharyngeal secretions
- Infective period:
  - Most infectious during catarrhal stage
  - Week of exposure to 3 weeks after paroxysmal stage
- Secondary attack rate ~ 90%
- Mode of transmission – droplet, direct contact
- Age of infections: <5 years

109. Ans. (a) Most infections during paroxysmal stage

No, pertussis is most infectious during catarrhal stage

110. Ans. (c) Erythromycin prophylaxis is indicated in the neonate

111. Ans. (a) Incubation period is 7-14 days; (d) Secondary attack rate in unimmunized person is 90%

Ref: K. Park, 24th ed. p 173-74

Whooping Cough (Pertussis) or "Hundred Day Cough"

- It is an acute infectious disease of infants and under 5 year children. Infants <6 months have highest mortality.
- Median age of infection is 20-30 months in developing country (50 months in developed country). Disease is not reported in older children, adolescent and adult
- *Source of infection*: Case of Pertussis. *Subclinical infection or chronic carrier state does not exist.*
- Overcrowding – Low socio economic status and Winter/ Spring month contributes to spread
- SAR (Secondary Attack Rate) is about 90% in unimmunized household contacts.
- *Incubation period* – 7-14 days (<3 weeks)[Q]

112. Ans. (a) Incubation period of 7-14 days

Ref: K. Park, 24th ed. p 174

MENINGOCOCCAL MENINGITIS

113. Ans. (a) Cases are important source of infection

Ref: K. Park, 25th ed. p 178–179

Meningitis:

- Most infections are due to A,B,C,X, W135, Y serogroups
- Shows seasonal trend – most cases from December – April
- Meningitis is endemic in India, with CFR of 6-7% in India
- Carriers are the most important source of infection
- Age group – maximum in 3-12 year old children
- Immunity acquired by subclinical infection, clinical disease or vaccination
- Incubation period – 2-10 days
- DOC –
  - Case of meningitis – penicillin
  - Carrier (established) state – Rifampicin
  - Close contacts (household contacts, direct health care providers, under medical supervision)
    - Rifampicin
    - Ciprofloxacin, ceftriaxone, azithromycin
  - Mass chemoprophylaxis (closed, medically supervised community)
    - Ciprofloxacin
    - Minocycline, spiramycin, ceftriaxone

114. Ans. (a) A

Ref -The Epidemiology of Meningococcal Disease in the United States. Lee H. Harrison, Clin Infect Dis. 2010 March 1; 50(S2).NIH,

Meningococcus

- It has 12 serotypes (characterized by differences in the polysaccharide capsule)
- Serotype A, B and C account for about 90% of meningococcal disease.
- Serotype A is responsible for the largest and most devastating meningococcal epidemics.
- Serotype B are a cause of endemic meningococcal disease
- Serotype C has occasionally caused epidemics. It frequently causes outbreaks

115. Ans. (b) Fatality in untreated cases is 60%

Ref: K. Park, 24th ed. p 175

Meningococcal Meningitis

- CFR of typical untreated cases = 80%. With early diagnosis and treatment, CFR declines to <10%.
- **Mode of transmission – D**roplet infection. (Portal of entry is nasopharynx).
- **Mass chemoprophylaxis** causes an immediate drop in the incidence rate of meningitis and in the proportion of carriers. It is recommended for closed and medically supervised communities.
- Drug of choice for mass chemoprophylaxis is Ciprofloxacin, Minocycline, Spiramycin and Ceftriaxone
- **Treatment**: Drug of choice for:
  - Cases is Penicillin
  - Carrier is Rifapicin
  - Contacts is Rifampicin, Ciprofloxacin, Ceftriaxone and Azithromycin

116. Ans. (b) Young adolescents

Ref: K. Park, 24th ed. p 176

Meningococcal Meningitis: About 50% of all cases occur in under 5 year children and 80-85% cases within 25 years of age

- Polysaccharide vaccine-
- Conjugate vaccine –
  - Monovalent (A) vaccine is recommended for people 1-29 year of age as single dose
  - Monovalent (C) vaccine is recommended for children ≥12 month (including teenagers and adults) as single dose. and 2 doses 2 month apart with a booster after 1 year in child 2-11 month.
  - Quadrivalent vaccine is recommended for children ≥2 year

Also Know......................

- No vaccine is available against group B Meningococcus

117. Ans. (b) 0.01%

WHO classification of meningococcal endemicity:

- Low endemicity: <2 cases per 100,000 poulations per year
- Moderate endemicity: 2–10 cases per 100,000 populations per year
- High endemicity: >10 cases per 100,000 populations per year

Also Know......................

- Epidemic is defined as more than 100 cases per 100,000 populations per year.

118. Ans. (a) ACW135Y

Ref: K. Park, 24th ed. p 176

TUBERCULOSIS

119. Ans. (b) High prevalence of immunized people

Ref: K. Park, 24th ed. p 196

Tuberculin testis. Its interpretation can lead to false conclusions in following conditions
- High coverage of BCG vaccination at birth
- Cross -sensitivity to atypical mycobacteria

120. Ans. (c) Resistant to INH and Rifampicin with or without resistant to other anti TB drugs

Ref: K. Park, 24th ed. p 189

Multi Drug Resistant TB (MDR-TB) *is defined as M. tuberculosis resistant to Isoniazid and Rifampicin with or without resistance to other drugs at a RNTCP-certified Culture and DST Laboratory.*

121. Ans. (d) 24-27 months

Ref: K. Park, 24th ed. p 199

Regimen of MDR TB

Intensive phase (IP)	Continuation phase (CP)
▪ **6 drug regimen-** Kanamycin, Levofloxacin, Ethionamide, Pyrazinamide, Ethambutol and Cycloserine **for** 6-9 months (Minimum 6 month)	▪ 4 drug regimen- Levovfloxacin, Ethionamide, Ethambutoland Cycloserine for 18 months
▪ If 4th or 5th month culture result remains positive, treatment is extended by 1 month. ▪ IP can be extended up to a maximum of 3 months	
RNTCP Regimen for MDR-TB: **6 (9) Km Lvx Eto Cs Z E/ 18 Lvx Eto Cs E** (Reserve/substitute drugs: PAS, Mfx, Cm) Total duration-24-27 months	

122. Ans. (d) All the above

Ref: K. Park, 24th ed. p 189

XDR TB case: *An MDR TB case whose recovered M. tuberculosis isolate is resistant to*
- At least Isoniazidand Rifampicin,
- A fluoroquinolone (Ofloxacin, Levofloxacin or Moxifloxacin) and
- A second-line injectable antiTB drug (Kanamycin, Amikacin or Capreomycin *at a RNTCP-certified Culture and DST Laboratory.*

Also Know......................

- MDR-TB patients diagnosed as XDR-TB is labelled an outcome of "Switched to regimen for XDR-TB".

123. Ans. (a) Chennai

Ref: K. Park, 24th ed. p 447

There are six NRL under the RNTCP
- National Tuberculosis Institute→ Bangalore
- National Institute of Respiratory Diseases (Formerly Tuberculosis Research Center) → Chennai
- National Institute of TB and Respiratory Diseases (Formerly LRS Institute of TB and Allied Diseases) → New Delhi
- National JALMA Institute for Leprosy →Agra
- Regional Medical Resource Center → Bhubaneshwar
- Bhopal Memorial Hospital and Research Center → Bhopal

124. Ans. (d) All of the above

Ref: K. Park, 24th ed. p 213

Tuberculosis and Diabetes

- Diabetes is an independent risk factor for TB. It accounts for 15% of all TB and 21% of smear positive TB
- Risk of progression from latent to active tuberculosis is 2-3 times higher in diabetic (Incidence increases)
- People with diabetes and TB are diagnosed very late.
- Risk of death during TB treatment and TB relapse after treatment is high in diabetics (Severity increases)

Also Know......................

- All TB patients should be screened for diabetes and All TB patients should be screened for diabetes, particularly in setting with high TB prevalence.

125. Ans. (b) To cure 100% of sputum positive TB...

Ref: K. Park, 24th ed. p 446

Stop TB Strategy

Vision → TB free world

Goal → Reduce global burden of TB by 2015 by ensuring all TB patients (including TB-HIV coinfected and Drug-resistant TB) benefit from universal access to high-quality diagnosis and patient centered treatment.

Targets

- By 2005 → Case detection rate >70% and Cure rate >85%.
- By 2015 → Reduce prevalence of and death due to TB by 50%. (Relative to 1990 levels i.e. Prevelance = 150 per 1 lakh or lower and Death = 15 per 1 lakh per year or lowerand number of people dying of TB ≤ 1 million including TB-HIV coinfected)
- By 2050 → Eliminate TB as a public health problem (<= 1 case per million population per year)

Components

- Pursue high-quality DOTS expansion and enhancement
- Address TB/HIV, MDR/XDR-TB and other challenges
- Contribute to health system strengthening
- Engage all care providers – PPM (Public Private Mix), International Standards for TB Care (ISTC)
- Empower people with TB, and communities
- Enable and promote research

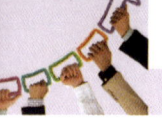

126. Ans. (d) New case

Ref: K. Park, 24th ed. p 189

Type of cases	
New	A patient who has never had treatment for TB or has taken anti-TB drugs for less than one month
Previously treated	A patient who received anti-TB drugs for one month or more in past
Treatment after loss to follow up (Previously Treatment after Default)	A patient previously treated for TB and declared lost to follow up at the end of their most recent course of treatment. (Sputum is sent for Culture and Drug Susceptibility Testing)
Failure	A patient who has been previously treated for TB but whose treatment failed at the end of his most recent course of treatment
Relapse	A TB patient who was declared cured or treatment completed at the end of his most recent course of treatmentand who is now diagnosed with a recurrent TB (Relapse or new TB reinfection)
Others	A patient who has been previously treated for TB but whose outcome after their most recent course of treatment is unknown or undocumented

127. Ans. (b) Sputum positive pulmonary TB

Ref: K. Park, 24th ed. p 449

128. Ans. (b) Prevalence rate

Ref: K. Park, 24th ed. p 188

129. Ans. (a) Prevalence of infection

Ref: K. Park, 24th ed. p 195

Positive Tuberculin test denotes hypersensitivity to a previous exposure of individual to tubercular protein.
- It is not *conclusive of the person suffering from disease.*
- It does not indicate susceptibility or resistance to TB.
- In child <2 yrs--tuberculin positive, is indirect evidence of an active TB lesion in the body even if it is not manifest.
- False positive result can occur in case of infection bynontuberculous mycobacteria or previous administration of BCG.

Negative Tuberculin Test is seen in

- Immune suppression eg:- Malignancy, Hodgkin's disease, HIV infection, malnutrition, viral infections (eg.measles, chicken pox etc)
- Immunosuppressive drugs therapy
- Incorrect injection of PPD.

130. Ans. (b) Tuberculin conversion index

Ref: K. Park, 24th ed. p 188

Incidence of infection: (*Annual Infection Rate* or *annual risk of TB*) or ***Tuberculin conversion index***:
- It is the number of people who are likely to get newly infected by Mycobacterium Tuberculosis from among the non -infected of the preceding survey during the course of one' year, expressed as percentage.
- It reflects the annual risk of being infected (or reinfected) in a given community.
- It also reflects the attacking force of TB in a community.
- In developing countries, every 1% of annual risk of infection corresponds to 50 new cases of smear-positive pulmonary tuberculosis, per year for 100,000 general population
- *It is one of the best indicators for evaluating TB problem, its trend* and impact of control measures
- In India, *Annual Infection Rate* =1.5%

131. Ans. (a) Sputum AFB positivity rate

Ref: K. Park, 24th ed.p-188

Incidence of TB disease in a community is measured in terms of Sputum smear positive (New or Relapse) TB cases in the population occurring in a year

132. Ans. (c) 2,00,000

Ref: K. Park, 24th ed. p 446

RNTCP Lab Network

Designed microscopy center (DMC):
- 1 per 1,00,000 population (50,000 in Tribal and hilly areas).
- Each DMC has a trained lab technician and MO

Tuberculosis unit (TU)
- 1 per 2,00,000 population
- Each TU has a senior treatment laboratory supervisor (STLS), senior treatment supervisor (STS) and Medical Officer TB

133. Ans. (b) 85%

Ref: K. Park, 24th ed. p-448

RNTCP: Objective

- Achieve *at least 85% cure rate of infectious cases*[Q] by DOTS
- Augment case finding by quality sputum microscopy to detect at least 70% estimated cases[Q]
- Most recent targets are to achieve 90% case detection and 90% cure rate for tuberculosis

134. Ans (d) Chronic alcoholics

Ref http://www.who.int/tb/challenges/ltbi/en/. Guidelines on the management of latent tuberculosis infection

Latent Tuberculosis Infection (LTBI)

- It affects about one-third of the world's population.
- Approximately 10% of people with LTBI develop active TB disease in their lifetime, with the majority developing it within the first five years after initial infection.
- Currently available treatments have an efficacy ranging from 60% to 90%.
- Systematic testing and treatment of LTBI in at-risk populations is a critical component of WHO's End TB Strategy

- **TST** (Tuberculin Skin Test) and **IGRAs** (Interferon-Gamma Release Assays) are the tests available for the diagnosis of LTBI.
- Risk of progression to active disease is considerably higher in infected individuals who belong to **specific high risk populations.**
  - HIV infection
  - Recent contact with an infectious patient,
  - Initiation of an anti-tumour necrosis factor (TNF) treatment
  - Receiving dialysis,
  - Receiving an organ or hematologic transplantation,
  - Silicosis,
  - Being in prison,
  - Being an immigrant from high TB burden countries,
  - Being a homeless person,
  - Being an illicit drug user.

WHO Recommended Regimen for the Treatment of LTBI is

- 6-month or 9-month isoniazid daily,
- 3-month rifapentine plus isoniazid weekly,
- 3- or 4-month isoniazid plus rifampicin daily,
- 3– or 4-month rifampicin alone daily

135. Ans. (c) Tuberculin test

Ref: K. Park, 24th ed. p 195

Mantoux test or Tuberculin test (Named after Charles Mantoux, a French physician)

- *It is a diagnostic tool for tuberculosis infection.*[Q]
- *It is the only way of estimating prevalence of TB infection in a population*
- Procedure: Intradermal injection of 5 TU of "PPD-RT-23 with Tween 80" in 0.1 mL on flexor surface of forearm.
- Interpretation: Read after 72 hours (3rd day) of Injection.
- Induration -10 mm or more is considered "***positive***". (≥20mm has greater chance of developing TB)
- Induration less than 6mm is considered " ***negative***"
- Induration 6 mm to 9 mm are considered "***doubtful***" - less risk of developing TB than those with ≥10 mm and ≤5 mm induration.

136. Ans. (a) Sputum smear positivity

Ref: K. Park, 24th ed. p 188

Epidemiological indices to measure Tuberculosis problem in a community:

- *Prevalence of infection*:
  - It is the percentage of individuals who show a +ve reaction to standard tuberculin test.
  - Age-specific prevalence is superior.
  - High BCG coverage at birth and cross-sensitivity to atypical mycobacteriae → cause prevalence to be over-estimated.
- *Incidence of infection*: (Annual Infection Rate)
  - *Percentage of non infected TB population acquiring new TB infection in a year*
  - It is the annual risk of being infected or reinfected with TB in a community
- *Prevalence of disease or case rate*:
  - Percentage of individuals whose sputum is +ve for tubercle bacilli on microscopic examination.
  - It is the best available practical index to estimate number of infectious cases or "case load" in a community.
  - Age -specific prevalence is a more relevant index.
- *Incidence of new cases*:
  - It is the percentage of new tuberculosis cases (confirmed by bacteriological examination) per 1,000 population occurring during one year.
  - It reveals the trend of problem in the community, including the impact of control measures.
  - Only of value in countries where a high proportion of new cases is detected and notification is reliable.
- *Prevalence of "suspect" cases*: based on X-ray examination of chest.
- *Prevalence of drug -resistant cases*: Culture and DST or CBNAAT
- *Mortality rate*: number of deaths from tuberculosis every year per 1,000 or 100,000 population.

Also Know.......................

- *Annual Infection Rate is one of the best indicators for evaluating TB problem and its trend* in community. Current AIR of India is 1.5%

137. Ans. (d) Children below 6 years

Ref: K. Park, 24th ed. p 207

Latest Updates

Indication for TB preventive chemotherapy:-

- Under 6 year age asymptomatic children (Active disease ruled out and Irrespective of BCG or Nutritional status), having contact with a smear positive case.
- HIV positive children (without active TB) having exposure to an infectious TB case or Tuberculin test positive (≥5 mm induration)
- All Tuberculin test positive children on immunosuppressive therapy (Nephrotic syndrome, Acute Leukaemia)
- Child born to mother diagnosed to have TB in pregnancy (Congenital TB ruled out). BCG can be given at birth

Drug of Choice – Isoniazid (10 mg/kg) daily x 6 month.

138. Ans. (c) Calculating probability of adverse drug reaction

Ref: Mahesh N. Belhekar et al A study of agreement between the Naranjo algorithm and WHO-UMC criteria for causality assessment of adverse drug reactions. Indian J Pharmacol. 2014 Jan-Feb; 46 (1; 24th ed. p: 117–120.

- It is for determining the likelihood of whether an adverse drug reaction (ADR) is actually due to the drug rather than the result of other factors.
- The probability is assigned via a score termed definite, probable, possible or doubtful.

139. Ans. (a) Incidence of infection

Ref: K. Park, 24th ed. p 188

140. Ans. (c) +++

Ref: K. Park, 24th ed. p 192

Also Know......................

- Number of AFB in a smear is an indicator of disease severity and patients infectivity

Number of Acid Fast Bacillus	Result
Nil per 100 oil immersion fields	0
1-9 per 100 oil immersion fields	Scanty (No. of AFB seen)
10-99 per 100 oil immersion fields	+
1-10 per oil immersion field	++
>10 per oil immersion field	+++

At least 10,000 Tubercle bacilli must be present in 1 mL of sputum for sputum smear microscopy to be positive

Also Know......................

- False Positive - Scratch on slide, Accidental transfer of AFB from a positive slide, Environmental mycobacteria contamination of smear, food particles/precipitate
- False Negative –Inadequate sample, Too long storage, faulty processing (fault in smear preparation, staining), wrong interpretation, misclassification.

141. Ans. (b) Inhalation

Ref: K. Park, 24th ed. p 191

Source of TB infection

- *Human- Sputum smear positive pulmonary TB patient (Untreated or Incompletely treated).*

Also Know......................

- *1 case of infectious pulmonary TB on an average infects 10-15 perons annually*

- *Bovine TB- Infected milk*

Transmission of TB: *Primarily airborne.*

- *It spreads from person to person by tiny microscopic droplets released when an active tuberculosis case coughs (maximum), sneezes, speaks, sings, or laughs or droplet nuclei*

Also Know......................

- *TB is not transmitted by fomites*

142. Ans. (c) For assessing Rifampicin resistance (e) Diagnosis of TB

Ref: K. Park, 24th ed. p 194

Xpert MTB/RIF

- It is a new fully automated molecular test for rapid diagnosis of TB and*Rifampicin drug resistance.*
- It *provides accurate results from unprocessed sputum samples in about 90 minutes*
- It *has minimal bio-safety requirements, training, and can be housed in non-conventional laboratories.*

Drug Susceptibility Test (In RNTCP)

Phenotypic- Evaluate if M. Tuberculosis grows in the presence of drug-containing media.	Genotypic- Looks for genetic mutations highly associated with phenotypic Resistance
▪ Solid egg-based Lowenstein-Jensen (LJ) media culture +DST ▪ Liquid culture (MGIT) + DST	▪ LPA ▪ CB-NAAT

143. Ans. (a) Prevent resistance

Ref: K. Park, 24th ed. p 198

Rationale for Multi Drug Therapy (MDT) in TB

- To cut transmission of TB infection in community (Bactericidal drugs).
- Early and complete cure of TB cases (Better compliance, Low cost, Reduced duration of treatment)
- To prevent emergence of drug resistance (Bacteriostatic Drugs)

144. Ans. (c) 10

Ref: K. Park, 24th ed. p 191

Also Know......................

- MDT for TB reduces infectivity by 80–90% within 48 hours.

145. Ans. (c) Patient is infected with mycobacterium

Ref: K park, 24th ed. p 195

146. Ans. (a) Ethambutol

Ref: K. Park, 24th ed. p 197

- *Rifampicin*→Most effective and Most bactericidal drug. It acts on "persisters", intra and extra cellular bacilli. 1st antitubercular drug to develop resistance
  - Adverse effect- Orange discolouration of urine, Hepatotoxicity, Gastritis, Nephrotoxicity, Thrombocytopenia, Purpura, Influenza like illness
  - Contraindicated in patients on protease inhibitor
- *Isoniazid* → 1st effective bactericidal drug used to treat TB. Adverse effect- Hepatotoxic, Peripheral neuropathy, Hyperglycemia, blood dyscrasia
- *Streptomycin* → Injectible anti TB drug, contraindicated in pregnancy. Adverse effect: vestibular damage.
- *Ethambutol* → causes optic neuritis (Red green colour blindness), peripheral neuropathy and GI toxicity. Contraindicated in children <6 year. Patients develops blue vision.

147. Ans. (b) Start category I immediately.

Ref: K. Park, 24th ed. p 199, 208

Management of TB in Special Situations

Situation	Management
Extremely ill patient (Haemoptysis, Pneumothorax, Massive pleural effusion) Cases requiring surgical intervention	▪ Hospitalization
Tuberculous meningitis	▪ Hospitalization. ▪ Ethambutol replaced with Streptomycin in intensive phase. ▪ Extension of Continuation phase by 3 months in both new and previously treated cases. ▪ Steroids are given initially and gradually tapered over 6–8 weeks.
Pregnancy and postnatal period	▪ Streptomycin (is absolutely contraindicated) is replaced by Ethambutol ▪ 2nd line drugs – Fluoroquinolones, Ethionamide, Protionamide are teratogenic and should not be used ▪ Breast feeding is to be continued in postnatal period ▪ Cough hygiene must be practiced by Lactating mother ▪ Preventive INH chemoprophylaxis for child
Patients with renal failure	▪ Dose adjustment for Streptomycin and Ethambutol, is needed according to creatinine clearance
Women on oral contraceptive pills	▪ Rifampicin decreases efficiency of OCP by increasing their metabolism. Increase in dose of OCP or switch over to alternate methods of contraception is advisable

Latest Updates

A child born to mother diagnosed to have TB in pregnancy (Congenital TB ruled out) must receive Isoniazid chemoprophylaxis (10 mg/kg/day) for 6 month. BCG can be given at birth even if INH chemoprophylaxis is planned

148. Ans. (d) Social and economic factors

Ref: Bruce G. Link etal, American Journal of Public Health. 2002 May; 92(5; 24th ed. p:730732,http://www.ncbi.nlm.nih.gov/pmc/articles/PMC1447154/

Mc Keown thesis States

- Enormous increase in population and dramatic improvements in health experienced by humans over the past 2 centuries, owe more to changes in economic and social conditions than to specific medical advances or public health initiatives.

149. Ans. (b) 1.33 per 100,000

Ref: K. Park, 24th ed. p 188

Incidence of TB = (No. of New cases/Susceptible Population) × 100000 = (22/164780) × 100000 = 1.33 per 100,000

150. Ans. (d) It is assessed by Tuberculin conversion in previously non vaccinated children.

Ref: K. Park, 24th ed. p 188

151. Ans. (c) 16-year-old with XDR TB resistant...

Ref: K. Park, 24th ed. p 448

Age selection criteria is age >18 years

- DOTS is given by peripheral health staff such as MPWs, or DOT 'Agent' - voluntary workers such as teachers, anganwadi workers, dais, ex-patients, social workers etc.
- DOT 'Agent' is paid incentive/honorarium of ₹150 per patient completing the treatment

INTESTINAL INFECTION

Poliomyelitis

152. Ans. (a) Type I virus

Ref: K. Park, 25th ed. p 222–229

- WPV type 2 is not detected since 1999
- WPV type 3 is not detected since Nov 2012
- Most epidemics were ported from WPV Type 1
- Switch from tOPV to bOPV in April-May 2016
- bOPV contains – P1 and P3
- FIPV (fractional IPV) is scheduled at 6- and 14-weeks intradermal injection, 0.1 mL in right upper arm
- AFP surveillance:
  - AFP reporting rate
    - Should be more than 1AFP case/100,000/year in all children <15 years of age sensitive indicator for ability to detect polio in community
  - Stool adequacy rate
    - Should be more than 80%
    - Indicator for operation efficacy of program
    - The stool sample should reach the laboratory within 72 hours of collection
- Surveillance Indicators
  - Completeness of reporting >80% of expected AFP surveillance
  - Sensitivity of surveillance >1 AFP/lac/year in age <15 years
  - Completeness of case investigation >80% adequate stool sample collection
  - Completeness of follow up >80% AFP cases should have the residual paralysis check at 60 days

Polio Epidemiology

- Most outbreaks due to polio type 1
- Man is the only reservoir of infection
- Most infections are subclinical
- Subclinical infections contribute to majority of cases of polio.
- It shows an iceberg phenomenon

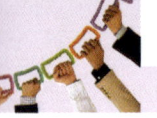

- Infective material: feces of the infected persons
- Period of communicability: most infectious 7-10 days before and after the onset of symptoms.
- More in males (3:1 for male: female ratio)
- Age: 50% of all cases are reported in infancy
- Shows seasonal variation: from June to September
- Mode of transmission: feco-oral route, direct contact and direct droplet spread
- Incubation period: 7-14 days (3-30 days)
- Clinical spectrum:
  - Inapparent infection ~ 90-95% of all infections
  - Abortive infection ~ 4-8% of all infections
  - Non-paralytic polio ~1% of infections
  - Paralytic polio <1% of all infections

153. Ans. (c) Females more commonly affected

154. Ans. (d) 1000

155. Ans. (c) Type 3

156. Ans. (d) 4-30 days

Ref: WHO Information sheet observed rate of vaccine reactions for polio vaccines; Park 25th ed. p 224

Vaccine associated paralytic poliomyelitis (VAPP) is defined as a case of AFP (Acute Flaccid Paralysis)

- With residual weakness at 60 days after onset of symptoms;
- A negative stool sample for wild poliovirus but positive for vaccine virus examined in a WHO accredited lab
- Evaluated and confirmed by an expert committee
- Onset of symptoms with VAPP occur 4–30 days following receipt of OPV or 4–75 days after contact with a recipient of OPV.
- In immunodeficient individuals (Hypogammaglobulinemia) VAPP may occur outside these windows.
- Incidence rate of VAPP is 4 cases per 1000,000 birth cohort per year. It is higher for 1st dose of OPV than for subsequent doses
- VAPP is more common in immunocompromised individuals
- No study has demonstrated transmission from a VAPP case resulting in another VAPP case.

Also Know.......................

Vaccine Derived Polio Virus (VDPV)

- VDPV is a live, attenuated strain of the virus contained in OPV, that has changed and reverted to a form capable of cause paralysis in humans and may develop the capacity for sustained circulation.
- VDPVs differ from the original Sabin strains in the vaccine by 1 to 15% of VP1 nucleotides.
- On rare occasions, in areas where populations are under-immunized, VDPVs can regain the ability to circulate in populations and can occasionally cause paralysis.
- Most circulating VDPV are type 2, followed by type 1 and type 3

Also Know.......................

- Low vaccination coverage results in VDPV. If a population is fully immunized, they will be protected against both VDPV and wild polioviruses.

157. Ans. (d) Type 3 is responsible for VAPP

Ref: K. Park, 24th ed. p 219

Poliomyelitis Virus has 3 serotypes - P_1, P_2 and P_3

- P_1 virus is most common cause of outbreaks of paralytic polio or polio epidemic.
- P_3 virus is most common cause of Vaccine Associated Pararlytic Polio (60%), followed by P_2 and P_1
- P_2 virus is most antigenic.
- Most infections are subclinical (95%), Paralytic polio is seen in (<1%)
- For every clinical case, there may be 1000 subclinical cases in children and 75 in adults
- No chronic carrier or animal source has been documented

158. Ans. (c) Serotype 3

Ref: K. Park, 24th ed. p 219

159. Ans. (d) 4 per 1000000 birth cohort

Ref: K. Park, 24th ed. p 219

160. Ans. (c) 60 days

Ref: AFP Surveillance manual (www.npsp.org); Park, 25th ed. p 223

In AFP Surveillance, examination for residual paralysis is done after 60 daysof onset of paralysis for

- AFP case with inadequate stool specimen and
- All positive WPV cases

161. Ans. (c) Mopping up is done in low risk districts

Ref: K. Park, 25th ed. p 228

Line listing of cases -It was initiated in 1989 with the following objectives

- To check for duplication of cases (same case reported more than once by different health facility visited by child)
- To screen children who developed poliomyelitis prior to the year of reporting
- To identify high risk pockets
- To document high risk age groups

Mopping up

- It is an end stage strategy for polio eradication, used when polio virus transmission is reduced to a few foci
- It involves door to door immunization (min 2rounds 4-6 week apart. In India 3 rounds)
- It is practiced in high risk districts, with known or suspected WPV circulation
- In addition to the district with WPV circulation, neighbouring district are also targeted.
- It is recommended to cover 2-5 million under 5 children in each mopping up

162. Ans. (d) There should be minimum 4 weeks interval between PPI...

Ref: K. Park, 24th ed. p 223-24

Pulse Polio Immunization

- Government of India conducted the *1st round of PPI, with 2 immunization days 6 weeks apart on 9th December 1995 and 20th January 1996.* It targeted all children under 3 years-of age.
- *In PPIs oral polio vaccine is given to all children 0-5 years of age, in the country in a week* (Booth + House to house visit + B team), *regardless of previous immunizationstatus.*[Q]
- Dose of OPV during PPIs are *extra doses that supplement and do not replace doses received during routine immunization services.*[Q]
- There is no minimum interval between PPI and scheduled OPV doses
- Bivalent OPV was introduced in PPI in 2009

163. Ans. (b) Polio

Ref: DK Taneja. Health Policies and Programmes in India p-194

The 107 Block Plan*- 66 blocks in UP and 41 blocks in Bihar were identified as high risk and were targeted for wiping out polio with special plans*

Objectives of the 107 Block Plan

- To ensure full strength and leadership of the Government of India
- Launch new and/or strengthen ongoing initiatives to address factors contributing to poliovirus transmission.
  - Interventions to improve water, hygiene and sanitation conditions
  - Village Health and Nutrition Days to deliver OPV to missed children and promote exclusive breastfeeding.
  - Reduce incidence of diarrhea by promotion of zinc/ORS
- Strengthen routine immunization services.
- Deliver the highest quality polio immunization activity in the 107 blocks
- Track performance and progress in HR blocks (Identify indicators, set targets, and report regularly on progress)
- Conduct research to refine strategies and optimize use of vaccines.

Note: 107 Block plan is an old strategy under the NPSP

164. Ans. (d) mVDPV

Ref: K. Park, 24th ed. p 219

VDPV (Vaccine Derived Polio Virus) are of 3 types
- cVDPV- Where person to person transmission occurs in community
- iVDPV- (Immunodeficiency associated VDPV). In person with primary immunodeficiency and prolonged VDPV infection
- aVDPV- (Ambiguous VDPV). Clinical isolates from a person with no known immunodeficiency or Sewage isolates of unknown source

165. Ans. (d) 12 weeks

Ref: K. Park, 24th ed. p 220

Infectious material for polio comprise–Faeces and Oropharyngeal secretion of an infected person
- In faeces virus is excreted for 2–3 week. Maximum for 3–4 month

Also Know......................

- Polio case is most infectious 7–10 days before and after onset of symptoms.

166. Ans. (b) (b) Pakistan; (d) Afganistan

Ref: K. Park, 24th ed. p 217

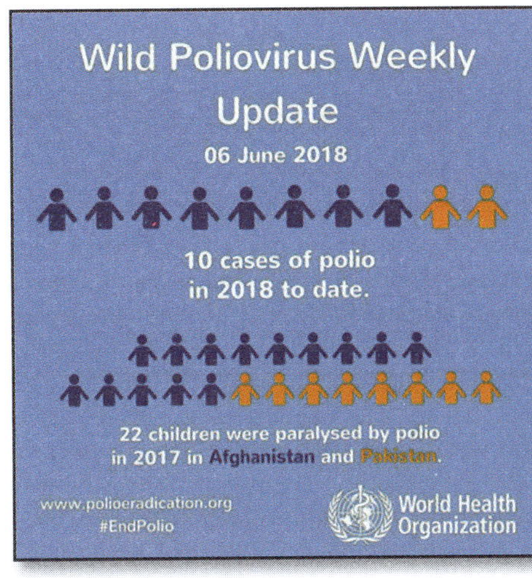

167. Ans. (b) Last polio case in India was reported in 13 january 2011

Ref: K. Park, 24th ed. p 217

168. Ans. (a) Type 3 is most common in India

Ref: K. Park, 24th ed. p 220, K. Park, 25th ed. p 230–242

HEPATITIS

169. Ans. (c) Anti HBc

Ref: K. Park, 25th ed. p 234

Lab marker for HAV infections:

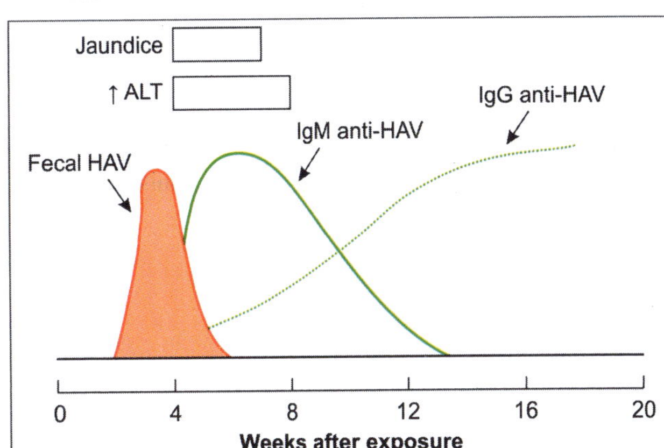

Lab marker for HBV infections:

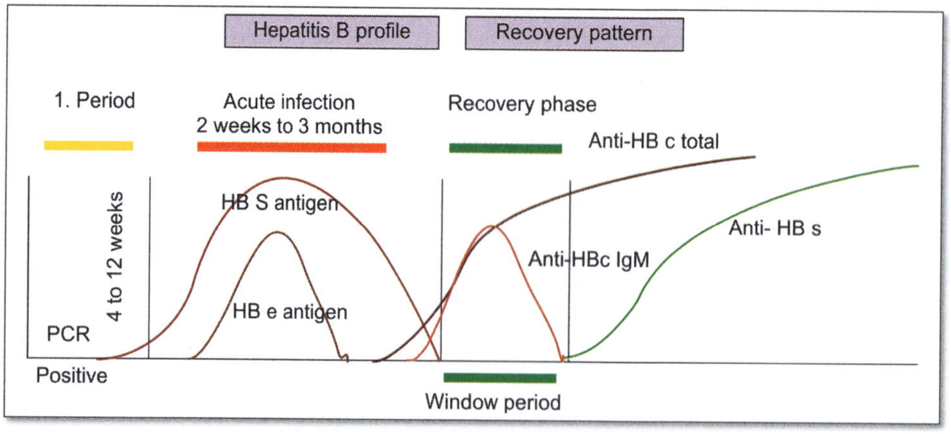

Antigen

- HBsAg (hepatitis B surface antigen) is the first serologic marker to appear in a new acute infection, which can be detected as early as 1 week and as late as 9 weeks, with an average of one month after exposure to the hepatitis B virus (HBV).
- HBsAg is detectable for a variable amount of time, along with the HBV DNA, though about 50% of persons will test HBsAg and HBV DNA negative 7 weeks after symptoms.
- HBeAg (hepatitis B e-antigen) is generally detectable in patients with a new acute infection; the presence of HBeAg is associated with higher HBV DNA levels, thus, increased infectiousness.

Antibody:

- Anti-HBs or HBsAb (hepatitis B surface antibody)
  - This antibody appears after roughly 4 weeks, after the disappearance of HBsAg.
  - It indicates the end of the acute phase and patient complete recovery from the infection.
  - The patient will develop immunity to HBV infection.
  - After vaccination, there is the appearance of HBsAb.
- Anti-HBc or HBcAb (hepatitis B core antibody) – this blood test remains positive indefinitely as a marker of past HBV infection.
  - This antibody appears after one month of infection.
  - In acute infection, this will be HBcAb-IgM type and later replaced by HBcAb-IgG type.
  - This antibody persists in circulation for several years.
  - This antibody will be present in chronic hepatitis cases.
  - In the window period when HBsAg is negative and still there are no HBsAb, then this is the antibody present in the patient.
  - HbcAb-IgM is the marker in the window period in acute infections.
  - This is also called as the window period marker.
- IgM anti-HBc – a positive blood test result indicates a person has a new acute hepatitis B infection. IgM anti-HBc is generally detectable at the time symptoms appear and declines to sub-detectable levels within 6 - 9 months. Note: An acute exacerbation (or liver flare) in a chronic HBV infection can also result in a positive anti-HBc IgM test result. So follow-up testing after 6 months is required.
- IgG anti-HBc – this blood test remains positive indefinitely as a marker of past HBV infection.
- HBeAb
  - The appearance of HBeAb is a sign of recovery.
  - This antibody shows the end of the acute phase.

170. Ans. (c) HBe Ag

171. Ans. (b) 6 months

Chronic HBV infection is defined as persistence of HBsAg for 6 motnhs or more after acute infection with HBV

172. Ans. (b) Communitisation

173. Ans. (c) HBV is a monovalent recombinant vaccine

Option	True/ false	Comment
Treatment for hepatitis B is started when the HBV DNA is >2000 IU/mL	F	No, the cases with HBV DNA <2000 are not treated irrespective of the HBsAg levels. Treatment is indicated for Levels >20,000 IU/mL
The assessment of cirrhosis is done when AST-to-platelet ration index of more than 10	F	No, the APRI score should be more than 2 indicated hepatic fibrosis and cirrhosis of liver
HBV is a monovalent recombinant vaccine	T	Yes correct.
Complete vaccination provides lifelong immunity for more than 95%	F	No, complete vaccination provides 95% coverage till 40 years of age, after which the protection reduces to lesser than 60% coverage by 60 years of age

174. Ans. (a) Water borne, (c) Fulminant infection in pregnancy

- Highest prevalence in south Asia and east Asia
- India has highest prevalence of genotype 1, HEV
- IP = mean of 40 days
- More common in young adults, age 15-40 years
- Fulminant hepatitis is more commonly associated with pregnancy and HEV infections, case fatality rate of up to 20%
- Diagnosis – IgM and IgG antibody in blood, RT-PCR may be done, but is expensive and not routinely used.
- Treatment: Usually self-limiting, prevention is most appropriate and effective approach.

175. Ans. (c) HBe Ag

Ref: K. Park, 24th ed. p 229

Also Know........................

- Appearance of HBsAg, HBeAg and DNA polymerase precede the onset of disease.

176. Ans. (a) Hepatitis A

Ref: K. Park, 23rd edition, p-211. Latin American Center for Perinatology/Women and ReproductiveHealth - Pan American Health Organization/World Health Organization

177. Ans. (a) Acute infectious hepatitis B

Ref: K. Park, 24th ed. p 229

178. Ans. (c) Active and infectious hepatitis B disease

Ref: K. Park, 24th ed. p 214

179. Ans. (b) IgM Anti HBc

Ref: K. Park, 24th ed. p 214

180. Ans. (c) Chronic Hepatitis B infection with high infectivity

Ref: K. Park, 24th ed. p-230

181. Ans. (d) E

Ref: S Lal, Textbook of community medicine, 4th edition, p-511

Outbreak of Hepatitis E

One of the most common cause of acute fulminant hepatitis among adults in Asia and Africa

Outbreak occur due to sewage contaminated drinking water

- 1954- New Delhi -40000 cases
- 1991- Kanpur -79000 cases

182. Ans. (a) Hepatits B vaccine + Immunoglobulin

Ref: K. Park, 24th ed. p 217

Simultaneous administration of Hepatitis B vaccine and Hepatitis B Immunoglobulin (HBIG) is more efficacious than HBIG alone

Ideal for

- Prophylaxis against accidental exposure to blood containing Hepatitis B virus
- Prevention of carrier state in newborn babies, born to carrier mother

Dose-HBIG -0.05-0.07 mL/kg as soon as possible (ideally within 24 hours) and Hepatitis B vaccine–1st dose (1 mL intramuscular) within 7 day of exposure (schedule being 0, 1 and 6 month

183. Ans. (a) HBsAg; (c) Anti – HBc; (d) HBeAg

Ref: K. Park, 24th ed. p 214

184. Ans. (c) 3 weeks

Ref: K. Park, 25th ed. p 231

Hepatitis A ("Infectious" hepatitis or epidemic jaundice) → is caused by Enterovirus type 72 of Picornaviridae family

- Disease is benign with complete recovery in several weeks.
- Infection is more frequent in children (mild or subclinical); clinical severity increases with age.
- Both sexes are equally susceptible
- Isolation period -3 weeks (23rd edition, p-120)
- *Reservoir of infection*: Cases (subclinical or symptomatic) No evidence of a chronic carrier state.
- Immunity after attack lasts for life. Most people in endemic areas acquire immunity via sub-clinical infection.
- **Modes of transmission** –Faeco oral (*major route*), Sexual (in homosexual)
- **Incubation period** –10 to 50 days. Length of I.P. is proportional to dose of virus ingested
- **Diagnosis** –
  - Demonstration of HAV particles (or specific viral antigens) in the faeces.
  - Demonstration of a rise in anti-HAV titre
  - Detection of IgM antibody to HAV in patient's serum; IgG signals past infection and immunity.
- Poor sanitation and overcrowding favour spread of infection (Water-borne/Food-borne) after heavy rain.
- **Prevention and containment**–
- **Control of reservoir:** Difficult. → Notification, complete bed rest, disinfection of Faeces/Fomites (0.5% Sodium hypochlorite).
- **Control of transmission:** Personal and community hygiene (Handwashing), Sanitary disposal of excreta, Purification of water (flocculation, filtration and chlorination), use of boiled water during epidemic.
- **Prevention of susceptible population:** (Traveller to endemic area, close contact of HAV patient)-HBIG **and** Vaccination

ACUTE DIARRHEAL DISEASE

185. Ans. (a) 245

Ref: K. Park, 24th ed. p 239

186. Ans. (d) 24 hours

Ref: K. Park, 24th ed. p 240

- Contents of ORS packet are dissolved in 1 L of drinking water.
- ORS solution should be made fresh and used within 24 hours. It should not be boiled or sterilised

Also Know.......................

- **Oral rehydration** was introduced by WHO in 1971. Mechanism of action -Oral glucose enhances intestinal absorption of salt and water, and corrects electrolyte and water deficit.

187. Ans. (c) To increase absorption of glucose

Ref: Textbook of PSM, Gupta and Mahajan, 4th ed p 218, Bull World Health Organ. 1986; 64 (1; 24th ed. p145-50

Sodium Citrate

- Makes the ORS salt more stable
- Reduces stool output
- Increases intestinal absorption of sodium and water.
- ORS-citrate is as successful as ORS-bicarbonate in terms of its ability to rehydrate, correct the acidosis, and maintain electrolyte concentrations

188. Ans. (b) 14 days

Ref: K. Park, 24th ed. p 236

Diarrhea is frequent passage (>3 times a day) of loose liquid or watery stools.

Also Know.......................

- Change in consistency is more important compared to number of stools.

Types

- Acute watery diarrhea- Caused by V. Cholerae, E. Coli and Rota virus. Major concern is dehydration. Lasts for a few hour to few days
- Dysentery (Visible blood in stool)- Caused by Shigella. Major concern is damage of intestinal mucosa, sepsis and malnutrition
- Persistent diarrhea- lasts ≥14 days. Concern is Malnutrition and serious non intestinal infection, dehydration may occur.
- Diarrhea with severe malnutrition – Concern is severe systemic infection, dehydration, heart failure Vitamin and mineral deficiency

189. Ans. (a) Sodium; (c) Glucose

Ref: K. Park, 24th ed. p 239

"Lactated Ringer's Solution" or "Hartmann's solution".

- It is a "***crystalloid***" solution, isotonic with blood & is intended for intravenous administration. (May be given subcutaneously).
- **pH is 6.5**
- Not suitable for maintenance therapy → sodium content (130 mEq/L) is too high, particularly for children and Potassium content (4 mEq/L) is too low.

Indications: Extracellular dehydration (vomiting, diarrhea, fistula, etc.), Hypovolemia (Hemorrhagic shocks, Burns), Perioperative electrolyte losses, Metabolic acidosis except lactic acidosis

Contraindications: Congestive Cardiac Failure, Hyper-hydration (predominantly extracellular), Hyperkalaemia, Hypercalcemia, Metabolic alkalosis

190. Ans. (d) 1:1

Ref: K. Park, 24th ed. p 239

191. Ans. (b) Moderate

Ref: K. Park, 24th ed. p 239

Mild diarrhea is characterised by 4-5% body weight loss and 40-50 mL /kg fluid deficit. Child appears thirsty, alert and restless

Severe diarrhea is characterised by ≥10% body weight loss and 100-110 mL /kg fluid deficit.

- Child appears drowsy, limp, cold, sweaty.
- Pulse is rapid and feeble (may be impalpable), BP is <80 mm Hg,
- Skin pinch retracts very slowly (>2 seconds), Tongue is dry, Anterior fontanelle is very sunken
- Urine output is little or none

192. Ans. (c) 800-1200 mL

Ref: K. Park, 24th ed. p 239

Patients should be given as much ORS solution as they want and signs of dehydration should be checked until they subside.

- Older children and adults should be given as much water as they want, in addition to ORS solution.
- Child <2 year age, a teaspoon of ORS is given every 1-2 min, with estimated amount to be given within 4 hour.
- In case of vomiting, ORS should be tried after about 10 min and given more slowly(1 spoonful every 2-3 min).
- Breast feeding should be continued during treatment with ORS in nursing women.
- Non-breastfed infants (<6 month age) should be given additional 100-200 mL of water in the first 4 hours.

Guidelines for ORT in first four hours

Age (used if weight is not known	<4-months	4-11 months	1-2 years	2-4 years	5-14 years	>15 years
Weight (kg)	Under 5	5-7.9	8-10.9	11-15.9	16-29.9	>30
ORS (mL)	200-400	400-600	600-800	800-1200	1200-2200	2200-4000

Intravenous rehydration–indicated only for initial rehydration of severely dehydrated patients (in shock or unable to drink)

- WHO recommends Ringer's lactate solution (Hartmann's solution) (**Best**) or Diarrhea Treatment Solution (DTS) or Normal saline (Poorest) for iv infusion

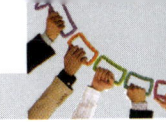

- Recommended dose of I.V. fluid is 100 mL/kg in 5 hour 30 min in Infants (30 mL/kg in 1st hour followed by 70 mL/kg in next 5hour) and 3 hour in older children (30 mL/kg in first 30 min followed by 70 mL/kg in next 2 hour 30 min)
- Initial rehydration should be fast (until pulse is easily palpable) If patient can drink ORS should be given about 5 mL/kg/hour. Rehydration must continue until all signs of dehydration have disappeared.

Also Know......................

- ORS packets are freely available at all primary health centers, sub-centers and Govt. hospitals.

193. Ans. (b) 600-800 mL

Ref: K. Park, 24th ed. p 239

194. Ans. (b) 245

Ref: K. Park, 24th ed. p 239

195. Ans. (d) 24 hours

Ref: K. Park, 24th ed. p 240

196. Ans. (b) 75

Ref: K. Park, 24th ed. p 239

CHOLERA

197. Ans. (b) Adenyl cyclase

Ref: K. Park, 24th ed. p 244

Vibrio Cholerae multiply in the intestinal lumen and produce an exotoxin that acts on the adenyl cyclase cyclic AMP system of mucosal cells of the small intestine and result diarrhea.

198. Ans. (d) Typhoid

Ref: K. Park, 24th ed. p 251

Disease	Doc For Chemoprophylaxis	Doc For Treatment
Plague	Tetracycline	Streptomycin
Diphtheria	Erythromycin	Penicillin or Erythromycin
Meningococcal meningitis	Ciprofloxacin, Minocycline, Spiramycin and Ceftriaxone	Penicillin
Cholera	Tetracycline	Tetracycline and Norfloxacin
Bacterial conjunctivitis	Erythromycin ointment	
Pertussis	Erythromycin	Erythromycin
Malaria	Doxycycline (For <6 week), Mefloquine (For >6 week)	
Influenza A	Zanamivir (If contraindicated then Rimantidine)	Zanamivir or Oseltamivir + Rimantidine
Influenza B	Oseltamivir OR Zanamivir	Oseltamivir OR Zanamivir

Contd...

199. Ans. (c) Measles

Ref: K. Park, 24th ed. p 156

200. Ans. (c) Due to O139 Strain; (e) Low proportion of adults in endemic regions

Ref: Cambridge International AS Level Biology, p 202

- Six pandemics of Cholera occurred between 1817 and 1923, caused by O1 strain (All of them originated from Bangladesh)
- Seventh pandemic began in 1961 in Indonesia, was caused by "El Tor" strain
- Eighth pandemic originated in Chennai (India) in 1992, caused by O139 strain of V. Cholerae.
- O139 is more virulent than El Tor and was reported in many adults (Exposure to El Tor does not offer immunity to O139)

201. Ans. (a) Safe water supply and sanitation

Ref: K. Park, 24th ed. p 246

Control of Cholera Outbreak: WHO Guidelines

- Verification of diagnosis (V. Cholerae O1 in patient stool) and Early case detection
- Setting up of treatment centers and rehydration therapy for cholera cases
- General sanitation measures at onset of outbreak
  - Safe water supply for all purpose
  - **Excreata disposal:** Provision of simple, cheap and effective excreta disposal system must be ensured
- **Food sanitation must be stressed:** Eating cooked hot food, Hygienic food handling techniques,
- **Disinfection:** Concurrent and Terminal. Disinfectant used is Cresol (RW coefficient ≥10) or Bleaching powder (33% Chlorine). Patient's stools/vomit/clothes/Items contaminated and latrine need to be disinfected
- **Chemoprophylaxis:** Tetracycline is the drug of choice. Mass chemoprophylaxis is not advised.
- **Vaccination:** Dukoral, Sanchol and mORCVAX. Protection commences at least 7 days after the last scheduled dose
- Health education -Most effective prophylactic measure (ORT, early reporting and prompt treatment, food hygiene, hand washing etc.)

202. Ans. (b) Few hours to 5 days

Ref: K. Park, 24th ed. p 245

Cholera

Reservoir of infection: Human (Case or Carrier)
Infective material: Stools and vomit of cases/carriers.
Infective dose: A very high dose

(1011 organisms) is needed to produce clinical disease in normal adults.

Period of communicability for:

- Case of cholera is 7-1 0 days.
- Convalescent carriers is 2-3 weeks.
- Chronic carrier is 1month to ≥10 years

Cholera is a notifiable locally, nationally and internationally (Notified to WHO within 24 hr)

Mild and asymptomatic cases play a significant role in maintaining endemic reservoir.

203. Ans. (a) Cresol

Ref: K. Park, 24th ed. p 247

Cresol with RW Coefficient >10 is ideal for disinfection of stool, especially in cholera

204. Ans. (d) Tetracycline

Ref: K. Park, 24th ed. p 247

Antibiotic	Children	Adult
Tetracycline BD × 3 days (**DRUG OF CHOICE**)	125 mg (4-13 year) and 50 mg (0-3 year)	500 mg
Doxycycline (Single dose)	6 mg/kg for children up to 15 year	300 mg

Antidiarrheals, Antiemetics, Antispasmodics, Cardiotonics and Corticosteroids should not be given

Also Know......................

- DOC in shigella dysentery is Trimethoprim and Sulphameth-oxazole, Acute Intestinal amoebiasis and giardiasis is Metro-nidazole.

205. Ans. (a) Cholera

Ref: K Park, Refer to Annexure for details

TYPHOID

206. Ans. (c) Man

Ref: K. Park, 24th ed. p 250

Typhoid Fever

Causative agent- S. Typhi. Infequently S Paratyphi A and B

Reservoir of infection: Man (cases and carriers) infectious as long as bacilli appear in stools or urine.

Source of infection:

- Primary → faeces and urine of cases/carriers;
- Secondary → contaminated water, food, fingers andfly

Typhoid Carrier

Average carrier rate is around 3%

- Convalescent carrier excrete bacilli for 6-8 week
- Chronic carriers (2-5% of cases) excrete bacilli for >1 year (or intermittently. Eg. "Typhoid Mary".) Organisms persist in gall bladder and biliary tract.[Q]
- Faecal carriers are more common than urinary carriers
- More cases occur in males than females.
- Carrier rate is more in females[Q]

207. Ans. (b) 10-14 days

Ref: K. Park, 24th ed. p 250

Typhoid Fever

- **Incubation period** –10-14 days.
- **Modes of transmission** – Faecal-oral route or urine-oral routes
- Natural infection does not always confer solid immunity. High antibody titre of O antigen is seen in diseased individuals and Flagellar antigen (H) in immunized individuals.

Control of Typhoid fever –3 lines of defence:

1. Control of reservoir

- Cases
  - Early diagnosis (Blood & Stools culture) and Notification
  - **Isolation:** (Preferable in a hospital) till 3 bacteriologically negative stools and urine reports are obtained on 3 separate days[Q]
  - **Treatment:** Ciprofloxacin is drug of choice.[Q]
  - Disinfection of stools and urine (5% cresol for at least 2 hours).
  - **Follow-up examination:** 3/4 month post discharge and at 12 month.
- Carrier
  - **Identification:** (Culture and Serological examination) 80% chronic carriers have Vi antibodies (Strong evidence)[Q]
  - **Treatment:** Ampicillin (4–6 g/day) + Probenecid (2 g/day) for 6 weeks and/or Surgery: Cholecystectomy Surveillance

2. Control of sanitation – (weakest link)

Protection and Purification of drinking water supply, Promotion of food hygiene + health education (Hand washing) Immunisation

Also Know......................

- Typhoid fever is the *index of general sanitation*[Q] in any country

FOOD POISONING

208. Ans. (d) Staph aureus

Ref: K. Park, 24th ed. p 253

Food poisoning	Incubation period (hours)
Staphylococcal Food poisoning	1–8
Botulinism	18–36
Cl. perfringens (welchii)	6–24 (peak 10 to 14 hours)
Bacillus cereus (Emetic)	1–6
Bacillus cereus (Diarrheaal)	12–24
Salmonellosis	12–24

AMOEBIASIS/ ASCARIASIS/ HOOK WORM INFECTION/ DRACUNCULIASIS

209. Ans. (a) Hookworms

Ref: K. Park, 22nd ed. p-221; 24th ed. p 221

210. Ans. (b) Hookworm infection – an important public health problem

Ref: K. Park, 22nd ed. p-221; 24th ed. p 221

***Chandler's index** is average number of hookworm eggs per gram of faeces for the entire community*[Q]

Average number of eggs per gram of stools	Indicates Hook worm infection is
▪ Below 200	Not of much significance
▪ 200-250	Potential danger
▪ 250-300	Minor public health problem
▪ Above 300	Major public health problem

211. Ans. (a) >300

Ref: K. Park, 24th ed. p 221

212. Ans. (a) Ankylostoma Duodenale

Ref: K Park 22nd ed. p-221; 24th ed. p 221

213. Ans. (c) No. of eggs of hookworm in 1 gram stool

Ref: K Park 22nd ed. p-221; 24th ed. p 221

214. Ans. (b) Monitoring individual treatment

Ref: K Park 22nd ed. p 221; 24th ed. p 221

Hookworm infection (*Necator Americanus* in South India and *Ancylostoma Duodenale* in North India)

- ***Chandler's index*** helps compare worm loads across different population groups and degree of reduction of egg output after mass treatment in closed communities
- ***Chandler's index*** is used to assess endemicity (Potential/ Minor/Major public health problem)

215. Ans. (b) DDT spray

Ref: K Park 24th ed. p 261

WHO Dracunculosis Eradication Strategy

- Safe drinking water supply (e.g. piped water)
- Control of Cyclops
- Health education-Boiling or Sieving of drinking water using a double thickness cotton cloth, Personal protection and prevention of water contamination by infected persons
- Surveillance (Active search for new cases)

Eradicated from India (last case in July 1996) in Feb 2000.[Q]

Reservoir of infection: An infected person harbouring gravid female

All individuals are susceptible to Multiple/Repeated infections

Disease is limited to tropical and subtropical regions. Larvae develop between 25°C–30°C (Not below 19°C).

Mode of transmission: Consumption of water containing cyclops (Harbouring infective stages of parasite).

Washing and Bathing in surface water (ponds- peak transmission between Jun-Sept) and step-wells (peak -March-May)contribute to infection.[Q]

Treatment: Mebendazole and Metronidazole limit inflammation and help remove worms. None of the drugs cures the disease or prevents transmission of disease.

RABIES

216. Ans. (d) Fatal only some cases

217. Ans. (b) 2 years

218. Ans. (d) All serotypes cause rabies

219. Ans. (b) Street virus

220. Ans. (a) Long incubation period

Rabies:

- Street virus: Variable incubation period of 20-60 days
- Fixed virus: Fixed incubation period of 4-6 days (shorter incubation period)
  - It does not form Negri bodies
  - It does not multiply in extra neural tissues
  - It is used for anti-rabies vaccine production

221. Ans. (b) Fixed virus

222. Ans. (a) 1

Lyssavirus 1 is a bullet shaped RNA containing virus from the family Rhabdoviridae – serotype 1. The other serotypes 2,3,4 are rabies related and cause rabies like illness in man and animals.

223. Ans. (a) Dogs

224. Ans. (d) Vampire bats

Bats are major source of infection in US and Canada.

225. Ans. (b) Aerosol transmission is quite common

Rabies

- Rabies is most common in age group 1-15 years (average cases are between age group 1-24 years of age)
- Transmission is by bite or scratch by infected animal. Direct transmission by inhalation is possible is but very rare.
- Human-to-human transmission of virus is only theoretically possible and never reported

226. Ans. (b) Severity of bite

227. Ans. (d) All of the above

228. Ans. (d) None of the above

There is no specific treatment for rabies.

The individual case management depends on specific case, severity of bite and other comorbidities:

- Isolation from any trigger factors as sound, light, thermal variations
- Relieve anxiety by sedatives
- Antispasmodics for severe muscular contractions – with curare like action
- Ensure hydration, diuresis
- Cardiorespiratory support systems

229. Ans. (c) Duck embryo vaccine (DEV)

Rabies vaccine:

2 major types of vaccines are available:

- Cell culture vaccine
- Embryonated (egg based) vaccine

Which of the following rabies vaccine is not available in India?

a. Semple vaccine
b. Suckling mouse brain vaccine
c. DEV
d. HDCV

230. Ans. (c) DEV

231. Ans. (d) All of the above

232. Ans. (b) Kills virus

233. Ans. (c) Can be given after exposure to infection

234. Ans. (c) Small Bite on thigh

235. Ans. (d) Toes

236. Ans. (d) All of the above

237. Ans. (b) 20 IU/Kg

238. Ans. (c) Foxes

Ref: https://www.cdc.gov/mmwr/preview/mmwrhtml/mm6214a3.htm

Baits laden with oral rabies vaccines are important for the management of wildlife rabies in the United States, Canada and other developed nations.

239. Ans. (b) Administer cell culture...

Ref: K. Park, 24th ed. p 296

Management of Exposure to a Suspect or Confirmed Rabid Animal

ARS should be given at the initiation of postexposure vaccination or as soon as possible but not beyond 7th day of initiation of postexposure vaccination

240. Ans. (c) 15 min

Ref: K. Park, 24th ed. p 296

Management of Rabid Animal Bite

Local wound management

- Cleaning/flushing the wound with soap and water (preferably under running tap water) for 15 min.
- Irrigation with catheter in case of punctured wound
- Chemical treatment: Viricidal agents alcohol and tincture iodine
- Wound should never be sutured immediately (if necessary, it should be done after 24–48 hours, applying minimum stitches and undercover of Anti Rabies Serum locally)

241. Ans. (d) Australia

Ref: K. Park, 24th ed. p 294

Rabies-free zone *is an area in which no case of indigenously acquired rabies in man or any animal species has been reported for 2 years*

- Australia, Cyprus, Japan, New Zealand, UK, China (Taiwan), Iceland, Ireland, Malta, Islands of Western Pacific, Liberian peninsula, Finland, Norway, Sweden are free from Rabies
- Maldives is the only country in the South East Asian region that is free of human or animal rabies.

Also Know.......................

- Water is the most effective natural barrier to rabies. In India, Lakshadweep & Andman and Nicobar islands are free of Rabies

242. Ans. (b) 3 mm/hour

Ref: Rajesh Bhatia, Rabies: the Killer Disease, p 42

243. Ans. (d) Days 0, 7

Ref: K. Park, 24th ed. p 297

Pre-exposure Prophylaxis (PEP)

- **Indication:** Persons at high risk of continual exposure (lab staff working with rabies virus, veterinarians, animal handlers and wild-life officers, Travellers with extensive outdoor exposure).
- Cell culture vaccine 1 mL/0.5 mL intramuscular or 0.1 mL intradermal on days 0, 7 days.
- Booster is recommended only for people who are at risk of continual exposure due to their occupation.
- Serological monitoring is done 6 monthly for people at risk of lab exposure to high concentration of live virus and 2 yearly in other individuals at risk of continual exposure e.g. veterinarians, animal handlers
- If titre of virus neutralizing antibodies in vaccinated individuals serum is less than 0.5 IU/mL, booster is recommended.

244. Ans. (b) Dog

Ref: K. Park, 24th ed. p 294

Rabies (Hydrophobia)

- *Causative agent* → Lyssavirus serotype 1 (*Neurotropic RNA virus*) of family Rhabdoviridae.

- Rabies in man is a *dead-end infection*
- *Only communicable disease of man that is always fatal.*
- ***Reservoirs of infection***:
  - *Urban rabies* (99% of human cases in India): *Dog, Cat* – (1 rabid dog involves an area of over 40 km in its span of clinical illness.)
  - *Wild-life rabies (Sylvatic form)* → ***Unidentified reservoir*** (Jackal, Fox, Hyena etc transmit infection to dogs and domestic animals). Man gets rabies by intrusion into wild -life cycle.
  - *Bat rabies*: Vampire bat is an host and vector of rabies in Latin American countries (e.g., Brazil, Venezuela, Mexico) and parts of U.S.A. Not reported in India
- ***Source of infection***: Saliva of rabid animals. (Dogs/cats → virus may be present in saliva for 3-4 days before onset of clinical symptoms, during course of illness till death.)
- **Mode of transmission** –
  - Animal bites, licks on abraded skin, mucosa, Aerosols (caves harbouring rabies infected bats and in laboratory)
  - Person -to -person: Rare. Transmission of rabies by corneal and organ transplants.
- **Incubation period** – Variable in man, commonly 3-8 weeks following exposure.
  - *Depends on site of bite, severity of bite, number of wounds, amount of virus injected, species of biting animal, protection provided by the clothing and treatment undertaken, if any.*[Q]
- **Clinical Features:**
  - Prodromal symptoms (Headache, malaise, sore throat and slight fever). About 80% patients complain of pain or tingling at the site of the bite
  - Followed by widespread excitation and stimulation of nervous system. (Involving in order Sensory → Motor → Sympathetic and CNS. The patient is intolerant to noise, bright light or a cold draught of air.
  - Hydrophobia (fear of water) is *pathognomonic of rabies.* Duration of illness is 2-3 days (Maximum 5-6 days)
- **Diagnosis** –
- Clinical → Based on history of rabid animal bite and characteristic signs and symptoms.
  - Antigen detection using immunof-luorescence of skin biopsy and virus isolation from saliva/other secretions.
- **Treatment:** No specific treatment. Case is managed by isolation in a quiet room, relieving anxiety and pain, hydration, diuresis and Intensive therapy (Respiratory and Cardiac support.)

245. Ans. (a) 20 IU/kg

Ref: K. Park, 24th ed p 297

Anti Rabies Serum (ARS)

- Dose: ***Equine ARS:*** 40 IU/Kg and Human Rabies immuno-globulin: (HRIG)-20 IU/Kg Single dose is given on day zero
- It prevents replication of virus at the site of bite and prolongs the incubation period
- All or as much as anatomically feasible amount of ARS is infiltrated into and around bite wound and the rest is given intramuscularly.
- ARS offers passive immunity and is recommended for all class III bites

246. Ans. (b) Hematogenous spread to brain

Ref: K. Park, 24th ed. p 294-95

Rabies virus multiplies in muscle or connective tissue at or near the site of inoculation and then enters peripheral nerve and ascends (centripetally) passively via nerve associated tissue space to brain. It then spreads via peripheral nerves (centrifufally) to other body parts

- CFR of Rabies is 100% (*Always fatal)*
- Rabies is contracted by bites of Dogs, Cats, Jackal, Wolves. It may be contracted from other animals → E.g., Monkey, Mongoose and Cattle (Horse, Sheep, Goat, Cow etc) Rodents –Domestic rat, mice, squirrel, hare & rabbit do not require antirabies treatment

247. Ans. (a) 2-2-2-0-0

Ref: WHO, Rabies position paper, 2018

The recent updated Rabies vaccination guidelines (WHO 2018) are:

- ONE week; 2 site; ID regime; Institut pasteur du cambodge regime; 2-2-2-0-0
- Two week; 1 site; IM regime; 4 dose; ESSEN regime; 1-1-1-1-0
- Three week; IM regime; 5 dose; ZAGREB regime; 2-0-1-0-1
- Four Week; ID regime; 8 dose; Thai Red Cross regime; 2-2-2-0-2

248. Ans. (b) 2

Ref: K. Park, 24th ed. p 294

249. Ans. (c) Fixed

Ref: K. Park, 24th ed. p 294

Street virus: Virus obtained from naturally occurring case of Rabies. Long incubation period (20-60 day) and cause disease in mammals

Fixed virus: Virus obtained by serial brain-to-brain passage of street virus in rabbits. It has a short, fixed and reproducible incubation period (4-6 days). It does not form Negri bodies and does not multiply in extra-neural tissues.

Also Know......................

- Fixed virus is used in preparation of Anti Rabies vaccine.

Latest Updates

Most cases of human rabies (99%) result from dog- bites.
Bite by all wild animals comprises class III exposure

SURFACE INFECTION

Trachoma

250. Ans. (b) Tetracycline

Ref: K. Park, 24th ed. p 327

Chemotherapy in Trachoma

- Mass treatment (Blanket treatment)
  - Indication – Prevalence of severe and moderate Trachoma in children under 10 years of age of >5%.

- Tetracycline (1% ointment- Treatment of choice) is given to all children, for 5 consecutive days each month or 60 consecutive days
- Alternative is Erythromycin

▪ Selective treatment – When prevalence is low to medium. Population is screened to find cases who are treated

251. Ans. (b) Tetracycline

Ref: K. Park, 24th ed. p 327

252. Ans. (d) 1-9 years

Ref: K. Park, 24th ed. p 326

Trachoma most *commonly affects children in the age group (2-5 years).*

▪ Prevalence of trachoma is assessed by screening children under 10 years of age for active trachoma.

Also Know......................

WHO recommendation for field diagnosis of Trachoma-cases must have at least 2 of the following diagnostic criteria

- Follicles on the upper tarsal conjunctiva
- Limbal follicles or their sequelae-Herbert's pits
- Conjunctival scarring (trichiasis, entropion)
- Vascular pannus on superior limbus

TETANUS

253. Ans. (d) None of the above

Ref. Park 25th pg 338

The clostridia spores are very resistant to:

▪ Phenols, cresols,
▪ Boiling, autoclaving for 10-15 mins at 120°C

The spores are best destroyed by:

▪ Autoclave – steam under pressure for at least 20 mins at 120 °C
▪ Gamma radiation

254. Ans. (d) None of the above

Reservoir: The natural habitat of tetanus is soil and dust

255. Ans. (c) <1 case per 1000 live births

Ref: K. Park, 25th ed. p 338

The elimination of Neonatal tetanus is defined as <1 case per 1000 live births in every district

256. Ans. (c) 7th day

The common cause is infection of the umbilical stump, the first symptom on 7th day – therefore also known as 8th day disease

257. Ans. (c) 4 degree C

258. Ans. (a) 250 IU

259. Ans. (d) Parasympathetic system

260. Ans. (b) Single dose of tetanus toxoid

Ref: K. Park, 25th ed. p 341

All wounds must be thoroughly cleaned immediately after injury for removal of foreign bodies, soil, dust, necrotic tissue (To abolish anaerobic conditions favouring germination of tetanus spores).

Immunisation status	Clean wound <6 hr old, Non penetrating/ Negligible Tissue damage	Other wounds
Complete course of TT or a booster dose within past 5 Years.	Nothing	Nothing
Complete course of TT or a booster dose more than 5 Years ago and less than 10 Years ago.	Toxoid 1 dose	Toxoid 1 dose
Complete course of TT or a booster dose more than 10 Years ago	Toxoid 1 dose	Toxoid 1 dose + human Tetanus Ig
Had not had a complete course of TT or Immunity status is unknown	Toxoid complete course	Toxoid complete course + human Tetanus Ig

When ATS is given, adrenaline solution 1 in 1000 for intramuscular injection in the dosage of 0.5 to 1 mL and hydrocortisone 100 mg for intravenous injection must be kept available.

261. Ans. (d) <0.1 per 1000

Ref: K. Park, 24th ed. p 328

Neonatal tetanus status of districts	Neonatal tetanus incidence rates	Immunization coverage in pregnant women with 2 doses or a booster dose of TT	Clean deliveries by trained personnel
High risk	>1/1000 live births or	<70% or	<50%
Control	<1/1000 live births	>70%	>50%
Elimination	<0.1/1000 live births	>90%	>75%

262. Ans. (b) Herd immunity present

Ref: K. Park, 24th ed. p 329

Tetanus

- *Causative agent* → Clostridium tetani (Gram-positive, anaerobic, spore bearing organism).
- *Reservoir* → Soil and dust. Bacilli is found in intestine of many herbivorous animal and man[Q]
- *Period of communicability*: None[Q]. Not transmitted from person to person.
- *Mode of transmission* – Contamination of wounds with tetanus spores.[Q]
- Majority of neonatal tetanus cases occur between July to September (Rainy season)
- Incubation period – 6-10 day
- Incidence is higher in males [Females are more exposed to risk (Delivery, Abortion)) and in rural areas.
- No age is immune unless protected by previous immunization.
    - Patients who recover from tetanus also need to be actively immunized
    - Immunity (<6 months) is transferred to baby from immunized mother during pregnancy.
    - *Herd immunity does not protect the individual*
- Tetanus bacilli produce a soluble ***exotoxin*** (lethal dose for a 70 kg man is about 0.1 mg) Its *principal action is to block inhibition of spinal reflexes.*
- Eliminantion is less than 0.1 case per 1000 births, with TT (2dose) coverage >90% and attended delivery >75%

Strategy for prevention of neonatal tetanus:

- Delivery by Skilled Birth Attendant or Institutional delivery (following "3 cleans" or "5 clean" or "7 clean"
- TT to all pregnant women (Unimmunized - 2 doses of TT (1st early in pregnancy and 2nd at least a month later, but 3 weeks before delivery, between 16-36 weeks), Previously immunized –(within 5 year) Booster dose.
- Antitoxin (750 IU) within 6 hours of birth to infants born to unimmunized mothers.
- Last TT dose given within 3 weeks of delivery- Does not guarantee protection of newborn (Protects future pregnancies).
- In developing countries, Golden rule is "No pregnant women be denied a dose of TT if she reports late in pregnancy"

263. Ans. (c) Seen commonly in winter and dry...

Ref: K. Park, 24th ed. p 329

LEPROSY

264. Ans. (a) 1 per 1000

Current Leprosy Stats (2017)

Prevalence	0.66 per 10,000 population
ANCDR (annual new case detection rate)	10.17 per lac population (reported as 9.73 for year 2018)
Grade II Disability%age	3.94

265. Ans. (a) Grows slowly in artificial media

Features of Lepra bacilli

- Acid fast bacilli which are found both intracellular and extracellular
- Found in clumps or clusters – called as Globi
- Affinity for Schwann cells and reticuloendothelial cells
- Most specific antigen is – phenolic glycolipid
- Highest in lepromatous leprosy
- Does not grow in artificial media

266. Ans. (d) All of the above

Mode of transmission:

- Droplet infection – via aerosols and nose as the portal of exit
- Contact transmission: Direct or indirect contact with soil, fomites, clothes, linen
- Other routes: Insect vectors (theoretical existence only)

267. Ans. (d) >95%

Ref: K. Park, 24th ed p-442

PIP Targets for 12 Plan Period (2012-13 – 2016-17) for Leprosy

Indicators	Targets
Prevalence rate less than 1 /10000	100% (642 districts)
Annual New Case Detection Rate (ANCDR) of less than 10/100,000	100% (642 districts)
Cure Rate for MB Leprosy	>95%
Cure Rate for PB Leprosy	>97%
Grade 2 disability rate in percentage of new cases	35% reduction (1.98%)
Stigma reduction	50% reduction over % reported by NSS

268. Ans. (b) 0.68

Ref: K. Park, 24th ed. p 333

Leprosy

- *Prevalence rate (as on 1st April 2014) was 0.68 per 10,000 population.*

Latest Updates

Elimination of Leprosy was attained: **Globally** in the year 2000, **India** *(at national level) in Dec 2005*

Leprosy is a highly infectious disease but of low pathogenicity.[Q]

Source of infection: All patients with "active leprosy" - Multibacillary cases (lepromatous and borderline lepromatous) (Most important)[Q]

Portal of exit:

- Nose (Sneeze or blowing)
- Ulcerated/broken skin of bacteriologically positive cases of leprosy.
- Intact skin via hair follicles.

Attack rates: Among household contacts of lepromatous cases → 4.4% to 12% (Show signs of leprosy within 5 year) despite treatment of the index case.

- Peak Incidence rates seen between 10–20 years of age
- A high prevalence of infection among children indicates that the disease is active and spreading.[Q]
- Both incidence and prevalence of leprosy are higher in males than in females.

Mode of transmission → Droplet infection, Contact transmission (Direct (skin to skin) and Indirect (contact with soil & fomites)), Insect vectors, Tattooing needle, Breast milk from lepromatous mother

269. Ans. (a) ASHA

Ref: K. Park, 24th ed. p

Major Initiatives Under NLEP (2012-13)

- Focus on new case detection, Treatment completion and Disability Limitation and Medical rehabilitation
- Strengthening of Medical Colleges and NGO for reconstructive surgery of leprosy affected people
- Incentive of Rs 5000 for each leprosy affected person from BPL family to undergo reconstructive surgery and Financial support of Rs 5000 per reconstructive surgery conducted for Govt institutions /PMR centers
- Intensive IEC for "Towards Leprosy Free India" –Early case reporting, treatment completion, reducing stigma/ discrimination, provision of quality services.
- Free medical facilities, counselling and MCR footwear
- ASHA to be involved in bringing out suspected leprosy cases from their villages for diagnosis and treatment at PHC and follow up of confirmed leprosy cases for treatment completion.

Also Know......................

- Incentive to ASHA – Rs 100 for each confirmed case brought by ASHA and On treatment completion Rs 200 per PB Leprosy case and Rs 400 per MB Leprosy case.

270. Ans. (b) 3.5

Ref: K. Park, 24th ed. p 337

Bacterial index (BI) *is the only objective way of monitoring benefit of treatment in Leprosy.*[Q]

It ranges from 0 to 6+ (Indicates density of Leprosy bacilli in smears (living/ solid staining and dead/fragmented))

WHO grading of smears for Bacteriological Index is as follows:

- Negative – No bacilli in any of the 100 oil immersion fields
- + → 1-10 bacilli, on average, in 100 oil immersion fields.
- + + → 1-10 bacilli, on average, in 10 oil immersion fields.
- + + + → 1-10 bacilli, on average, in each oil immersion fields.
- + + + + 10-100→bacilli, on average, in each oil immersion fields.
- + + + + + → 100-1000 bacilli, on average, in each oil immersion fields.
- + + + + + + → More than 1000 bacilli, on average, in each oil immersion fields.

Bacterial index is calculated by totaling the index from each site examined and dividing the total by number of sites examined

BI = 1+1+6+6/ 4 = 3.5

271. Ans. (b) 1 per 10000 population

Ref: K. Park, 24th ed. p 441

272. Ans. (a) Clofazimine included in..., (c) Grenz zone is...; (e) MBL recommended...

Ref: K. Park, 24th ed. p 337, 341

Recommended treatment regimens

Age group	Drug	Dosage and frequency	Duration	
			MB	PB
Adult	Rifampicin	600 mg once a month	12 months	6 months
	Clofazimine	300 mg once a month and 50 mg daily		
	Dapsone	100 mg daily		
Children (10–14 years)	Rifampicin	450 mg once a month	12 months	12 months
	Clofazimine	150 mg once a month, 50 mg daily		
	Dapsone	50 mg daily		
Children <10 years old or <40 kg	Rifampicin	10 mg/kg once month	12 months	6 months
	Clofazimine	6 mg/kg once a month and 1 mg/kg daily		
	Dapsone	2 mg/kg daily		

Note: The treatment for children with body weight below 40 kg requires single formulation medications since no MDT combination blister packs are available. For children between 20 and 40 kg, it would be possible to follow the instructions of the Operational Manual, Global Leprosy Strategy 2016–2020 on how to partly use (MB–Child) blister packs for treatment (60).

Also Know......................

- MDT is not contraindicated in patients with HIV infection and is safe during pregnancy.

273. Ans. (d) Diagnosis of leprosy

Ref: K. Park, 24th ed. p 336

Application of Lepromin Test

- *To assess resistance or immune status (CMI) of individuals to leprosy*
  - ***Positive*** → *(Majority)* escape clinical disease or develop paucibacillary disease (Minority)
  - ***Negative*** → *High risk of developing progressive multibacillary Leprosy*
- *To classify type of disease.*
  - ***Positive*** → Tuberculoid, ***Negative*** → Lepromatous, ***Variable***→Indeterminate/Dimorphous
- *To assess prognosis*
  - *Positive* → Good prognosis, *Negative*→Bad prognosis
- *To assess response to treatment*:
  - Conversion of Lepromin negative to lepromin positive during treatment is good response to treatment

Drawback:

- False positive results, Negative result in Lepromatous and near Lepromatous case, *Not a diagnostic test*[Q]

Lepromin skin test: 0.1 mL of lepromin, is injected intradermally into inner aspect of forearm. It has *2 types of reaction –*

Early or Fernandez reaction	Late or Mistuda reaction
▪ Read at 48 to 72 hours. ▪ Redness and induration at site of inoculation appears in 24-48 hour and disappears in 3-4 days. ▪ *It is delayed hypersensitivity reaction to soluble constituents of leprosy bacilli.*[Q] ▪ *Positive Test - Diameter of red area>10 mm (Indicates previous exposure and infection).* ▪ *Early reaction is superior to late reaction.* ▪ *Positive in patients with tuberculoid and borderline tuberculoid leprosy.*	▪ Read at 21 days ▪ A nodule appears 7-10 days after injection and maximum at 3-4 weeks. ▪ It is cell mediated immune response to bacillary component of antigen. ▪ *Positive Test – Nodule >5mm diameter (Indicates the person has not been previously sensitized by exposure to lepromin bacilli)*

Also Know......................

- ***Most infants <6 month are lepromin negative; some become positive by end of 1st year.***[Q] *BCG vaccination converts lepra reaction from negative to positive in a large proportion of individuals*[Q]

274. Ans (a) Leprosy

Ref: K. Park, 24th ed. p 336-37

"***Case" of leprosy*** *is a person showing clinical signs of leprosy with or without bacteriological confirmation of diagnosis and who has not yet completed a full course of treatment with MDT.* The definition is used to estimate the prevalence of leprosy.

Paucibacillary leprosy *(60% of all leprosy cases)*:A person having 1-5 skin lesions and/or only one nerve involvement.

- Bacterial index <2 (TT, BT of **Ridley and Jopling classification.**)

Multibacillary leprosy: A person having 6 or more skin lesions and/or more than 1 nerve involvement.

- Bacterial index >2) (BB,BL,LL of **Ridley and Jopling classification.**)

Classification Used in Leprosy

Ridley and Jopling	Indian (Dharmendra's index)	Madrid
Tuberculoid (TT)	Intermediate (Bacteriologically - ve)	Indeterminate
Borderline Tuberculoid (BT)	Tuberculoid (Bacteriologically - ve)	Tuberculoid: flat: raised
Borderline (BB)	Borderline	Borderline Lepromatous
Borderline Lepromatous (BL)	Lepromatous (Bacteriologically +ve)	Lepromatous
Lepromatous (LL)	Pure Neuritic type (Bacteriologically - ve)	

275. Ans. (b) <1 per 10000

Ref: K. Park, 24th ed. p 333

Leprosy

- Elimination is prevalence rate <1 case per 10,000 population[Q]

Also Know......................

- *Leprosy prevalence rate more than 1 per 10,000 is considered a public health problem.*[Q]

276. Ans. (d) 0.69

Ref: K. Park, 24th ed. p 333

277. Ans. (b) Lepromatous leprosy

Ref: K. Park, 24th ed. p 342

Also Know......................

- ***Lepra reaction*** can occur before initiation of MDT, during or after treatment with MDT has been completed. It can be both mild or severe. Only severe reaction are treated with corticosteroids

Type I (Reversal Reaction- A delayed hypersensitivity reaction)	Type II (Erythema nodosum- Antigen antibody reaction)
Occurs in both Paucibacillary and Multibacillary cases (BT,BB,BL)	Occurs only in Multibacillary cases (BL and LL)

Contd...

Type I (Reversal Reaction- A delayed hypersensitivity reaction)	Type II (Erythema nodosum- Antigen antibody reaction)
Skin lesions get reddish, swollen, warm, tender and painful. New lesions may appear	Subcutaneous nodules (red tender, painful) appear in crops, B/L symmetrical on face/arms/leg and subside on their own in few days without treatment also
High risk of permanent damage to peripheral nerve trunks (enlarged, tender, painful and loss of function)	Nerves may be affected (Not as common or severe)
Other organs are not involved	Organs (Eyes, Testis, Kidney etc) may be affected
General symptoms (Fever, joint pain etc.) are uncommon	General symptoms do occur

Treatment: (Moderate to severe) → Bed rest, Rest to affected nerve by splint, analgesic, prednisolone. *Clofazimine is added for ENL* (Not more than 12 months).

278. Ans. (b) It is a diagnostic test

Ref: K. Park, 24th ed. p 338

279. Ans. (a) Uterus

*Ref: K. Park, 23rd edition p-316, Blaustein's pathology of the female genital tract By Ancel Blaustein, Robert J. Kurman., p- 680 **

Leprosy (Hansen's Disease)

- It affects mainly the peripheral nerves.
- It also affects the skin, muscles, the eye, bones, testes and internal organs.
- Leprosy rarely involves female genital tract. Ovary is the most common gynaecologic site involved*.
- It is clinically characterised by one or more of the following **cardinal features**:
  - Hypopigmented patches
  - Partial/Total loss of cutaneous sensation in affected areas (earliest sensation affected is light touch)
  - Presence of thickened nerves
  - Presence of acid -fast bacilli in the skin or nasal smears

Signs of advanced disease are → presence of nodules or lumps in the skin of the face and ears; plantar ulcers; loss of fingers or toes, nasal depression, foot drop, claw toes and other deformities

280. Ans. (b) Leprosy

Ref: K. Park, 24th ed. p 344

Leprosy → *Mass chemoprophylaxis is not recommended as a public health measure.*

SEXUALLY TRANSMITED DISEASE (STD)

281. Ans. (c) White

Ref: K. Park, 24th ed p-352

282. Ans. (d) Metronidazole and fluconazole

Ref: K. Park, 24th ed. p 352

283. Ans. (d) Notification

Ref: K. Park, 24th ed. p 357

Methods of early case detection in STD control program are:

- **Screening**:
  - Testing of apparently healthy volunteers from general population
  - High priority is given to screening of special groups, viz. pregnant women, blood donors, industrial workers, army, police, refugees, prostitutes, convicts, restaurant and hotel staff, etc.
- **Contact tracing:**
  - Sexual partners of diagnosed patients are identified, located, investigated, and treated.
  - One of the best methods of controlling the spread of infection.
  - Patients are interviewed for their sexual contacts by specially trained staff using telephone or other rapid means of communication.
  - Contacts are persuaded to attend a STD clinic for examination and treatment.
  - If prevalence is low, contact tracing is expensive.
- **Cluster testing**:
  - Patients are asked to name other persons of either sex who move in the same socio-sexual environment.
  - These persons are then screened (e.g., blood testing).
  - It doubles the number of cases found.

284. Ans. (c) Scabies

Ref: K. Park, 24th ed. p 819

Scabies is transmitted by close contact with an infested person and contaminated clothes

- Causative agent -Itch mite (Sarcoptes scabiei): Female parasite burrows into epidermis, breeds and causes itch
- **Site of lesions:** Hands and wrist (63%), extensor aspect of elbows (10.9%). Axillae, buttocks, lower abdomen, feet and ankles, palms in infants are all common sites
- All members of the affected household are simultaneously treated whether or not they appear to be infested.
  - Before starting treatment patient is given a good scrub with soap and hot water.
  - **Benzyl benzoate**: (25%) is applied to entire body below chin including soles. In babies, head is also treated. It is reapplied after 12 hours and after a further 12 hours bath is given and all undercloth, clothes and sheets are changed/washed.
  - **HCH**: 0.5 to 1.0% strength in coconut oil or any vegetable oil or vanishing cream.
  - **Tetmosol**: 5% solution - 3 daily applications
  - **Sulphur ointment**: 2.5% to 10% daily for 4 days
- Mass chemoprophylaxis in population is not recommended.

Also Know......................

- Mass Chemoprophylaxis is given in-Lymphatic Filariasis (DEC), Plague (Tetracycline), Yaws, Trachoma (Tetracycline)

AIDS

285. Ans. (a) 2 hours

Ref: MoHFW, National technical guidelines on ART, NACO - 2018

HIV-Postexposure prophylaxis should be started as early as possible (ideally within 2 hour) in all individuals, who had an exposure with a potential for HIV transmission.

As postexposure prophylaxis (PEP) for HIV has its greatest effect if begun within 2 hours of exposure, it is essential to act immediately. There is little benefit if >72 hours have lapsed but PEP can still be used if the health care worker presents after 72 hours of exposure. The prophylaxis needs to be continued for 4 weeks.

Postexposure Prophylaxis is Recommended in
- Parenteral exposure
- Mucous membrane exposure- Splash of blood on eye/nose/ oral cavity
- Sexual exposure

Also Know......................

- Blood, Blood stained saliva, breast milk, genital secretions, Cerebrospinal fluid, Amniotic/Rectal/Peritoneal/Synovial/ Pleural/Pericardial fluids – on exposure pose risk of HIV infection.
- Tear, Sweat, Urine, Non blood stained saliva do not pose risk of HIV infection

286. Ans. (a) HAART (Best Option)

Ref: Vertical Transmission Rate is Low When Pregnant Women Get HIV Therapy. Vol-40, Issue 3, Sep 2008, p-184-85

Most effective approach to prevent vertical HIV infection in children
- Prevention among women of childbearing age
- Prevention of unwanted pregnancies among HIV-infected women 2016

287. Ans. (b) When prevalence in high risk...

Ref: K. Park, 24th ed. p 452

288. Ans. (b) Concentrated HIV epidemic

Ref: K. Park, 24th ed. p 362

289. Ans. (d) >1% in pregnant women

Ref: K. Park, 24th ed. p 362

290. Ans. (b) Avahan programme

Ref: K. Park, 24th ed. p 437

Avahan Program [(India AIDS Initiative)] is a Bill and Melinda Gates Foundation initiative started in 2003

Goals:
- Build an HIV prevention model at scale in India
- Catalyze others to take over and replicate the model
- Foster and disseminate learnings within India and worldwide

Target-*Individuals with great vulnerability to HIV infection* (Sex worker, MSM, injectable drug abusers and truck drivers at risk) in 6 high prevalence states.

Approach → Community outreach + Empowerment + Condom programming + STI/HIV testing services

291. Ans. (a) HIV

Ref: K. Park, 24th ed. p 344

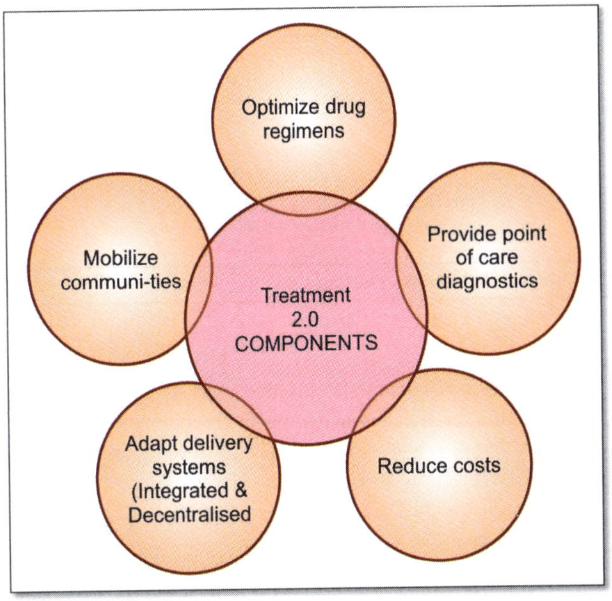

292. Ans. (c) STD/RTI

Ref: K. Park, 24th ed. p 457

RTI/STI services have been branded by NACO as Suraksha Clinics

293. Ans. (a) Homosexual men

Ref: K. Park, 24th ed. p 456

High Risk Group for AIDS Comprise
- Male homosexuals and Bisexuals
- Heterosexual partners (Including prostitutes and Clients of sex workers)
- I.V. drug abusers
- Blood transfusion recipients and Haemophiliacs
- Clients with STD

294. Ans. (c) 50%

Ref: IYCF Counselling, 4in 1 Course, Trainers Guide, April 2013, p-193

ART at Birth (Tab Nevirapine 200 mg to Mother 4 hour prior to delivery and Infant Syrup Nevirapine 2mg/Kg body weight within 72 hour of birth) reduces HIV transmission by 30-50%

295. Ans. (b) 1983

Ref: K. Park, 24th ed. p 451

1st case of AIDS in South-East Asia Region (SEAR) of WHO was reported from Thailand in 1984.

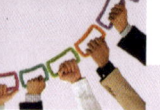

- 1st case of HIV in India was detected in Chennai→ 1986
- 1992 → NACP I launched, NACO was set up.
- 1999 → NACP II launched, SACS –State AIDS Control Society were established
- 2002 → National AIDS control policy and National Blood policy were adopted
- 2004 → ART initiated
- 2006 → National Council on AIDS constituted and National policy on pediatric ART formulated
- 2007 → NACP III launched
- 2012-2017 → NACP IV launched

Latest Updates

2012- People Living with HIV AIDS- 35.2 million (Global), India-20.89 lakh (Adult prevalence-0.27%)

296. Ans. (c) 15-30%

Ref: K. Park, 23rd ed. p 347, Ref. IYCF Counselling, 4in 1 Course, Trainers Guide, April 2013, p-192

All babies born to HIV positive mothers do not get HIV infection (even in absence of any intervention)

- About 63% babies born to HIV positive mothers never get HIV infection from them
- Parent to child transmission rate of HIV at birth is about 20-25%
- Risk of transmission to unborn child via placenta is 7%
- Infection can occur as early as the first 12-15 week of gestation or early second trimester.Q
- About 15% infants are infected at time of delivery and another 15% of infants are likely to develop HIV if the mother practices breast feeding for 2 years

297. Ans. (a) 2 hours

Ref: K. Park, 24th ed. p 371

298. Ans. (b) Vitamin A supplementation

Ref: IYCF Counselling, 4in 1 Course, Trainers Guide, April 2013, p-193

Factors Affecting Parent to Child Transmission	Measures to cut down mother to child HIV transmission
▪ Recent Infection of HIV ▪ Severity of HIV infection ▪ Infection with other STD (HIV transmission risk increases by 8-10 times) ▪ Obstetric procedures ▪ Duration of breast feeding ▪ Mixed feeding ▪ Condition of breast ▪ Condition of baby mouth ▪ Provision of ART	▪ Early diagnosis and Cure of STD ▪ Invasive procedures (Artificial rupture of membrane, Episiotomy) should be avoided ▪ Caesarean Section ▪ Mixed feeding to infant (Breast milk + Other milk) should be avoided ▪ ART to mother and Nevirapine in infant ▪ Treatment of breast condition s – Nipple sore, fissure, bleeding ▪ Treatment of oral ulcers in infant and avoiding feeding till corrected

299. Ans. (c) HIV C

Ref: Human Immunodeficiency Virus Type 1 Subtype Distribution in the Worldwide Epidemic: Pathogenetic and Therapeutic Implications L. Buonaguro, M. L. Tornesello, and F. M. Buonaguro. JOURNAL OF VIROLOGY, 2007, Vol. 81, No. 19, p-10209; 24th ed. p

Human immunodeficiency virus type 1 (HIV-1) is the causative agent of AIDS

Globally most prevalent HIV-1 genetic forms are subtypes A, B, and C, with subtype C accounting for almost 50% of all HIV-1 infections worldwide

300. Ans. (d) All of above

Ref: K. Park, 24th ed. p

WHO case definition for AIDS surveillance →An adult or adolescent (>12 years of age) is considered to have AIDS if at least 2 of the following major signs are present in combination with at least 1 of the minor signs and if these signs are not known to be due to a condition unrelated to HIV infection.

- Major signs –
  - Weight loss - 10% of body weight
  - Chronic diarrhea for more than 1 month
  - Prolonged fever for more than 1 month' (intermittent or constant)
- Minor signs –
  - Persistent cough for more than 1 month
  - Generalized pruritic dermatitis
  - History of herpes zoster
  - Oropharyngeal candidiasis
  - Chronic progressive or disseminated herpes simplex infection
  - Generalized lymphadenopathy
- Presence of generalized Kaposi sarcoma or cryptococcal meningitis is sufficient for diagnosis of AIDS for surveillance purpose.
- For patients with tuberculosis, persistent cough for >1 month should not be considered as a minor sign

301. Ans (d) All of the above

Ref: J Kishore, National Health Programs of India, 11th edition, p-331

HIV sentinel surveillance (Done by NACO and Ministry of Health and Family Welfare since 1998)

- To determine level of HIV infection in general population and High risk group
- To understand trends of HIV epidemic in general population as well as high risk groups
- To understand the geographical spread of HIV infection and to identify emerging pockets
- To provide information for prioritising of program resources and evaluation of program impact
- To estimate HIV prevalence and burden in the country

MISCELLANEOUS

302. Ans. (b) Body fluids

Ref: K. Park, 24th ed. p 364

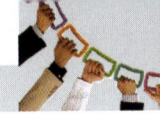

Modes of Transmission

- Direct contact with blood, organ, body secretion/fluids of infected animals.
- Human to Human via blood or body fluids of an infected symptomatic person or exposure to objects (needles) contaminated with infected secretions.

Also Know.......................

- Ebola virus is not transmitted via air, water or food or by sexual transmission

303. Ans. (b) Effective vaccine with 82% protective efficacy

Ref: K. Park, 24th ed. p 184

304. Ans. (b) Leptospirosis

Ref: K. Park, 24th ed. p 823

Diseases Associated with Rodents

Bacterial → Plague, Tularaemia, Salmonellosis	Viral → Lassa fever, Haemorrhagic fever, Encephalitis
Rickettsial → Scrub typhus, Murine typhus, Rickettsial pox	Parasitic → Hymenolepis diminuata, Leishmaniasis, Amoebiasis, Trichinosis, Chagas disease
Others → Rat bite fever, Leptospirosis, Histoplasmosis, Ring worm etc.	

305. Ans. (d) Permethrin

Ref: Howard I. Maibach, Farzam Gorouhi, Evidence Based Dermatology. p-413

Drug of Choice in Scabies

Condition	Drug of Choice
Crusted scabies	Ivermectin
Innate and acquired immunodeficiency	Ivermectin
Newborn	Crotamiton or Permethrin under strict medical supervision
Infants	Crotamiton or Permethrin
Children	Ivermectin
Pregnancy	Permethrin
Lactation	Benzyl benzoate under strict medical supervision

306. Ans. (d) Shigella flexneri

Ref: Oxford Textbook of Medicine, Volume 1, p-494

- **Shigella dysenteriae type1 is the most virulent form of shigella**
- Shigella flexneri is the most common isolate in developing country. It results in severe bloody diarrhea/dysentery
- Shigella boydii prevalent in Indian subcontinent but not elsewhere. It causes a mild disease
- Shigella sonnei is the most common isolate in developed country

307. Ans. (b) Floods

Ref: K. Park, 24th ed. p 309

Leptospirosis

- It is a zoonosis and most widespread of the disease transmissible from animal to man
- Out breaks occur after heavy rainfall and consequent floodings
- Source of infection: Urine of infected animals
- Reservoir: Rats (R. Norvegicus, Mus musculus).

308. Ans. (c) Incubation period is less than 48 hours
(e) Oseltamivir is quite...

Ref: K. Park, 24th ed. p 374

RNTCP

309. Ans. (d) 1%

310. Ans. (b) Sputum microscopy

311. Ans. (c) Incidence of new cases

312. Ans. (c) 8 wks

313. Ans. (d) INH & Rifampicin

314. Ans. (d) WHO recommends Danish 1331 strain for vaccine production

315. Ans. (b) Failure case

316. Ans. (b) Father

Ref: K. Park, 24th ed. p 200

DOTS is given by DOTS provider →Peripheral health staff (MPW), voluntary worker (Teacher), AWW, dais, ex patients and social workers etc.

- DOT provider cannot be a family member.
- A DOT provider is provided an incentive of Rs 150 for each patient completing the treatment

317. Ans. (d) High cost

Ref: National Strategic Plan for TB elimination 2017–2025, March 2017

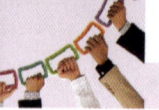

SWOT Analysis of RNTCP Program

	Strengths	Weakness
Internal factors	▪ High level political and administrative commitment ▪ Deliberate efforts to move away form routine and set goals, target, strategies and actions to match. ▪ Availability of new drugs, regimens, diagnostics, approaches and strategies to end TB.	▪ Diverse TB epidemiology in India ▪ TB program structure unable to cope with growing demands for ending TB ▪ Limited human resource at the contral TB division ▪ Private sector involvement in public heath actions related to TB control is not commensurate to its size and dominances in TB care
	Opportunities	**Threats**
External factors	▪ Aggressive research agenda ▪ In-country innovations and pilots with potential for replications and scale up. ▪ SDGs and End TB strategy provide ambitious targets to aim for by the national efforts	▪ Amplification of drug resistance. ▪ Insufficient budgetary outlay for health ▪ Variable implementation capacity, capability and ownership of the stats. ▪ Loss of independent, third party, technical assistance from development partners

318. Ans. (c) 85%

Ref: K. Park, 24th p-445

Objectives of RNTCP Program: → To achieve and maintain:
- Cure rate of at least 85% among newly detected smear-positive (infectious) pulmonary TB cases[Q]
- Case detection of at least 70% of the expected new smear positive PTB cases in a community.

319. Ans. (d) Pyrazinamide

Ref: K. Park, 24th ed. p 189

320. Ans. (b) Reduction in default case rate to <10% for new case and <5% for reinfection cases

Ref: Technical and Operational Guidelines for TB Control in India 2016, Mohfw, India

321. Ans. (a) a, b

Ref: Manual of Standard Operating Procedures (SOPs; 24th ed. p, Culture of M.Tuberculosis and DST on solid Medium. RNTCP -2009

Sputum specimen collected from a suspected TB Case has 2 specimen cards with suffix a (spot), and b (early morning) Chance of detecting smear positive case with spot sample is -80% and morning sample is 93%

322. Ans. (c) 30 day

Ref: Guidelines for TB Notification, NIKSHAY, MOHFW, GOI

NIKSHAY: Is a case based web enabled TB surveillance system (launched in May 2012)
- It was developed by the Central TB division in collaboration with National informatics Center
- As per GOI notification 7th May 2012- TB is a Notifiable disease (mandatory for all healthcare providers)
- On diagnosis or initiation of anti-TB treatment of a TB case, reporting to nodal public health authority to be done at least on monthly basis

323. Ans. (c) 2 (HRZE) + 4 (HRE)

As per latest 2019 RNTCP recommendations, both the categories I and II will have treatment regime as:
2 HRZE + 4 HRE – as daily doses.

324. Ans. (c) Tuberculosis

Ref: K. Park, 24th ed. p 448

325. Ans (c) Category 2, Blue

Recent 2019 recommendation is same treatment for cat 1 and cat 2

326. Ans. (a) Rifampicin; (b) Any one Fluoroquinolone; (c) INH; (d) Kanamycin

Ref: K Park, 23rd ed. p 199 http://www.who.int/tb/challenges/mdr/tdrfaqs/en/

327. Ans. (d) Mycolic acid

Ref: http://tbcindia.nic.in/pdfs/Training%20manual%20M%20tuberculosis%20C%20DST.pdf

- Acid fastness in Mycobacterium Tuberculosis is due to the presence Mycolic acid

Latest Updates

Other bacteria containing mycolic acids- e,g, Nocardia, also exhibit Acid fastness.

328. Ans. (c) Non DOTS based therapy

Ref: http://tbcindia.nic.in/pdfs/Training%20Module%20for%20Medical%20Practitioners.pdf; 24th ed. p

Non-DOTS Regimen under RNTCP

- Needed in rare and exceptional situation. Examples include:
  - Adverse reactions to Rifampicin and/or Pyrazinamide
  - "New" patients who refuse DOTS despite all efforts
- A maximum of 1% of patients may get non-DOTS treatment in an RNTCP area.
- Justification for initiating non-DOTS should be specified in "Remarks" column of treatment card and TB register.
- Regimen - 2 SHE followed by 10 HE (Total duration = 12 month)

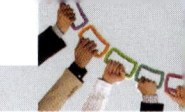

- Dose administered per day in the regimen are: Isoniazid - 300 mg, Ethambutol - 800 mg, Streptomycin - 750 mg (500 mg for those >50 years of age).
- Those weighing less than 30 kg, dose is calculated as per body-weight.

329. Ans. (a) 150 mg

Treatment Plan for Drug sensitive TB – Adults
The dose for drugs in Fixed dose combination FDC tablets is: HRZE - 75/150/400/275 (mg/tablet)

330. Ans. (a) 1 Sample out of 2 positive

Refer to the new diagnostic algorithm for diagnosis of TB

331. Ans. (a) 2 HRZE + 4 HRE

332. Ans. (a) RNTCP

Ref: K. Park, 24th ed. p 445

In 1992- Govt. of India, WHO and SIDA reviewed the National TB Program implementation and formulated the RNTCP with inclusion of DOTS

333. Ans. (b) Bedaquiline is drug of choice for Rifampicin resistant TB

Tuberculosis cases are now classified into 2 categories on basis of treatment received

- New case: A TB patient (pulmonary or extrapulmonary) who has never had treatment for TB or has taken anti-TB drugs for less than 1 month.
  - It includes new smear positive or negative pulmonary TB and extrapulmonary TB cases
  - It includes all cases previously classified as category I and III
- Previously treated: A person diagnosed to have TB and had antitubercular treatment for >1 month in past and is again diagnosed to have TB.
  - It includes Relapse, Failure and Default (Category II)
- However, the recent update is: NO separate treatment regime for category II. Both category I and II will receive the same treatment regime

For Mono drug – isoniazid resistance: the regime is 6 months of Lfx R Z E
Bedaquiline is given only for specific cases as:

- MDR TB with resistance to all FQs
- MDR TB with resistance to all SLIs
- All FQ and All SLI resistant
- All FQ and any SLI resistant
- Any FQ and all SLI resistant
- Any FQ and Any SLI resistant
- Treatment failure of Cat IV –MDR
- XDR-TB
- Treatment failure for XDR TB
- MDR/RR-TB patients with extensive pulmonary lesions, advanced disease and others deemed at higher baseline risk for poor outcome

Also Know.......................

- **Transferred in** - A TB patient received for treatment in a Tuberculosis Unit, after starting treatment in another TB unit where s/he has been registered.
- **Transferred out** - A TB patient who has been transferred to another area register and treatment results are not known
- **Treatment after default** - A patient, who has received treatment for TB for 1 month or more from any source and returns for treatment after having defaulted i.e., not taken anti-TB drugs consecutively for 2 months or more and found to be smear-positive.
- **Failure** - Any TB patient who is smear-positive at 5 months or more after initiation of treatment
- **Relapse** - A TB patient who was declared cured or treatment completed by a physician and who reports back to the health facility and is now found to be sputum smear positive
- **Treatment completed** - Initially smear negative patient who received full course of treatment or smear positive patient who completed treatment with negative smear at end of intensive phase, but no or only one negative smear during continuation and none at treatment end.
- **Cured** - Initially smear positive patient who completed treatment and had negative smear result at least on 2 occasions (1 at treatment completion)

334. Ans. (a) 1 out of 2 sputum positive

Ref: K. Park, 24th ed. p 192

335. Ans. (a) To avoid emergence of resistance

Ref: K. Park, 24th ed. p 188

Rationale for Multi Drug Therapy (MDT) in TB

- To cut transmission of TB infection in community (Bactericidal drugs).
- Early and complete cure of TB cases (Better compliance, Low cost, Reduced duration of treatment)
- To prevent emergence of drug resistance (Bacteriostatic Drugs)

336. Ans. (c) Both

The case finding in RNTCP is essentially passive, i.e. the patients themselves present to the health professional to get screened for Tuberculosis.
Recent advance: Recently – house to house active case detection has been started in few states to compliment the case finding activity and ensure – END TB 2025.

337. Ans. (e) Achievement of at least 70% cure rate

Ref: K Park, 24th ed. p 445, J Kishore, National Health Programe, 11th edition, p-110

RNTCP objectives is to achieve and maintain:

- Cure rate of at least 85% among newly detected smear-positive pulmonary tuberculosis cases[Q]
- Case detection of at least 70% of expected new smear positive PTB cases in a community[Q]
- Case finding in RNTCP is passive.[Q]

- Sputum smear microscopic examination is the method of choice[Q] .It is done in a RNTCP Designated Microscopy Centers (1 for every 1 lakh population[Q]).
- DOTS is given by DOTS provider →Peripheral health staff e.g MPW or voluntary worker e.g. Teacher, AWW, dais, ex patients and social workers etc.
- National programmes on Malaria, TB, Kalazaar, Filaria are horizontally integrated under NRHM

Recent update: In few states, the ACTIVE CASE detection for TB has been started from 2017–2018 onwards

NACP

338. Ans. (d) Lamivudine + Tenofovir for 4 weeks

The postexposure prophylaxis

- Should be started best within 2 hours, not later than 72 hours
- The regimes are

Dosages of drugs for PEP for Adults	Recommendations for PEP	Duration
Tenofovir (300) + Lamivudine (300)- One tablet once daily	One tablet immediately within 2 hours of accidental exposure either at day or night time	Next day one tablet once a day, continue for 4 weeks
Lopinavir (200) + Ritonavir (50)-Two FDC tablets twice daily	Two tablets immediately within 2 hours of accidental exposure either at day or night time	Next day two tablets twice daily, continue for 4 weeks
If Lopinavir/ritonavir is not available or cannot be used, Tenofovir (300) + Lamivudine (300) + Efavirenz (600) may be given 2 hours after dinner before going to bed daily for four weeks		

339. Ans. (b) AIDS

Ref – NACO (2015; 24th ed. p . National Integrated Biological and Behavioural Surveillance (IBBS; 24th ed. p, India 2014-15. New Delhi: NACO, MOHFW, GOI

National Integrated Biological and Behavioural Surveillance

- **It is** the largest bio-behavioural study of its kind in the world
- It was implemented in six population groups -- Female Sex Workers (FSW), Men who have Sex with Men (MSM), Injecting Drug Users (IDU), Transgender (TG), Migrants and Currently Married Women (CMW) in high outmigration districts.
- It was a community based cross-sectional survey using probability-based sampling.
- Blood specimens were collected using Dried Blood Spot (DBS) method.
- HIV testing approach was Unlinked Anonymous Testing with informed consent.
- All positive and 2% of negative specimens were re-tested at NARI, Pune under external quality assurance.

340. Ans. (d) None of above

Ref: K. Park 24th ed. p 370

ART is initiative irrespective of the CD4 count.

341. Ans. (b) 30 November 2006

Ref: K. Park, 24th ed. p 156

342. Ans. (b) NACP

Ref: K. Park, 24th ed. p 456

Link Worker Scheme-NACP

Objective is to reach out to HRG and vulnerable population via link worker with

- Information and knowledge on prevention and risk reduction of HIV and STI
- Condom promotion and distribution
- Referral and follow up linkages for various services
- Counseling, testing and treatment of STI and opportunistic infections
- Creating an enabling environment for PLHIV and their families
- Reducing stigma and discrimination

343. Ans. (b) Estimation of total cases in hospitals

Ref: K. Park, 24th ed. p 452

Objectives of HIV Sentinel Surveillance

- To understand the levels and trends of the HIV epidemic among the general population, bridge populations as well as high risk groups in different states
- To understand the geographical spread of the HIV infection and to identify emerging pockets
- To provide information for prioritization of programme resources and evaluation of programme impact
- To estimate HIV Prevalence and HIV burden in the country

HIV Sentinel Surveillance – A annual cross sectional survey of risk group (same place – fixed sentinel sites over a few year) is done using unlinked anonymous serological testing procedure.

Population	Sentinel sites	Sample size
High risk groups-IDU, MSM FSW,TG Targeted Interventions projects		250
Bridge populations	STD Clinic and Targeted Interventions projects	250
General population	Antenatal clinic	400

- Consecutive sampling is used
- **Targeted interventions projects:** Dried Blood Spot is collected, whereas from STD Clinic and Antenatal clinic- Serum sample is collected

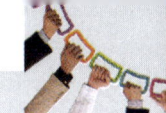

344. Ans. (d) Kit 4 - Red

Ref: K. Park, 23rd ed. p 438, Operational Guidelines for STI/RTI

345. Ans. (b) Yellow

Ref: K. Park, 25th ed. p 363–472

Symptom	Syndrome	Causative Organism	Kit and Colour code
Lower abdominal pain	Lower abdominal pain	Gonorrhoea, Chlamydia, Myco-plasma gardnerella, Anaerobic bacteria (bacteroids, eg. gram positive cocci)	Kit 6 (Yellow)

Syndromic Management of RTI/STI

- It is diagnosis based on the identification of **syndromes** (a combination of the symptoms the client reports and the signs the health care provider observes
- The recommended treatment is effective for all the diseases that could cause the identified syndrome
- Provides single-dose treatment as far as possible
- It is comprehensive (includes patient education and counselling)

Advantage	Disadvantage/ Limitations
▪ Fast—patient is diagnosed and treated in one visit ▪ Highly effective for selected syndromes, especially urethral discharge and genital ulcer disease (GU(d). Also good for lower abdominal pain/PID. ▪ Relatively inexpensive since it avoids use of lab tests	▪ Not useful in asymptomatic individuals ▪ Over-treatment if patient has only one STI that causes a syndrome ▪ Financial cost of over-treatment, side-effects
▪ No need for patient to return for lab results ▪ All possible STIs causing signs and symptoms are treated at once ▪ Scientifically tested in many part of the world ▪ Easy for health workers to learn and practice for patients ▪ Integrated into other primary health care services more easily ▪ Can be used by providers at all levels ▪ It standardizes treatment regimens	▪ Increases potential for creation of antibiotic resistance especially if full course is not completed ▪ Not effective in some cases such as vaginal discharge

NATIONAL HEALTH POLICY & NATIONAL POPULATION POLICY

346. Ans. (d) Dengue

Ref: K. Park, 24th ed. p 910

NLEP

347. Ans. (d) >90%

Ref - NLEP, Programme Implementation Plan (PIP; 24th ed. p, Central Leprosy Division, MOHFW

National Leprosy Eradication Programme (Programme Implementation Plan 2012-2017)

Objectives

- Elimination of leprosy i.e. prevalence <1 case per 10,000 population in all districts of the country.
- Strengthen Disability Prevention and Medical Rehabilitation of persons affected by leprosy.
- Reduction in the level of stigma associated with leprosy.

Leprosy has been Eliminated from India

Indicator	Targets (Mar 2017)
Prevalence Rate (PR) <1/10,000	642 Districts (100%)
Annual New Case Detection Rate (ANCDR) <10/100000 population	642 Districts (100%)
Cure rate MultiBacillary Leprosy Cases (MB)	>95%
Cure rate PauciBacillary Leprosy Cases (PB)	>97%
Gr.II disability rate in percentage of New cases	35% reduction 1.98%
Stigma reduction	50% Reduction over the percentage reported by NSS

348. Ans. (b) 9 months

Ref: K. Park, 24th ed. p 341

For chemotherapy Leprosy cases are classified into 2 groups:
Paucibacillary leprosy (1-5 skin lesions) (Includes Indeterminate (I), Tuberculoid (TT) and borderline tuberculoid (BT) in the Ridley-Jopling classification)
Multibacillary leprosy (>5 skin lesions) (Includes LL, BL, BB cases in Ridley-Jopling classification)

349. Ans. (d) Minocycline

Ref: K. Park, 24th ed. p 341

MDT for Leprosy is available free of cost at all health care facilities in blister packs containing drugs for 28 days

Indicators in Leprosy Eradication Program

Epidemiological - To evaluate effectiveness of programme

- **Incidence rate** → Most sensitive index of transmission of disease.[Q] Only index for measuring the effectiveness of measures taken & is useful in monitoring the success of a control programme.[Q]
- **Prevalence** → Is a measure of "case load" and is useful in planning treatment services.[Q]

Core indicators for monitoring progress -
- Number and rate of new case detected per 1 lakh population per year.
- Rate of new cases with grade II disabilities per 1 lakh population per year
- Treatment completion/cure rate

Indicators for evaluating case detection
- Proportion of children (<15 years) among newly detected cases (Signals active & recent transmission of disease, useful in calculating drug requirement).
- Proportion of multibacillary cases among newly detected cases.
- Proportion of females among newly detected cases.

Indicator for assessing quality of services
- Proportion of new cases verified as correctly diagnosed
- Proportion of treatment defaulters
- Relapse rate (one of the best indicators of the efficacy of the drug regimen)

350. Ans. (c) 5 years

Ref: K. Park, 24th ed. p 344

As per current recommendation -Follow up (or Clinical Surveillance post completion of treatment is essential to assure Long term success of treatment and early detection of relapse
- Paucibacillary Leprosy → 1 clinical examination per year for Minimum 2 years post completion of treatment
- Multibacillary Leprosy → 1 clinical examination per year for Minimum 5 years post completion of treatment

Accompanied MDT: To help irregular patients with interruption in treatment because of inability to attend health facility regularly or due to geographical distance.[Q]
- Patients are given more doses of MDT in case he/she is not likely to come for next collection after proper counseling.
- Any responsible person from family or village can collect MDT, if patient is unable to come

351. Ans. (d) Dapsone, Rifampicin, Clofazimine

Ref: K. Park, 24th ed. p 340

352. Ans. (d) 1983

Ref: K. Park, 24th ed. p 441

National leprosy control program - 1955
National leprosy eradication program - 1983
MDT was started in - 1982

353. Ans. (c) Post-treatment surveillance of paucibacillary leprosy

Ref: K. Park, 24th ed. p 344

NATIONAL POLIO ERADICATION PROGRAMME

354. Ans. (c) 0-5 yrs

Ref: K. Park, 24th ed. p 223

Pulse Polio Immunization – (PPI)

- 1st round of PPI was carried out on 9th Dec 1995 and 20th Jan 1996 among all children under 3 years-of age irrespective of their immunization status.
- Later age group was increased from under 3 to under 5 years.
- In PPIs oral polio vaccine is given to all children 0-5 years of age, in the country in a week (Booth + House to visit + B team), regardless of previous immunization status.[Q]
- No minimum interval exists between PPI and scheduled OPV doses
- Bivalent OPV vaccine was introduced in PPI during 2009.

Also Know........................

- Dose of OPV in PPIs are extra doses (They supplement routine immunization and do not replace it)[Q]

355. Ans. (d) To identify high risk population

Ref: K. Park, 24th ed. p 223

356. Ans. (c) 60 days

Ref: K. Park, 24th ed. p 219

357. Ans. (b) 60 days

Ref: K. Park, 24th ed. p 219

358. Ans. (a) 0- 5 years children

Ref: K. Park, 24th ed. p 224

ARTHROPOD-BORNE DISEASE

359. Ans. (a) Lamivudine is drug of choice

Ref: K. Park, 24th ed. p 163

Dengue Hemorrhagic Fever **(DHF)** *is caused by infection with more than one dengue virus*[Q]. [1st infection sensitizes the patient and 2nd produces an immunological reaction]

Criteria for clinical diagnosis of DHF

- **Grade I**-Fever - acute onset, high, continuous lasting 2 to 7 days, Positive tourniquet test (i.e. >20 petechiae/ 2.5 cm2)
- **Grade II -Features of Grade I + Any** hemorrhagic manifestations
  - Petechiae, Purpura, Ecchymosis
  - Epistaxis, Gum bleeding
  - Hematemesis and/or Melena
    Including at least a positive tourniquet test (i.e. >20 Petechiae per 2.5 cm^2)
- Enlargement of liver

Laboratory Diagnosis

- Thrombocytopenia (100,000/mm3 or less)
- Hemoconcentration -(Hemotocrit ≥20% of base line value)
- Hypo-proteinemia, Ascites

Diagnosis is established → If 1st two clinical criteria plus Thrombocytopenia and Hemoconcentration or Haematocrit ≥20% of base line value is present

Dengue Shock Syndrome (DSS)→ shows all clinical features of DHF + shock
- **Grade III:** Features of Grade I & II + Circulatory failure → Rapid and weak pulse, narrowing of pulse pressure (≤ 20 mm Hg) or hypotension with cold clammy skin and restlessness.
- **Grade IV:** Features of Grade I, II & III +Profound shock with undetectable BP and pulse, Pleural effusion

- 30% DHF cases develop DSS by 2nd or 5th day & result in death in 12-24 hours

360. Ans. (b) Dengue fevers

Ref: Mahajan and Gupta, Textbook of Preventive and Social Medicine, 4th Edition

361. Ans. (d) Reappearance of sexual stage parasitemia after treatment

Ref: Biodiversity of Malaria in the world, p-39

Relapse refers to reactivation of hypnozides after a quiscent period of variable duration. It occurs in P. vivax and ovale.

Malaria Recrudescence

- It is a type of treatment failure due to → Drug resistance, unusual pharmacokinetics in individual, incorrect treatment
- It refers to an attack of malaria due to multiplication of parasites, the load of which was below the clinical threshold.
- It is seen in P. malariae and less frequently in drug resistant Plasmodium falciparum
- Artesunate or its derivatives are associated with high Malaria recrudescence 10-50%. Artemether has least and artesunate has maximum chances.

Also Know......................

- Reoccurrence of malaria is due to either by Reinfection or Recrudescence or Relapse.

362. Ans. (d) Endogenous

Ref: K. Park, 24th ed. p 274

363. Ans. (b) 10-20 days

Ref: K. Park, 24th ed. p-274

Extrinsic Incubation period is 10-20 days, depending upon conditions of atmospheric temperature and humidity

364. Ans. (c) Serotype 4 is more dangerous than other serotypes

Ref: K. Park, 24th ed. p 261-67

Classical Dengue or "Break-Bone Fever"

- An acute viral infection, caused by 4 serotypes (1, 2, 3 and 4) of dengue virus.
- *Reservoir of infection → man and mosquito.*
- Transmission cycle is "***Man-mosquito-Man***".
- *Aedes aegypti is the main vector.*^{Q}
- All ages and both sexes are susceptible to dengue fever.
- *Children usually have a milder disease than adults.*^{Q}
- Incubation period of 3 to 10 days (commonly 5-6 days).

Dengue Fever Clinical Features

- Sudden onset with chills and high fever (39-40°C). Fever lasts for about 5 days, rarely >7 days after which recovery is usually complete although convalescence may be protracted
- Intense headache, severe muscle and joint pain (***Break bone fever***)
- Retroorbital pain and photophobia
- Fever is typically followed by remission of the few hours to 2 days (biphasic curve)
- Eruptions appear in (80%) of cases and lasts for 1-2 days.
- Lymph node are frequently enlarged
- Case fatality rate is extremely low.

Infection with one Dengue serotype gives immunity against that particular serotype and partial protection against others.

MALARIA

365. Ans. (d) P. malariae

Ref: K. Park, 24th ed. p 277

Clinical Features of Malaria

- Peaks of fever coincide with release of successive broods of merozoites into the bloodstream.
- Typical attack has 3 distinct stages, i.e. Cold stage [1 hour], Hot stage [2-6 hours] and Sweating stage [2-4 hours] followed by an afebrile period. May not always be observed.
- Febrile paroxysms occur periodically every 48 hrs [72 hours in P. malariae].

366. Ans. (b) Regular spray with 3 rounds of malathion

Ref: K. Park, 24th ed. p 437

Insecticides of Choice for IRS

- *2 rounds of DDT* [1g/m^{2}]^{Q} in transmission season
- If the vector is refractory to DDT, 3 rounds of Malathion [2 g/m^{2}]^{Q} in transmission season
- *If the vector is refractory to DDT and Malathion, 2 rounds of synthetic pyrethroids* [0.25 g/m^{2}] *at 6 week* interval

Also Know......................

- *Areas with API ≥5 is to be covered with LLIN and Areas with API between 2-5 is to be covered by conventional nets treated with insecticides and Indoor Residual Spray.*

367. Ans. (c) Malaria and dengue in rural area

Ref: K. Park, 24th ed. p 437

Under NVBDCP, Integrated Vector Management (IVM) is done by using identical vector control methods to control

- Malaria and leishmaniasis in Urban area
- Malaria and Dengue in Rural areas

Objective is to achieve cost effectiveness and synergy.

IVM includes safe use of insecticides and monitoring of insecticide resistance.

Integrated vector management techniques include

- Measures to control adult mosquito -Indoor residual spray (IRS).
- Personal protection measures -Insecticide Treated Bed Nets (ITNs) and Long Lasting Insecticidal Nets (LLINs)
- Antilarval measures –Chemical, Biological and Environmental measures

368. Ans. (c) If Pf proportion is <50%

Ref: K. Park, 23rd ed. p 418

Recommendation of Technical Advisory Committee on IRS for Malaria [2002]

- *Spray on priority in areas with API ≥5,* where ABER is 10% or more, taking subcenter as unit.
- *Spray on priority in areas with SPR ≥5%,* where ABER is below 10%
- Spray on priority areas with proportion of P. falciparum cases >50%
- Spray on priority in areas with API <5 or SPR <5% in case of drug resistant foci, project areas with population migration and aggregation
- Spray on priority in case of epidemics

369. Ans. (b) Malaria prevention

Ref: K. Park, 24th ed. p 438

BCC is a key supportive strategy for Malaria prevention and treatment. It is aimed at

- Early identification of signs and symptoms of malaria
- Early treatment from appropriate service provider
- Protection of children and pregnant women
- Adherence to treatment regime
- Use of ITN and LLIN
- Acceptance of IRS

370. Ans. (d) Spleen rate

Ref: K. Park, 24th ed. p 277

Malaria rates	Definition	Use
Spleen rate	Percentage of children between 2 -10 year of age showing enlargement of spleen	Measures malaria endemicity [or prevalence] Hyperendemic – Spleen rate <10% Mesoendemic – Spleen rate 11-50% Hyperendemic – Speen rate >50%; (Adults over 25%) Holoendemic – Spleen rate in children >75% (Adult <25%)
Parasite density index	Density of parasite in a sample of well-defined group of population. . Only '+'ve slides are included in denominator	Measures average degree of parasitemia
Infant parasite rate	Percentage of infants showing malaria parasites in their blood films	Most sensitive index of recent transmission of malaria in a locality. Used to asses impact of control operations

Contd...

Malaria rates	Definition	Use
Annual parasite incidence (API)	API = (Confirmed cases during one year/ Population under surveillance) x 1000	Measure of malaria incidence in a community.
Annual blood examination rate(ABER)	ABER = (Number of slides examined/ Population) x 100	Index of operational efficiency [Minimum prescribed is 10% of the population in a year]
SPR/SFR	Slide positivity rate and slide falciparum rate	Information on trend of malaria transmission
Human blood index	Proportion of freshly-fed female Anopheline mosquitoes whose stomach contains human blood	It indicates the degree of anthrophilism

Also Know......................

Malariometric Measures

- Preeradication Era → Spleen rate, Average enlarged spleen, Parasite rate, Parasite density index and Infant parasite rate
- Eradication Era → API, ABER, SPR, SPF.

371. Ans. (d) Annual blood examination rate

Ref: K. Park, 24th ed. p 261

372. Ans. (d) Artesunate weekly, 1 day before arrival

Ref: K. Park, 24th ed. p 284

Malaria Chemoprophylaxis (to be complemented with personal protection and other methods)

- **Indication** → Selective groups [Military and Para-military forces, labor forces, travellers from nonendemic area for long stay in high *P. falciparum* endemic areas]
- ***Short term chemoprophylaxis* (up to 6 weeks):** All drugs to be taken strictly on time and continued for 4 weeks after the last possible exposure to infection
  - Doxycycline: 100 mg OD for adults and 1.5 mg/kg OD for children started 2 days before travel
  - Not recommended for pregnant women and children <8 years. Dose in children >8 year is to be based on body weight
  - Chloroquine: 300 mg (base) once weekly or 100 mg (base) OD for 6 days a week. Initiated a week before arrival
  - Mefloquine 250 mg weekly. Initiated 2-3 week before arrival
- *Chemoprophylaxis for longer stay* (>6 weeks)
  - Mefloquine: 250 mg weekly for adults, administered 2 weeks before, during and 4 weeks after exposure.
  - Chloroquine (300 mg weekly/100 mg OD) + Proguanil (100 mg OD) – (Screening for retinal changes to be done 6 month after 5 year (weekly regimen) and 3 year (daily regimen)

373. Ans. (d) Source reduction

Ref: K. Park, 24th ed. p 809-10

Anti-Larval Measures for Mosquito Control

- *Environmental Control or Source reduction-yield permanent results*
  - Minor engineering methods [(E.g. Filling, leveling, drainage of breeding places and water management (such as intermittent irrigation)]
  - Rendering water unsuitable for mosquito breeding. [Changing salinity of water].
- *Chemical Control*
  - Mineral oil, Paris green and synthetic insecticide [Fenthion, Chlorpyrifos, and Abate]
- *Biological Control*
  - Larvivorous fish -Gambusia affinis and Lebister reticulatus (Barbados Millions)
  - Toxorhynchites splendens (Predator Mosquito) for Aedes aegypti
  - Used in burrow pits, sewage oxidation ponds, ornamental ponds, cisterns and farm ponds. Effective only when used in conjunction with other methods.

374. Ans. (a) Main vector in urban and industrial areas

Ref: K. Park, 24th ed. p 227

Anopheles Fluviatilis

- Propagate malaria at lower densities (efficient vector)
- Highly anthropophilic (high preference for human blood)
- Breed in moving water

Also Know......................

- Anopheles culicifacies is the main vector in rural area and Anopheles stephensi in urban and industrial areas.

375. Ans. (c) Primaquine is contraindicated in infants and...

Ref: K. Park, 24th ed. p 279

376. Ans. (d) All the above

Ref: K. Park, 24th ed. p 436

Malaria Surveillance in India

- Active case detection (ACD) is done fortnightly in rural areas, blood smear is collected by MPWs during home visits
- Passive cases detection (PCD) is done in fever cases reporting to peripheral health institutions (SC/PHC), ASHAs and secondary /tertiary level health institutions.
- Sentinel surveillance is being established in high endemic districts

377. Ans. (b) Artemisinin

Treatment of Malaria in Pregnancy

- P. falciparum cases
  - 1st Trimester: Quinine
  - 2nd and 3rd Trimester: ACT [Artemisinin Combination Therapy]
  - ***P. vivax cases*** → Chloroquine

378. Ans. (b) Artesunate

Ref: K. Park, 24th ed. p 284

379. Ans. (d) Primaquine

Ref: K. Park, 24th ed. p 284

380. Ans. (c) 10-14 days

Ref: K. Park, 24th ed. p 276

Incubation period→ is length of time between infective mosquito bite and 1st appearance of clinical signs.

Duration of Incubation period varies with species of parasite in natural infections:

- ***12 (9-14) days*** for falciparum malaria
- ***14 (8-17) days*** for vivax malaria
- ***28 (18-40) days*** for quartan malaria
- ***17 (16-18) days*** for ovale malaria.

381. Ans. (a) Malaria

Ref: K. Park, 24th ed. p 103

Biological Transmission is of 3 Types

- *Propagative*: Agent only multiplies in vector, there is no change in form, e.g., Plague bacilli in rat flea
- *Cyclopropagative*: Agent changes in form and also multiplies e.g., Malaria parasites in mosquito
- *Cyclodevelopmental*: Agent undergoes chonly development but no multiplication, e.g., Microfilaria in mosquito.

382. Ans. (a) 1.5 million annually; (b) Quinine drug of choice in severe malaria in pregnancy; (e) Falciparum malaria is most common type

Ref: K. Park, 24th ed. p 271-286

383. Ans. (a) Drug Resistance in host

Ref: http://wwwnc.cdc.gov/eid/article/4/3/98-0313_article.htm, Nchinda TC. Malaria: A Reemerging Disease in Africa.Emerging Infectious Diseases, Sep 1998. Macxy-Rosenau, Public health and preventive medicine, 15th edition, p-383.

Factors Contributing to Resurgence of Malaria

- Emergence and rapid spread of drug-resistant malaria parasites [Antigenic variations in parasite could be possible mechanism]
- Emergence of insecticide-resistant vectors [Vector resistance to DDT]
- Change in international priorities and support –Integration of malaria control activities into basic health services. Change in approach to horizontal and decentralized program.
- Frequent armed conflicts and civil unrest, forcing large populations to settle under difficult conditions, sometimes in areas of high malaria transmission
- Migration of nonimmune populations from nonmalarious parts to areas of high transmission, for agriculture, commerce and trade etc.
- Changing rainfall patterns and water development projects [dams and irrigation canals], that create new mosquito breeding sites

- Adverse socioeconomic conditions, reduced health budget and gross inadequacy of funds for drugs
- High birth rates leading to a rapid increase in the susceptible population under 5 years of age
- Change in behavior of vectors, particularly in biting habits.

384. Ans. (c) June

Ref: K. Park, 24th ed. p 438

Antimalaria month is observed every year in **June** (Before onset of monsoon and transmission season)

It seeks to increase awareness levels, encourage community participation and consolidate intersectoral collaboration.

LYMPHATIC FILARIASIS

385. Ans. (b) Infectivity rate

386. Ans. (b) DEC - 6 mg/Kg/day x 12 days

Treatment for filaria (Mf positive persons)
DEC – 6mg /kg/day for 12 doses to be completed in 2 weeks
+
Albendazole 400 mg stat (for age more than 2 years)
+
Ivermectin (150-200 mcg/kg of BW)

387. Ans. (a) Microfilaria

388. Ans. (b) All of the above

Ref: K. Park 25th ed. p 302

389. Ans. (a) DEC + Albendazole

Ref: K. Park, 24th ed. p 439

Strategy for Elimination of Lymphatic Filariasis

- Annual Mass Drug Administration-
  - Initiated in 2004 by Govt of India.
  - Single dose of DEC + Albendazole is to be administered to all (except pregnant women and child <2 year) for 5 year to interrupt the transmission
- Home based management of lymphedema and hydrocele operations in identified CHC/

District hospitals/Medical College.

Also Know......................

- Goal set in the National Health Policy 2002 is Elimination of Lymphatic Filariasis by 2015.
- Elimination of Lymphatic Filariasis means – Microfilaria carrier <1% and Subsequent born children are free from adult filaria worm in body. By 2020, all endemic countries are expected to be free of transmission or enter post MDA surveillance

390. Ans. (c) Filaria

Ref: K. Park, 24th ed p-291

Mass Chemoprophylaxis is recommended for the following diseases

- Filaria [DEC]
- Plague [Tetracycline]
- Yaws [Penicillin]
- Trachoma [Tetracycline]

391. Ans. (c) Larvae are deposited on skin surface where they cannot survive

Ref: K. Park, 24th ed. p 287-89, 439

Also Know......................

- Man is the definitive host and Mosquito the intermediate host of Bancroftian and Brugian filariasis.
- Adult worm is found in lymphatic system of man and do not multiply in humans (life span is about ≥15 years)
- Adult female worm (viviparous) gives birth to about 50,000 Microfilaria/day that enter blood circulation via lymphatics
- Mosquito picks up the micro filarial, where it undergoes only development
- Mode of transmission–Bite of infected Culex mosquito (parasite is deposited near site of bite enters via the punctured skin or penetrates skin by itself to reach the lymphatic system.

YELLOW FEVER

392. Ans. (b) Flavivirus

393. Ans. (d) Monkeys

394. Ans. (b) Fatality rate >90%

Ref: K. Park, 25th ed p 308–309

- Yellow fever, has clinical spectrum like other hemorrhagic diseases. The clinical spectrum varies from asymptomatic cases to severe disease involving hepatic and renal involvement.
- The case fatality also ranges from 30% to as high as up to 80%
- Reservoir of infection:
  - Forest areas: Monkeys and mosquitoes
  - Urban areas: Humans
- Modes of transmission:
  - Jungle yellow: Fever – monkey → mosquito → monkey/ humans/ other animals
  - Intermediate yellow fever:
    - Humid/semi humid parts
    - Small scale epidemics in villages or small areas
    - Infect both monkeys and humans
    - Most common type of outbreak in Africa
  - Urban yellow fever: large epidemics occur when infected people introduce the virus into densely populated areas with people who are non-immune
- Period of Communicability:
  - Humans: blood is infectious for the first 3-4 days of illness
  - Mosquitoes: Infective after completing an extrinsic incubation period of 8-12 days.
    - Once the mosquito becomes infective it remains so for the whole life.
    - Transovarian transmission is also seen in few cases
- One attack gives life-long immunity

395. Ans. (a) Aedes

396. Ans. (b) 3–10 days

397. Ans. (a) Aedes aegypti index

Is the percentage of houses and their premises in a well-defined area, showing actual breeding of aedes Aegypti larvae. this index should not be more than 1% in towns and seaports in endemic areas.

398. Ans. (d) Breteau index

$$\text{Breteau index} = \frac{\text{number of containers positive for aedes larvae}}{\textit{number of houses checked}} \times 100$$

399. Ans. (c) 0.5 ml subcutaneous dose

400. Ans. (b) 10–12 days

401. Ans. (d) None of the above

402. Ans. (c) Yellow Fever

Ref: W. John W. Morrow, Nadeem A. Sheikh. Vaccinology: Principles and Practice

Mass Vaccination is done for Meningitis and Yellow Fever if risk factors for epidemic are present

403. Ans. (d) Validity of certificate of vaccination begins 10 days after vaccination and extends till 5 years

Ref: K. Park, 24th ed. p-299-301

Yellow fever reference centers in India are: NIV, Pune and Central Research Institute, Kasauli

404. Ans. (b) 10 days

Ref: K. Park, 24th ed. p 310

Yellow Fever Vaccination

- Route – Subcutaneous at the insertion of deltoid
- Dose - 0.5 mL (single dose) for all age group
- Vaccine is live attenuated freeze dried (17D strain
- Immunity- Begins to appear by 7th day of vaccination and lasts >35 years or lifelong.
- Amendment to the period of validity of the international certificate of vaccination against yellow fever, which is now extended to the life of the person vaccinated, WHO update July 2016.
- Control strategy -Rapid immunization of the population at risk.

Also Know......................

- Cholera and Yellow fever vaccine should be given ≥3 weeks apart.

405. Ans. (c) Validity of vaccine 6 years

Ref: K. Park, 25th ed. p 308–310

Yellow Fever

- It is an exotic zoonotic disease in India.
- *Causative agent*[Q] → Group B Arbovirus (Flavivirus fibricus) [Togavirus family].
- *Reservoir* → Monkey in forest areas and Man in urban area
- *Vector* → Aedes aegypti[Q]
- *Incubation Period*[Q] → Intrinsic 3-6 days, Extrinsic 8-12 days
- *Immunity* → One attack confers lifelong immunity. Infants born of immune mothers are protected up to 6 months of life.
- *Clinical features* → Hemorrhagic fever (black vomit, epitaxis, malena), hepatic and renal manifestations. Spectrum of disease varies from clinically indeterminate to severe cases.
- ***Case fatality rate*** → up to 80% in severe cases.[Q]
- India is a yellow fever receptive area- i.e. Yellow fever virus does not exist but conditions favorable for transmission exist -population is unvaccinated and susceptible, Vector Aedes aegypti found, Climatic conditions are favorable, Reservoir monkey is susceptible)
- Period of communicability: First 3 to 4 days of illness.
- Vaccine -**17D vaccine** is a Live attenuated, Freeze dried vaccine.
- All travellers (including infants) exposed to risk of yellow fever or passing via endemic zones of yellow fever must possess a valid International certificate of vaccination.
- *Quarantine* → A traveller without valid international certificate of vaccination is placed on quarantine in a mosquito proof ward for 6 days.

406. Ans. (d) Lifelong

Ref: K. Park, 24th ed. p 301

Amendment to the period of validity of the international certificate of vaccination against yellow fever, which is now extended to the life of the person vaccinated, WHO update July 2016.

407. Ans. (b) 1%

Ref: K. Park, 24th ed. p 301

Aedes aegypti Index

- *It is a house index used by WHO for surveillance of Aedes mosquito.*
- *It is the percentage of houses and their premises, in a limited well-defined area, that show actual breeding of Aedes aegypti larvae*

Also Know......................

- *Aedes aegypti index must be <1% in towns and seaports in endemic areas to ensure freedom from yellow fever*

408. Ans. (d) Lifelong, starting from 10 days after vaccination

Ref: K. Park, 24th ed. p 301

JAPANESE ENCEPHALITIS

409. Ans. (d) In endemic areas, vaccination is given to cover children 1-9 years age

Ref: K. Park, 24th ed. p 303, 132

Japanese Encephalitis Vaccine

SA14-14-2 vaccine *is a cell culture derived lyophilised (freeze dried) live attenuated vaccine*

- *Efficacy is 99% with single dose*
- *2 doses are being administered in Routine Immunization in endemic areas – 1st between 9-12 months and 2nd between 16-24 months of age.(Along with Measles 2nd dose)*
- *Contraindication –Infants <6 months, Pregnancy, AIDS or immunosuppressive illness, Anaphylaxis to previous dose, hypersensitivity to Kanamycin/Gentamycin/Gelatin, Fever (>38.5°C)*
- In endemic areas, vaccination is given to cover children 1-15 years age

410. Ans. (a) Pigs – mosquito

Ref: K. Park, 24th ed. p 302

Japanese encephalitis (JE) is a mosquito-borne encephalitis [zoonotic disease] caused by group B arbovirus (Flavivirus).

- The cycles of JE transmission are:
  - Pig - Mosquito – Pig
  - The Ardeid bird - Mosquito - Ardeid bird
- JE is transmitted to man by the bite of infected ***Culicine mosquitoes*** → *C. tritaeniorhynchus*[Q] *[Most important vector in South India], C. vishnui* and *C. gelidus*
- Man is an incidental "***dead-end***" host. *Man to man transmission has not been recorded.*[Q]
- Pigs act as "amplifiers" of virus.
- Cattle and buffaloes act as "mosquito attractants."

Control of JE –

- ***Vector control***:
  - Aerial or Ground fogging with Ultra-Low-Volume (ULV) insecticides (e.g. Malathion, Fenitrothion) in villages where cases are reported and surrounding uninfected villages within 2-3 km radius.
  - Villages surrounding infected villages are to be kept under surveillance.
  - Use of mosquito nets is advocated.
- ***Vaccination***:
  - *Live attenuated vaccine*- SA 14-14-2.

411. Ans. (c) Pigs

Ref: K. Park, 24th ed. p 303

Pig is Considered as an "Amplifier" of JE Virus

- It is a major vertebrate hosts for JE virus (About 100% of pigs may be infected with JE virus at places).
- Infected pigs do not manifest any overt symptoms of illness, but circulate the virus.

Also Know......................

- Horses are the only domestic animals known to shows signs of encephalitis due to JE virus.

412. Ans. (a) Culex

Ref: K. Park, 24th ed. p 302-03

JE is transmitted to man by the bite of infected ***Culicine mosquito's*** → *C. tritaeniorhynchus*[Q], C. vishnui and C. gelidus

- Mosquitoes breed in irrigated *rice fields*[Q][Most important site], shallow ditches and pools.
- Culex mosquitoes are zoophilic (Feed mainly on vertebrate host).
- Female mosquitoes get infected on feeding a viraemic host and can transmit virus to other hosts (after 9-12 days incubation period)

413. Ans. (c) Japanese Encephalitis

Ref: K. Park, 24th ed. p 303

Mosquito-borne diseases in India	
Anopheles	Malaria, filaria (not in India)
Culex	Bancroftian filariasis, Japanese encephalitis, West Nile fever, Viral arthritis (epidemic/polyarthritis)
Aedes	Yellow fever (not in India) Dengue, Dengue hemorrhagic fever, Chikungunya fever, Chikungunya hemorrhagic fever, Rift valley fever, Filaria (not in India)
Mansonoides	Malayan (Brugian) filariasis Chikungunya fever

414. Ans. (b) Mosquito bite always results in disease

Ref: K. Park, 24th ed. p 303

Japanese Encephalitis (JE)

- Majority of cases (about 85%) occur in under 15 years age children.
- Mosquito bite does not always results in disease
- Ratio of overt disease to inapparent infection varies from 1:250 to 1: 1000 (22nd edition, K Park).
- CFR ranges between 20-40%. Average period between onset of illness and death is about 9 days.
- *Incubation period in man* varies from 5-15 days.[Q]

KFD AND CHIKUNGUNYA FEVER

415. Ans. (d) Chikungunya

Comment:

- Alphavirus: Chikungunya virus (CHIKV), is a member of the genus Alphavirus, and family Togaviridae
- Flavivirus: This genus includes the West Nile virus, dengue virus, tick-borne encephalitis virus, yellow fever virus, JE virus, Zika virus and several other tick borne viruses which may cause encephalitis

416. Ans. (c) Infected pigs manifest disease

417. Ans. (b) Rice fields

418. Ans. (b) Single dose, booster not needed

419. Ans. (c) Karnataka

420. Ans. (b) Haemaphysalis

Haemaphysalis is the tick. Ticks could be further classified as soft ticks or hard ticks, but both ticks may transmit KFD

421. Ans. (c) Ardeid birds

The birds belonging to family *Ardeidae* are commonly called as ardeid birds or the 'Herons'. They are implicated in maintenance of the KFD virus in the environment

422. Ans. (a) Aedes

Ref: K. Park, 24th ed. p 306

423. Ans. (d) Chikungunya is transmitted by...

Ref: K. Park, 24th ed. p 306

Arbovirus Prevalent in India are

- **GROUP A (Alpha virus):** Sindbis, Chikungunya
- **GROUP B (Flavi virus):** Dengue, KFD, JE, West Nile

424. Ans. (a) Chikungunya fever; (b) West nile fever; (c) JE; (d) Sandfly fever

Ref: K. Park, 24th ed. p 302

PLAGUE

425. Ans. (c) Tatera indica

Rattus rattus – is the domestic rat

Bandicota bengalensis – is the lesser bandicoot rat. They are considered a pest in the cereal crops and gardens of India and Sri Lanka, and emit pig-like grunts when attacking

Mus booduga : Is the Little Indian field rat

Tatera indica: Is the wild rodent or Indian gerbil. These are light brown/rusty colored with typical bounding gait.

426. Ans. (b) X. cheopis Index

Ref: K. Park, 24th ed. p 311

- ***Cheopis index***[Q] is average number of X. cheopis per rat. [Specific flea index]
- **X. Cheopis index** >1 indicates *potential explosiveness of plague outbreak*[Q]

Also Know......................

Other Flea indices used to evaluate effectiveness of a spray operations

- ***Total flea index***: Average number of fleas of all species per rat.
- ***Specific percentage of fleas***: Percentage of different species of fleas found on rats.
- ***Burrow index*** average number of free-living fleas per species per rodent burrow.

427. Ans. (c) Rat flea

Ref: K. Park, 25th ed. p 320–324

Plague

- *Causative agent* – Yersinia Pestis[Q]
- *Reservoir of infection*: Wild rodents. *In India, Tatera indica is the main reservoir.*[Q]
- *Source of infection* – Infected rodents and fleas and a case of pneumonic plague.
- *Vectors* → Rat flea [X. Cheopis]. Both sexes of flea bite and transmit the disease.
- Infected fleas may live up to 1 year, certain species survive in burrow microclimate for as long as 4 years.
- All ages and both sexes are susceptible. No natural immunity. Immunity after recovery is relative.
- **Mode of transmission–B**ite of an infected flea, direct contact with infected animal tissue or droplet infection
- ***Incubation period***- Bubonic and septicemic plague 2-7 days[Q]. Pneumonic plague is 1 to 3 days.
- *Bubonic plague* - Most common type of plague, *Pneumonic plague* is the most infectious and Septicaemic plague is rare

Chemoprophylaxis is indicated for all contacts. Drug of choice is Tetracycline.[Q] [500 mg 6 hourly × 5 days]

Also Know......................

- Plague occurs in *enzootic, epizootic, sporadic and epidemic forms.* In SEAR, natural foci exist in India, Indonesia, Myanmar

428. Ans. (b) Cheopis Index

Ref: K. Park, 25th ed. p 321

429. Ans. (b) Cheopis index

Ref: K. Park, 25th ed. p 321

430. Ans. (a) Plague

Ref: Harrison 17th edition, chapter-214 p- 1345

U.S. Centers for Disease Control and Prevention (CDC) classifies potential biologic threats into 3 categories.

- Category A → Highest-priority pathogens. [Anthrax, Botulinism, Plague, Small pox, Tularemia, Viral hemorrhagic fevers, Ebola, Marburg]
  - Easily disseminated or transmitted from person to person
  - Result in high mortality and have potential for major public health impact
  - May cause public panic and social disruption
  - Require special action for public health preparedness.
- Category B → 2nd highest priority pathogens [Brucellosis, Epsilon toxin of *Clostridium perfringens*, Food safety threats (e.g., *Salmonella* spp., *Escherichia coli* 0157:H7, *Shigella*), Glanders, Melioidosis, Psittacosis, Q fever, Typhus fever]
  - Moderately easy to disseminate
  - Moderate morbidity rates and low mortality rates
  - Require specifically enhanced diagnostic capacity.
- Category C → 3rd highest priority. [Nipah, hantavirus, SARS coronavirus, and pandemic influenza]
  - Emerging pathogens, to which the general population lacks immunity
  - Could be engineered for mass dissemination in future
  - Potential for high morbidity and mortality, and major public health impact.

Here, we have 3 category A agents as options. However answer is a. Plague because

- When used as aerosol, it has highest mortality [about 100% >smallpox(10-30%) and botulinism (60-100%)
- Secondary cases also occur by person to person transmission.
- Whole of the world population is susceptible [no routine vaccination done]

RICKETTSIAL DISEASES

431. Ans. (a) Tetracycline

Ref: Park 25th ed. p 326

432. Ans. (d) Q fever

Control measures for Q-fever-

- Drug of choice – doxycycline
- Pasteurization of milk to inactivate the causative agent
- Hygienic environment in cattle sheds
- Coxiella vaccine – inactivated vaccine

433. Ans. (a) R. prowazeki

Comment:

Diseases	Rickettsial agent	Insect vectors	Mammalian reservoirs
▪ **Typhus groups** • Epidemic typhus	*R. prowazekii*	Louse	Humans
• Murine typhus	*R. typhi*	Flea	Rodents
• Scrub typhus	*R. tsutsugamushi*	Mite*	Rodents
▪ **Spotted fever group** • Indian tick typhus	*R. conorii*	Tick*	Rodents, dogs
• Rocky mountain spotted fever	*R. rickettsii*	Tick*	Rodents, dogs
• Rickettsial pox	*R. akari*	Mite*	Mice
▪ **Others** • Q fever	*C. burnetii*	Nil	Cattle, sheep, goats
• Trench fever	*Rochalimaea quintana*	Louse	Humans

434. Ans. (c) Q Fever

All Rickettsial disease are characterized by fever, skin rash, hepato-splenomegaly <u>Except</u> Q fever (coxiella burnetti infection)

Indian Tick Typhus

Reservoir of infection: Tick [Transovarial and Transstadial transmission]

Man is an accidental host

Mode of transmission –Bite of an infected tick or Contamination of skin with crushed tissues or feces of an infected tick

Incubation period: 3 - 7 days

Clinical features –

Eschar at the site of bite.

Acute onset of fever [2 to 3 weeks], malaise and headache. Maculopapular rash starting from the extremities (ankles & wrist), then moving centripetally to involve the rest of the body.[Q]

Control measures –

Treatment: Broad spectrum antibiotics

Personal prophylaxis: Avoiding Tick infested areas, Disinfection of dogs, inspection of body for ticks for those exposed to the risk of infection.

435. Ans. (d) Scrub typhus

436. Ans. (b) Not reported in India

Scrub typhus

- Most widespread
- Rickettsia tsutsugamushi
- Reservoir – trombiculid mite (leptotrombidium delinese and L. akamushi)
- Transovarian transmission
- Larvae stage of the mite is both the vector and reservoir of infection
- Incubation 10-12 days
- Clinical feature:
  - High grade fever with rash on 5-6th day of illness.
  - Blackened eschar (scab) at the location of the mite bite
- Diagnosis: Weil Felix reaction with proteus strain OXK
- DOC – tetracycline

437. Ans. (c) Tick borne infection

Q. fever does not have an arthropod vector

438. Ans. (c) Scrub typhus

439. Ans. (a) Rocky Mountain Spotted Fever

Ref: K. Park, 24th ed. p 316

440. Ans. (a) Rickettsia prowazekii and Louse

Ref: K. Park, 24th ed. p 316

441. Ans. (d) R. tsutsugamushi

Ref: K. Park, 24th ed p-317

Scrub Typhus is the *most widespread disease caused by Rickettsiae in man*

- *Causative agent → Rickettsia tsutsugamushi.*
- *Reservoir* → Trombiculid mite. Larva act both as a reservoir (Transovarian transmission) and as a vector for humans and rodents.
- ***Mode of transmission*** *– By bite of infected larval mites.*[Q]

442. Ans. (c) Crushing of louse on body

Ref: K. Park, 24th ed. p-318

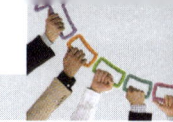

443. Ans. (a) Louse

Ref: Vagabond's Leukomelanoderma, Lambert M. Surhone, Miriam T. Timpledon VDM Publishing, 2010

Vagabond's disease-is a cutaneous disorder caused body lice (Pediculus corporis) that lay their eggs in the seams of cloth

444. Ans. (b) Mite

Ref: K. Park, 24th ed. p 317

In Scrub Typhus, direct man-man transmission does not occur.

Features	Scrub typhus	Murine typhus	Indian tick typhus	Epidemic typhus	Rickettsialpox	Rocky mountain fever	Q fever
Agent	Rickettsia	R. moser	R. conorii	R. Prowazekii	R. akari	R. rickettsii	Coxiella burnetii
Reservoir	Mite	Commensally rats	Ticks	Man	Domestic rodents	Wild rodents	Cattle
Insect vector	Mite	Flea	Tick	Louse	Mite	Tick	–
IP	10–12	1–2 weeks	3–7 days	1–2 weeks	7–9 weeks	5–7 days	2–3 weeks
Eschar	Present	Absent	Present	Absent	Present	Present	Absent
Rash	Centrifugal	Centrifugal	All over body	Centrifugal	All over body	Centripetal	No rash
Treatment	Tetracycline	Tetracycline	Doxy	Tetra	Doxy	Doxy	Doxy
Remark	Most common rickettsial infection	Also knows as endemic typhus	Atypical measles	–	Atypical chicken pox	–	Transmitted by aerosol

445. Ans. (b) Flea

Ref: K. Park, 24th ed. p 317

Endemic or Murine Typhus

Reservoir→Rats (Rattus rattus and R. norvegicus).
Mode of transmission → Inoculation into skin of faeces of infected fleas and Inhalation of dried infective faeces.
No direct man to man transmission.
Vector → Flea (Once infected, remains so for life).
Transmission cycle:
Rat → Rat flea → Rat → Rat flea
Rat → Rat flea → Man
Incubation period – 1 to 2 weeks (Average 12 days)
Weil Felix reaction with Proteus OX-19 becomes positive in the 2nd week.
Treatment: Tetracycline is drug of choice.
Control of fleas: Residual insecticides (e.g., BHC, malathion) and Rodent control measures.

446. Ans. (a) Louse

Ref: K. Park, 24th ed. p 316

447. Ans. (b) Q fever

Ref: K. Park, 24th ed. p 316

Q fever

Causative agent - Coxiella burnetii.
Vector & Reservoir- ***Ticks***

Cattle, Sheep, Goats, Ticks & some wild animals are natural reservoirs.

- **Mode of transmission:**
  Inhalation of infected dust [contaminated by urine/ feces of diseased animals] or aerosols. [most important route]
  Entry via abrasions, conjunctiva
  Ingestion of contaminated foods
- **Incubation period** - 2 to 3 weeks
- **Clinical features** – Acute onset with fever, chills, general malaise and headache.
  No rash or local lesion.[Q] [All other rickettsial diseases have rash]
  Infection may be asymptomatic
- **Control measures –**
  Treatment: Tetracyclines [Orally up to 5 days after remission of fever]
- ***Preventive measures:*** Pasteurization or boiling of milk, sanitary cattle sheds, disinfection & disposal of infectious products.
  - *No arthropod is involved in transmission of Q fever to Man*[Q].

448. Ans. (b) Adult mite feeds on vertebrate host

Ref: K. Park, 24th ed. p 317

Scrub Typhus

- ***Mode of transmission***–*By bite of infected larval mites.*[Q] The transmission cycle may be as below:
  - Mite → Rats and mice → Mite → Rats and mice
  - Mite → Rats and mice → Mite → Man
- No direct person to person transmission
- **Incubation period** - 10-12 days

- **Clinical features** – Resemble epidemic typhus. Acute onset with chills and fever (104°-105° F), headache, malaise, prostration. A *macular rash appears around the 5th day of illness. Generalized lymphadenopathy and lymphocytosis* are common. **Eschar** a punched-out ulcer covered with a blackened scab is characteristic.[Q]
- Weil Felix reaction is strongly positive with the Proteus strain OXK.
- *Treatment*: **Drug of choice is** Tetracycline.
- *Vector control:* Clearing the vegetation where rats and mice live; application of insecticides [lindane or chlordane] to ground and vegetation
- Personal prophylaxis: Impregnating clothes and blankets with Benzyl benzoate, Application of mite repellents (diethyltoluamide) to exposed skin surfaces
- No vaccine exists at present.

NVBDCP

449. Ans. (a) Albendazole; (b) DEC; (c) Ivermectin

Ref: K. Park, 24th ed. p 439

Revised Strategy under NVBDCP for Filaria

Annual Mass Drug Administration of a single dose of 2 medicines to entire at-risk population to interrupt transmission of disease:

- Albendazole (400 mg) with Diethyl Carbamazine citrate (DEC) (6 mg/kg).
- Recently, Ivermectin has also been added as triple drug therapy for mass elimination of Lymphatic Filariasis.
- The World Health Organization (WHO) and GoI is recommending an alternative three drug treatment to accelerate the global elimination of lymphatic filariasis - a disabling and disfiguring neglected tropical disease. The treatment, known as IDA, involves a combination of ivermectin, diethylcarbamazine citrate and albendazole. It is being recommended annually in settings where its use is expected to have the greatest impact.

Population Excluded

- Children below two years,
- Pregnant women
- Seriously ill persons in affected areas.

Morbidity Management comprises

- Home based management of lymphedema cases
- Up-scaling of hydrocele operations in the identified CHCs/ District hospitals/ medical colleges.

450. Ans. (b) Abate

Ref - http://nvbdcp.gov.in, Urban Malaria Scheme. Norbert Becker, Dusan Petric, Mosquitoes and Their Control, 2nd edition, p-457

Urban Malaria Scheme Programme

Chemical larvicides used

- Temephos (Trade name–Abate) - Disadvantage-Disagrreable smell
- Bti (WP and 12 AS)

Biological Control (Larvivorous Fish)

- Gambusia and Guppy (If chemical control is not feasible).

Also Know......................

Insecticide Approved as Safe for use in Potable Water (WHO ICPS 1992)

- Temephos
- Permethrin
- Methoprene
- Products based on B. thuringiensis israelensis

451. Ans. (a) API <1 per 1000

Ref: Strategic Plan for Malaria Control in India -2012-2017, NVBDCP, MOHFW,GOI

Strategic Plan for Malaria Control in India [2012-2017]

Mission: To reduce morbidity and mortality due to malaria and improving the quality of life, thereby contributing to health and alleviation of poverty in the country

Goals

- Screen all fever cases suspected for malaria (60% through quality microscopy and 40% by Rapid Diagnostic Test)
- Treat all P. falciparum cases with full course of effective ACT and primaquine and all P. vivax cases with 3 days chloroquine and 14 days primaquine
- Equip all health Institutions (PHC level and above), especially in high-risk areas, with microscopy facility and RDT for emergency use and injectable artemisinin derivatives
- Strengthen all district and sub-district hospitals in malaria endemic areas as per IPHS with facilities for management of severe malaria cases.

Objective: To achieve by the end of 2017, API <1 per 1000 Population

452. Ans. (c) Annual incidence <10 per 1000

Ref: Strategic Plan for Malaria Control in India -2012-2017, NVBDCP, MOHFW,GOI

453. Ans. (c) 4 mg/kg daily Artesunate × 3 day + Sulfadoxine and Pyrimethamine...

Ref: K. Park, 24th ed. p 279

National Malaria Diagnosis and Treatment Guideline 2013

P. falciparum cases→Artemisinin based Combination Therapy (ACT-SP)** + Primaquine: 0.75 mg/kg body weight on day 2

**Artesunate 4 mg/kg body weight daily for 3 days + Sulfadoxine 25 mg/kg body weight and Pyrimethamine 1.25 mg/kg on day 1

454. Ans. (c) Malaria, Dengue, Kala azar

Ref: K. Park, 24th ed. p 432

NVBDCP was launched in 2003-04

- It includes prevention and control of vector borne diseases – Malaria, Filaria, Kala-azar, Japanese Encephalitis, Dengue and Chikungunya
- Directorate NVBDCP is nodal agency for planning, policy making, technical guidance, monitoring and evaluation of program implementation under NRHM

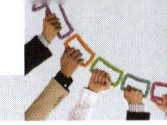

Also Know.......................

3 Pronged Strategy for NVBDCP

- Disease management Early diagnosis and complete treatment, Strengthening referral services, Epidemic preparedness and rapid response
- Integrated vector management (Indoor Residual spray in High Risk Area, Insecticide Treated Bednet, Larvivorous Fish, Anti larval measures, source reduction and minor environmental engineering)
- Supportive intervention – BCC, Public Private Partnership, Intersectoral Convergence, Human recourse development, Research

455. Ans. (a) Early detection of malaria illness

Ref: J Kishore, National Health Programmes of India, 11th ed. p-269; 24th ed. p 269

Roll Back Malaria (RBM)

Aim: Reduce the burden of malaria by 50% by 2010

Priority Technical Strategies under RBM comprise

- Prompt access to effective treatment
- Promote use of insecticide-treated bed nets and improved vector control
- Prevention and management of malaria in pregnancy
- Improved response to malaria in epidemics and complex emergencies- Health system strengthening and capacity building

456. Ans. (a) ACT only

Ref: K. Park, 24th ed. p 279

Malaria Diagnosis and Treatment Guideline 2013

Latest Updates

Treatment of uncomplicated malaria

No more presumptive treatment[Q]. All fever cases suspected to be malaria must be investigated by microscopy or RDT.

P.vivax cases → *Chloroquine:* 10mg/kg on day 1 and 2 and 5mg/kg on day 3. + *Primaquine** 0.25 mg/kg body weight daily for 14 days. (*contraindicated in pregnancy, G6PD deficiency)

P.Falciparum cases→Artemisinin based Combination Therapy (ACT-SP)** + Primaquine: 0.75 mg/kg body weight on day 2

(**Artesunate 4 mg/kg body weight daily for 3 days
+ Sulfadoxine 25 mg/kg body weight) and Pyrimethamine
1.25 mg/kg on day 1)

- ***Mixed infection [P. falciparum + P. vivax]***–ACT-SP × 3 days + *Primaquine* 0.25 mg /kg body weight daily for 14 days.

In North Eastern states

- ***P. falciparum cases***-ACT-AL (Coformulated tablet of Artemether (20 mg) + Lumefantrine (120 mg) as per age specific schedule) + Primaquine: 0.75 mg/kg body weight on day 2
- ***Mixed infection [P. falciparum + P. vivax]***–ACT-AL × 3 days + *Primaquine* 0.25 mg /kg body weight daily for 14 days.

Treatment of malaria in pregnancy

P. falciparum cases→1st Trimester: Quinine, 2nd and 3rd Trimester: ACT

P. vivax cases → Chloroquine

Treatment of resistant cases

- Resistance is suspected if full treatment, shows no response in 72 hour.
- Treatment-Oral Quinine +Tetracycline/Doxycycline

Treatment of severe malaria

- Artesunate: 2.4 mg/kg IV or IM on admission, then at 12 h and 24 h and then once a day or
- Artemether: 3.2 mg/kg body weight IM on admission and then 1.6 mg/kg per day or
- Arteether: 150 mg IM daily for 3 days in adults only or
- Quinine: 20 mg/kg body weight on admission (IV or IM) followed by maintenance dose of 10 mg/kg body weight 8 hourly.

457. Ans. (c) Primaquine is contraindicated in infants and pregnant women

Ref: K. Park, 24th ed. p 284-85

Contraindication of Primaquine- Infants, Pregnant women, Patients with G6PD deficiency

458. Ans. (d) 300 mg once/week

Ref: K. Park, 24th ed. p 284-85

Chemoprophylaxis (to be complemented with personal protection and other methods)

- **Indication** → Selective groups [Military and Para-military forces, labor forces, travellers from nonendemic area for long stay in high P. falciparum endemic areas]
- Short term chemoprophylaxis (up to 6 weeks) – All drugs to be taken strictly on time and continued for 4 weeks after the last possible exposure to infection)
  - Doxycycline: 100 mg OD for adults and 1.5 mg/kg OD for children started 2 days before travel
    Not for pregnant women and children <8 years (Dose in children >8 year is based on body weight
  - Chloroquine – 300 mg (bas(e) once weekly or 100 mg (bas(e) OD for 6 days a week. Initiated a week before arrival
  - Mefloquine 250 mg weekly. Initiated 2-3 week before arrival
- Chemoprophylaxis for longer stay (>6 weeks)
  - Mefloquine: 250 mg weekly for adults, administered 2 weeks before, during and 4 weeks after exposure.
  - Chloroquine (300 mg weekly/100 mg O(d) + Proguanil (100 mg O(d) – (Screening for retinal changes to be done 6 month after 5 year (weekly regimen) and 3 year (daily regimen)

459. Ans. (c) Quinine

Ref: K. Park, 24th ed. p 283

Parenteral (Initial 48 hour –Minimum)	Quinine -20 mg salt /Kg body weight (i.v. or im divided doses) on admission*, followed by maintenance dose 10 mg /kg x TDS (Infusion rate <5 mg/kg/hour) Or Artesunate -2.4 mg/kg (IV or IM) on admission, 12 hour, 24 hour and then once daily Or Artemether- 3.2 mg. kg body weight i.m. on admission followed by 1.6 mg/kg/day Or Arteether- 150 mg /day IM for 3 days (only for adults)
Follow up treatment (Patient can take medicines orally) – Follows initial parenteral treatment	Quinine -10mg salt /Kg body weight x TDS + Doxycycline 100 mg OD ** Or ACT SP × 3 days + Primaquine (single dose on day 2) **North Eastern States**-ACT AL × 3 days + Primaquine (single dose on day 2)

**Not to be administered if Quinine has been given previously*
***Clindamycin 10 mg/kg BD for 7 days to be used in place of Doxycycline in pregnant women and children <8 year age*

460. Ans. (c) 1

Ref: K. Park, 24th ed. p

Annual Parasite Incidence (API) is a measure of malaria incidence in a community based on active and passive surveillance with cases confirmed by blood examination

$$\text{API} = \frac{\text{Confirmed case in a year}}{\text{Population under surveillance}} \times 1000 = \frac{100}{100000} \times 1000 = 1$$

Also Know...................

- API ≥2 per 1000 population – Signifies High risk area.V

Annual blood examination rate (ABER)

$$= \frac{\text{Number of slides examined}}{\text{Population}} \times 100$$

AEBR is an index of operational efficiency. Minimum prescribed ABER is 10%.

461. Ans. (c) Developing newer insecticides

Ref: J Kishore,National Health Programmes of India, 11th ed. p-269

462. Ans. (a) Zika virus disease

Ref: K. Park, 24th ed. p 432

463. Ans. (c) Anti-larval measures

Ref: K. Park, 24th ed. p 433

Urban malaria scheme, was launched in 1971 to reduce and interrupt malaria transmission in Towns and Cities

- It emphasized on vector control by antilarval measures and drug treatment
- As per the recommendation of Expert Committee on Malaria- All urban areas with a population >50000 and SPR (Slide Positivity Rat(e) of ≥5% is to be covered under Urban malaria scheme

464. Ans. (b) API

Ref: K. Park, 24th ed. p 434

Current Strategy aims for malaria elimination (No indigenous transmission i.e. API <1)

Based on endemicity, states have been classified into 3 categories

Category 1	States with API <1 and all districts in the state are with API <1
Category 2	States with API <1 and one or more districts reporting API >1
Category 3	States with API >1

ARI

465. Ans. (b) 3-5

- In children Under 5 years, average 3-5 ARI attacks may happen per child/year.
- Leading cause for disability due to hearing loss due to Otitis media as sequel
- 18% of all under five deaths were due to pneumonia (2017 India health profile)

466. Ans. (b) Staphylococcus pyogenes

Remember:

▪ Paroxysmal cough	B. pertussis
▪ Secondary infections	Staph aureus
▪ Community acquired pneumonia	Strep pneumoniae
▪ Acute exacerbation of chronic bronchitis	Strep pneumoniae
▪ Acute pharyngitis/tonsillitis	Strep pyogenes
▪ Common cold	Rhino virus/corona virus
▪ Croup	Parainfluenza virus
▪ Atypical pneumonia	Q. Fever, psittacosis
▪ Pneumonia like illness + Diarrhea	Legionnaire's pneumonia

467. Ans. (a) Chest in drawing

Tachypnoea:

- Age <2 months more than 60 breaths/minute
- Age 2 months – 12 months more than 50 breaths/minute
- Age 1 year – 5 years more than 40 breaths/minute

For Age Months – 5 years

		No pneumonia – cough or cold	Pneumonia	Severe pneumonia
Signs	Chest indrawing	No	No	Yes
	Tachypnea	No	Yes	Yes
	Recurrent wheezing	No	No	Yes (treat urgently)
Treatment		Home care + follow up and if cough for more than 30 days – refer for assessment	Advise antibiotic + home care + follow up within 1-2 days	Refer urgently + give first dose antibiotic

For Age <2 Months

		Very severe Disease	Severe Pneumonia	No pneumonia – cough or cold
Signs	Danger signs	Inability to feed, convulsions, abnormal sleepy, stridor, wheeze, fever		
	Chest indrawing	Severe chest indrawing	Severe chest indrawing	No severe chest indrawing
	Tachypnea	Not a criterion for classification	Fast breathing >60 breaths/min	No fast breathing
Treatment		Refer urgently + Give first dose antibiotic + Keep baby warm	Refer urgently + Give first dose antibiotic + Keep baby warm	Advise home care + Keep baby warm + breast feed frequently + close Follow up

468. Ans. (d) Pneumonia

Ref: K. Park, 24th ed. p 18081

469. Ans. (b) Severe pneumonia

Ref: K. Park, 24th ed. p 181

470. Ans. (c) Frequent breastfeeding

Ref: K. Park, 24th ed. p-180-81

Since, there is no chest indrawing and no fast breathing (Respiratory rate >60/min in infants <2 months), hence this case comes under No Pneumonia.

Management: Home care and frequent breastfeeding

471. Ans. (c) Antibiotic with home care

Ref: K. Park, 24th ed. p-180-81

Respiratory Rate -58/min (Fast Breathing as >50/min)

No Chest in drawing.

Hence, this case comes under pneumonia

Management: Home care, Antibiotic, Antipyretic Treatment and Follow up

472. Ans. (d) Very severe pneumonia

Ref: K. Park, 24th ed. p 181

Here the child has a weight 5 kg (Indicative of severe malnutrition- where typical signs of pneumonia are masked). Hence, it is a case of very severe pneumonia

473. Ans. (c) Oxygen saturation

Ref: K. Park, 24th ed. p 181

474. Ans. (b) Chest indrawing

Ref: K. Park, 24th ed. p 181

475. Ans. (c) >50/min

Ref: K. Park, 24th ed. p 180

OTHER INFECTIONS

476. Ans. (a) B. melitensis

Ref: K. Park, 25th ed. p 317

Four species infect humans:

Brucella melitensis	most virulent, infects goats, sheep
B. abortus	less virulent, primarily infects cattle
B. suius	intermediate virulence, infects pigs
B. canis	parasite in dogs

477. Ans. (d) All of the above

Brucellosis primarily affects adult farmers, shepherds, butchers, lab workers

478. Ans. (a) Contact infection

Mode of transmission:

- Most common route is by direct contact infection with infected blood, urine, vaginal discharge, aborted fetuses and other routes
- Infection may also spread by ingestion of milk or dairy products infected with Brucella infection
- Airborne spread is also possible but requires a very heavy contamination of the cattle shed area for inhalation of the pathogen.

479. Ans. (a) Tetracycline

Control and treatment measures:

- Treatment: Tetracycline 500 mg 6 hourly for 3 weeks
- Pasteurization of milk
- Vaccination – human live vaccine of B. abortus 19-BA strain
- Prevent direct contact with infected animals

480. Ans. (b) B. abortus

481. Ans. (d) Corneal transplantation

Modes of transmission

- Trachoma is known to be a familial disease - when one case is detected its almost certain that there will be other cases in the family members.
- In areas with trachoma endemicity, eye to eye transmission is most frequent route.
- Eye to eye transmission may occur by direct or indirect contact with ocular discharges from the infected persons using fomites as towels, fingers or others.
- Eye seeking flies – (Musca spp.) may play a small role in transmission of trachoma

482. Ans. (a) T solium

T. Solium causes human cysticercosis. The intermediate host is pig.
Treatment: Morning, empty stomach -
Praziquantel 10 mg/kg single dose +
Niclosamide 2gms, single dose

483. Ans. (a) Man

Parasite	Definitive host	Intermediate host
T. saginata	Human	Cattle
T. solium	Human	Pig

Incubation period: 8-14 weeks

484. Ans. (c) Pig

485. Ans. (d) Cattle

Ref: Park 25th ed. p 330

Hydatid disease:

- Caused by Metacystode stage of the intestinal tapeworm – echinococcus
  - E. granulosus – cause Hydatidosis 'unilocular' type of echinococcosis
  - E. multilocularis – in northern hemisphere, cause 'alveolar' type of echinococcosis
  - E. oligarthus – in central and south America
  - E. vogeli – in central and south America, cause polycystic Hydatidosis
- Life cycle – dog sheep cycle is maintained, with human as accidental or intermediate host
- Mode of transmission: by ingestion of eggs of echinococcosis inadvertently with food or unwashed vegetables
- Diagnosis
  - X-ray – location of the cyst
  - ELISA
- Treatment:
  - Surgical removal – PAIR – Puncture – Aspiration – Injection – Re-aspiration (+/- drainage)
  - Mebendazole has been tried with good success in many cases

486. Ans. (d) All of the above

487. Ans. (b) AP &. Tamil Nadu

488. Ans. (b) Cutaneous

Leishmaniasis

- Visceral Leishmaniasis: known as kala azar
  - Endemic in 7 countries – Brazil, Ethiopia, India, Kenya, Somalia, South Sudan and Sudan
- Cutaneous leishmaniasis: is the most common form
  - Prevalent in 6 countries – Afghanistan, Algeria, Brazil, Columbia, Iran, Syria

- Mucocutaneous leishmaniasis – leads to total or partial destruction of the mucus membrane
  - Endemic in Peru, Ethiopia, Brazil

In India Kala azar is endemic is: Bihar, Jharkhand, West Bengal and Uttar Pradesh

489. Ans. (a) P. argentipes

Vector for Leishmaniasis

Phlebotomus argentipes	Kala azar (visceral leishmaniasis)
Phlebotomus papatasii	Sand fly fever, oriental sore, cutaneous leishmaniasis
Phlebotomus sergentii	Oriental sore, cutaneous leishmaniasis
Phlebotomus punjabiensis	Sandfly fever

490. Ans. (a) L. donovani

491. Ans. (a) DDT

492. Ans. (b) Partially blocked flea

493. Ans. (c) Tetracycline

494. Ans. (a) Gastroenteritis

495. Ans. (d) Designated microscopy center

RNTCP Organogram

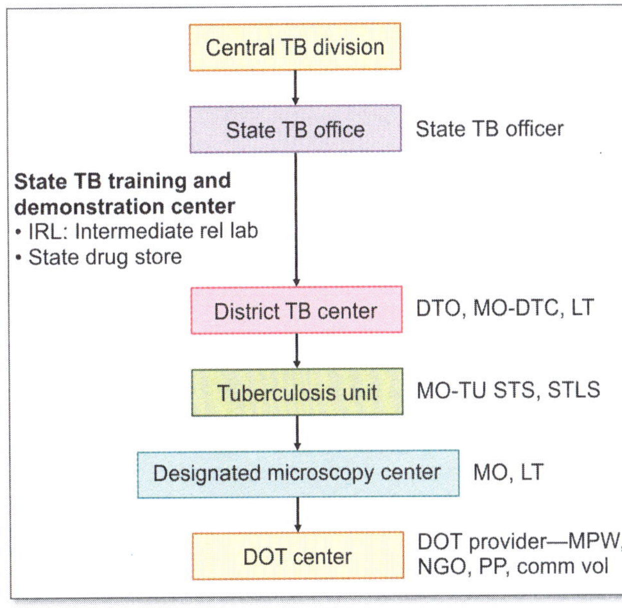

496. Ans. (c) Nikshay

Nikshay

- **NIKSHAY**- is a case based web enabled TB surveillance system *(launched in May 2012)*
- As per GOI notification 7th May 2012- TB is a *Notifiable disease* (mandatory for all health care providers)
- Serological tests are not receommended for diagnosis of TB in India
  - Nirbhaya – is a SOS social safety mobile app
  - Nischay – is a field testing kit for pregnancy

497. Ans. (c) Assam

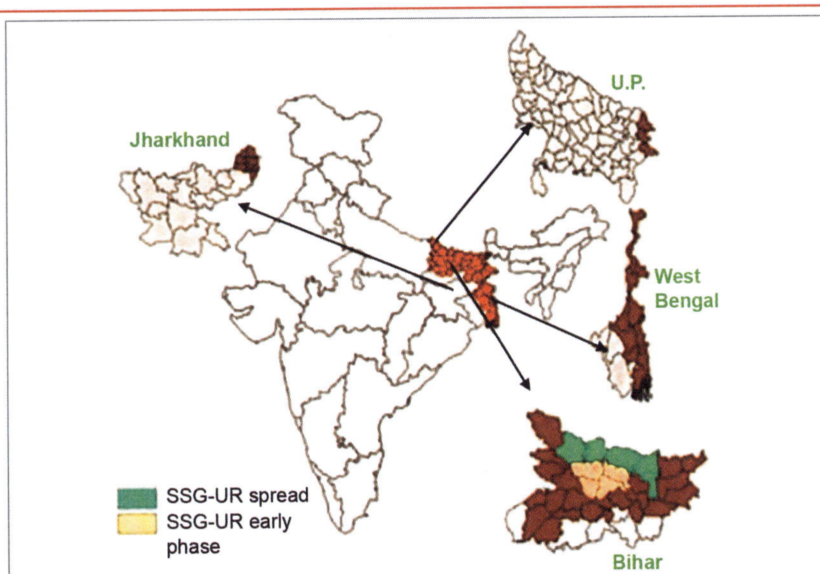

- Endemic in eastern States of India namely Bihar, Jharkhand, Uttar Pradesh and West Bengal
- Mostly poor socio-economic groups of population primarily living in rural areas are affected

498. Ans. (b) 9.7/1,00,000 population

Ref: http://nlep.nic.in/pdf/Sparsh2018_guidelines_2Jan18_F.pdf, http://nlep.nic.in/pdf/Final%20NewsLetter%20July-%20Sept%202018.pdf

Leprosy Survey Report 2016-2017 Data

- A total of 88166 leprosy cases are on record as on 1st April 2017, giving a Prevalence Rate (PR) of 0.66 per 10,000 population
- A total of 1,35,485 new cases were detected during the year 2016-17, which gives Annual New Case Detection Rate (ANCDR) of 10.17 per 100,000 population
- Grade II disabled cases have been prevented by achieving the Grade II disability rate 3.87% during 2016-17.
- A total of 11792 child cases were recorded, indicating the Child Case rate of 8.7%

499. Ans. (c) 28 September

World Leprosy Day	30 January
World TB Day	24 March
World Malaria Day	25 April
World Health Day	7 April
World Dengue Day	16 May
World Heart Day	29 September

500. Ans. (c) MDA is done after a filariasis survey in all age groups

Target

L. Filariasis Elimination by 2020

- Five to **6 rounds of annual MDA** [Q] are required to interrupt transmission of LF.
- Each round of MDA should be 'effective' i.e. **at least 65% treatment coverage** [Q] should be accomplished. (ideally more than 80%)
- After MDA, the evidence for interruption of transmission is generated through implementation of the first transmission assessment survey (TAS 1) among **children of 6-7 year age** [Q] in each district.
- If the number of infected children found in TAS 1 is less than the threshold number (which is approximately **2% Ag or Ab prevalence** [Q]), then the MDA is stopped.
- After stopping the MDA, post-MDA surveillance is initiated. This consists of two more rounds of TAS (TAS 2 and TAS 3).
- Simultaneously, the chronic disease burden should be estimated in all endemic districts, plans for delivery of care to chronic patients developed and each chronic patient provided minimum package of care.
- When all districts in a country complete TAS 3 successfully and minimum package of care is delivered to all patients with chronic disease, the country is deemed to have eliminated LF.
- Then the country prepares LF elimination dossier for validation of elimination of LF.

LF Situation in India

- W. bancrofti is the predominant parasite, prevalent in all endemic states and transmitted by Cx. quinquefasciatus except (in Andaman and Nicobar alone, the vector is Ae. niveus.
- B. malayi is also prevalent in the country, but only in the state of Kerala, and is transmitted by Mansonia species.
- Nationally, 98% of the infections are due to infection with W. bancrofti.

Mass Drug Administration

- The MDA is done AFTER conducting the survey. The survey is done in 4 sentinel sites and 4 random sites collecting total 4000 slides
- MDA is done using Albendazole 400 mg single dose and DEC@ 6mg
- The recommended strategy to interrupt transmission of LF is annual single dose mass drug administration (MDA) in all districts and areas endemic for LF.
- The drugs used in MDA programme are a combination of DEC (6 mg/kg body weight) + ALB (400 mg) in endemic areas free from onchocerciasis prevalence

Diagnosis of LF

- Until now, BinaxNOW filariasis was the only immune-chromatographic test available for bancroftian filariasis.
- A new test for rapid diagnosis – FTS (filariasis strip test) is designed to detect in human blood the antigen of the W. bancrofti.
- The FTS is now recommended and used for mapping, monitoring and evaluation activities.

Treatment for LF

- Triple drug regime is given for filariasis treatment. Consists of ivermectin, albendazole and Diethyl carbmazine (DEC).

501. Ans. (b) RNTCP

RBRC – Random blinding, Random checking: is done for Internal Quality assurance of the laboratory diagnostics for tuberculosis under RNTCP

10% of the positive and negative slides are randomly selected and cross checked for diagnostic matching

502. Ans. (d) Viral isolation is the gold standard

Viral isolation is not feasible and done only for research purpose. PCR is diagnostic and gold standard

503. Ans. (d) 500 IU

Tetanus immune globulin (TIG) is recommended for persons with tetanus. TIG can only help remove unbound tetanus toxin. It cannot affect toxin bound to nerve endings. A single intramuscular dose of 500 units is generally recommended for children and adults, with part of the dose infiltrated around the wound if it can be identified. Intravenous immune globulin (IVIG) contains tetanus antitoxin and may be used if TIG is not available.

Tetanus Toxoid

- Formalin-inactivated tetanus toxin
- Schedule
  - Three or four doses plus booster
  - Booster every 10 years
- Efficacy
  - Approximately 100%
- Duration
  - Approximately 10 years

- Should be administered with diphtheria toxoid as DTaP, DT, Td, or Tdap

Guideline for Tetanus Prophylaxis (NHM, MoHFW)

- Assess and categorize the patient based on previous TT exposure
- Advise for the prophylaxis

Category	Category criteria	Wound <6 hours old Clean, non-penetrating and negligible tissue damage	All other wounds
Category A	Has had complete dose of TT or booster in last 5 years	Nothing required	Nothing required
Category B	Has had complete dose of TT or booster more than 5 years but less than 10 years.	TT/Td 1 dose	TT/Td 1 dose
Category C	Has had complete dose of TT or booster more than 10 years ago	TT/Td 1 dose	TT/Td 1 dose + TIG
Category D	Has never had complete TT dose or status unknown	TT/Td complete dose	TT/Td complete dose + TIG

504. Ans. (c) 1500 mg

Refer to the standard treatment regime for the P. Falciparum infections

Dosage Chart for Treatment of Falciparum Malaria with ACT-SP

Age group (years)	1st day		2nd day		3rd day
	AS	SP	AS	PQ	AS
0–1* Pink blister	1 (25 mg)	1 (250 + 12.5 mg)	1 (25 mg)	Nil	1 25 (mg)
1–4 Yellow blister	1 (50 mg)	1 (500 + 25 mg each)	1 (50 mg)	1 (7.5 mg base)	1 (50 mg)
5–8 Green blister	1 (100 mg)	1 (750 + 37.5 mg each)	1 (100 mg)	2 (7.5 mg base each)	1 (100 mg)
9–14 Red blister	1 (150 mg)	2 (500 + 25 mg each)	1 (150 mg)	4 (7.5 mg base each)	1 (150 mg)
15 & above White blister	1 (200 mg)	2 (750 + 37.5 mg each)	1 (200 mg)	6 (7.5 mg base each)	1 (200 mg)
* SP is not to be prescribed for children <5 months of age and should be treated with alternate ACT * ACT-AL is not to be prescribed for Children weighing less than 5 kg.					

Extra edge:

For Prophylaxis

Short term doxycycline 100 mg for all time of stay till 4 wks before the last exposure

Long term with mefloquine

505. Ans. (a) It's time

506. Ans. (c) Nipah virus

Ref: Park 25th ed. p 310

In this image, we can notice infection starts from flying bats to fruits/human which further spreads to others and to animals. This is a typical life cycle for NIPAH virus.

NIPAH is a zoonotic disease, with Large fruit bats (genus *Pteropus)* (Flying foxes) as natural reservoirs. Pigs on the other hand acts as an intermediate and amplifying host after contact with infected bats or their secretions.

The infection is transmitted as:

- Pig to human
- Bat to human
- Human to human

507. Ans. (a) Onset of catarrhal symptoms to 3 days after rash

Ref: Park 25th ed. p 162

Measles

- Also known as 14-day fever or First disease
- It shows a seasonal trend (peaks in winter/spring)

- Peak age –
  - 6 months to 3 years developing countries
  - Over 5-year children in developed countries
- Period of isolation for measles
- Reservoir – humans
- Transmission – airborne
- Period of communicability – 4 days before rash and 4 days after rash
- Clinical feature:
  - Incubation period 10-14 days
  - Prodrome stage – 2-4 days – fever, coryza, Koplik spots
  - Eruptive phase (204 days after prodrome), persists for 6-7 days
- Isolation: onset of catarrhal stage at least for 3-4 days of rash (best till 7 days of rash)

508. Ans. (b) Maraviroc, (d) Darunavir

Ref: National technical guidelines for HIV. NACO 2018.

The HIV entry to CD4 cells is by a series of events consisting of:

- The binding of HIV surface protein gp120 to the CD4 receptor
- A conformational change in gp120, which both increases its affinity for a co-receptor and exposes gp41
- The binding of gp41 to a co-receptor either CCR5 or CXCR4 *(Meraviroc, Enfuviritde)*
- The penetration of the cell membrane by gp41, which approximates the membrane of HIV and the T cell and promotes their fusion
- The entry of the viral core into the cell

Entry Inhibitors

CCR5 inhibitors: Maraviroc prevents an interaction with gp41 protein. It is also referred to as a "chemokine receptor antagonist"

Fusion inhibitor: Enfuvirtide binds to gp41 and interferes with its ability to approximate the two membranes.

Monoclonal Antibody

Ibalizumab: It is Recombinant humanized monoclonal antibody. It blocks HIV-1 from infecting CD4+ T cells by binding to domain 2 of CD4 and interfering with post-attachment steps required for the entry of HIV-1 virus particles into host cells and preventing the viral transmission that occurs via cell-cell fusion

Integrase inhibitor: Raltegravir

509. Ans. (a) Congenital anomalies is more when 1st trimester infection; (d) Higher chances of herpes zoster in infancy; (e) Higher chances of microcephaly in infants born to VZV exposed mothers

Ref: Park 25th Page 158

Option	T/F	Comment
Congenital anomalies is more when 1st trimester infection	T	Yes, correct. 0.5-2% of children born to mothers with VZV during first 20 weeks of gestation develop infection
Highest chances of anomalies are with last trimester infection	F	No, not correct
Max chances of transmission when 4 days before to 3 days after Pregnancy	F	No, not correct
Higher chances of herpes zoster in infancy	T	Yes, correct
Higher chances of microcephaly in infants born to VZV exposed mothers	T	Yes, correct, the other complications are: cutaneous scars, Low birth weight, limb atrophy, microphthalmia, chorioretinitis, deafness and cerebro-cortical atrophy

Contd...

510. Ans. (a) Dose is 10-20 mcg at 0,1,6 months during pregnancy; (b) In case of accidental exposure to Hepatitis B infected blood in a pregnant female, the HBIG is given in dose of 0.05 ml/kg within 6 hours of accidental exposure

Park 25ed, Pg 235-236

Option	T/F	Comment
Dose is 10-20 mcg at 0,1,6 months during pregnancy	T	Yes correct. pregnancy or lactation is NOT a contraindication for HBV vaccine
In case of accidental exposure to Hepatitis B infected blood in a pregnant female, the HBIG is given in dose of 0.05 ml/kg within 6 hours of accidental exposure	T	Yes correct
To prevent effectively prevent the perinatal transmission of HBV infection, the birth dose Hep B vaccine should be given within 7 days of birth	F	No, the HBV vaccine should be given within 24 hours of birth (and not 7 days of birth)
Both Hep B Vaccine and HBIG is contraindicated in pregnancy	F	No, not correct
HBIG (Hep B Immunoglobulin) may be given while HepB vaccine is contraindicated in pregnancy	F	No, not correct

Note: Hep B Vaccine should not be frozen. The temperature for storage is 2-8°C

511. Ans. (a) Detects DNA sequence by PCR; (c) Investigation for detection of TB infection and rifampicin resistance

Ref: Park 25th ed, Pg 197

Detects DNA sequence by PCR

- Investigation for detection of HIV infection

- Investigation for detection of TB infection and rifampicin resistance
- Results obtained within 48 hours
- Based on assessment of growth index and O_2 utilization in a specialized media

Option	T/F	Comment
Detects DNA sequence by PCR	T	Yes, correct
Investigation for detection of HIV infection	F	No, GeneXpert is for MTB detection and not HIV
Investigation for detection of TB infection and rifampicin resistance	T	Yes correct
Results obtained within 48 hours	F	No, the results are obtained within 2 hours (or 90 mins)
Based on assessment of growth index and O_2 utilization in a specialized media	F	No, it is based on PCR and nucleic acid detection.

GeneXpert MTB/Rif

- Detects DNA sequence specific for Mycobacterium tuberculosis (MTB) AND rifampicin resistance by polymerase chain reaction (PCR)
- Mechanism
  - It is based on the principle of Nucleic acid Amplification (NAA)
  - Concentrates TB bacilli from sputum sample, isolates the genetic material and amplifies the genomic DNA using PCR
  - Detects for RNA Polymerase beta (rpoB) gene in MTB – which is commonly responsible for rifampicin resistance in MTB
- The results are processed within 90 mins

Other Methods

BACTEC 460 TB Method

- C-14 labelled palmitic acid in 7H12 medium is used
- Based on principle of measurement of CO_2 production and expressed in terms of growth index – detects the live replicating bacilli load

MGIT 960 MTB Detection Method

- Growth detection is based on metabolic O_2 utilization in a MTB growth indicator tube (MGIT)

512. Ans. (a) Soil transmitted helminthiasis, (b) Lymphatic filariasis, (c) Trachoma, (d) Meningococcal infection

Ref: Park 25th ed. Pg 256, 179, 337

Option	T/F	Comment
Soil transmitted helminthiasis	T	Yes, mass chemoprophylaxis with albendazole is given.
Lymphatic filariasis	T	Yes, mass chemoprophylaxis with DEC is given
Trachoma	T	Yes, a prevalence of more than 5% severe and moderate trachoma in children under 10 years is an indication for mass treatment.
Meningococcal infection	T	Yes, mass chemoprophylaxis with ciprofloxacin is done
Cholera	F	No, mass chemoprophylaxis is not advised for whole community

Mass treatment for trachoma: application of 1% tetracycline ointment to all children as:

- Twice daily for 5 days each month for 6 months
- Once daily for 10 days each month for 6 months

513. Ans. (b) Azithromycin, (c) Cefixime

Clinical condition	Kit to be prescribed	Drugs included	Image
Urethral or anorectal or cervical discharge	KIT 1: Grey	Tab azithromycin 1 g (1 tab) Tab cefixime 400 mg (1 tab)	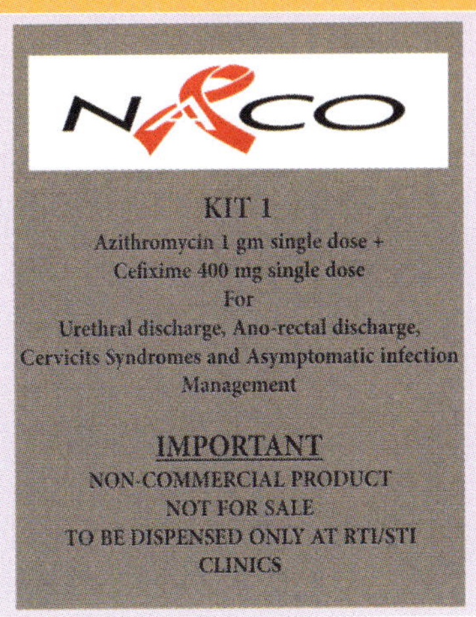

Contd...

Clinical condition	Kit to be prescribed	Drugs included	Image
Vaginal discharge (vaginitis)	KIT 2: Green	Tab secnidazole 1 g (2 tab) Tab fluconazole 150 mg (1 tab)	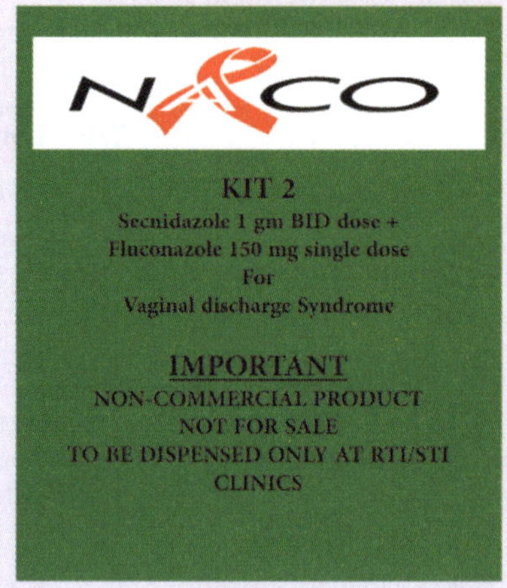
Genital ulcer diseases (nonherpetic)	KIT 3: White	Inj. benzathine penicillin 2.4 MU (1 vial) + tab Azithromycin 1 g (Kit also contains 10 mL disposable syringe + 21 gauge needle + 1 vial of 10 mL sterile water	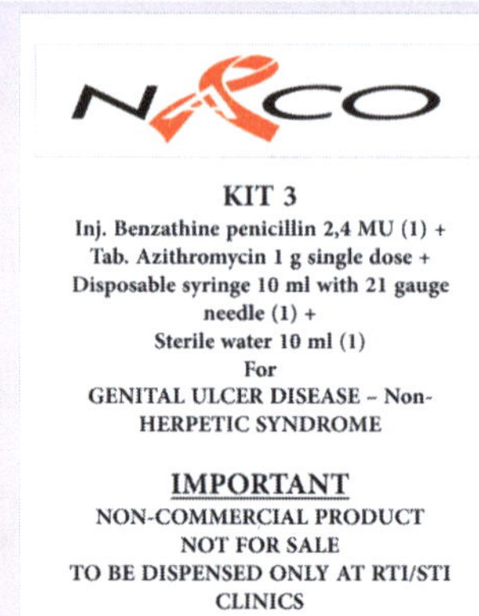
Genital ulcer disease (nonherpetic) in patient allergic to penicillin	KIT 4: Blue	Tab doxycycline 100 mg (1 tab BD for 15 days) Tab azithromycin 1 g × 1 tab	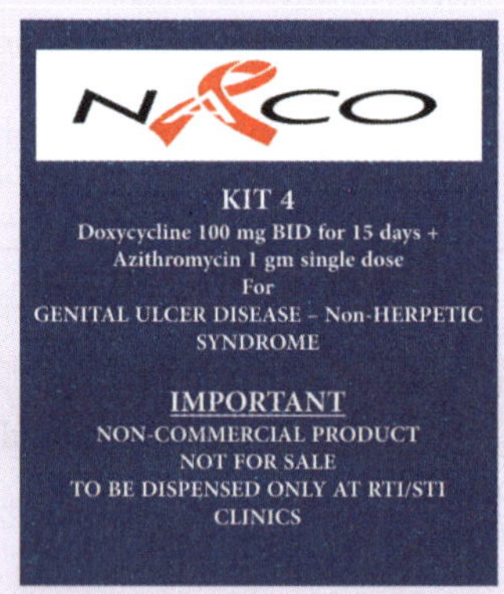
Genital ulcer disease	KIT 5: Red	Tab acyclovir 400 mg × 1 tab TDS × 7 days	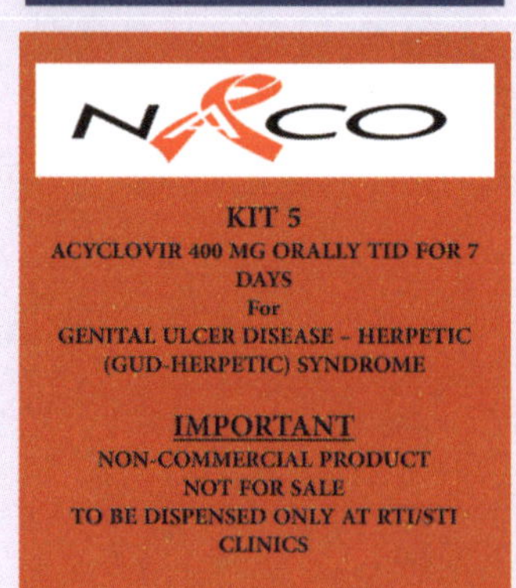

Contd...

Clinical condition	Kit to be prescribed	Drugs included	Image
Lower abdominal pain (pelvic inflammatory disease)	KIT 6: Yellow	Tab cefixime 400 mg × 1 tab Tab metronidazole 400 mg × (1 BD 14 day) Tab doxycycline 100 mg (1 BD 14 days)	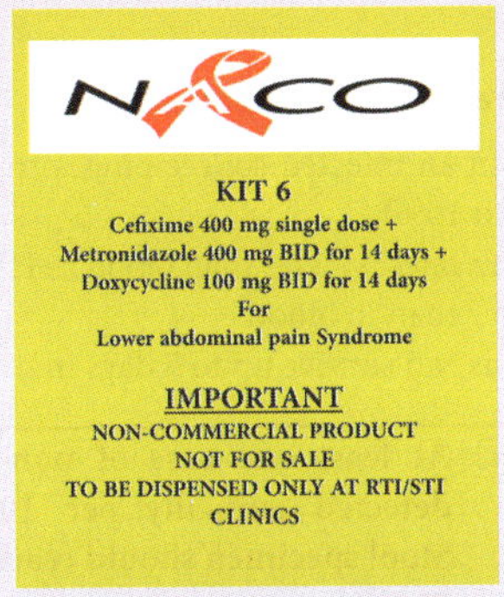
Inguinal Bubo	KIT 7: Black	Tab doxycycline 100 mg (1 BD × 21 days) Tab azithromycin 1 g × 1 tab	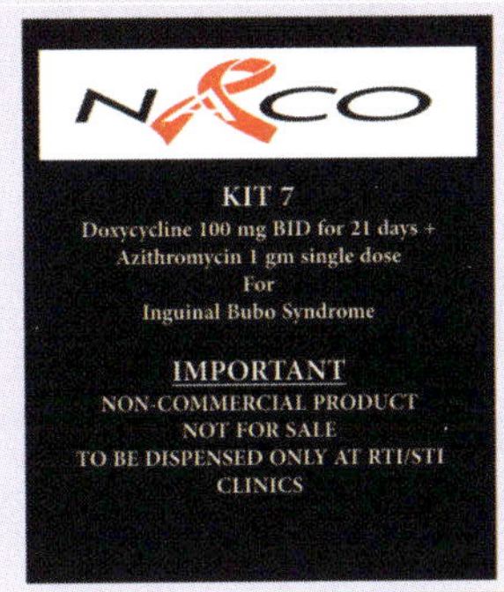

514. Ans. (a) Fever >38°C, (c) Tachycardia >90bpm, (e) $PaCO_2$ <32 mmHg

Criteria for SIRS are considered to be met if at least 2 of the following clinical findings are present:

- Temperature higher than 38°C (100.4°F) or lower than 36°C (96.8°F)
- Tachycardia (higher than 90 beats/min)
- Tachypnoea (higher than 20 breaths/min) or with $PaCO_2$ lower than 32 mm Hg
- Leucocytosis (>12,000/μL) or TLC <4000 /μL or with >10% immature band forms (indicates severe systemic infection)

Note that a patient can have a severe infection without meeting SIRS criteria; conversely, SIRS criteria may be present in the setting of many other illnesses not caused by an infectious process (see the image below).

Spectrum of SIRS – Systemic Inflammatory Response Syndrome

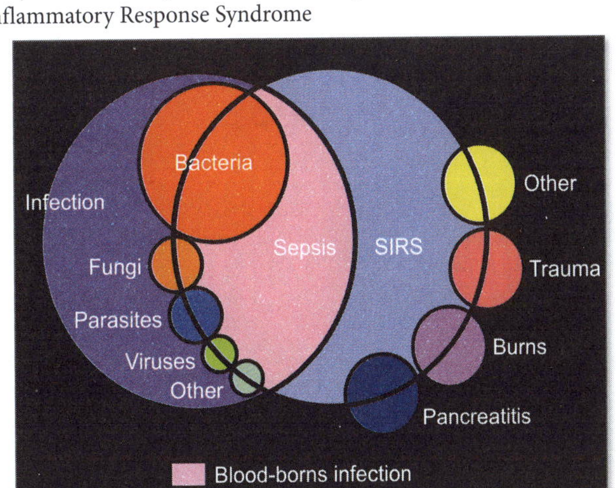

Good to remember; normal values for blood gas:

- Arterial blood pH of 7.38 – 7.42
- Partial pressure of oxygen (PaO_2) - 75 – 100 mmHg
- Bicarbonate - (HCO_3) – 22 – 28 mEq/L
- Partial pressure of carbon dioxide ($PaCO_2$) - 38 – 42 mmHg
- Oxygen saturation (SaO_2) – 94 – 100%

515. Ans. (b) 10%

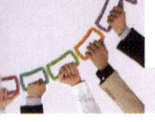

Ref: Blood-Borne Diseases Surveillance Protocol for Ontario Hospitals-2012

General Risk of Transmission

- From an infected source ranges from 6 to 30% (average of up to 10%)
- From bites is lesser than blood as HBV is 1000–10,000 times lower than in blood
- Virus can survive up to 7 days in dried blood sample also

516. Ans. (c) At least one case of non-polio AFP should be detected annually per 100000 population; (d) Stool specimen should reach the laboratory within 72 hours

Ref. Park 25th ed. Pg 223

True options: CD
False options: ABE

Options	T/F	Comment
Surveillance only till 5 years of age	F	No, it is till 15 years of age
Sample collected for suspected AFP even after 15 years	F	No, it is till 15 years of age
At least one case of non-polio AFP should be detected annually per 100000 population	T	Yes, correct at least 1 case/100,000 per year is to be reported
Stool specimen should reach the laboratory within 72 hours	T	Yes correct. the first stool sample should be within 48 hours of reporting and second stool sample within 14 days of first sample. The samples should reach the laboratory within 72 hours of collection
At least 80% should have follow up after 60 days from the last stool sample	F	Not correct. residual paralysis is done at 60 days after onset of paralysis

Contd...

517. Ans. (a) KFD, (c) Babesiosis

Ref. Park 25th Ed. pg 836

Sudeep AB, Gurav YK, Bondre VP. Changing clinical scenario in Chandipura virus infection. Indian J Med Res. 2016;143(6):712–721. doi:10.4103/0971-5916.191929

KFD is tick borne viral hemorrhagic fever.

Kyasanur forest disease (KFD) virus ecology

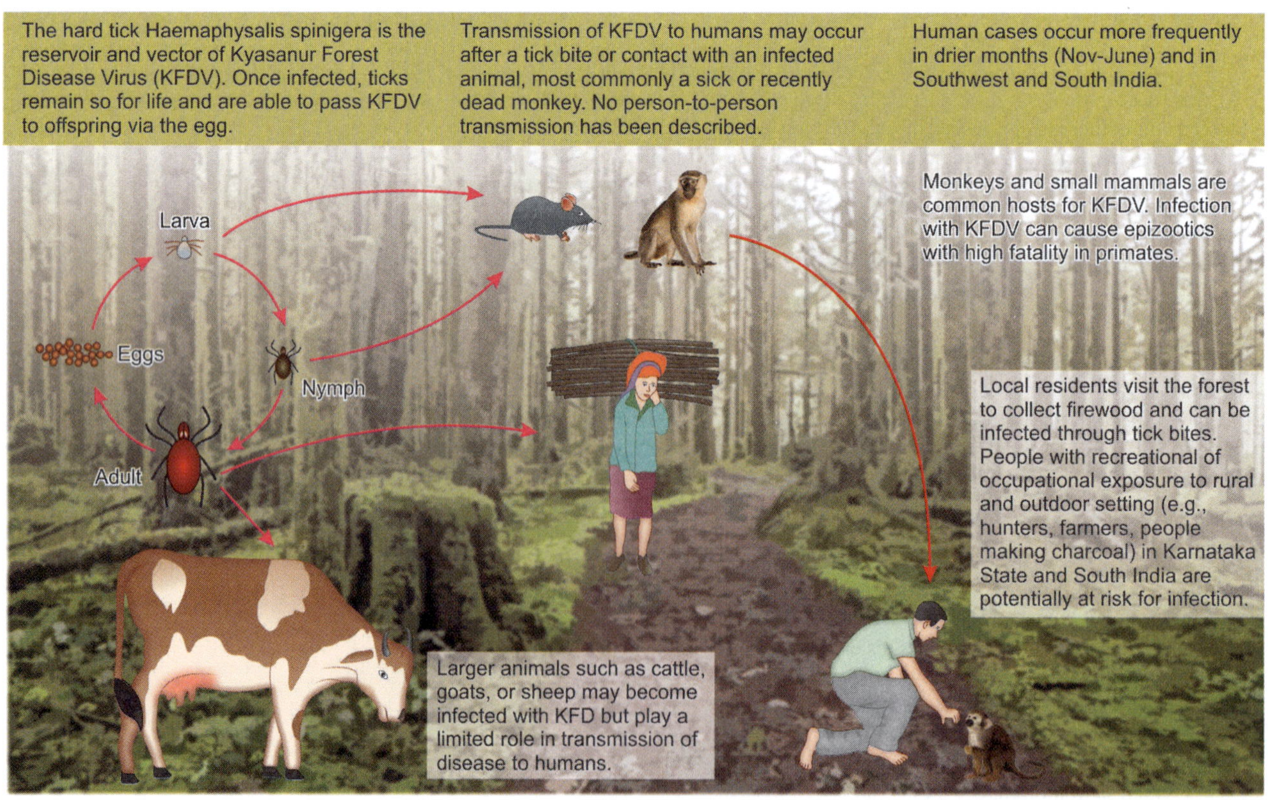
The hard tick Haemaphysalis spinigera is the reservoir and vector of Kyasanur Forest Disease Virus (KFDV). Once infected, ticks remain so for life and are able to pass KFDV to offspring via the egg.
Transmission of KFDV to humans may occur after a tick bite or contact with an infected animal, most commonly a sick or recently dead monkey. No person-to-person transmission has been described.
Human cases occur more frequently in drier months (Nov-June) and in Southwest and South India.
Larva
Eggs
Nymph
Adult
Monkeys and small mammals are common hosts for KFDV. Infection with KFDV can cause epizootics with high fatality in primates.
Local residents visit the forest to collect firewood and can be infected through tick bites. People with recreational of occupational exposure to rural and outdoor setting (e.g., hunters, farmers, people making charcoal) in Karnataka State and South India are potentially at risk for infection.
Larger animals such as cattle, goats, or sheep may become infected with KFD but play a limited role in transmission of disease to humans.

Babesiosis is spread by the bite of an infected blacklegged (or deer) tick, *Ixodes scapularis*. It can also be spread by transfusion of contaminated blood and possibly from an infected mother to her baby during pregnancy or delivery. Babesiosis is not spread from person to person.

Sandfly Transmits

Phlebotomous argentipes	Kala Azar
Phlebotomous papatasii	Sandfly fever/Oriental sore/ CHPV
Phlebotomous sergentii	Oriental sore
S. Punjabiensis	Sandfly fever

Chandipura virus (CHPV) is transmitted by phlebotomine sandflies. The *Phlebotomus papatasi* showed their potential not only to replicate the virus but also to transmit the virus through vertical, venereal and horizontal routes. Other transmitting vectors are *P. argentipus*, and *Sergentomyia* spp. from various sources and literature reviews.

518. Ans. (d) Apron; (b) Gloves; (c) Eyewear; (a) Facemask

Ref: https://www.cdc.gov/hai/pdfs/ppe/PPE-Sequence.pdf; https://www.who.int/csr/disease/ebola/remove_ppequipment.pdf

The CDC and WHO guidelines have minor differences, but the concept for correct use of Personal protective equipment (PPE) is universal and is summarized as below:

- The sequence for **putting ON the PPE** for protection of body parts is
  - Apron/gown → Mask/Respirator → EYE goggles/Face mask → Gloves

The sequence is as shown in the image below:

Sequence for putting on Personal Protective Equipment (PPE)

The type of PPE used will vary based on the level of precautions required, such as standard and contact, droplet or airborne infection isolation precautions. The procedure for putting on and removing PPE should be tailored to the specific type of PPE.

1. **Gown**
- Fully cover torso from neck to knees, arms to end of wrists, and wrap around the back
- Fasten in back of neck and waist

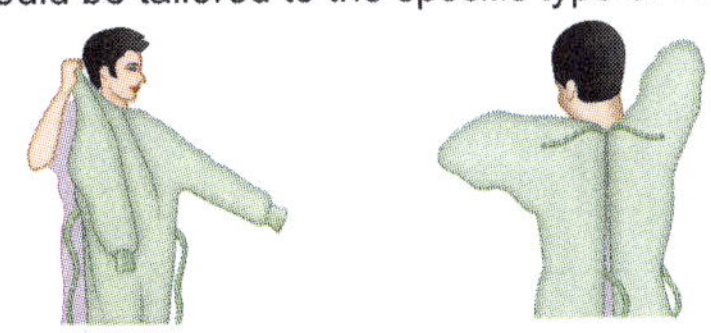

2. **Mask or respirator**
- Secure ties or elastic bands at middle of head and neck
- Fit flexible band to nose bridge
- Fit snug to face and below chin
- Fit snug to face and below chin
- Fit-check respirator

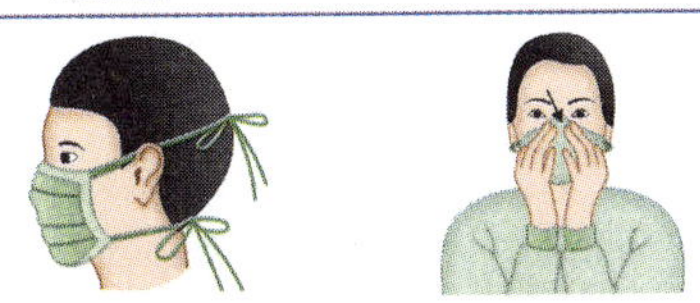

3. **Goggles or face shield**
- Place over face and eyes and adjust to fit

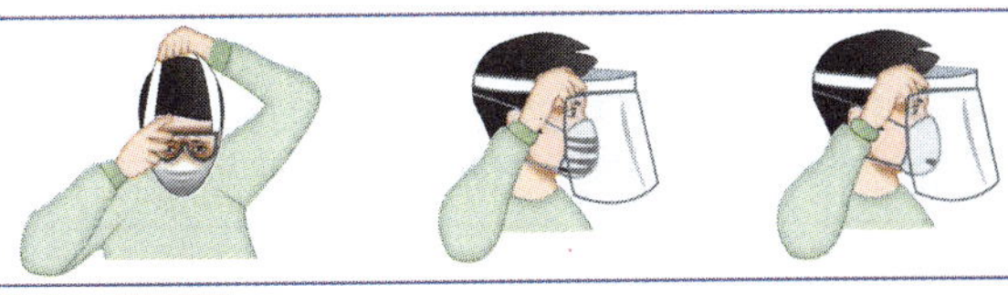

4. **Gloves**
- Extends to cover wrist of isolation gown

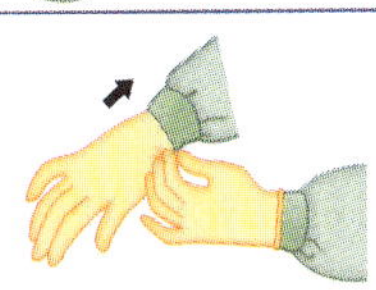

- The recommendations for **REMOVING the PPE** for protection of health care workers is
  - Remove ALL PPE except the face mask/respirator BEFORE exiting the patient's room
  - Remove the face mask/respirator AFTER exiting and closing the door of patient's room
  - The sequence for removal of PPE is
  - Gown and Gloves → Eye Goggles*/face shield → mask/ respirator → hand hygiene

*Untie the lower string of goggles first

The sequence is as shown in the image below:

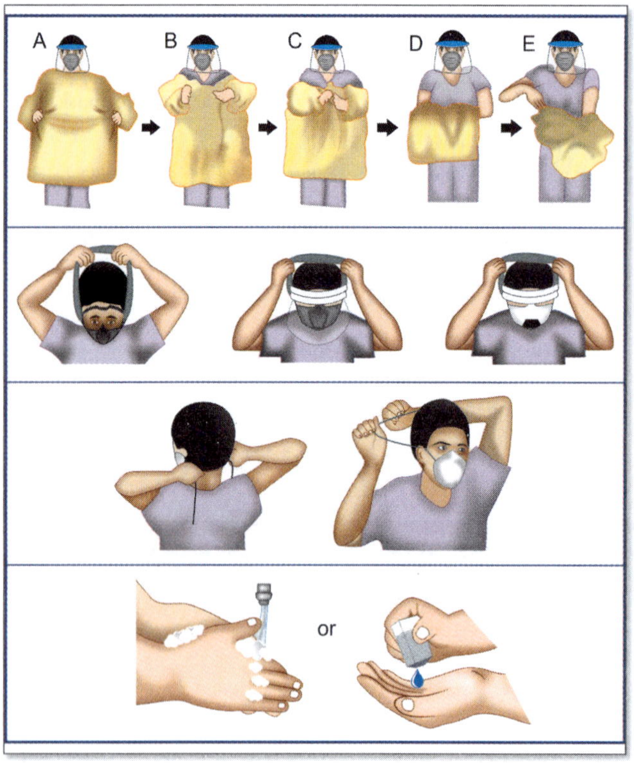

Sequence for Removal of PPE

Note:

- Gloves >Overshoes cover >Gown >HAND HYGEINE >Goggles (from behind) >Face Mask/Respirator (untie lower string followed by upper String) >HAND HYGEINE
- Remove all PPE except the respirator/face mask before exiting the patient room. Remove the facemask/respirator after exiting the patient room and closing the door.

519. Ans. (a) Japanese encephalitis

Ref: Park 25th Ed. Pg 312

JE Life Cycle

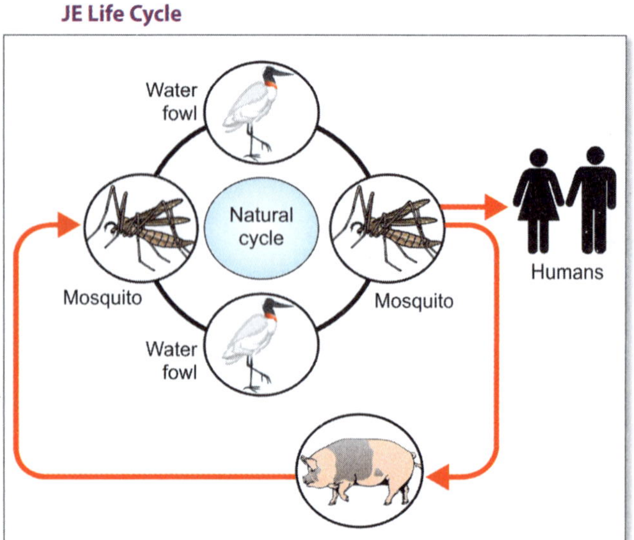

Life cycle of Japanese encephalitic

The life cycle of JE viruses is:

- Pig → mosquito → Pig
- Ardeid birds → mosquito → ardeid birds

520. Ans. (b) Erythromycin

Ref: Park 25th Ed. Pg 174

The carriers should be treated with 10 days oral course of erythromycin which is the most effective drug for the treatment of carriers

521. Ans. (c) Annual parasite index

Ref: Park 25th Ed. Pg 287

Malariometric Indicators

- Annual parasite Incidence (API)
  - It tells about the burden or Prevalence of malaria
  - Sophisticated for measure of incidence of malaria
  - It is the main target//impact indicator
  - API >2 is high risk Malaria endemic areas
  - Formula

$$\text{API} = \frac{\text{No. of blood smears found positive for malaria parasite}}{\text{Population covered under surveillance}} \times 1000$$

- Annual Blood Examination Rate (ABER):
  - Indicator for operational efficacy of the program
  - Proxy indicator for prevalence of fever in the area/country
  - Target is to achieve an ABER of >10%

$$\text{ABER} = \frac{\text{No. of blood smears collected during the year}}{\text{Population covered under surveillance}} \times 1000$$

- Slide positivity Rate (SPR)
  - Indicator for impending outbreak

$$\text{SPR} = \frac{\text{No. of blood smears found positive for malaria parasite}}{\text{Number of smears examined}} \times 1000$$

- Annual Falciparum Incidence (AFI)
  - Indicator for falciparum malaria as a public health problem

$$\text{AFI} = \frac{\text{No. of blood smears found positive for Pl.falciparum malaria parasite}}{\text{Population covered under surveillance}} \times 1000$$

522. Ans. (b) 20000-1000000 IU

Ref: Park 25th Ed. Pg 174

Treatment of Diphtheria Cases

- Give Diphtheria antitoxin without delay
- Route – IM or IV
- Dose: 20,000 – 100,000 Units – depending on the severity of the disease
  - Mild cases – 20,000 – 40,000 unit
  - Moderate cases – 40,000 – 60,000 units
  - Severe cases – 80,000 – 100,000 units

523. Ans. (b) Face shield

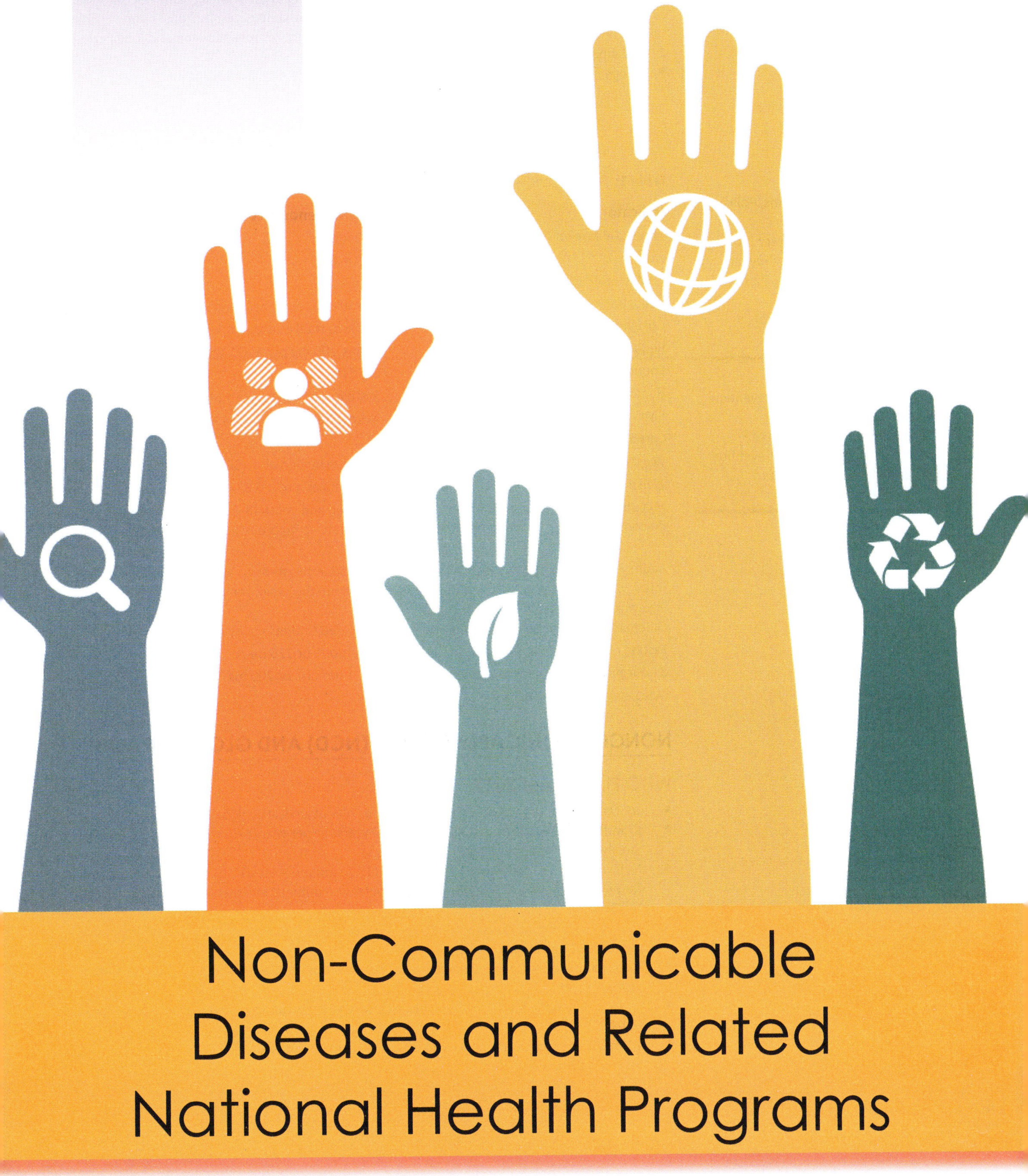

Non-Communicable Diseases and Related National Health Programs

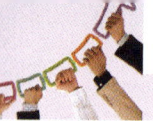

Chapter Outline

INTRODUCTION AND RECOMMENDED INDICATORS IN NONCOMMUNICABLE DISEASES

- *Chronic disease* is defined as impairment or deviation from normal, with one or more of following characteristics—Permanent, residual disability, result from nonreversible pathological alteration, require special training of patient for rehabilitation and long period of supervision and care.
- Gaps in natural history of noncommunicable diseases (NCD) occurs due to:
  - Absence of a known agent
  - Multifactorial causation
  - Long latent period
  - Indefinite onset.

Table 1: Recommended levels for selected indicators applicable to NCD

Indicators	Recommended/cut of valves
Threshold level of cholesterol	220 mg/dL
HDL	>40 mg/dL
Cholesterol/HDL ratio	<3.5
Reduction of fat intake	20–30% of total energy intake[Q]
Consumption of saturated fats	<10% of total energy intake[Q]
Reduction of dietary cholesterol	Below 100 mg per 1000 Kcal/day
Reduction of salt intake	5 g daily or less
Hypertension (diagnosed if)	Systolic blood pressure ≥140 and diastolic >90
BMI	Normal range—18.50–24.99
Corpulence index (To rule out obesity)	<1.2
Waist circumference (classified as obese if)	>102 cm in men and >88 cm in women
Waist:-to-lrip ratio (WHR) (Recommended)	< 1 in males and < 0.85 in females
Minimum physical exercise for adults (Recommended)*	Children and youth (5–17 years)—60 minutes of moderate to vigorous intensity physical activity daily
Adults (18–64 years)—At least 150 minutes of moderate-intensity aerobic physical activity (brisk walking, jogging, gardening) spread throughout the week, or at least 75 minutes of vigorous-intensity activity Older adults—same amount of physical activity tailored to their ability and circumstances	
Fasting plasma glucose (diabetes)	≥7 mmol/L or 126 mg/L
2 hour postprandial venous plasma glucose	>11.1 mmol/L or 200 mg/L

*WHO. Global Report on Diabetes. 2016

NONCOMMUNICABLE DISEASE (NCD) AND GLOBAL HEALTH

WHO Fact Sheet 2017

- NCDs kill 40 million people each year (About 70% of all deaths globally).
- 17 million people die from a NCD before 70 years age per year (87% are "premature" deaths, mostly in low- and middle-income countries).
- NCD Deaths—Cardiovascular diseases (17.7 million—Most), Cancers (8.8 million), Respiratory diseases (3.9 million), and diabetes (1.6 million) together account for 81% of all NCD deaths.
- Tobacco use, physical inactivity, the harmful use of alcohol and unhealthy diets all increase the risk of dying from a NCD.
- Management of NCD—Key components are detection, screening and treatment, as well as palliative care
- Tobacco accounts for 7.2 million deaths every year (including exposure to second-hand smoke).
- 4.1 million annual deaths are due to excess salt/sodium intake.

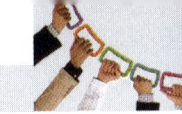

- More than 50% of the annual deaths attributable to alcohol are from NCDs, including cancer.
- 1.6 million deaths annually can be attributed to insufficient physical activity.

STEPS Approach by WHO

The WHO has developed a STEP-wise approach towards surveillance of noncommunicable diseases with following features:

- It is a sequential process of gathering comparable and sustainable NCD risk factor information at country level.
- Developed by WHO as part of a global surveillance strategy in response to growing need for country-level trends in noncommunicable diseases.
- It uses a standard survey instrument and a methodology that can be adapted to different country resource settings and help to build country capacity.
- Countries can use STEPS information for monitoring within—country trends and also for making between—country comparisons and plan for disease prevention through population-level risk factor reduction.
- It focuses on a minimum number of risk factors that predict the major noncommunicable diseases.
- WHO STEPS, have been developed to help low and middle income countries get started.
- Standardized data from representative populations of specified sample size is collected to ensure comparability over time and across locations.
- **Step 1 (Questionnaire-based measurements)** → Gathers information on risk factors (socio-demographic features, tobacco use, alcohol consumption, physical inactivity and fruit/vegetable intake) from the general population by questionnaire.
- **Step 2** → Includes simple physical measurements [height, weight, waist circumference (for obesity) and blood pressure] needed to examine risk factors that are physiologic attributes of the human body.
- **Step 3** → Includes taking blood samples for measuring lipid and glucose levels.

Global Framework for Noncommunicable Disease—2020 (2017 Updates)

- A 25% relative reduction in risk of premature mortality from cardiovascular diseases, cancer, diabetes, or chronic respiratory diseases
- At least 10% relative reduction in the harmful use of alcohol
- A 10% relative reduction in prevalence of insufficient physical activity
- A 30% relative reduction in mean population intake of salt/sodium
- A 30% relative reduction in prevalence of current tobacco use
- A 25% relative reduction in the prevalence of raised blood pressure or contain the prevalence of raised blood pressure, according to national circumstances
- Halt the rise in diabetes and obesity
- At least 50% of eligible people receive drug therapy and counseling (including glycemic control) to prevent heart attacks and strokes
- An 80% availability of the affordable basic technologies and essential medicines, including generics, required to treat major noncommunicable diseases in both public and private facilities

Comprehensive approach (Multi Sectoral) is needed to lessen impact of NCD

High impact essential NCD interventions can be delivered through a primary health care approach to strengthen early detection and timely treatment.

CORONARY HEART DISEASE (CHD)

- Manifestations: Angina pectoris of effort, MI, irregularities of heart, cardiac failure and sudden death.
- Myocardial infarction is specific to CHD (Not angina pectoris or sudden death).
- CHD is a modern epidemic and has a variable natural history. Death may occur in 1st episode or after a long history.
- CHD is expected to be the single most important cause of death in India by 2015.
- Life style changes have led to high prevalence of CHD in urban areas (6.4%) compared to rural areas (2.5%)

138 High Yield Points

- Cardiovascular diseases are responsible for about 25 % of DALYs lost due to NCD in South-East Asia Region (SEAR) countries.
- Incidence of CVD is higher in urban areas than in rural areas.
- CVD deaths are reported at a relative early age in developing countries compared to developed countries.
- Disorder of unknown cause and progressive course is termed **"Degenerative Disorder"**

85 Must Remember

Metabolic risk factors contributing to increased risk of NCDs:

- Raised blood pressure (19% of global deaths are attributed)
- Overweight/obesity
- Hyperglycemia
- Hyperlipidemia

86 Must Remember

Cardiovascular disease (48%), Cancer (21%), Chronic respiratory disease (12%) and Diabetes (3.5%) are largest contributors to mortality and morbidity due to NCDs globally

94 Good to Remember

- 63% of global deaths in 2008 were due to NCD.
- In India, NCD accounted for about 53% deaths.

139 High Yield Points

NCD management interventions are essential for achieving the global target of a 25% relative reduction in the risk of premature mortality from NCDs by 2025, and the SDG target of a one-third reduction in premature deaths from NCDs by 2030.

Must Remember

- Males are at higher risk than females.
- Individuals at special risk include smokers, alcoholics (>75 g/day), family history of CHD, diabetes and obesity and use of OCP in young women

High Yield Points

- Serum cholesterol of 220 mg/dl or more (Threshold level) is an important risk factor for CHD
- Total "Cholesterol/HDL ratio" less than 3.5 is recommended as a clinical goal for CHD prevention. HDL cholesterol is protective against occurrence of CHD and serum HDL level >40 mg/dL is recommended

- In developing countries (e.g. India), CHD is reported a decade earlier (51–60 years[Q]) compared to developed countries.
- Community prevalence of CHD is 6.5% and 4.8% in urban men and women and 2.3% and 1.7% in rural men and women respectively.

Table 2: Risk factors for coronary heart disease (CHD)

Non modifiable	Modifiable
Age, male sex, family history, genetic factors, personality (Type A), race, menopause	Smoking, high BP, elevated serum cholesterol, diabetes, obesity, sedentary habit and stress

The new AACE/ACE guidelines classifies atherosclerosis risk into 5 categories for LDL Goals.

- **Category 1: Extreme-risk**
  - Established or recent hospitalization for acute coronary syndrome, coronary, carotid, or peripheral vascular disease, 10-year risk >20%.
  - Diabetes or CKD stages 3/4 with one or more risk factors
  - Goals:
    - LDL < 55 mg/dL
    - Non-HDL < 80 mg/dL
    - Apolipoprotein B (apoB) < 70 mg/dL
- **Category 2: Very high-risk goals**
  - Established or recent hospitalization for acute coronary syndrome, coronary, carotid, or peripheral vascular disease, 10-year risk >20%.
  - Diabetes or CKD stages 3/4 with one or more risk factors.
  - Goals:
    - LDL < 70 mg/dL
    - Non-HDL < 80 mg/dL
    - ApoB < 80 mg/dL
- **Category 3: High risk**
  - Two or more risk factors and 10-year risk 10% to 20%.
  - Diabetes or CKD stages 3/4 with no other risk factors.
  - Goals:
    - LDL < 100 mg/dL
    - Non-HDL < 130 mg/dL
    - ApoB < 90 mg/dL
- **Category 4. Moderate Risk**
  - Two or more risk factors and 10-year risk <10%.
  - Goals: Same as category 3
- **Category 5:**
  - Two or more risk factors and 10-year risk <10%.
  - Low-risk goals:
    - LDL < 130 mg/dL
    - Non-HDL < 160 mg/dL
    - ApoB not relevant)

Recommended Prevention Strategy for CHD

Population strategy → To shift the risk-factor distribution in direction of "biological normality".

- *Dietary changes or Prudent diet*:
  - Reduction of fat intake to 20–30% and saturated fats intake to less than 10% of total energy intake[Q]
  - Reduction of dietary cholesterol to below 100 mg per 1000 kcal/day
  - Increase in complex carbohydrate consumption (i.e., vegetables, fruits, legumes etc.)
  - Avoidance of alcohol consumption
  - Reduction of salt intake to ≤ 5 g/day
- *Primordial prevention* (Prevent emergence and spread of CHD risk factors and life styles in populations (developing countries) where they have not yet appeared or become endemic)
  - Smoke free society

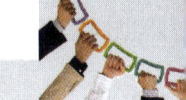

- Increase in physical activity
- Reduction of mean population blood pressure levels, Prudent diet (reduced salt intake and avoidance of a high alcohol intake) and weight control

High risk strategy: Individuals identified as having high risk are brought under preventive care and motivated to take positive action against all the identified risk factors.

American Heart Association ACLS Guidelines for Acute Coronary Syndrome

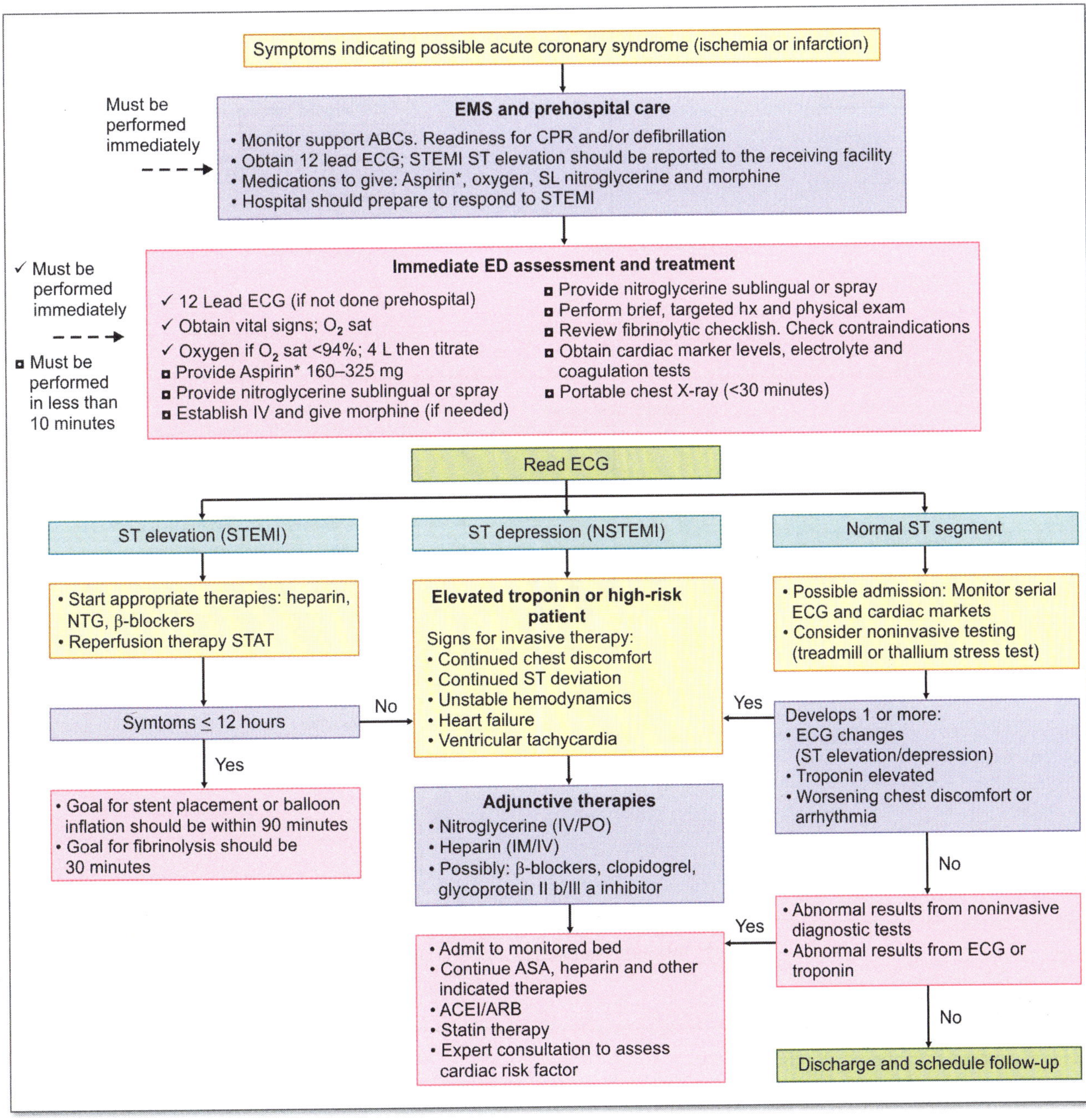

Symptoms indicating possible acute coronary syndrome (ischemia or infarction)
Must be performed immediately
EMS and prehospital care
• Monitor support ABCs. Readiness for CPR and/or defibrillation
• Obtain 12 lead ECG; STEMI ST elevation should be reported to the receiving facility
• Medications to give: Aspirin*, oxygen, SL nitroglycerine and morphine
• Hospital should prepare to respond to STEMI
✓ Must be performed immediately
◘ Must be performed in less than 10 minutes
Immediate ED assessment and treatment
✓ 12 Lead ECG (if not done prehospital)
✓ Obtain vital signs; O2 sat
✓ Oxygen if O2 sat <94%; 4 L then titrate
◘ Provide Aspirin* 160–325 mg
◘ Provide nitroglycerine sublingual or spray
◘ Establish IV and give morphine (if needed)
◘ Provide nitroglycerine sublingual or spray
◘ Perform brief, targeted hx and physical exam
◘ Review fibrinolytic checklish. Check contraindications
◘ Obtain cardiac marker levels, electrolyte and coagulation tests
◘ Portable chest X-ray (<30 minutes)
Read ECG
ST elevation (STEMI)
ST depression (NSTEMI)
Normal ST segment
• Start appropriate therapies: heparin, NTG, β-blockers
• Reperfusion therapy STAT
Symtoms ≤ 12 hours
No
Yes
• Goal for stent placement or balloon inflation should be within 90 minutes
• Goal for fibrinolysis should be 30 minutes
Elevated troponin or high-risk patient
Signs for invasive therapy:
• Continued chest discomfort
• Continued ST deviation
• Unstable hemodynamics
• Heart failure
• Ventricular tachycardia
Adjunctive therapies
• Nitroglycerine (IV/PO)
• Heparin (IM/IV)
• Possibly: β-blockers, clopidogrel, glycoprotein II b/III a inhibitor
• Admit to monitored bed
• Continue ASA, heparin and other indicated therapies
• ACEI/ARB
• Statin therapy
• Expert consultation to assess cardiac risk factor
• Possible admission: Monitor serial ECG and cardiac markets
• Consider noninvasive testing (treadmill or thallium stress test)
Yes
Develops 1 or more:
• ECG changes (ST elevation/depression)
• Troponin elevated
• Worsening chest discomfort or arrhythmia
No
Yes
• Abnormal results from noninvasive diagnostic tests
• Abnormal results from ECG or troponin
No
Discharge and schedule follow-up

Fig. 1: AHA ACLS acute coronary syndrome algorithm

Adapted from: Jeffery Media Productions 2016 Amsterdam EA, Wenger NK, Brindis RG, et al. 2014 AHA/ACC guideline for the management of patients with non-ST-elevation acute coronary syndromes. Circulation. 2014 Jan 1:CIR-0000000000000134

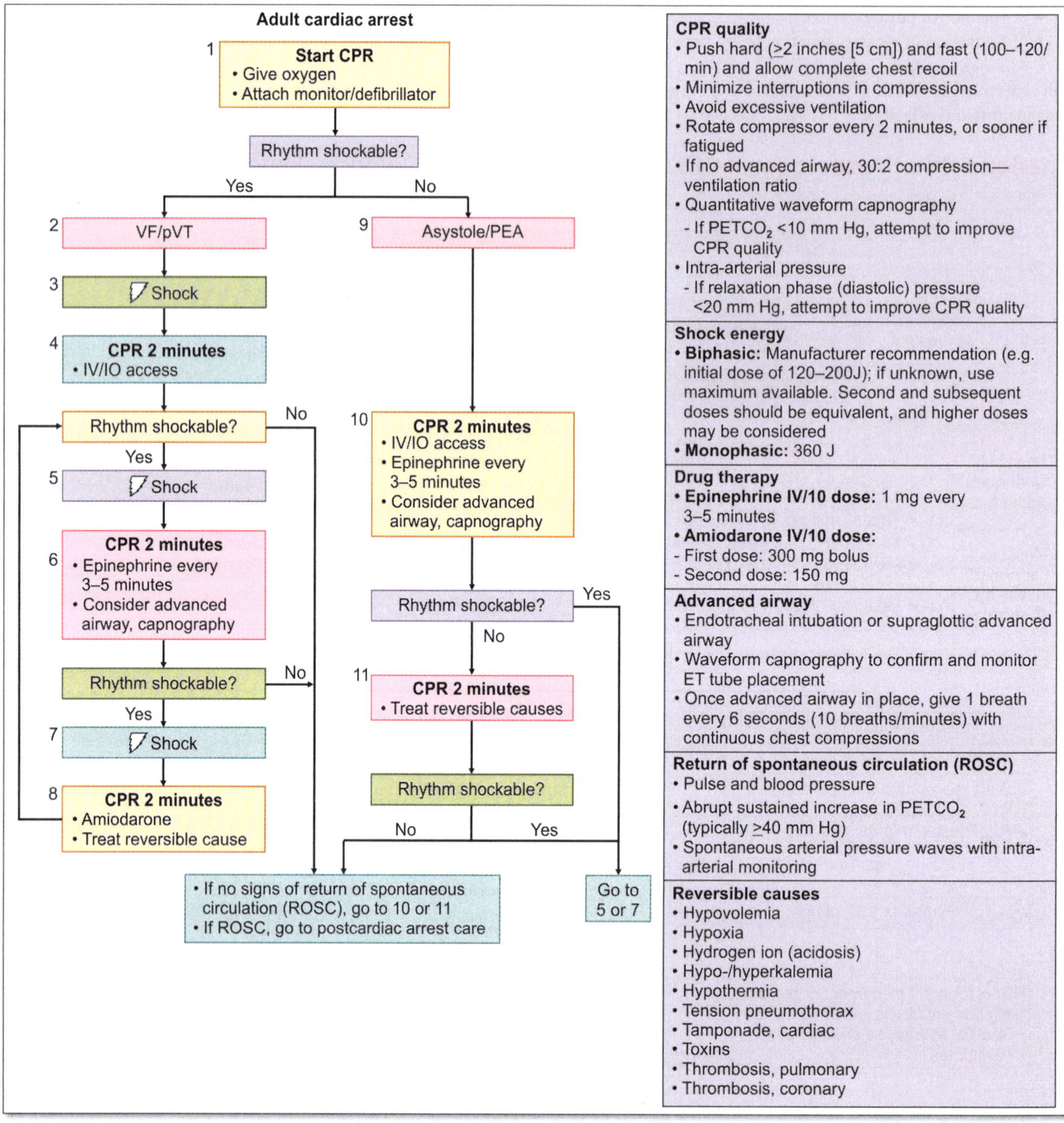

Adult cardiac arrest
1 Start CPR
• Give oxygen
• Attach monitor/defibrillator
Rhythm shockable?
Yes
No
2 VF/pVT
3 Shock
4 CPR 2 minutes
• IV/IO access
Rhythm shockable?
No
Yes
5 Shock
6 CPR 2 minutes
• Epinephrine every 3–5 minutes
• Consider advanced airway, capnography
Rhythm shockable?
No
Yes
7 Shock
8 CPR 2 minutes
• Amiodarone
• Treat reversible cause
9 Asystole/PEA
10 CPR 2 minutes
• IV/IO access
• Epinephrine every 3–5 minutes
• Consider advanced airway, capnography
Rhythm shockable?
Yes
No
11 CPR 2 minutes
• Treat reversible causes
Rhythm shockable?
No
Yes
• If no signs of return of spontaneous circulation (ROSC), go to 10 or 11
• If ROSC, go to postcardiac arrest care
Go to 5 or 7
CPR quality
• Push hard (≥2 inches [5 cm]) and fast (100–120/min) and allow complete chest recoil
• Minimize interruptions in compressions
• Avoid excessive ventilation
• Rotate compressor every 2 minutes, or sooner if fatigued
• If no advanced airway, 30:2 compression—ventilation ratio
• Quantitative waveform capnography
- If PETCO2 <10 mm Hg, attempt to improve CPR quality
• Intra-arterial pressure
- If relaxation phase (diastolic) pressure <20 mm Hg, attempt to improve CPR quality
Shock energy
• Biphasic: Manufacturer recommendation (e.g. initial dose of 120–200J); if unknown, use maximum available. Second and subsequent doses should be equivalent, and higher doses may be considered
• Monophasic: 360 J
Drug therapy
• Epinephrine IV/10 dose: 1 mg every 3–5 minutes
• Amiodarone IV/10 dose:
- First dose: 300 mg bolus
- Second dose: 150 mg
Advanced airway
• Endotracheal intubation or supraglottic advanced airway
• Waveform capnography to confirm and monitor ET tube placement
• Once advanced airway in place, give 1 breath every 6 seconds (10 breaths/minutes) with continuous chest compressions
Return of spontaneous circulation (ROSC)
• Pulse and blood pressure
• Abrupt sustained increase in PETCO2 (typically ≥40 mm Hg)
• Spontaneous arterial pressure waves with intra-arterial monitoring
Reversible causes
• Hypovolemia
• Hypoxia
• Hydrogen ion (acidosis)
• Hypo-/hyperkalemia
• Hypothermia
• Tension pneumothorax
• Tamponade, cardiac
• Toxins
• Thrombosis, pulmonary
• Thrombosis, coronary

Fig. 2: Advanced cardiac life support guidelines

HYPERTENSION

It is the most common cardiovascular disorder:

Updated Classification of Hypertension

2018 ESC/ESH Guidelines for the management of arterial hypertension

Table 3: Classification of office blood pressure[a] and definitions of hypertension grade[b]

Category	Systolic (mm Hg)		Diastolic (mm Hg)
Optimal	<120	and	<80
Normal	120–129	and/or	80–84

Contd...

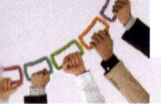

Category	Systolic (mm Hg)		Diastolic (mm Hg)
High normal	130–139	and/or	85–89
Grade 1 hypertension	140–159	and/or	90–99
Grade 2 hypertension	160–179	and/or	100–109
Grade 3 hypertension	≥180	and/or	≥110
Isolated systolic hypertension[b]	≥140	and	<90

BP = Blood pressure; SBP = systolic blood pressure
a. BP category is defined according to seated clinic BP and by the highest level or BP, whether systolic or diastolic
b. Isolate systolic hypertension is graded 1, 2, or 3 according to SBP value in the ranges indicated
The same classification is used for all ages from 16 years

Rule of Halves

Hypertension is an iceberg disease

It is evident from general community surveys that out of the total general population only about half of population were aware about the hypertensive condition, out of which only half were being treated and out of the treated, only half were actually being adequately treated.

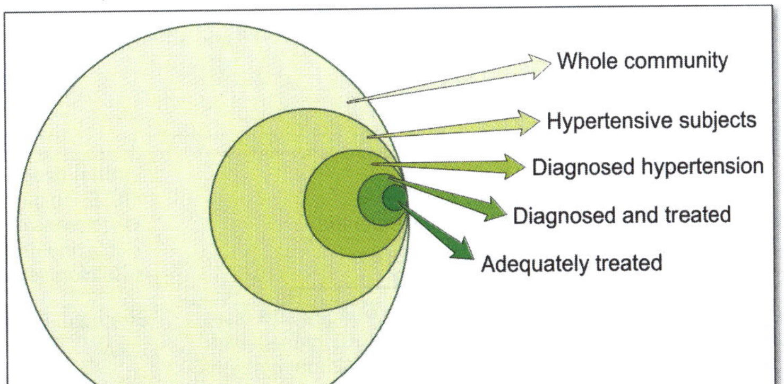

Hypertension in community

Hypertension Prevalence in India

- As per NFHS 4 data, with criteria of SBP ⩾ 140 and DBP ⩾ 90
  - Females 11%
  - Males 15%

Tracking of Blood Pressure

The blood pressure of the individuals are being followed up over a period of years from early childhood to adult life, the individuals with lower pressure will tend to remain as lower and continue on the same "track". This phenomenon of persistence of blood pressures is known as tracking of hypertension. It is **applied to adolescents and younger age group children** who may be at risk of development of hypertension may be screened and the lower BP recording are kept on track to remain as lower BP recordings

Risk Factors for Hypertension

- **Nonmodifiable risk factors**
  - Age
  - Gender
  - Genetic factors
  - Ethnicity
- **Modifiable risk factors**
  - Obesity
  - Higher—Salt intake, alcohol intake, Saturated fat intake
  - Lower—Dietary fibers intake
  - Physical activity
  - Heart rate
  - Socio economic status
  - Environmental stress
  - Other factors – most common cause for secondary hypertension – use of OCPs by females

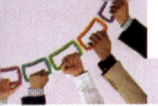

Approaches to Prevention of Hypertension

Primary Prevention

Population strategy

- Reduction of salt intake (Average < 5 g/day)
- Moderate fat intake
- Avoidance of a high alcohol intake (Not more than 2 drinks/day (1 oz or 30 mL ethanol) in men and 1 drink/day in women/light weight person)
- Restriction of energy intake appropriate to body needs.
- **Weight reduction:** Maintain normal body weight (BMI, 18.5–24.9)
- **Exercise promotion:** Regular physical activity (30 min/day on most days of the week)
- **Behavioral changes:** Reduction of stress and smoking, modification of personal life-style, yoga and transcendental meditation.
- **Health education:** On all risk factors and related health behavior.
- Self-care or patient participation.

High risk strategy: To prevent attainment of levels of BP at which start of treatment would be considered in high risk groups.

Secondary Prevention

- **Early case detection:** Screening the population.
- Treatment to maintain a blood pressure below 140/90, and ideally a BP of 120/80 and attention to other risk factors such as smoking and elevated blood cholesterol levels
- Maintain patient compliance

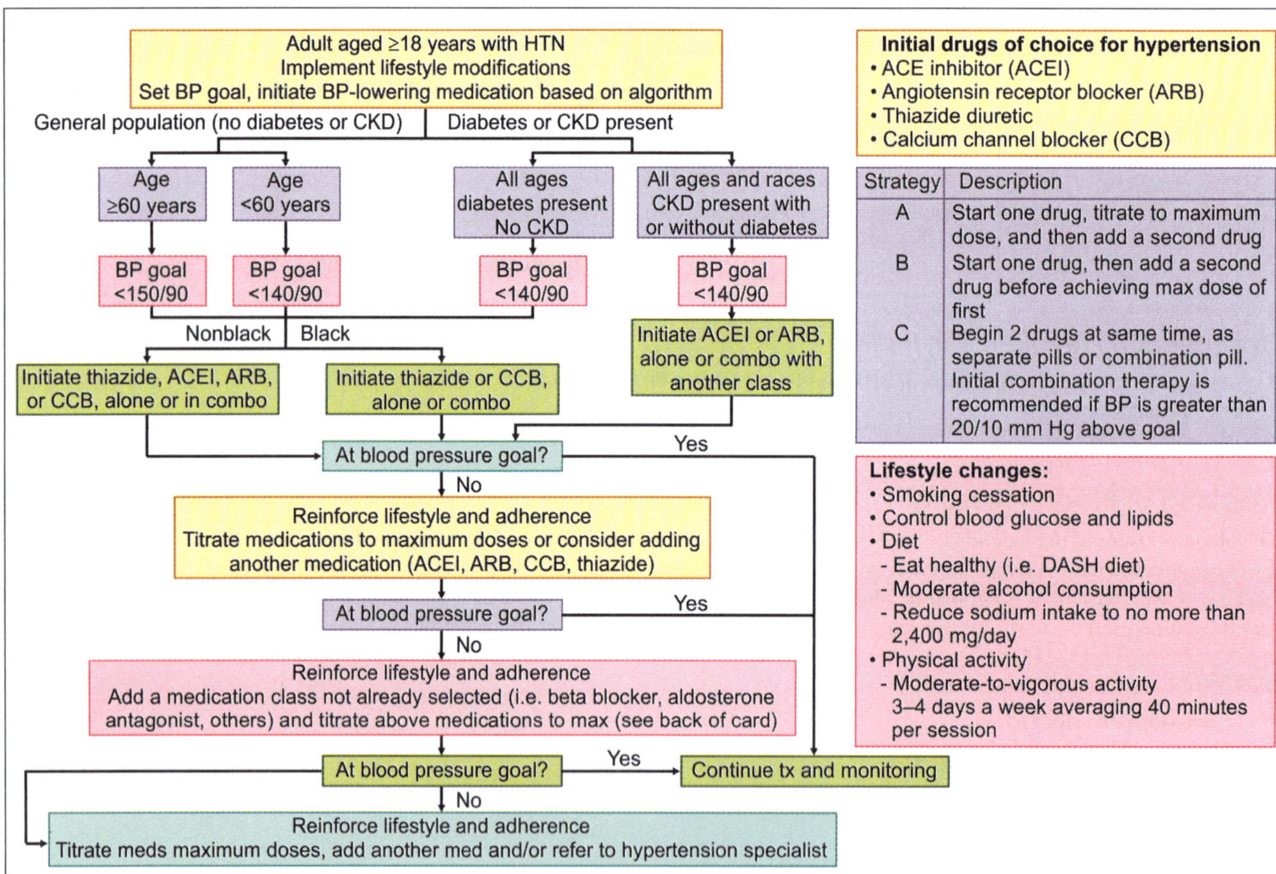

Fig. 3: JNC 8 hypertension guideline

(The most prevalent form of malnutrition) Reference: James PA, Ortiz E, et al. 2004 evidence-based guideline for the management of high blood pressure in adults: (JNCS). JAMA. 2014 Feb 5;311(5):507-20

Card developed by Cole Glenn, Pharm. D, and James L Taylor, Pharm. D

OBESITY

(The most prevalent form of malnutrition)

Criteria used for assessment of obesity are

Body weight: Conventionally +2 SD from median weight for height is taken as a cut-off point for obesity.

$$\text{Body mass index } \textbf{\textit{(Quetelet's index)}} = \frac{\text{Weight (kg)}}{\text{Height}^2\text{ (m}^2\text{)}}$$

$$\textbf{\textit{Ponderal index}} = \frac{\text{Height (cm)}}{\text{Cube root of body weight (kg)}}$$

$$\textbf{\textit{Brocca index}} = \text{height (cm)} - 100$$

$$\textbf{\textit{Lorentz's formula}} = \text{Height (cm)} - 100 - \frac{\text{Height (cm)} - 150}{\text{2 (for women) or 4 (for men)}}$$

$$\textbf{Corpulence index} \text{ (should not exceed 1.2)} = \frac{\text{Actual weight}}{\text{Desirable weight}}$$

Skinfold thickness (using Herpenden Callipers at 4 sites—mid triceps, and biceps, sub scapular and supra iliac) Sum $\geq$ 50 in girls and $\geq$ 40 in boys. A rapid and *"non invasive" method, but* poor repeatability, standards for subcutaneous fat do not exist for comparison, measurements is difficult in extreme obesity

Waist circumference: $\geq$102 cm in men and $\geq$88 cm in women worldwide. Indian population >90 cm in male and $\geq$80 cm in female indicate obesity

Waist: Hip ratio (WHR) >1 in males and >0.85 in females indicate obesity

Waist: Height ratio—Cut off is 0.5

Table 4: Classification of obesity

Classification of obesity based on BMI	Global	Asians	Indians
Under weight Grade 1–(17–18.49), II–(16–16.99), III (<16)	<18.50	<18.50	<18.50
Normal range	**18.50–24.99**	**18.50–22.99**	**18.50–22.99**
Overweight–Preobese Obese class I Obese class II Obese class III	$\geq$25.00 25.00-29.99 30.00-34.99 $\geq$40.00	$\geq$23.00 23.00-26.99 $\geq$27.00	$\geq$23.00 23.00-24.99 $\geq$25.00

Obesity can be

- Android obesity (abdominal fat distribution)—More serious
- Gynoid obesity (fat distributed more evenly and peripherally around the body (less serious).

Measures for Prevention/Control of Obesity

- Dietary changes:
  - Proportion of energy-dense foods such as simple carbohydrates and fats should be reduced
  - Fiber content in the diet should be increased.
  - Adequate levels of essential nutrients in low energy diets (1000 kcal daily model for an adult).
  - Regular physical exercise

DIABETES

- It is an "Iceberg Disease" characterized by a state of chronic hyperglycemia, resulting from a diverse etiologies, environmental and genetic, acting jointly.
- Population in India has an increased susceptibility to diabetes mellitus. Prevalence is higher in urban areas.
- More than 80% diabetic deaths occur in low and middle income countries.

88 **Must Remember**

- As per 2012 estimates, more than 40 million children under 5 years age were overweight (About 30 million in developing and 10 million in developed countries).
- At least 3.4 million adults die each year as a result of being overweight or obese.

141 **High Yield Points**

Total body water, Total body potassium and Body density are more accurate measurements of body fat[Q]

Waist: Height ratio is the best indicator of cardiovascular risk. It is age and sex independent

95 **Good to Remember**

- BMI is age independent and applicable for both sexes[Q]
- BMI >50 is referred to as **Super Obesity** and >40 as **morbid obesity**

89 **Must Remember**

India is the World's diabetes capital. The International Diabetes Federation (IDF) estimates that by 2030, 8.4% of India's adult population will have diabetes

Table 5: Types of diabetes and characteristics

Type 1 DM	Most severe form of the disease	▪ Abrupt onset ▪ Usually seen in individuals <30 years of age ▪ It is lethal unless promptly diagnosed and treated ▪ Immune-medicated in over 90% of cases and idiopathic <10% cases ▪ Usually associated with ketosis in untreated state ▪ Occurs mostly in children (Highest incidence 10–14 years) but occasionally in adults ▪ Circulating insulin is virtually absent, plasma glucagon is elevated and pancreatic b cells fail to respond to insulinogenic stimuli ▪ Exogenous insulin is required
Type 2 DM	More common than type 1 DM	▪ Gradual onset ▪ Occurs mainly in middle-aged and elderly ▪ Mild, slow to ketosis and compatible with long survival if given adequate treatment

Table 6: Levels of evidence for risk factors in diabetes and metabolic diseases

Level of evidence	Protective factors	Risk factors
Convincing	Physical activity weight reduction	▪ Overweight and obesity ▪ Abdominal obesity (malnutrition) ▪ Physical inactivity ▪ Maternal diabetes including gestational diabetes, alcoholism
Probable	Non starch polysaccharide	▪ Saturated fat, IUGR
Possible	Omega 3 fatty acid, low glycemic index food, exclusive breast feed	▪ **Viral infections:** Rubella, mumps and human coxsackie B4 ▪ **Chemical agents:** Alloxan, streptozotocin, VALCOR, high intake of cyanide producing foods (e.g., cassava and certain beans) ▪ **Stress:** ▪ **Low dietary Fiber** (Minimum recommended daily intake 20 g)

Table 7: WHO recommended diagnostic criteria for diabetes mellitus

	Diabetes	Impaired glucose tolerance	Impaired fasting glucose
Fasting plasma glucose	≥7 mmol/L or 126 mg/L	<7 mmol/L or 126 mg/L	6.1–6.9 mmol/L or 110 mg/L- 125 mg/L
Venous Plasma Glucose 2 hours after 75 g oral glucose load	>11.1 mmol/L or 200 mg/L	≥7.8 and <11.1 mmol/L or 140–200 mg/L	<7.8 mmol/L or <140 mg/L

Diabetes screening: Blood sugar level 2 hours after 75 g oral glucose alone or with fasting value is recommended for epidemiological surveys.

Glycosylated Hemoglobin (HbA_1C)

- It is a long-term index of glucose control, i.e. previous 2–3 months
- Should be estimated half-yearly

The best level of prevention for diabetes and other life style diseases is—Primordial prevention—life style modification.

RHEUMATIC HEART DISEASE (RHD)

- Rheumatic fever (RF) is a hypersensitivity reaction to streptococcal throat infection (Group A beta haemolytic streptococci, Serotype M5)[Q] occurring in 1–3% of patients and affects connective tissues in heart and joints.
- Recently coxsackie B-4 virus has been suggested as a causative factor and streptococcus as a conditioning agent.
- It is a disease of childhood and adolescence (5–15 years) and affects both sexes equally.

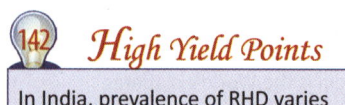

142 *High Yield Points*

In India, prevalence of RHD varies between 5 and 7 per 1000 children age 5–15 years.[Q]

- Affects connective tissues in the heart and joints
- RF is a social disease linked to poverty, overcrowding, poor housing, inadequate health services etc. It declines sharply when the standard of living is improved.
- ***High-risk groups:*** School age children (5–15 years), slum dwellers and those living in closed community (e.g., barracks).
- **Evaluation of RF control program:** Prevalence of RHD in the age group 6–14 years (school children) is considered the best indicator. Survey is recommended at 5-year intervals on a sample size of 20000–30,000

WHO Criteria for Diagnosis of Rheumatic Fever and RHD (Revised Jones Criteria)—2002–03

Major manifestations[Q] → Carditis; polyarthritis; chorea; erythema marginatum; subcutaneous nodules.

Minor Manifestations[Q]

- Clinical → Fever, Polyarthralgia
- Laboratory → Elevated acute phase reactants (erythrocyte sedimentation rate or leukocyte count)
- Evidence of a Preceding Streptococcal Infection within the last 45 days
  - ECG (prolonged P-R interval)
  - Elevated or rising antistreptolysin-O or other streptococcal antibody or
  - Positive throat culture
  - Rapid antigen test for group A streptococci
  - Recent scarlet fever

Table 8: Diagnostic categories and criteria of rheumatic fever

Diagnostic categories	Criteria
Primary episode of RF	2 major or 1 major and 2 minor manifestations plus evidence of a preceding group A streptococcal infection.
Recurrent attack of RF in a patient without established RHD (Infective endocarditis excluded)	2 major or 1 major and 2 minor manifestations plus evidence of a preceding group A streptococcal infection
Recurrent attack of RF in a patient with established rheumatic heart disease	Two minor manifestations plus evidence of a preceding group A streptococcal infection

Prevention of RHD

- *Primary (High risk approach):* Single IM dose of Benzathine Benzylpenicillin (Adult 1.2 million unit, Child 6 lakh unit) or Oral Penicillin V or G for 10 days).
- In case of allergy to penicillin, erythromycin is the drug of choice.
- *Secondary (Prevention of recurrence):* Patients with RF are given- Single IM dose of Benzathine Benzylpenicillin- (Adult 1.2 million unit, Child 6 lakh unit) at 3 weeks interval for 5 years or till 18 years of age.
- In case of Carditis -Penicillin is given for 10 years after last attack or until 25 year of age.
- More severe valvular disease or post-valve surgery lifelong treatment is needed.
- *Non-medical measures*: Improving living conditions, Breaking poverty-disease-poverty cycle. Improvements in socioeconomic conditions (particularly better housing).

Must Remember

- RF is the most common cause of heart disease in the 5–30 years age-group worldwide
- Mitral stenosis is most common cardiac lesion in RHD[Q] (Most common in children is mitral regurgitation[Q]).
- Other manifestations are carditis, cardiomegaly, CHF

CANCER

Table 9: Most common cancer and its mortality

Cancer mortality—In decreasing order–Most common (Top row) and least common (Bottom row)	Globally			India		
	Male	Female	Both sex	Male	Female	Both sex
	Lung	Breast	Lung	Lung	Breast	Breast
	Liver	Lung	Liver	Lip, oral cavity	Cervix uteri	Cervix uteri
	Stomach	Colorectal	Stomach	Stomach	Colorectal	Lung
Cancer Incidence (In decreasing order)	**Globally**			**India**		
	Male	Female	Both sex	Male	Female	Both sex
	Lung	Breast	Lung	Lung, lip, oral cavity	Breast	Breast
	Prostate	Colorectal	Breast	Stomach	Cervix uteri	Cervix uteri
	Colorectal	Lung	Colorectal	Colorectal	Colorectal	Lip, oral cavity

- Risk of getting cancer and death is more in males compared to females
- About 25% of cancers in developing countries are associated with chronic infections, e.g. Hepatitis B (liver cancer), HPV (cervical cancer) and *Helicobacter pylori* (stomach cancer).
  - Cervical cancer is associated with poor genital hygiene, early consummation of marriage, multiple pregnancies and contact with multiple sexual partners.
- Breast cancer is related to late marriage, birth of first child at a later age, fewer children and shorter periods of breastfeeding which are common among educated urban women.

96 Good to Remember

Methods of Cancer Screening

- Mass screening
- Mass screening at single sites and
- **Selective screening:** (Examination of those people thought to be at special risk)

Breast Cancer

Possible reasons for rise in incidence:

- Late marriage
- Late birth of the first child
- Fewer children
- Shorter duration of breastfeeding

Screening techniques include:

Table 10: Screening tools for breast cancer

Screening techniques	Advantages	Disadvantages
Breast self-examination	Easy to perform and may detect early cancers	Effectively as screening tool is not established
Palpation by physician		Unreliable for large, heavy breasts
Thermography	Advantage of no exposure to radiation	Not sensitive tool
Mammography (maybe recommended in some guidelines after age of 35 years)	▪ Most sensitive tool ▪ Most specific tool	▪ Radiation exposure (up to 500 mR – milli roentgen) ▪ Highly technical, and sophisticated device requirement ▪ False positive results may be found on further biopsy

Note: Women under 35 years of age should not have X-rays unless they are symptomatic or a family history of early onset of breast cancer.

91 Must Remember

- Screening for early detection of carcinoma breast constitutes secondary prevention.

Prevention of Breast Cancer

Primary prevention: Elimination of risk factors and promotion of cancer education.
Secondary prevention: Early diagnosis for treatment and follow-up (to detect recurrence early and to detect cancer in the opposite breast at an early stage).

WHO 3 STEP Ladder in Pain Management in Cancer (WHO Pain Relief Ladder)

Step 1 – Nonopioids (Aspirin, Paracetamol, etc.)
Step 2 – Mild opioids (Codeine) + NSAIDs Adjuvants (to calm fear and anxiety)
Step 3 – Strong opioids (Morphine) + NSAIDs + Adjuvants (to calm fear and anxiety)
Drugs are to be given at 3–6 hours interval

Cancer of the Cervix

It is the second most common cancer in females (after breast cancer)

Natural Course of History of Ca Cervix

- Normal epithelium ↔ dysplasia ↔ cancer in situ → invasive cancer
- Carcinoma in situ persists for a long time, which may regress without treatment of progress to invasive cancers
- Invasive cancer spreads through the lymph nodes and direct extension to the pelvic organs

Risk factors:
- Age—maximum incidence in age group 25–45 years
- Genital warts
- Multiple sexual partners
- Early marriage
- Prolonged use of OCP's with high estrogen component
- Poor genital hygiene

Primary prevention:
- Improved personal hygiene, birth control
- HPV vaccine
- Cervarix is designed to prevent infection from HPV types 16 and 18, that cause about 70% of cervical cancer cases. Cervarix also contains AS04, a proprietary adjuvant that has been found to boost the immune system response for a longer period of time
- Gardasil-9 is a vaccine for use in the prevention of HPV strains - 6, 11, 16, 18, 31, 33, 45, 52, 58. It is FDA approved for prevention of anal cancer and associated precancerous lesions due to human papillomavirus.

Secondary prevention:
- Screening by VIA, PAP smears

Recommendations:
- All females should have PAP smear test at the beginning of sexual activity and then every 3 years there after
- PAP smear requires sophisticated testing methods, hence for primary care—cost effective method is:
  - Visual inspection with 5% acetic acid (VIA)
  - Visual inspection post application of Lugol's iodine (VILI)
  - Visual inspection with 5% acetic acid with magnification (VIAM)

143 *High Yield Points*

Visual inspection with 5% acetic acid:
- Perform visual inspection after application of 5% acetic acid solution (5 mL acetic acid mixed with 95 mL of distilled water)
- The VIA test is considered as positive with detection of:
  - Well-defined opaque aceto-white close to the squamo columnar junction
  - Well-defined circumorificial aceto-white lesions
  - Dense aceto-whitening of ulceroproliferative growth on cervix

Lung Cancer

Globally it is the most common cancer with high fatality.
Risk factors:
- Smoking—most dangerous is:
  - Tar (carcinogenic)
  - Carbon monoxide and nicotine (cardiovascular effects, coagulopathies)

Screening for Ca lung:
- Chest X-ray
- Sputum cytology

Oral Cancer

It is one of the common cancers among both sexes globally.

Risk factors:
- Tobacco
  - Most common form of tobacco chewing in India is 'betel quid'—consisting of betel leaf, areca nut, lime, tobacco
- Alcohol
- Precancerous lesions as leukoplakia, erythroplakia.

144 *High Yield Points*

Table 11: Predisposing customs/habits leading to cancer

Habits/Customs	Cancer
Smoking	Lung cancer
Alcoholism	Liver cancer
Sun bath	Skin cancer
Pan, zarda, tobacco chewing	Oropharyngeal cancer
Reverse smoking	Oropharyngeal cancer
Low fiber diet	Colon cancer
High fat intake	Breast cancer
Promiscuous behavior (Multiple sex partners)	Cervical cancer
Use of hot pot in winter	Kangri cancer
Smoked fish	Stomach cancer
Beer consumption	Rectal cancer
Aniline dye	Bladder cancer

STROKE

Rapidly developed clinical signs of focal disturbances of cerebral functions **lasting more than 24** hours or leading to death with no apparent cause other than vascular origin

TIA (transient ischemic attack): signs of focal disturbances which last for **less than 24 hours**

Stroke Profile in India

- Crude death rate of stroke in India – 54.2 / 100,000 population
- Higher younger population is affected in India
- Common causes include:
  - Rheumatic heart disease
  - Ischemic stroke
  - Arteriopathies
  - CNS infections – meningitis, encephalitis

Risk Factors

- Primary factor: Hypertension
- Secondary factors:
  - Hyperlipidemia
  - Diabetes
  - Cardiac anomalies
- **Host factors:**
  - Age – higher age
  - Gender – higher in males > females
  - Personal history: Obesity, smoking and other life style related risk factors

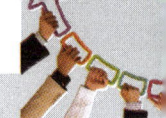

SNAKE BITE

It is a public health problem in females, children, farmers in poor and rural communities in low and middle income countries.

- Most of the snake bites are from non-venomous snakes
- Most of the deaths due to snake bites have been reported from Africa followed by Asia and Latin America.

First Aid in Snake Bite

- Immobilize the limb
- Alcoholic beverages or stimulants are **Not recommended** as they may act as vasodilators and promote the absorption of the snake venom
- Remove any tight clothing which may constrict the bitten site
- Incision of the bitten area or application of ice is NOT recommended
- Early transportation of patient to the nearest medical facility is recommended

Antivenom

- Developed by French physician, Albert Calmette
- Is the only DEFINITIVE treatment for snake bite
- Antivenoms are usually polyvalent and may be effective for multiple snake types
- Most of the available antivenoms are usually area specific – depending on the types of snake in that specific area
- Most common side effect of antivenom: anaphylaxis

ORAL HEALTH

Background

- These are the **most common non communicable disease**
- Key indicator for overall health, wellbeing and quality of life

Oral Health in India

- The Oral diseases burden was assessed in India with help of government infrastructure and capacity. Two large scale surveys have been conducted in India as:
  - National oral health survey and fluoride mapping (2003)
  - Oral health India report (2007)
- The burden of oral disease in India can be summarised for exam as follows:

Disease	Prevalence
Dental caries	40-45 %
Periodontal disease	> 90% (with advanced stage in ~40%)
Malocclusion	30% among children
Edentulousness	20-30% in age > 65 years
Oral cancer	12.6 per lac population
Cleft lip/cleft palate	1.7 per 1000 Live births
Dental fluorosis	Endemic in 230 districts in 19 states of India

Risk Factors

- Modifiable risk factor (life style, tobacco, alcohol consumption)
- Diabetes mellitus linked in reciprocal way with development and progression of oral diseases

Oral Diseases

Various diseases, local and systemic have a serious impact on oral health and quality of life. Most common oral diseases of public health importance are discussed below:

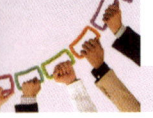

- Dental caries
  - Microbial biofilm (plaque) covers the tooth surface and converts the free sugars from food to chemical acid which dissolves tooth enamel and dentine over time
  - **Common public health issues**: cavities, pain, sickness absenteeism, poor quality of life, tooth loss, systemic infections
- Periodontal diseases (gum diseases)
  - Mainly due to tobacco and poor oral hygiene and bad oral habits
  - **Common public health issues:** periodontitis (11th most prevalent disease globally), gingivitis, bleeding
- Edentulousness (tooth loss)
  - Leading cause for higher YLD (years lived with disability) with higher age group
- Oral cancer:
  - Male are more commonly affected than females
  - Tobacco, alcohol and areca nut- are most common cause for oral cancer
  - HPV infection is also linked to higher chances of oral cancer among the high risk population.
- Oral-dental trauma – global prevalence of oral trauma is ~ 20%
- Noma
  - It is a necrotizing disease which affects children age 2-6 years
  - Commonly in children with malnutrition, under-weight for age, weak immune status
  - Starts as soft tissue sore in gums which later develops into ulcerative necrotizing gingivitis which progresses rapidly
  - High case fatality of upto 90%
  - Key feature to prevent disability due to Noma and related oral infections: screening, early diagnosis and prompt treatment
- Cleft lip/palate:
  - These are heterogenous disorders which affect 1-2 children per 1000 Live births
  - Risk factors
    - Genetic predisposition
    - Poor maternal nutrition, tobacco consumption, alcohol intake and obesity during pregnancy

Prevention of oral diseases: The prevention for oral diseases could be the best way to combat the menace for this most common morbidity affecting all age groups and affecting the quality of life. The preventive measures may include the following as:

- Promoting health dietary habits (low sugar, high fruit and vegetables intake)
- Reduce smoking / tobacco use
- Encourage protective equipment while in sports, during travel
- Maintaining low level fluoride in oral cavity
  - Consumption Of Adequately Fluoridated Water Supply
  - Regular use of toothpaste with 1000-1500 ppm of fluoride

The MoHFW has launched a 'National oral health program' in year 2014-2015 for integrated and comprehensive oral health in India

NATIONAL HEALTH PROGRAMS/POLICIES RELATED TO NCD

NATIONAL CANCER REGISTRY PROGRAM

- Launched by the Indian Council of Medical Research (ICMR) with a network of cancer registries across the country in December 1981.

The main objectives of this program were:

- To generate reliable data on the magnitude and patterns of cancer
- Undertake epidemiological studies based on results of registry data
- Help in designing, planning, monitoring and evaluation of cancer control activities under the National Cancer Control Program v(NCCP)
- Develop training programs in cancer registration and epidemiology.

97 Good to Remember

Personal hygiene and circumcision can have a protective role in cervical and penile cancer respectively.

NATIONAL PROGRAM FOR PREVENTION AND CONTROL OF CANCER, DIABETES, CARDIOVASCULAR DISEASES AND STROKE (NPCDCS)

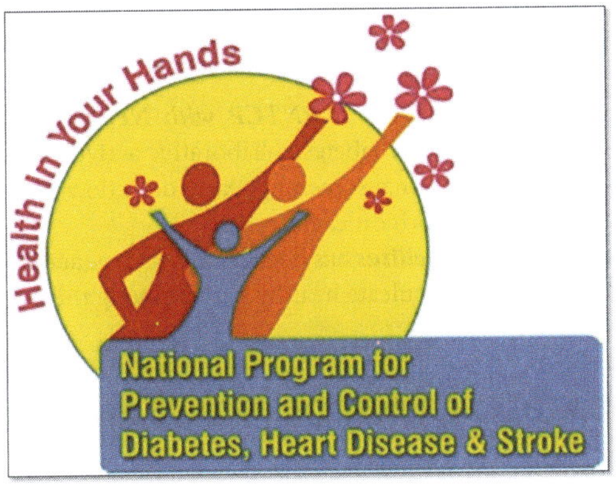

Fig. 4: Emblem of NPCDCS

Package of Services

- ***Home based care:*** 1 Nurse appointed under the program has to make home visits to bed ridden patients with diabetes, stroke etc. (1 village per week)
- ***Subcentre:*** Health promotion for behavior change and counseling, opportunistic screening (BP/Blood sugar), early identification of warning signals of common cancer, referral
- ***PHC:*** All the above services at SC + Clinical diagnosis and treatment of simple cases of hypertension and diabetes
- ***CHC/FRU:*** All above services at PHC + Early diagnosis by clinical and laboratory investigations, management of common CVD, diabetes, stroke
- ***District hospital:*** Early diagnosis of CVD, diabetes, cancer and higher investigations, medical management of cases and intensive care, follow-up cancer chemotherapy, Rehabilitation/physiotherapy services + above services at CHC/FRU
- ***Medical college:*** Mentoring district hospital, early diagnosis and management of diabetes, CVD etc, training and operational research
- ***Tertiary cancer center:*** Mentoring district hospital, comprehensive cancer care, training and operational research.
  - For the cancer component, there is the tertiary care cancer centers (TCCC) scheme, which aims at setting up/strengthening of 20 state cancer institutes (SCI) and 50 TCCCs for providing comprehensive cancer care in the country.
  - Under the scheme there is provision for giving a 'one time grant' of ₹120 crore per SCI and ₹45 crore per TCCC, to be used for building construction and procurement of equipment, with the Center to State share in the ratio of 60:40 (except for North-Eastern and Hilly States, where the share is 90:10).

Other Initiatives under the Program

- ***Population-based screening*** of common NCDs like diabetes, hypertension and common cancers under NHM in 100 districts of the country in the first phase. This will utilize the services of ASHA and Health-staff (Staff Nurse/ANM, etc.) of the existing primary health care system in screening of NCD risk factors as well as early detection and referral of NCDs.
- Guidelines for prevention and management of ***chronic obstructive pulmonary disease (COPD) and chronic kidney disease (CKD)*** are being included under the program to prevent and manage the chronic respiratory and kidney diseases respectively, which are also major causes of death due to NCDs.
- Pilot project on '***Integration of AYUSH with NPCDCS***' has been initiated in six districts, namely Bhilwara (Rajasthan), Gaya (Bihar), Surendranagar (Gujarat) under Central Council for Research in Ayurvedic Sciences (CCRAS); Lakhimpur Kheri (Uttar Pradesh) under Central Council for Research in Unani Medicine (CCRUM); and Krishna (Andhra Pradesh)

> 145 *High Yield Points*
>
> **AMRIT Pharmacy**
>
> ***A***ffordable ***M***edicine and ***R***eliable ***I***mplants for ***T***reatment - aims to reduce expenditure by patients on treatment for cancer and cardiac diseases. The *GoI* has opened retail outlets for sale of drugs and implants at highly discounted rates. It is implemented by government owned Hindustan lifecare limited (HLL) across country

and Darjeeling (West Bengal) under Central Council for Research in Homeopathy (CCRH). Besides health promotion and patient management services at the NCD/Lifestyle Clinics, training on Yoga are also provided through an integrated Yoga program. The government is planning to expand NPCDCS-AYUSH integration project to more districts of the country.

- Pilot intervention has been initiated for the ***prevention and control of rheumatic fever and rheumatic heart disease*** under the platforms of NPCDCS and Rashtriya Bal Swasthya Karyakram (RBSK), in three select districts (Gaya in Bihar, Firozabad in Uttar Pradesh and Hoshangabad in Madhya Pradesh).
- Another initiative is the integration of ***RNTCP with NPCDCS,*** wherein the "National Framework for Joint Tuberculosis-Diabetes collaborative activities" has been developed for a national strategy for 'bi-directional screening', early detection and better management of Tuberculosis and Diabetes co-morbidities in India.
- An application called ***Diabetes mellitus*** has been launched to generate awareness, to promote adherence of treatment and to inculcate healthy habits among the masses with special focus on target groups.

98 Good to Remember

As per Global Adult Tobacco Survey (GATS) 2009–10, conducted in the age group of 15 years and above 47.8% men and 20.3% women consume tobacco in some form or other.

NATIONAL TOBACCO CONTROL PROGRAM

The National Tobacco Program was launched in 2007–08 under 11th Five-Year Plan.

Objectives

- Public awareness/mass media campaigns for awareness building and behavior change.
- Establishment of tobacco product testing laboratories, to build regulatory capacity, as required under COPTA, 2003.
- Mainstreaming the program component as a part of the health delivery mechanism under the National rural Health Mission framework.
- Mainstreaming research and training on alternate crops and livelihood in collaboration with other nodal Ministries.
- Monitoring and evaluation including surveillance, e.g. Global Adult Tobacco Survey (GATS) India.

Tobacco Cessation Centers (TCCs) would also be established to help people quit tobacco consumption in any form.

BLINDNESS AND "NPCB & VI"

146 High Yield Points

Blindness is defined by WHO as—"visual acuity of less than 3/60 (Snellen) or its equivalent" or "inability to count fingers in daylight at a distance of 3 meters".[Q]

The definition of Blindness under the national program for control of blindness (NPCB) is hereby modified in line with WHO Definition:

- Presenting distance visually acuity less than 3/60 (20/400) in the better eye and limitation of field of vision to be less than 10 degrees from center of fixation.

Latest Updates

Table 12: Revised category of visual impairments

Category*	Visual acuity worse than	Visual acuity equal to or better than
0-mild or no visual impairment		6/18
1-moderate visual impairment	6/18	6/60
2-severe visual impairment (economic blindness)	6/60	3/60
3-blindness (social blindness)	3/60	1/60 or count fingers at 1 meter
4-blindness (manifest blindness)	1/60 or count fingers at 1 meter	Perception of light
5-blindness (absolute blindness)	No perception of light	
9	Undetermined or unspecified	

*Low vision in previous classification has been replaced with categories

Main Causes of Blindness

Cataract	(62.6%)
Refractive error	(19.70%)
Corneal blindness	(0.90%)
Glaucoma	(5.80%)
Surgical complication	(1.20%)
Posterior capsular opacification	(0.90%)
Posterior segment disorder	(4.70%)
Others	(4.19%)

99 Good to Remember

Estimated National Prevalence of Childhood Blindness/Low vision is 0.80 per thousand.

NPCB and VI-National Program for Control of Blindness and Visual Impairment

Goal

- To reduce the prevalence of blindness from 1.4% to 0.3% by 2020.

Objectives

- To reduce backlog of avoidable blindness by identification and cure at different levels of health care (Cataract surgery rate of 400 operations per lakh population)
- To develop comprehensive universal quality eye care services in every district to prevent visual impairment (Construction of 50 pediatric ophthalmic units-Target 11th Five-Year Plan)
- To develop additional human resources for providing eye care services and strengthen infrastructure
- To emphasize on research for prevention of visual impairment and blindness
- To secure participation of voluntary organizations/private practitioners in delivery of eye care.
- To enhance community awareness on eye care and stress on prevention
- Strengthening and upgradation of regional institutes of ophthalmology and medical colleges.

147 High Yield Points

As per 2006-07 survey prevalence of blindness was 1.0 %[Q]

Revised Strategies under NPCB

- Strengthen services for other causes of blindness [Corneal blindness (Corneal transplantation), refractive errors, follow-up of cataract operated persons and treatment of other conditions like glaucoma][Q]
- Shift from the eye camp approach to a fixed facility surgical approach[Q]
- Shift from conventional surgery to IOL implantation
- Expand World Bank project activities like construction of eye OT and wards at district level, training of eye surgeons in modern cataract and other eye surgeries and supply of equipment etc.
- Strengthen participation of voluntary organizations, earmark geographic areas to NGOs and Government hospitals to avoid duplication of effort and improve performance of Government units.
- Enhance coverage of eye care services in tribal and under-served areas.

Vision 2020: The Right to Sight

- It is a global initiative by WHO launched in 1999 to reduce avoidable (preventable and curable) blindness by the year 2020.
- Government of India adopted 'Vision 2020: The right to sight' under NPCB in 2001.

148 High Yield Points

- WHO has identified 5 major blinding conditions for immediate attention: Cataract, Childhood blindness, Trachoma, Refractive errors and onchocerciasis.[Q]

Target Disease under 'Vision 2020

In India,

- Cataract
- Childhood blindness

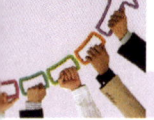

- Trachoma
- Refractive errors
- Dorneal blindness
- Diabetic retinopathy
- Glaucoma.[Q]

Table 13: Proposed structure for vision 2020, NPCB

Level of health care	Proposed structure	Services
Primary	Vision Centres—**20,000**	Primary eye care, school eye screening, refraction test and prescription of glass, screening and referral
Secondary	Service Centres—**2000**	Facility for refraction, cataract and other common surgery, referral
Tertiary	**Training Centres**—200	Tertiary eye care—retinal surgery, corneal transplantation, glaucoma surgery Training and CME
	Centres for excellence—**20**	Professional leadership, strategy making, CME, laying standards and quality assurance and research

School Vision Screening Program

- All children age 10–14 years are screened for refractive error by trained teachers once a year.
- Child unable to read the 6/9 line with any eye is sent to ophthalmic assistant at CHC for refraction test[Q]
- School teachers can identify 80–90% of children with low vision.
- Child needing spectacle is provided free spectacles by opticians contracted by NPCB[Q]

National Program for Prevention of Nutritional Blindness, 1970

- Administration of massive doses of vitamin A periodically
- 1st dose (1 lakh units) is given at nine months of age along with measles vaccination.[Q]
- 2nd dose (2 lakh units) is given along with DPT/OPV booster doses.[Q]
- Subsequent doses (2 lakh units each) are given at six months intervals up to 5 years of age.

Sick Children

- Children suffering from measles → 1 dose of vitamin A, if not received in previous 1 month
- Children suffering from malnutrition → 1 extra dose of vitamin A

NATIONAL PROGRAM FOR PREVENTION AND CONTROL OF DEAFNESS

Objectives

Long-Term Objective

To reduce total disease burden by 25% by end of XI Five-Year Plan[Q]

Immediate Objective

- To prevent avoidable hearing loss due to disease or injury
- Early identification, diagnosis and treatment of ear problems causing hearing loss
- Medically rehabilitate all persons/all age groups suffering from deafness
- Strengthen intersectoral linkages
- Develop institutional capacity for ear care (providing equipment, material and training personnel)

149 *High Yield Points*

Hearing loss is the 2nd leading cause of "Years Lived with Disability" (1st being depression)[Q] In India, 6.3% people suffer from significant auditory impairment.

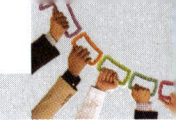

ACCIDENTS

Capacity Building for Trauma Care Facilities in Government Hospitals on National Highways

- This Program was started on pilot mode under the 9th and 10th Five-Year Plan as "Pilot Project for strengthening emergency facilities along the highways".
- During the 11th Plan, the program was named as "Assistance for capacity building for trauma care for upgradation and strengthening of emergency facilities in Government hospitals located on National Highways"
- The scheme was extended to the 12th Plan period as "Capacity building for developing Trauma Care Facilities in Government Hospitals on National Highways", for development of 85 new trauma care facilities.
- Designated hospitals are upgraded for providing trauma care facilities.
- The trauma care network has been so designed that no trauma victim has to be transported for more than 50 km to a designated hospital having trauma care facilities. For this purpose an equipped basic life support ambulance is to be deployed by NHAI (Ministry of Road Transport and Highways) at a distance of 50 km on the designated National Highways.

The criteria for identification of State Government Hospitals on the National Highways during the 12th Five-Year Plan

- Connecting two capital cities.
- Connecting major cities other than capital city
- Connecting ports to capital city
- Connecting industrial townships with capital city
- During the 12th Five-Year Plan, preference was given to states which were not covered during 11th Five-Year Plan, and to the Hilly and North Eastern states.

92 Must Remember

- *Road traffic accidents*—Rank 1st among all fatal accidents. Rate of death in RTA is 1.2 per 1000 vehicles (2011).
- *Drowning*—is 3rd leading cause of unintentional injury/death. It accounts for 7% of all injury-related deaths.

150 High Yield Points

Haddon Matrix is useful for preventing Road traffic accidents and crash injuries. It is a strategic method for understanding of possible reasons for crash as human, equipment and environmental factors attributing to causation of road crashes.

NATIONAL PROGRAM FOR PREVENTION AND MANAGEMENT OF BURN INJURIES (NPPMBI)

The **National Program for Prevention and Management of Burn Injuries** (NPPMBI) is an initiative by the Directorate General of Health Services, Ministry of Health and Family Welfare to strengthen the preventive, curative and rehabilitative services for burn victims.

Goal

- To reduce incidence, mortality, and disability due to burn injuries.
- To improve the awareness among the general masses and vulnerable groups especially the women, children, industrial and hazardous occupational workers.
- To establish adequate network of infrastructural facilities along with trained personnel for burn management and rehabilitation.
- To carry out research for assessing behavioral, social and other determinants of burn injuries in our country for effective need based program planning for burn injures, monitoring and subsequent evaluation.

Burn Unit

- The proposed Burn Unit would approximately require 400 sq. meters.
- Burn Units comprising of 6 beds (4 general beds + 2 Acute Care beds + Other Facilities required) will be established in District Hospitals where such facilities do not exist.
- Where they already exist, the same will be augmented through addition/alteration/ renovation so as to ensure that they have the required number of beds.
- The Burn Unit will be provided with equipment required for treatment and rehabilitation of burns injury patients.

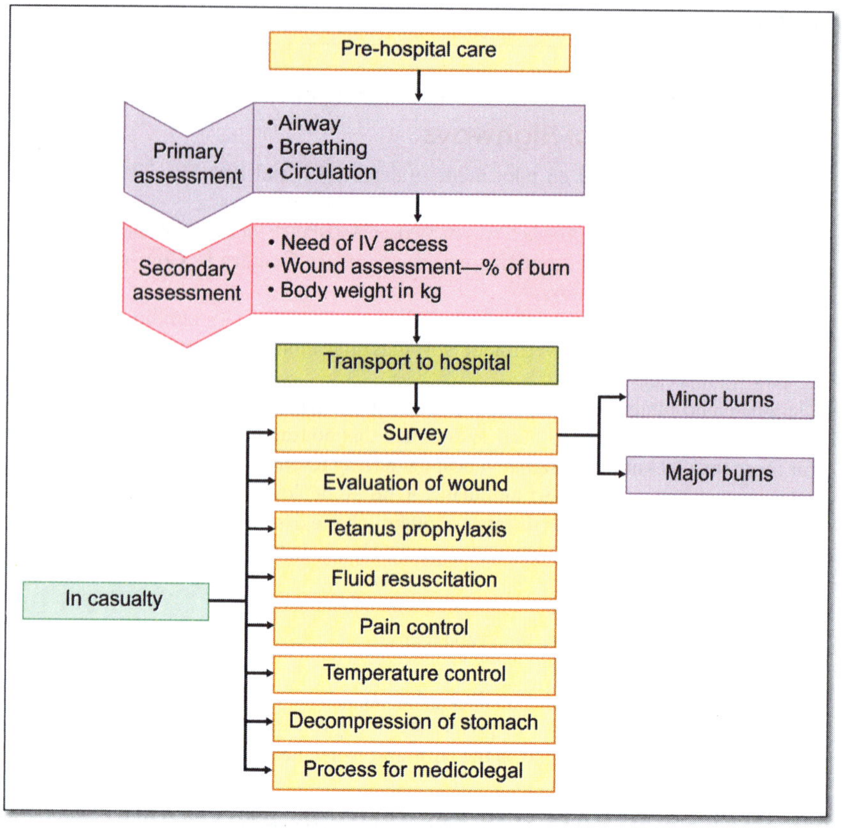

Fig. 5: Management of burns

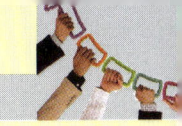

Image-Based Question

1. The image shown in figure depicts WHO-World No Tobacco day theme: Get ready for?

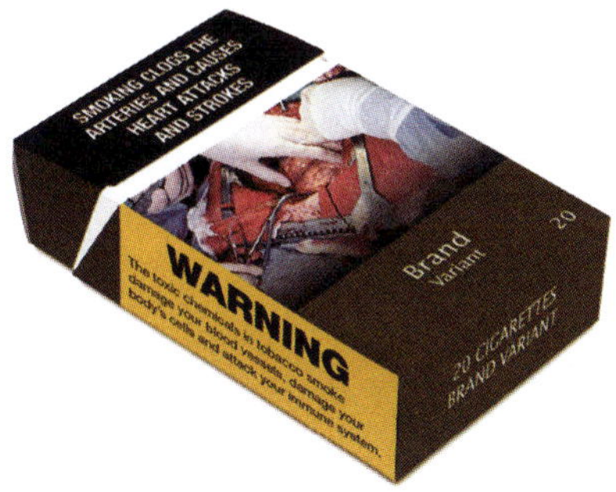

a. Plain packaging
b. Aggressive packaging
c. Minimum packaging
d. Standard packaging

Answer of Image-Based Question

1. Ans. (a) Plain packaging

Multiple Choice Questions

1. WHO global target for prevention and control of non-communicable disease by 2025, is to decrease hypertension by: *(Recent Question 2018)*
a. 25% b. 35%
c. 55% d. 75%

2. BMI level for men which is considered as lethal is: *(Recent Question 2018)*
a. 11
b. 13
c. 12
d. 15

3. Which cancer is preventable by vaccine?
a. Ovarian CA b. Cervix CA
c. Breast CA d. Uterus CA

4. Rule of halves is related to the following disease:
a. Hypertension
b. Coronary heart disease
c. Obesity
d. Blindness

5. Most common cancer in India: *(Recent Question 2017)*
a. Lung b. Stomach
c. Breast d. Cervix

6. Obesity can be measure from: *(Recent Question 2017)*
a. Mid triceps thickness
b. Biceps thickness
c. Thickness of calf
d. Chest diameter

INTERNATIONAL CLASSIFICATION OF DISEASE

7. Neoplasms are included in the following chapter of ICD-10
a. I b. II
c. X d. XX

DESCRIPTIVE EPIDEMIOLOGY

8. Rural and Urban difference in prevalence is seen in all of the following, except: *(Recent Question 2017)*
a. Lung cancer b. Tuberculosis
c. Mental Illness d. Chronic Bronchitis

HYPERTENSION/CHD/RHD

9. Physical activity like brisk walking for 30 minutes a day will reduce systolic BP by approximately
a. 10–20 mm Hg
b. 5–10 mm Hg
c. 2–4 mm Hg
d. None of the above

10. Rule of halves is related to the following disease:
a. Hypertension
b. Blindness
c. Obesity
d. CHD

11. Tracking of blood pressure means:
a. Keeping a track of a person with hypertension for follow-up
b. Keeping a track of the relatives of a hypertensive for screening
c. BP levels of individuals are followed up early childhood into adult life
d. Checking BP at regular intervals once hypertension is diagnosed

12. DASH approach of hypertension includes: *(Recent Question 2017)*
a. Fruits only
b. Vegetables and fruits only
c. Pulses and nuts only
d. Vegetables, fruits, whole grain and low fat diet

13. DASH is the acronym for?
a. Domestic approach to safeguard hepatitis
b. Dietary approach to stop hyperlipidemia
c. Dietary approach to stop hypertension
d. Domestic approach to stop hypertension

14. Diet recommended in hypertension is:
a. Fruits, vegetables and low salt
b. Fruits, vegetables, low fat dairy product
c. Proteins, fibres and low salt
d. Carbohydrates, fibres and low salt

15. Jai Vigyan mission mode project is related to the control of:
a. Coronary heart disease b. Rheumatic heart disease
c. Stroke d. Road traffic accidents

16. Single most useful test for identifying individuals at high risk of coronary heart disease: *(Recent Question 2016)*
a. Serum cholesterol b. Blood pressure
c. Blood sugar d. Serum homocysteine

17. Best method of prevention of CHD:
a. Primordial prevention b. Primary prevention
c. Secondary prevention d. Tertiary prevention

18. In the prevention of CHD, in smoking intervention strategies, the goal is:
a. Smoke free society b. Safer cigarette
c. Nicotine chewing gum d. Reducing smoking frequency

19. The clinical goal for CHD prevention is a "Cholesterol/HDL" ratio less than: *(Recent Question 2016)*
a. 3.0 b. 3.5
c. 4.0 d. 4.5

20. Consumption of the following does not alter the risk of cardiovascular diseases:
a. Vitamin E supplements
b. Linoleic acid
c. Trans-fatty acids
d. Low to moderate alcohol intake

21. Tracking of BP implies
a. BP increase with age
b. BP decreases with age
c. BP of hyoptensive patients becomes hypertensive
d. BP of hyoptensive patients remain hypotensive

Ans.

1. a
2. b
3. b
4. a
5. c
6. a
7. b
8. b
9. c
10. a
11. c
12. d
13. c
14. b
15. b
16. b
17. a
18. a
19. b
20. a
21. d

Most Recent Questions of 2019-18 are given at the end of MCQs

22. Inability to perform any work without discomfort is:
a. NYHA 1 b. NYHA 2
c. NYHA 3 d. NYHA 4

23. Best known large study program for coronary heart disease is: ***(Recent Question 2016)***
a. Framingham study b. North Karelia study
c. Stanford study d. Oxford study

24. Modifiable risk factors for hypertension is:
a. Ethnicity b. Age
c. Sex d. Obesity

25. Not included among major criteria in acute rheumatic fever is:
a. Erythema marginatum
b. Polyarthralgia
c. Chorea
d. Pancarditis

26. Not a dietary modification in high risk cardiovascular disease group is? ***(Recent Question 2016)***
a. LDL cholesterol less than 100 mg/dL
b. Avoidance of alcohol
c. Saturated fat intake limited to 7% of total calories
d. Salt intake less than 5 g/day

27. Following are major criteria of Jones in Rheumatic Fever except:
a. Pancarditis b. Arthritis
c. Chorea d. Elevated ESR

28. Which of the following is maximally associated with occurrence of coronary heart disease?
a. HDL b. LDL
c. VLDL d. Chylomicron

29. STEPS is done for: ***(Recent Question 2016)***
a. Surveillance of risk factors of non-communicable disease
b. Surveillance of incidence of non-communicable disease
c. Surveillance of evaluation of treatment of non-communicable disease
d. Surveillance of mortality from non-communicable disease

30. WHO STEPS approach is used for?
a. Noncommunicable diseases
b. Communicable diseases
c. Immunodeficient disease
d. Auto immune disease

31. True about cardiovascular diseases (CVD): ***(PGI May 2010)***
a. Urban and rural areas have equal incidence
b. RHD is an important cause of CVD
c. Primordial prevention is best strategy
d. Coronary heart disease cause 25% of total death
e. In developing countries, the CHD risk is higher in rural areas

CANCER

32. The present strategy of initial screening of cervical cancer:
a. Pap smear
b. Cervical biopsy
c. High vaginal swab
d. Visual inspection after application of freshly prepared 5% acetic acid solution

33. Carcinoma resulting in maximum mortality among women in India is?
a. Lungs b. Breast
c. Ovary d. Cervix-uteri

34. Most common malignant tumor occurring among adult males in India is: ***(Recent Question 2016)***
a. Lung cancer b. Oropharyngeal carcinoma
c. Gastric carcinoma d. Colorectal carcinoma

35. All of the following are early warning signals of cancer except:
a. Persistent cough
b. Lump or hard area in breast
c. Unexplained weight gain
d. Change in wart/mole

36. Tobacco is responsible for ___% of oral cancer
a. 100% b. 40%
c. 90% d. 60%

37. The most common cancer, affecting both males and females worldwide is: ***(Recent Question 2016)***
a. Cancer of the pancreas b. Buccal mucosa cancer
c. Lung cancer d. Colorectal cancer

38. Globally most common cancer is:
a. Colorectal cancer b. Bladder cancer
c. Lung cancer d. Oropharyngeal cancer

OBESITY

39. Quetelet's index is calculated by:
a. Weight (kg)/Height^2(m)
b. Height (cm)/Cube root of body weight (kg)
c. Height (cm) –100
d. Actual weight/desirable weight

40. BMI of 25-29.99 indicates:
a. Normal weight
b. Preobese
c. Obese class I
d. Obese class II

41. Normal body mass index: ***(Recent Question 2016)***
a. 16.00 – 18.49 b. 18.50 – 24.99
c. 25.00 – 29 .99 d. 30.00 – 34.99

42. Waist-hip ratio greater than___ indicates abdominal fat accumulation in men:
a. 0.85 b. 1.0
c. 1.25 d. 1.5

43. Normal waist to hip ratio in females is:
a. Less than 0.85 b. 0.90
c. 0.95 d. More than 1

44. Calculate the BMI of a person weighing 64 kg and height 160 cm:
a. 20 b. 24
c. 25 d. 32

45. Ponderal index is calculated by:
a. Height (cm)/cube root of body weight (kg)
b. Height (cm) - 100
c. Ht(cm)- 100-(Ht(cm)-150/2 (women) or 4 (men))
d. Actual weight/desirable weight (should not exceed 1.2)

46. A patient is called obese if BMI is:
a. 20-30 b. >25
c. >30 d. >40

Ans.

22. d
23. a
24. d
25. b
26. a
27. d
28. b
29. a
30. a
31. b, c, d
32. d
33. b
34. a
35. c
36. c
37. c
38. c
39. a
40. b
41. b
42. b
43. a
44. c
45. a
46. c

Most Recent Questions of 2019-18 are given at the end of MCQs

47. Overweight is BMI:
a. 25-29.99 b. 15-15.8
c. 18.5-24.99 d. 30-34.99

48. BMI for normal weight: *(Recent Question 2015)*
a. 18.5-27.99 b. 18.5-24.99
c: 23.0-24.99 d. >30

49. Which index of obesity does not include height?
a. BMI b. Ponderal index
c. Brocca's index d. Corpulence index

50. What will be the BMI of a male whose weight is 89 kg and height is 172 cm:
a. 27 b. 30
c. 33 d. 36

BLINDNESS

51. Refractive errors are the second major cause of blindness in India after cataract. Children, who are the particularly vulnerable are screened under NPCB by school eye screening program. In the program, what is the cut off for abnormal vision? *(Recent Question 2015)*
a. 6/6 b. 6/9
c. 6/12 d. 6/18

52. The goal of NPCB was to reduce blindness prevalence in India from 1.4% to:
a. 1% b. 0.8%
c. 0.5% d. 0.3%

53. Most common cause of blindness in India is
a. Cataract b. Refractive error
c. Diabetic retinopathy d. Corneal pathology

54. As per national survey causes of blindness in India in increasing order are:
a. Corneal opacity, glaucoma, refractive error, cataract
b. Glaucoma, refractive error, corneal opacity, cataract
c. Refractive error, glaucoma, corneal opacity, cataract
d. Cataract, refractive error, glaucoma, corneal opacity

55. Under NPCB eye donation fortnight is organized during:
a. January and February b. April and may
c. August and September d. November and December

56. As per WHO, a person with visual acuity of 6/60 in right eye and 3/60 in left eye is classified as:
a. Mild visual impairment
b. Moderate visual impairment
c. Severe visual impairment
d. Blindness

57. As per NPCB, cut off for blindness is a vision of:
a. <3/60 in worse eye *(Recent Question 2015)*
b. <6/60 in better eye
c. <3/60 in better eye
d. <6/60 in worse eye

58. As per WHO definition of high prevalence of night blindness does not include?
a. Night blindness > 1
b. Conjunctival xerosis >0.5%
c. Corneal ulceration > 0.01%
d. Corneal scarring > 0.05%

59. Blindness rate in India due to refractive errors:
a. 62.6% *(Recent Question 2014)*
b. 19.7%
c. 8%
d. 6.2%

60. Disease not included in vision 2020, India is:
a. Cataract
b. Glaucoma
c. Diabetic retinopathy
d. Onchocerciasis

61. If blindness is surveyed using schools as compared to populations surveys, then estimation of prevalence of blindness will have: *(Recent Question 2014)*
a. Overestimation
b. Underestimation
c. Remains same
d. None of them is used for evaluation

62. Disability certificate is given for poor vision if visual acuity is 4/60, in tune of visual impairment as a percentage:
a. 1 b. 0.4
c. 0.3 d. 0.75

63. WHO defines blindness if the visual activity is less than:
a. 3/60
b. 18/38
c. 9/60
d. 6/6

ROAD TRAFFIC ACCIDENT

64. A person who is killed in a road traffic accident is defined as any person who was killed outright or who died within how many days as a result of the accident:
a. 7 days
b. 14 days
c. 30 days
d. 42 days

65. Suicide rate in India, as per the NCRB report 2014 is:
a. 11 per 100,000 population
b. 10.6 per 100,000 population
c. 11.2 per 100,000 population
d. 11.4 per 100,000 population

66. Most common means of committing suicide in India, as per
a. Poisoning *(Recent Question 2014)*
b. Hanging
c. Self-immolation
d. Drowning

67. Haddon matrix is concerned with:
a. Hypertension
b. Maternal and child mortality
c. Prevention of injury
d. Communicable disease

68. In India causing maximum death among the following is:
a. Drowning *(Recent Question 2013)*
b. Road traffic accident
c. Burns
d. Poisoning

Ans.
47. a
48. b
49. d
50. b
51. b
52. d
53. a
54. d
55. c
56. c
57. c
58. b
59. b
60. d
61. b
62. d
63. a
64. c
65. b
66. b
67. c
68. b

Most Recent Questions of 2019-18 are given at the end of MCQs

MISCELLANEOUS

69. NOT true about counterfeit medicines is: *(Recent Question 2013)*
- a. No active ingredients
- b. Wrong ingredient
- c. Correct packaging
- d. Right active ingredient in wrong dose

70. Drug monitoring in India is carried out by:
- a. Central Drugs Standard Control Organization
- b. Central Drug Research Institute
- c. Indian Standards Organization
- d. Central Drug Laboratory

71. Rheumatic Heart Disease can be prevented by:
- a. Treatment of Respiratory Infections in Children
- b. Vaccination against Streptococcus
- c. Screening among school children
- d. All the above

72. In India, most common cause of cervical cancer is:
- a. HPV 31, 45
- b. HPV 6, 11
- c. HPV 31, 33
- d. HPV 16, 18

73. Vision 2020 "The right to sight" includes all except:
- a. Trachoma
- b. Measles induced blindness
- c. Cataract
- d. Onchocerciasis

74. Obesity is defined as if BMI is: *(Recent Question 2013)*
- a. 20
- b. 50
- c. 40
- d. 30

75. Broca's Index is:
- a. Weight – 100 = Height
- b. Height – 100 = Weight
- c. Weight/Height
- d. Weight/Height^2

76. All are primordial prevention strategies against Coronary Heart Disease *(Recent Question 2013)*
- a. Regular physical activity
- b. Management of diabetes and hypertension
- c. Prevention of Tobacco use
- d. Taking healthy balanced diet

NPCB

77. Not a criteria for diagnosis of blindness under NPCB is
- a. Vision of ≤ 6/60 with best possible correction
- b. Vision < 4/60 in better eye
- c. Inability to count fingers from a distance of 20 feet
- d. Diminution in field of vision to 20°

78. NPCB was launched in the year:
- a. 1975
- b. 1976
- c. 1983
- d. 1963

79. Under National Program for Control of Blindness, District blindness control society is headed by: *(Recent Question 2013)*
- a. District program manager
- b. District eye surgeon
- c. District collector
- d. District health officer

80. Number of vision centers under vision 2020, national program for control of blindness are:
- a. 20
- b. 200
- c. 2000
- d. 20000

81. In SAFE strategy, S stands for:
- a. Surgery
- b. Syringing
- c. Streptomycin
- d. All of the above

82. Follow-up of cataract operation in national blindness control program is done by: *(Recent Question 2013)*
- a. Active surveillance
- b. Passive surveillance
- c. Sentinel surveillance
- d. Routine check-up

NPCDCS

83. National cancer awareness day is observed on:
- a. 7th November
- b. 1st December
- c. 4th April
- d. 25th July

84. National program for prevention and control of cancer, diabetes, cardiovascular disease and stroke (NPCDCS), true is
- a. Separate center for stroke, DM, cancer
- b. Implementation in some 5 states over 10 districts
- c. District hospital has specialized facilities
- d. Sub center has facility for diagnosis and treatment

85. True about national program for prevention and control of cancer, diabetes, cardiovascular diseases and stroke is:
- a. Home based care is not required
- b. Implementation is some 5 states over 10 districts
- c. Separate center for stroke, DM
- d. CHC has facilities for diagnosis and treatment of CVD, diabetes

86. What is the new change in National Program on Prevention and control of diabetes, cardiovascular disease and stroke?
- a. Opportunistic screening
- b. Awareness of lifestyle and behavior related diseases
- c. Specialized units at medical colleges
- d. Integration with national cancer control program

MISCELLANEOUS

87. The National Program that came into existence during 11th Five-Year Plan is *(Recent Question 2013)*
- a. National cardiovascular diseases and stroke control program
- b. National diabetes and cancer control program
- c. National cancer control program
- d. National program for prevention and control of cancer, diabetes, cardiovascular diseases and stroke

Ans.

69. c
70. a
71. c
72. d
73. b
74. d
75. b
76. b
77. b
78. b
79. c
80. d
81. a
82. c
83. a
84. c
85. d
86. d
87. d

Most Recent Questions of 2019-18 are given at the end of MCQs

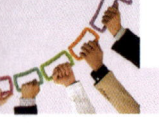

Most Recent Questions (2019-2018)

88. Under the national program for prevention and management of burn injuries, the burn units should be: *(AIIMS Nov 2017)*
a. 3 bedded
b. 6 bedded
c. Available at every CHC
d. Available at every district hospital

89. Metabolic syndrome c/f *(PGI Nov 2018)*
a. Hypertension
b. Increase HDL
c. Increase Triglycerides
d. Increase blood glucose
e. Increased ASL/ALT

90. Which of the following is/are the primary prevention strategies for hypertension *(PGI Nov 2018)*
a. Weight reduction
b. Adopting DASH diet
c. Physical exercise
d. Early case detection
e. Tracking of hypertension

91. For cervical cancer, which of the following is true statement: *(PGI Nov 2018)*
a. Human papilloma virus is the most common cause of cervical cancer in India
b. Highest incidence is in females age 25- 65 years
c. All females age 30 years and above should get cervix cancer screening every 5 years in primary health care setting
d. PAP smear is screening test of choice for CA Cervix at a field centre or primary health centre
e. HPV vaccine may be given to males to prevent HPV transmission and cervical cancer in females

92. Primary prevention for Hypertension are all except: *(PGI May 2018)*
a. Early diagnosis
b. Treatment with Anti-hypertensive drug
c. Low salt intake
d. Reduction in weight
e. Regular exercise

93. According to Commission on chronic illness (1957) chronic illness was defined as impairment with: *(AIIMS May 2019)*
a. Of more than 3 months duration
b. With residual disability
c. With irreversible pathological alteration
d. With significant impairment

Ans.

88. b
89. a, c, d
90. a, b, c, e
91. a, c
92. a, b
93. a

Answers with Explanations

1. Ans. (a) 25%

2. Ans. (b) 13

BMI cut off in lethal range:
For females: < 12
For males < 13

Note:

- Females have greater body stores of fat than males, and this can be used as a source of energy for a much longer period (fat is more energy dense than protein)
- The contribution of fat energy to total energy expenditure is greater in the female, resulting in a greater conservation of protein
- Females appear better able to mobilise adipose tissue from most sites in the body

3. Ans. (b) Cervix CA

Ref: K. Park, 24th ed. p 133

4. Ans. (a) Hypertension

Ref: K. Park, 24th ed. p 392

5. Ans. (c) Breast

Ref: K. Park, 24th ed. p 401

6. Ans. (a) Mid triceps thickness

Ref: K. Park, 24th ed. p 418

INTERNATIONAL CLASSIFICATION OF DISEASE

7. Ans. (b) II

Ref: K. Park, 24th ed. p 54

DESCRIPTIVE EPIDEMIOLOGY

8. Ans. (b) Tuberculosis

Ref: K. Park, 24th ed. p 71

Rural/urban variations in disease prevalence:

- Higher prevalence in urban area→ Chronic bronchitis, accidents, lung cancer, cardiovascular diseases, mental illness and drug dependence.
- Higher prevalence in rural area→ Skin diseases, zoonotic diseases and soil-transmitted helminths.

Reasons for variations in disease prevalence:

- Differences in population density, social class.
- Deficiencies in medical care
- Levels of sanitation, education and environmental factors.

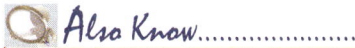

Also Know

Tuberculosis is prevalent in both urban and rural population.

HYPERTENSION/CHD/RHD

9. Ans. (c) 2–4 mm Hg

Ref: K. Park, 24th ed. p 395

Life Style Modifications Leading to Systolic BP Reduction

Recommendation	Approximate Reduction in Systolic BP (in mm Hg)
Weight reduction (BMI 18.5-24.9)	5-20/10 kg weight loss
DASH diet	8-14
Dietary sodium intake of ≤ 100 mEq/day (2.4 g Sodium or 6 g Sodium Chloride)	2–8
Regular physical activity (E.g. brisk walk for ≥30 min/day on most days of the week)	4–9
Alcohol consumption ≤2 drinks/day in males and ≤ 1 drinks/day in females (1 oz = 30 mL ethanol)	2–4

10. Ans. (a) Hypertension

Ref: K. Park, 24th ed. p 392

Rule of halves: Hypertension is an Iceberg Disease

- About ½ of the hypertensive subjects in general population of most developed countries are aware of the condition
- About ½ of those aware get treated
- About ½ of those treated are adequately treated

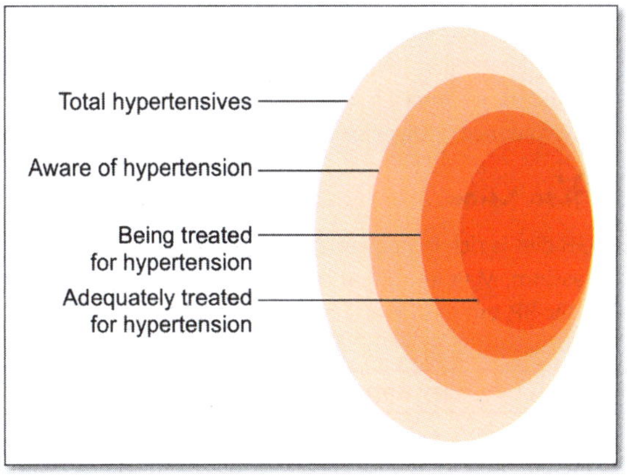

11. Ans. (c) BP levels of individuals are followed up early childhood into adult life

Ref: K. Park, 24th ed. p 393

Tracking of Blood Pressure

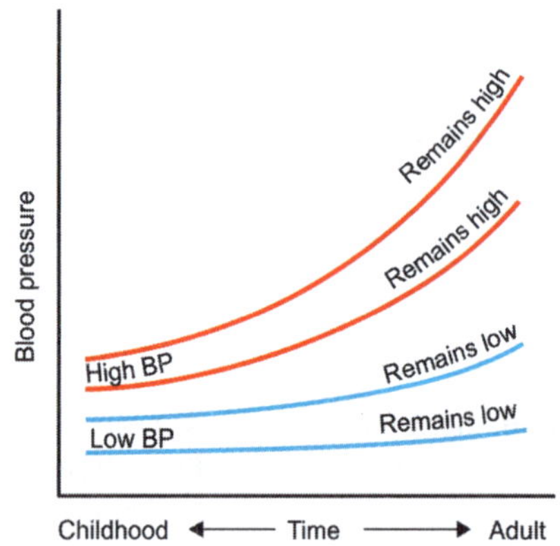

- It is used to identify children and adolescents "at risk" of developing hypertension in future.
- Follow up of blood pressure levels of individuals from early childhood into adult life, reveals that those individuals whose BP were initially high, continue in the same "track" as adults.
- This phenomenon of persistence of rank order of BP is described as "tracking".

12. Ans. (d) Vegetables, fruits, whole grain and low fat diet

Ref: Community Medicine with Recent Advances, AH Suryakanta, 3rd edition, p- 534

DASH- (Dietary Approach to Stop Hypertension) is a dietary approach to control hypertension. It recommends
- Avoidance of saturated fat
- Inclusion of MUFA (Mono Unsaturated Fatty Acid), PUFA (Poly Unsaturated Fatty Acid) in diet
- Inclusion of fresh fruits (Specially potassium rich fruits like Banana, Orange) and Vegetables (Carrot, Spinach, Mushroom, potato) in daily diet.
- Whole grain flour (instead of white flour)
- Inclusion of nuts, seeds or legumes (dried peas or beans) daily
- Moderate quantity of protein (Fish or poultry is preferred, Red meat avoided)
- Avoidance of sugar sweetened beverages and added fat

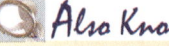

Also Know......................

- DASH diet is rich in nutrients, fiber and electrolytes (Calcium, Potassium, Magnesium). It results in 8-14 mm Hg fall in systolic BP, but has no effect on body weight.

13. Ans. (c) Dietary Approaches to Stop Hypertension

Ref: K. Park, 24th ed. p 395

14. Ans. (b) Fruits, vegetables, low fat dairy product

Ref: K. Park, 24th ed. p 3955

15. Ans. (b) Rheumatic heart disease

Ref: K. Park, 24th ed. p 397

Jai Vigyan Mission Mode project on Community Control of RF/RHD in India has 4 main components
- To study the epidemiology of streptococcal sore throats
- Establish registries for RF and RHO
- Vaccine development for streptococcal infection
- Conducting advanced studies on pathological aspects of RF and RHO.

16. Ans. (b) Blood pressure

Ref: K. Park, 24th ed. p 387

Blood pressure and serum cholesterol estimation are useful for identifying individuals at high risk of coronary heart disease
- A small (2–3 mm Hg) reduction in average BP of entire population is likely to produce a large reduction in the incidence of cardiovascular complications

Individuals at special risk include smokers, family history of CHD, diabetes and obesity and use of OCP in young women

17. Ans. (a) Primordial prevention

Ref: K. Park, 24th ed. p 388

Primordial prevention involves prevention of emergence and spread of CHD risk factors and life styles in populations where they have not yet appeared or become endemic. It involves
- Smoke free society
- Regular physical activity
- Prudent diet (reduced salt intake and avoidance of a high alcohol intake) and weight control

Primordial prevention is the best method of prevention of CHD

18. Ans. (a) Smoke free society

Ref: K. Park, 24th ed. p 386

Smoking and CHD

- Degree of risk of CHD is directly related to number cigarettes smoked per day
- Smoking is synergistic with other risk factors (e.g. Hypertension, elevated serum cholesterol)
- Goal is to achieve a smoke-free society by means effective information and education activities, legislative restrictions, fiscal measures and smoking cessation programs.

19. Ans. (b) 3.5

Ref: K. Park, 24th ed. p 387

20. Ans. (a) Vitamin E supplements

Ref: K. Park, 24th ed. p 388, 650-51

21. Ans. (d) BP of hypotensive patients remain hypotensive

Ref: K. Park, 24th ed. p 393

22. Ans. (d) NYHA 4

Ref: Humbert M, Sitbon O, Simonneau G. Treatment of pulmonary arterial hypertension. N Engl J Med. 2004;351:1425-1436

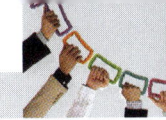

NYHA stands for "New York Heart Association" functional classification of pulmonary hypertension

NYHA 1	▪ No limitation of physical activity. ▪ Ordinary physical activity does not cause undue Dyspnea/Fatigue, Chest pain or near Syncope.
NYHA 2	▪ Slight limitation of physical activity. Comfortable at rest ▪ Ordinary physical activity causes undue Dyspnea/Fatigue, Chest pain or near Syncope.
NYHA 3	▪ Marked limitation of physical activity. Comfortable at rest. ▪ Less-than-ordinary physical activity causes undue Dyspnea/Fatigue, Chest pain or near Syncope
NYHA 4	▪ Inability to carry out any physical activity without symptoms. Patients manifest signs of right heart failure ▪ Dyspnea and/or fatigue may be present at rest. Discomfort is increased by any physical activity.

23. Ans. (a) Framingham study

Ref: K. Park, 24th ed. p 389-90

Framingham Study initiated in 1948 by United States Public Health Service is one of the best known Cohort study[Q]

- It helped in establishing CHD risk factors and their relative importance.
- Elevated serum cholesterol, smoking, hypertension and sedentary habits were established as major risk factors.

Other Intervention Trials for CHD

Trials	Objective
Stanford Heart Disease Prevention Program, California-1972	Determine whether community health education can reduce risk of cardiovascular disease
North Karelia Project, Finland-1972 (Multiple risk factor intervention trial)	Reduce high level of risk factors for CVD and To promote early diagnosis, treatment and rehabilitation in CVD patient.
Oslo Study, Norway-1973	To know if lowering serum lipids and cessation of smoking can reduce incidence of 1st attack of CHD, in males 40–50 years
Multiple Risk Factor Intervention Trial (MRFIT), USA	To know impact of interventions- cessation of smoking, control of BP and Diet modification on CHD mortality
Lipid Research Clinics, USA	To test if reduction of serum cholesterol can prevent CHD
Secondary prevention trials	To prevent subsequent coronary attack or sudden death)

24. Ans. (d) Obesity

Ref: K. Park, 24th ed. p 393

Risk Factors for Hypertension

Modifiable	Nonmodifiable
▪ Obesity ▪ High salt intake ▪ High saturated fat intake ▪ Low Dietary Fiber intake ▪ Alcohol ▪ Lack of physical activity ▪ Environmental stress ▪ Socioeconomic status* ▪ OCP (High estrogen)	▪ Age (BP rises with age) ▪ Sex ▪ Genetic (Polygenic inheritance) ▪ Ethnicity (Black communities have higher BP)

**Among countries in post-transitional stage of economic and epidemiological change- High BP is seen in lower socioeconomic class. Whereas in countries in transitional or pre-transitional phase, high BP is seen in upper socioeconomic class*

25. Ans. (b) Polyarthralgia

Ref: K. Park, 24th ed. p 399

2002-2003 WHO Criteria for Rheumatic fever and RHD Diagnosis

26. Ans. (a) LDL Cholesterol less than 100 mg/dL

Ref: K. Park, 24th ed. p 388

Suggested dietary modification for prevention of CHD.

- Reduce fat intake to 20-30% of total energy intake
- Consumption of saturated fats limited to less than 10% of total energy intake.
- Reduce of dietary cholesterol intake to less than 100 mg per 1000 kcal per day
- Increase consumption of complex carbohydrates (i.e., vegetables, fruits, whole grains and legumes)
- Avoid alcohol consumption
- Reduce salt intake to ≤ 5 g daily

27. Ans. (d) Elevated ESR

Ref: K. Park, 24th ed. p 399

28. Ans. (b) LDL

Ref: K. Park, 24th ed. p 387

CHD and Serum Cholesterol

- Risk of CHD rises steadily with serum cholesterol concentration (220 mg/dL or more)
- LDL is associated with CHDQ and VLDL with peripheral vascular disease (e.g., Intermittent claudication).
- HDL > 40 mg/dL is protective against development of CHD.
- Total Cholesterol/HDL ratio less < 3.5 is the recommended clinical goal for CHD prevention.
- Plasma apolipoproteinA-I (Major HDL protein) and apolipoprotein-B (major LDL protein) levels are better predictors of CHD than HDL or LDL cholesterol respectively.

29. Ans. (a) Surveillance of risk factors of non-communicable disease

Ref: www.who.int/entity/chp/steps/en. Bulletin of WHO

STEP wise approach to NCD risk factor surveillance

30. Ans. (a) Noncommunicable diseases

Ref: www.who.int/entity/chp/steps/en. Bulletin of WHO

31. Ans. (b, c, d) RHD is an important cause of CVD (c) Primordial prevention is best strategy (d) Coronary heart disease cause 25% of total death

Ref: K. Park, 24th ed. p 883-388

Cardiovascular diseases are world's largest killers, claiming 17.3 million lives every year (Modern Epidemic)

- Over 80% of CVD deaths occur in low and middle income countries
- Coronary heart disease cause 25% of total death in Industrialized countriesQ (Male 30% > Female 25%)
- Cardiovascular diseases are responsible for about 25% of DALYs lost due to NCD in SEAR countries. (IHD causes 40% of DALYs lost, Cerebrovascular diseases 19%, RHD 6%, Inflammatory heart diseases 6% and others 29%).
- Incidence of cardiovascular diseases is more in urban areas.
- In developing countries (e.g. India) CHD is reported a decade earlier (51-60 year) compared to developed countries.
- Primordial prevention is the most cost effective strategy.

CANCER

32. Ans. (d) Visual inspection after application of freshly prepared...

Ref: K. Park, 24th ed. p 405

Screening of Cervical Cancer

- Present strategy—Visual Inspection after application of freshly prepared 5% Acetic acid solution with/without magnification (VIA or VIAM)
- Well defined opaque acetowhite lesions close to squamocolumnar junction or well-defined circumorificial acetowhite lesion or dense acetowhite ulceroproliferative growth on cervix constitute a positive test

Also Know......................

- All women should have a Pap test (cervical smear) at beginning of sexual activity and then every 3 years thereafter

33. Ans. (b) Breast

Ref: K. Park, 24th ed. p 402

34. Ans. (a) Lung Cancer

Ref: K. Park, 24th ed. p 402

35. Ans. (c) Unexplained weight gain

Ref: K. Park, 24th ed. p 404

Early warning signals (Danger signals) of cancer are:

- Lump/Hard area in the breast
- Change in a wart or mole
- Unexplained weight loss
- Excessive blood loss (Monthly periods or outside usual dates)
- Blood loss (Any natural orifice)
- Persistent change in digestive and bowel habits
- Persistent cough or hoarseness
- Swelling or sore that does not heal

36. Ans. (c) 90%

Ref: K. Park, 24th ed. p 406

Approximately 90% of oral cancers in South East Asia are linked to tobacco chewing and tobacco smoking. Alcohol has a synergistic effect in tobacco users.

- Most common form of tobacco chewing in India is betel quid.
- 2012 estimated incidence of Oral cancer was 10 cases per 1,00,000 populations for males and 4 per 100000 population in females. The estimated mortality was about 6.7 per 100,000 in males and 3 per 100,000 in females.
- Precancerous lesions (Leukoplakia, erythroplakia) can be detected about 15 years prior to their change to an invasive carcinoma.

Also Know......................

- Epidermoid carcinoma of hard palate is associated with the habit of reverse smoking of cigar (chutta)

37. Ans. (c) Lung cancer

Ref: K. Park, 24th ed. p 401

38. Ans. (c) Lung cancer

Ref: K. Park, 24th ed. p 401

OBESITY

39. Ans. (a) Weight (kg)/Height2 (m 2)

Ref: K. Park, 24th ed. p 417

$$\textbf{Body Mass Index } (\textbf{\textit{Quetelet's index}}) = \frac{\text{Weight (kg)}}{\text{Height}^2\text{ (m)}}$$

Body mass index (BMI) is a simple index commonly used to classify underweight, overweight and obesity in adults.

- BMI values are age-independent and the same for both sexes.Q
- BMI does not distinguish between weights associated with muscle and weight associated with fat.
- Percentage of body fat mass increases with age up to 60–65 years in both sexes (higher in women than in men of equivalent BMI.)

40. Ans. (b) Preobese

Ref: K. Park, 24th ed. p 417

41. Ans. (b) 18.50 – 24.99

Ref: K. Park, 24th ed. p 417

42. Ans. (b) 1.0

Ref: K. Park, 24th ed. p 418

A Waist-hip ratio *(WHR) > 1.0 in men and > 0.85 in women indicates abdominal fat accumulation.*[Q]

43. Ans. (a) Less than 0.85

Ref: K. Park, 24th ed. p 418

44. Ans. (c) 25

Ref: K. Park, 24th ed. p 417

45. Ans. (a) Height (cm)/cube root of body weight (kg)

Ref: K. Park, 24th ed. p 418

46. Ans. (c) >30

Ref: K. Park, 24th ed. p 417

47. Ans. (a) 25-29.99

Ref: K. Park, 24th ed. p 417

48. Ans. (b) 18.5-24.99

Ref: K. Park, 24th ed. p 417

49. Ans. (d) Corpulence index

Ref: K. Park, 24th ed. p 418

50. Ans. (b) 30

Ref: K. Park, 24th ed. p 417

BLINDNESS

51. Ans. (b) 6/9

Ref: Sunderlal Textbook of PSM, 4th ed, p-641

52. Ans. (d) 0.3%

Ref: K. Park, 23rd ed. p 439; 24th ed. p 458

Prevalence of blindness in India (2006- National Survey on Blindness) is 1% and estimated childhood blindness/low vision is 0.8 per 1000

- Goal is to reduce prevalence of blindness to 0.5% by 2010 and 0.3% by 2020

53. Ans. (a) Cataract

Ref: K. Park, 24th ed. p 420

Most Common Causes of Blindness in India

- Cataract (62.6%)
- Refractive error (19.7%)
- Glaucoma (5.8%)
- Posterior segment pathology (4.7%)
- Surgical complication (1.2%)
- Corneal opacity /Posterior capsular opacification (0.9%).
  - Globally most common cause of blindness is Cataract followed by Glaucoma

Also Know.......................

- **Retinopathy of Prematurity** (ROP) is an important emerging cause of childhood blindness. Prematurity and Low birth weight are important risk factors for ROP.

54. Ans. (d) Cataract, refractive error, glaucoma, corneal opacity

Ref: K. Park, 24th ed. p 420

55. Ans. (c) August and September

Ref: K. Park, 24th ed. p 459

National Eye donation fortnight is organized from 25th August to 8th September

- Objective- To promote eye donation and eye banking
- Gujarat, Tamil Nadu, Maharashtra, Andhra Pradesh are leading states

56. Ans. (c) Severe visual impairment

Ref: K. Park, 24th ed. p 419

- Vision less than 6/60 or less in better eye, with correction and/or visual field <10°central = Legal blind

57. Ans. (c) Less than 3/60 in better eye

58. Ans. (b) Conjunctival Xerosis >0.5%

Ref: WHO - Xerophthalmia and night blindness for the assessment of clinical vitamin A deficiency in individuals and populations. WHO_NMH_NHD_EPG_14.4

Prevalence criteria for determining the public health significance of Xerophthalmia and Vitamin A deficiency in children (6 months to 6 years)

Indicator	Minimum prevalence, %
Night blindness (XN)	>1
Bitot spots (X1B)	>0.5
Corneal xerosis/corneal ulceration/ keratomalacia (X2/X3A/X3B)	>0.01
Corneal scar (XS)	>0.05

Prevalence of night blindness to define a public health problem and its level of importance among children aged 24–71 months

	Degree of public health problem, %		
	High	Moderate	Severe
Prevalence of night blindness	0.01–0.99	1- 4.9	5 or more

59. Ans. (b) 19.7%

Ref: K. Park, 24th ed. p 420

60. Ans. (d) Onchocerciasis

Ref: K. Park, 24th ed. p 422

61. Ans. (b) Underestimation

Ref: K. Park, 24th ed. p 420

- If blindness is surveyed using schools as against population surveys – It would lead to underestimation of prevalence of blindness in country (Prevalence of blindness in childhood is very less i.e<0.08%).

62. Ans. (d) 0.75

Ref: Disability assessment and certification Guidelines and explanations, National Institute for Orthopaedically Handicapped

Category of visual impairment	Better Eye	Worse Eye	Percentage of Impairment
0	6/9–6/18	6/24-6/36	20%
1	6/18–6/36	6/60–Nil	40%
2	6/40–4/60 or Field of vision 10°-20°	3/60–Nil	75%
3,4,5,	3/60-Nil or Field of vision 10°	Finger Count at 1 feet -Nil	100%

63. Ans. (a) 3/60

Ref: K. Park, 24th ed. p 419

WHO defined blindness as "*Visual acquity <3/60 (Snellen) or its equivalent (inability to count fingers in day light at a distance of 3 meters).*"

ROAD TRAFFIC ACCIDENT

64. Ans. (c) 30 days

Ref: K. Park, 24th ed. p 423

"Killed" in a road traffic accident is defined as death of any person outright or within 30 days as a result of the accident

Mortality in RTA is assessed in terms of

- Proportional mortality rate,
- Deaths per million population
- Death rate per 1000 (or 100,000) registered vehicles per year
- Accidents (fatalities) per number of vehicles per kilometer or passengers per kilometer
- Deaths of vehicle occupant~ per 1000 vehicles per year
- Morbidity in a RTA is measured in terms of "serious injuries" and "slight injuries"

Also Know......................

- **"Abbreviated Injury Scale"** is used to assess the seriousness of the injury

65. Ans. (b) 10.6 per 100,000 population.

Ref: NCRB Report 2014. http://ncrb.nic.in/

- Number of suicides in the country during the decade (2004–2014) recorded an increase of 15.8%
- Number of suicides in 2014 were 1,31,666 and rate of suicide was 1.06 per lakh population
- Rate of suicides is showing declining trend since 2010
- Number of male victims were more than females in all means of suicides except 'Fire/Self-immolation'.
- Highest suicides were reported in Maharashtra, followed by Tamil Nadu and West Bengal (i.e. 12.4%, 12.2% and 10.9% respectively of total suicides)
- In male—maximum suicides were committed by self-employed, followed by daily wagers
- In females maximum suicides were committed by housewives followed by students and self-employed
- Government servants accounted for 1.7% of total suicide victims as compared to 4.7% victims from Private Sector Enterprises.

66. Ans. (b) Hanging

Ref: NCRB Report 2014. http://ncrb.nic.in

Percentage of means/mode adopted by victims to commit suicide

SL	Means/mode adopted	Percentage and number	
		2014	2015
(1)	(2)	(3)	(4)
1. Consuming sleeping pills		0.5% (714)	0.5% (645)
2. Drowning		5.6% (7,426)	5.4% (7,267)
3. Fire/self immolation		6.9% (9,122)	7.2% (9,558)
4. Firearms		0.4% (507)	0.4% (469)
5. By hanging		41.8% (55, 050)	45.6% (60, 952)
6. By poison		26.0% (34, 254)	27.9% (37, 232)
7. By self infecting injury		0.4% (566)	0.4% (572)
8. By jumping		1.1% (1,408)	1.8% (2,382)
9. By coming under running vehicles/trains		2.6% (3,387)	2.5% (3,338)
10. By touching electric wire		0.6% (752)	0.7% (954)
11. By other means		14.0% (18,480)	7.7% (10,254)
Total		100.0	100.0

Data from NCRB (national crime records bureau) 2015 update

Also Know......................

- **Herbicide poisoning** is second most common method of suicide in India and it is associated with high morbidity and mortality. Among different herbicidal poisonings the most predominantly found poisonings are paraquat and glyphosate. These compounds are highly toxic and their poisonings require proper management techniques. High fatality is seen in these cases which are mainly due to its inherent toxicity and lack of effective treatment. Common symptoms of these poisonings includes gastrointestinal corrosive effects with mouth and throat, epigastric pain and dysphagia, acid-base imbalance, pulmonary edema, shock and arrhythmia.

67. Ans. (c) Prevention of injury

Ref: Rajiv Bhalawar, Textbook of Community Medicine, p 638

Haddon Matrix

	Host Factors (Intrinsic or Extrinsic)	Agent of Energy or Vehicle (Mechanical/ Thermal/ Electrical/ Chemical)	Physical Environment	Social Environment
Pre-Event				
Event				
Post Event				

Haddon's Matrix combines the elements of an epidemiology triangle (host, agent, and environment) and levels of prevention (Pre-accident, during accident and postaccident) to explain the causation and prevention of accidents.

It assess the contributory factors from the perspective of:

- Host or Human Factors (Intrinsic – Age, sex preexisting medical condition or Extrinsic – Fatigue, Alcohol)
- Agent of Energy or Vehicle (Motor vehicle, electric wire, animals)
- Physical Environment (Good roads, street light)
- Social Environment (enforcement of seat belt laws, efficient traffic policing)

It combines the contributory factors with time phases

- Pre-Event: Factors affect the host before occurrence of the event.
- Event: Factors related to the crash or accident
- Post-Event: Factors related to the Post-Event Phase

68. Ans. (b) Road traffic accident

Ref: K. Park, 24th ed. p 424

Accidents and injuries in India in decreasing order.

1. Road traffic accidents it is the most common cause of fatal accident in India comprising of (2.1% of all causes of death.
2. Work related injuries
3. Falls
4. Drowning
5. Poisoning
6. Burn or Fire
7. Violence

MISCELLANEOUS

69. Ans. (c) Correct packaging

Ref: Current Scenario of Spurious and Substandard Medicines in India: A Systematic Review, Indian J Pharm Sci. 2015 Jan-Feb; 77(1): 2-7. AN Khan, RK Khar

International Medical Products Anti-counterfeiting Taskforce (IMPACT) of World Health Organization defines SFFC (Spurious/Falsely-labeled/Falsified/Counterfeit) medicines as

- Medicines deliberately and fraudulently mislabeled with respect to identity and/or source
- Medicines with correct ingredients or with the wrong ingredients, without active ingredients, with insufficient or too much active ingredient
- Medicines with fake packaging.

70. Ans. (a) Central Drugs Standard Control...

Ref: http://www.cdsco.nic.in/

The Central Drugs Standard Control Organization (CDSCO) is the Central Drug Authority for discharging functions assigned to the Central Government under the Drugs and Cosmetics Act.

- Regulatory control over the import of drugs
- Approval of new drugs and clinical trials
- Meetings of Drugs Consultative Committee (DCC) and Drugs Technical Advisory Board (DTAB)
- Approval of certain licenses as Central License Approving Authority is exercised by the CDSCO.

Also Know...

- Regulation of manufacture, sale and distribution of drugs is primarily the concern of the State authorities.
- Central Authorities are responsible for approval of New Drugs, Clinical Trials, laying down standards for Drugs, control over the quality of imported drugs, coordination of the activities of State Drug Control Organizations and providing expert advice
- Drug Controller General of India is responsible for approval of licenses of specified categories of Drugs such as blood and blood products, IV Fluids, Vaccine and Sera.

71. Ans. (c) Screening among school children

Ref: K. Park, 23rd ed. p 380-81; 24th ed. p- 399; Julie Munden, Disease Management for Nurse Practitioners, p-126

72. Ans. (d) HPV 16,18

Ref: Practical Management of Gynecological Problems - Page 190 K. Kaarthigeyan, Cervical cancer in India and HPV vaccination Indian J Med Paediatr Oncol. 2012 Jan-Mar; 33(1): 7–12.

HPV serotypes 16 and 18 account for nearly 76.7% of cervical cancer in India.

Worldwide, HPV-16 and 18 contribute over 70% of all cervical cancer cases HPV-16 50–60% and HPV-18 in at least 10–12%).

73. Ans. (b) Measles induced blindness

Ref: K. Park, 23rd ed. p 404

74. Ans. (d) 30

Ref: K. Park, 23rd ed. p 399

75. Ans. (b) Height – 100 = Weight

Ref: K. Park, 23rd ed. p 399

76. Ans. (b) Management of diabetes and hypertension

Ref: K. Park, 24th ed. p 388

NPCB

77. Ans. (b) Vision < 4/60 in better eye

Ref: NPCB, MOHFW, GOI (http://npcb.nic.in/index1.asp?linkid=55)

Blindness under the "National Program for Control of Blindness and Visual Impairment" (Earlier -National Program for Control of Blindness) is defined as:

- Presenting distance visually acuity less than 3/60(20/400) in the better eye
- Limitation of field of vision to be less than 10 degrees from center of fixation

78. Ans. (b) 1976

Ref: K. Park, 24th ed. p 439

NPCB: National Program for Control of Blindness was launched in the year 1976

Also Know......................

New Initiatives under NPCB in 12th Five year plan

- Setting up of 400 Multipurpose District Mobile Ophthalmic Units (₹30 lakh per unit) in district hospitals.
- Distribution of 10 lakh spectacles (₹100 per spectacle) to geriatric population suffering from presbyopia.

79. Ans. (c) District collector

Ref: Website – NPCB http://npcb.nic.in/writereaddata/mainlinkfile/File106.pdf; 24th ed. p Sunderlal Textbook of PSM, 4th edition, p-639-40

Composition of District Blindness Control Society (Maximum 15 members comprising not more than 8 ex-official members)

- Chairman: District Collector/Magistrate
- Vice-Chairman: Chief Medical Officer
- Member Secretary: District Program Manager
- Technical advisor: Chief Ophthalmic Surgeon or HOD Ophthalmology of Medical College
- Members – Medical superintendent, District Education Officer, Project Director DRDA, Ophthalmic surgeon of Mobile eye unit, President IMA, 3 representative of NGO, District mass media officer and practicing ophthalmic surgeons

Functions of DBCS

- To estimate the magnitude and spread of blindness in the district by village wise active case finding
- To periodically review and monitor implementation of the district action plan
- To coordinate activities of Govt., Non Govt. and NGO
- To motivate people for eye donations

Also Know......................

Composition of State Health Society

- Chairman: State Mission Director/Secretary, Vice Chairman: Director Health Services and Member Secretary: Joint/Dy. Director (from state cadre).

80. Ans. (d) 20000

Ref: K. Park, 24th ed. p 460

81. Ans. (a) Surgery

Ref: Sunderlal Text book of PSM, 4th ed. p-642; 24th ed. p 642

SAFE strategy for control of Trachoma:

S → Surgery for entropion or trichiasis
A → Antibiotics (Oral Azithromycin)
F → Facial hygiene
E → Environmental modification (sanitation)

Latest Updates

WHO Simplified Trachoma Grading Scale (Based on clinical examination with a loupe (X-2-2.5) or Examination of conjunctival slides with loupe)

- TF (Trachomatous Inflammation –Follicular)- ≥ 5 follicles on upper tarsal conjunctiva
- TI (Trachomatous Inflammation-Intense)-Inflammatory thickening of upper tarsal conjunctiva obscuring >50% of deep tarsal vessels.

82. Ans. (c) Sentinel surveillance

Ref: NPCB Document, GOI, DK Taneja, Health Policies and Programmes in India,13th ed. p-390; 24th ed. p 390

Latest Updates

25 Sentinel surveillance units have been established in department of ophthalmology and PSM in medical college in India for assessment of:

- Beneficiary profiles
- Visual outcome based on cataract surgery records
- Follow up of operated cases
- Ocular morbidity data

NPCDCS

83. Ans. (a) 7th November

Ref: K. Park, 24th ed. p 279

84. Ans. (c) District hospital has specialized facilities

Ref: K Park, 23rd ed. p 471 -73. DK Taneja, Health Policies and Programmes in India,13th ed. p-400

85. Ans. (d) CHC has facilities for diagnosis and treatment of CVD, diabetes

Ref: K Park, 23rd ed. p 471 -73. DK Taneja, Health Policies and Programmes in India, 13th ed. p-400

86. Ans. (d) Integration with national cancer control program

Ref: K Park, 23rd ed. p 471 -73. DK Taneja, Health Policies and Programmes in India,13th ed. p-400; 24th ed. p 493

Revised NPCDCS (12th Plan)

- NCD Flexi-pool under NRHM
- All interventions of the NPCDCS up to District level and below are integrated within NRHM.
- Separate tertiary cancer care component.

MISCELLANEOUS

87. Ans. (d) National Program for prevention and control of cancer, diabetes, cardiovascular diseases and Stroke

Ref: K. Park, 24th ed. p 493

88. Ans. (b) 6 bedded

The burn unit in a District hospital will have 6 beds (4 general beds + 2 acute care beds) and other facilities. In order to prevent infection, there will be packaged type air cooled/water cooled units with requisite number of air changers

89. Ans. (a) Hypertension, (c) Increase Triglycerides, (d) Increase blood glucose

Metabolic syndrome features are:

- Large waist — A waistline that measures at least 35 inches (89 cms) for women and 40 inches (102 cms) for men
- High triglyceride level — 150 mg/dL, or 1.7 mmol/L, or higher
- Low HDL cholesterol — Less than 40 mg/dL (1.04 mmol/L) in men or less than 50 mg/dL (1.3 mmol/L) in women
- Increased blood pressure — 130/85 mmHg or higher
- Elevated fasting blood sugar — 100 mg/dL (5.6 mmol/L) or higher

90. Ans. (a) Weight reduction, (b) Adopting DASH diet, (c) Physical exercise, (e) Tracking of hypertension

Prevention of Hypertension

Prevention of Hypertension – strategies are:

- Primary strategies
  - Population strategy
    - DASH diet/nutrition
    - Weight reduction
    - Physical exercise/self-care/behavioural changes
  - High risk strategy
    - Tracking of hypertension
- Secondary prevention
  - Early case detection
  - Treatment for hypertension
  - Compliance and adequacy of treatment

91. Ans. (a) Human papilloma virus is the most common cause of cervical cancer in India, (c) All females age 30 years and above should get cervix cancer screening every 5 years in primary health care setting

Ref: Park 25th ed. Pg 417

Cancer Screening Guidelines, FOGSI 2018

Option	T/F	Comment
Human papilloma virus is the most common cause of cervical cancer in India	T	Yes, correct. more than 95% of all cases have been found to have associated HPV infection
Highest incidence is in females age 25- 65 years	F	No, the peak incidence of cases is from 25-45 years of age and then the incidence gradually lowers with advancing age
All females age 30 years and above should get cervix cancer screening every 5 years in primary health care setting	T	Yes correct (refer FOGSI 2018 guidelines)
PAP smear is screening test of choice for CA Cervix at a field centre or primary health centre	F	No, at PHC or low resource setting, VIA (visual inspection with acetic acid) is the method of choice for initial screening for Ca Cervix
HPV vaccine may be given to males to prevent HPV transmission and cervical cancer in females	F	No, HPV vaccine may be given to males, but to prevent higher risk for genital warts, penile cancer, and anal cancers in men

Cervical Cancer Screening protocol – FOGSI 2018

	Good resource setting	Limited resource setting
Modality	HPV testing ▪ Primary HPV testing\ ▪ Co-testing (HPV & Cytology) Cytology Colposcopy and biopsy VIA	VIA (visual inspection with acetic acid) Colposcopy ± Biopsy

	Good resource setting	Limited resource setting
Target Age Group (years)	25 - 65	30 - 65 (In postmenopausal women, screening with VIA may not be as effective)
Age to start (years)	Cytology at 25 Primary HPV Testing/ Co-testing at 30 years	30 years
Frequency	Primary HPV Testing or Co-testing - every 5 years Cytology – every 3 years	Every 5 years (at least 1-3 times in a lifetime)
Age to stop	▪ 65 years with consistent negative results in last 15 years ▪ Women with no prior screening should undergo tests once at 65 years and, if negative, they should exit screening.	
Follow-up method after treatment; interval	HPV testing (preferred) or Cytology 12 months	VIA (12 monthly)
Screening in hysterectomized women	▪ Following hysterectomy in which cervix was removed for benign causes : no need for screening, unless there is history of previous cervical intraepithelial neoplasia ▪ Absence of cervix must be confirmed by clinical records or examination ▪ If indications for hysterectomy unclear, screening may be performed at clinician's discretion	
F/up with CIN in hysterectomy HPE report	Need to be screened with HPV at 6 months and 18 months	

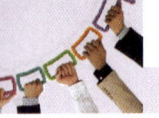

92. Ans. (a) Early diagnosis, (b) Treatment with Anti-hypertensive drug

Ref: Park 25th, pg: 406

Option	T/F	Remarks
▪ Early diagnosis	False	No, primary prevention – is to remove the risk factors and to prevent the disease. early case detection, treatment and compliance to treatment constitute secondary level of prevention.
▪ Treatment with Anti-hypertensive drug	False	No, primary prevention – is to remove the risk factors and to prevent the disease
▪ Low salt intake	True	Yes, primary prevention – is to remove the risk factors and to prevent the disease. Low salt intake is preventive measure for Hypertension
▪ Reduction in weight	True	Yes, primary prevention – is to remove the risk factors and to prevent the disease. Life style modification, exercise and reduction in weight is preventive measure for hypertension
▪ Regular exercise	True	No, primary prevention – is to remove the risk factors and to prevent the disease. Regular exercise will help prevent hypertension

Primary Prevention

- Nutritional changes
- Weight reduction
- Exercise promotion
- Behavioral changes
- Health education and self care

Secondary Prevention

- Early case detection
- Treatment
- Compliance to treatment

93. Ans. (a) Of more than 3 months duration

Chronic illness has been defined by various organizations with different criteria, grossly leading to a common point of chronicity and non-communicability of the condition.

U.S. National Center for Health Statistics

- The Chronic diseases are those - lasting 3 months or more. Chronic diseases generally cannot be prevented by vaccines or cured by medication, nor do they just disappear

WHO Defines Chronic Illness as

- These not transmitted from person to person.
- They are of long duration and generally slow progression.
- The four main types have been classified as
  - Cardiovascular diseases
  - Cancers
  - Chronic respiratory conditions
  - Metabolic disease as diabetes

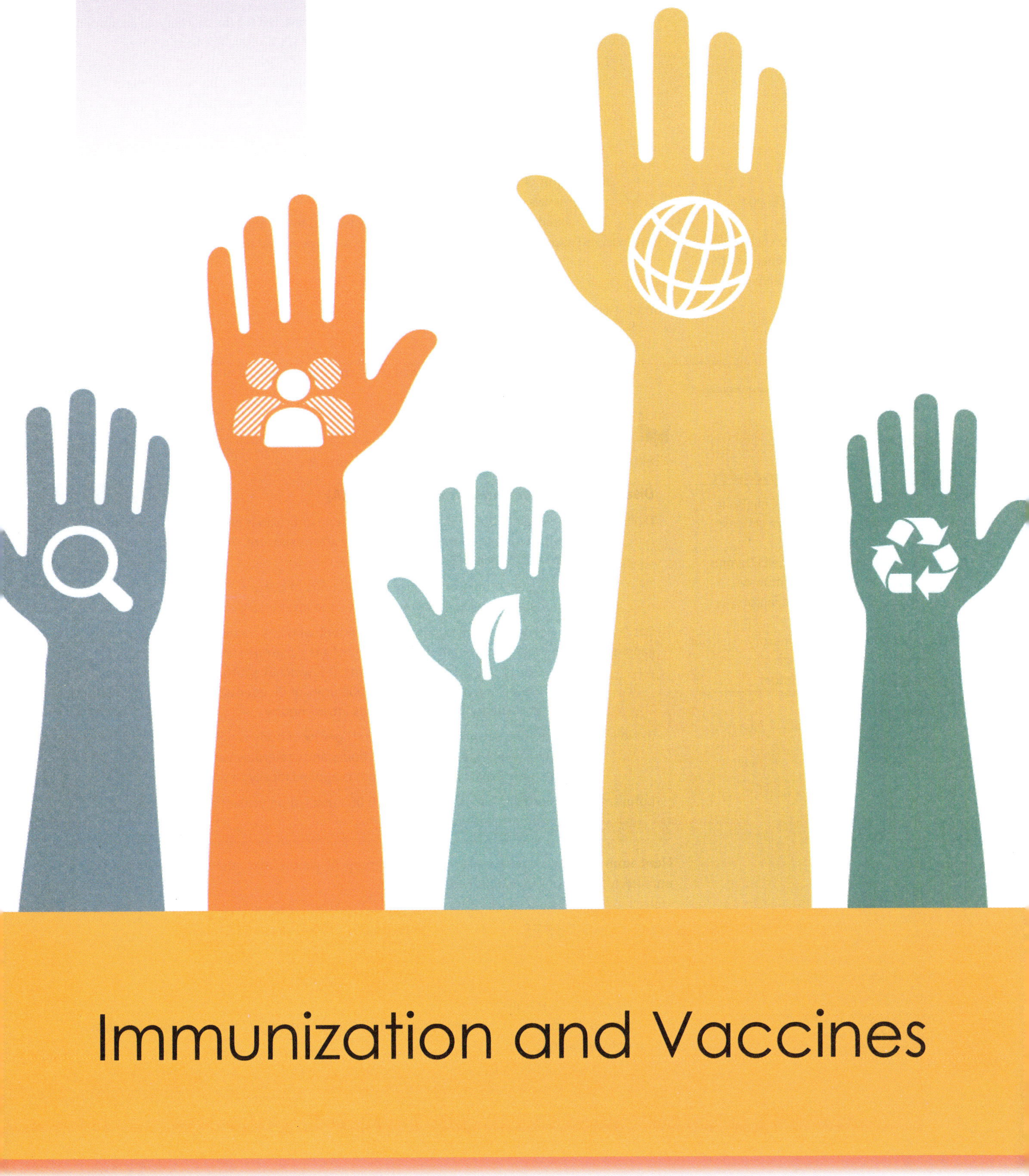

Immunization and Vaccines

Chapter Outline

93 Must Remember

- **Humoral immunity:** B-Cell (Bone marrow) mediated, Five classes: IgM, IgG, IgA, IgE, IgD
- **Cellular immunity:** T-cell (Thymus derived) mediated immunity, Includes the cytotoxic factors, antigen recognition cells, mononuclear inflammatory reactions, secretion of immunological mediators

151 High Yield Points

The proportion of immune individuals in a population above which a disease may no longer exist is known as ***herd immunity threshold***

IMMUNITY

Active Immunity

The immune response

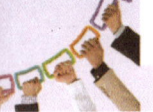

- **Primary immune response:** When an antigen is administered for the first time to an animal or human who is never exposed, there is production of antibodies. The features are:
  - Latent period of 3–10 days
  - IgM antibody arises first followed by IgG (if the antigenic stimulus was sufficient)
  - It is the fundamental mechanism for production of the memory cells
- **Secondary immune response:** Arises following the primary immune response. The features are:
  - Shorter latent period
  - Production of antibody is rapid
  - Higher levels and abundant antibody
  - The elicited antibody has higher capacity to bind to the antigen

* The accelerated response is probably due to the previous sensitization and the immunological memory

Passive Immunity

Administration of 'ready-made' antibodies

- Rapid establishment of immunity
- Temporary immunity
- No education of the Reticuloendothelial cells – no immunological memory

94 Must Remember

Table 1: Passive immunization procedures with antisera

Disease	Passive immunization (ANTISERA)
Diphtheria	A dose of 500–1,000 of IU of diphtheria antitoxin is given intramuscularly to susceptible contacts immediately after exposure. Protection does not last more than 2–3 weeks
Tetanus	The usual prophylactic dose is 1,500 units of horse A.T.S. given subcutaneously or intramuscularly, soon after injury
Gas gangrene	A polyvalent antitoxin is used. A patient who has sustained a wound possibly contaminated with spores of gas gangrene should receive a dose of 10,000 IU of Cl. perfringens. (Cl. welchii) antitoxin, 5,000 units of Cl. septicum antitoxin and 10,000 units of Cl. edematiens antitoxin, intramuscularly, or in urgent cases intravenously
Rabies	Antirabies serum in a dose of 40 IU per kg of body weight should be given intramuscularly within 72 hours and preferably within 24 hours of exposure. A part of the antiserum is applied locally to the wound
Botulism	When botulism is suspected, 10,000 units of polyvalent antitoxin are recommended every 3–4 hours

Herd immunity: Vaccination of a particular group of people may provide protection to the unprotected or unvaccinated individuals

VACCINE TYPES

Live Vaccines

BCG, Measles, and oral polio

- Prepared from live attenuated organisms (*cannot induce full-blown disease but retain immunogenicity*)

- ***Not be administered to*** *people with* immunodeficiency diseases, leukemia, lymphoma or malignancy or on therapy with corticosteroids, alkylating agents, antimetabolic agents, or radiation.[Q]
- Live vaccines are contraindicated in pregnancy unless the risk of infection exceeds the risk of harm to the fetus.
- Immunity is achieved with a single dose (except polio vaccine)[Q] and is durable.
- Live vaccines must be properly stored to retain effectiveness.

Inactivated or Killed Vaccines

- Safe but *less efficacious than live vaccines.*
- *Require a primary series of 2 or 3 doses of vaccine to produce an adequate antibody response* and in most cases "*booster*" injections are required.
- Duration of immunity following the use of inactivated vaccines varies from months to many years.
- *Only absolute contraindication* is severe local or general reaction to a previous dose.

Subunit Vaccine

(Prepared from extracted cellular fractions).

- High efficacy and safety

Types of subunit Vaccine

- **Toxoids (Detoxicated Toxins):** E.g. Diphtheria, Tetanus, Anthrax
- **Protein Vaccine:** Influenza vaccine (Hemagglutinin and Neuraminidase) and acellular pertussis vaccines
- **Recombinant protein vaccine:** Antigens are expressed on *E. coli*, yeast, mammalian cells, etc

Advantage and disadvantage

- **Advantage:** Safe
- **Disadvantage:** Less immunogenic and need an adjuvant to enhance efficacy E.g. Hepatitis B, HPV Vaccine.

Table 2: Types of vaccine and their viral and bacterial infections

Vaccine	Viral	Bacterial	Rickettsial
Live attenuated	Polio (OPV/Sabin), Yellow fever Measles, Mumps, Rubella, Influenza, JE (SA 14-14-2) Varicella, Rotavirus	BCG, Typhoid (oral) Plague	Epidemic typhus
Killed	Polio (Salk/IPV), KFD, Influenza, Hepatitis B and A, Japanese encephalitis, Rabies	Typhoid (IM), Plague, Cholera, Pertussis, Cerebrospinal Meningitis	Typhus
Toxoid		Diphtheria, Tetanus, Anthrax	
Protein		Acellular Pertussis, Influenza (HA and NA)	
Polysaccharides		Pneumococcal vaccine, Meningococcal vaccine, Typhoid (Vi), Hib	
Recombinant	Hepatitis B, HPV	Cholera Toxin B, Lyme disease	

Mixed Formulation Vaccine

DPT, DT, DP, MMR → Simplify administration, reduces costs and minimize number of contacts of patient with health system.

Polyvalent vaccines → Vaccines (e.g., polio, influenza) prepared from 2 or more strains of same species.

Autogenous vaccine → It is applied when the organism in the vaccine is obtained from the same patient.

Freeze-dried vaccines (e.g., BCG, yellow fever, and measles) are more stable preparations than liquid vaccines.

100 **Good to Remember**

2 live vaccines can be given simultaneously at different sites or with an interval of at least 3 weeks[Q].

101 **Good to Remember**

Live vaccines are more potent than the killed vaccines

152 **High Yield Points**

- **Polysaccharide vaccines:** Antibody is produced against capsular polysaccharide of pathogenic bacteria. **Disadvantage:** Serotype specific immune response.
  Hib, Salmonella typhimurium, Meningococcal vaccine, Pneumococcal vaccine
- **Conjugate vaccines:** Polysaccharide antigen is chemically linked to a protein recognized by T cell. **Advantage:** More Effective in children < 2 years age. **Disadvantage:** Serotype specific. E.g. Pneumococcal vaccine, Men ACWY

Immunoglobulins Used in Public Health

Table 3: Sources of immunoglobulins

Human Immuno-globulins	Human normal Ig	Hepatitis A, Measles, Rabies, Tetanus, Mumps
	Human specific Ig	Hepatitis B, Varicella, Diphtheria
Non-human (Antisera)	Bacterial	Diphtheria, Tetanus, Gas gangrene, Botulism
	Viral	Rabies

Administration of antisera may occasionally give rise to serum sickness and anaphylactic shock

VACCINE CONSTITUENTS

Adjuvants

Adjuvant (Immune enhancer) promote a stronger immune response to the antigen).

- Inactivated and subunit vaccines usually require an adjuvant.
- Reduce amount of antigen per dose of vaccine and number of dose needed to attain full immunity
- MF59, AS03, AF03 are oil (Squalene) in water emulsion used as adjuvant in pandemic influenza vaccines and newer vaccines.
- Aluminum hydroxide, Aluminum phosphate and Potassium aluminum sulfate (Alum) used as adjuvant in Diphtheria, Tetanus, Pneumococcal, hepatitis (A and B) vaccines.

153 *High Yield Points*

Table 4: Human vaccine adjuvants

Name	Class	Components	Vaccine
Alum	Mineral salts	Aluminum phosphate, aluminum hydroxide	Diphtheria, tetanus, pneumococcus, HAV, HBV, anthrax, tick-borne encephalitis, MenC, HPV
MF59	Oil-in-water emulsion	Squalene, Tween 80, Span 85	Seasonal and pandemic influenza
AS03	Oil-in-water emulsion	Squalene, Tween 80, α-tocopherol	Pandemic influenza
AF03	Oil-in-water emulsion	Squalene, Montane 80, Eumulgin B1PH	Pandemic influenza
Virosomes	Liposomes	Phospholipids, cholesterol, HA	Seasonal influenza, HAV
AS04	Alum-absorbed TLR4 agonist	Aluminum hydroxide, MPL	HBV, HPV
RC-529	Alum-absorbed TLR4 agonist	Aluminum hydroxide, synthetic MPL	HBV

Abbreviations: HAV, hepatitis A virus; HBV, hepatitis B virus; HPV, human papillomavirus; Men, meningococcus, MPL, monophosphoryl liped A; TLR, toll-like receptor

Other Constituents

- **Excipient** are inert substances other than active ingredient included in the manufacturing process or contained in a finished pharmaceutical product.
- **Preservatives** → Stop unwanted microbial contamination of vaccines.
  - Example: Phenoxyethanol (Most commonly used preservative), Phenol and Thiomersal.
- **Stabilizers** → Inhibit chemical reactions and prevent components separating or sticking to vial during transport and storage
  - Examples: Lactose, Sucrose, Amino acids (glycine) and their salts (Monosodium glutamate), Albumin, Gelatin
- **Buffers** → Resist changes in pH, adjust tonicity and maintain osmolarity.
  - Most commonly used buffer is sodium chloride (table salt).
- **Diluents** → Liquid used to dilute a vaccine to proper concentration prior to administration
  - Distilled water – Measles; Normal saline – BCG; Phosphate buffer – JE Vaccine

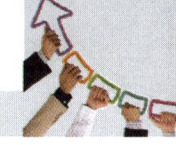

- **Surfactants or emulsifiers** → Wetting agents that alter the surface tension of a liquid and lower the tension between two liquids
    - Example: Polysorbate 80 (Tween)
- **Residuals** → Minute quantities of substances, used during manufacturing or production process of individual vaccines
- Antibiotics:
    - Neomycin/or polymyxin B used in varicella (chickenpox) vaccines, some influenza vaccines, DTPa, IPV and MMR vaccine –To prevent bacterial contamination of tissue culture cell in which virus is cultivated
    - Gentamicin is used in some influenza vaccines
    - Streptomycin/Neomycin in IPV
- Other products used in manufacturing of vaccine are—Cell culture fluids, egg proteins, yeast, antibiotics, inactivating agents (Formaldehyde, glutaraldehyde)

STRAINS OF VACCINE

Table 5: Vaccines and their strains

Vaccine	Strain
Rubella	RA 27/3
Measles	Edmonston-Zagreb (Aerosolized), Schwarz and Moraten (Heat Stable)
OPV/IPV	P1 and P3
Mumps	Jeryl Lynn, RIT 4835, L Zagreb, Leningrad-3, Urabe
JE Vaccine	SA-14-14-2, Nakayama (killed vaccine)
Chicken pox/ varicella	OKA
Yellow fever	17 D
BCG	Danish 1331
Typhoral	Ty 21A
Potential vaccine-HIV	Modified Vaccine Ankara (MVA), Recombinant Adeno Associated Virus (RAAV), AIDSVAX
Dengue Vaccine-Dengvaxia	CYD-TDV
Malaria vaccine	RTS, S/AS01

154 ***High Yield Points***

Marc Koska invented nonreusable K1 auto disable syringe

VACCINATION UPDATE—2016-2018

- The successful elimination of polio and **polio free certification** of India and SEARO on 27th March, 2014 is a public health milestone which is a credit for the entire health workforce. India's commitment to a world free of polio is reiterated by the introduction of IPV as an additional dose along with the 3rd dose of OPV on 30th November, 2016.
- **Rotavirus vaccine** has been approved by the Government of India for inclusion into the UIP with the phase 1 launch of the vaccine in 4 states (Himachal Pradesh, Odisha, Andhra Pradesh and Haryana) in February, 2016.
- **Rubella vaccine** has been approved for introduction as MR vaccine, thus replacing the measles containing vaccine first dose (MCV1) at 9 months and second dose (MCV2) at 16–24 months.

Pipeline vaccines
Campylobacter jejuni
Chagas disease
Chikungunya
Dengue

Contd...

95 ***Must Remember***

eVIN:

- Electronic Vaccine Intelligence Network (eVIN) is India's solution for ensuring effective management of the immunization supply chain

Immunization Surveillance

- **Fully immunized child:** Fully immunized if s/he has received all the due vaccines up to 1 year of age
- **Complete immunization**: A child is to be considered as completely immunized if s/he has received all the due vaccines up to 2 years of age

Pipeline vaccines
Enterotoxigenic *Escherichia coli*
Enterovirus 71 (EV 71)
Group B Streptococcus (GBS)
Herpes simplex virus
HIV-1
Human Hookworm disease
Leishmaniasis disease
Malaria
Nipah virus
Nontyphoidal salmonella disease
Norovirus
Paratyphoid fever
Respiratory syncytial virus (RSV)
Schistosomiasis disease
Shigella
Staphylococcus aureus
Streptococcus pneumoniae
Streptococcus pyogenes
Tuberculosis
Universal influenza vaccine

155 *High Yield Points*

Vaccine requirement:

- Vaccine beneficiary are estimated as per demographic data and actual head count
- The permissible wastage for vaccine is 10–50%, being maximum for BCG (50%), measles and JE (25%)
- The vaccine multiplicative factor:
  - BCG–2
  - Measles, JE - 1.33
  - Hep B, DPT, OPV, Rotavirus vaccine (RVV), IPV, Pentavalent vaccine, Tetanus toxoid - 1.11

156 *High Yield Points*

- Mission Indradhanush (MI) = 7 times vaccination to under five child, for VPD's (vaccine preventable diseases)
- Intensified Mission Indradhanush (IMI) –7 working days in a month, starting 7th every month, excluding Sunday, holiday and immunization days.

MISSION INDRADHANUSH—UPDATE 2016

The Government of India has launched Mission Indradhanush on 25 December 2014 as a special drive to vaccinate all unvaccinated and partially vaccinated children and pregnant women by 2020 under the Universal Immunization Program.

Focus: To achieve a vaccination coverage of more than 90% by 2020.

Strategy

- Planning at community level
- Communication and social mobilization
- Training of professionals
- Accountability and surveillance
- For 6 VPD prevention for all children under 2 years and pregnant females
- Measles, TB, Hepatitis B, Diphtheria, Polio, Pertussis, Tetanus (+additional diseases: Influenza, Rotavirus, Japanese encephalitis, Rubella)

To implement this: Intensified mission Indradhanush (IMI) was launched in 'selected states and districts' to achieve the **target of more than 90% immunization coverage by December 2018**. IMI will cater to left outs and drop outs in selected districts and some urban areas.

Intensified Mission Indradhanush (IMI) is for:

- Urban slums with migratory population
- Nomadic sites (brick kilns, construction sites, other migrant settlements-fisherman villages, riverine areas with shifting populations, underserved and hard-to-reach populations-forested and tribal populations, hilly areas, etc).
- Areas with low routine immunization coverage identified through measles outbreaks, cases of diphtheria and neonatal tetanus in the last two years.

NATIONAL IMMUNIZATION SCHEDULE

Table 6: National immunization schedule

Ideal age	Vaccine	Special comments
At birth (for institutional deliveries)	BCG and OPV -0 dose, Hep B (birth dose)	▪ OPV -0 dose can be given till 15 days after birth ▪ Hep B (Within 24 hours)
At 6 weeks	BCG (if not given at birth), OPV-1, Pentavalent Vaccine-1 and Rotavirus-1* fIPV-1@, PCV-1***	▪ BCG can be given up to 1 year of age. ▪ **Rotavirus vaccine**- Dose is 5 drops, Storage conditions similar to OPV (Up to district level -20°C and below district 2–8°C), No Open Vial policy (open vial to be discarded in 4 hours), it can be initiated maximum by 1 year age
At 10 weeks	OPV-2, Pentavalent Vaccine-2 and Rotavirus-2*,	▪ Interval between 2 doses should not be less than one month ▪ Pentavalent Vaccine protects against – Diphtheria, Pertussis, Tetanus, Hepatitis B, *H. Influenza* type B associated Pneumonia and Meningitis
At 14 weeks	OPV-3, Pentavalent Vaccine-3* and Rotavirus-3*, fIPV-2@ PCV-2***	▪ If 2nd or 3rd dose in an immunization is delayed, immunization schedule need not be started all over again
At 9 months (complete)	Measles – 1/MR Vaccine, Vit A, JE-1**, PCV-B	▪ Along with Vitamin A- 1st dose 9th month, 2nd 18 month, 3rd to 9th dose at 6 monthly intervals till 5 years of age
At 16–24 months	DPT Booster, OPV Booster, 2nd dose Measles-2/MR-2, 2nd dose of JE vaccine**	
At 5 years	DPT booster	▪ 2nd dose of DPT should be given at 1-month interval if there is no clear history or documented evidence of previous immunization with DPT
At 10 and at 16 years	Td Vaccine$ (tetanus diphtheria toxoid)	▪ 2nd dose of TT vaccine should be given at 1-month interval if there is no clear history or documented evidence of previous immunization with DPT, DT or TT vaccines
National Immunization Schedule (Pregnant Women)		
As early as possible in pregnancy (16 weeks)	Td -1 or Booster	1 dose if previously vaccinated with 2 doses of TT one month apart in the last 3 previous year
One month after TT -1 and ideally before the last month of gestation	TT-2	Interval between 2 doses should not be less than 1 month

**Rotavirus vaccine- At present in Andhra Pradesh, Himachal Pradesh, Odisha and Haryana from 2016.*
***JE vaccination in 110 JE endemic districts.*
****Pneumococcal Vaccine – to be scaled up to whole of the country*
@IPV given as fractional dose (0.1 mL) intradermal route (Right upper arm deltoid)

- Measles-Rubella (MR) vaccination campaign was started in 2016 from few states and scaled up to the whole country
- MCV-1/MR-1 vaccine has also been started in few states in India

$ - Td vaccine is the most recent update in the UIP 2019. TT is now being replaced with TD vaccine for children and pregnant females

Catch-up vaccination can be given up till:

- Measles, Vitamin A and OPV is to be given maximum by 5 years,
- BCG, Pentavalent and Rotavirus (initiation) by 1 year
- Hepatitis B birth dose is given only within 24 hours
- DPT given maximum by 7 years

Table 7: Important vaccines – (Type, dose, route, site, protection offered)

Vaccine	Type	Dose	Route	Site	Till age	Protects against
OPV (Vial -20 doses)	Live attenuated vaccine	2 drops	Oral	Mouth	5 years (OPV 0 Dose within 15 days of age	Poliomyelitis
IPV#	Killed vaccine	0.5 mL	Intramuscular	—		Poliomyelitis
BCG (Diluent: 1 mL sodium chloride; Vial - 10 doses)	Live attenuated freeze-dried vaccine – (Danish 1331 strain)	0.1 mL (0.05 mL for less than 1 month)	Intradermal	Left Upper arm	Till one year of age	Childhood tuberculosis (Meningeal, Military)
DPT (Vial-10 doses) (replaced by Pentavalent vaccine**)	Killed vaccine	0.5 mL	Intramuscular	Outer Mid-thigh (Antero-lateral side of mid-thigh)	Till 7 years of age	Diphtheria, Pertussis, Tetanus
Hepatitis B	Killed Subunit vaccine	0.5 mL	Intramuscular	Outer Mid-thigh (Antero-lateral side of mid-thigh)	Till 1 year of age (Hep B 0 dose – birth dose- to be given within 24 hours of birth)	Hepatitis B
Measles (Diluent: 2.5 mL double distilled water) Vial -5 doses	Live attenuated freeze-dried vaccine Edmonston-Zagreb Strain	0.5 mL	Subcutaneous	Right Upper arm	Till 5 years of age	Measles
TT- (Vial-10 doses)	Toxoid	0.5 mL	Intramuscular	Upper arm (Deltoid)	—	Tetanus
JE Vaccine@	Live attenuated vaccine	0.5 mL	Subcutaneous	Left Upper arm	Till 15 years of age	Japanese encephalitis
HPV vaccine	Inactivated vaccine (Virus Like particle)	0.5 mL	Intramuscular	Upper arm (Deltoid)	—	Cervical cancer
Rotavirus vaccine†	Live attenuated	5 drops	Oral	Mouth	Till 1 year of age	Rotavirus diarrhea
Haemophilus influenzae type B	Killed Subunit vaccine	0.5 mL	Intramuscular	Upper arm	Till 1 year of age	*Haemophilus Influenzae type B* meningitis and pneumonia
Pneumococcal PCV13	Killed Subunit vaccine	0.5 mL	Intramuscular	Upper arm	Till one year of age	Pneumococcal pneumonia and meningitis
MR vaccine##	Live attenuated	0.5 mL	Subcutaneous	Right upper arm	9 months to 15 years	Measles + rubella
Pentavalent vaccine**	—	0.5 mL	Intramuscular	(Anterolateral side of mid-thigh – LEFT	Till 1 year of age	Diphtheria + Pertussis + Tetanus + H Influenza B + Hepatitis B
Td vaccine*	Toxoid	0.5 mL	Intramuscular	Upper arm	2 doses of TT, 4 weeks apart (Note – only one Td dose if complete Td 2 doses was taken within last 3 years)	

*Give Td-2 or Booster doses before 36 weeks of pregnancy. However, give these even if more than 36 weeks have passed. Give Td to a woman in labor, if she has not previously received Td.

**Pentavalent vaccine is introduced in place of DPT and Hep B 1, 2 and 3

† Rotavirus vaccine has been introduced in initially 4 states – Andhra Pradesh, Haryana, Himachal Pradesh and Odisha.

IPV – fractional dose (0.1 mL) intradermal at ages 6 weeks and 14 weeks introduced in select states (Intramuscular or Subcutaneous)

##MR vaccine has been recommended and approved for introduction in place of measles vaccine in the UIP schedule. **If first dose delayed beyond 12 months ensure minimum 1 month gap between 2 MR doses.**

@JE vaccine has been introduced in select endemic districts. **If first dose delayed beyond 12 months ensure minimum 3 months gap between 2 JE doses.**

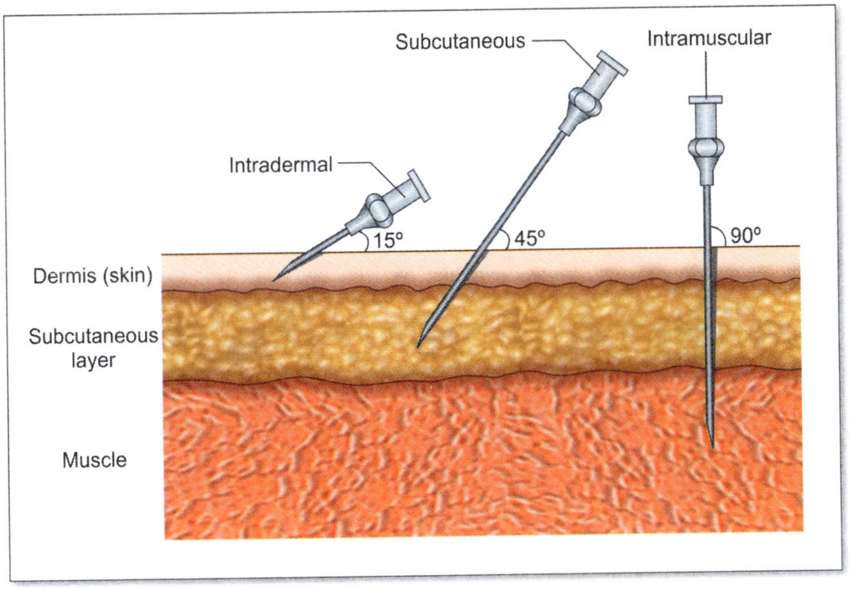

Fig. 1: Needle position and route of administration

157 ***High Yield Points***

Correct site of vaccine – quick recall
- **BCG:** Upper arm **LEFT**
- **DPT and Hep B:** Anterolateral aspect (outer side) of midthigh **LEFT**
- **Pentavalent:** Anterolateral aspect of mid-thigh **LEFT**
- **IPV:** Anterolateral aspect of mid-thigh **RIGHT**
- **Measles/MR:** Upper arm **RIGHT**
- **TT:** Upper arm **RIGHT**
- **JE:** Upper arm **LEFT**

IMMUNIZATION AND GLOBAL HEALTH

Table 8: Other WHO recommended vaccines

All children	Age at 1st dose	Number of Primary doses	Interval	Booster
IPV	6 weeks	4	4 weeks	
H. influenza type B	6 weeks (Minimum) with DPT 1 and 24 months (Maximum)	3	4 weeks (Minimum)	
Pneumococcal	6 weeks (Minimum) with DPT 1	3	4 weeks (Minimum)	
Rotavirus vaccine	6 weeks (Minimum) with DPT 1 and 15 weeks (Maximum)	2 (Rotarix) or 3 (Rotateq)	4 weeks (Minimum), No later than 24 weeks of age	
HPV	9–13 years old girls	3	Between 1st and 2nd 6 months (Minimum – 5 months)	
Recommended in endemic regions				
JE	Mouse brain derived → 6 months	2	4 weeks (Minimum)	
	Live attenuated→ 8 months Live attenuated→ 9 months	1		
Yellow fever	9–12 months with measles	1		
Tick Borne Encephalitis	≥1 year (FMSE-IMMUM and ENCEPUR) ≥1 year (FMSE-IMMUM and ENCEPUR)		Between 1st and 2nd 1–3 months 2nd and 3rd -5–12 months, booster-1 Every 3 years Between 1st and 2nd 1–7 months, 2nd and 3rd -12 months, booster-1 Every 3 years	
Recommended in high risk population				
Typhoid	Vi polysaccharide → 2 years (Minimum)	1		Every 3 years

Contd...

All children	Age at 1st dose	Number of Primary doses	Interval	Booster
	Ty 21a capsule → 5 years (Minimum)	3 or 4	1 day between 1st and 2nd, 2nd-3rd and 3rd and 4th	Every 3–7 years
Meningococcal (Polysaccharide)	2 years (Minimum)	1		
Hepatitis A	1 year (Minimum)	2	6–18 months between 1st and 2nd	
Cholera	Dukoral → 2 years (Minimum)	3 (2-5 years age) 2 (> or = 6 years)	At least 7 days, <6 weeks (Maximum)	Every 6 months Every 2 years
	Shancol and mORCVAX → 1 year (Minimum)	2	14 days	After 2 year
Dengue	CYD-TDV-9 year (Minimum)	3	6 months (Between the 1st and 2nd, 2nd and 3rd	
Mumps	12–18 months with measles vaccine	2	1 month (Minimum) to school entry	

Table 9: Global vaccine action plan 2011–2020

Goal	Target by 2015	Target by 2020
World free of poliomyelitis	Interrupt wild polio virus transmission globally (by 2014)	Certification of poliomyelitis eradication (by 2018)
Meet global and regional elimination targets	▪ Neonatal tetanus eliminated in all WHO regions ▪ Measles eliminated in at least four WHO regions ▪ Rubella congenital rubella syndrome eliminated in at least two WHO regions	
Meet vaccination coverage targets in every region, country and community	Reach 90% national coverage and 80% in every district or equivalent administrative unit with three doses of diphtheria-tetanus-pertussis-containing vaccines	Reach 90% national coverage and 80% in every district or equivalent administrative unit with all vaccines in national programs, unless otherwise recommended
Develop and introduce new and improved vaccines and technologies	At least 90 low-income and middle-income countries have introduced one or more new or underutilized vaccines	▪ All low income and middle-income countries have introduced one or more new or underutilized vaccines ▪ Licensure and launch of vaccine or vaccines against one or more major currently nonvaccine preventable disease ▪ Licensure and launch of at least one platform delivery technology
Exceed the millennium development Goal 4 target for reducing child mortality	Reduce by two thirds, between 1990 and 2015. the under-five mortality rate (target 4A)	Exceed the millennium development Goal a Target 4A for reducing child mortality

HIGH YIELD POINTS AND NEWER VACCINES

BCG

- Prevents severe form of TB and bladder cancer
- **0.05 mL BCG dose is given to child at birth:** Because the skin of the newborn is very thin and intradermal injection with 0.1 mL may break the skin or lead to abscess formation
- BCG is given till 1 year of age as by age 1 year there could be natural acquiring of the TB immunity or a subclinical infection.

Pentavalent Vaccines

- Pentavalent vaccine is a vaccine that contains five antigens (diphtheria + pertussis + tetanus + hepatitis B + Haemophilus influenzae type b).
- As per the National Immunization Schedule, three doses of pentavalent vaccine are to be administered. The first dose is given only after a child is 6 weeks old. The second and third doses are given at 10 and 14 weeks of age, respectively. There is no booster dose recommended under UIP
- **Note:** Pentavalent vaccine should be started for any child aged more than 6 weeks and can be started up to 1 year of age.
- Minimal side effects as redness, pain or swelling
- The Hep B zero dose (at birth) and DPT Booster at 16–24 months will continue as per schedule

Rotavirus Vaccine

- Recommended in countries with diarrheal deaths accounting for more than or equal to 10% of mortality in under 5 years children.
- Schedule 1st dose (RotaTeq or Rotarix) is administered at age 6–15 weeks.
- Maximum age for administering the last dose of either vaccine should be 32 weeks.
- 2 doses of Rotarix be administered with 1st and 2nd dose of DTP rather than with 2nd and 3rd doses.
- It has to be a part of a comprehensive strategy (Hygiene and sanitation, zinc, ORS, Improved case management) to control diarrheal diseases.
- Route oral, given till 1 year of age
- Rotavirus vaccines are live attenuated

Three formulations are available:
Rotarix, RotaTeq, Rotavac

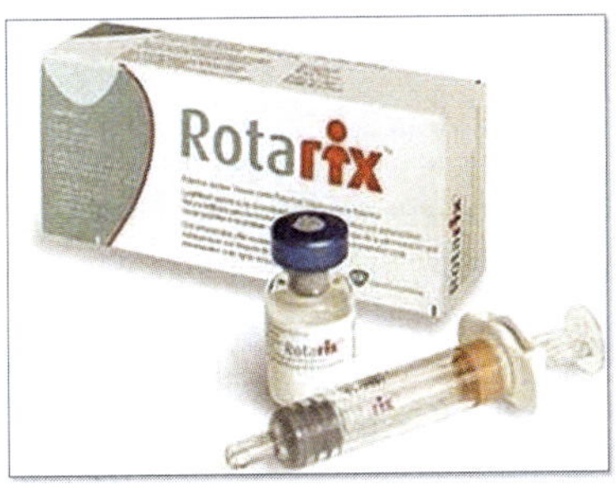

Fig. 2: Rotarix

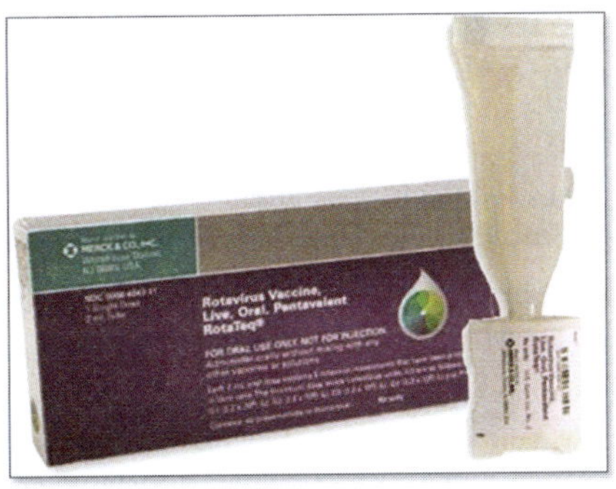

Fig. 3: RotaTeq

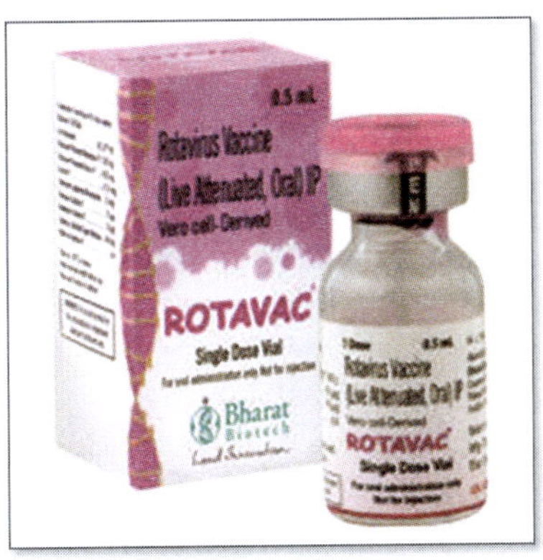

Fig. 4: Rotavac

Hepatitis B Vaccine

- **Plasma derived vaccine:** (Formalin inactivated sub-unit viral vaccine)
  - Dose = 1.0 mL (20 micrograms of HBsAg in an **alum adjuvant**)
  - Given in 3 doses at 0, 1 and 6 months by intramuscular injection.

- Booster doses may be given after 3–5 years.
- Both pre-exposure and post-exposure administration has been recommended.
- Advisable to give specific anti-HBs immunoglobulin, with or before the 1st vaccine dose, in post exposure cases.
- Pre-exposure prophylaxis is indicated in countries with a high prevalence of HBV infection.
- It has no effect on HBsAg carriers

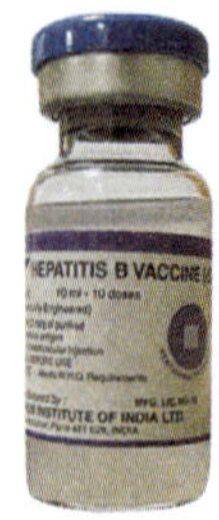

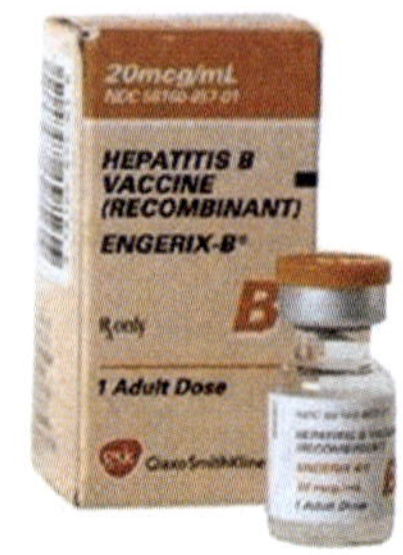

Figs 5 and 6: Hepatitis B vaccine

- **RDNA-yeast derived vaccine**
  - As immunogenic, safe and effective as the plasma-derived vaccine and is more cost-effective.
  - Dose for adult is 10-20 mg initially (depending on formulation) and again at 1 and 6 months
  - Deltoid muscle is preferred for injection.
  - Newborn and pediatric dose is one-half the adult dose. Booster is not routinely recommended.

Pneumococcal Pneumonia Vaccine

Pneumococcal Conjugate Vaccine (PCV 13)

- For vaccination of children
- Constitutes a diphtheria crm197 protein – works as a carrier protein for conjugate vaccine

Pneumococcal Polysaccharide Vaccine (PPV23)

- Polysaccharide nonconjugate vaccine containing capsular antigens of 23 serotypes.
- Not recommended for Children <2 years of age and immune compromised individuals.
- Recommended for those who had splenectomy or have sickle-cell disease, chronic diseases of heart, lung, liver or kidney; diabetes mellitus, alcoholism, generalized malignancies, organ transplants etc.
- In some industrialized countries (USA) it is routinely advised for everyone aged above 65 years
- Dose = 0.5 mL (contains 25 micrograms of purified capsular polysaccharide from each 23 serotypes)
- Primary immunization single intramuscular dose in deltoid muscle or as subcutaneous dose.
- It can be administered at same time as other vaccine by separate injection in another arm.
- Minor adverse reactions (Transient redness and pain at injection site) occur in 30–50% of those vaccinated, more commonly with subcutaneous administration; Local reactions more common in recipients of 2nd dose.

102 Good to Remember

- The PCV 7 (Pneumococcal Conjugate Vaccine) is almost out of the market
- Currently used are PCV 10 and PCV 13 – both are preservative free and are freeze sensitive

PCV Schedule

- 2p+1 = 2 primary and 1 booster dose (6 weeks, 14 weeks and 9 months)
- 3p+0 = 3 primary and no booster dose (6, 10, 14 weeks)

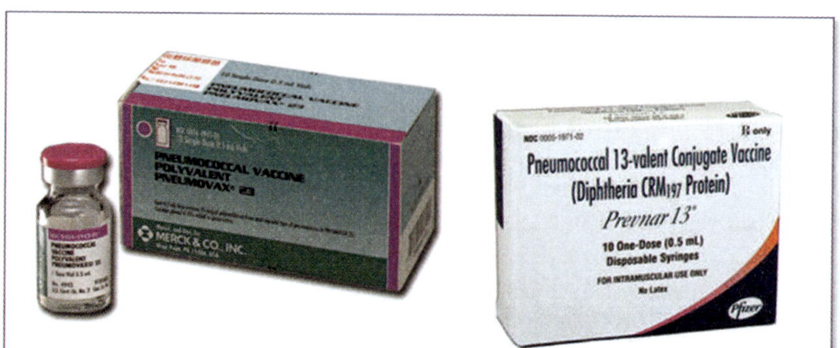

Fig. 7: Pneumococcal polysaccharide vaccine

Dengue Vaccine—Dengvaxia (CYD-TDV)

- CYD-TDV is a live recombinant tetravalent dengue vaccine
- It has been evaluated as a 3-dose series on a 0/6/12 months schedule in Phase III clinical studies.
- It has been registered for use in individuals 9–45 years of age living in endemic areas.
- April 2016, WHO Strategic Advisory Group of Experts (SAGE) on Immunization recommended introduction of the vaccine only in geographic settings (national or subnational) with high endemicity.

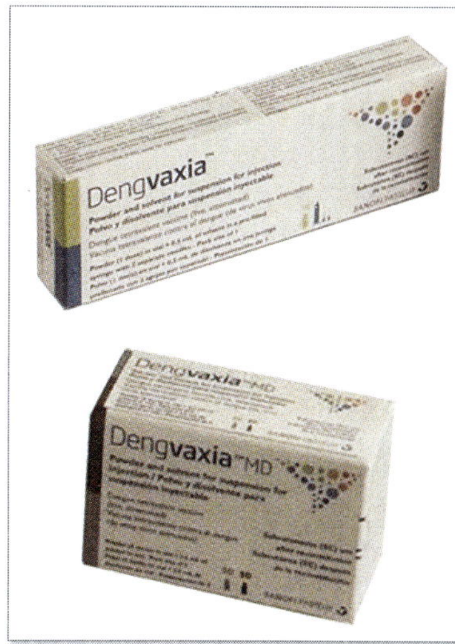

Fig. 8: Dengue vaccine

Malaria Vaccine (RTS, S/AS01)

- It is the first malaria vaccine to have completed pivotal Phase 3 testing.
- RTS, S is a vaccine against *Plasmodium falciparum*
- It offers no protection against *P. vivax malaria*
- The vaccine is being considered as a complementary malaria control tool in Africa

Details for RTS, S vaccine (Mosquirix™):

RTS, S is a scientific name given to this malaria vaccine candidate and represents its composition.

- The 'R' stands for the central repeat region of Plasmodium (P.) falciparum 'circumsporozoite protein (CSP);
- The 'T' for the T-cell epitopes of the CSP;
- The 'S' for hepatitis B surface antigen (HBsAg).

These are combined in a single fusion protein ('RTS') and co-expressed in yeast cells with free HBsAg.

The 'RTS' fusion protein and free 'S' protein spontaneously assemble in 'RTS,S' particles.

The vaccine is administered via intramuscular injection (preferably to the deltoid region), over 3 dosing periods, each 1 month apart, which is consistent with administration of other WHO EPI vaccines. The product is stable for 3 years when stored at temperatures between 2 and 8°C, but must be used within 6 hours of reconstitution

Rubella Vaccine (RA 27/3)

- It is a live attenuated vaccine.
- Prevents subclinical superinfection with wild virus.
- Administered in a single dose of 0.5 mL subcutaneously.
- Mild reactions occur in some subjects.
- Vaccine-induced immunity lasts 14–16 years and probably lifelong.
- Contraindication → Infancy and pregnancy
- Recipients of the vaccine are advised not to become pregnant over the next 3 months.
- Available as equally effective combined measles, mumps and rubella (MMR) vaccine.

Vaccination Strategy for Eradication of Congenital Rubella Syndrome

1st priority → Vaccinate nonpregnant women of childbearing age (15–34 or 39 years of age).[Q]
2nd priority → Interrupt transmission by vaccinating all children currently aged 1–14 years
3rd priority → Then revert to routine universal immunization of all children at age 1 (using combined MR or MMR vaccine.

Measles-Rubella (MR) Vaccine Campaign

- Measles-Rubella vaccination campaign is a special campaign to vaccinate all children of 9 months to <15 years of age group with one additional dose of MR vaccine.

Focus: This additional campaign dose will boost the immunity of child and protect the entire community by eliminating transmission of measles and rubella.

Target: Vaccination of 100% children:

The campaign dose will be administered to all children falling between the age group of 9 months to <15 years of age, irrespective of any past history of disease or vaccination the child should receive both routine doses of Measles and Rubella vaccines at 9–12 months and 16–24 months of age, irrespective of any Measles-Rubella vaccination campaign dose in the past.

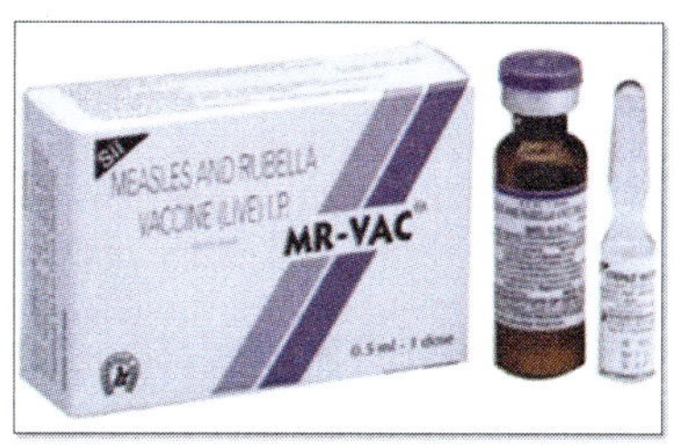

Fig. 9: Measles-Rubella vaccine

Inactivated (Salk) Polio Vaccine

- It has wild polio virus strains → Mahoney (Salk type-1), MEF-1 (Salk type 2) and Saukett (Salk type 3), grown in vero cell/human diploid cell and inactivated by formaldehyde
- It contains at least 40, 8, 32 antigen units of types 1,2 and 3 respectively
- It is a killed vaccine administered via subcutaneous, intradermal or intramuscular route
- OPV can be given as booster after an initial course of IPV.[Q]
- Recent update (Source Immunization for medical officers 2017) –
  - IPV is administered as single dose at 14 weeks, intramuscular anterolateral right thigh
  - IPV is also launched as 'fractional IPV' at 6, 14 weeks intradermal injection –right upper arm

Disadvantage

- Unsuitable in case of an epidemic (Immunity is not rapidly achieved) injections are to be avoided as they are likely to precipitate paralysis
- Costlier and difficult to manufacture compared to OPV
- IPV induces humoral antibodies (IgM, IgG and IgA serum antibodies) but does not induce intestinal or local gut immunity and hence does not cause prevention of transmission of virus from person to person

Advantages

- Safe to administer to persons with immune deficiency diseases, persons undergoing corticosteroid and radiation therapy, over 50 years age receiving vaccine for 1st time and in pregnancy.
- Negligible chances of any serious adverse reactions or vaccine-associated paralytic polio (VAPP)
- IPV is not as heat sensitive like OPV and does not require stringent conditions during storage and transportation; It has a longer shelf life.

bOPV Vaccine

- Key dates for the national switch day (April 25th 2016)
  - **April 1st:** tOPV would not be available after this date.
  - **April 11th:** bOPV would be available in private market but it is not to be opened or used before 25th April.
  - **April 25:** Polio Switch Day, when tOPV would be completely withdrawn and replaced by bOPV in both routine immunization and polio campaigns.
  - **9th May:** National Validation Day when India would be declared free of tOPV.
- Shifting from the trivalent OPV to the Bivalent (P1 and P3) OPV

Cholera Vaccine

- Dukoral (WC-rBS):
  - Monovalent vaccine based on formalin and heat killed whole cells (WC) of *V. cholerae* 01 and recombinant B subunit.
  - Used as 3 mL vaccine vial with bicarbonate buffer (to prevent gastric degradation)
- Sanchol and mORCVAX – do not have the B subunit and does not require buffer
- **Euvichol:** Same as sanchol. FDA approved in 2015.

Td Vaccine (Update 2019)

- WHO prequalified Td vaccine
- VVM 30
- Shelf life: 24-36 months ; Preservative: Thiomersal
- Td is freeze and heat sensitive, Shake test is applicable
- Open vial policy is applicable to Td vaccine.
- TT is replaced with Td at 10 and 16 years and for pregnant females

Leprosy Vaccine

- BCG vaccine offers variable, partial protection towards leprosy
- Mycobacterium Indicus Pranii (previously called as Mycobacterium w) has been used with reasonable efficacy and effectivity in various trials.
  - Incidentally, MIP (Mycobacterium Indicus Pranii) has also shown effect on treatment for cutaneous warts
  - MIP clears also the bacilli resident in peripheral nerves restoring normal sensitivity

COLD CHAIN

Introduction and Equipment Used

***Cold chain** is a system of storage and transport of vaccines at low temperature from manufacturer to the actual vaccination site.*

158 *High Yield Points*

Cold chain—equipment	Levels
Walk in cold rooms (WIC)**	Regional level
Deep freezers (300 L) and ILRs (300/240 L)*	All districts and WIC locations
Small deep freezer and ILR (140 L) set*	PHCs, Urban Family Planning Centers and Postpartum Centers
Cold boxes, vaccine carrier, day carrier	Outreach centers, peripheral centers

*Store vaccine for 1 month.
**Store vaccines up to 3 months and serve 4–5 districts

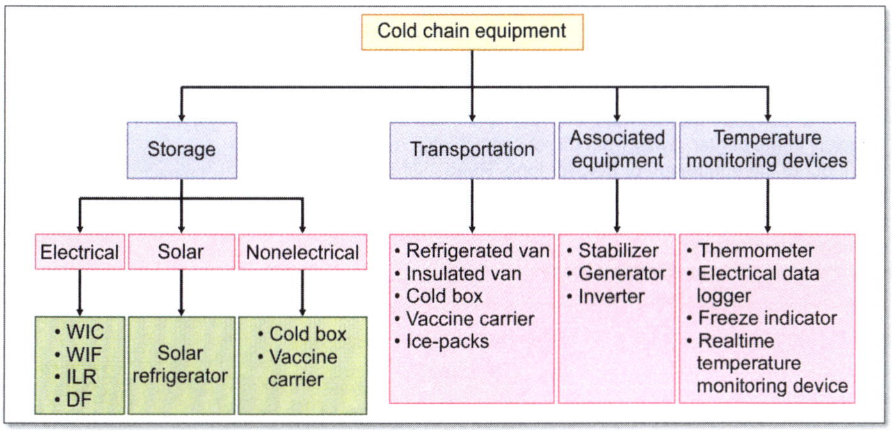

Fig. 10: Overview of cold chain equipment

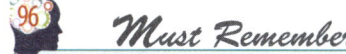

- No vaccine storage is done below PHC level (i.e. Subcenter)
- Deep freezer – may maintain a temperature of –20°C to –40°C,
- ILR maintain a temperature of +2°C to +8°C
- Temperature is to be monitored twice daily using dial thermometer. Maximum chance of Cold chain failure is at subcenter level and below
- Diluent are kept in the cold chain 24 hours before the scheduled immunization session.

96 *Must Remember*

- Deep freezers are used for making ice packs. OPV and Measles vaccines can be stored in Deep Freezer.
- Ideally vaccines need to be kept in the ILR as per instructions (T series vaccine at top and Polio/ Measles at bottom).
- ILR can maintain temperature with a minimum of 8 hour of uninterrupted electricity

Thermosensitivity of Vaccines

Table 10: Heat, light and freeze sensitivity of vaccine

Vaccine	Exposure to heat/light	Exposure to cold	Temperature at PHC
Heat and light sensitive vaccines			
BCG	Relatively heat stable, but sensitive to light	Not damaged by freezing	+2°C to +8°C
OPV	Sensitive to heat	Not damaged by freezing	+2°C to +8°C
Measles	Sensitive to heat and light	Not damaged by freezing	+2°C to +8°C
Freeze sensitive vaccines			
DPT	Relatively heat stable	Freezes at –3°C (Should not be frozen)	+2°C to +8°C
Hepatitis B	Relatively heat stable	Freezes at –0.5°C (Should not be frozen)	+2°C to +8°C
DT	Relatively heat stable	Freezes at –3°C (Should not be frozen)	+2°C to +8°C
TT	Relatively heat stable	Freezes at –3°C (Should not be frozen)	+2°C to +8°C
At the PHC level, all vaccines are kept in the ILR for a period of one month at temperature of +2°C to +8°C			

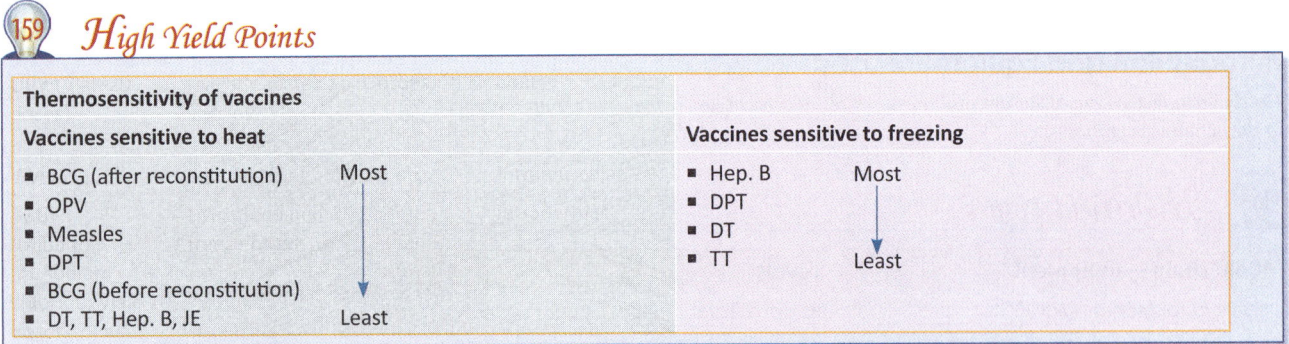

159 *High Yield Points*

Thermosensitivity of vaccines

Vaccines sensitive to heat		Vaccines sensitive to freezing	
▪ BCG (after reconstitution)	Most	▪ Hep. B	Most
▪ OPV	↓	▪ DPT	↓
▪ Measles		▪ DT	
▪ DPT		▪ TT	Least
▪ BCG (before reconstitution)			
▪ DT, TT, Hep. B, JE	Least		

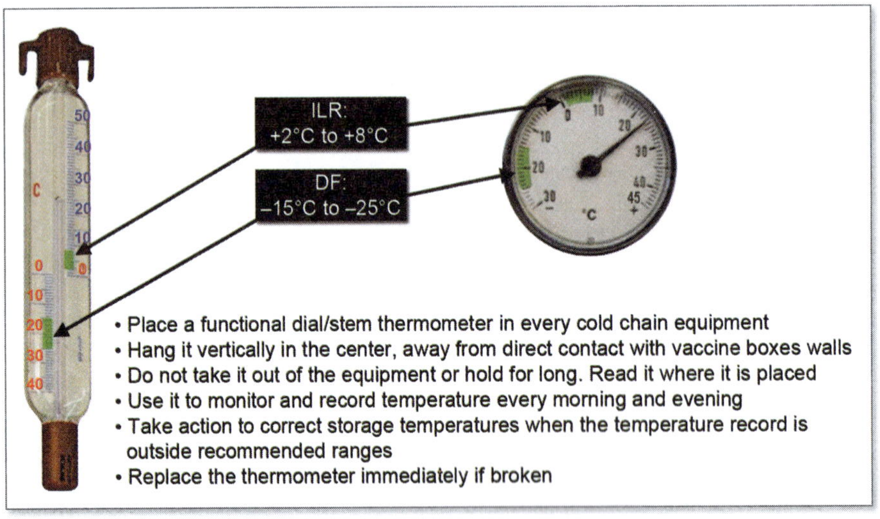

ILR:
+2°C to +8°C
DF:
–15°C to –25°C
• Place a functional dial/stem thermometer in every cold chain equipment
• Hang it vertically in the center, away from direct contact with vaccine boxes walls
• Do not take it out of the equipment or hold for long. Read it where it is placed
• Use it to monitor and record temperature every morning and evening
• Take action to correct storage temperatures when the temperature record is outside recommended ranges
• Replace the thermometer immediately if broken

Fig. 11: Temperature maintenance–dial thermometer

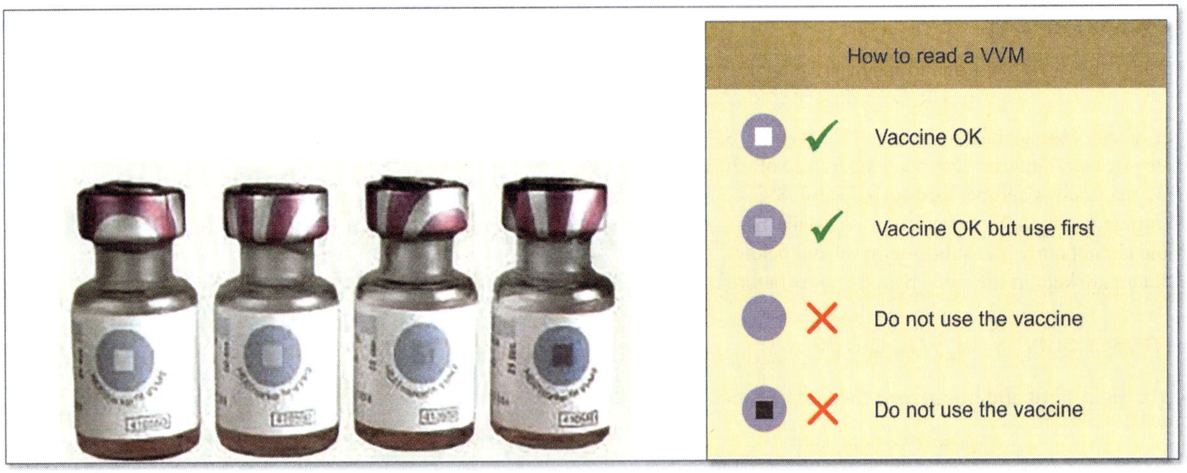

Fig. 12: How to read a VVM

Open Vial Policy—2015

It allows reuse of partially used vials of vaccines under UIP in subsequent sessions (Fixed and Outreach) up to 28 days (Reducing wastage) subject to fulfilling the following conditions:

- Expiry date is not passed
- VVM has not reached discard point
- Aseptic technique used to withdraw doses
- Vaccine stored at appropriate temperature during transport and storage

- Vaccine vial septum not submerged in water or contaminated
- All vials must have the date and time of opening recorded
- It applies to DPT, TT, Hepatitis B, OPV and Liquid Pentavalent
- It is not applicable for BCG, Measles and JE vaccine and rotavirus vaccine.

Shake Test

It is used to check if freeze-sensitive vaccines (e.g. Pentavalent, PCV10, TT or Hep. B) have been subjected to freezing temperatures likely to damage them.

Steps

- Prepare a frozen control vial (Same type, batch number and manufacturer as the vaccine to be tested frozen for at least 10 hours at –10°C) and then let it thaw.
- Choose the suspected frozen test vial
- Shake the control and test vials vigorously for 10–15 seconds.
- Allow the vials to rest on a table side by side

If the vaccine in the suspected test vial shows a much slower sedimentation rate than the vaccine in the frozen control vial, we conclude that the test vaccine has most probably not been frozen and can be used.

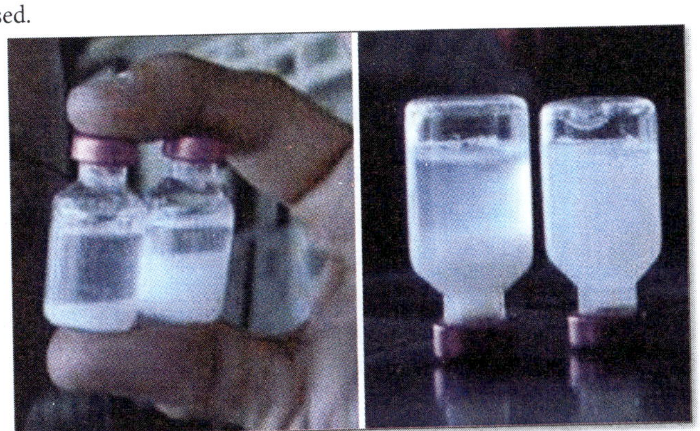

Fig. 13: Shake test to check freeze-sensitive vaccines

> **160 High Yield Points**
>
> Under the open vial policy **(OVP)**, any open vaccine vial returned from the field has to be used within 4 weeks (28 days) from the date of opening, provided the vaccine vial monitor **(VVM)** is in usable condition, vaccine has not been frozen and is within expiry date. The vaccines that come under this policy are **Hep B**, **OPV**, **DPT**, pentavalent, **TT** and **IPV**.

ADVERSE EVENTS FOLLOWING IMMUNIZATION (AEFI)

It is any untoward (unfavorable or unintended) medical occurrence presenting as sign, abnormal laboratory results or symptom following immunization but not necessarily having a causal relationship with use of the vaccine.

Table 11: 2012 Council for international organizations of medical sciences (CIOMS) and WHO revised classification of AEFI

Type of AEFI	Reason
Product related	An AEFI due to inherent property of the vaccine product
Quality related	An AEFI due to quality defect in the vaccine or its administration device
Immunization error (Program error)	A preventable AEFI due to inappropriate vaccine handling, prescription or administration. Once product has left the manufacturer/packaging site. For example, inadequate cold chain or nonsterile injections → Local suppuration abscess, Sepsis or Toxic Shock syndrome or Blood borne viral infection
Anxiety related	An AEFI due to anxiety (Not related to vaccine content). E.g. Fainting, Clonic seizure, breath holding, facial flush and cyanosis, hyperventilation
Coincidental	An AEFI due to any reason other than the vaccine product, immunization error or immunization anxiety

Table 12: AEFI regarding vaccine

Vaccine	Reaction	Onset interval	Rate/doses*
BCG	▪ Suppurative lymphadenitis BCG, ▪ Osteitis disseminated ▪ BCG infection	▪ 2–6 months ▪ 1–12 months ▪ 1–12 months	▪ 1 to 10/10,000 ▪ 1 to 700/1,000,000 ▪ 0.19 to 1.56/1,000,000
Oral poliomyelitis	VAPP	4–30 days	2 to 4/1,000,000
Hepatitis B	Anaphylaxis	0–1 hour	1.1/1,000,000
Hib	None		
Pertussis (DwPT)/ Pentavalent vaccine	▪ Persistent (>3 hours) inconsolable screaming seizures ▪ Hypotonic, hypo responsive episode (HHE), ▪ Anaphylaxis ▪ Encephalopathy	0–24 hours 0–3 days 0–24 hours 0–2 days	<1/100 1 to 2/1000 20/1,000,000 0 to 1/1,000,000
Tetanus toxoid	▪ Brachial neuritis ▪ Anaphylaxis	▪ 2–28 days ▪ 0–1 hour	▪ 5 to 10/1,000,000 ▪ 1 to 6/1,000,000
Measles/MMR/MR	▪ Febrile seizures ▪ Thrombocytopenia ▪ Anaphylaxis ▪ Encephalopathy	▪ 6–12 days ▪ 15–35 days ▪ 0–1 hour ▪ 6–12 days	3/1000 3/10,000 ~1/1,000,000 <1/1,000,000
Rotavirus	Intussusception	3–14 days	1 to 2/100,000

*Rates of AEFI per number of doses

161 *High Yield Points*

- All vaccine recipients' must be kept under observation for at least 20 minutes following injection.
- Highest expected frequency of minor vaccine reaction is with – Meningococcal vaccine (71%), DPT and Hepatitis A (50%)

97 *Must Remember*

Anaphylactic shock is a severe rapid onset (within 1 hour) allergic reaction involving multiple body systems characterized by circulatory collapse with or without bronchospasm and/or laryngospasm usually following administration of antisera or vaccine (with traces antibiotics)

ANAPHYLACTIC SHOCK

Table 13: Differences between fainting and anaphylaxis

	Fainting	Anaphylaxis
Onset	Usually at the time or soon after the injection	Usually some delay, between 5 to 30 minutes, after injection
Systemic		
Skin	Pale, sweaty, cold and clammy	Red, raised and itchy rash; swollen eyes, face, generalized rash
Respiratory	Normal to deep breaths	Noisy breathing from airways obstruction (wheeze or stridor)
Cardiovascular	Bradycardia, transient hypotension	Tachycardia, hypotension
Gastrointestinal	Nausea, vomiting	Abdominal cramps
Neurological	Transient loss of consciousness, relieved by supine posture	Loss of consciousness, not relieved by supine posture

Serious AEFI is life threatening and may result in death, inpatient hospitalization or prolongation of existing hospitalization, persistent or significant disability, congenital anomaly.

Anaphylaxis Treatment Protocol

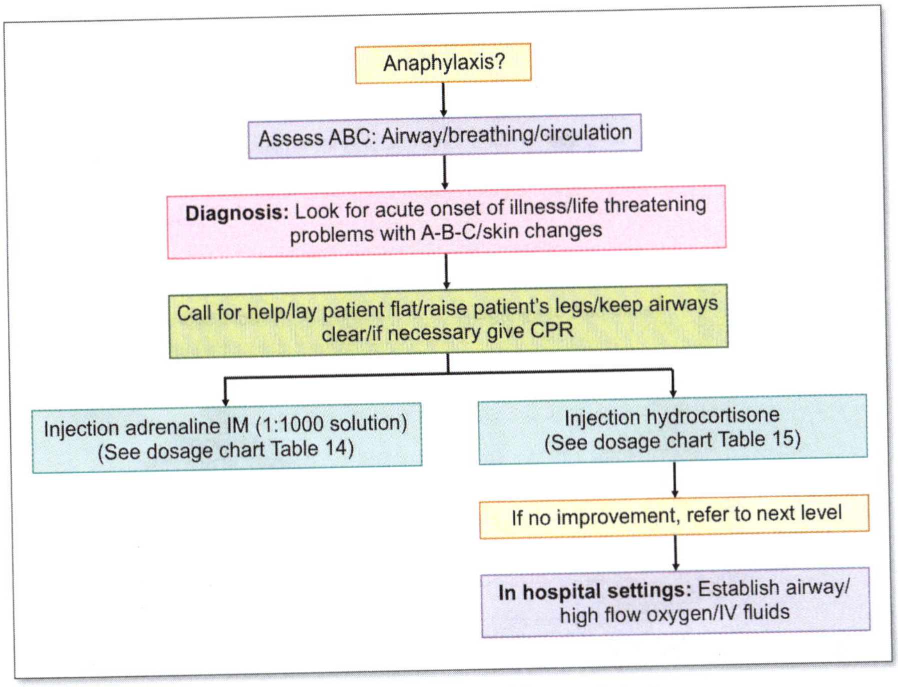

Fig. 14: Treatment protocol for anaphylaxis

> **162 High Yield Points**
>
> There is weekly reporting mechanism for any serious AEFI at the **district level**

Adrenaline Dosage

Adrenaline dosage: 1:1000 adrenaline (epinephrine) at a dose of 0.01mL/kg up to a maximum of 0.5 mL injected intramuscularly (or subcutaneously in very mild cases)

Table 14: Injection adrenaline (1:1000) dosage chart IM

Age	Dosage
Less than 2 years	0.0625 mL (1/16 of a mL)
2–5 years	0.125 mL (1/8 of a mL)
6–11 years	0.25 mL (1/4 of a mL)
11+ years	0.5 mL (1/2 of a mL)

Table 15: Injection hydrocortisone (IM or slow IV): Dosage chart

Age	Dosage
Less than 6 months	25 mg
6 months to 6 years	50 mg
6–12 years	100 mg
>12 years	200 mg

VACCINE DISPOSAL

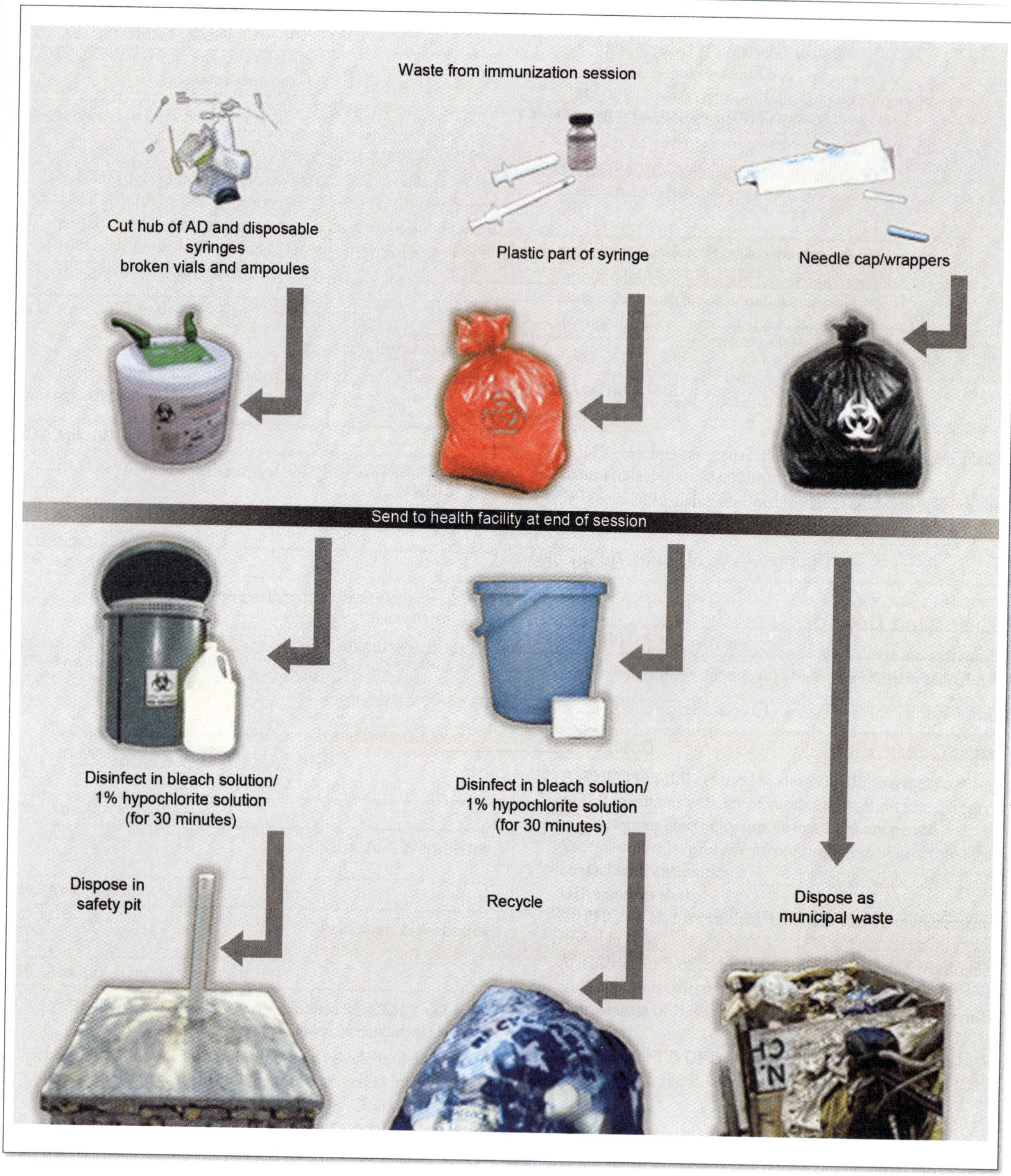
Waste from immunization session
Cut hub of AD and disposable syringes broken vials and ampoules
Plastic part of syringe
Needle cap/wrappers
Send to health facility at end of session
Disinfect in bleach solution/ 1% hypochlorite solution (for 30 minutes)
Disinfect in bleach solution/ 1% hypochlorite solution (for 30 minutes)
Dispose in safety pit
Recycle
Dispose as municipal waste

Fig. 15: Vaccine disposal

Image-Based Questions

1. Identify the scientist in figure?

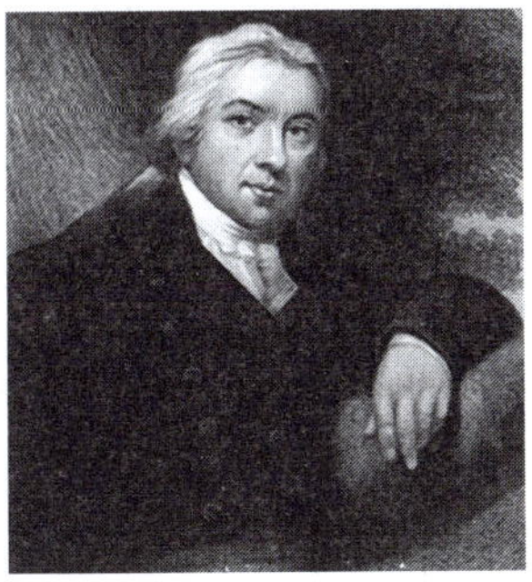

a. Edward Jenner
b. Alexander Fleming
c. John Snow
d. Louis Pasteur

2. Injection technique shown in figure is used to administer?

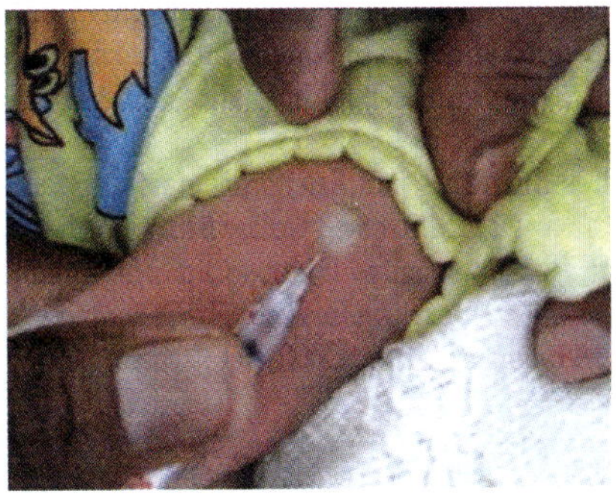

a. BCG
b. Measles
c. Hepatitis B
d. Japanese Encephalitis

Answers of Image-Based Questions

1. **Ans. (a) Edward Jenner**

2. **Ans. (a) BCG**

Multiple Choice Questions

1. Which of the following vaccine vials can be used? *(AIIMS Nov 2017)*

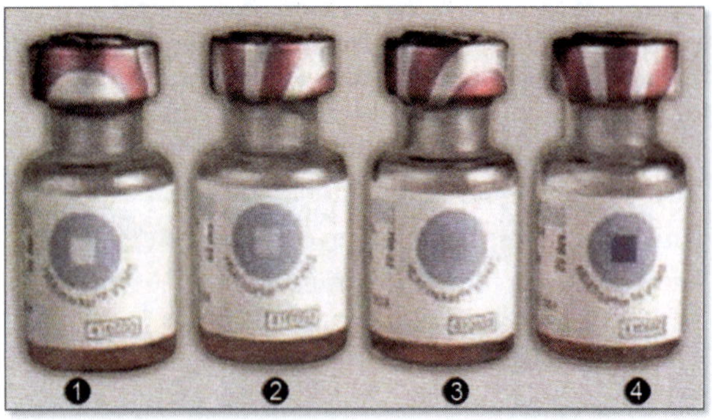

a. 1, 2 can be used
b. 3, 4 can be used
c. 1, 2, 3 can be used
d. Only 1 can be used

2. All of the following vaccine preventable diseases are covered under Mission Indradhanush except: *(AIIMS May 2017)*
a. Measles b. Tuberculosis
c. Hepatitis B d. Meningococcal meningitis

3. Vaccine contraindicated in AIDS patient: *(PGI May 2017)*
a. MMR vaccine b. Hepatitis A vaccine
c. Varicella vaccine d. Hib vaccine
e. DPT vaccine

4. 9-valent HPV vaccine covers which type(s) HPV strain: *(PGI May 2017)*
a. 6, 11 b. 16, 18
c. 31, 33 d. 41, 35
e. 42,58

5. True statement about IPV vaccine: *(PGI May 2017)*
a. Given through IM/SC route
b. Given through Intradermal route
c. Does not require stringent conditions
d. Dose is- 0.1 mL/dose
e. Dose is -0.5 mL/dose

6. Varicella zoster immunization is given to all except:
a. Contacts with varicella zoster
b. To the newborn and pregnant female who was exposed 6 weeks before delivery
c. All HIV positive patients
d. Patients with varicella zoster

7. What is the measles vaccine dose? *(Recent Question 2017)*
a. 0.1 cc b. 0.5 cc
c. 0.01 cc d. 1.0 cc

8. Reconstituted JE vaccine may be given up till:
a. 2 hours
b. 4 hours
c. 24 hours if stored at 2-8°C
d. Till one month if stored at 2-8°C

DISCOVERIES AND CONTRIBUTIONS

9. Smallpox vaccine was developed by:
a. Louis Pasteur b. Robert Koch
c. Joseph Lister d. Edward Jenner

10. The term vaccination was coined by: *(Recent Question 2015)*
a. Hippocrates b. Louis Pasteur
c. Edward Jenner d. Alexander Fleming

11. Edward Jenner died in: *(Recent Question 2013, 2012)*
a. 1749 b. 1775
c. 1823 d. 1920

12. Smallpox vaccine was invented by:
a. Louis Pasteur b. Edward Jenner
c. Paul Eugene d. John Snow

INFECTIOUS DISEASE EPIDEMIOLOGY

13. Postexposure vaccination is given in:
a. Typhoid b. Rabies
c. Mumps d. Rubella

GENERAL VACCINE

14. As per vaccine vial monitoring, a vial is discarded when?
a. When the inner square becomes equal in color
b. When the inner square becomes deeper in color
c. When inner square is lighter in color
d. When inner square fades away

15. Vaccine is not available in the following form: *(Recent Question 2016)*
a. Recombinant DNA b. Prion
c. Toxoid d. Live attenuated

16. Which of the following vaccines is most sensitive to heat? *(Recent Question 2016)*
a. Oral polio vaccine b. BCG vaccine
c. DPT vaccine d. Measles vaccine

17. Which of the following vaccine should not be given to an elderly man:
a. Measles b. H. influenza
c. Tetanus Toxoid d. Pneumococcal

18. Which of the following vaccine should not be given in patient with Egg allergy:
a. Measles b. Influenza
c. MMR d. Varicella

19. Which of the following is the most common cause of vaccine failure:
a. Improper administration b. Inappropriate manufacturing
c. Maternal antibodies d. Improper storage

20. Which of the following vaccines is/are contraindicated in pregnancy?
1. Rubella 2. Hepatitis-B
3. Diphtheria

Choose the correct answer among the following:
a. 1 only b. 2 and 3 only
c. 1 and 3 only d. 1, 2 and 3

Ans.

1. a
2. d
3. a,b,c
4. a,b,c
5. a,c,e
6. d
7. b
8. b
9. d
10. c
11. c
12. b
13. b
14. a
15. b
16. a
17. a
18. a
19. c
20. a

Most Recent Questions of 2019-18 are given at the end of MCQs

21. Which of the following is the first recombinant vaccine to be cloned in yeast: *(Recent Question 2016)*
a. Hepatitis B b. Rubella
c. Typhoid d. Measles

22. Salk vaccine is:
a. Live vaccine
b. Live attenuated vaccine
c. Killed vaccine
d. Toxoid

23. Parents of a 6-week girl child want to give her a vaccine other than National Immunization schedule. Which vaccine(s) need to be given: *(Recent Question 2015)*
a. Hib, Mumps
b. Typhoid, Rotavirus, MMR
c. Rotavirus, Yellow fever
d. Pneumococcal vaccine

24. Live attenuated vaccines are:
a. Measles, Mumps, Hepatitis B, Varicella
b. Measles, Mumps, BCG, Plague
c. Measles, Mumps, BCG, Varicella
d. Measles, Rubella, Hepatitis B, Plague

25. Storage time for reconstituted JE vaccine is
a. 2 hours b. 24 hours
c. 1 hour d. 4 hours

26. Reconstructed Japanese encephalitis vaccine at 2–8 degrees can be stored up to how many hours:
a. 1 b. 2
c. 3 d. 4

27. Vaccine not given at birth: *(Recent Question 2015)*
a. BCG
b. DPT
c. OPV
d. Hepatitis B

28. Killed vaccine is:
a. Hepatitis A
b. Measles
c. OPV
d. BCG

29. Which is a live vaccine: *(Recent Question 2014)*
a. BCG
b. Salk
c. DPT
d. Tetanus toxoid

30. Additional component of UIP PLUS does not include:
a. Hepatitis B vaccine
b. Safe motherhood
c. Acute respiratory infections
d. Diarrhea management

31. Which vaccine is contraindicated in pregnancy:
a. Rubella
b. Diphtheria
c. Tetanus
d. Hepatitis B

32. Which of the following vaccines can result thrombocytopenia: *(Recent Question 2014)*
a. MMR vaccine
b. Typhoid vaccine
c. Influenza vaccine
d. Hib vaccine

33. Syringes and glassware are sterilized by:
a. Irradiation
b. Autoclave
c. Hot air oven
d. Glutaraldehyde

34. MMR vaccine is recommended at the age of:
a. 9–12 months b. 15–18 months
c. 2–3 years d. 10–19 years

35. At the Primary Health Center (PHC) level, vaccine are stored in the
a. Cold box b. Deep freezer
c. Ice lined refrigerator d. Walk in cold room

36. Which vaccine is/are not contraindicated in pregnancy? *(PGI Pattern Question)*
a. Rubella
b. Varicella
c. Hepatitis B
d. Measles
e. Rabies

37. Strain used for Mumps vaccine is: *(Recent Question 2014)*
a. Jeryl Lynn
b. Edmonston
c. DANISH 1331
d. OKA

38. Which type of vaccine is MMR?
a. Live attenuated b. Killed
c. Toxoid d. Subunit

39. Under UIP program which of the following vaccines is administered at 9 months of age?
a. DPT-1
b. BCG
c. Measles
d. Hepatitis B-1

40. According to latest guidelines of vaccination, which of the following is applicable at the age of 5 years?
a. DT booster + vitamin A
b. DT
c. DPT + OPV
d. DPT + vitamin A

41. Hepatitis B vaccine, dose scheduled in adult (in months):
a. 0, 1, 2 months
b. 0, 1, 3 months
c. 0, 6, 12 months
d. 0, 1, 6 months

42. Protection level of tetanus anti-toxin is:
a. >0.01 IU/mL
b. >0.5 IU/mL
c. >1.0 IU/mL
d. >5 IU/mL

43. Which of the following is NOT a cholera vaccine?
a. Ty21 A
b. CVD-103-Hgr
c. WC-Rbs
d. mORC-Vax

44. Mass vaccination is ineffective in:
a. Measles b. Poliomyelitis
c. Tetanus d. None of the above

45. Trivalent oral polio vaccine contains, type 3 virus:
a. 100,000 TCID 50 b. 200,000 TCID 50
c. 300,000 TCID 50 d. 400,000 TCID 50

Ans.

21. a
22. c
23. None
24. c
25. d
26. d
27. b
28. a
29. a
30. a
31. a
32. a
33. c
34. b
35. c
36. c, e
37. a
38. a
39. c
40. d
41. d
42. a
43. a
44. c
45. c

Most Recent Questions of 2019-18 are given at the end of MCQs

46. Rabies vaccine for pre exposure prophylaxis is given at:
a. 0, 3, 7 days
b. 0, 3, 7, 14 days
c. 0, 3, 7, 14, 30 days
d. 0, 7 days

47. Newborn child with HIV + and symptomatic, which vaccine will be given: *(Recent Question 2013)*
a. Measles
b. OPV vaccine
c. BCG
d. Live JE

48. Live attenuated vaccine can be given to: *(Recent Question 2015)*
a. Children under 8 years
b. HIV patients
c. Patients on steroids
d. Patients on radiation

49. Mass immunization is indicated in the following except:
a. Leprosy
b. Tuberculosis
c. Pneumococcal pneumonia
d. Influenza

BCG

50. BCG is given over: *(Recent Question 2015)*
a. Volar aspect of left forearm
b. Dorsal aspect of left forearm
c. Left deltoid
d. Right deltoid

DPT/TT

51. A man falls from bike and sustains an injury to his foot. TT was last taken 12 years ago. What would you recommend?
a. Nothing required
b. TT 1 dose
c. TT 1 dose + Human Tetanus Immunoglobulin
d. TT complete course + Human Tetanus Immunoglobulin

52. A 8-month-old child had history of unusual cry and convulsions following previous vaccination after BCG, DPT, OPV-1 and Hepatitis B. Now parents have brought the child for next dose of vaccination. Which vaccine is contraindicated here ?
a. DT
b. DPT
c. Measles
d. Hepatitis B

53. Preferred vaccine for a 12 year old child is:
a. DT
b. DPT
c. dT
d. DTaP

54. Which disease is prevented by giving booster dose to a 5-6 years old child? *(Recent Question 2014)*
a. Measles
b. BCG
c. DT
d. DPT

OPV AND IPV

55. VAPP develops in how many days following OPV administration: *(Recent Question 2014)*
a. 7–14
b. 60–90
c. 20–70
d. Immediately

56. True about polio vaccination is all except:
a. Follow up of AFP every 30 days
b. Salk contains three types of polio virus
c. Pulse polio virus are extra and supplemental
d. Oral polio vaccine provides intestinal immunity also

57. Which of the following is *not* true about Oral Polio Vaccine:
a. Induces both local and systemic immunity
b. Maternal antibody is completely protective
c. Live attenuated vaccine
d. Requires subzero temperature for long-term shortage

58. Vaccine derived polio virus outbreaks are mostly due to:
a. Type 1 virus
b. Type 2 virus
c. Type 3 virus
d. All of the above

59. OPV bivalent vaccine contains:
a. P1 and P2
b. P1 and P3
c. P2 and P3
d. P1, P2 and P3

MEASLES

60. Strain of virus not used in measles vaccine is: *(Recent Question 2013)*
a. Edmondson Zagreb strain
b. Schwartz strain
c. Jeryl Lynn strain
d. Moraten strain

61. MMR vaccine given at the age of :
a. 0 month
b. 15–18 months
c. 2–3 years
d. 5 years

62. What is the measles vaccine dose?
a. 0.1 cc
b. 0.5 cc
c. 0.01 cc
d. 1.0 cc

63. In measles outbreak, measles vaccine can be given within:
a. 2–3 months
b. 3–5 months
c. 2–7 months
d. 6–9 months

NEWER VACCINE

64. The trivalent influenza vaccine contains all strains of influenza virus except: *(Recent Question 2013)*
a. H1N1
b. H3N2
c. H2N1
d. Influenza B

65. Vi Polysaccharide can be first given at the age of
a. 6 months
b. 12 months
c. 18 months
d. 24 months

66. Dokoral, Sanchol, Morcvax are used in manufacture of
a. Typhoid vaccine
b. Cholera vaccine
c. Influenza vaccine
d. Swine flu vaccine

67. Following is Hib conjugate vaccine
a. Capsular polysaccharide
b. Cell wall polysaccharide
c. Capsular polysaccharide with carrier
d. PRP with carrier

68. Dose of Rubella immunoglobulin is:
a. 5 mL
b. 10 mL
c. 20 mL
d. 40 mL

69. True regarding SA-14-14-2 Japanese Encephalitis vaccine is
a. Diploid cell culture inactivated
b. Killed vaccine
c. Lifelong immunity
d. Primary schedule consists of 2 doses

Ans.

46. d
47. a
48. a
49. a
50. c
51. d
52. b
53. c
54. d
55. a
56. a
57. b
58. b
59. b
60. c
61. b
62. b
63. d
64. c
65. d
66. b
67. d
68. c
69. d

70. True regarding cervical cancer vaccine is/are: *(PGI Nov 2013)*

a. Bivalent and quadrivalent
b. Given to married women 20-45 years age group
c. Most common subtype are 16, 18
d. Two doses given
e. Gives 100% protection

71. Which cancer is preventable by vaccine:

a. Ovarian CA b. Cervix CA
c. Breast CA d. Uterus CA

72. Which of the following Human Papilloma Virus subtypes are not covered by quadrivalent anti-cervical cancer vaccine?

a. Type 6 b. Type 7
c. Type 11 d. Type 16
e. Type 18

73. True about HPV vaccination: *(Recent Question 2013)*

a. Given in woman of age group 25-40 years
b. Primary immunization consists of 2 dose
c. Efficacy >70% for cervical cancer
d. Two types of vaccine are available in the market
e. Protect against HPV 16 and 18

74. True statement about Vi polysaccharide vaccine is:

a. Has many serious systemic adverse reaction
b. Has many serious local side effects
c. Has many contraindication
d. Can be administered with yellow fever and hepatitis A vaccine

75. Immunoprophylaxis of leprosy includes:

a. BCG
b. MMR
c. ICRC bacillus
d. Anthrax vaccine
e. Mycobacterium 'W'

76. Ty 21a is a vaccine for: *(Recent Question 2013)*

a. Cholera b. TB
c. Pertussis d. Typhoid

77. Which one of the following is not included in the mission Indradhanush scheme of vaccine?

a. TB b. Diphtheria
c. Japanese encephalitis d. Mumps

78. Which of the following vial may be used by the health worker for polio immunization: *(AIIMS Nov 2017)*

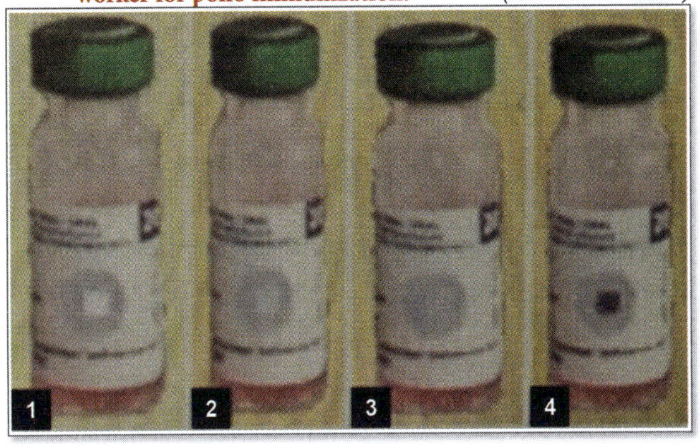

a. 1 & 2 b. 1, 2 and 3
c. 3 & 4 d. 2, 3 and 4

79. Strain used for JE Vaccine is: *(AIIMS Nov 2017)*

a. Live vaccine, SA-14-14-2 strain
b. Killed Vaccine, SA 14-14-2 strain
c. Live Vaccine, RA 27 strain
d. Killed vaccine, RA 27 strain

80. Which of the following is true regarding mission Indradhanush *(AIIMS Nov 2017)*

a. 5 visits till 5 years b. 5 visits till 7 years
c. 7 visits till 5 years d. 7 visits till 7 years

81. Immunization of preschool children with diphtheria toxoid results in: *(AIIMS Nov 2017)*

a. Detectable antitoxin for about 10 years.
b. Protection against diphtheria carrier state.
c. Frequent adverse reactions
d. Protection against infection of the respiratory tract by Corynebacterium diphtheria.

82. What is true regarding "intensified mission Indradhanush" *(AIIMS Nov 2017)*

a. It is targeting the rural and BPL families
b. It is for launch of the pentavalent vaccine
c. It does not include Injectable inactivated polio vaccine
d. It is targeting urban slums with nomadic population

Most Recent Questions (2019-2018)

83. All of the following vaccine given under universal program of immunization India; except: *(AIIMS Nov 2018)*

a. Rota virus b. Influenza
c. Adult JE d. Measles and Rubella

84. The test used to identify frozen vaccine is:

a. Shake test b. Habel test *(AIIMS Nov 2018)*
c. Shick test d. Test

85. Which of the following parameters is used to determine the sensitivity of vaccine due to heat? *(AIIMS May 2018)*

a. VVM b. VCM
c. VMV d. VMM

86. Mw vaccine is made from: *(AIIMS May 2019)*

a. M. Bovis
b. M. Welchii
c. M. indicus pranii
d. M. Tuberculosis

87. Which of the vaccine strain changed every year: *(Recent Question 2019)*

a. Measles b. Mumps
c. Polio d. Influenza

Ans.

70. a, c
71. b
72. b
73. c, d, e
74. d
75. a, c, e
76. d
77. d
78. a
79. a
80. c
81. a
82. d
83. b
84. a
85. a
86. c
87. d

Answers with Explanations

1. Ans. (a) 1, 2 can be used

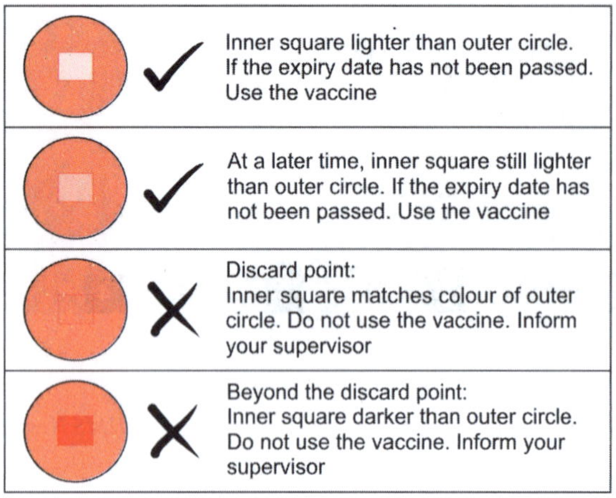

Inner square lighter than outer circle. If the expiry date has not been passed. Use the vaccine
At a later time, inner square still lighter than outer circle. If the expiry date has not been passed. Use the vaccine
Discard point: Inner square matches colour of outer circle. Do not use the vaccine. Inform your supervisor
Beyond the discard point: Inner square darker than outer circle. Do not use the vaccine. Inform your supervisor

2. Ans. (d) Meningococcal meningitis

3. Ans. (a) MMR vaccine; (b) Hepatitis A vaccine; (c) Varicella vaccine

4. Ans. (a) 6, 11; (b) 16, 18; (c) 31, 33

- Human papilloma virus (HPV) types 6, 11, 16, 18, 31, 33, 45, 52, and 58
- Ages 15 through 26 years: 0.5 mL IM as a 3-dose series at 0, 2, and 6 months

Indications in boys and men

- Anal cancer caused by HPV types 16, 18, 31, 33, 45, 52, and 58
- Genital warts (condyloma acuminata) caused by HPV types 6 and 11
- Following precancerous or dysplastic lesions caused by HPV types 6, 11, 16, 18, 31, 33, 45, 52, and 58
- Anal intraepithelial neoplasia (AIN) grades 1, 2, and 3

Indications in females:

- Cervical, vulvar, vaginal, and anal cancer caused by human papillomavirus (HPV) types 16, 18, 31, 33, 45, 52, and 58
- Genital warts (condyloma acuminata) caused by HPV types 6 and 11

5. Ans. (a) Given through IM/SC route; (c) Does not require stringent conditions; (e) Dose is -0.5 ml/dose

6. Ans. (d) Patients with varicella zoster

Ref: K. Park, 24th ed. p 156

7. Ans. (b) 0.5 cc

Ref: K. Park, 24th ed. p 132

8. Ans. (b) 4 hours

Ref: K. Park, 23rd ed. p 481; http://www.who.int/immunization_standards/vaccine_quality/pq266_je_1dose_biologicale/en/

Note: JE vaccine is under the open vial policy along with measles, MR, rotavirus vaccine and BCG

DISCOVERIES AND CONTRIBUTIONS

9. Ans. (d) Edward Jenner

Ref: K. Park, 24th ed. p 6

Smallpox vaccine (1st vaccine) was discovered by Edward Jenner (1749–1823[Q]) of Great Britain, in 1796.

- Edward Jenner also coined the term "vaccination"[Q].
- Smallpox is the only disease to be eradicated[Q].
- Measles, Tetanus, Guinea worm and Endemic goiter are targets for eradication.[Q]

10. Ans. (c) Edward Jenner

Ref: K. Park, 24th ed. p 6

11. Ans. (c) 1823

Ref: K. Park, 24th ed. p 6

12. Ans. (b) Edward Jenner

Ref: K. Park, 24th ed. p 6

INFECTIOUS DISEASE EPIDEMIOLOGY

13. Ans. (b) Rabies

Ref: K. Park, 24th ed. p 296

Postexposure Prophylaxis is Indicated in

- *Hepatitis B and HIV (ART)*
- *Measles (immunized within 2 days of exposure)*
- *Varicella (Varicella Zoster Immunoglobulin within 72 hours of exposure)*
- *Rabies*
- *Tetanus*

*Mnemonic : **HMVRing** Tone*

GENERAL VACCINE

14. Ans. (a) When the inner square becomes...

Ref: K. Park, 23rd ed. p 110

VVM is a label containing a heat-sensitive material placed on a vaccine vial. It registers cumulative heat exposure over time.

Stages of VVM	
Stage 1	The inner square is lighter than the outer circle
Stage 2	The inner square is still lighter than the outer circle
Stage 3 – Discard Point	The color of the inner square matches that of the outer circle. **Vaccine should not be used**
Stage 4 – Beyond the Discard Point	The color of the inner square is darkerthan the outer circle. **Vaccine should not be used**

Stage 1 and 2 vaccine can be used, if the expiry date has not passed.

15. Ans. (b) Prion

Ref: K. Park, 24th ed. p 108

16. Ans. (a) Oral polio vaccine

Ref: K Park 24th ed. p 114, Immunization Handbook for MO, Department of Health and Family Welfare, p-40.

Also Know........................

Vaccine sensitivity to heat *→ BCG (after reconstitution) (Most sensitive) > OPV > Measles> DPT > BCG (before reconstitution) > DT > TT > Hepatitis B> JE (least sensitive)*
Light sensitive vaccines *→ BCG, Measles*
Vaccine sensitive to freezing *→ Hepatitis B (Most) > DPT > DT> TT (Least)*

- *Reconstituted BCG, measles and JE vaccines are the most sensitive to heat and light.*
- *Other than reconstituted vaccine OPV is the most heat sensitive vaccine.*

17. Ans. (a) Measles

Ref: Vaccines for older adults. Lam S1, Jodlowski TZ. Consult Pharm. 2009, 24 (5:380-91)

Vaccines Recommended for Elderly Population

- **H. Influenza inactivated vaccine** (High-risk groups -Health care staff and caretakers, adults ≥50 years, and those with comorbidities that increase the risk of influenza complications.)
- **Pneumococcal vaccine** (elderly ≥65 years of age and those with certain medical conditions). One-time revaccination is offered to elderly who initially received the vaccine before 65 years age and at least five years passed since the initial vaccination.
- **Zoster vaccine** (All elderly ≥60 years of age unless contraindications or precautions exist)
- Tetanus booster (Td or Tdap) every 10 years in adults who have completed the primary series
- Diphtheria and Pertussis

Also Know........................

- Hepatitis A and B, MMR, Meningococcal and Hib vaccine is contraindicated in elderly with medical conditions or lifestyles that put them at higher risk of these disease.

18. Ans. (a) Measles

Ref: Vaccine Safety, Canadian Immunization Guide.http://www.phac-aspc.gc.ca/publicat

Following vaccines contain trace amounts of residual egg and chicken protein and can result in Hypersensitivity reactions among recipients.

- MMR vaccine
- Varicella vaccine
- Influenza vaccines
- Tick-borne encephalitis vaccine
- Rabies vaccine
- Yellow fever vaccine

19. Ans. (c) Maternal antibodies

Ref: Measles and Poliomyelitis: Vaccines, Immunization, and Control, Edouard Kurstak, p-80

Types of Vaccine Failure	Cause
Primary – Failure of Serological Response to Vaccine	▪ Vaccine administered at too young an age (Maternal Antibodies interfere with vaccination)- Most Common cause
	▪ Related to vaccine potency (Inappropriate manufacturing, Cold chain failure, Immunodeficiency, Concurrent illness/Malnutrition, Improper administration –Dose/Site/Route etc.
Secondary- Loss of vaccine offered protection in individuals who had earlier shown seroconversion	▪ Not well known – Coadministration of vaccine and immunoglobulin could be a possible cause

20. Ans. (a) 1 only

Ref: CDC –General recommendations for vaccine use in Pregnant Women -www.cdc.gov/vaccines/pubs/preg-guide.htm#tdap

Vaccination in Pregnancy

- Recommended- Tdap, Influenza (Inactivated)
- Recommended (If indicated)-Polio, Td, Meningococcal, Hepatitis A, Hepatitis B
- Not Recommended -HPV
- Contraindicated-Varicella, Zoster, MMR, Influenza (LAIV)

Vaccine Contraindications

Group	Vaccines
Pregnant women	Varicella, Zoster, MMR, Influenza (LAIV)
Infant	Pneumococcal, Influenza (LAIV), Meningococcal, Yellow Fever
HIV (symptomatic)*, Immunosuppressed and Corticosteroid therapy	All live vaccine

**BCG can be administered. Asymptomatic HIV–All vaccines can be administered*

21. Ans. (a) Hepatitis B

Ref: K. Park 24th ed. p 110

Hepatitis B recombinant vaccine cloned in yeast was the 1st recombinant (cloned) viral vaccine licensed for use in 1986

22. Ans. (c) Killed vaccine

Ref: K. Park, 24th ed. p 108

23. Ans. None

Ref: National Immunization Schedule, Govt of India

Vaccines recommended for a 6 week child are: BCG (if not given at birth), OPV-1, Pentavalent Vaccine (HiB component present) and Rotavirus Vaccine* (*At present in Andhra Pradesh, Himachal Pradesh, Orissa and Haryana from 2016), fractional IPV,* Pneumococcal vaccine

24. Ans. (c) Measles, Mumps, BCG, Varicella

Ref: K. Park, 24th ed. p 108

There is both live attenuated vaccines and killed vaccine against plague

25. Ans. (d) 4 hours

Ref: Immunization handbook for MO, Department of Health and Family Welfare, p-41

Reconstituted vaccine should be discarded after 4 hours

26. Ans. (d) 4

Ref: Immunization Handbook for MO, Department of Health and Family Welfare, p-41

27. Ans. (b) DPT

Ref: K. Park, 24th ed. p 132

Vaccine recommended at birth (for institutional deliveries)	BCG and OPV -0 dose, Hep B

28. Ans. (a) Hepatitis A

Ref: K. Park, 24th ed. p 108

29. Ans. (a) BCG

Ref: K. Park, 24th ed. p 108

30. Ans. (a) Hepatitis B vaccine

Ref: Textbook of Paediatric Nursing, Assuma Beevi.T.M, 1st ed. p-41, UNICEF. Org/ immunization/ index_immunization plus.html

UIP Plus is use of immunization as a vehicle to deliver a set of essential and cost effective maternal and child interventions

- *It includes – Universal Immunization + CSSM, ARI control program, Oral Rehydration Therapy and Vitamin A supplementation, Malaria prophylaxis*

31. Ans. (a) Rubella

Ref: K. Park, 23rd ed. p 103, Guideline for vaccinating pregnant woman 2013, CDC

- *Vaccines contraindicated in Pregnancy are-Influenza (LAIV), MMR, Varicella, Zoster, BCG*
- *Not Recommended – HPV*
- *May be used if otherwise indicated- Rabies, MPSV4, Td, MCV4, Hepatitis A and B*

MMR Vaccine is contraindicated in pregnant women because of possible teratogenic effects of Rubella component.

- *Can be given to seronegative married nonpregnant women, who are advised to avoid pregnancy in next 3–4 months*

Also Know......................

- **Contraindication to Live vaccines**[Q] Pregnancy, Immunodeficiency disease (Leukemia, Lymphoma, Malignancy) and Immunodeficiency state (Immunosuppresive drug and radiation therapy).

32. Ans. (a) MMR vaccine

Ref: K. Park, 24th ed. p 123

MMR vaccine can cause thrombocytopenia (serum platelet count of less than 50,000/mL)

- Leads to bruising and/or bleeding (mild and self-limiting) and occasionally steroid or platelets may be needed.

33. Ans. (c) Hot air oven

Ref: K. Park, 24th ed. p 137

34. Ans. (b) 15-18 months

Ref: K. Park, 24th ed. p 131

35. Ans. (c) Ice lined refrigerator

Ref: K. Park, 24th ed. p 115

At PHC level, ILR are used to store all UIP vaccine

- ILR maintains potency of vaccine with minimum 8 hours of continuous electricity supply in a 24 hours period

Vaccines must be protected from sunlight and prevented from contact with antiseptics.

UIP requires that:

At PHC → Not more than 1-month vaccine requirement is stored in ILR

At District → Not more than 3 months vaccine requirement and supplies is stored in WIC

Temperature of ILR is to be maintained strictly between +2°C to + 8°C

Vaccines like TT, DPT, DT, and diluents are kept in the basket provided with the ILR. Never to be kept on the floor of ILR.

Also Know......................

- Vaccines in ILR are kept in the following order (from top to bottom) → Hepatitis B, DPT, TT, BCG, Measles and OPV at bottom
- Hepatitis B, DPT, TT, DT, Typhoid, and diluents should **never be allowed to freeze.**

36. Ans. (c) Hepatis B; (e) Rabies

Ref: K. Park, 24th ed. p 128

- Live attenuated vaccines are contraindicated in pregnancy. E.g. Measles, Varicella
- Rubella vaccine has a possible teratogenic effect hence contraindicated in pregnancy
- Rabies and Hep B are killed vaccines → hence can be given in pregnancy

37. Ans. (a) Jeryl Lynn

Ref: K. Park, 24th ed. p 162

38. Ans. (a) Live attenuated

Ref: K. Park, 24th ed. p 108

39. Ans. (c) Measles

Ref: K. Park, 24th ed. p 132 Refer Annexure 3.1

40. Ans. (d) DPT + Vitamin A

Ref: K. Park, 24th ed. p 132

41. Ans. (d) 0, 1, 6 months

Ref: K. Park, 24th ed. p 130, CDC website

42. Ans. (a) >0.01 IU/mL

Ref: K. Park, 24th ed. p 330

Tetanus prevention–Aim is to vaccinate whole community *(all age group) and ensure protective level of tetanus anti-toxin as 0.01 IU/mL throughout life.*

Tetanus Toxoid

- Immunity persists for 10 or more years.
- **CDC recommends** booster of TT every 10 years
- In India, TT schedule in adults having not received the primary course of immunization consists of 2 doses of TT adsorbed (0.5 mL, injected into the arm) given at intervals of 1–2 months.
- Longer the intervals between 2 doses, better is the immune response.
- 1st booster dose (third in order) should be given a year after the initial two doses.
- Additional booster dose is given 5 years after the 3rd dose in developing countries.

Also Know........................

- Infants born to mothers who had not received 2 doses of TT-Antitoxin (750 IU) is given within 6 hours of birth.

43. Ans. (a) Ty21 A

Ref: K. Park, 24th ed. p 248

Typhoid Vaccine (Ty 21a)

- Used for typhoid prophylaxis
- Requires storage at 2–8°C
- Capsules are licensed for use in individuals aged ≥5 years; Liquid vaccine in individuals aged >2 years
- Schedule → 1st, 3rd and 5th day. Repeated every 3 years for people living in endemic area and every year for people traveling from nonendemic to endemic countries
- 3-dose regimen, offers protective immunity 7 days after last dose
- It may be given simultaneously with other live vaccines (OPV, cholera and yellow fever or MMR)
- Proguanil and antibacterial drugs should be stopped from 3 days before until 3 days after giving Ty21a.
- It is likely to be less efficacious if administrated at time of ongoing diarrhea
- It can be administered to HIV-positive, asymptomatic individuals provided CD4 count is >200/mm^3;
- Contraindication → Congenital or acquired immuno-deficiency, treatment with immunosuppressive and antimitotic drugs, acute febrile illness and acute intestinal infection

44. Ans. (c) Tetanus

Ref: K. Park, 24th ed. p 330. Mass vaccination: Global aspects-progress and obstacles. Stanley A Plotkins, P-3

Reasons for Mass Immunization

- *To improve the herd immunity in a setting of existing or likely potential outbreak, to reduce morbidity and mortality*
- *To accelerate efforts for disease control by rapidly increasing vaccination coverage*
- *To improve herd immunity to meet international targets for eradication and mortality reduction*

Also Know........................

- In Tetanus – Herd immunity does not protect the individual, whereas it is protective in polio and measles

45. Ans. (c) 300,000 TCID 50

Ref: K. Park, 24th ed. p 221

OPV (Sabin) is a Live attenuated vaccine that contains 3,00,000, 1,00,000 and 3,00,000 TCID 50 of type 1, 2 and 3 live attenuated poliovirus respectively

46. Ans. (d) 0, 7 days

Ref: K. Park, 24th ed. p 297

According to the latest Rabies pre-exposure prophylaxis guidelines (WHO rabies guidelines 2018) the vaccine is given as

- Site intramuscular injection on day 0, 7
- Site intruder alert injections on day 0, 7

47. Ans. (a) Measles

Ref. Infectious Disease in Children and Newer Vaccines, TK Ghosh, 1st ed., p-142, Nancy R. Immunization for children with HIV /AIDS, BIPAI

- All inactivated vaccines are safe in HIV
- In HIV positive asymptomatic patients (not immuno-deficient)- Live vaccine are safe
- **Vaccines contraindicated In HIV positive symptomatic patients (Immunodeficient –CD4 Count <15%)**-BCG, OPV, Mumps Rubella, Japanese Encephalitis, Rotavirus, Yellow Fever, Varicella zoster
- **Vaccines that can be given in HIV positive symptomatic patients (Immunodeficient)**- DPT, Hepatitis A and B, Pneumococcal and Meningococcal Vaccine

Also Know........................

- Exception - Measles vaccine is a live vaccine recommended even in symptomatic

48. Ans. (a) Children under 8 years

Ref: K. Park, 24th ed. p 108

Live vaccines: (e.g., BCG, Measles, Oral polio) prepared from live attenuated organisms induce a full-blown disease but retain immunogenicity

Live attenuated vaccine cannot be given to **persons with**

- Immune deficiency diseases,
- Leukemia
- Lymphoma or malignancy
- Therapy with corticosteroids, alkylating agents, antimetabolic agents, or radiation.[Q]
- Pregnancy unless risk of infection exceeds the risk of harm to the fetus.

49. Ans. (a) Leprosy

Ref: Mass vaccination : Global aspects- progress and obstacles. Stanley A Plotkins, P-3

BCG

50. Ans. (c) Left deltoid

Ref: K Park 22nd ed. p-196

BCG Vaccine is Light Sensitive

Phenomena after vaccination:

2-3 weeks → A papule develops at site of vaccination. It increases in size and reaches a diameter of about 4 to 8 mm in 5 weeks. It then subsides or breaks into a shallow ulcer, usually covered with a crust. Healing occurs spontaneously within 6 to 12 weeks leaving a permanent, tiny, round scar, typically 4-8 mm in diameter. This is a normal reaction.

Individual becomes **Mantoux-positive** after a period of 8 weeks, but sometimes about 14 weeks are needed.[Q]

Complications

Ulceration and suppurative lymphadenitis (1–10%)

Osteomyelitis

Disseminated BCG infection (Least)

Contraindications:

Generalized eczema, infective dermatosis, hypogammaglobulinemia and history of deficient immunity.

BCG Protective efficacy → 0 to 80 percent **Duration of protection** → 15 to 20 years.

DPT/TT

51. Ans. (d) TT complete course + Human Tetanus Immunoglobulin

Ref: K. Park 24th ed. p 331

Here, there is no indication regarding the receipt of complete course of Toxoid or Immune status. Also, being a Road Traffic Accident the injury would not be clean

Immunization status	Clean wound < 6 hours old, Non penetrating/ Negligible Tissue damage	Other wounds
Complete course of TT or a booster dose within past 5 years	Nothing	Nothing
Complete course of TT or a booster dose more than 5 years ago and less than 10 years ago	Toxoid 1 dose	Toxoid 1 dose
Complete course of TT or a booster dose more than 10 years ago	Toxoid 1 dose	Toxoid 1 dose + human Tetanus Ig
Had not had a complete course of TT or Immunity status is unknown	Toxoid complete course	Toxoid complete course + human Tetanus Ig

- When ATS is given, adrenaline solution 1 in 1000 for intramuscular injection in the dosage of 0.5 to 1 mL and hydrocortisone 100 mg for intravenous injection must be kept available.

52. Ans. (b) DPT

Ref: K. Park, 24th ed. p 172

Contraindications to DPT Vaccine

- Seriously ill child,
- History of severe reaction (collapse or shock, persistent screaming episodes, temperature >40°C, convulsions, other neurological symptoms and anaphylactic reactions) after a previous dose. In such cases subsequent immunization with DT only is recommended

53. Ans. (c) dT

Ref: K. Park, 24th ed. p 172

- **Children** >**7 years age** who have not received DPT, 2 doses of DT vaccine, 4 weeks apart, with a booster dose 6 months to 1 year later is recommended.

- **Children >12 years of age and adults,** dT (No more than 2 Lf of Diphtheria toxoid per dose)2 doses at an interval of 4 to 6 weeks, followed by a booster 6 to 12 months after the 2nd dose is given. Alternatively, for primary immunization of adults, FT or TAF may be used (cause fewer reactions).

54. Ans. (d) DPT

Ref: K. Park, 24th ed. p 132

DPT Vaccine: Combined triple antigen vaccine against 3 diseases, viz., Diphtheria, Pertussis and Tetanus.

- *A great gain administratively.*[Q]
- *Pertussis component in DPT enhances the potency of the Diphtheria toxoid.*[Q]
- *Acellular pertussis vaccine is highly immunogenic and with fewer adverse effects.*
  - **Type** - Plain and Adsorbed (Adsorbed on aluminum phosphate or hydroxide.[Q])
  - DPT vaccines should not be frozen. They should be stored in a refrigerator between 4^0 to 8° C. [Q]
  - DPT vaccine has 25-30 Lf of Diphtheria toxoid and 5-10 Lf of Tetanus toxoid.
  - 3 doses of DPT (0.5 mL) at an interval of 4 weeks, with 1st dose at 6 weeks after birth is considered optimal for primary immunization.
  - 2 booster injection at 1.5 years and 5 years are recommended (can be given till 7 years)
  - Route and site: Deep i.m. injection in mid anterolateral aspect of thigh (especially for infants).
  - Reactions: Fever and mild local reactions are common.
  - **ANTISERA** - the mainstay of passive prophylaxis and treatment of Diphtheria.
- *Prophylactic: 500 to 2000 units by subcutaneous or intramuscular injection*
- *Therapeutic: 10,000 to 30,000 units by IM injection or 40,000 to 100,000 units by i.v. in 2 divided doses with an* interval of 1.5 to 2 hours.
  - Most serious complication → are neurological and primarily due to pertussis component.

OPV AND IPV

55. Ans. (a) 7–14

Ref: WHO Information sheet observed rate of vaccine reactions for polio vaccines

VAPP- Case definition includes the following:

- A case of acute flaccid paralysis with residual weakness at 60 days after onset of symptoms;
- A negative stool sample for wild poliovirus but positive for vaccine virus as examined in a WHO accredited lab
- Evaluation and confirmation of the case by an expert committee (WHO 1998).
  - Onset of symptoms with VAPP occur 4–30 days following receipt of OPV or 4–75 days after contact with a recipient of OPV.
  - In immunodeficient individuals (Hypogammaglobulinemia) VAPP may occur outside these windows.
  - Rate of VAPP (one case per 700,000 to one case per 3.4 million first doses).is higher for the 1st dose of OPV than for subsequent doses
  - WHO estimates VAPP risk at 2–4 cases per million birth cohort. VAPP is more common in immunocompromised individuals
  - No study has demonstrated transmission from a VAPP case resulting in another VAPP case.

56. Ans. (a) Follow up of AFP every 30 days

Ref: K. Park, 24th ed. p 219

In AFP surveillance: Follow up is done after 60 days of onset of paralysis.

57. Ans. (b) Maternal antibody is completely ...

Ref: K. Park, 24th ed. p 221

Oral Polio Vaccine (OPV)

- It is a live attenuated vaccine (contains 3 Lakh, 1 Lakh and 3 Lakh TCID 50 of type 1, 2 and 3 live attenuated poliovirus respectively)
- OPV and Measles (**Mnemonic** – **P**rime **M**inister) vaccine are very sensitive to heat and require stringent conditions for storage and transport. OPV can be stored in freezers (Sub Zero temperature) for long durations
- OPV induces both systemic and intestinal or local immunity
- OPV is associated with VAPP → 1 case per million vaccine recipient and 1 case per 5 million doses of vaccine among close contact of vaccine recipients
- OPV zero dose is given at birth in all institutional deliveries (Maternal antibody is not completely protective)

58. Ans. (b) Type 2 virus

Ref: WHO Information sheet observed rate of vaccine reactions for polio vaccines

Vaccine Derived Polio Virus (VDPV)

Also Know......................

- VDPV is a live, attenuated strain of the virus contained in OPV, that has changed and reverted to a form capable of cause paralysis in humans and may develop the capacity for sustained circulation.
- VDPVs differ from the original Sabin strains in the vaccine by 1 to 15% of VP1 nucleotides.
- On rare occasions, in areas where populations are under-immunized, VDPVs can regain the ability to circulate in populations and can occasionally cause paralysis.
- Most circulating VDPV are type 2 followed by Type 1 and type 3
- Oral polio vaccine protects against VDPVs and is used to contain outbreaks.
- Low vaccination coverage results in VDPV. If a population is fully immunized, they will be protected against both VDPV and wild polioviruses.

59. Ans. (b) P1 and P3

Ref: Global Polio Eradication Initiative www.polioeradication.org

Bivalent Oral Polio Vaccine– is a live attenuated vaccine with Wild Polio virus strains (Type 1 and 3)

In PPI, 2 rounds 4-6 weeks apart are carried out in low transmission season of polio, i.e. Nov-Feb.

Dose of OPV in PPIs are extra doses (Supplement not replace the dose received during routine immunization)

Children must receive all their scheduled doses and PPI doses

There is no minimum interval between PPI and scheduled OPV doses

MEASLES

60. Ans. (c) Jeryl Lynn strain

Ref: Community Medicine Recent Advances –Suryakanta, 3rd ed., p-319

61. Ans. (b) 15–18 months

Ref: K. Park, 24th ed. p 132

MMR is a Mixed or Combined Vaccine→It simplifies administration, reduce costs and minimize number of contacts of patient with health system. It is administered at 15-18 month

62. Ans. (b) 0.5 cc

Ref: K. Park, 24th ed. p 132

63. Ans. (d) 6–9 months

Ref: K. Park, 24th ed. p 259

WHO Expanded Program on Immunization recommends measles immunization at 9 months age.[Q]

- Age can be lowered to 6 months if there is measles outbreak in the community.
- For infants immunized between 6 to 9 months of age, a 2nd dose should be administered as soon as possible after the child reaches age of 9 months provided at least 4 weeks have elapsed since last dose.
- In countries where the incidence of measles has declined, the age of immunization is being raised to 15 months in order to avoid the blocking effect of persistent transplacentally acquired antibody

Latest Updates

In India, a 2nd dose of measles vaccine (between 16–24 months of age) has been added to the national immunization schedule.

Also Know......................

Measles vaccine

- Live attenuated, lyophilized freeze dried tissue culture vaccine.[Q]
- Reconstituted vaccine is administered in a single subcutaneous dose of 0.5 mL in right upper arm[Q]
- Diluent used is distilled water[Q] and must be kept cold at 4-8°C.
- Reconstituted vaccine should be kept on ice and used within 1 hour.
- Recently measles vaccine has been adapted for aerosol administration.

Also Know......................

- Vaccine provide immunity to even severely malnourished children. Immunity is for life.
- Single dose of the vaccine offers 95% protection.
- Postexposure prophylaxis → To susceptible contacts (9-12 months age) given within 3 days of exposure.
- Contraindications: Pregnancy, acute illnesses, deficient cell mediated immunity, use of steroids/immunosuppressive drugs.
- Adverse effects: Toxic shock syndrome (TSS)
- Combined measles vaccine: MMR.

Latest Updates

Measles and HIV→ Measles vaccine is advocated for RI to potentially susceptible, asymptomatic HIV +ve children or Symptomatic HIV +ve not severely immunocompromised. 1st dose is offered as early as 6 months.

Toxic shock syndrome is preventable and reflects poor quality of immunization services (A vial used for >1 session on same or next day)

Symptoms → Severe watery diarrhea, vomiting and high fever within hours of measles vaccination.

All infants vaccinated from contaminated vial are affected

NEWER VACCINE

64. Ans. (c) H2N1

Ref:-Key Facts About Seasonal Flu Vaccine, CDC http://www.cdc.gov/flu/protect/keyfacts.htm

Quadrivalent flu Vaccine (Influenza A H1N1 and H3N2 virus and 2 Influenza B virus)

- It is an improvement over Trivalent Flu vaccine. In addition to protection against (Influenza A H1N1 and H3N2 virus) it offers protection against 2 strains of Influenza B virus (as against 1 strain in Trivalent vaccine). It is not 100% protective, but reduces risk
- Injectible vaccine can be given to children as young as 6 months of age. It is inactivated vaccine
- Nasal spray vaccine (LAIV4) is approved for people 2–49 years of age who do not have contraindications to the nasal spray vaccine. It is live attenuated vaccine
- LAIV4 is contraindicated in pregnant women, immunosuppressed persons, persons with egg allergy and children 2–4 years with H/O asthma or who have had a wheezing episode noted in the medical record within the past 12 months, or for whom parents report that a health care provider stated that they had wheezing or asthma within the last 12 months.
- LAIV4 should not be administered to persons who have taken influenza antiviral medications within the previous 48 hours.
- Persons who care for severely immunosuppressed persons who require a protective environment should not receive LAIV4, or should avoid contact with such persons for 7 days after receipt

- Contraindications- Severe allergic reaction to any vaccine component, including egg protein, or after previous dose of any influenza vaccine.
- Precautions: Moderate to severe acute illness with or without fever; history of Guillain-Barré syndrome within 6 weeks of receipt of influenza vaccine.

65. Ans. (d) 24 months

Ref: K Park 24th ed. p 252

VI Polysaccharide Vaccine

- It is a subunit vaccine composed of purified Vi capsular polysaccharide from Ty2 S. Typhi strain.
- It does not elicit adequate immune responses in children <2 years and is licensed for individuals ≥2 years
- Vaccine is administered subcutaneously or intramuscularly
- 1 dose (25 mg of antigen) of vaccine confers protection 7 days after injection.
- Re-vaccination is recommended every 3 years
- It can be co-administered with other vaccines (Yellow fever, hepatitis A and RI vaccines)
- Recommended storage temperature is 2-8°C

66. Ans. (b) Cholera vaccine

Ref: K. Park, 24th ed. p 248

Cholera Vaccine	Minimum age at 1st dose	Doses (Primary Series)	Interval between doses	Booster
Dukoral- *Oral monovalent killed whole cell (Vibrio Cholerae O1 and recombinant (Sub Unit B) vaccine Protection starts 1 week after the last dose*	2 years	3 (2-5 year age)	≥7 days is (minimum) and <6 weeks (maximum) If the interval between doses is delayed > 6 week- Primary immunization is restarted	Every 6 months (if gap after primary vaccination exceeds 6 month – primary series is repeated
		2 (Adult and Child ≥6 years)	≥7 days is (minimum) and < 6 week (maximum) If the interval between doses is delayed >6 week- Primary immunization is restarted	Every 2 years if gap after primary vaccination exceeds 2 years – primary series is repeated
Shancol and mORCVAX (bivalent 1-year oral vaccine-0139 and O1)		2	14 days	After 2 years

67. Ans. (d) PRP with carrier

Ref: –Haemophilus b Conjugate vaccines for prevention of H. Influenza. www.cdc.gov/mmwr/preview/mmwrhtml/00041736.htm

Hib Conjugate Vaccine

- Polyribosylribitol Phosphate (PRP) Capsule of Hib is the major virulence factor
- Conjugate vaccines are Conjugation of PRP with T – cell dependent protein antigens
- 3 types of Conjugate vaccine are licensed for use with older children –HbOC, PRP-OMP, PRP-D
- Conjugate vaccine differ by protein carrier, polysaccharide size, method of chemical conjugation

68. Ans. (c) 20 mL

Ref: K. Park, 24th ed. p 113

Disease causing agent	Dose of immunoglobulin	Recommendation
Rubella	20 mL	Women exposed in early pregnancy (Optional)
Hepatitis A	0.02- 0.05 mL/kg body weight (3.2-8.0 mg /kg body weight)	Recommended for prevention in Family contacts, Institutional outbreak, Travellers
Hepatitis B	0.05 mL -0.07 (8-11mg/kg) mL/kg body weight	Recommended for prevention in percutaneous/mucosal exposure, Newborns with HBsAg positive mothers. Optional in case of sexual contact with acute Hep B case
Hepatitis C	0.05 mL /kg (8 mg/kg) body weight	Optional in case of percutaneous/mucosal exposure
Varicella Zoster	15–25 Unit/kg body weight (min 125 units)	Recommended for prevention in immunosuppressed contacts of acute cases or newborn contact
Measles	0.25 mL/ kg body weight (0.5 mL/ kg in immune-suppressed)	Recommended for prevention in Infants or immune-suppressed contacts of acute cases exposed within last 6 days
Rh isoimmunization	1 vial (200–300 ug) per 15 mL of Rh+ blood exposure	Recommended for prevention in Rh (D) –VE mother with Rh +ve infant, Transfusion of Rh +ve blood to Rh –ve mother

69. Ans. (d) Primary schedule consist of 2 doses

Ref: K. Park, 23rd ed. p 286. Infectious Diseases in Children and Newer Vaccine. 1st ed. p- 180

SA14-14-2 vaccine

- *It is a cell culture derived live attenuated vaccine for Japanese Encephalitis developed by a US Company (VacGen)*
- *It is a lyophilized (freeze dried vaccine) to be used within 2 hours of reconstitution*
- *Dose – 0.5 mL, Route – Subcutaneous, Site- Upper arm*
- *Based on stable neuro attenuated strain of JE virus (SA 14-14-2) grown on hamster kidney cell culture*
- *Efficacy 99% with single dose*
- *Contraindication – Pregnancy, AIDS or immunosuppressive illness, Anaphylaxis to previous dose, hypersensitivity to Kanamycin/Gentamycin/Gelatin, Fever (>38.5°C)*

70. Ans. (a) Bivalent and quadrivalent; (c) Most common subtype are 16, 18

Ref: 24th ed. p 133. WHO Position paper on HPV Vaccine

HPV Vaccines

- *Prophylactic only*, do not clear existing HPV infections or treat HPV related disease.
- *Recommended for* young adolescent girls (10–14 years) before onset of sexual activity to prevent cervical precancer and cancer
- *Quadrivalent vaccine* (licensed in 2006, contains virus like particles (VLP) for HPV 6,11,16 and18)
- *Schedule* – Baseline- 2 and 6 months (Minimum interval of 4 week between 1st and 2nd and 12 week between 2nd and3rd dose)
- *Bivalent vaccine* (Licensed 2007, contains virus like particles (VLP) for HPV 16 and18)
- *Schedule* - Baseline, 1 and 6 months
- Vaccine is available as sterile suspension in single use glass vials or single use prefilled syringe
- Storage – maintained at 2–8°C and not frozen.
- Dose – 0.5 mL
- Route – Intramuscular injection
- Efficacy = 92% (the efficacy applies to 70% of cancer caused by HPV 16and 18B, not all cervical cancer

71. Ans. (b) Cervix CA

Ref: 24th ed. p 134,. WHO Position paper on HPV Vaccine; www.cancer.gov

Cancer Vaccine -2 Types

- Preventive (Prophylactic) – HPV Vaccine and Hepatitis B Virus Vaccine
- Treatment (Therapeutic) – Vaccine for Prostate cancer

72. Ans. (b) Type 7

Ref: 24th ed. p 134. WHO Position paper on HPV Vaccine

73. Ans. (c) Efficacy >70% for cervical cancer; (d) Two types of vaccine are available in the market; (e) Protect against HPV 16 and 18

Ref: WHO position paper on HPV vaccine. No. 15,2009,84,p-117-132, Adult Immunization. CD Alert. Monthly Newsletter of National Center for Disease Control. DGHS, GoI. Feb-Mar. 2011. Vol. 14:2

74. Ans. (d) Can be administered with yellow fever and hepatitis A vaccine

Ref: K Park 24th ed. p 252

Vi Polysaccharide Vaccine

- Re-vaccination is recommended every 3 years
- It can be co-administered with other vaccines (Yellow fever, hepatitis A and RI vaccines)
- No contraindications, except for previous severe hypersensitivity reaction to vaccine components
- It is safe for HIV-infected individuals, induction of protective antibodies is directly correlated to levels of CD4 positive T-cells.
- No serious adverse event and minimum local side effects.

75. Ans. (a) BCG; (c) ICRC bacillus; (e) Mycobacterium 'W'

Ref: K. Park, 24th ed. p 344, Various Journals – Mentioned

Vaccines Available for Leprosy

- **BCG** – Worldwide
- **ICRC bacilli cultivable**-(India)
- **Mycobacterium 'W'** cultivable (India)
- **Mycobacterium habana**- cultivable (India)

30 January, 1998 (50th anniversary of Mahatma Gandhi's death) India announced approval of the 1st commercially available leprosy vaccine → **Leprovac** (Manufactured by Cedilla Pharmaceuticals in Ahmedabad, → contains a heat killed, fast growing, nonpathogenic mycobacterium called Mycobacterium w.)

76. Ans. (d) Typhoid

Ref: K. Park, 24th ed p252

77. Ans. (d) Mumps

Mumps is not a part of the National immunization schedule, under mission Indradhanush scheme. Other vaccines are part of the NIS. For details, pls refer to table below

National Immunization Schedule (NIS) for Infants, Children and Pregnant Women

Vaccine	When to give	Dose	Route	Site
For Pregnant women				
TT-1	Early in pregnancy	0.5 ml	Intra-muscular	Upper Arm
TT-2	4 weeks after TT-1*	0.5 ml	Intra-muscular	Upper Arm
TT-Booster	If received 2 TT doses in a pregnancy within the last 3 yrs*	0.5 ml	Intra-muscular	Upper Arm
For Infants				
BCG	At birth or as early as possible till one year of age	0.1ml (0.05 ml until 1 month age)	Intra-dermal	Left upper arm
Hepatitis B-Birth dose	At birth or as early as possible within 24 hours	0.5 ml	Intra-muscular	Antero-lateral side of mid-thigh
OPV-0	At birth or as early as possible within the first 15 days	2 drops	Oral	Oral
OPV 1, 2 & 3	At 6 weeks, 10 weeks & 14 weeks (OPV can be given till 5 years of age)	2 drops	Oral	Oral
Pentavalent 1, 2 & 3	At 6 weeks, 10 weeks & 14 weeks (can be given till one year of age)	0.5 ml	Intra-muscular	Antero-lateral side of mid-thigh
Rotavirus#	At 6 weeks, 10 weeks & 14 weeks (can be given till one year of age)	5 drops	Oral	Oral
IPV	Two fractional dose at 6 and 14 weeks of age	0.1 ml	Intra dermal two fractional dose	Intra-dermal: Right upper arm
Measles /MR1st Dose$	9 completed months-12 months. (can be given till 5 years of age)	0.5 ml	Sub-cutaneous	Right upper Arm
JE – 1**	9 completed months-12 months.	0.5 ml	Sub-cutaneous	Left upper Arm
Vitamin A (1st dose)	At 9 completed months with measles- Rubella	1 ml (1 lakh IU)	Oral	Oral
For Children				
DPT booster-1	16-24 months	0.5 ml	Intra-muscular	Antero-lateral side of mid-thigh
Measles/MR 2nd done $	16-24 months	0.5 ml	Sub-cutaneous	Right upper Arm
OPV Booster	16-24 months	2 drops	Oral	Oral
JE-2	16-24 months	0.5 ml	Sub-cutaneous	Left Upper Arm
Vitamin A*** (2nd to 9th dose)	16-18 months. Then one dose every 6 months up to the age of 5 years.	2 ml (2 lakh IU)	Oral	Oral
DPT Booster-2	5-6 years	0.5 ml.	Intra-muscular	Upper Arm
TT	10 years & 16 years	0.5 ml	Intra-muscular	Upper Arm

Note: The recent NIS has update on
All TT vaccines to be replaced with Td Vaccine

78. Ans. (a) 1 & 2

The discard point of the vaccine is when the same color is there for the outer circle and inner square

79. Ans. (a) Live vaccine, SA-14-14-2 strain

Live attenuated vaccine (SA 14-14-2 strain). The first dose is given subcutaneously at the age 8 months, followed by a booster dose at 2 years of age. In some areas, an additional booster is offered at 6–7 years of age. However, protection for several years may be achieved with a single dose of this vaccine, and in many countries one dose without subsequent boosters is recommended.

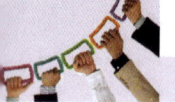

80. Ans. (c) 7 visits for immunization till 5 years

As per National Immunization Schedule the children can get the vaccines at birth, at 6, 10 and 14 weeks and then at 9 months. The booster doses are given at 16-24 months and then at 5 years of age. (7 visits till 5 years)

The ultimate goal of Mission Indradhanush is to ensure full immunization with all available vaccines for children up to two years and pregnant women.

The Mission is strategically designed to achieving high quality routine immunization coverage while contributing to strengthening health systems that can be sustained over years to come. In the last few years, India's full immunization coverage has increased only by 1% per year. The Mission has been launched to accelerate the process of immunization and achieve full immunization coverage for all children in the country.

The Mission Indradhanush, depicting seven colours of the rainbow, targets to immunize all children against seven vaccine preventable diseases, namely:

- Diphtheria
- Pertussis
- Tetanus
- Tuberculosis
- Polio
- Hepatitis B
- Measles.

In addition to this, vaccines for Japanese Encephalitis (JE) and Haemophilus influenzae type B (HIB) are also being provided in selected states.

81. Ans. (a) Detectable antitoxin for about 10 years.

Diptheria toxoid alone or in combination with pertussis vaccine and tetanus toxoid induces protective levels of antitoxin that persists for around 10 years. Boosters are required every 10 years.

Antitoxin antibody do not prevent infection of the respiratory tract with C.diptheriae and do not prevent the development of carrier state.

The antibodies are directed against the exotoxin produced by bacteria and not against the bacteria themselves.

Adverse reactions from the toxoid are infrequent in infants and young children but are more common in adults. Thus administration of reduced dose of toxoid is recommended for children over 6 yrs of age and adults. The reduced dose is symbolized as 'd' and may be combined with tetanus toxoid as 'Td'.

82. Ans. (d) It is targeting urban slums with nomadic population

Mission Indradhanush

For 7 VPD (Vaccine preventable disease) prevention for all children under 2 years and pregnant females

Measles, TB, Hepatitis B, Diphtheria, Polio, Pertussis, Tetanus (+additional diseases: Influenza, Rota virus, Japanese Encephalitis, Rubella)

To implement this – Intensified Mission Indradhanush was lunched in 'selected states and districts' to achieve the target of more than 90% immunization coverage by December 2018. IMI will cater to left outs and drop outs in selected districts and some urban areas.

IMI (Intensified mission indradhanush) – is for

- Urban slums with migratory population
- Nomadic sites (brick kilns, construction sites, other migrant settlements-fisherman villages, riverine areas with shifting populations, underserved and hard-to-reach populations-forested and tribal populations, hilly areas, etc.
- Areas with low routine immunization coverage identified through measles outbreaks, cases of diphtheria and neonatal tetanus in the last two years.

Note:

- MI (mission Indradhanush) = 7 times vaccination to under five children, for 7 VPD's (vaccine preventable diseases)
- IMI (Intensified Mission Indradhanush) – 7 working days in a month, starting 7th every month, excluding Sundays, holidays and immunization days.

83. Ans. (b) Influenza

The new vaccines added into national immunization schedule are:

- Pentavalent vaccine
- Rotavirus vaccine
- Bivalent OPV (bOPV) vaccine
- f-IPV (fractional IPV)
- Pneumococcal Conjugate vaccine
- JE Live vaccine*
- Td vaccine (replace TT Vaccine)
- MR Vaccine (replace Measles vaccine) $

*JE vaccine is given only in the selected JE endemic districts. It is for all children age < 15 years. recently, the GoI has also initiated the adult JE vaccine on pilot project basis in few states apart from the ongoing JE vaccination strategy for children.

$MR vaccine is replacing the previous Measles II vaccine and recently in selected states Measles I vaccine is also replaced with MR vaccine as MR campaign is accelerated throughout the country

84. Ans. (a) Shake test

Shake Test

It is used to check for the efficacy for the freeze-sensitive vaccine

It is done for Pentavalent, TT, DPT, Td, Hepatitis B vaccines

85. Ans. (a) VVM

Ref: K. Park, 25th ed., Pg. 120; https://mohfw.gov.in/basicpage/immunization-handbook-medical-officers2017

Vaccine Vial Monitor

It is a chemical indicator device attached to the vaccine vial or the ampule. VVM can measure the cumulative heat exposure of the vaccine while its journey through the cold chain.

The VVM may be at different locations on the vial, as:

- VVM on the side or the label of the vaccine – means that the vaccine vial once opened can be kept for subsequent use upto 28 days or till the VVM is applicable

- VVM is on the top/cap/neck of ampule – means that the vaccinator should check and then open the vaccine, but once opened it must be discarded at the end of session or within 6 hours, whichever is first. These vaccines are not under the open vial policy.

Note: Open vial policy does not apply to BCG, Measles, Measles/rubella, JE and Rotavirus vaccine how to read a VVM:

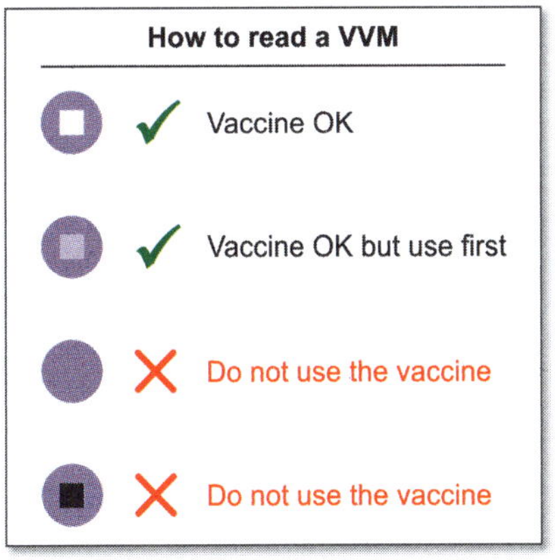

How to read a VVM
Vaccine OK
Vaccine OK but use first
Do not use the vaccine
Do not use the vaccine

86. Ans. (c) M. indicus pranii

Ref. Yadav, A.R., Mohanty, K.K. and Sengupta, U. (2017) ICRC Bacillus a Vaccine Candidate Strain (C-44) Is Coated with Human IgG. Open Journal of Immunology, 7, 45-50.; Singh S, Chouhan K, Gupta S. Intralesional immunotherapy with killed Mycobacterium indicus pranii vaccine for the treatment of extensive cutaneous warts . Indian J Dermatol Venereol Leprol 2014;80:509-14

Leprosy Vaccine

- A vaccine approved for use was MIP (mycobacterium Indicus Pranii) vaccine (also called as Mw vaccine). review of literature shows that it is also used for genital and other multiple cutaneous warts.
- Another candidate vaccine is Indian Cancer Research Center (ICRC), bacillus strain (C-44) for leprosy

87. Ans. (d) Influenza

Ref: Park 25th Ed. Pg 171

NOTES

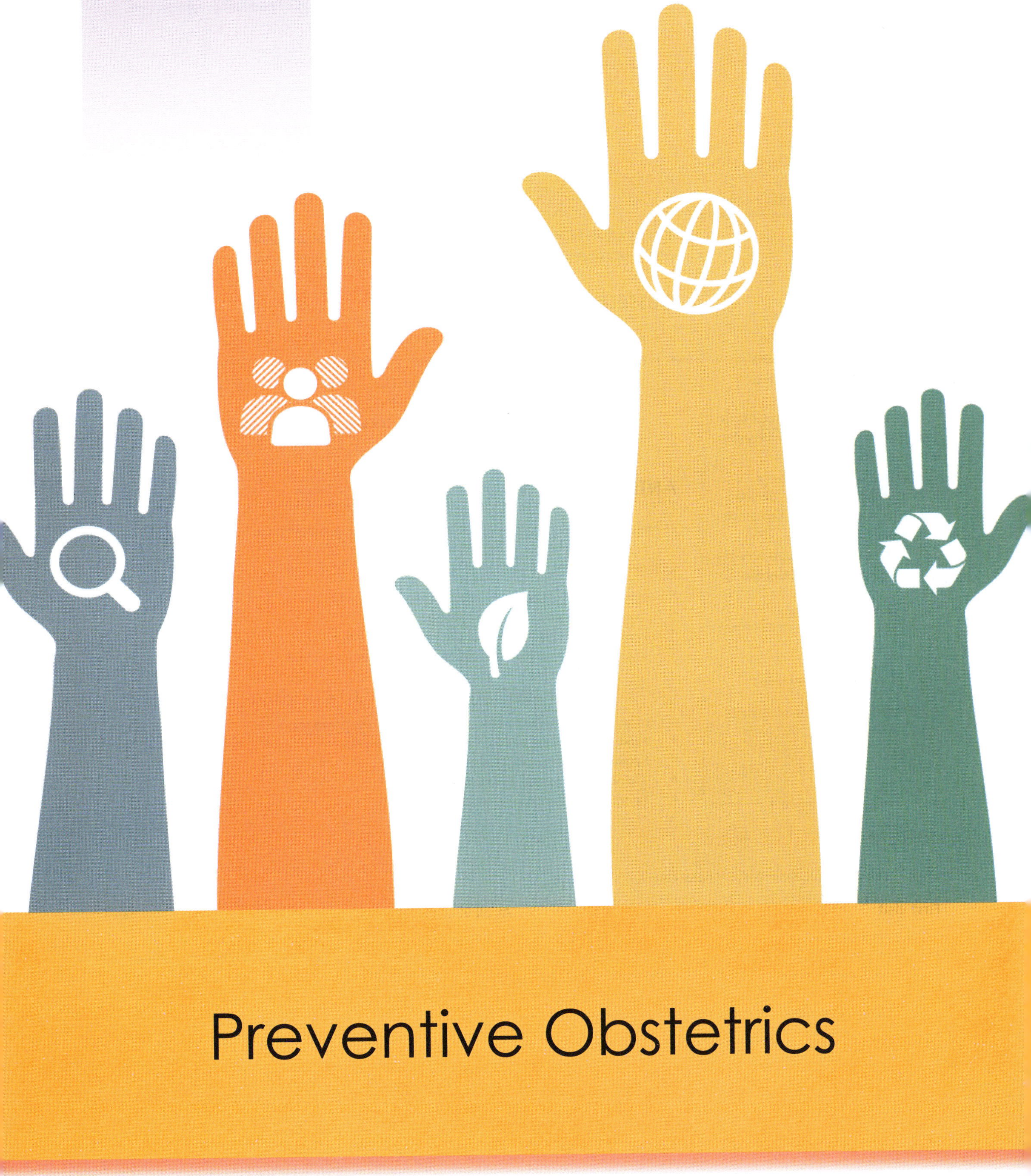

Preventive Obstetrics

Chapter Outline

Services of the Mothers
- Obstetric Care
- Antenatal Care
  - Nutritional Recommendations
  - GDM Screening
- Intranatal Care
- Postnatal Care
- Maternal Mortality
- Protocols for Management of Obstetric Emergencies

Schemes Related to MCH in India
- RCH Program
- Anemia Mukt Bharat Guidelines

163 High Yield Points

Emergency Obstetric Care (EmOC) at First referral unit (FRU)
- ***Basic EmOC***- Skilled health personnel [all CHC and 50% PHC 24 × 7] who can provide parenteral antibiotics, anticonvulsant and oxytocic drug
  - Manual removal of retained products
  - Assisted vaginal delivery
- ***Comprehensive EmOC***- Skilled health personnel who can provide full Basic EmOC plus
  - Safe blood transfusion services
  - Surgical services [Cesarean section]
  - Anesthetic services.

103 Good to Remember

Specific Infections to be screened during ANC:
- HepB
- HIV
- VDRL

SERVICES TO THE MOTHERS

- **Preconceptional care:** Females are educated regarding planned parenthood, institutional delivery and services, medical supervision during pregnancy and genetic counseling
- **Obstetric care:** Care of the female during the physiological process of reproduction.

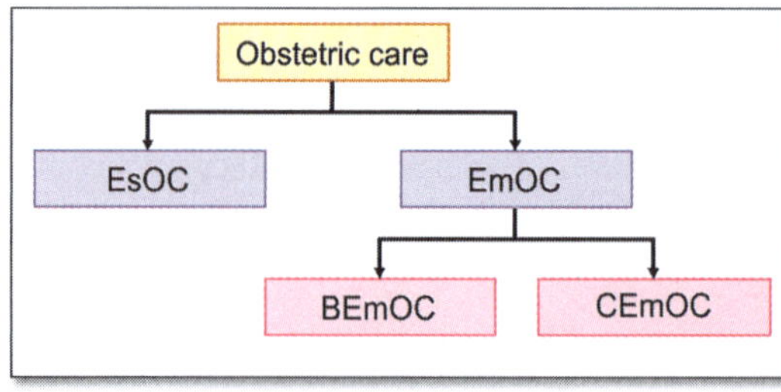

Fig. 1: Hierarchy chart

Abbreviations: EsOC, essential obstetrics care; EmOC, emergency obstetrics care, BEmOC, basic emergency obstetrics care; CEmOC, comprehensive emergency obstetrics care

OBSTETRIC CARE

- **Essential obstetric care:** Care of female before, during and after delivery
- **Emergency obstetric care:** Care of female anytime in emergency before or during the process
  - **Basic emergency obstetric care:** Care of the female before/during the process of delivery
  - **Comprehensive emergency obstetric care:** Care for the maternal and child health as a combined package.

ANTENATAL CARE

Minimum obstetric care to be made available to all pregnant women.

Objectives

- Helps to identify the complications of pregnancy in time
- Ensures good and quality management
- Ensures healthy outcomes for the mother and baby
- Important for well-being of the mother and her fetus/child

Guidelines for ANC under NRHM 2014 Update

A minimum of 4 antenatal visits are made during the pregnancy:
- **First visit:** As soon as possible or before 12 weeks
- **Second visit:** Between 14 and 26 weeks
- **Third visit:** Between 28 and 34 weeks
- **Fourth visit:** Between 36 weeks and term

Antenatal Care Visits Protocol

Table 1: Protocol guidelines for antenatal care visits

First visit	At all visits
▪ Pregnancy detection test ▪ Fill up mother and child protection (MCP) card and ANC register ▪ Give filled up MCP card and safe motherhood booklet to the women ▪ Past and present history of any illness/complications in this or previous pregnancy	▪ Physical examination ▪ Abdominal palpation for fetal growth, fetal lie and auscultation of fetal heart sound

Contd...

First visit	At all visits
▪ Physical examination (weight, BP, respiratory rate and check CVS/Respiratory system, breast, pallor, jaundice and edema) ▪ Two doses of inj. TT 4 weeks apart whenever pregnancy is detected **Investigation** ▪ Hb%, urine examination ▪ Blood group including Rh factor ▪ RPR/VDRL, HBsAg, HIV screening ▪ RDK test for malaria (in endemic areas) **Information for pregnant woman and her family** ▪ Encourage institutional delivery/ensure delivery by identification of SBA (Skilled Birth Attendant) ▪ Explain entitlement under JSSK and JSY ▪ Identify the nearest functional PHC/FRU for delivery ▪ High risk pregnancy to be attended in district hospital and medical college ▪ Preidentification of referral transport and blood donor	**Investigation** ▪ Hemoglobin estimation ▪ Urine exam for protein, sugar and micro exam ▪ At 24–28 weeks blood sugar (OGCT)*–2nd or 3rd visit **Counselling for** ▪ Adequate rest, nutrition and balanced diet ▪ Recognition of danger signs during pregnancy, labor and after delivery or abortion and signs of normal labor ▪ Initiation of breastfeeding immediately after birth ▪ Counseling for small family norm ▪ Use of contraceptives (birth spacing or limiting) after birth/ abortion * OGCT-Oral glucose challenge test

Supplementation in Pregnancy

- Folic acid tab 400 mg daily in 1st trimester
- Iron folic acid table daily from 14 weeks onwards
- For anemic women, iron folic acid tab twice daily

Nutritional Recommended of the Mother

Table 2: Recommended additional daily nutritional allowances (pregnancy and lactation)

Group	Energy (kcal/day)	Protein* (g/day)	Fat (g/day)	Calcium (mg/day)**	Iodine mcg/day	Vitamin A IU/day
Pregnancy	+ 350	RDA + 23	30	1,200 (i.e. RDA + 600)	250–260	900
Lactation (0–6 months)	+ 600	RDA + 19	30	1200 (i.e. RDA + 600)	290 mcg	
Lactation (6–12 months)	+ 520	RDA + 13				

* RDA = 1 g/kg body weight/day
**RDA = 600 mg/day

GDM Screening 2017-2018 Guidelines

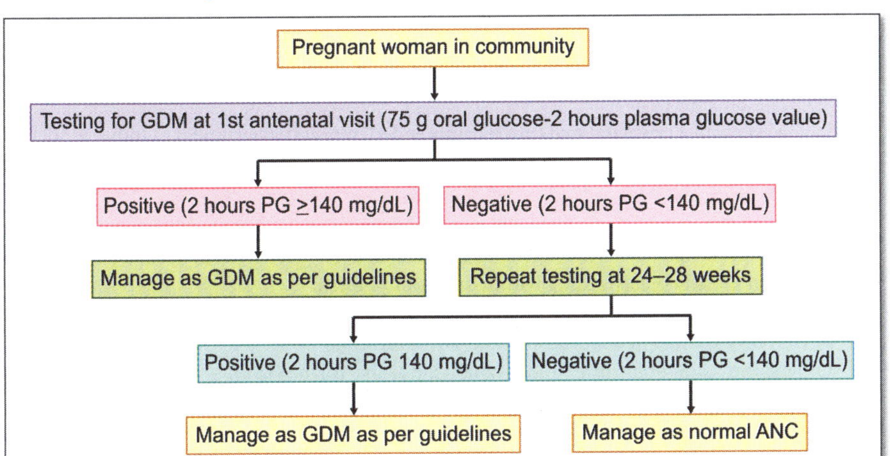

164 High Yield Points

'Weight height product index (WHPI)' is used to assess the nutritional status of the mother.

$$\text{WHPI} = \frac{\text{Current weight (kg)} \times \text{Height (cm)}}{\text{Expected weight (kg)} \times \text{Height (cm)}} \times 100$$

WHPI = Less than 100 indicates malnutrition.

165 High Yield Points

Special micronutrient requirement in pregnancy:

	Normal	Pregnancy
Iodine	150 mcg/ day	260 mcg/ day
Vitamin A	600 IU/day	900 IU/day

104 Good to Remember

- A pregnancy in total duration consumes about 60,000 kcal over and above normal metabolic requirements
- On an average, a normal healthy woman gains about 11-12 kg of weight during pregnancy.
- 50 to 60% of Indian women belonging to low socioeconomic groups are anemic in 3rd trimester of pregnancy

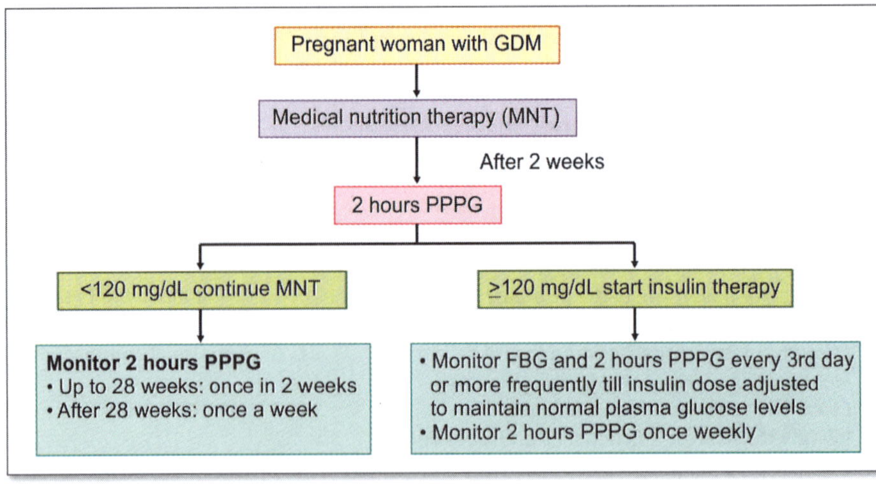

Tetanus toxoid in pregnancy:

- Two doses of tetanus toxoid (TT) for unknown immunization status of pregnant women. The first dose is administered as soon as pregnancy is detected and the second dose is administered after 4 weeks
- If the mother received 2 TT doses in the last pregnancy and gets pregnant again within 3 years, then only one dose of TT is recommended and that dose is called *booster dose.*

98 Must Remember

Contents of Disposable Delivery kit
- Gauze piece (7.5 cm × 1 m) - 1
- Ligatures - 2
- Razor blade (ISI) - 1
- Soap (10 g) - 1
- Antiseptic lotion - 10 mL
- Cotton - 10 g

INTRANATAL CARE

- Assistance during delivery: Institutional delivery or safe delivery at home by skilled birth attendant.

  '5 cleans' in conduct of delivery[Q] important in prevention of neonatal tetanus-
  - Clean hands
  - Clean surface for delivery
  - Clean cut
  - Clean tie
  - Clean cord – no application

'7 clean' → '5 Clean' + Clean Water + Clean Towel (for hand wiping)

105 Good to Remember

Complications of Postpartum Period
- Puerperal sepsis, Thrombophlebitis, Secondary hemorrhage (6 hours-6 weeks after delivery), Urinary tract infection and mastitis.

POSTNATAL CARE

- It is the care of the mother and baby after delivery
- It ensures complete well-being of the mother and baby
- Elements of postnatal care
  - 0 & 3rd day at the health facility both for the mother and new-born and
  - Direction to the ANM of the concerned area for ensuring 7th & 42nd day postnatal home visits.
  - 3 additional visits for a low birth weight baby (less than 2500 gm) on 14th day, 21st day and on 28th day.

  Minimum 4 postnatal visits are recommended by GoI (Government of India) guidelines

1st check-up	1st day of delivery
2nd check-up	3rd day of delivery
3rd check-up	7th day of delivery
4th check-up	6 weeks after delivery

- Initiation of early breastfeeding within one hour of birth.
- Counseling on nutrition, hygiene, contraception, essential new born care (As per Guidelines of GOI on Essential new-born care) and immunization.
- Others: Provision of facilities under Janani Suraksha Yojana (JSY).
- Tracking of missed and left out PNC.

PNC protocol under NRHM 2014 update

Table 3: Service provision during check ups

	Mother	Newborn
Ask	▪ Heavy bleeding ▪ Breast engorgement	▪ Confirm passage of urine (within 48 hours) and stool (within 24 hours) ▪ For convulsions, diarrhea and vomiting
Observe and check	▪ Pallor, pulse, BP and temperature ▪ Urinary problems and perineal tears ▪ Excessive bleeding (PPH) ▪ Foul smelling discharge (Puerperal sepsis)	▪ Activity, color and congenital malformation ▪ Temperature, jaundice, cord stump and skin for pustules ▪ Breathing, chest in drawing ▪ Suckling by the baby during breastfeeding
Counsel for	▪ Danger signs ▪ Correct position of breastfeeding and care of breast and nipples ▪ Exclusive breastfeeding for 6 months ▪ Nutritious diet and calcium rich foods ▪ Maintaining hygiene and use of sanitary napkins ▪ Choosing contraceptive method	▪ Keeping the baby warm ▪ No bathing on first day ▪ Keep the cord stump clean and dry ▪ Additional check-up for the low birth weight babies ▪ On importance of routine immunization ▪ Danger signs in baby
Do	▪ Hb% estimation ▪ Give iron and folic acid (IFA) supplementation to the mother for 3 months	▪ Give 0 dose BCG, OPV, Hepatitis B ▪ Give inj. Vitamin K 1 mg IM

- **Postnatal visits by ASHA [under the—home based neonatal care (HBNC) scheme]**
  - **Institutional delivery:** (Six visits)- Day 3, 7, 14, 21, 28 and 42. *(If cesarean delivery, then visit by ASHA on day 3 is omitted, so number of ASHA visits are 5)*
  - **Home delivery:** (Seven visits)- Day 1, 3, 7, 14, 21, 28, and 42
- **Family planning services**
  - PPIUCD (Postpartum IUCD insertion)
  - Copper T may be fitted within 48 hours after delivery or after 6 weeks postdelivery
  - If the family has been completed, female is motivated for permanent sterilization.

MATERNAL MORTALITY

The most essential indicator or maternal health care is maternal mortality ratio (MMR). It is also the most sensitive indicator of delivery services under health care in an area.

Causes of Maternal Mortality

Direct cause account for 80% of maternal deaths globally and about 66% maternal deaths in India[Q].

- ***Direct cause:*** Is death due *to obstetric complications* of Pregnancy/Labor/Puerperium or from interventions/omissions/incorrect treatment or from a chain of events resulting from any of the above
  - Obstetric hemorrhage (25% Globally, 38 % in India)
  - Puerperal sepsis (15%- Globally, 11% in India)
  - Unsafe abortion (13%- Globally, 8% in India)
  - Hypertensive disorders (12%- Globally, 5% in India)
  - Obstructed labor (8%- Globally, 5% in India)
  - Others - Ectopic pregnancies, embolism, due to interventions (8%- Globally)
- ***Indirect cause:*** Death from pre-existing disease or disease acquired in pregnancy (other than direct obstetric causes) aggravated by physiological effect of pregnancy.
- Social factors are maternal age (optimal age 20–30 years), birth interval (Short birth intervals increase risk) and Parity (High parity).

Table 4: Maternal health statistics

Indicators	India Stats (NFHS 4 – 2015-2016)
Maternal Mortality Ratio (MMR)	130/lac LB Assam – 237 Kerala – 46 (Target for MMR < 100/lac by 2020)

Contd...

166 *High Yield Points*

Maternal Mortality

- *Maternal Mortality Ratio (MMR)* is number of maternal death due to complications of pregnancy, childbirth or within 42 days of delivery from "puerperal causes" in a given area during a given year per 1000 live births in the same area and year

106 *Good to Remember*

Maternal mortality rate is number of maternal deaths in a given period per 100, 000 women of reproductive age group (15-49 years).[Q]

167 *High Yield Points*

- Indirect causes, anemia is the leading cause responsible for about 19% maternal death in India.

107 Good to Remember

- **RHIME (Representative, Re-sampled, Routine Household Interview of Mortality with Medical Evaluation)** is a method of verbal autopsy- introduced in SRS (Sample Registration System) 2000.
- **MAPEDIR**: Maternal and perinatal death inquiry and response is through investigation of social, biological and medical events leading to maternal or perinatal death.

108 Good to Remember

Maternal Death Surveillance and Response: The MDSR system is a continuous cycle of identification, notification, and review of maternal deaths followed by actions to improve quality of care and prevent future deaths.

168 High Yield Points

LAQSHYA- approach for quality assessment of services and manpower for MCH services in public sector

Indicators	India Stats (NFHS 4 – 2015-2016)
Maternal mortality rate@	8.8
Adult life time risk of maternal death #	0.3%
TT coverage in pregnancy	89%
ANC coverage (4 ANC Visits)	59%
Institutional deliveries	79%
Delivery by trained personnel	89% rural, 75% rural
Postnatal check up (Within 2 days of delivery)	81.4%
Crude birth rate	India -20.4 (Rural -22.7, Urban -17.4)
Total fertility rate	2.2, Target -2.1 (by 2017-12th Five year plan)
Couple protection rate	53.5, Target -65 (by 2017-12th Five year plan)

@ The life time risk is defined as the probability that at least one women of reproductive age (15-49) will die due to child birth or puerperium assuming that chance of death is uniformly distributed across the entire reproductive span. The formula is:

$$\text{Lifetime risk} = (1 - \frac{\text{maternal mortality rate}}{100{,}000})$$

Maternal mortality rate = number of maternal deaths among females age group 15-49 years (per lakh)

Approach to Reducing MMR

- **'Delay' Model Leading to Maternal Deaths**: Maternal deaths is due to:
  - Delay in seeking care
  - Delay in transport to appropriate health facility
  - Delay in provision of adequate care.
- **Adult lifetime risk of maternal death** is probability of a woman dying in her reproductive life span because of maternal cause.
  Lifetime risk = [Maternal mortality rate] × [length of reproductive period]
- Continuum of care approach begins before pregnancy and extends through child birth and into baby's childhood. It forms the basis of RMNCH+A strategy initiated in 2013.
- Risk approach seeks to screen out "high risk" cases at the earliest from a large group of antenatal mothers and arrange for them skilled care, while continuing to provide appropriate care for all mothers[Q].

Laqshya

- Under MoHFW
- **Focus:** Improving Quality of Labour room and maternity operation theatre
- **Outcome:** Improve quality of care for pregnant women in labour room, maternity Operation Theatre and Obstetrics intensive care units (ICUs) and High Dependency Units (HDUs)
- **Implementation:** All Medical College Hospitals, District Hospitals and First Referral Unit (FRU), and Community Health Center (CHCs)
- **Beneficiary:** Every pregnant woman and new-born delivering in public health institution

High-Risk Pregnancies

- Elderly primigravida (Age 30 years and more)
- Short statured primigravida (Height 140 cm and less)
- Malpresentation (Breech, Transverse lie, etc.)
- Antepartum hemorrhage
- Threatened abortion
- Preeclampsia and eclampsia
- Anemia
- Twins
- Hydramnios
- Previous still-birth
- Intrauterine death
- Manual removal of placenta
- Elderly grand multipara

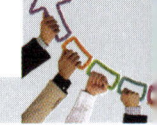

- Prolonged pregnancy (14 days after expected date of delivery)
- History of previous cesarean or instrumental delivery
- Pregnancy with other diseases, cardiovascular disease, kidney disease, diabetes, tuberculosis, liver disease, etc.
- History of three or more spontaneous consecutive abortion
- History of infertility

Danger Signs in Pregnancy

- Any bleeding per vaginum during pregnancy or heavy vaginal bleeding (>500 mL) during delivery or postpartum
- Severe headache with blurred vision
- Convulsion or loss of consciousness
- Labor lasting for more than 12 hours
- Preterm labor
- Premature rupture of membrane
- Severe abdominal pain
- Failure to deliver placenta within 30 minutes of delivery
- Associated medical conditions like diabetes, heart disease and asthma

PROTOCOL FOR MANAGEMENT OF OBSTETRIC EMERGENCIES (EMOC)

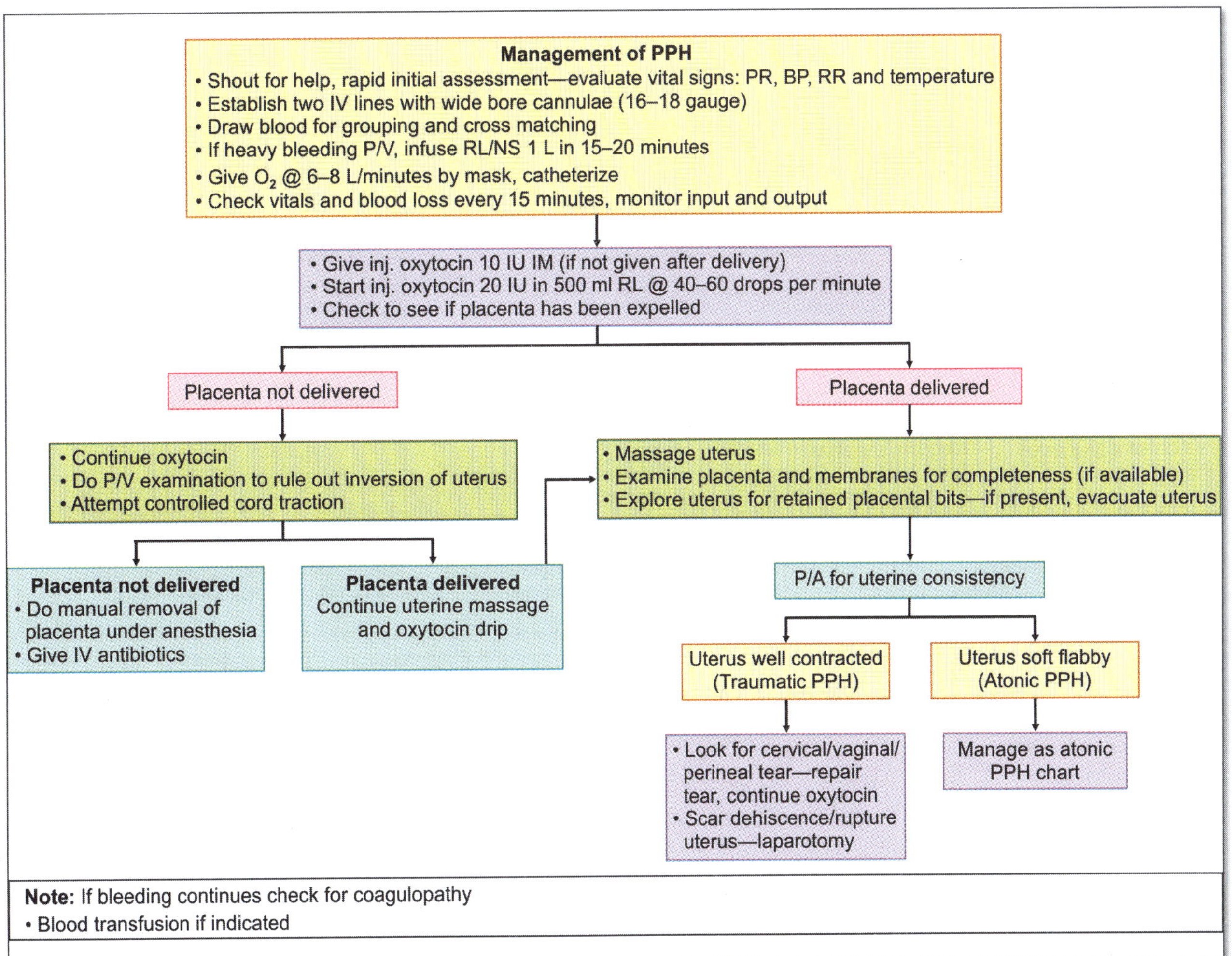

Management of PPH
• Shout for help, rapid initial assessment—evaluate vital signs: PR, BP, RR and temperature
• Establish two IV lines with wide bore cannulae (16–18 gauge)
• Draw blood for grouping and cross matching
• If heavy bleeding P/V, infuse RL/NS 1 L in 15–20 minutes
• Give O_2 @ 6–8 L/minutes by mask, catheterize
• Check vitals and blood loss every 15 minutes, monitor input and output
• Give inj. oxytocin 10 IU IM (if not given after delivery)
• Start inj. oxytocin 20 IU in 500 ml RL @ 40–60 drops per minute
• Check to see if placenta has been expelled
Placenta not delivered
Placenta delivered
• Continue oxytocin
• Do P/V examination to rule out inversion of uterus
• Attempt controlled cord traction
• Massage uterus
• Examine placenta and membranes for completeness (if available)
• Explore uterus for retained placental bits—if present, evacuate uterus
Placenta not delivered
• Do manual removal of placenta under anesthesia
• Give IV antibiotics
Placenta delivered
Continue uterine massage and oxytocin drip
P/A for uterine consistency
Uterus well contracted (Traumatic PPH)
Uterus soft flabby (Atonic PPH)
• Look for cervical/vaginal/ perineal tear—repair tear, continue oxytocin
• Scar dehiscence/rupture uterus—laparotomy
Manage as atonic PPH chart
Note: If bleeding continues check for coagulopathy
• Blood transfusion if indicated

Fig. 2: Management of postpartum hemorrhage
Source: NHM Operational Guidelines

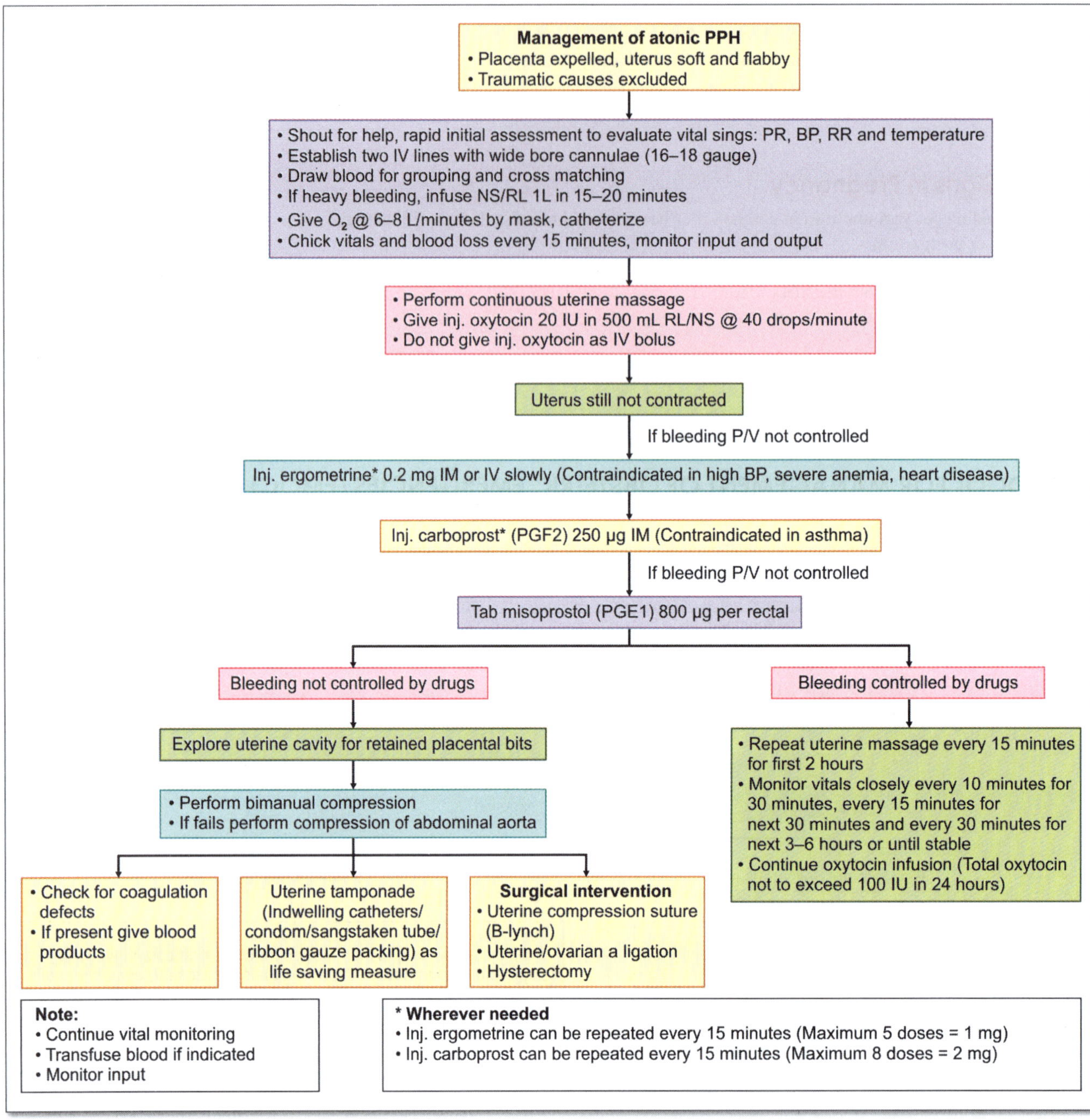
Management of atonic PPH
• Placenta expelled, uterus soft and flabby
• Traumatic causes excluded
• Shout for help, rapid initial assessment to evaluate vital sings: PR, BP, RR and temperature
• Establish two IV lines with wide bore cannulae (16–18 gauge)
• Draw blood for grouping and cross matching
• If heavy bleeding, infuse NS/RL 1L in 15–20 minutes
• Give O_2 @ 6–8 L/minutes by mask, catheterize
• Chick vitals and blood loss every 15 minutes, monitor input and output
• Perform continuous uterine massage
• Give inj. oxytocin 20 IU in 500 mL RL/NS @ 40 drops/minute
• Do not give inj. oxytocin as IV bolus
Uterus still not contracted
If bleeding P/V not controlled
Inj. ergometrine* 0.2 mg IM or IV slowly (Contraindicated in high BP, severe anemia, heart disease)
Inj. carboprost* (PGF2) 250 μg IM (Contraindicated in asthma)
If bleeding P/V not controlled
Tab misoprostol (PGE1) 800 μg per rectal
Bleeding not controlled by drugs
Bleeding controlled by drugs
Explore uterine cavity for retained placental bits
• Perform bimanual compression
• If fails perform compression of abdominal aorta
• Repeat uterine massage every 15 minutes for first 2 hours
• Monitor vitals closely every 10 minutes for 30 minutes, every 15 minutes for next 30 minutes and every 30 minutes for next 3–6 hours or until stable
• Continue oxytocin infusion (Total oxytocin not to exceed 100 IU in 24 hours)
• Check for coagulation defects
• If present give blood products
Uterine tamponade (Indwelling catheters/ condom/sangstaken tube/ ribbon gauze packing) as life saving measure
Surgical intervention
• Uterine compression suture (B-lynch)
• Uterine/ovarian a ligation
• Hysterectomy
Note:
• Continue vital monitoring
• Transfuse blood if indicated
• Monitor input
* Wherever needed
• Inj. ergometrine can be repeated every 15 minutes (Maximum 5 doses = 1 mg)
• Inj. carboprost can be repeated every 15 minutes (Maximum 8 doses = 2 mg)

Fig. 3: Management of postpartum hemorrhage with uterine atony

Source: NHM Operational Guidelines

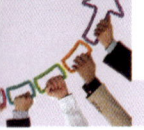

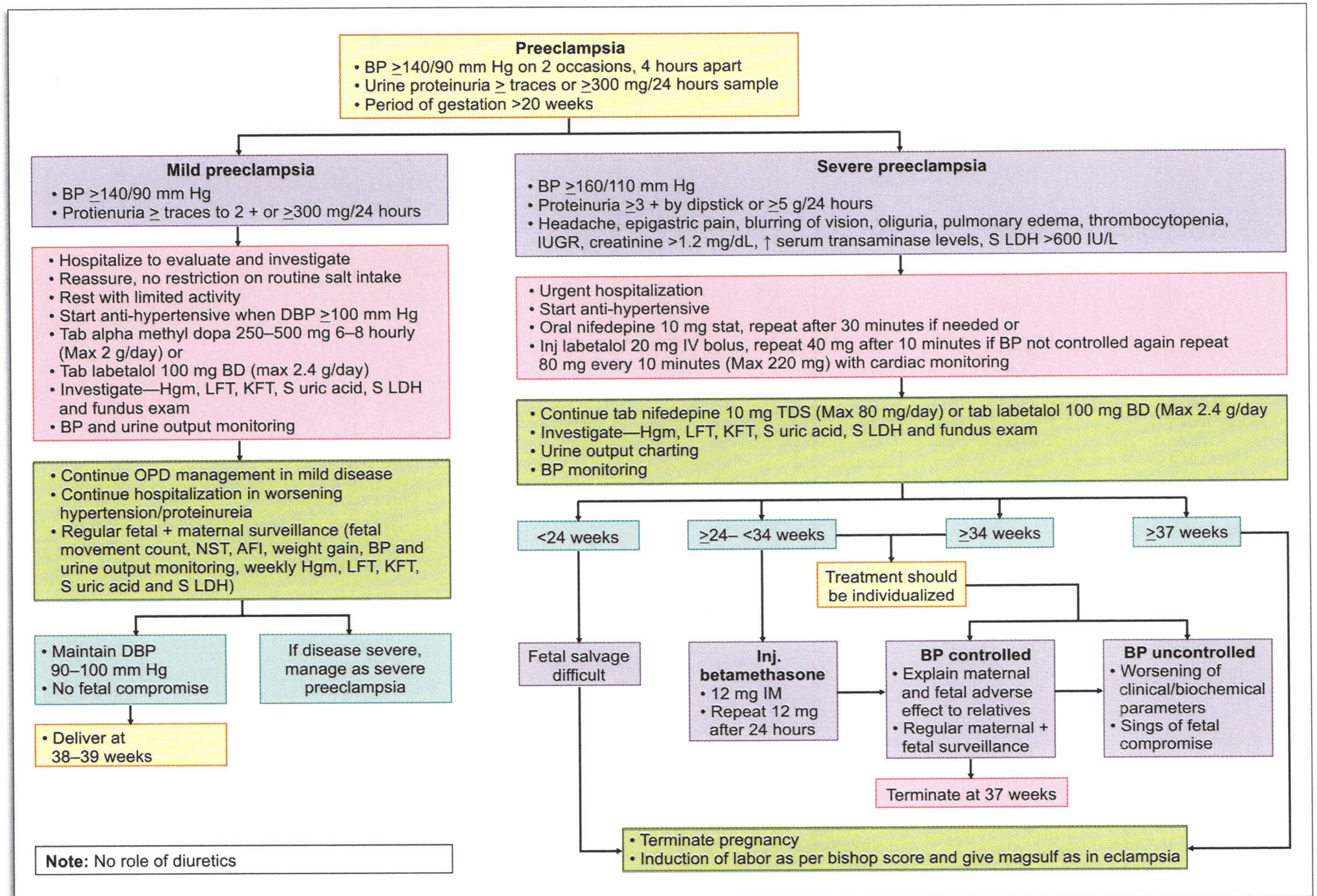

Preeclampsia
• BP ≥140/90 mm Hg on 2 occasions, 4 hours apart
• Urine proteinuria ≥ traces or ≥300 mg/24 hours sample
• Period of gestation >20 weeks
Mild preeclampsia
• BP ≥140/90 mm Hg
• Protienuria ≥ traces to 2 + or ≥300 mg/24 hours
• Hospitalize to evaluate and investigate
• Reassure, no restriction on routine salt intake
• Rest with limited activity
• Start anti-hypertensive when DBP ≥100 mm Hg
• Tab alpha methyl dopa 250–500 mg 6–8 hourly (Max 2 g/day) or
• Tab labetalol 100 mg BD (max 2.4 g/day)
• Investigate—Hgm, LFT, KFT, S uric acid, S LDH and fundus exam
• BP and urine output monitoring
• Continue OPD management in mild disease
• Continue hospitalization in worsening hypertension/proteinureia
• Regular fetal + maternal surveillance (fetal movement count, NST, AFI, weight gain, BP and urine output monitoring, weekly Hgm, LFT, KFT, S uric acid and S LDH)
• Maintain DBP 90–100 mm Hg
• No fetal compromise
If disease severe, manage as severe preeclampsia
• Deliver at 38–39 weeks
Note: No role of diuretics
Severe preeclampsia
• BP ≥160/110 mm Hg
• Proteinuria ≥3 + by dipstick or ≥5 g/24 hours
• Headache, epigastric pain, blurring of vision, oliguria, pulmonary edema, thrombocytopenia, IUGR, creatinine >1.2 mg/dL, ↑ serum transaminase levels, S LDH >600 IU/L
• Urgent hospitalization
• Start anti-hypertensive
• Oral nifedepine 10 mg stat, repeat after 30 minutes if needed or
• Inj labetalol 20 mg IV bolus, repeat 40 mg after 10 minutes if BP not controlled again repeat 80 mg every 10 minutes (Max 220 mg) with cardiac monitoring
• Continue tab nifedepine 10 mg TDS (Max 80 mg/day) or tab labetalol 100 mg BD (Max 2.4 g/day
• Investigate—Hgm, LFT, KFT, S uric acid, S LDH and fundus exam
• Urine output charting
• BP monitoring
<24 weeks
≥24– <34 weeks
≥34 weeks
≥37 weeks
Treatment should be individualized
Fetal salvage difficult
Inj. betamethasone
• 12 mg IM
• Repeat 12 mg after 24 hours
BP controlled
• Explain maternal and fetal adverse effect to relatives
• Regular maternal + fetal surveillance
BP uncontrolled
• Worsening of clinical/biochemical parameters
• Sings of fetal compromise
Terminate at 37 weeks
• Terminate pregnancy
• Induction of labor as per bishop score and give magsulf as in eclampsia

Fig. 4: Management of preeclampsia at primary care

Source: NHM Operational Guidelines

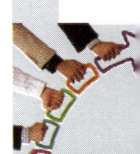

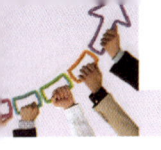

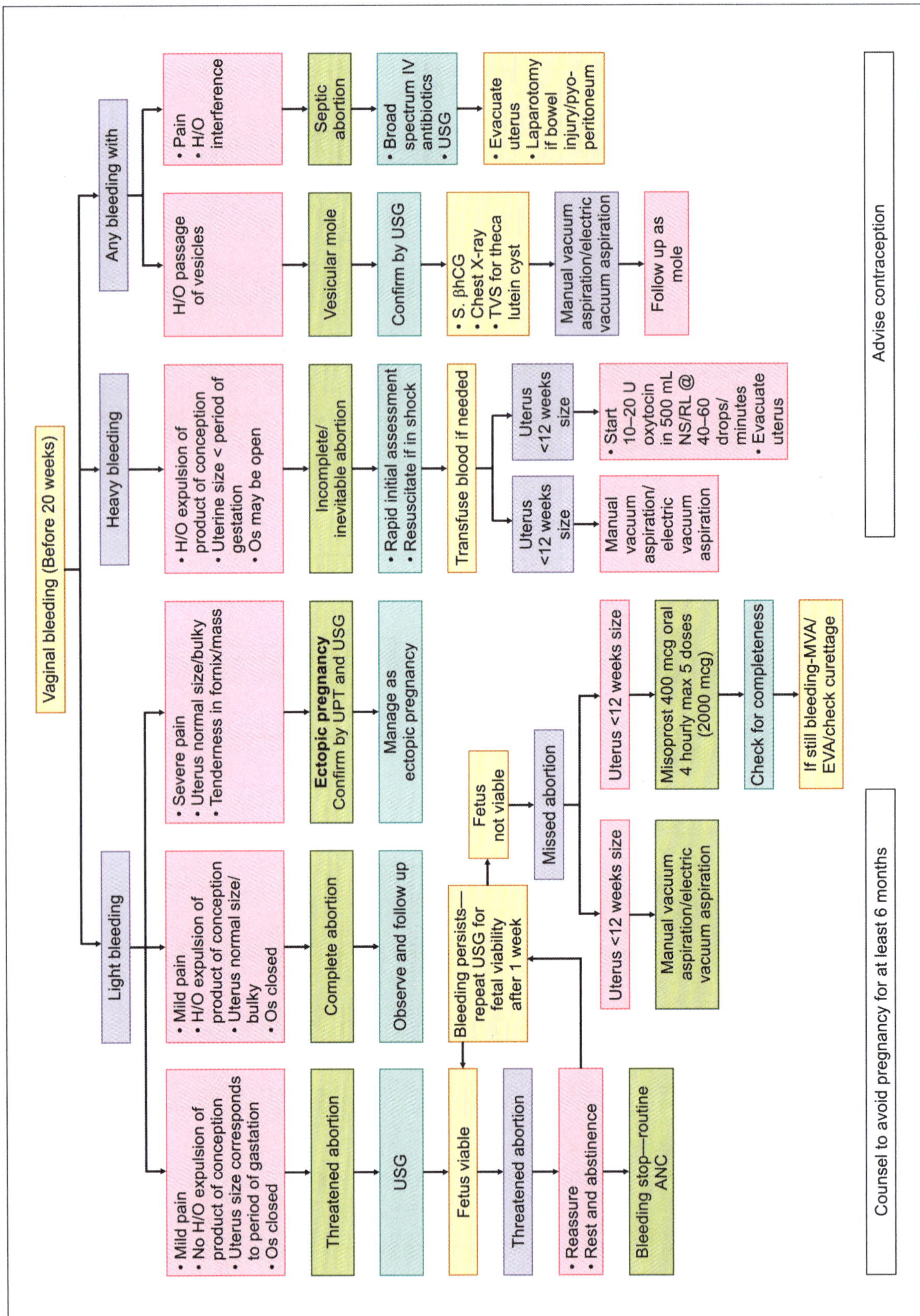

Vaginal bleeding (Before 20 weeks)
Light bleeding
Heavy bleeding
Any bleeding with
• Mild pain
• No H/O expulsion of product of conception
• Uterus size corresponds to period of gastation
• Os closed
• Mild pain
• H/O expulsion of product of conception
• Uterus normal size/ bulky
• Os closed
• Severe pain
• Uterus normal size/bulky
• Tenderness in fornix/mass
• H/O expulsion of product of conception
• Uterine size < period of gestation
• Os may be open
H/O passage of vesicles
• Pain
• H/O interference
Threatened abortion
Complete abortion
Ectopic pregnancy
Confirm by UPT and USG
Incomplete/ inevitable abortion
Vesicular mole
Septic abortion
USG
Observe and follow up
Manage as ectopic pregnancy
• Rapid initial assessment
• Resuscitate if in shock
Confirm by USG
• Broad spectrum IV antibiotics
• USG
Fetus viable
Bleeding persists—repeat USG for fetal viability after 1 week
Fetus not viable
Transfuse blood if needed
• S. βhCG
• Chest X-ray
• TVS for theca lutein cyst
• Evacuate uterus
• Laparotomy if bowel injury/pyo-peritoneum
Threatened abortion
Missed abortion
Uterus <12 weeks size
Uterus <12 weeks size
Manual vacuum aspiration/electric vacuum aspiration
• Reassure
• Rest and abstinence
Uterus <12 weeks size
Uterus <12 weeks size
Manual vacuum aspiration/ electric vacuum aspiration
• Start 10–20 U oxytocin in 500 mL NS/RL @ 40–60 drops/ minutes
• Evacuate uterus
Follow up as mole
Bleeding stop—routine ANC
Manual vacuum aspiration/electric vacuum aspiration
Misoprost 400 mcg oral 4 hourly max 5 doses (2000 mcg)
Check for completeness
If still bleeding-MVA/ EVA/check curettage
Counsel to avoid pregnancy for at least 6 months
Advise contraception

Fig. 5: Management of vaginal bleeding before 20 weeks

Source: NHM Operational Guidelines

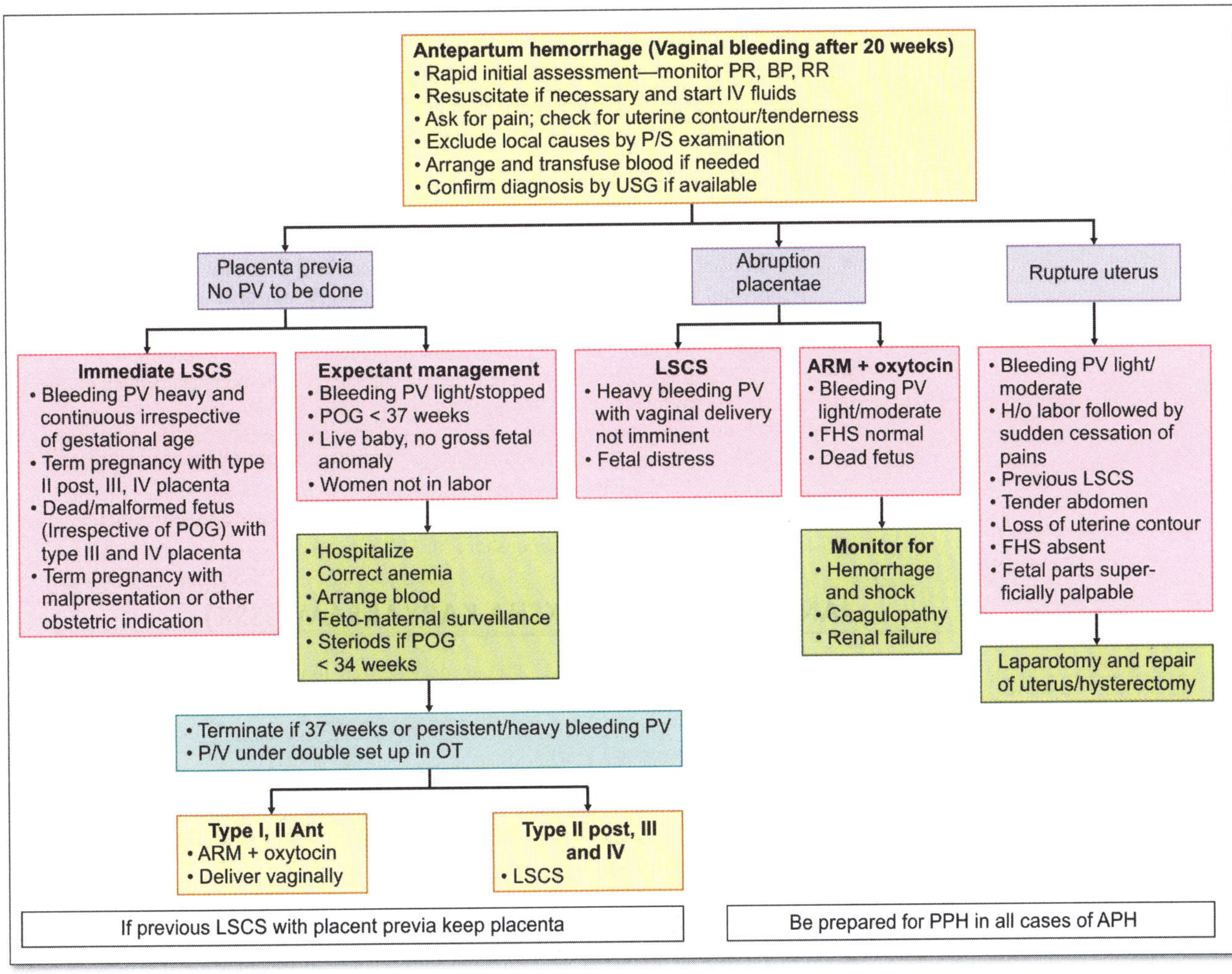

Antepartum hemorrhage (Vaginal bleeding after 20 weeks)
• Rapid initial assessment—monitor PR, BP, RR
• Resuscitate if necessary and start IV fluids
• Ask for pain; check for uterine contour/tenderness
• Exclude local causes by P/S examination
• Arrange and transfuse blood if needed
• Confirm diagnosis by USG if available
Placenta previa
No PV to be done
Abruption placentae
Rupture uterus
Immediate LSCS
• Bleeding PV heavy and continuous irrespective of gestational age
• Term pregnancy with type II post, III, IV placenta
• Dead/malformed fetus (Irrespective of POG) with type III and IV placenta
• Term pregnancy with malpresentation or other obstetric indication
Expectant management
• Bleeding PV light/stopped
• POG < 37 weeks
• Live baby, no gross fetal anomaly
• Women not in labor
LSCS
• Heavy bleeding PV with vaginal delivery not imminent
• Fetal distress
ARM + oxytocin
• Bleeding PV light/moderate
• FHS normal
• Dead fetus
• Bleeding PV light/ moderate
• H/o labor followed by sudden cessation of pains
• Previous LSCS
• Tender abdomen
• Loss of uterine contour
• FHS absent
• Fetal parts superficially palpable
• Hospitalize
• Correct anemia
• Arrange blood
• Feto-maternal surveillance
• Steriods if POG < 34 weeks
Monitor for
• Hemorrhage and shock
• Coagulopathy
• Renal failure
Laparotomy and repair of uterus/hysterectomy
• Terminate if 37 weeks or persistent/heavy bleeding PV
• P/V under double set up in OT
Type I, II Ant
• ARM + oxytocin
• Deliver vaginally
Type II post, III and IV
• LSCS
If previous LSCS with placent previa keep placenta
Be prepared for PPH in all cases of APH

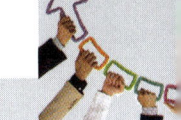

Fig. 6: Management of vaginal bleeding after 20 weeks (Antepartum hemorrhage)

Source: NHM Operational Guidelines

SCHEMES RELATED TO MOTHER AND CHILD HEALTH IN INDIA

PRADHAN MANTRI SURAKSHIT MATRITVA ABHIYAN (PMSMA)

- The Pradhan Mantri Surakshit Matritva Abhiyan has been launched by the Ministry of Health & Family Welfare (MoHFW), Government of India on November 4, 2016. The program aims to provide assured, comprehensive and quality antenatal care, free of cost, universally to all pregnant women on the 9th of every month.
- PMSMA guarantees a minimum package of antenatal care services to women in their 2nd / 3rd trimesters of pregnancy at designated government health facilities
- The program follows a systematic approach for engagement with private sector which includes motivating private practitioners to volunteer for the campaign developing strategies for generating awareness and appealing to the private sector to participate in the Abhiyan at government health facilities.

Objectives:

- Ensure at least one antenatal checkup for all pregnant women in their second or third trimester by a physician/specialist
- Improve the quality of care during antenatal visits. This includes ensuring provision of the following services:
  - All applicable diagnostic services
  - Screening for the applicable clinical conditions
  - Appropriate management of any existing clinical condition such as Anemia, Pregnancy induced hypertension, Gestational Diabetes etc.
  - Appropriate counseling services and proper documentation of services rendered
  - Additional service opportunity to pregnant women who have missed antenatal visits

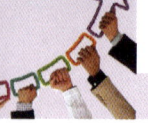

- Identification and line-listing of high risk pregnancies based on obstetric/medical history and existing clinical conditions.
- Appropriate birth planning and complication readiness for each pregnant woman especially those identified with any risk factor or comorbid condition.
- Special emphasis on early diagnosis, adequate and appropriate management of women with malnutrition.
- Special focus on adolescent and early pregnancies as these pregnancies need extra and specialized care

Strategy:

- A minimum package of antenatal care services (including investigations and drugs) would be provided to the beneficiaries on the **9th day of every month** at identified public health facilities (PHCs/CHCs, DHs/urban health facilities etc) in both urban and rural areas in addition to the routine ANC at the health facility/outreach.
- Fixed day assured, comprehensive and quality antenatal care to pregnant women on the 9th of every month
- Special antenatal check-up to pregnant women in their second or third trimesters at Government health facilities by Gynecologists/Physicians with support from private sector doctors to supplement the efforts of the Government sector.

"***IPledgeFor9***" - Achievers Awards have been devised to celebrate individual and team achievements and acknowledge voluntary contributions for PMSMA in states and districts across India.

JANANI SHISHU SURAKSHA KARYAKRAM (JSSK)

- JSSK was launched on June 1, 2011 to provide free and cashless service in Government hospitals (rural and urban) to
  - Pregnant women
  - Sick infant (up to 1 year)
- Includes free medical services, free laboratory services, free treatment, free transport to and from the hospital. The JSSK program basically guarantees services/entitlements and eliminates out of pocket expenses of pregnant women and Sick newborn.

Free entitlements under JSSK include

- Free and cashless delivery and cesarean operation
- Free treatment of sick-newborn up to 1 year
- Exemption from user charges, free drugs, consumables and diagnostics
- Free diet during stay in the health institutions—3 days for normal delivery and 7 days in case of caesarean section
- Free provision of blood
- Free transport: Home to health institutions, between facilities in case of referral and drop back from Institutions to home after 48 hours stay

JANANI SURAKSHA YOJANA

- It is a safe motherhood intervention under NRHM, launched on April 12, 2005 to replace NMBS.
- It is a 100% Central government funded scheme
- States are categorized as LPS (very low institutional delivery) and HPS.

Goals:[Q]

- To reduce MMR and IMR
- To increase institutional delivery among BPL families.

Table 5: Eligibility for cash assistance under JSY[Q]

LPS-UP, MP Jharkhand, Bihar, Uttarakhand, Rajasthan, Chhattisgarh, Assam, Jammu and Kashmir and Odisha	▪ All pregnant women including SC/ ST women delivering in a govt. health center i.e. SC/PHC/CHC/FRU/District hospital or accredited Private Institution. Irrespective of age and parity. ▪ BPL certification is not mandatory for delivery at a government health center
HPS	▪ All pregnant women from BPL/SC/ST families irrespective of age and parity (8th May 2013)

Latest Updates

- ASHA package is of INR ₹600 in rural area (₹300 for ANC and INR ₹300 for facilitating institutional delivery) and INR ₹400 in urban areas (INR ₹200 for ANC and ₹200 for facilitating institutional delivery).
- Assistance for mother in case of home delivery-is INR ₹500 per delivery up to 2 live birth irrespective of age and parity. BPL certificate is a must.
- If facilities for managing obstetric complication are not available
  - Assistance up to INR ₹1500/case is available to hire services of Private facilities
- Cash disbursement to beneficiaries is to be disbursed at time of delivery or around 7 days before delivery by ASHA.
- AADHAR enabled cash payment has also been introduced.

Table 6: Revised cash assistance under JSY[Q]-2018

Category	Rural			Urban		
	Mother	ASHA	Total	Mother	ASHA	Total
LPS	1400	600	2000	1000	400	1400
HPS	700	600	1300	600	400	1000

INDIRA GANDHI MATRITVA SAHYOG YOJANA

- Conditional cash transfer is done to pregnant and lactating mother to improve their nutritional and health status
- ***Aim:*** To compensate partly for wage-loss to pregnant and lactating women prior to and after delivery of child
- ***Objective:*** Short-term – Income support (cash incentive), Long-term: Behavior and attitudinal change.
  - Approved on a pilot basis in 52 districts across the country and is to be implemented via ICDS.

YASHODA/MAMTA PROGRAM

- Introduced in 2008 under NIPI (Norway India Partnership Initiative) in MP, Bihar, Odisha and Rajasthan.
- Yashoda (local women trained and deputed by district health authorities at CHC/Dist. hospital with 24 hours delivery services) works as birth companion and provides congenial environment for mother and new born, assisting in pre and postdelivery care.
- She gets Rs 100/child mother cohort (Maximum 3000-3500 per month).

MAA

Mother's Absolute affection - 2016

Goal: To promote, protect and support breastfeeding practices through health systems

Components:

- Awareness generation – via mass media
- Community level interventions:
  - Capacity building of ASHA workers, ANMs, AWWs
  - Community-based discussions and interpersonal communication
- Health system strengthening: Capacity building of ANMs/nurses for lactation support
- Monitoring and evaluation

REPRODUCTIVE AND CHILD HEALTH (RCH)

Districts have been divided into three categories, A,B,C based on 2 parameters[Q]

- CBR
- Female literacy rate.

Maternal Health Services in RCH

Essential Obstetric Care

- Early registration of pregnancy (12–16 weeks)
- Minimum 4 ANC checkups by ANM/ MO
- TT immunization and IFA, deworming

- Institutional delivery and safe delivery at home
- Referral to FRU for obstetric emergency
- Four postnatal checkups.

Emergency Obstetric Care

- Basic and Comprehensive emergency obstetric care.
    - 24 hours safe delivery.
    - Safe MTP services
    - Spacing (at least 3 years) between children.

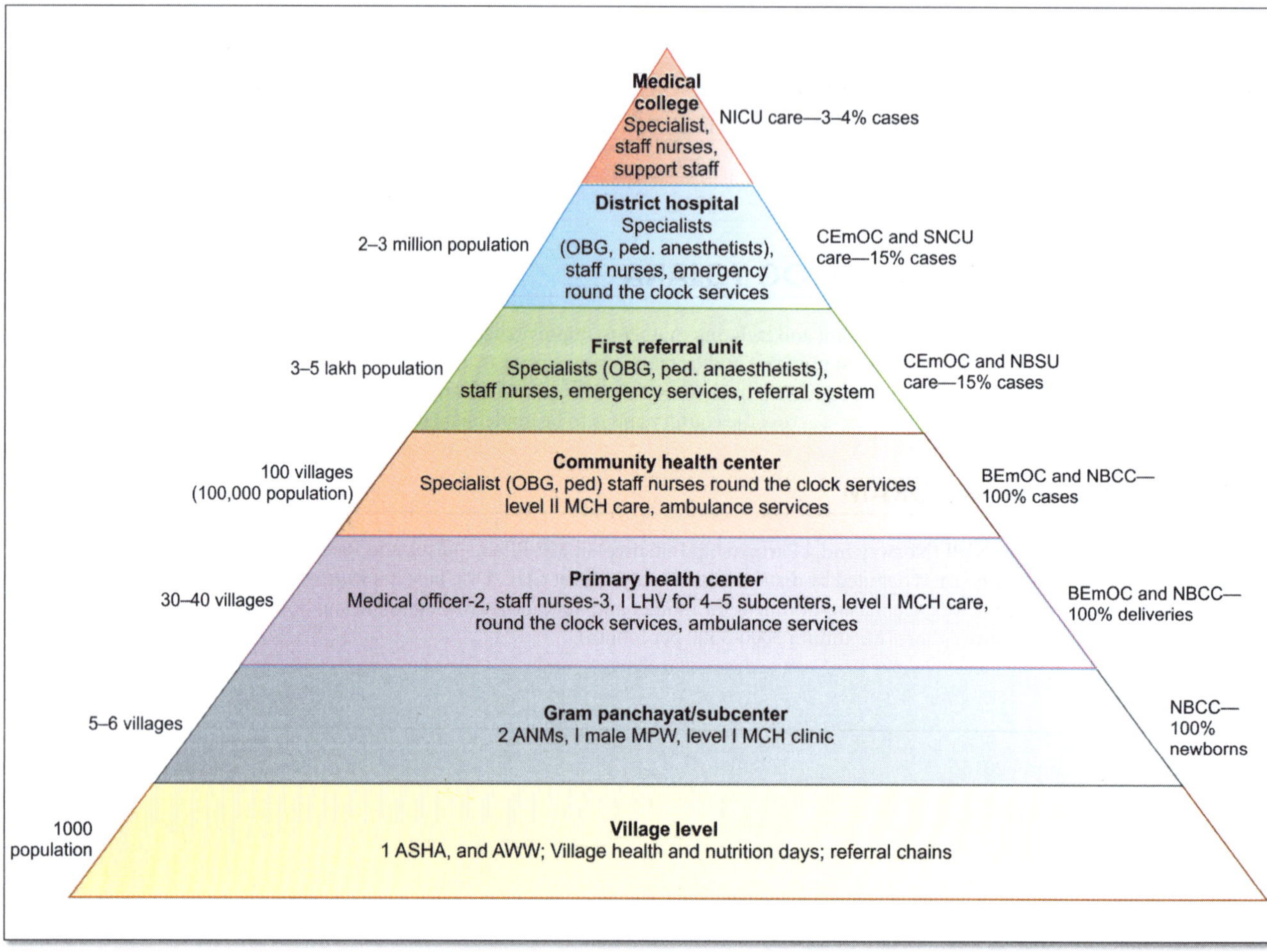

Fig. 7: Obstetric care model in India

Abbreviations: **NBCC**, newborn care corner; **BEmOC**, basic emergency obstetric care; **CEmOC,** comprehensive emergency obstetric care; **NBSU**, newborn stabilization unit (for details – refer chapter – preventive pediatrics); **NICU**, neonatal intensive care units; **SNCU**, Sick newborn care units; ***Newborn and Child Care Services in RCH,*** *Refer to Chapter "Preventive Pediatrics"*

RMNCH+A

(Refer to Chapter "Preventive Pediatrics")

- Reproductive. Maternal, neonatal, child health + adolescent health
- Gives an inclusive life package services for mother and child health

Table 7: Calcium supplementation to the pregnant/lactating female

When	How many	By whom	Where
Second ANC	12 strips (@ 15 tablets per strip)	ANM	ANC clinic/ VHND
Third ANC	12 strips (@ 15 tablets per strip)	ANM	ANC clinic/ VHND
At the time of zero dose of polio for the infant	12 strips (@ 15 tablets per strip)	ANM	Immunization clinic/VHND
At the time of third dose of Diphtheria, Pertussis, and Tetanus (DPT) for the infant	12 strips (@ 15 tablets per strip)	ANM	Immunization clinic/VHND

Abbreviation: *VHND, village health and nutrition day

ANEMIA MUKT BHARAT (2018) GUIDELINES

Vision

To decrease anemia prevalence in the country

Strategy

6 × 6 × 6 strategy – "**SOLID BODY – SMART MIND**" Campaign
6 beneficiaries
6 interventions
6 institutional mechanisms

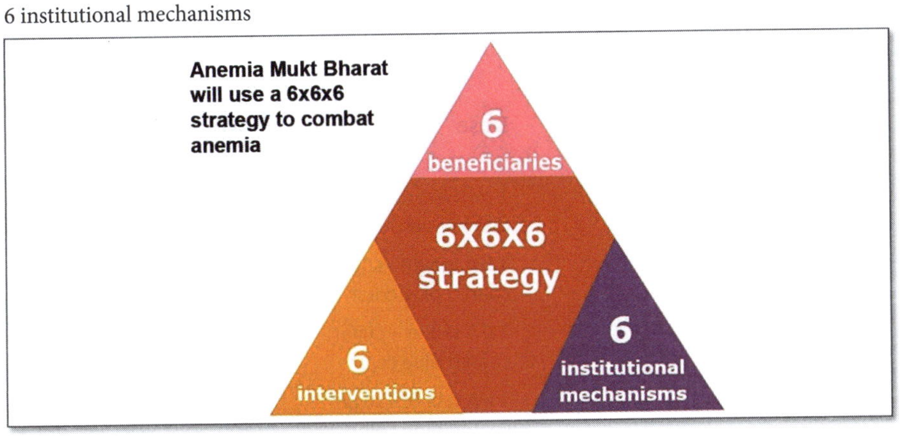

6 Targets for 'Anemia Mukt Bharat'

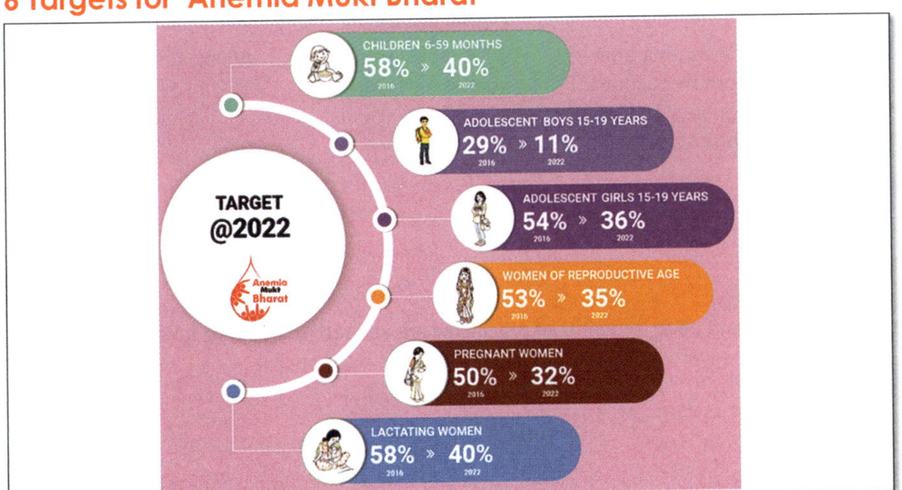

Must Remember

Calcium Supplementation during Pregnancy and lactation-

- All pregnant and lactating women to be counseled about intake of calcium-rich foods.
- Oral swallowable calcium tablets to be taken twice a day (total 1g calcium/day) starting from 14 weeks of pregnancy up to six months postpartum.
- One calcium tablet should be taken with the morning/afternoon meal and the second tablet with the evening/night meal. It is not advisable to take both calcium tablets together as > 800 mg calcium interferes with iron absorption.
- Calcium tablets should not be taken empty stomach since it causes gastritis.
- Calcium and Iron Folic Acid (IFA) tablets should not be taken together since calcium inhibits iron absorption. IFA tablets should be taken preferably two hours after a meal.
- Each calcium tablet should contain 500 mg elemental calcium and 250 IU vitamin D3. The preferred formulation for calcium is calcium carbonate. The rationale for inclusion of Vitamin D is to enhance the absorption of calcium.

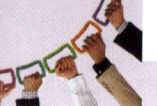

6 Eligible Beneficiaries

- Children — 6–59 month
- School age children — 5–9 years
- Adolescent boys# + girls — 10–19 years
- Reproductive age females$ — 20–24 years
- Pregnant females
- Lactating females

#adolescent boys: From school

Adolescent girls–from the school and girls under kishori shakti yojana, anganwadi centers

$reproductive age group females under the mission parivar vikas

6 Institutional Mechanisms

- Inter-ministerial coordination
- National anemia mukt bharat unit
- National center of excellence and advance research on anemia control
- Convergence with other ministries
- Strengthen supply chain and logistics
- Anemia mukt bharat dashboard and digital portal

6 Interventions

- Prophylactic iron and Folic acid supplementation
- Deworming
- Intensified behavior change communication campaigns
- Testing of anemia using digital methods and point of care treatment
- Iron and folic acid fortified food through the national funded programs
- Addressing non nutritional causes of anemia–malaria, hemoglobinopathies, fluorosis

Prophylactic iron and Folic acid supplementation (2018–guidelines)

Eligible beneficiary@	Age group	Dosing schedule	Dose	Iron + Folic acid composition
Children	6–59 months	Biweekly	1 ml IFA syrup from 50 mL auto-dispenser bottle	20 mg elemental iron + 100 mcg folic acid
Children	5–9 years	Weekly	1 IFA tablet - sugar coated pink color	45 mg elemental iron + 400 mcg folic acid
Adolescent boys	10–19 years – school going	Weekly	1 IFA tablet – sugar coated blue color	60 mg elemental iron + 500 mcg folic acid
Adolescent girls	10–19 years – school going and out of school	Weekly	1 IFA tablet – sugar coated blue color	60 mg elemental iron + 500 mcg folic acid
Women of reproductive age group	Under mission parivar vikas	Weekly	1 IFA tablet – sugar coated red color	60 mg elemental iron + 500 mcg folic acid
Pregnant females and lactating mothers	Pregnant + lactating (0-6 months)	Daily starting from 4th month throughout pregnancy and for 180 days postpartum#	1 IFA tablet – sugar coated red color	60 mg elemental iron + 500 mcg folic acid

#180 days before delivery + 180 days after delivery

@**Note:**

- IFA prophylaxis is withheld for
  - Acute illness (fever, diarrhea, pneumonia)
  - Known case of thalassemia major (recurrent transfusions)
- Females in reproductive age in preconception age group and up to 3 months of pregnancy are advised for **400 mcg folic acid tablets**

Deworming dose and regime (2018 - guidelines)

National deworming day program: Biannual deworming is done on 10 February and 10 August every year

Age category	Age	Dose and regime
Children	12–24 months	½ tablet (200 mg) biannual dose
Children	24–59 months	1 tablet – 400 mg Biannual dose
Children	5–9 years	
School going adolescent boys and girls	10–19 years	
Out of school adolescent girls	10–19 years	
Reproductive age group females	20–49 years	
Pregnant and lactating females	Lactating female 0–6 months	1 tablet 400 mg, Single dose in 2nd trimester

Must Remember

Calcium Supplementation during Pregnancy and Lactation

- All pregnant and lactating women to be counseled about intake of calcium-rich foods.
- Oral swallowable calcium tablets to be taken twice a day (total 1 g calcium/day) starting from 14 weeks of pregnancy up to six months postpartum.
- One calcium tablet should be taken with the morning/afternoon meal and the second tablet with the evening/night meal. It is not advisable to take both calcium tablets together as > 800 mg calcium interferes with iron absorption.
- Calcium tablets should not be taken empty stomach since it causes gastritis.
- Calcium and Iron Folic Acid (IFA) tablets should not be taken together since calcium inhibits iron absorption. IFA tablets should be taken preferably two hours after a meal.
- Each calcium tablet should contain 500 mg elemental calcium and 250 IU vitamin D3. The preferred formulation for calcium is calcium carbonate. The rationale for inclusion of Vitamin D is to enhance the absorption of calcium.

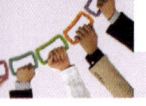

Multiple Choice Questions

1. **All of the following facilities are provided to pregnant women under Janani Shishu Suraksha Karyakram (JSSK), except:** *(Recent Question 2017)*
   a. Free family planning kit
   b. Free blood if required
   c. Free diet up to 7 days for caesarian section
   d. Free transportation from home to institution

NRHM

2. **A lady comes to the clinic with her 15-day-old child with fever, runny nose and cough. Under which program can she avail free transport to the hospital:**
   a. JSSK
   b. Indira Gandhi Matritva Sahyog Yojana
   c. F-IMNCI
   d. Home-based Care
3. **All of the following facilities are provided to pregnant women under Janani Shishu Suraksha Karyakram (JSSK), except:** *(Recent Question 2017)*
   a. Free diet up to 7 days for caesarian section
   b. Free blood if required
   c. Free transportation from home to institution
   d. Free family planning kit
4. **Janani Suraksha Yojana (JSY) is a safe motherhood intervention under the National Rural Health Mission (NRHM) implemented with the objective of reducing maternal and neonatal mortality by promoting institutional delivery among poor pregnant women. The scheme was launched in which year:**
   a. 2001 b. 2005
   c. 2006 d. 2008
5. **All of the following are features of Janani Suraksha Yojana, except:** *(Recent Question 2017)*
   a. It promotes institutional deliveries
   b. Anganwadi acts as link between pregnant woman and Government
   c. Cash assistance is given to mothers for high and low performing states
   d. It is a 100% Central Govt. sponsored scheme
6. **Cash assistance under Janani Suraksha Yojana is given to all of the following women, except:**
   a. Urban women below poverty line
   b. Rural women above 19 years of age
   c. Up to 2 live births in low performing states
   d. SC/ST pregnant women in high performing states
7. **All are true about Janani Shishu Suraksha Karyakram (JSSK), except:**
   a. Free diet to mother during hospital stay
   b. Free delivery
   c. Free transport from home to hospital and back
   d. Free treatment of sick infants up to 2 years
8. **Janani suraksha yojana includes:**
   a. Tetanus immunization b. Institutional deliveries
   c. Iron supplementation d. Abortions
9. **'JSY' stands for:** *(Recent Question 2016)*
   a. Janani Suraksha Yojana b. Janani Samridhi Yojana
   c. Janani Swarojgar Yojana d. Janani Sampooma Yojana

RCH

10. **Under RMNCH +A strategy, goals for 2017 are all, except:**
    a. Reduction of MMR to 100
    b. Reduction of IMR to 25
    c. Reduction of TFR to 2.1
    d. Reduction of anemia in adolescent at 6% annually
11. **"Plus" in RMNCH +A Strategy stands for:**
    a. Reproductive health b. Adolescent health
    c. Vaccination d. Maternal Health
12. **Which of the following is not done under RMNCH+A**
    a. Linking of maternal health to reproductive health
    b. Linking home and community based services to facility based care
    c. Private sector involvement
    d. Referral to PHC/CHC
13. **Under RMNCH+A strategy, which of the following does not apply to adolescent:** *(Recent Question 2016)*
    a. Iron supplementation
    b. Pneumonia management
    c. School Health examination
    d. Nutritional education
14. **All of the following are components of RCH-1, except:**
    a. Vande Mataram scheme
    b. Client approach to health care
    c. Child survival and safe motherhood
    d. Family planning
15. **Not true about vande mataram scheme:**
    a. For providing safe motherhood services
    b. An MBBS or OG specialist can volunteer
    c. Free treatment in private clinics
    d. IFA tablets, OC pills, TT inj are provided to Vande Mataram clinics by the district medical officers
16. **RCH program includes:** *(Recent Question 2016)*
    a. CSSM plus school health
    b. CSSM plus family planning
    c. CSSM plus ORS
    d. CSSM plus pneumonia control
17. **Components of RCH elaborated include:**
    a. Prevention of STD b. Family planning
    c. Child survival d. All of the above
18. **RCH phase 2 does not include:**
    a. Immunization of pregnant women
    b. Treatment of STD/RTI
    c. Feed to malnourished children
    d. Early registration of pregnancy up to 12-16 weeks
19. **Under RCH program, intervention done in selected districts:** *(Recent Question 2016)*
    a. Immunization b. Treatment of STD
    c. ORS therapy d. Vitamin A supplementation

Ans.

1.	a
2.	a
3.	d
4.	b
5.	b
6.	c
7.	d
8.	b
9.	a
10.	d
11.	b
12.	c
13.	b
14.	a
15.	c
16.	b
17.	d
18.	c
19.	b

Most Recent Questions of 2019-18 are given at the end of MCQs

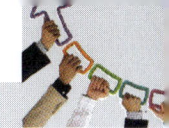

MISCELLANEOUS

20. All are the indications of therapeutic termination of pregnancy except *(Recent Question 2015)*
a. Cardiac disease in NYHA Gr IV
b. Chronic severe glomerulonephritis
c. Cervical malignancy
d. Thyroid disorder

PREVENTIVE OBSTETRICS

21. Registration of pregnancy within 12 weeks is the prime responsibility of:
a. Anganwadi worker b. ASHA
c. ANM d. MPW

22. Risk approach in MCH care is a:
a. Screening tool b. Diagnostic tool
c. Clinical guide d. Managerial tool

23. A pregnant woman, who has been immunized against tetanus last year, comes for the first antenatal check-up at 16 weeks. Number of doses of tetanus toxoid required for her: *(Recent Question 2015)*
a. None b. 1
c. 2 d. 3

24. If the same woman (mentioned in the previous question) delivers a healthy male baby. She becomes pregnant after 1 year. Number of doses of tetanus toxoid required for her:
a. None b. 1
c. 2 d. 3

25. Birth rate in a population of 5000 is 30 per 1000 population. Calculate the total number of expected pregnancies:
a. 20 b. 135
c. 150 d. 165

26. The following laboratory investigations are available at a sub-center to a pregnant women, except:
a. Pregnancy detection test
b. Hb examination
c. VDRL
d. Rapid malaria test

27. All are true regarding management of a Rh-negative pregnant women, except: *(Recent Question 2015)*
a. If the women is Rh negative and the husband is Rh positive, her RH-anitbody levels are tested at 28 weeks and 34–36 weeks of gestation
b. Rh anti-D immunoglobulin is given at 28 weeks of gestation so that sensitization during the first pregnancy can be prevented
c. If the baby is Rh-positive, Rh anti-D lg is given again within 72 hours of delivery
d. Rh anti-D lg need not be given after abortion

28. MCH care is assessed by:
a. Maternal mortality rate b. Birth rate
c. Maternal mortality ratio d. Anemia in pregnancy

29. In a town there are 2500 live birth in last six month. During same period there is death of 5 women due to peripartum infection, 5 due to electrocution, 2 due to obstructed labor and 3 due to PPH. What is the MMR:
a. 4 per 1000 live birth b. 6 per 1000 live birth
c. 40 per 1000 live birth d. 60 per 1000 live birth

30. Minimum number of ANC visits during pregnancy should be: *(Recent Question 2014)*
a. 3 b. 5
c. 4 d. 6

MATERNAL MORTALITY

31. Most common cause of maternal death in India is:
a. Infection b. Eclampsia
c. Anaemia d. Bleeding

32. Least common cause of maternal mortality in India:
a. PPH b. Sepsis
c. Anemia d. CHF

33. "Maternal death" is death of a woman during pregnancy or at the time of delivery or postdelivery up to:
a. 14 Weeks b. 6 Weeks
c. 10 Weeks d. 8 Weeks

34. MMR for India (2016-2017) is: *(Recent Question 2014)*
a. 155 b. 167
c. 219 d. 370

35. Maternal mortality rate definition include all, except:
a. Death in pregnancy
b. Death during pregnancy
c. Death within 6 weeks post delivery
d. Death within 6 months post delivery

36. Maternal Mortality Ratio is calculated by:
a. Maternal deaths/ live birth
b. Maternal deaths/ 1000 live births
c. Maternal deaths/ 100,000 live births
d. Maternal deaths/ 100,000 populations

37. Maternal mortality rate is defined as:
a. Maternal death per 1000 total births
b. Maternal death per 1000 live births
c. Maternal death per 1000 women
d. Maternal death per 1000 women of reproductive age

38. Maternal Mortality Ratio (MMR) is expressed as:
a. Per 100,000 live births b. Per 1000 live births
c. Per 100,000 births d. Per 1000 population

39. Denominator in Maternal Mortality Rate is:
a. Total number of live births
b. Total number of births
c. Total number of married women in reproductive age group
d. Mid-year population

40. About Maternal Mortality Rate which of the following is true: *(Recent Question 2013)*
a. It is a rate not ratio
b. Numerator includes complications related death up to 42 days after pregnancy
c. Denominator includes stillbirth and abortions
d. Expressed as rate per 1000 live birth

MISCELLANEOUS

41. Essential component of kangaroo mother care comprise all, except: *(Recent Question 2013)*
a. Skin-to-skin positioning of a baby on the mother's chest
b. Adequate nutrition through breast-feeding
c. Domiciliary care
d. Support for the mother and her family in caring for the baby

Ans.
20. d
21. c
22. d
23. b
24. a
25. d
26. c
27. d
28. c
29. a
30. c
31. d
32. d
33. b
34. b
35. d
36. c
37. a
38. a
39. c
40. b
41. c

Most Recent Questions of 2019-18 are given at the end of MCQs

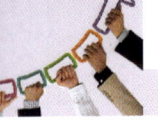

42. A 5 × 5 matrix is
a. RCH II
b. RMNCH+A
c. Nat immunization schedule
d. JSSK

43. Which of the following is correct regarding survey based color coded score cards?
a. Green – less than 20% of national average for mortality, fertility
b. Yellow – less than 30% of the national average
c. Red – more than 10% of the national average for mortality indicators
d. Includes pregnancy care, child birth, postnatal & maternal care, reproductive age group care

Most Recent Questions (2019-2018)

44. Syphilis screening test in pregnant women is/are: ***(PGI Nov 2018)***
a. RPR
b. VDRL
c. Dark ground microscopy
d. TPHA
e. Fluorescent Treponema Antibody Absorption Test

45. Which of the following is true for gestational diabetes mellitus screening during pregnancy? ***(PGI Nov 2018)***
a. The criteria for GDM screening is Fasting blood glucose ≥ 126 mg/dl
b. The criteria for GDM screening is 2 step OGTT ≥ 140 mg/dl
c. The first GDM Screening is done in 1st antenatal visit
d. A trial for Medical nutrition is given for 2 weeks to all cases of GDM in pregnancy
e. The treatment target is to keep the 2 hr Post prandial Plasma glucose ≤ 140 mg/dl

46. What all conditions can commonly occur in baby a result of uncontrolled diabetes in mother. ***(PGI Nov 2018)***
a. Intrauterine death
b. Fetal macrosomia
c. Discordant twins
d. Open neural tube defect
e. Chromosomal abnormalities

47. Program for increasing quality of labor room care: ***(AIIMS May 2019)***
a. LaQshya program
b. Janani Shishu suraksha karyakram
c. Ayushman bharat scheme
d. PM Surakshit Matritva Abhiyan

48. Under RMNCH program peripheral level of planning is done at: ***(Recent Question 2019)***
a. Anganwadi
b. Subcenter
c. District level
d. PHC level

49. Vaccine contraindicated in pregnancy: ***(Recent Question 2019)***
a. Rabies
b. Hep A
c. Hep B
d. Varicella

Ans.
42. b
43. a
44. a, b
45. b, c, d
46. a, b
47. a
48. c
49. d

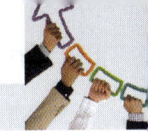

Answers with Explanations

1. Ans. (a) Free family planning kit

Ref: K. Park, 23rd ed. p 456; DK Taneja, Health Policies and Programs in India,13th ed. p 111

NRHM

2. Ans. (a) JSSK

Ref: K. Park, 23rd ed. p 456, DK Taneja, Health Policies and Programs in India,13th edition, p-111

Janani Shishu Suraksha Karyakram [JSSK] Refer To theory

3. Ans. (d) Free family planning kit

Ref: K. Park, 23rd ed. p 456, DK Taneja, Health Policies and Programs in India,13th edition, p-111

Also Know.......................

- JSSK guarantees services/ entitlements and eliminates out of pocket expenses of pregnant women and Sick newborn

4. Ans. (b) 2005

Ref: K. Park, 24th ed. p 475

Janani Suraksha Yojana

Refer to theory

5. Ans. (b) Anganwadi acts as link between pregnant woman and Government

Ref: K. Park, 24th ed. p 475

Cash Assistance Under JSY[Q] [Revised from 8th May 2013]

Category	Rural			Urban		
	Mother	Asha	Total	Mother	Asha	Total
LPS	1400	600	2000	1000	400	1400
HPS	700	600	1300	600	400	1000

6. Ans. (c) Up to 2 live births in low performing states

Ref: K. Park, 24th ed. p 475

Eligibility for cash assistance under JSY

Refer To Theory

7. Ans. (d) Free treatment of sick infants up to 2 years

Ref: K. Park, 23rd ed. p 456, DK Taneja, Health Policies and Programs in India,13th edition, p 111

8. Ans. (b) Institutional deliveries

Ref: K. Park, 24th ed. p 475

9. Ans. (a) Janani Suraksha Yojana

Ref: K. Park, 24th ed. p 45

RCH

10. Ans. (d) Reduction of anemia in adolescent at 6% annually

Ref: K. Park, 24th ed. p 483-84

In line with the RMNCH +A strategy, goals set for the 12th Five-Year Plan (2012-2017) are

- Reducing the IMR to 25 per 1,000 live births.
- Reducing the MMR to 100 per 100,000 live births.
- Reducing the TFR to 2.1.
- Increasing the child sex ratio in the 0-6 year age group to 950.

11. Ans. (b) Adolescent Health

Ref: K. Park, 24th ed. p 483

Refer to theory

12. Ans. (c) Private sector involvement

Ref: K. Park, 24th ed. p 483

13. Ans. (b) Pneumonia management

Ref: K. Park, 24th ed. p 485-86

Refer to theory

14. Ans. (a) Vande Mataram scheme

Ref: K. Park, 24th ed. p 472, 475

- **Vande Matram scheme:** The scheme envisages provision of free out-patient department (OPD) services, including antenatal check-up of all pregnant women and family planning counseling to new mothers regularly by the government and private doctors at their facility on the 9th of every month
- The public health facilities of the Government would also observe the 9th of every month as 'Vande mataram Day' and provide priority to expectant mothers.
- It was an old scheme started in year 2003–2004 before the implementation of the NRHM, which now has an integrated approach

15. Ans (c) Free treatment in private clinics

Ref: K. Park, 24th ed. p 475

Refer to Theory

16. Ans. (b) CSSM plus family planning

Ref: K. Park, 23rd ed. p 452, DK Taneja, Health Policies and Programs in India,13th edition, p 115

17. Ans. (d) All of the above

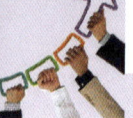

Ref: K Park, 23rd ed. p 454, DK Taneja, Health Policies and Programs in India,13th edition, p 115

18. Ans. (c) Feed to malnourished children

Ref: K. Park, 24th ed. p 474

19. Ans. (b) Treatment of STD

Ref: K. Park, 24th ed. p 472

RCH program was based on Differential Approach (Inputs varied across districts)

- All districts received care components
- Weaker districts got more support
- Advanced districts got more sophisticated facilities

Interventions in all district	Intervention in selected district
▪ CSSM interventions ▪ IEC activities ▪ Implementation of Target Free Approach ▪ RTI/STD clinics at district hospital (if not available) ▪ Safe abortion services at PHC ▪ Target Free Approach ▪ High Quality training	▪ Screening and treatment of RTI/STD at subdivisional level ▪ Emergency Obstetric Care at select FRU ▪ Essential Obstetric care at PHC ▪ Additional ANM at Sub Center in weak district
▪ Enhanced community participation ▪ Adolescent health and reproductive hygiene ▪ Special RCH project for Urban slums	▪ Improved delivery and emergency care services, IUD insertion at Sub Center ▪ Facility of referral transport

MISCELLANEOUS

20. Ans. (d) Thyroid disorder

Ref: K. Park, 24th ed. p 540

(Refer to text in Chapter demography/MTP Act)

PREVENTIVE OBSTETRICS

21. Ans. (c) ANM

Ref: K. Park 24th ed. p 558

Registration of pregnancy within 12 weeks and ANC check-up is primary responsibility of ANM.

22. Ans. (d) Managerial tool

Ref: K. Park, 24th ed. p 561

Risk approach is a managerial tool that seeks to screen out "high risk" pregnancies at the earliest from a large group of antenatal mothers and arrange for them skilled care, while continuing to provide appropriate care for all mothers

23. Ans. (b) 1

Ref: K. Park 24th ed. p 563

TT Immunisation in Pregnancy

Previous Immunization Status	Number of Doses	Timing
Not Immunized	2 [Minimum 1 month interval between 2 doses]*	1st dose at 16 to 20 Weeks and 2nd dose at 20–24 Weeks.
Immunized	1 [Booster]	Preferably 1 month before expected date of delivery

**No pregnant woman should be denied even 1 dose of TT, if she is seen late in pregnancy*

24. Ans. (a) None

Ref: K. Park 24th ed. p 563

Booster dose provides cover for subsequent pregnancies during next 5 years.

Also Know......................

- TT should not be given at every successive pregnancy. (Risk of Hyper immunization and side effects).

25. Ans. (d) 165

Ref: K. Park 24th ed. p 559

Expected number of live births (A)

$$= \frac{\text{Birth rate (per 1000 population} \times \text{population of the area)}}{1000}$$

All pregnancies may not result in a live birth (About 10% of pregnancy may terminate as abortions/ stillbirths).

So, Total number of expected pregnancies = Expected number of live births (A) + 10% of A*

= (30 × 5000)/1000 + 10% of (30 × 5000)/1000

= 150 + 15 =165

Also Know......................

- In any given month, approximately half of the pregnancies estimated should be in records.

26. Ans. (c) VDRL

Ref: K. Park 24th ed. p 561

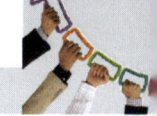

LAB Investigation facilities available at Primary level of Health care	
Sub Center	**PHC (Facilities in addition to that at Sub center)**
▪ Pregnancy detection test ▪ Hemoglobin estimation ▪ Urine test for albumin and sugar ▪ Rapid malaria test	▪ Blood group and Rh ▪ VDRL/RPR ▪ HIV testing ▪ Rapid malaria test (If not available at Sub Center) ▪ Blood Sugar ▪ HBsAg for Hepatitis B infection

27. Ans. (d) Rh anti-D lg need not be given…

Ref: K. Park 24th ed. p 563

Management of a Rh-negative Pregnant Women

- Rh antibody levels in a Rh negative women with Rh positive husband should be tested at 28 weeks and 34-36 weeks of gestation
- Rh anti-D immunoglobulin is given at 28 weeks to avoid sensitization during first pregnancy
- If the baby delivered is Rh-positive, Rh anti-D immunoglobulin is given again within 72 hours of delivery
- Rh anti-D immunoglobulin also need to be administered after abortion

Also Know……………………

- In India, Incidence of hemolytic disease due to Rh factor is 1 per 400-500 live birth.

28. Ans. (c) Maternal mortality ratio

Ref: K. Park, 24th ed. p 593

Indicators of MCH care are

- Maternal Mortality Ratio
- Perinatal mortality rate
- Neonatal mortality rate
- Post Neonatal mortality rate
- Infant mortality rate
- 1-4 year mortality rate
- Under 5 mortality rate
- Child survival rate

29. Ans. (a) 4 per 1000 live birth

Ref: K. Park, 24th ed. p 593

Maternal death—is defined as death of a woman while pregnant or within 42 days of termination of pregnancy, irrespective of duration and site of pregnancy, from any cause related to or aggravated by pregnancy or its management but not from accidental or incidental causes.[Q]

Total maternal deaths = 15
Total live birth = 2500
Accidental death = 5 (due to electrocution)
Hence for formula, the maternal deaths are 10

Maternal mortality ratio: (MMR) = [Total maternal deaths/ total live birth] * 1000 = 10/2500 × 1000 = 4 per 1000 live birth

30. Ans. (c) 4

Ref: K. Park, 24th ed. p 558

Ideal ANC visits →Once a month in first 7 months; 2 times per month in 8th month and once a week in 9th month (If everything is normal).

Minimum ANC visits Target	Timings
1st	Within 12 weeks or as soon as pregnancy is suspected (Registration by ANM and ANC Checkup)
2nd	14-26 week
3rd	28-34 week (ANC Check up by Medical Officer)
4th	36 week -Term

MATERNAL MORTALITY

31. Ans. (d) Bleeding

Ref: K. Park, 24th ed. p 595,597

Refer to theory

Also Know……………………

- Highest vulnerability of maternal death is in the post partum period [50–70%]
- About 45% of maternal deaths occur in the first 24 hour after delivery
- More than 66% of all maternal deaths occur in first week post delivery.
- About 11–17% of maternal deaths occur during child birth

32. Ans. (d) CHF

Ref: K. Park, 24th ed p-597

33. Ans. (b) 6 Weeks

Ref: K. Park, 24th ed. p 593

Maternal death is defined as "Death of a woman while pregnant or within 42 days of termination of pregnancy, irrespective of duration and site of pregnancy, from any cause related or aggravated by pregnancy or its management but not from accidental or incidental cause"[Q]

Also Know……………………

***Late maternal death** is* death of a woman from direct or indirect obstetric causes after 42 days and within a year of termination of pregnancy.

34. Ans. (b) 167 per 100,000 live births

Ref: K. Park, 23rd ed. p 519

35. Ans. (d) Death within 6 months post delivery

Ref: K. Park, 24th ed. p 593

Maternal mortality rate is number of maternal deaths (*due to complications of pregnancy, child birth or within 42 days of delivery from puerperal cause)* in a given time period per 100000 women of reproductive age in the same time period[Q]

36. Ans. (c) Maternal deaths/ 100,000 live births

Ref: K. Park, 24th ed. p 593

Refer to theory

37. Ans. (a) Maternal death per 100,000 live births

Ref: K. Park, 24th ed. p 593

In developed country, MMR has declined significantly-so multiplying factor of 100,000 is used instead of 1000 to avoid fractions

38. Ans. (a) Per 100,000 live births

Ref: K. Park, 24th ed. p 593

39. Ans. (c) Total number of married women in reproductive age group

Ref: K. Park, 24th ed. p 593

40. Ans. (b) Numerator includes complications related death up to 42 …

Ref: K. Park, 24th ed. p 593

- ***Pregnancy Related Death*** is defined as death of a woman while pregnant or within 42 days of termination of pregnancy, irrespective of the cause of death.

MISCELLANEOUS

41. Ans. (c) Domiciliary care

Ref: K. Park, 24th ed. p 572

Essential Elements of Kangaroo Mother Care (KMC) are

- Skin to Skin contact of a baby on mother's chest between her breasts
- Exclusive Breast feeding
- Ambulatory care - Early discharge and follow up
- Support for mother and her family in care of the baby

Also Know........................

- KMC was initiated by Dr Hector Martinez and Edzar Rey in 1979 in Colombia for LBW newborns.

KMC is indicated for hemodynamically stable LBW babies weighing 1800-2000 gm

KMC is to be given immediately after birth and 24 hours a day (Position can be altered once in 2 hour to feed or change diapers)

Parameters Monitored in KMC

- Temperature- 6 hourly (2 hourly for sick baby)
- Respiration
- Feeding –Every 90 min to 120 min
- Growth – Weight gain of about 40gm/day (15-20 gm/kg body weight/day)
- Well-being – Danger signs monitored
- Compliance

42. Ans. (b) RMNCH+A

5 × 5 matrix: RMNCH+A

Targets – 12th FYP (Five Year Plan)

- Reduction of Infant Mortality Rate (IMR) to 25 per 1,000 live births by 2017
- Reduction in Maternal Mortality Ratio (MMR) to 100 per 100,000 live births by 2017
- Reduction in Total Fertility Rate (TFR) to 2.1 by 2017

Also introduces new initiatives like the use of Score Card to track the performance, National Iron + Initiative to address the issue of anemia across all age groups and the Comprehensive Screening and Early interventions for defects at birth , diseases and deficiencies among children and adolescents.

Some Background Data

In India, 22% babies born each year have LBW, which has been linked to maternal under-nutrition and anaemia among other causes. The mother's condition before pregnancy is a key determinant of its outcome; half of adolescents (boys and girls) have below normal body mass index (BMI) and almost 56% of adolescent girls aged 15–19 years have anaemia.

- Most common cause for maternal mortality in India – Post-partum hemorrhage
- Most common cause for Post-partum hemorrhage in females
  - Unskilled labor
  - Trauma during labor
  - Secondary causes as anemia
- Most common cause of Neonatal mortality in India - prematurity
- Most common cause of Infant mortality in India - Low birth weights and prematurity
- Most common cause of Under-five mortality in India
  - Malnutrition (m/c due to Low birth weights and prematurity)
  - Infections (because of under-weight for age)

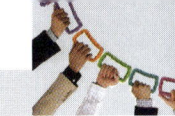

Reproductive care		Pregnancy and child birth care	Newborn and childcare	
Clinical	▪ Comprehensive abortion care ▪ RTI/STI case management ▪ Postpartum IUCD and sterilization; interval IUCD procedures ▪ Adolescent friendly health services	▪ Skilled obstetric care and immediate newborn care and resuscitation ▪ Emergency obstetric care ▪ Preventing parent to child Transmission (PPTCT) of HIV ▪ Postpartum sterilisation	▪ Essential newborn care ▪ Care of sick newborn (SNCU, NBSU) ▪ Facility-based care of childhood illnesses (IMNCI) ▪ Care of children with severe acute malnutrition (NRC) ▪ Immunisation	
	Reproductive health care	**Antenatal care**	**Postnatal care**	**Child health care**
Outreach/Sub center	▪ Family planning (including IUCD insertion, OCP and condoms) ▪ Prevention and management of STIs ▪ Peri-conception folic acid supplementation	▪ Full antenatal care package ▪ PPTCP	▪ Early detection and management of illnesses in mother and newborn ▪ Immunisation	▪ First level assessment and care for newborn and childhood illnesses ▪ Immunisation ▪ Micro-nutrient supplementation
Family & Community	▪ Weekly IFA supplementation ▪ Information and counselling on sexual reproductive health and family planning ▪ Community based promotion and delivery of contraceptives ▪ Menstrual hygiene	▪ Counselling and preparation for newborn care, breast feeding, birth preparedness ▪ Demand generation for pregnancy care and institutional delivery (JSY, JSSK)	▪ Home-based newborn care and prompt referral (HBNC scheme) ▪ Antibiotic for suspected case of newborn sepsis ▪ Infant and Young Child Feeding (IYCF), including exclusive breast feeding and complementary feeding ▪ Child health screening and early intervention services (0–18 years) ▪ Early childhood development ▪ Danger sign recognition and care-seeking for illness ▪ Use of ORS and Zinc in case of diarrhoea	
	Intersectoral: Water, sanitation, hygiene, nutrition, education, empowerment			

43. Ans. (a) Green – less than 20% of national average for mortality, fertility

The score cards for MCH are based on HMIS – health management and information systems

It Takes into Account

- Mortality indicators
- Fertility indicators
- Nutrition indicators
- Immunization
- Diarrhoea
- Pneumonia
- Service delivery indicators

For all Mortality, Nutrition and Fertility Indicators

- **Green:** Less than 20% of national average
- **Yellow:** Within 20% below or above the national average
- **Red:** More than 20% of the national average

All Other Indicators

- Green > 20% of national average
- **Yellow:** Within 20% below and above the average
- **Red:** Less than 20% of the national average

44. Ans. (a) RPR, (b) VDRL

Ref: National guidelines on prevention, management and control of RTI/STI, MoHFW(2018); 65-67

Syphilis In Pregnancy

- Infection to mother through sexual contact
- To baby – transplacental
- Highest risk of transmission to foetus is T1 – T3

Diagnosis of Syphilis

Screening of Syphilis

The current nontreponemal tests for syphilis are Venereal Disease Research Laboratory (VDRL) and rapid plasma reagin (RPR) test. RPR test is most suitable for the primary health care setup

Confirmation of Syphilis

Treponemal tests, such as Treponema pallidum hemagglutination test (TPHA), fluorescent Treponema antibody absorption test (FTAAbs), micro-hemagglutination assay for antibodies to Treponema pallidum (MHATP), if available, can be used to confirm nontreponemal test results.

Interpretation of RPR Test

Infection	RPR Titre
▪ Active infection	1:8 or higher
▪ Latent infection	1:4
▪ False positive	1:4
▪ Treatment response	2 fold decline in the titre

If RPR Positive

- Enquire if the woman and her partner have received proper treatment.
- If not, treat woman and partner for syphilis with benzathine penicillin.
- Treat newborn with benzathine penicillin.
- Follow-up newborn in 2 weeks.
- Counsel on safer sex.

45. Ans. (b) The criteria for GDM screening is 2 step OGTT ≥ 140 mg/dl, (c) The first GDM Screening is done in 1st antenatal visit, (d) A trial for Medical nutrition is given for 2 weeks to all cases of GDM in pregnancy

Ref. National guidelines for diagnosis & Management of Gestational Diabetes Mellitus. MoHFW (2014).

Option	T/F	Comment
The criteria for GDM screening is Fasting blood glucose ≥ 126 mg/dl	F	No, the GDM screening is based on 2 step OGTT criteria
The criteria for GDM screening is 2 step OGTT ≥ 140 mg/dl	T	Yes correct
The first GDM Screening is done in 1st antenatal visit	T	Yes correct. 1st screening is done in 1st ANC visit, followed by repeat screening (if negative on first) at 24-28 weeks
A trial for Medical nutrition is given for 2 weeks to all cases of GDM in pregnancy	T	Yes, correct
The treatment target is to keep the 2 hr Post prandial Plasma glucose ≤ 140 mg/dl	F	No, the target is to keep PPPG ≤ 120 mg/dl

GDM Diagnosis Guidelines 2018

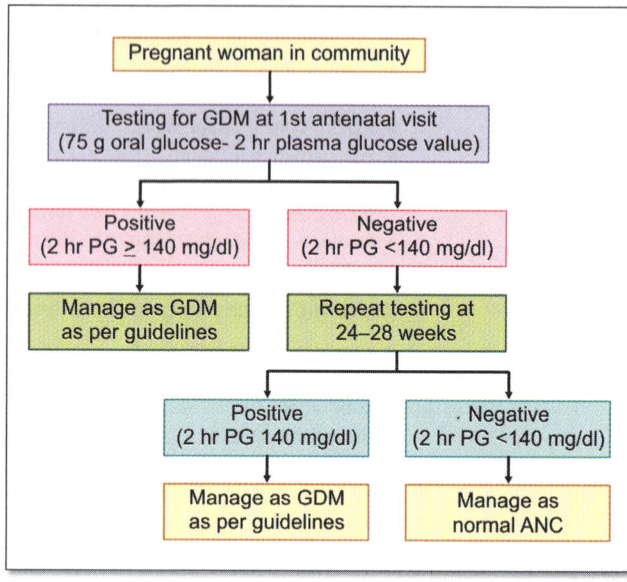

The treatment Target is

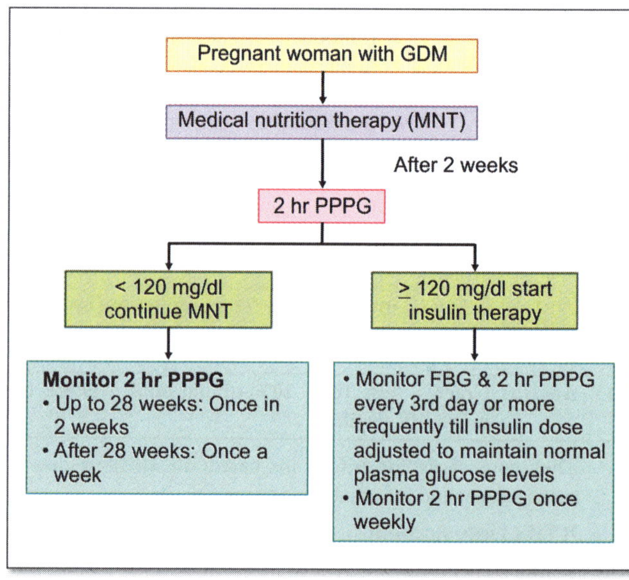

Thus, GDM is managed initially with MNT and if it is not controlled with MNT, insulin therapy is added to the MNT.

46. Ans. (a) Intrauterine death, (b) Fetal macrosomia

The evidence suggests the following risks for baby and mother due to uncontrolled diabetes in mother.

Maternal risk	Fetal risk
▪ Polyhydramnios ▪ Pre-eclampsia ▪ Prolonged labour ▪ Obstructed labour ▪ Caesarean section ▪ Uterine atony ▪ Postpartum haemorrhage ▪ Infection	▪ Spontaneous abortion ▪ Intra-uterine death ▪ Stillbirth ▪ Congenital malformation ▪ Shoulder dystocia ▪ Birth injuries ▪ Neonatal hypoglycaemia ▪ Infant respiratory distress syndrome

Other risks as given in MCQ options as twins, Neural tube defects and chromosomal abnormalities – may occur as separate events, but GDM does not predispose or increase the risk for same.

47. Ans. (a) LaQshya program

LaQshya

Under MoHFW

- **Focus:** Improving Quality of Labour room and maternity operation theatre
- **Outcome:** improve quality of care for pregnant women in labour room, maternity Operation Theatre and Obstetrics Intensive Care Units (ICUs) and High Dependency Units (HDUs)
- **Implementation:** all Medical College Hospitals, District Hospitals and First Referral Unit (FRU), and Community Health Center (CHCs)
- **Beneficiary:** Every pregnant woman and new-born delivering in public health institutions

48. Ans. (c) District level

Ref: Park 25th Ed. Pg 501

RMNCH+A

Focus

- Include adoloscents
- Link MCH with adolescent health, gender preconception, HIV
- Comprehensive care including primary, secondary and tertiary care

Plan

- Coverage complete at the HPD's (High priority districts)
- Use the RMNCH + A 5 × 5 matrix framework – based on 5 components of health and 5 subcomponents of focus areas

Main Goals

- Decrease IMR < 25 per 1000 live births
- Decrease MMR < 100 per 100,000 live births
- Reduce TFR < 2.1

49. Ans. (d) Varicella

Ref: https://www.cdc.gov/vaccines/pregnancy/index.html

Vaccine in Pregnancy

Varicella / Zoster Vaccine

- Zoster vaccine should not be administered to pregnant women. Additionally, Zostavax is not licensed for the age groups that include women of traditional childbearing ages
- Because the effects of the varicella virus on the fetus are unknown, pregnant women should not be vaccinated. Nonpregnant women who are vaccinated should avoid becoming pregnant for 1 month after each injection

Rabies

- Because of the potential consequences of inadequately managed rabies exposure, pregnancy is not considered a contraindication to post exposure prophylaxis. If the risk of exposure to rabies is substantial, pre-exposure prophylaxis also might be indicated during pregnancy. Rabies exposure or the diagnosis of rabies in the mother should not be regarded as reasons to terminate the pregnancy

Hepatitis A

- The safety of hepatitis A vaccination during pregnancy has not been determined; however, because hepatitis A vaccine is produced from inactivated HAV, the theoretic risk to the developing fetus is expected to be low. The risk associated with vaccination should be weighed against the risk for hepatitis A in pregnant women who might be at high risk for exposure to HAV

Hepatitis B

- Pregnancy is not a contraindication to HepB vaccination. Pregnant women who are identified as being at risk for HBV infection during pregnancy (e.g., having more than one sex partner during the previous 6 months, been evaluated or treated for an STD, recent or current injection drug use, or having had an HBsAg-positive sex partner) should be vaccinated

NOTES

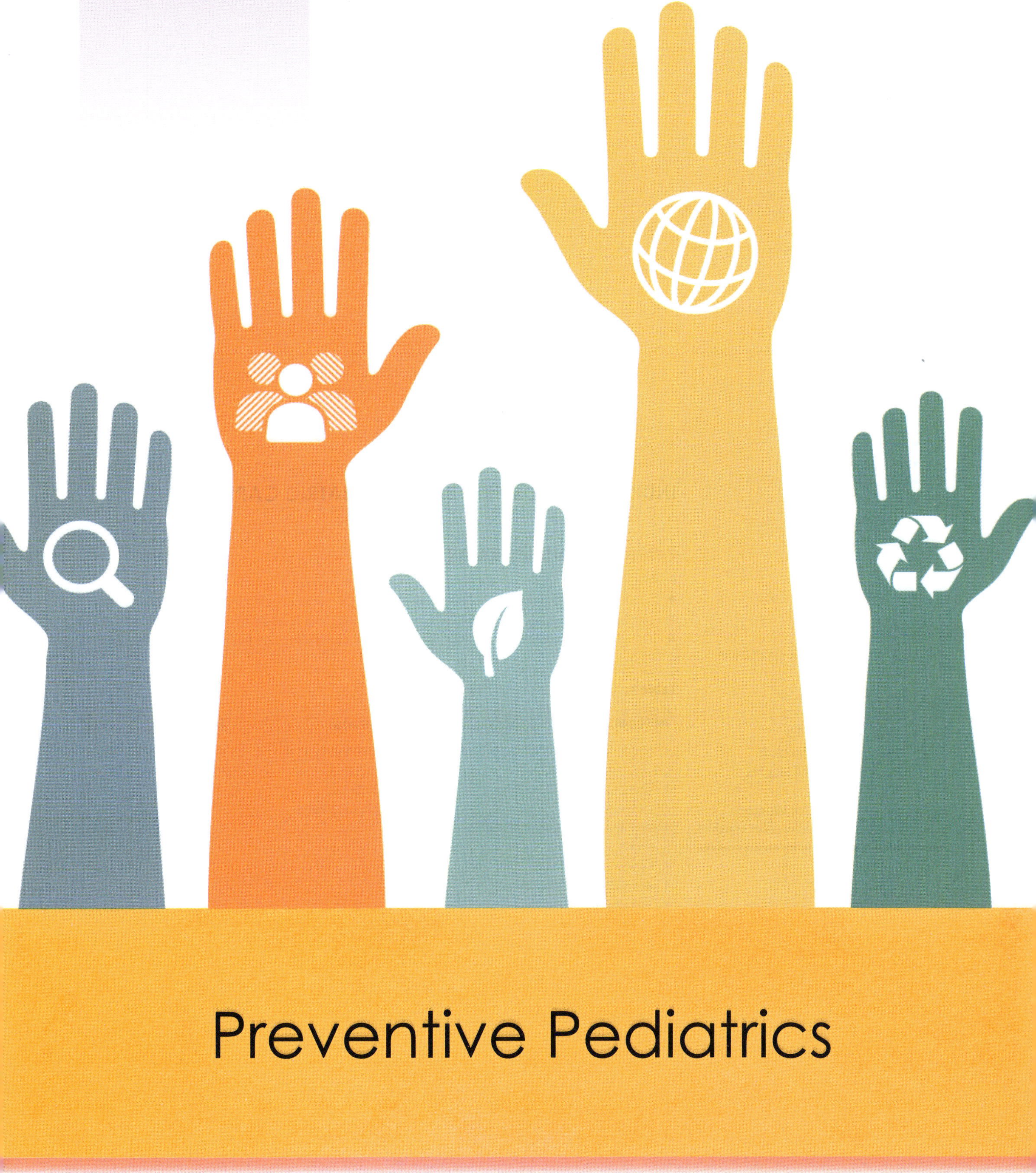

Preventive Pediatrics

Chapter Outline

GESTATION CHART

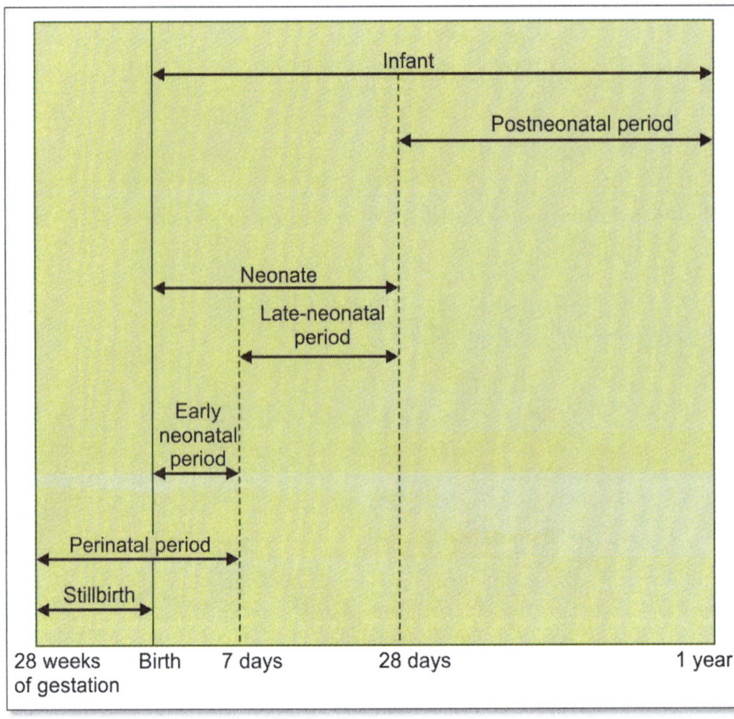

Fig. 1: Gestation chart

INDICATORS FOR PREVENTIVE PEDIATRIC CARE

Perinatal Mortality Rate (PNMR)

Perinatal mortality includes *late fetal deaths*, *live births* and *early neonatal deaths* with:

- Minimum birthweight of 1000 g (equivalent to 28 weeks of gestation) - Preferred criterion
- If the birthweight is not available, a gestational age of at least 28 weeks
- If both birthweight and gestational age are not available, body length (crown to heel) of at least 35 cm.

Table 1: Causes of perinatal mortality

Antenatal	Intranatal	Postnatal
▪ Maternal hypertension, cardiovascular disease and diabetes ▪ Uterine myomas, Endometriosis, Ovarian tumors ▪ Uterine anomalies, incompetent cervix ▪ Congenital defects ▪ Malnutrition and anemia ▪ Toxemias of pregnancy and tuberculosis ▪ Endocrine imbalance and inadequate uterine preparation ▪ Blood incompatibilities ▪ Antepartum hemorrhages ▪ Advanced age of mother	▪ Birth injury and asphyxia ▪ Obstetric complications	▪ Prematurity ▪ Respiratory distress syndrome ▪ Congenital anomalies ▪ Respiratory and GI infections

Infant Mortality Rate (IMR)Q

- It is the number of infant deaths in a given area in a year per 1000 live births in the same area and year.
- It is regarded worldwide as the most important indicator of health status of a community, level of living of people and effectiveness of MCH services.Q
- Neonatal deaths contribute 70% to infant mortality.Q

$$\textbf{Infant mortality rate (IMR)}^{Q} = \frac{\textit{Number of deaths of children less than 1 year of age in a year}}{\textit{Number of live births in the same year}} \times 1000$$

Table 2: Causes of infant mortality

Neonatal mortality (0-4 weeks)	Low birthweight (LBW-most Common), Birth injury, congenital anomaly, hemolytic disease, placenta/cord conditions, diarrhea, acute respiratory infection (ARI), neonatal tetanus
Postneonatal mortality (>4 week-1 year)	Diarrhea, ARI, other communicable disease, malnutrition, congenital anomaly, accidents
Overall (0-1 year)	LBW (Most common—57%), ARI (17%), diarrhea, congenital anomaly, cord infection, birth trauma, others

Principal Causes of Infant Mortality

- Developing countries → LBW and combined effects of infection (e.g., diarrhea, ARI) and malnutrition.
- Developed countries → Congenital anomalies, anoxia and hypoxia.
- Neonatal mortality rate is 24 per 1000 live birth [neonatal deaths comprise 67.6% of Infant deaths]
- Early neonatal Mortality is 18 per 1000 live birth [52% of Infant death and 75% of neonatal deaths] 10% of children born in India do not survive till 5 years of age. 50% of under 5 death occur in neonatal period
- Under 5 mortality rate in India is 39 per 1000 live birth 1/3rd of death in under 5 year children is due to preventable infectious diseases
- Infants constitute 3% of the total population in IndiaQ
- Neonatal mortality is higher in boys worldwide [Newborn boys are biologically more fragile than girls]
- Infant deaths account for 13% of total deaths
- About 50% of childhood deaths in India are attributable to malnutrition.

Neonatal Mortality Rate (NNMR)

It is number of neonatal deaths in a given year per 1000 live births in same year.Q

$$\textbf{NMR} = \frac{\textit{Number of deaths of within 28 days of birth in a year}}{\textit{Total live births in the same year}} \times 1000$$

The neonatal mortality rate of India is 24/1000 live birth SRS 2016-18

169 *High Yield Points*

- **Infant mortality rate:** Best indicator for health status of a population of effectiveness of MCH services. It is the overall general indicator for health status and is an important component in the physical quality of life index (PQLI)
- **Perinatal mortality rate:** Good indicator for health care services
- **MMR:** Good indicator for the delivery services in a population
- **U5MR (Under 5 Mortality Rate):** Good indicator for development of a country in terms of political, economic, health and other external variables. It is a variable for the Global Hunger Index—an indicator for evaluation by the UNICEF

170 *High Yield Points*

National Data: SRS 2018
- Infant mortality is 34/1000 live births
- TFR = 2.2
- MMR = 130/100,000 live births

101 **Must Remember**

- **Most common cause of:** neonatal mortality in India is low birthweight and prematurity (35%)[Q]
- **Most common cause of:** early neonatal mortality in India is prematurity and congenital anomaly
- **Most common cause of:** late neonatal mortality in India is diarrhea, tetanus

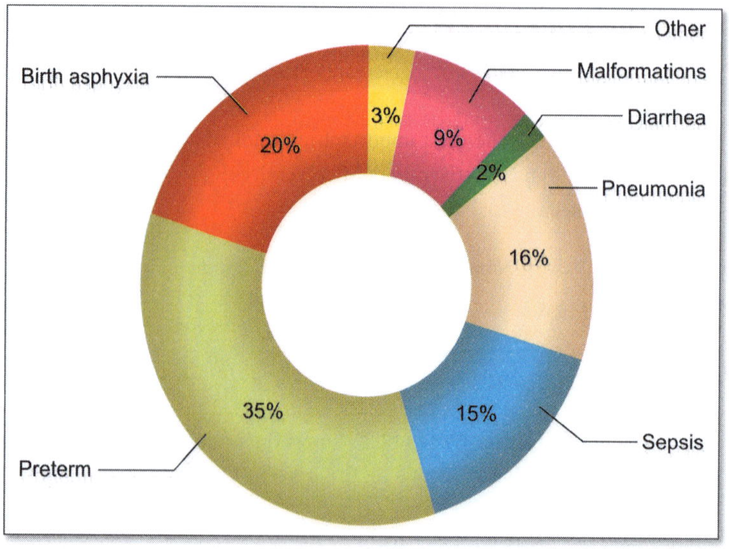

Fig. 2: Causes of neonatal deaths in India

Source: Liu et al, Lancet 2012 Statistical report

102 **Must Remember**

Under-5 Mortality Rate
Considered by UNICEF as the best single indicator of overall social development and well-being of entire society[Q] and not only of the state of nations children.

Under-5 Mortality Rate

- It is the annual deaths of children under 5 years of age, expressed as a rate per 1000 live births.
- It is the probability of dying between birth and 5 years of age.[Q]

$$\text{U5MR} = \frac{\textit{Number of deaths of children less than 5 year of age in a given year}}{\textit{Number of live births in the same year}} \times 1000$$

Stillbirth Rate (SBR)

- It is the death of a fetus weighing 1000 g (equivalent to 28 weeks of gestation or more) occurring in a year per 1000 total births (live births plus stillbirths).

$$\textbf{Stillbirth Rate} = \frac{\textit{Fetal deaths weighing more than 1000 g in a year}}{\textit{Total birth [Live + Stillbirths] in same year}} \times 1000$$

1–4 Years Mortality Rate (Child Death Rate)

- It is the number of deaths in children aged 1–4 years per 1000 children in the same age group in a given year.

$$\text{Child death rate} = \frac{\textit{Number of deaths of children aged 1–4 years during a year}}{\textit{1000 Total number of children aged 1–4 years at the middle of the year}} \times 1000$$

103 **Must Remember**

Child death rate excludes infant mortality. It is a more refined indicator of social situation in a country than IMR

Child Survival Index (Child Survival Rate Per 1000 Births)

It is the proportion of children who survive till the age of 5 years.
It is calculated as:

$$\text{Child survival index} = \frac{1000 - \text{under 5 mortality rate}}{10}$$

Low Birthweight (LBW)

It is birthweight less than 2.5 kg (up to and including 2499 g), with measurement being done within 1st hour of life,[Q]

- LBW babies can be preterm or small-for-date
- *Small-for-date (SFD)* babies are those that weigh less than 10th percentile for the gestational age
- SFD babies show retarded intrauterine fetal growth.[Q]
- SFD babies may be born at term or preterm.
- SFD babies have a high risk of death (PEM and infections).
- Factors associated with occurrence of SFD babies:
  - Maternal → Malnutrition, severe anemia, heavy physical work during pregnancy, hypertension, malaria, toxemia, smoking, low economic status, short maternal stature, young age, high parity and close birth spacing, low education status etc.
  - Placental → Placental insufficiency and placental abnormalities
  - Fetal → Fetal abnormalities, intrauterine infections, chromosomal abnormality and multiple gestation.

171 *High Yield Points*

LBW is the single most important factor influencing child survival. IMR is 20 times higher in LBW babies.

India Newborn Action Plan (INAP) 2016

Table 3: INAP–National Targets

Target	Current	2020	2025	2030
Impact targets				
NMR (per 1000 live births)	24	21	15	<10
SBR (per 1000 live births) (As per UNICEF Global Data)	22	17	13	<10
Coverage targets				
Safe delivery (institutional + home delivery by SBA [%])	79	95	95	95
Initiation of breastfeeding within one hour of birth (%)	–	90	90	90
Women with preterm labor receiving at least one dose of antenatal corticosteroids (%)	–	90	95	95
Babies born in health facilities with birth asphyxia received resuscitation (%)	–	90	95	95
Babies received complete schedule of home visits under HBNC by ASHA (%)	–	75	95	95
Newborn with sepsis in the community received gentamicin by ANM (%)	–	75	75	75
Newborn discharged from SNCU followed until age one (%)	–	50	75	75
Newborn with low birthweight/Prematurity managed with KMC at facility (%)	–	50	75	90

Abbreviations: NMR, neonatal mortality rate; SBR, still birth rate; SBA, skilled birth attendant; HBNC, home based neonatal care; SNCE, special newborn care unit; KMC, Kangaroo mother care

172 *High Yield Points*

The INAP targets are:
- single digit NMR and SBR by 2030

NEONATAL AND INFANT CARE

Neonatal Care

- **Rooming in**- Keeping baby's bed near to mother soon after birth.
- **Warm Chain**- Keeping the newborn on the mother's bed in close physical contact all the time to keep warm.

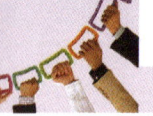

- **Kangaroo Mother Care**- Baby is placed on the chest of the mother having skin-skin contact and covered with a cloth or dupatta. It is usually given to premature preterm babies to prevent hypothermia.

Table 4: Apgar score

Sign	Score		
	0	1	2
Color	Blue	Body pink extremities blue	Completely pink
Heart rate	Absent	<100	>100
Respiratory effort (cry)	Absent	Slow and irregular (feeble cry)	Good cry
Muscle tone (Movements of limbs)	Flaccid	Sluggish	Active
Reflex response	No response	Grimace	Good (cry)
Grading	Severe depression 0–3	Mild depression 4–6	No depression 7–10

A newborn with Apgar score less than 5 is ‘at–risk newborn who needs immediate special attention.

Neonatal Screening

- It is done to detect infants with treatable genetic, developmental and other abnormalities and to provide their parents with genetic counseling. [Secondary level of prevention]
- Neonatal hypothyroidism → Most common disorder that is screened[Q]
- Rh incompatibility → Coombs test on infants of all Rh negative mothers
- Sickle cell and other hemoglobinopathy (e.g., Thalassemia, G6PD deficiency)
- Congenital dislocation of hip

Other diseases amenable to screening:

Congenital Hypothyroidism	Mental retardation, Poor Growth and Neurological Capabilities	T3, T4, TSH
Congenital Adrenal Hyperplasia	Ambiguity of genitalia, salt wasting diseases, Hyponatremia, Hypovolemia	17-Hydroxy Progesterone
Glucose 6 Phosphate Dehydrogenase deficiency	Anemia, Neonatal Jaundice, Hemolysis	G6PD
Galactosemia	Liver failure, Sepsis, Mental retardation. If unchecked can lead to death	Gal-1-P/Galactose
Phenylketonuria	Severe mental retardation, microcephaly, epilepsy	Phenylalanine Guthrie test
Cystic Fibrosis	▪ Chronic Obstructive Lung Disease with thick secretions and recurrent infections ▪ Pancreatic insufficiency leading to digestive problems ▪ Persistent coughing and poor weight gain	Immunoreactive Trypsinogen
Hemoglobinopathies – Thalassemia, Sickle Cell	Chronic Hemolytic Anemia	Hemoglobin
Maple Syrup Urine Disease	▪ Increased leucine levels lead to Mental Retardation ▪ Difficulty in walking, speech, seizure and death	Leucine
Biotinidase deficiency	Seizures, rash, hearing loss and developmental delay	Biotinidase

Danger Signs in the Newborn

- Refusal of feeds
- Increased drowsiness (lethargy)
- Cold to touch
- Difficult or rapid breathing
- Convulsions
- Persistent vomiting
- Jaundice at birth
- Blue coloration of the extremities.

Infant Care

Infant Feeding

- Breastfeeding is the ideal and best feeding for the newborns.
- **Foremilk** is low in fat, and high in lactose, protein, vitamin, minerals and water.
- **Hind milk** is rich in fat and supplies more energy.
- **Preterm milk** (in a mother with preterm baby) is rich in protein, minerals (Na and Cl), immunoglobulins and lactoferrin than mature milk.
- **Exclusive breastfeeding**- Feeding the mother's milk only and no other drinks or water or foods are given to the newborns. ORS, vitamin, mineral and medicines are allowed. It is done for the first 6 months.
- **Complimentary feeding** should be started from 6th month onwards only.
- **Predominantly breastfeeding:** Mostly breast milk + sometimes water, juice, sweetened water and tea
- **High partial:** >80% of infant feed is breast milk
- **Medium partial:** Only 20–80% of infant feed is breast milk
- **Low partial:** < 20% of infant feed is breast milk
- **Token feeding:** Breastfeeding from either one or both breasts for less than 15 minutes per day.
- **Prelacteal food:** Any fluid or food given before colostrums
- **Postlacteal food:** Fluid or food given after breastfeeding has started (within 3 days of birth)

Breastfeeding

Under usual situation –
Milk secretion (average): 450–600 mL/day
Energy: 70 kcals/100 mL of milk
Protein content: 1.1 g/100 mL of milk

Breastfeeding – Signs of Good Attachment

- Baby's chin is touching the breast
- Baby's mouth is wide open and lower lip turned outwards
- More areola is visible above the baby's mouth than below.

Breastfeeding guidelines:

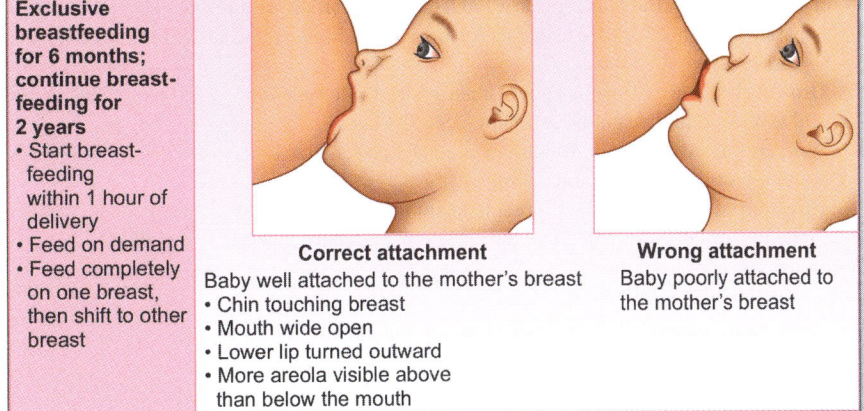

Exclusive breastfeeding for 6 months; continue breast-feeding for 2 years
- Start breast-feeding within 1 hour of delivery
- Feed on demand
- Feed completely on one breast, then shift to other breast

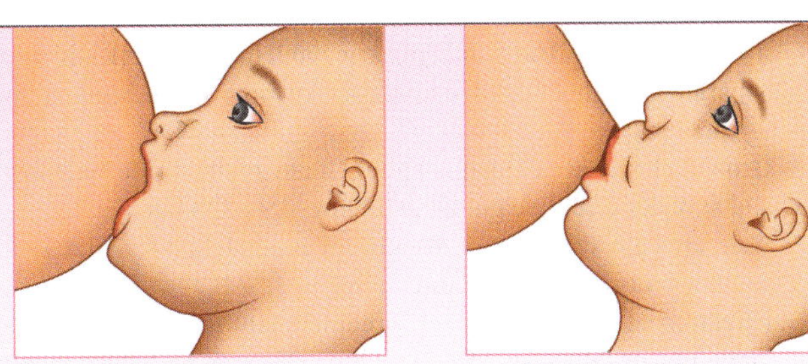

Correct attachment
Baby well attached to the mother's breast
- Chin touching breast
- Mouth wide open
- Lower lip turned outward
- More areola visible above than below the mouth

Wrong attachment
Baby poorly attached to the mother's breast

Fig. 3: Proper breastfeeding

173 High Yield Points

Breastfeeding must be initiated within ½ an hour to 2 hours after birth. In case of cesarean section, feeding should be initiated in about 4 hours.

104 Must Remember

An average Indian woman secretes about 400–600 mL (av. 500 mL) of milk per day.

109 Good to Remember

- *Preterm baby:* Born after 28 completed weeks of pregnancy and before 37 completed weeks (between 196 to 259 days).
- *Term baby:* Born after 37 completed weeks and before 42 completed weeks (between 259 to 294 days). Normal gestation period is 40 weeks = 280 days.
- *Post-term baby (Postmaturity):* Born after 42 completed weeks of pregnancy (after 294 days).

Nutritional Needs for Infants on Artificial Feeds

- Energy requirement: Average 100 kcal per kg - approx. 150 mL per kg bodyweight each day
- Protein requirement:
  - 2 g/kg bodyweight during 1st six months
  - 1.5 g/kg for the next 6 months
- Carbohydrate requirement: 10 g/kg bodyweight/day
- Infant require feed approx. 6-8 times per day

Quantity per feed:

- Cow milk is the recommended milk in case breastfeed is not available
- Cow milk should be diluted during the first two months to decrease the solute load on the infant kidneys

Table 5: Nutritional needs of infants according to their weight

Particular	Weight–3 kg	Weight–4 kg	Weight–5 kg	Weight–6 kg
Cow milk (mL)	70	100	150	180
Water (mL)	20	20	0	0
Sugar (g)	5	10	10	10
Kcal	64	103	135	153
Protein	2.1	3.0	4.5	5.4

GROWTH AND DEVELOPMENT OF CHILD

Table 6: Height and weight increments according to age

Age	Height increments	Weight increments
1 year	25 cm	0-3 months-200 g/Week, 4-6 months -150 g/Week, 7-9 months -100 g/ Week, 10-12 month -50 g/Week
2 years	12 cm	2.5 kg
3 years	9 cm	2.0 kg
4 years	7 cm	2.0 kg
5 years	6 cm	2.0 kg

110 Good to Remember

Birthweight of the baby

3500–2500 g	Normal birthweight (Av = 2.7 to 2.9 kg)
2500–2000 g	LBW
2000–1000 g	Very low birthweight
<1000 g	Extremely LBW

Growth Charts

New WHO Child Growth Standards

- It was adopted by India in February 2009, for use in NRHM and ICDS.
- Separate growth charts are available for boys (Blue border) and girls (Pink border) below 5 years of age.
- Growth chart have a normal zone (Green zone), Undernutrition zone (below -2SD- Yellow) and severely underweight zone (below -3SD-Orange)
- Standards are available for Weight for Age, Height for Age, Weight for Height, BMI for Age and 6 motor development indicators
- Direction of growth curve is more important than position of dots.[Q]
- Flattening or fall of growth curve indicates growth failure *[Earliest sign of PEM [Q]]*

Uses of Growth Chart

- Growth monitoring. [Physical growth and development]
- Diagnostic tool to identify "high risk" children.
- Planning and policy making
- Educational tool: To educate and actively involve mother in growth monitoring of her child.

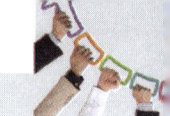

- Tool for action: Aids health worker to choose the required intervention and makes referral easier
- To evaluate effectiveness and impact of a program for improving child growth and development
- Teaching aid.

ICDS Growth Chart

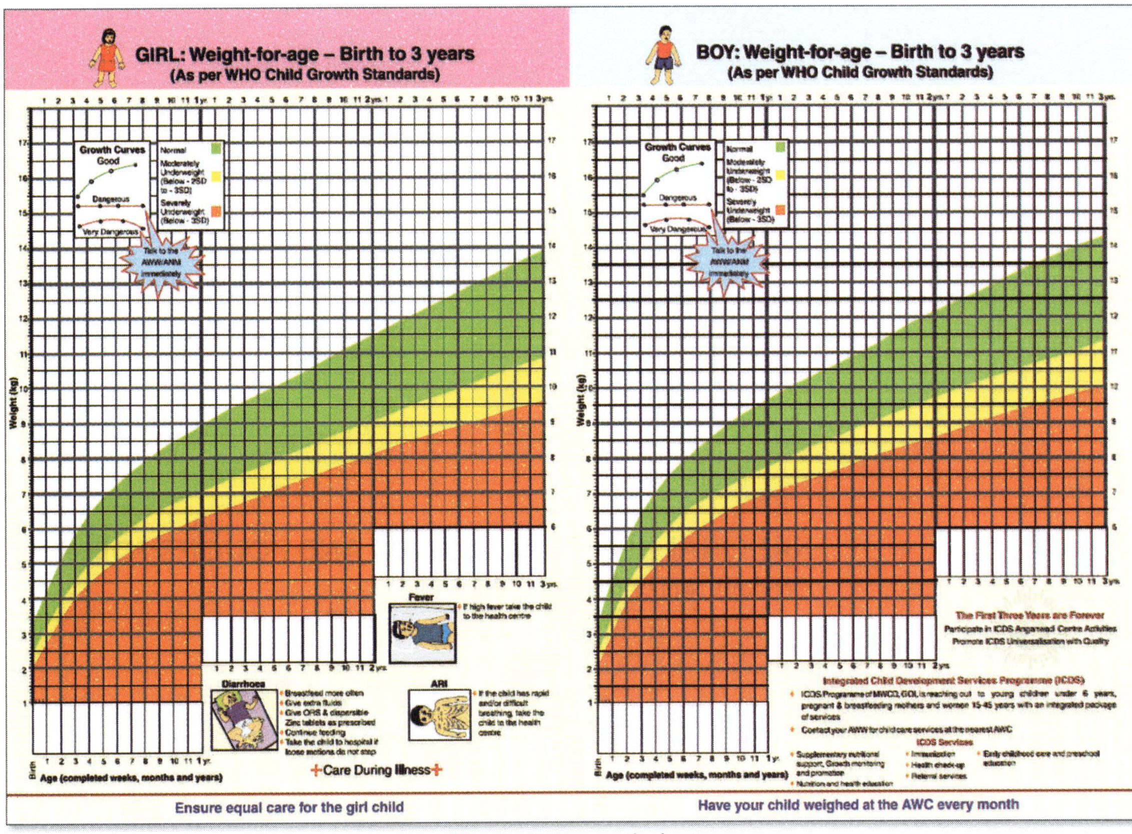

Fig. 4: ICDS growth chart

- The ICDS Growth chart has three curves
  - Upper reference curve
  - Lower reference curve -1 – at (-) 2 SD
  - Lower reference curve 2 – at (-) 3 SD

Malnutrition

Indicators of Malnutrition

- Stunting or Dwarfism (chronic malnutrition) → Low height for age[Q]
- Wasting or emaciation (acute malnutrition) → Low weight for height.[Q]
- Underweight → Low weight for age (Acute on chronic or mixed malnutrition).[Q]
- Birthweight of a healthy baby doubles by 5 month, trebles by 1 year and quadruples by 2 years.
- Weight should ideally be recorded once monthly (in infants), once every two month (2nd year) and once every three month (3rd -5th year)

Gomez classification:

- Based on weight for age
  - Mild malnutrition: 76-90% of expected weight
  - Moderate malnutrition: 61-75% of expected weight
  - Severe malnutrition: <60% of expected weight

The Gomez classification originally classifies based on Harvard (or Boston) standards, which eventually have been standardized according to the countries and ethnicity

Presently, most clinics are using the modified Gomez classification:

174 *High Yield Points*

- Weight gain <500 mg/month between birth and 3rd month indicates malnutrition.
- Mid Upper Arm Circumference (MUAC) → >13.5 cm (normal), 12.5-13.5 cm (moderate malnutrition), and <12.5 cm (Severe malnutrition).[Q]

105 *Must Remember*

Head and chest circumference

- Chest circumference overtakes head circumference by 9 months of age.[Q]
- It is delayed in severe malnutrition

Weight for height and MUAC are age independent indicators of nutritional status

Table 7: Modified Gomez classification

Nutritional status	Wt. as % age of the standard wt.
Normal	More than 80%
Grade 1	71–80%
Grade 2	61–70%
Grade 3	51–60%
Grade 4	≤50%

The **Waterlow's classification**: is used to determine the duration and severity of malnutrition based in two different indicators:

- Height for age
- Weight for height

The cut-off for the indicator W/H or H/A is at least 2 standard deviations below (-2SD) the median of the NCHS (WHO) growth standards.

Table 8: Waterlow's classification

H/A \ W/H	>m – 2SD	<m – 2SD
>m – 2SD	Normal	Wasted
<m – 2SD	Stunted	Wasted and stunted

where, m = Median, SD = Standard Deviation, H/A = Height for Age, W/H = Weight for Height

175 *High Yield Points*

GOBI Program (UNICEF)

- **G** = Growth promotion,
- **O** = ORT (Oral rehydration therapy)
- **B** = Breastfeeding
- **I** = Immunization.

GOBIFFF → GOBI was later extended with 3 F

- **F** = female fertility or family planning
- **F** = Female nutrition
- **F** = Female education (Litaracy)

NATIONAL HEALTH PROGRAMS AND POLICIES FOR INFANT AND CHILD CARE

Under-5 Clinic

- Offer a package of preventive, promotive, curative, referral and educational services to -under five children

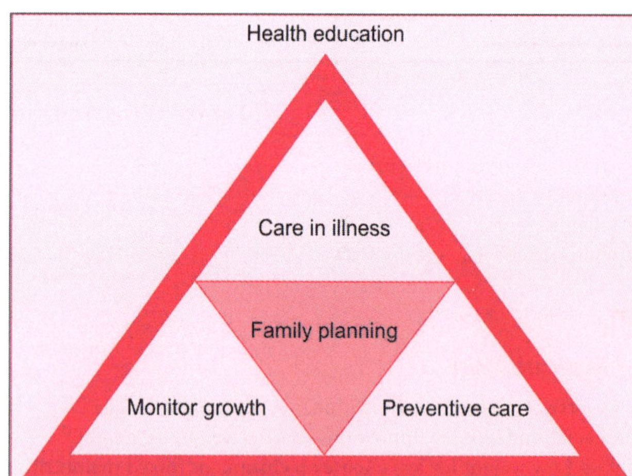

Fig. 5: Under five's clinic objectives

Objectives

- Care in illness – (Apex of the symbol)[Q]
- Diagnosis and treatment of illness (Physical/Mental/Congenital/Acquired) and disorders of growth/development
- X-ray and laboratory services
- Referral services

Preventive Care

- Immunization against Vaccine Preventable Diseases

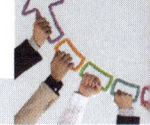

- Nutritional surveillance
- Health check-up every 3–6 months.
- Oral rehydration

Growth monitoring using Growth chart

Family planning: [Triangular area in center of symbol[Q]]

Health education: [Border around the symbol that touches all the other areas[Q]].

School Health Services

Health services to school children (5-15 years).

Juvenile Delinquency

- All deviations from normal behavior.
- An offence committed by a child, a boy below 16 years or a girl below 18 years of age.

RMNCH+A Strategy

- It is based on provision of comprehensive care through the 5 pillars, or thematic areas
  - Reproductive health
  - Maternal health
  - Neonatal health
  - Child health
  - Adolescent health
- **Guiding principles:** Equity, Universal Care, Entitlement, and Accountability.

The "plus" within the strategy focuses on:

- Including adolescence as a distinct life stage
- Linking maternal and child health to reproductive health, family planning, adolescent health, HIV, gender, and preconception and prenatal diagnostic techniques
- Linking home- and community-based services to facility-based care
- Ensuring linkages, referrals and counter-referrals between and among health facilities at primary (PHC), secondary (CHC), and tertiary levels (district hospital).

> 176 *High Yield Points*
>
> **Health Outcome Goals Established in the 12th Five Year Plan**
>
> - Reduction of Infant Mortality Rate (IMR) to 25 per 1,000 live births by 2017
> - Reduction in Maternal Mortality Ratio (MMR) to 100 per 100,000 live births by 2017
> - Reduction in Total Fertility Rate (TFR) to 2.1 by 2017

RMNCH+A 5 × 5 Matrix

- 5 × 5 Matrix for high impact RMNCH+A Interventions to be implemented with high coverage and high quality.

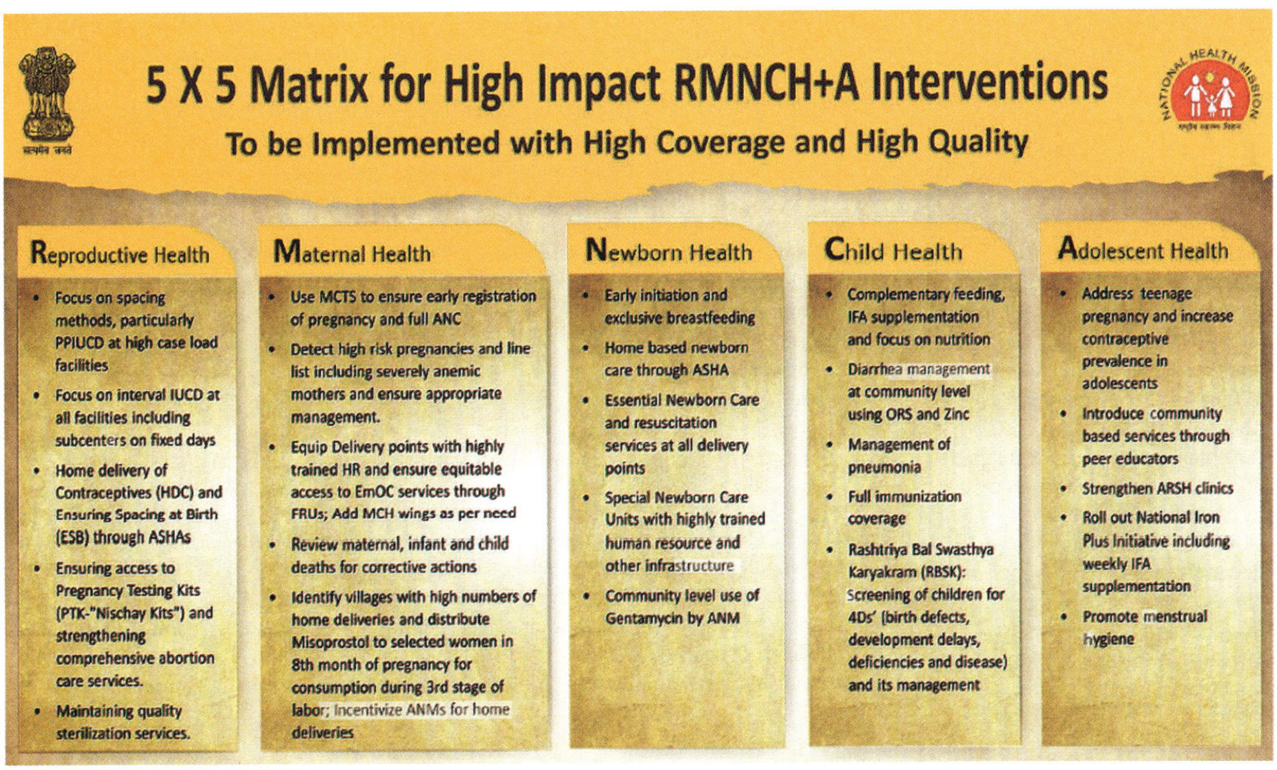

5 X 5 Matrix for High Impact RMNCH+A Interventions
To be Implemented with High Coverage and High Quality
Reproductive Health
Focus on spacing methods, particularly PPIUCD at high case load facilities
Focus on interval IUCD at all facilities including subcenters on fixed days
Home delivery of Contraceptives (HDC) and Ensuring Spacing at Birth (ESB) through ASHAs
Ensuring access to Pregnancy Testing Kits (PTK-"Nischay Kits") and strengthening comprehensive abortion care services.
Maintaining quality sterilization services.
Maternal Health
Use MCTS to ensure early registration of pregnancy and full ANC
Detect high risk pregnancies and line list including severely anemic mothers and ensure appropriate management.
Equip Delivery points with highly trained HR and ensure equitable access to EmOC services through FRUs; Add MCH wings as per need
Review maternal, infant and child deaths for corrective actions
Identify villages with high numbers of home deliveries and distribute Misoprostol to selected women in 8th month of pregnancy for consumption during 3rd stage of labor; Incentivize ANMs for home deliveries
Newborn Health
Early initiation and exclusive breastfeeding
Home based newborn care through ASHA
Essential Newborn Care and resuscitation services at all delivery points
Special Newborn Care Units with highly trained human resource and other infrastructure
Community level use of Gentamycin by ANM
Child Health
Complementary feeding, IFA supplementation and focus on nutrition
Diarrhea management at community level using ORS and Zinc
Management of pneumonia
Full immunization coverage
Rashtriya Bal Swasthya Karyakram (RBSK): Screening of children for 4Ds' (birth defects, development delays, deficiencies and disease) and its management
Adolescent Health
Address teenage pregnancy and increase contraceptive prevalence in adolescents
Introduce community based services through peer educators
Strengthen ARSH clinics
Roll out National Iron Plus Initiative including weekly IFA supplementation
Promote menstrual hygiene

Fig. 6: 5 × 5 Matrix for RMNCH + interventions

Table 9: Strengthening health system and cross cutting interventions

Health systems strengthening	Cross cutting interventions
▪ Case load based deployment of HR at all levels ▪ Ambulances, drugs, diagnostics, reproductive health commodities ▪ Health Education, demand promotion and behavior change communication ▪ Supportive supervision and use of data for monitoring and review, including scorecards based on HMIS ▪ Public grievances redressal mechanism; client satisfaction and patient safety through all round quality assurance	▪ Bring down out of pocket expenses by ensuring JSSK, RBSK and other free entitlements ▪ ANMs and Nurses to provide specialized and quality care to pregnant women and children ▪ Address social determinants of health through convergence ▪ Focus on un-served and underserved villages, urban slums and blocks ▪ Introduce difficult area and performance based incentives

Newborn and Child Care Services in Reproductive and Child Health (RCH) Program

Essential newborn care:
- Resuscitation of newborn with asphyxia
- Prevention of hypothermia
- Prevention of infection
- Referral of sick newborn
- IMNCI
  - Evidence based syndromic approach to management of common childhood illness, with rational effective and affordable use of drugs and diagnostic tools.
- Cover—Possible bacterial infection, Diarrhea/Dysentery, Jaundice, Malnutrition, ARI, Malaria, Measles, Ear infection and Anemia.[Q]
- Immunization:
  - Vaccination against 6 VPD
  - Hepatitis B to be introduced in phased manner.
  - Prevention and control of anemia and vitamin A deficiency.
- ORS → 150 packets 2 times a year are supplied to all subcenters as part of drug kit.
- Emphasis on Exclusive breastfeeding during first six months. Semisolids to start after 6 months.

RCH II → All First Referral Units (FRU) are to be made operational for providing emergency and essential obstetric care.
- Sub district level CHC, Postpartum center [PPC] and upgraded PHC are designated as FRU.
- The minimum services to be provided by a fully functional FRU are:
  - 24-hour delivery services including normal and assisted deliveries;
  - Emergency obstetric care including surgical interventions like cesarean sections.
  - New-born care and emergency care of sick children
- Full range of family planning services including laparoscopic services
- Safe abortion services
- Treatment of STI/RTI
- Blood storage facility
- Essential laboratory services
- Referral (transport) services

111 *Good to Remember*

To be able to perform the full range of FRU function, a health facility must have the following:
- Minimum bed strength of 20-30. Relaxed to 10-12 beds in difficult areas [North-East states and underserved areas of EAG states]
- A fully functional operation theater and labor room
- An area earmarked and equipped for newborn care in the labor room and in the ward
- A functional laboratory
- Blood storage facility
- 24-hour water supply and electricity supply
- Arrangements for waste disposal
- Ambulance facility

Integrated Management of Neonatal and Childhood Illness [IMNCI]

Integrated Management of Neonatal and Childhood Illness - Indian version of IMCI[Q]

The major highlights and differences are:
- Inclusion of 0-7 days age (Early neonatal period) in the program.[Q]
- National guidelines on malaria; anemia, vitamin A supplementation and immunization schedule are incorporated.
- Training of the health personnel begins with sick young infant's up to 2 months.

- Shorter duration of training (8 days) with proportion of training time devoted to sick young infant and sick child is almost equal[Q]
- Provision of home based care by AWW/ANM. It also has a basic health worker module.
- IMNCI aims to prevent morbidity and mortality from 5 major childhood conditions –
  - Diarrhea
  - ARI and ear problems (including Otitis media)
  - Malaria
  - Measles
  - Malnutrition

Child at the Health Facility is:

- Checked for danger signs:
  - Convulsions
  - Lethargy, unconsciousness, inability to drink or breastfeed and vomiting.
- Assessed for main symptoms
  - Cough/difficulty breathing
  - Diarrhea
  - Fever
  - Ear problems
- Assessed for nutrition and immunization status and potential feeding problems

Child is checked for other problems:

Table 10: Classified and treated according to color-coded treatment schedule

Pink	Urgent referral	Prereferral treatment is given
Yellow	Treatment at outpatient health facility	Local infection is treated, oral drugs are given, caretaker is advised and follow-up is done
Green	Home management	Caretaker is counseled on how to give oral drugs, treat local infections at home, continue feeding and when to return immediately and for follow up.

Home-based Newborn Care (HBNC)

Objectives

- To provide essential newborn care to all newborn and prevent complication
- Early identification and special care of preterm and low birthweight newborn
- Early identification sick newborn and appropriate care
- Support adoption of healthy practices by the family
- Build confidence of mother and develop skills in her to safeguard her health and of the newborn

ASHA has to make home visits to all newborns as per a schedule up to 42 days of life.

- ***Institutional delivery:*** 6 visits—Day 3, 7, 14, 21, 28, 42
- ***Home delivery***: 7 visits—Day 1, 3,7, 14, 21, 28, 42

Home visits include: Weighing the newborn, measuring temperature, ensuring warmth, supporting exclusive breastfeeding, identifying problems related to breastfeeding and counseling, promote handwashing, providing skin, cord and eye care, ensuring prompt identification of danger signs for mother and baby, health promotion and counseling on key messages on newborn care, discouraging unhealthy practices, counseling on family planning

ASHA is paid an incentive of ₹250 one time after 45 days of delivery subject to:

- Recording of weight of the newborn in mother and child protection card
- Ensuring BCG, 1st dose of OPV and DPT vaccination
- Registration of birth
- Both mother and newborn are safe at 42 days of the delivery

She is paid ₹50 for monthly follow-up visits of low birthweight babies (2 years) and newborns discharged from SNCU (1 year)

If a woman delivers at her maternal house and returns to her husband's house, 2 ASHAs undertake.

HBNC visits, HBNC incentive of ₹250 is divided (each ASHA who completes 3 visits or more is entitled to ₹125. If an ASHA undertakes <3 visits, she is not entitled to HBNC incentive.

Facility-based Newborn Care (FBNC)

Table 11: Facility based newborn care model and services offered

	Newborn care corner (at all delivery points)	Newborn stabilization units (FRUs/CHCs)	Special newborn care unit (Sub district/district)
Care at birth	▪ Resuscitation, provision of warmth, prevention of infection early initiation of breastfeeding, weighing the newborn	▪ Resuscitation, provision of warmth prevention of infection, early initiation of breastfeeding ▪ Weighing the newborn	▪ Resuscitation, provision of warmth, prevention of infection, early initiation of breastfeeding and weighing the newborn
Care of normal newborn	▪ Breastfeeding/feeding support	▪ Breastfeeding/feeding support	▪ Breastfeeding/feeding support
Care of sick newborn	▪ Identification and prompt referral of 'at risk' and 'sick' newborn	▪ Management of low birth weight infants ≥1800 g with no other complication ▪ Phototherapy for newborns with hyperbilirubinemia ▪ Management of newborn sepsis stabilization and referral of sick newborns and those with very low birth weight (rooming in) referral services	▪ Managing of low birth weight infants <1800 g ▪ Managing all sick newborns (except those requiring mechanical ventilation and major surgical interventions) ▪ Follow-up of all babies discharged from the unit and high risk newborns referral services

Source: Facility-based newborn care: Operational guidelines 2011, Ministry of Health and Family Welfare, Government of India

FBNC Infrastructure Requirements

Table 12: Requirements infrastructure for facility-based newborn care

	Newborn care corner (at all delivery points I PHCs, CHCs, and DHs)	Newborn stabilization corner (FRUs/CHCs)	Special newborn care unit (sub district/ district)
Beds	I	4	12–20
Area (sq. feet)	20–30 sq. feet	200 sq. feet	Min. 1200 sq. feet (100 sq. feet/extra bed)
Location	Within labor room and OT	Close to the labor room	Vicinity of labor room
Civil work	None or minimum	Power supply, water supply lighting, floor spaces and walls	Power supply, floor spaces, walls, water supply, lighting temperature
Equipment	Radiant warmer and resuscitation kits	Radiant warmers resuscitation kit, weighing scale, phototherapy unit	Same as NBSU, plus oxygen hoods, oxygen concentrator, syringe pump (desirable: irradiance meter, multi sign monitor, transport incubator)
Personnel			
Specialist	0	0	1
Doctor	1	1	3
Nurses	1	4	10
ANMs	1	–	–
NBCC: FRUs and DHs: Also set up NBCC in operation theaters, where cesarean sections are conducted **NBSU:** In addition 2 beds in the postnatal ward should to be dedicated for rooming in **SNCU:** 12 beds for catering to 3000 deliveries per year and 4 beds may be added for each 1,000 deliveries—additional space for step-down unit (at least 30% of SNCU beds, e.g. for 12 bedded unit, 4 beds for step down are required)			

Source: Facility-based newborn care: Operational guidelines 2011, Ministry of Health and Family Welfare, Government of India

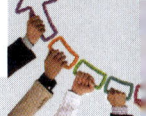

Criteria for Admission/Upgradation to SNCU

- Birth weight <1.8kg or >4.0 kg
- Perinatal asphyxia
- Apnea or gasping
- Refusal to feed
- Respiratory distress (Rate >60/min or grunt/retractions)
- Severe jaundice (appears <24 hrs/stains palms or soles/lasts >2 weeks)
- Hypothermia (<36.4°C) or hyperthermia (>37.5°C)
- Central cyanosis
- Shock (Cold periphery with CFT >3 sec and weak and fast pulse) coma, convulsion or encephalopathy
- Abdominal distension
- Diarrhea/Dysentery
- Bleeding
- Major malformations

Neonatal Resuscitation Guidelines

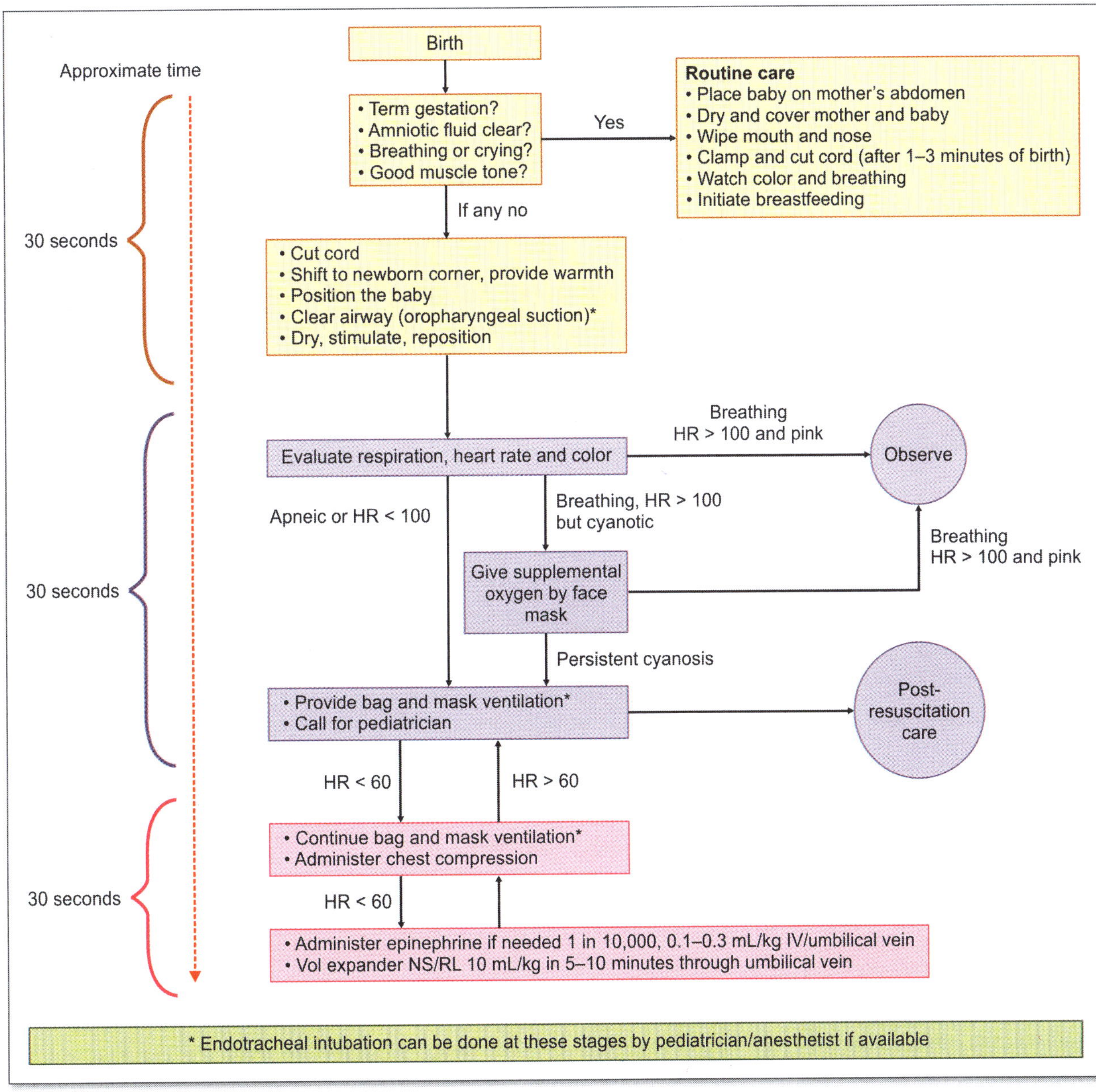

Fig. 7: Neonatal resuscitation guidelines

Baby-Friendly Hospital Initiative (BFHI)

Ten steps to successful breastfeeding promoted by WHO and UNICEF:

- A written breastfeeding policy routinely communicated to all health care staff in the hospital
- Trained health care staff
- All pregnant women are to be made aware about the benefits and management of breastfeeding
- Help mothers initiate breastfeeding within 1 hour of birth.[Q]
- Show mothers how to breastfeed and how to maintain lactation, even if separated from their infants.
- No food or drink other than breast milk to the infant, unless medically indicated
- "Rooming in" to be practiced (i.e. mothers and infants are kept together 24 hours a day).
- Breastfeeding on demand
- No pacifiers or artificial nipples to infants
- Establishment of breastfeeding support groups and refer mothers to them on discharge.

Mother's Absolute Affection (MAA)

- MAA programme was launched on 5th August 2016 to bring undiluted focus on:
  - Promotion of breastfeeding
  - Provision of counseling services for breastfeeding
  - Supporting breastfeeding through health systems.
- Major components of MAA
  - Community awareness generation
  - Strengthening interpersonal communication through ASHA
  - Skilled support for breastfeeding at delivery points in public health facilities
  - Monitoring and award/recognition.

Infant Milk Substitutes, Feeding Bottles and Infant Foods (Regulation of Production, Supply and Distribution) Act, 1992. (IMS Act)

106 **Must Remember**

Violation of the Act can lead to fine up to ₹5,000/- or imprisonment up to 3 years or both.

The Act prohibits:

- Advertising to public about commercial baby foods
- Free samples to mothers
- Promotion in hospitals
- Gifts or samples to health workers
- Financial inducement to any person to promote the sale of such foods
- Commission on sales to employees
- Payment of any kind to a health worker, working for the sales of such foods.

Intensified Diarrhea Control Fortnight (IDCF)

107 **Must Remember**

IDCF day in India:

Recent one was from 12 June to 24 June 2017.

- The Ministry of Health and Family Welfare has launched the Intensified Diarrhea Control Fortnight (IDCF) in order to intensify efforts to reduce child deaths due to diarrhea.
- ORS to be made available in the household when needed at the time of diarrhea.
- ORS corners to be operational at health facilities to demonstrate the way to prepare the ORS mixture.
- ORS corners to administer ORS and Zinc to children in need during diarrhea.

Important Component of the IDCF

- IEC activities to create awareness and generate demand
- Intensified community awareness campaigns on hygiene
- Promotion of ORS and Zinc therapy at the state, district and village levels
- **Target:** About 10 crore children <5 years of age across the country.

112 **Good to Remember**

India's first National Deworming Day took place on the 10th February 2015, during which the Indian Government publicly committed to deworming 140 million children nationwide.

National Deworming Day (NDD)-10 February and 10 August

- Largest ever single-day public health campaign in the world targeting children at risk of parasitic worm infection, through schools and Anganwadi centres.

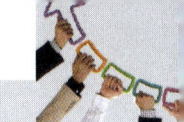

- **Target population:** Children in age group of 1-5 (8 crore) and 6-19 years (19 crore) respectively across 561 districts of the country
- Over 900,000 education and health workers administer tablet Albendazole.

Weekly Iron and Folic Acid Supplementation (WIFS)

- It is an evidence based program
- **Goal** is to break the inter-generational cycle of anemia
- **Objective**: To reduce the prevalence and severity of anemia in adolescent (10-19 years).
- **Target groups:** School going adolescent girls and boys (6th to 12th class) enrolled in government/government aided/municipal schools and out of school adolescent girls.

Intervention

- Administration of supervised weekly iron folic acid supplements of 100 mg elemental iron and 500 ug folic acid using a fixed day approach.
- Screening of target groups for moderate/severe anemia and referring these cases to an appropriate health facility.
- Biannual deworming (Albendazole 400 mg), six months apart, for control of helminthic infestation.
- Information and counseling for improving dietary intake and for taking actions for prevention of intestinal worm infestation.
- Convergence of key stake holder ministries *Ministry of Women and Child Development* and *Ministry of Human Resource Development* is an essential part of implantation plan of the WIFS program.
- **Key convergent areas include:** Joint program planning, capacity building of nodal service providers including Medical Officers, Anganwadi Worker (AWW) Staff Nurses, School teachers, monitoring and a comprehensive communication component.

Vitamin K Prophylaxis in Newborns

- Includes all newborns delivered in the facilities at all levels (both public and private)
- All newborns weighing >1000 g should be given 1 mg of vitamin K IM.
- For babies weighing less than 1000 g, a dose of 0.5 mg is recommended.

Site: Anterolateral aspect of the thigh, intramuscular injection

Time: Soon after delivery, ensuring skin-to-skin contact with mother and initiation of breastfeeding. Not later than 24 hours of birth.

Preparation to be used: Injection vitamin K1 (Phytonadione): [1 mg/1 mL and 1 mg/0.5 mL]

Rashtriya Bal Swasthya Karyakram (RBSK)

- Rashtriya bal swasthya karyakram for children age group 0-18 years. 0-6 years age group are specifically managed at District Early Intervention Center (DEIC) level while for 6-18 years age group, management of conditions is done through existing public health facilities. DEIC acts as referral linkages for both the age groups.
- 4 D's- Diseases, deficiencies, defects, delays

Table 13: Selected health conditions for child health screening and early intervention services

Defects at birth	Deficiencies
▪ Neural tube defect ▪ Down's syndrome ▪ Cleft lip and palate/cleft palate alone ▪ Talipes (club foot) ▪ Developmental dysplasia of the hip ▪ Congenital cataract ▪ Congenital deafness ▪ Congenital heart diseases ▪ Retinopathy of prematurity	▪ Anemia especially severe anemia ▪ Vitamin A deficiency (Bitot spot) ▪ Vitamin D deficiency (Rickets) ▪ Severe acute malnutrition ▪ Goiter

Contd...

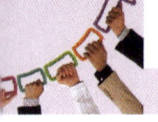

Diseases of childhood	Developmental delays and disabilities
▪ Skin conditions (scabies, fungal infection and eczema) ▪ Otitis media ▪ Rheumatic heart disease ▪ Reactive airway disease ▪ Dental conditions	▪ Vision impairment ▪ Hearing impairment ▪ Neuro-motor impairment ▪ Motor delay ▪ Cognitive delay ▪ Language delay
▪ Convulsive disorders	▪ Behaviour disorder (Autism) ▪ Learning disorder ▪ Attention deficit hyperactivity disorder
Congenital hypothyroidism, sickle cell anemia, Beta thalassemia (Optional)	

Target Group Covered

Category	Age group
Babies born at health facility and home	Birth to 6 weeks
Pre-school children in rural area and urban slums	6 weeks to 6 years
Children enrolled in classes 1st to 12th in Government and Government aided schools	6-18 years

RBSK stats (source: operational guidelines 2014)

- Birth defects — 64.3 infants/1000 LB
  - Cardiovascular — 7.9/1000
  - NTD — 4.7/1000
  - G6PD — 2.4/1000
  - Down's syndrome — 1.3/1000
- Deficiencies
  - Underweight — 43% among under 5 years
  - Anemia — 70% among under 5 years
- Diseases
  - Rheumatic heart disease — 1.5/1000 among school age group
  - Reactive airway disease — 4.7 percent

Rashtriya Kishor Swasthya Karyakram (RKSK)

Target group age groups 10–14 years and 15–19 years with universal coverage.

Objectives

Table 14: Objectives of target age group with universal coverage

Improve nutrition	▪ Reduce prevalence of malnutrition among adolescent girls and boys (including overweight/obesity) ▪ Reduce the prevalence of iron-deficiency anemia (IDA) among adolescent girls and boys
Enable sexual and reproductive health	▪ Improve knowledge, attitudes and behavior, in relation to SRH ▪ Reduce teenage pregnancies ▪ Improve birth preparedness, complication readiness and parenting support for adolescent parents
Enhance mental health	▪ Address mental health concerns of adolescents
Prevent injuries and violence	▪ Promote favorable attitudes for preventing injuries and violence (including GBV) among adolescents
Prevent substance	▪ Increase adolescents' awareness of the adverse effects and consequences of substance misuse
Address conditions for NCDs	▪ Promote behavior change in adolescents to prevent NCDs such as cancer, diabetes, cardiovascular diseases and strokes

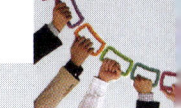

Table 15: Strategies under rashtriya kishore swasthya karyakram (RKSK)

Community based interventions	▪ Peer education (PE) ▪ Quarterly adolescent health day (AHD) ▪ Weekly iron and folic acid supplementation program (WIFS) ▪ Menstrual hygiene scheme (MHS)
Facility based interventions	▪ Strengthening of adolescent friendly health clinics (AFHC)
Convergence	▪ Within health and family welfare –FP, MH (including VHND), RBSK, NACP, National Mental Health Program, NCDs and IEC ▪ With other departments/schemes –WCD (ICD, KSY, BSY, SABLA), HRD (AEP, MDM), Youth affairs and sports (Adolescent Empowerment scheme), National service scheme, NYKS, NPYAD
Social and behavior change communication with focus on inter personal communication	

School Health

Vision:
- Decrease morbidity as goiter, malnutrition, dental caries

Strategy:
- Regular screening of school children by teacher

School norms:
- 40 students/classroom with area allocation >10 sq ft per child
- 1 urinal/60 students
- 1 latrine/100 students
- Minus type desk for students

School Vision Screening Program

- All children age 10–14 years are screened for refractive error by trained teachers once a year
- Child unable to read the 6/9 line with any eye is sent to ophthalmic assistant at community health center (CHC) for refraction test[Q]
- School teachers can identify 80–90% of children with low vision
- Child needing spectacle is provided free spectacles by opticians contracted by NPCB[Q]

SABLA—Rajiv Gandhi Scheme for Empowerment of Adolescent Girls

- Launched on 19th November 2010, targeted toward out of school girls
- Aim is to improve health and nutrition of adolescent girls and to equip them on family welfare, health, hygiene etc.
- 100% Central Government funded except for nutrition provision, that is shared by central and state government on 50:50 basis
- Implementation is by the state government and Anganwadi center is focal point for delivery of services
- It emphasizes on convergence of various schemes /program for adolescent girls (i.e. health, education, youth affair, PRI, Labor etc.)

Nutrition component Take home ration or Hot cooked food—11-14 years—Out of school girls and 14–18 years–All girls.

Non-nutrition component: It is for out of school girls provided 2-3 times per week.

- 11–14 years →
  - IFA, Health checkup and referral services
  - Nutrition and health education
  - Counseling/guidance on family welfare
  - Adolescent reproductive and sexual heal (ARSH)
  - Child care and home management
  - Life skill education and accessing public services.

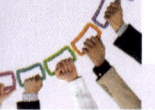

108 Must Remember

Health problems of school children:
- **Malnutrition,**
- **Infectious diseases**
- **Intestinal parasites**
- **Diseases of skin, eye and ear**
- **Dental caries.**

- 16-18 years →
  - Vocational training
  - For school going adolescent girls 11-18 years, non-nutritional component (except vocational training) is provided 2 times per month in school days and 4 times a month in vacations.

ACTS AND LEGISLATIONS FOR CHILDREN IN INDIA

Rights of Child – Under Indian Constitution

Universal children's Day – 14 November
Article 24: Prohibits employment of children below age 14 years in factories
Article 39: Prevents abuse of children of tender age
Article 45: Provides free and compulsory education for all children until 14 years of age

Juvenile Justice (Care and Protection of Children) Act 2000 (Amendment 2006)

- Defines juvenile/child as a person who has not completed 18 year of age.[Q]
- It addresses:
  - Juveniles in conflict with law [child alleged to have committed an offence]
  - Children in need of care and protection. [Neglected, abused, abandoned, victims of war or natural calamity]
  - Offences against children listed in the act are cognizable and punishable.

Children Act, 1960 India (Amended in 1977)

- Covers neglected and destitute, socially handicapped, uncontrollable, victimized and delinquent children
- It provides for their care, maintenance, welfare, training, education and rehabilitation.

Juvenile Justice (Care and Protection of Children) Act, 2015

- It came into force on 15 January 2016
- It replaces Indian juvenile delinquency law, Juvenile Justice (Care and Protection of Children) Act, 2000
- Juveniles in conflict with Law aged 16–18 years, involved in Heinous Offences, can be tried as adults.

National Commission for Protection of Child Rights, 2006

- Is statutory body notified under an Act of Parliament?
- It enquires into complaints and takes suo motu notice of matters relating to deprivation of child's rights and nonimplementation of laws providing for protection and development of children.

113 Good to Remember

- ***Trafficking*** refers to relocation of a child away from his family, community and support network. It results in isolation and vulnerability to exploitation.
- About 1.2 million children are affected by trafficking every year[Q]

The Protection of Children from Sexual Offences (POCSO) Act 2012

- It is applicable to the whole of India.
- It defines a child as any person below the age of 18 years and provides protection to all children <18 years from sexual abuse.
- It also intends to protect the child through all stages of judicial process and gives paramount importance to the principle of "best interest of the child".
- Offences against children covered under this Act
  - Penetrative and aggravated penetrative sexual assault
  - Sexual and aggravated sexual assault
  - Sexual harassment
  - Using a child for pornographic purposes
- It recognizes that the intent to commit an offence, even when unsuccessful needs to be penalized.
- The punishment for the attempt to commit is up to half the punishment prescribed for the commission of the offence.

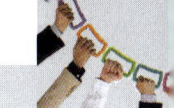

- It suggests that any person, who has an apprehension that an offence is likely to be committed or has knowledge that an offence has been committed, has a mandatory obligation to report the matter i.e. media personnel, staff of hotel/lodges, hospitals, clubs, studios, or photographic facilities.
- Failure to report attracts punishment with imprisonment of up to six months or fine or both.
- It is now mandatory for police to register an FIR in all cases of child abuse.
- A child's statement can be recorded even at the child's residence or a place of his choice and should be preferably done by a female police officer not below the rank of sub-inspector.
- The child's medical examination can be conducted even prior to registration of an FIR. The IO has to get the child medically examined in a government hospital or local hospital within 24 hours of receiving information about the offence with consent of the child or parent or a competent person whom the child trusts and in their presence.
- Child Welfare Committees (CWC) needs to be reported within 24 hours of recording the complaint.
- State Commissions for Protection of Child Rights (SCPCR) has been empowered with the responsibility of monitoring the implementation of the provisions of the POCSO Act 2012, to conduct inquiries and to report the activities undertaken under the POCSO Act 2012, in its annual report.
- Some child-friendly procedures envisaged:
  - At night no child to be detained in the police station.
  - The statement of the child to be recorded as spoken by the child.
  - Frequent breaks for the child during trial.
  - Child not to be called repeatedly to testify.
- For offences under this Act the burden of proof is shifted on the accused
- To prevent misuse, punishment has been provided for false complaints or false information with malicious intent.

Global Strategy for Women, Children and Adolescent Health (2016–2030)

Survive - End Preventable Deaths

- Reduce MMR <70 per 100,000 live births
- Reduce Neonatal Mortality Rate <12 per 1,000 live births in every country
- Reduce under-five mortality to 25 per 1,000 live births in every country
- End epidemics of HIV, TB, malaria, neglected tropical diseases and other communicable diseases
- Reduce by one third premature mortality from noncommunicable diseases and promote mental health and well-being

Thrive - Ensure Health and Well-Being

- End all forms of malnutrition and address the nutritional needs of children, adolescent girls, and pregnant and lactating women
- Ensure universal access to sexual and reproductive health-care services (including for family planning) and rights
- Ensure all girls and boys have access to good quality early childhood development
- Substantially reduce pollution-related deaths and illnesses
- Achieve universal health coverage, financial risk protection and access to quality essential services, medicines and vaccines.

Transform - Expand Enabling Environments

- Eradicate extreme poverty
- Ensure all girls and boys complete free, equitable and good-quality primary and secondary education
- Eliminate all harmful practices and all discrimination and violence against women and girls
- Achieve universal and equitable access to safe and affordable drinking water and to adequate and equitable sanitation and hygiene
- Enhance scientific research, upgrade technological capabilities and encourage innovation
- Provide legal identity for all, including birth registration
- Enhance the global partnership for sustainable development.

Image-Based Question

1. The logo depicted in figure represents:

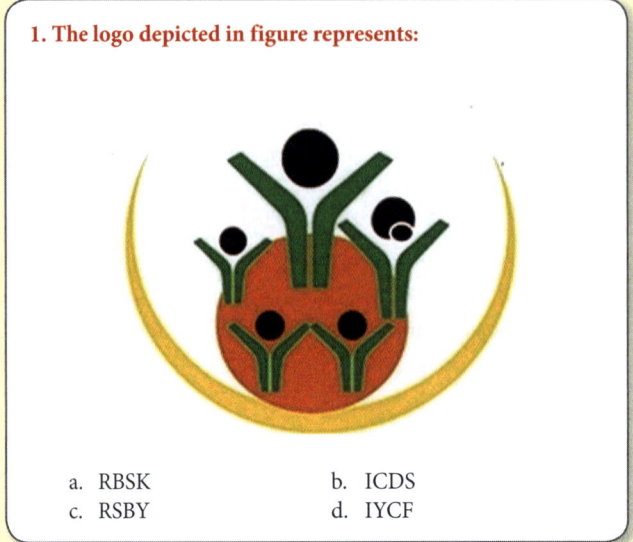

a. RBSK
b. ICDS
c. RSBY
d. IYCF

Answer of Image-Based Question

1. Ans. (c) RSBY

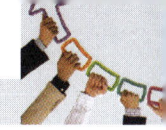

Multiple Choice Questions

1. **Total osmolarity of reduced osmolality ORS:**
   a. 215 mmol/L b. 220 mmol/L
   c. 225 mmol/L d. 245 mmol/L
2. **In a District hospital, the requirement of special newborn care beds is:** *(Recent Question 2017)*
   a. 30 b. 16
   c. 8 d. 4
3. **A newborn care corner (NBCC) is:**
   a. Newborn care center is a primary health center
   b. A space in the delivery room in any health facility
   c. Specialized Newborn units in referral centres
   d. A mobile unit with a team specialized in Newborn care
4. **IMNCI target group is:** *(Recent Question 2017)*
   a. Up to 5 years b. Up to 10 years
   c. Up to 15 years d. Up to 20 years
5. **Breastfeeding week is celebrated in:**
   a. 1st week of March b. 1st week of August
   c. 1st week of July d. 1st December

RCH

6. **Under IMNCI program in outpatient health facility all for the following are danger signs except:**
   a. Convulsions b. Difficult breathing
   c. Vomiting d. Lethargy
7. **Which of the following is not a part of RCH II strategy?**
   a. 24 × 7 PHC b. PCPNDT Act
   c. Blood storage facility d. Institutional delivery
8. **A newborn care corner (NBCC) is:**
   a. Newborn care center in a Primary Health Center
   b. A space in the delivery room in any health facility
   c. A mobile unit with a team specialized in Newborn care
   d. Specialized Newborn units in referral centres
9. **Newborn care corner is present in:**
   a. OPD b. NICU
   c. Labor room d. Ward side room
10. **Navjat Shishu Suraksha Karyakram (NSSK) is a program aimed to train health personnel in:**
    a. Basic Newborn care and resuscitation
    b. Emergency obstetric care
    c. Screening of newborn for hereditary services
    d. Examination of Newborn for congenital anomalies
11. **All of the following are true about a Special Newborn Care Unit except** *(Recent Question 2017)*
    a. To provides special care for sick newborns (all cares including assisted ventilation)
    b. Any facility with >3000 deliveries per year should have an SNCU
    c. Minimum recommended number of beds for SNCU at a district hospital is 12
    d. A 12 bedded unit requires 4 additional adult beds for step down
12. **Under HBNC, ASHA has to make how many numbers of home visits to a baby born in home delivery:**
    a. 3 b. 4
    c. 6 d. 7
13. **A patient treated at home is allotted which color code according to IMNCI coding:**
    a. Pink b. Red
    c. Green d. Yellow
14. **IMNCI target group is:** *(Recent Question 2017)*
    a. Up to 5 years b. Up to 10 years
    c. Up to 15 years d. Up to 20 years
15. **IMNCI differs from IMCI in all except:**
    a. Malaria and anemia are included
    b. 0–7 days infants are included
    c. Sick neonates are preferred over sick older children
    d. Treatment is aimed at more than one disease (condition) at a time

LOW BIRTHWEIGHT (LBW)

16. **Very pre-term babies are those born before/between**
    a. 32–37 weeks b. 28 – 32 weeks
    c. <28 weeks d. <24 weeks
17. **As per WHO low birthweight is defined as:**
    a. Birthweight less than 2.5 kg
    b. Birthweight <10th percentile
    c. Gestational age <34 weeks
    d. Gestational age <28 weeks
18. **Prevalence of low birthweight in India is:**
    a. 19% b. 28%
    c. 30% d. 32%
19. **By international agreement, low birthweight has been defined as a birthweight when measured within the first hour of life is:** *(Recent Question 2017)*
    a. Less than 2000 g
    b. Less than 2500 g
    c. Less than 2800 g
    d. Less than 3000 g
20. **Which of the following does not indicate poor nutrition in children?** *(Recent Question 2016)*
    a. Low birthweight
    b. Infection
    c. Hemoglobin <11 g%
    d. Malnutrition

PERINATAL MORTALITY

21. **An index of extent of pregnancy wastage is reflected by**
    a. Maternal mortality rate
    b. Perinatal mortality rate
    c. Neonatal mortality rate
    d. Infant mortality rate
22. **Perinatal mortality rate includes**
    a. Still births + early neonatal deaths per 1000 live births
    b. Still births + neonatal deaths per 1000 births
    c. Intrapartum deaths + early neonatal deaths per 1000 live births
    d. Intrapartum deaths + neonatal deaths per 1000 births

Ans.

1. d
2. b
3. b
4. a
5. b
6. b
7. b
8. b
9. c
10. a
11. a
12. d
13. c
14. a
15. c
16. b
17. a
18. a
19. b
20. a
21. b
22. a

Most Recent Questions of 2019-18 are given at the end of MCQs

23. As per WHO guidelines, for international comparisons or perinatal mortality rate, the denominator should be
a. Total live births weighing >1000 g
b. Live birth + late fetal death
c. Live birth + early fetal death
d. Baby born with birthweight >1500 g

24. Perinatal death is up to: *(Recent Question 2016)*
a. 24 hours postpartum
b. 1 week postpartum
c. 28 days postpartum
d. 1 month postpartum

25. Still birth rate is:
a. Death of a fetus weighing 1000 g or more in one year per 1000 total births
b. Death of a fetus weighing 1000 g or more in one year per 1000 live births
c. Death of a fetus weighing 1000 g or more in one year per 1000 still births
d. Any of the above

26. Best indicator of obstetric and neonatal care available around the time of birth is: *(Recent Question 2016)*
a. Infant mortality rate
b. Under 5 mortality rate
c. Still birth rate
d. Perinatal mortality rate

27. Denominator in perinatal mortality rate:
a. Mid-year population
b. Total pregnant women
c. Total live births
d. Total live births plus still births

28. Perinatal mortality includes all except:
a. Late fetal death
b. Early neonatal death
c. Late neonatal death
d. All are included

29. Perinatal mortality rate includes: *(Recent Question 2016)*
a. Deaths within first week of life
b. Abortions, stillbirths, deaths within first week of life
c. Deaths from 28 weeks to with first week of life
d. Deaths within one month of life

30. Extended definition of perinatal mortality includes crown heel length of:
a. >15 cm at birth
b. >25 cm at birth
c. >35 cm at birth
d. >45 cm at birth

31. Perinatal mortality includes death:
a. After 28 weeks of gestation
b. First 7 days after birth
c. Both
d. From period of viability

NEONATAL MORTALITY RATE

32. Most common cause of late neonatal mortality:
a. Acute respiratory infections
b. Diarrheal diseases
c. LBW and prematurity
d. Congenital anomalies

33. Most common cause(s) of early neonatal mortality:
a. Acute respiratory infections
b. Diarrheal disease
c. LBW and prematurity
d. Congenital anomalies

34. In a certain population, there were 4050 births in the last one year. There were 50 still births. 50 infants died within 7 days whereas 150 died in the late neonatal period. What is the neonatal mortality rate: *(Recent Question 2016)*
a. 12/1000
b. 50/1000
c. 38/1000
d. 62/1000

35. Leading cause of neonatal mortality in India is:
a. Infections
b. Birth asphyxia/trauma
c. Diarrhea
d. Prematurity and congenital malformation

36. Which of the following is the least likely cause of neonatal mortality in India: *(Recent Question 2016)*
a. Severe infections
b. Congenital malformations
c. Prematurity
d. Birth asphyxia

37. The current neonatal mortality is
a. 28 b. 30
c. 33 d. None

INFANT MORTALITY RATE

38. IMR for India is:
a. 27/1000 mid-year population
b. 34/1000 live births
c. 27/1000 live births
d. 34/1000 mid-year population

39. All the following features contribute to high risk babies, except: *(Recent Question 2016)*
a. Babies of working mother
b. Birth order of 4 or more
c. Artificial feeding
d. Weight less than 70% of the expected weight

40. Most important indicator of health status in a country and effectiveness of MCH services in particular:
a. Child survival index
b. Human development index
c. Infant mortality rate
d. Maternal mortality rate

41. In a community of 100,000 population 105 children were born in a year out of which 5 was still births, and 2 died within 6 months after birth and another 2 died within next six months. The IMR is: *(Recent Question 2016)*
a. 40 b. 90
c. 120 d. 150

42. Apart from IMR other important indicator for socio-economic health:
a. Maternal mortality rate
b. Perinatal mortality rate
c. Under-5 mortality rate
d. Neonatal mortality rate

Ans.

23. a
24. b
25. a
26. d
27. c
28. c
29. c
30. c
31. a
32. b
33. c
34. b
35. d
36. b
37. d
38. b
39. b
40. c
41. a
42. c

Most Recent Questions of 2019-18 are given at the end of MCQs

43. **Infant mortality rate is:**
a. Death of infants per 1000 pregnant women
b. Death of infants per 1000 births
c. Death of infants per 1000 live births
d. Death of infants per 1000 population

44. **Most common cause of infant mortality in India is:** *(Recent Question 2015)*
a. Low birthweight
b. Respiratory disease
c. Diarrheal disease
d. Congenital anomalies

45. **Most common cause of infant mortality in India is:**
a. LBW b. Injury
c. ARI d. Tetanus

46. **Infant mortality does not include:**
a. Early neonatal mortality
b. Perinatal mortality
c. Post neonatal mortality
d. Late neonatal mortality

CHILD MORTALITY

47. **Most common cause of 1–4 years mortality in developed countries:** *(Recent Question 2015)*
a. Accidents
b. Congenital anomalies
c. Diarrheal diseases
d. Child abuse

48. **Most common cause of death among under 5 years children worldwide is** *(Recent Question 2015)*
a. Congenital anomalies
b. Accidents
c. Diarrheal diseases
d. Pneumonia

49. **Most important cause of under 5 mortality in India:**
a. Respiratory infection b. Diarrhea
c. Prematurity d. Accidents

50. **In India a child is:** *(Recent Question 2015)*
a. <8 years b. <10 years
c. <14 years d. <18 years

51. **Health status of a child under 5 years of age will be adversely affected by all of the following except:**
a. Malnutrition
b. Low birthweight
c. Maternal Hb of 11 g%
d. Infections

52. **Child survival index is calculated by:**
a. 1000- IMR/10
b. IMR – 1000/10
c. 1000- U5MR /10
d. U5MR – 1000/10

GROWTH CHART

53. **Weight of a healthy baby usually doubles by**
a. 3 months b. 5 months
c. 9 months d. 1 year

54. **Height of a newborn doubles by the age of:**
a. 5 months b. 1 years
c. 4 years d. 5 years

55. **In the 'Milestones of Development' 'Listening' comes under which type of development?** *(Recent Question 2015)*
a. Language
b. Adaptive
c. Personal –Social
d. Motor

56. **Best indicator of long-term nutritional status in children is:**
a. Mid arm circumference b. Weight for height
c. Height for age d. Weight for age

57. **In Gomez's classification, a child with 88% of normal weight for age will be classified as having:**
a. Severe malnutrition
b. Moderate malnutrition
c. Mild malnutrition
d. No malnutrition

58. **Best indicator for growth measurement is**
a. Height b. Weight
c. Arm circumference d. None

59. **Types of growth charts used by Anganwadi workers for growth monitoring** *(Recent Question 2014)*
a. NCHS b. IAP
c. MGRS d. CDC

60. **Road to health card or the growth chart was first designed by**
a. Edwin Chadwick b. David Morley
c. Gopalan d. CE Winslow

61. **In WHO "Road to Heath" chart, upper and lower limit of represents**
a. 30 percentile for boys and 3 percentile for girls
b. 50 percentile for boys and 3 percentile for girls
c. 30 percentile for boys and 5 percentile for girls
d. 50 percentile for boys and 5 percentile for girls

62. **Feature of a healthy school environment is:** *[Recent Question 2015]*
a. Minus type desk
b. Light from front
c. 5 square feet area per student
d. A class room can accommodate up to 80 students

63. **Maximum recommended number of students in a school class room**
a. 30 b. 35
c. 40 d. 50

BREASTFEEDING

64. **Mother friendly childbirth initiative was launched in**
a. India b. Britain
c. Australia d. USA

65. **Breastfeeding week is celebrated in:**
a. 1st week of March b. 1st week of July
c. 1st week of August d. 1st December

66. **All are included in Kangaroo Mother care except:**
a. Skin to skin contact
b. Early discharge and follow up
c. Free nutritional supplements
d. Exclusive breastfeeding

67. **Compared with unprocessed cow's milk, human breast milk contains more of:**
a. Lipids b. Proteins
c. Minerals d. Carbohydrates

Ans.

43. c
44. a
45. a
46. b
47. a
48. d
49. c
50. d
51. c
52. c
53. b
54. c
55. a
56. c
57. c
58. b
59. c
60. b
61. b
62. a
63. c
64. d
65. c
66. c
67. d

68. In normal delivery, breastfeeding should be started within:
a. ½ hour of delivery
b. 1 hour of delivery
c. 4 hours of delivery
d. 6 hour of delivery

69. Calcium in human milk is (mg/100 g):
a. 200
b. 100
c. 70
d. 28

MISCELLANEOUS

70. Article 24 of our Constitution *(Recent Question 2014)*
a. Prohibits employment of children below the age of 14 in factories
b. Prevents abuse of children of tender age
c. Provides for free and compulsory education for all children until they complete the age of 14 years
d. Provides safety for women

71. Most common congenital anomaly in North India is: *(Recent Question 2014)*
a. Club foot
b. Cleft lip
c. Cleft palate
d. Neural tube defects

72. National plan of action for children (NPAC). Defines a child as a person up to the age of:
a. 12 years
b. 15 years
c. 16 years
d. 18 years

73. Components of Ujjwala Scheme include all of the following except: *(Recent Question 2014)*
a. Rescue
b. Remuneration
c. Repatriation
d. Rehabilitation

74. As per the UN Convention on Child Rights, children have the following rights?
1. Right to expression
2. Right to recreation
3. Right to name a nationality

Choose the correct answer from the responses given below:
a. 1 and 2
b. 2 and 3
c. 3 only
d. None

75. Which of the following states is used as Yardstick-of-health in India is *(Recent Question 2013)*
a. Tamil Nadu
b. Kerala
c. Uttar Pradesh
d. Gujarat

76. Ujjwala scheme is for the prevention of:
a. Child abuse
b. Child trafficking
c. Child labor
d. Child marriage

77. A place where children are kept in care of doctor and psychiatrist is: *(Recent Question 2013)*
a. Borstals
b. Foster home
c. Remand home
d. Orphanage

78. Which Of the following constitutional article is not related to children rights?
a. 39
b. 45
c. 46
d. 24

79. The 4 D's of Rashtriya Bal Swasthya Karyakram include all of the following except:
a. Deficiencies
b. Developmental delays
c. Diarrhoeal diseases
d. Defects at birth

Most Recent Questions (2019-2018)

80. Neonatal mortality rate target for 2030 *(JIPMER Nov 2018)*
a. 12
b. 15
c. 9
d. 25

81. Assessment of the developmental delay and early intervention is under which program: *(JIPMER Nov 2018)*
a. JSSK
b. JSY
c. Rashtriya Bal Swasthya Karyakram
d. Ayushman Bharat

82. To call it as fast breathing in a child of 6 months of age, the respiratory rate should be more than: *(Recent Question 2019)*
a. 40
b. 50
c. 60
d. 30

83. A 2-year-old boy with Vitamin A deficiency is treated with: *(Recent Question 2019)*
a. 1 lakh IU on days 0,1,6
b. 2 Lakh IU on days 0,1,6
c. 2 lakh IU on days 0,1,14
d. 1 lakh IU on days 0,1,14

84. Based on WHO criteria, severe acute malnutrition is defined as: *(Recent Question 2019)*
a. Weight for age < 2 standard deviation
b. Weight for age < 3 standard deviation
c. Weight for age < 1 standard deviation
d. Weight for height < 1 standard deviation

Ans.
68. b
69. d
70. a
71. d
72. d
73. b
74. b
75. b
76. b
77. c
78. c
79. c
80. c
81. c
82. b
83. c
84. b

Most Recent Questions of 2019-18 are given at the end of MCQs

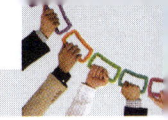

Answers with Explanations

1. Ans. (d) 245 mmol/L

Ref: K. Park, 24th ed. p 239

2. Ans. (b) 16

Ref: K. Park, 24th ed. p 478

The number of beds in SNCU should be 12–20

3. Ans. (b) A space in the delivery room in any...

Ref: K. Park, 24th ed. p 478

4. Ans. (a) Up to 5 years

Ref: K. Park, 24th ed. p 481

5. Ans. (b) 1st week of August

Ref: J Kishore, National Health Program of India., 11th ed. p 929

RCH

6. Ans. (b) Difficult breathing

Ref: K. Park, 24th ed. p 481

IMNCI is an initiative to prevent morbidity and mortality from 5 major childhood conditions – Diarrhea, ARI and ear problems (including Otitis media), Malaria, Measles and Malnutrition. It is Indian adaptation of IMCI

Refer to theory for Details

7. Ans. (b) PCPNDT Act

Ref: K. Park, 24th ed. p 474

RCH -2 Strategies Includes

- Essential obstetric care[Q]
- Emergency obstetric care
- Essential newborn care
- Prevention/ management of RTI/STI and AIDS
- Family planning and MTP services (at PHC)

Also Know...

New Initiatives were

- Training of MBBS doctors in life saving anesthetic skills for emergency care
- Setting up of blood storage facility at FRU

8. Ans (b) A space in the delivery room in...

Ref: K. Park, 24th ed. p 478

Newborn Care Corner (NBCC)

- NBCC is a space within the delivery room in any health facility where immediate care is provided to all newborns at birth.
- NBCC are 1 bedded facility attached to the labor room and Operation Theater (OT)
- It is MANDATORY for all health facilities where deliveries are conducted to have a NBCC

Also Know...

Special Newborn Care Units (SNCU)

- It is 12-20 bedded unit and requires 4 trained doctors and 10-12 nurses for round the clock services.
- Norm – Minimum one SNCU in each district

Newborn Stabilization Units (NBSUs)

- It is established at community health centres /FRUs.
- NBSU are 4 bedded units with trained doctors and nurses for stabilization of sick newborns.

9. Ans. (c) Labor room

Ref: K. Park, 24th ed. p 478

10. Ans. (a) Basic Newborn care and resuscitation

Ref: K. Park, 24th ed. p 481

Navjat Shishu Suraksha Karyakram (NSSK)

- It aims to train health personnel in basic newborn care and resuscitation at every delivery point
- It addresses issue like prevention of hypothermia/infection, early initiation of breastfeeding and basic newborn resuscitation.

11. Ans (a) To provides special care for sick...

Ref: K. Park, 24th ed. p 478

Special Newborn Care Unit (SNCU)

- It is a neonatal unit in the vicinity of labor room to provide special care for sick newborns.
- It provides all care except assisted ventilation and major surgery.
- Any facility with >3,000 deliveries per year should have an SNCU (District hospitals/ some sub-district hospitals)
- Minimum number of beds for an SNCU at a district hospital is 12. (For >3,000 deliveries per year, 4 beds should be added for each 1,000 additional deliveries).
- A 12 bedded unit will require 4 additional adult beds for the step down.

Level of health facility	Health Facility	For all newborns	Sick newborns
MCH Level 1	PHC & Sub Center	NBCC	Referral
MCH Level 2	CHC/FRU	NBCC	NBSU
MCH Level 3	District hospital	NBCC	SNCU

12. Ans. (d) 7

Ref: K. Park, 24th ed. p 480

Home-based Newborn Care (HBNC)

Refer to theory for Details

Latest Updates

ASHA has to make home visits to all newborns as per a schedule up to 42 days of life.

- Institutional delivery – 6 visits—Day 3, 7, 14, 21, 28, 42
- Home delivery: 7 visits—Day 1, 3, 7, 14, 21, 28, 42

13. Ans. (c) Green

Ref: K. Park, 24th ed. p 481

Green	Home management	Caretaker is counseled on how to give oral drugs, treat local infections at home, continue feeding and when to return immediately and for follow up.

14. Ans. (a) Up to 5 years

Ref: K. Park, 24th ed. p 481

IMNCI - Children are divided into 2 major categories.

- Young infants → Up to 2 months
- Children → 2 months to 5 years.

15. Ans. (c) Sick neonates are preferred over sick older children

Ref: K. Park, 24th ed. p 478

Also Know.......................

- **IMNCI PLUS** = Skilled care at birth + IMNCI with inpatient care + Immunization.

LOW BIRTHWEIGHT (LBW)

16. Ans. (b) 28 – 32 weeks

Ref: K. Park, 24th ed. p 571

On basis of gestational age babies are classified into 3 groups

- ***Preterm***: Born before 37 completed weeks of gestation (less than 259 days).
- Extreme preterm (<28 weeks), Very preterm (28 to <32 weeks), Moderate/ Late (32–37 weeks)
- ***Term***: Babies born between 37 completed weeks to less than 42 completed weeks (259 to 293 days) of gestation.
- ***Post-term***: Babies born at 42 completed weeks or thereafter (≥294 days of gestation).

Also Know.......................

- Preterm babies have normal intrauterine growth and can catch up growth by good neonatal care.
- Prematurity is the most important cause of neonatal and 2nd most common cause of under 5 death in children

Cause → Multiple birth, acute infections, hard physical work, hypertensive disorders of pregnancy etc.

Prevention comprises good prenatal screening/care, discouragement of adolescent pregnancy and treatment of hypertension

17. Ans. (a) Birthweight less than 2.5 kg

Ref: K. Park, 24th ed. p 570

As per WHO, birthweight of 2.5 kg is the demarcation line between LBW and mature baby.

- *In most parts of India, the mean birth-weight is between 2.7 kg and 2.9 kg.*[Q]

Also Know.......................

- ***Risk factors for LBW*** **are**: Malnutrition, Infection and Unregulated fertility

18. Ans. (a) 19%

Ref: K. Park, 24th ed. p 676

Prevalence of low birthweight among newborns in India is 18.6% *[Compared to about 4% in developed countries, 15% Globally]*

- LBW is associated with mental retardation, perinatal and infant mortality (1/3rd of all infant death) and morbidity, high cost of special and intensive care, socioeconomic underdevelopment.

Latest Updates

India contributes to 40% of global burden of LBW babies

Prevention of Low Birthweight

Direct Intervention	Indirect Intervention
▪ **Identify** women "at risk" and reduce risk ▪ **Increase food intake:** Supplementary feeding, IFA tablets, food fortification ▪ **Control infection:** Diagnosis and Treatment e.g., Malaria, UTI, CMV, toxoplasmosis, rubella and syphilis ▪ **Early detection and treatment of medical disorders:** Hypertension, toxemia and diabetes.	▪ Family planning, cessation of smoking, sanitation measures ▪ Improved health and nutrition of young girls ▪ Socio-economic upliftment ▪ Maternity leave with full wages and child benefits

Treatment: LBW babies (<2 kg or 2-2.5 kg) need intensive care (in NICU) comprising (a) Incubatory care, adjustment of temperature, humidity and oxygen supply. (b) **Feeding:** Breast milk (by nasal catheter) (c) Prevention of infection.

19. Ans. (b) Less than 2500 g

Ref: K. Park, 24th ed. p 570

By international agreement, low birthweight is *birthweight less than 2.5 kg, measured preferably within 1st hour of life*[Q]

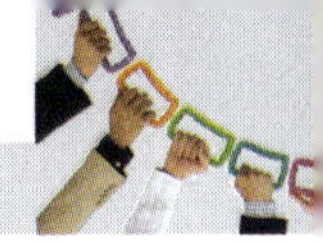

Also Know......................

- LBW is the single most important factor influencing child survival. IMR is 20 times higher in LBW babies.

20. Ans. (a) Low birthweight

Ref: K. Park, 24th ed. p 570

LBW is a consequence of maternal malnutrition, ill health and unregulated fertility.

Also Know......................

- ***Other adverse consequences of maternal malnutrition are*** -Maternal depletion, Anemia, Toxemias of pregnancy and Postpartum hemorrhage.

PERINATAL MORTALITY

21. Ans. (b) Perinatal mortality rate

Ref: K. Park, 24th ed. p 599

PMR is an indicator of

- Extent of pregnancy wastage
- Quality and Quantity of available health care for mother and child

Also Know......................

- **Perinatal mortality rate** is a yardstick for measurement of obstetric and pediatric care before and around time of birth[Q]

22. Ans. (a) Still births + early neonatal deaths per 1000 live births

Ref: K. Park, 24th ed. p 599

Perinatal mortality rate in country with poor vital records of stillbirth)

$$\frac{\text{Late fetal deaths } (\geq 28 \text{ weeks gestation or stillbirths}) + \text{Early neonatal death (1st week) in a year}}{\text{Live births in the same year}} \times 1000$$

PMR in countries with well-established vital records

$$\frac{\text{Late fetal deaths } (\geq 28 \text{ weeks gestation or stillbirths}) + \text{Early neonatal death (1st week) in a year}}{\text{Live births in the same year + Late fetal death in the same year}} \times 1000$$

23. Ans. (a) Total live births weighing >1000 g

Ref: K. Park, 24th ed. p 599

PMR (For International comparisons)[Q]

$$\frac{\text{Late fetal and early neonatal deaths weighing} > 1000 \text{ g at birth}}{\text{Total live births weighing more than 1000 g at birth}} \times 1000$$

24. Ans. (b) 1 week postpartum

Ref: K. Park, 24th ed. p 599

25. Ans. (a) Death of a fetus weighing 1000 g or more in one year per 1000 total births

Ref: K. Park, 24th ed. p 598

Still birth is death of a fetus weighing 1000 g (equivalent to 28 weeks of gestation) or more.[Q]

Still Birth Rate

$$\frac{\text{Fetal deaths weighing more than 1000 g in a year}}{\text{Total birth [Live + Still births] in same year]}} \times 1000$$

Prevention comprises early diagnosis and treatment of → Infections in pregnancy, High blood pressure and its complications, Rh incompatibility, diabetes and premature rupture of the membrane

26. Ans. (d) Perinatal mortality rate

Ref: K. Park, 24th ed. p 599

27. Ans. (c) Total live birth

Ref: K. Park, 24th ed. p 599

Denominator in Perinatal Mortality Rate is Total live births
Denominator in Still Birth Rate is Total birth [Live + Still births]

28. Ans. (c) Late neonatal death

Ref: K. Park, 24th ed. p 599

Perinatal deaths comprise *-Late fetal deaths (≥28 weeks gestation or stillbirths) + Early neonatal death (1st week) in a year*

29. Ans. (c) Deaths from 28 weeks to with first week of life

Ref: K. Park, 24th ed. p 599

30. Ans. (c) >35 cm at birth

Ref: K. Park, 24th ed. p 599 newborn

Refer to Notes

31. Ans. (a) After 28 weeks of gestation

Ref: K. Park, 24th ed. p 599

NEONATAL MORTALITY RATE

32. Ans. (b) Diarrheal diseases

Ref: K. Park, 24th ed. p 601

Causes of early neonatal mortality (1st week of life) → Prematurity, Congenital anomalies and asphyxia
Causes of late neonatal mortality (After 1st week of life) → Infection (Diarrhea, Tetanus)

33. Ans. (c) LBW and prematurity

Ref: K. Park, 24th ed. p 601

34. Ans. (b) 50/1000

Ref: K. Park, 24th ed. p 600

Neonatal Mortality Rate *(NMR) is number of neonatal deaths in a given year per 1000 live births in same year.*[Q]

$$\frac{\text{Number of deaths within 28 days of birth in a year}}{\text{Total live births in the same year}} \times 1000$$

Number of birth = 4050
Number of still birth = 50
Early neonatal death = 50
Late neonatal death = 150
Neonatal deaths = 200

So, Number of live birth = 4050 – 50 = 4000
NMR = [200/ 4000] × 1000 = 50/1000 live births

35. Ans. (d) Prematurity and congenital malformation

Ref: Park, 24th ed. p 602

Causes of Neonatal Mortality in India

- Low birthweight and prematurity (35%)
- Birth injury and asphyxia (20%)
- Acute respiratory infections (Pneumonia)- (16%)
- Sepsis (15%)
- Congenital anomalies (9%)
- Other (Hemolytic diseases of newborn, placental/cord anomalies, diarrhea, Tetanus)-5%

Also Know......................

- Neonatal mortality is higher in boys compared to girls

36. Ans. (b) Congenital malformations

Ref: Park, 24th ed. p 602

Latest Updates

In India, in first 7 days of life - About 75% of neonatal deaths and 50% of maternal deaths occur.

37. Ans. (d) None

Refer to theory

INFANT MORTALITY RATE

38. Ans. (b) 34/1000 live births

Refer to theory

39. Ans. (b) Birth order of 4 or more

Ref: K. Park, 24th ed. p 570

"At Risk" Infants Comprise

- Birthweight <2.5 kg
- Twins
- Birth order 5 or more
- Infants on Artificial feeding
- II and III degree malnutrition (Weight <70% of expected weight)
- Failure to gain weight in 3 successive months
- Child with PEM, Diarrhea
- Babies of working mother and Single parent

40. Ans. (c) Infant mortality rate

Ref: K. Park, 24th ed. p 603

Infant mortality rate is the number of infant deaths in a given area in a year per 1000 live births in the same area and year.

Also Know......................

- IMR is the most important indicator of health status of a community, level of living of people and effectiveness of MCH services.

41. Ans (a) 40

Ref: K. Park, 24th ed. p 603

$$\text{Infant mortality rate} = \frac{\text{Number of deaths of children less than 1 year of age in a year}}{\text{Number of live births in the same year}} \times 1000$$

The total births = 105
Still births = 5
So, the live births = 105 – 5 = 100

Number of deaths within 6 months = 2
Number of deaths within next 6 months = 2
Total infant (up to 1 year) deaths = 4

So, IMR = 4/100 * 1000 = 40 per thousand

42. Ans. (c) Under-5 mortality rate

Ref: K. Park, 23r d ed. p-571; 24th ed. p 608

Under-5 Mortality Rate or **Child Mortality Rate** is annual number of deaths in children under 5 years of age per 1000 live births.

It is considered by UNICEF as the best single indicator of social development and well-being.

43. Ans. (c) Death of infants per 1000 live births

Ref: K. Park, 24th ed. p 603

44. Ans. (a) Low birthweight

Ref: Park, 24th ed. p 605

Major cause of infant mortality in India are → Low Birthweight and prematurity (57%) followed by infections of respiratory tract (17%), diarrhea (4%) and congenital anomalies (5%).

Latest Updates

Developing country – LBW, infection and malnutrition are major cause whereas in developed country – Congenital anomaly is major cause.

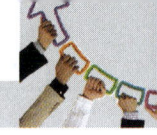

45. Ans. (a) LBW

Ref: Park, 24th ed. p 605

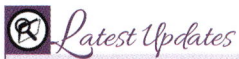

Latest Updates

IMR is a universally accepted indicator of health status of a community, level of living of people and effectiveness of MCH services[Q]

46. Ans. (b) Perinatal mortality

Ref: K. Park, 24th ed. p 598

CHILD MORTALITY

47. Ans. (a) Accidents

Ref: K. Park, 24th ed. p 608

1-4 Years Mortality Rate (Child Death Rate) is defined as number of deaths in children aged 1-4 years per 1000 children in the same age group in a given year.

Major causes of death in 1-4 years age group are:

- Developing countries – Diarrhea [***Most common***[Q]], Respiratory infections, Malnutrition; Infectious diseases (e.g., Measles, Whopping cough), Other febrile diseases, Accidents and Injuries.
- Developed countries: Accidents, congenital anomalies, malignant neoplasms, influenza and pneumonia

48. Ans. (d) Pneumonia

Ref: K. Park, 24th ed. p 609

Under-5 Mortality Rate or **Child Mortality Rate** is annual number of deaths in children under 5 years of age per 1000 live births.

Causes of Under 5 Mortality

- **Global** → Pneumonia (13%), Preterm birth complication (13%), Diarrhea (9%), Intrapartum complication (9%), Malaria (7%), Neonatal sepsis, Meningitis, Tetanus (6%)
- **India** → Prematurity (24%), Pneumonia (13%), Intrapartum complication (11%), Diarrhea (10%)

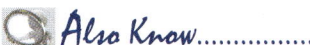

Also Know......................

- 50% of under 5 deaths globally are attributed to undernutrition.
- About 44% of all under 5 deaths occur in the neonatal period
- About one third of under 5 deaths are caused by infectious diseases
- India contributes 25% of under 5 deaths globally per year.

Every Newborn Action Plan – Targets

- *Ending preventable newborn deaths by 2035 (10 or fewer newborn deaths per 1000 live birth and continuous reduction in death and disability)*
- *Ending preventable still birth by 2035 (10 or fewer still birth per 1000 live birth and narrow gap in equity)*

49. Ans. (c) Prematurity

Ref: K. Park, 24th ed. p 611

50. Ans. (d) <18 years

Ref: K Park 24th ed. p 622

National Plan of Action for Children (NPAC), 2005 defines child as a person up to 18 years of age

51. Ans. (c) Maternal Hb of 11 g %

Ref: K. Park, 24th ed. p 609

Major health problems affecting children under 5 years of age are: LBW, Malnutrition, Infection, Parasite infestations, poisoning, accidents and behavioral problems

- *UNICEF considers Under 5 Mortality rate as single best indicator of social development and well-being*

52. Ans. (c) 1000- U5MR /10

Ref: K. Park, 24th ed. p 612

Child Survival Index (Child survival rate per 1000 births) is the proportion of children who survive till the age of 5 years

$$\textit{Child survival rate} = \frac{[1000 - U_5 MR]}{10} \times 1000$$

Latest Updates

Child survival rate of India = 94.7[Q]

GROWTH CHART

53. Ans. (b) 5 months

Ref: K. Park, 24th ed. p 578

Birthweight of a healthy baby doubles by 5 months, triples by 1 year and quadruples by 2 years

54. Ans. (c) 4 years

Ref: K. Park, 24th ed. p 579

Age	Height Increments
1 year	25 cm
2 years	12 cm
3 years	9 cm
4 years	7 cm
5 years	6 cm

- Average length of a healthy baby at birth is 50 cm. It doubles by 4 years of age.
- Boys gain about 20 cm and girls 16 cm in height during growth spurt. 98% of final height is achieved by 16.5 years in girls and 17.75 years in boys in India

55. Ans. (a) Language

Ref: K. Park, 24th ed. p 580

Age	Milestone	Type of development
6-8 weeks	Looks at mother and smiles	Socio personal
3 months	Head holding	Motor
4-5 months	Listening	Language
	Reach out for objects	Adaptive
	Recognizes mother	Socio personal
6-8 months	Sit with support	Motor
	Experimenting with noises	Language
	Hand to hand transfer of objects	Adaptive
	Enjoying Hide and Seek	Socio personal
9-10 months	Crawling	Motor
	Releases objects	Adaptive
	Stranger anxiety	Socio personal
10-11 months	Stand with support	Motor
	First words	Language
12-24 months	Walks wide base	Motor
18-21 months	Walks narrow base and starts to run	Motor
	Joins words	Language
	Begins to explore	Adaptive
24 months	Runs	Motor
	Forms short sentences	Language
	Dry by day	Socio personal

56. Ans. (c) Height for age

Ref: K. Park, 24th ed. p 578, 677

Indicators of Nutritional Status in Children

- ***Stunting or Dwarfism*** (chronic malnutrition) → Low height for age[Q]
- ***Wasting or emaciation*** (acute malnutrition) → Low weight for height.[Q]
- ***Underweight*** → Low weight for age.[Q]
- **MUAC** (Mid Upper Arm Circumference) → >13.5 cm (normal), 12.5–13.5 cm (moderate malnutrition), and <12.5 cm (Severe malnutrition).[Q]

Also Know......................

- Height for age is a stable measurement of growth and signals long-term nutritional status or chronic malnutrition.

57. Ans. (c) Mild malnutrition

Ref: K. Park, 23rd ed. p 640)

Gomez' classification is based on weight retardation (i.e. Weight for age (%) = (weight of the child/weight of a normal child of same age) × 100).

Weight for age (%)	Nutritional Status
90–110%	Normal
75–89% (1st Degree)	Mild malnutrition
60–74% (2nd Degree)	Moderate malnutrition
Under 60% (3rd Degree)	Severe malnutrition

Normal reference child is in the 50th centile of the Boston standards

Disadvantages

- Cut off point of 90% of reference is high
- It is difficult to know if the low weight is due to a sudden acute episode of malnutrition or chronic undernutrition

Also Know......................

- Gomez classification has a prognostic value for hospitalized children.

58. Ans. (b) Weight

Ref: K. Park, 24th ed. p 578

Measurement of weight and rate of weight gain are best parameters for assessing physical growth.

59. Ans. (c) MGRS

Ref: K. Park, 24th ed. p 581-82

In 2009, NRHM and ICDS, Government of India adopted WHO Child Growth Standards 2006, also known as MGRS (Multicenter Growth Reference Study Standards)

60. Ans. (b) David Morley

Ref: K. Park, 24th ed. p 580

Growth chart was designed by *David Morley*[Q] and modified afterwards by WHO.

61. Ans. (b) 50 percentile for boys and 3 percentile for girls

Ref: K. Park, 20th ed. 468

Earlier WHO growth chart based on NCHS (National Center for Health Statistics, USA) standards had 2 reference curves.

- Upper reference curve represented the median (50th percentile) for boys
- Lower reference curve represented the 3rd percentile for girls.

The space between the 2 growth curves was referred to as the "road-to-health". It could be used for both sexes

62. Ans. (a) Minus type desk

Ref: K Park, 24th ed. p 616

Minimum Standards for a Healthy School Environment in India:

- ***Location:*** It should be away from busy places i.e. cinema/ mall complex, factory, railway track, market places etc. and should have proper approach roads. It should be properly fenced and free from hazards
- ***Site:*** It should be on a high land, not subject to inundation or dampness and with proper drainage.
- **Area** - 10 acres of land for higher elementary and 5 acres for primary schools with an additional 1 acre per 100 students. Public park or Playground should be made available to students.
- ***Structure:*** Nursery and secondary schools should ideally be single storied. Exterior walls should be heat resistant and 10 inch (minimum) in thickness.
- ***Class Room*** should have attached verandas, A class *should not have more than 40 students (per capita space not be less than 10 sq. ft.*[Q])
- ***Furniture*** should be suited to age of students. Single desks (Minus Type) and chairs with proper back rests are recommended
- ***Doors and windows:*** *Combined door and window area should be at least 25% of floor space*[Q] and area of ventilators should not be less than 2% of floor area. Windows should be broad with the bottom sill, at a height of 2'-6" from the floor level and on different walls (for cross ventilation)
- ***Color***: Inside walls of the class room should be white
- ***Lighting:*** *Class rooms should have sufficient natural light (from left and not from the front).*
- ***Water supply*** should be independent, continuous, safe and potable water.
- ***Eating facilities:*** A separate room should be provided for midday meals and local vendors should not be allowed inside school premises.
- ***Lavatory:*** Separate for boys and girls. 1 *urinal for 60 students and 1 latrine for 100 students.*[Q]

63. Ans. (c) 40

Ref: K Park, 24th ed. p 616

BREASTFEEDING

64. Ans. (d) USA

Ref: http://www.motherfriendly.org/mfci/

Mother Friendly Childbirth Initiative was launched in the USA by CIMS (Coalition for Improving Maternity Services)

- **Mission:** To promote an evidence-based mother, baby and family-friendly model on prevention and wellness, with focus on substantially reducing costs.

Ten Steps of the Mother-Friendly Childbirth Initiative

- Unrestricted access to birth companion of choice, emotional and physical support (Skilled /Professional midwifery care)
- Accurate descriptive and statistical information to public on its practices/procedures for birth care
- Provide culturally competent care
- Freedom to walk, move about, assume positions of her choice during labor and birth for birthing woman. Lithotomy position is discouraged.
- Clearly defined policies and procedures for collaborating and consulting in perinatal period with other maternity services, including communicating with the original caregiver
- Linking the mother and baby to appropriate community resources, including prenatal and postdischarge follow-up and breastfeeding support.
- Educate staff on nondrug pain relief
- Encourage mothers/families (including sick or premature newborns/infants with congenital problems) to touch, hold, breastfeed, and care for their babies to the extent compatible with their conditions.
- Discourages nonreligious circumcision of the newborn.
- Strives to achieve WHO-UNICEF Ten Steps of BFHI to promote successful breastfeeding.

65. Ans. (c) 1st week of August

Ref: J Kishore, National Health Program of India., 11th ed. p-929

World Breastfeeding Week – 1st -7th August
Eye Donation Fortnight – 25th August-8th September
National Nutrition Week – 1st -7th September

66. Ans. (c) Free nutritional supplements

Ref: K Park, 23rd edition p-537, Suryakanta, Community Medicine Recent Advances, 3rd Ed. p-579; 24th ed. p 572

67. Ans. (d) Carbohydrate

Ref: K. Park, 24th ed. p 574

Advantages of Human Milk

- *Human milk has more lactose (useful for brain development) compared to other milks.*[Q]
- *Human milk has low protein content*[Q] [3 times less than cow's milk]
- *Human milk has more Cysteine, Taurine (essential for premature), Tryptophan and less Methionine* than cow's milk.
- *Breast milk is better digested and utilized for growth,* compared to cow's milk protein
- *Breast milk contains anti -infective proteins -Antibody (Ig A), Lysozyme, Lactoferein*
- *Human milk is rich in fats*[Q](35-50% of total energy value). Content of *essential PUFA- linoleic acid and alpha linoleic acid is higher compared to* cow's milk.
- *Human milk contains more vitamin A and C*[Q] than cow's milk. *Vitamin D in human milk is in water-soluble form.*[Q]
- *Human milk is rich in copper, selenium and cobalt* than cow's milk. Iron is less, but has *better bioavailability* [Coefficient of uptake of iron = 70%]
- *Human milk contains less sodium*[Q] than cow's milk (Avoids unnecessary strain on infant's kidneys.)

- *Human milk has less calcium*[Q] than cow's milk, *but it is much better absorbed* (High Calcium/Phosphorus ratio aids better *uptake of calcium* than cow's milk.)

Also Know......................

- **Artificial feeding** (Breast-milk substitutes) Indications → Failure of breast milk secretion, Severe illness or death of mother, emergency or HIV positive mother

68. Ans. (b) 1 hour of delivery

Ref: K. Park, 24th ed. p 568,573

Current Recommendation for Breastfeeding

- *Initiate breastfeeding within 1 hour of birth*
- *Exclusively breastfeeding* ***on demand*** *up to 6 months of age and continued to breast feed till 2 years of age.*[Q]
- *Timely initiation of complementary feeding after 6 months age.*[Q]
- *First milk* or *"colostrum"* rich in *anti-infective* protein, vitamin A and other nutrient must be fed.
- *Integrate IYCF practices with other national health programs*

69. Ans. (d) 28

Ref: K. Park, 24th ed. p 668

MISCELLANEOUS

70. Ans. (a) Prohibits employment of children below the age of 14 in factories

Ref: K Park 24th ed. p 586

Constitutional Provisions to Children

- ***Article 14***: Equality before the law or the equal protection of laws
- ***Article 15***: Nothing shall prevent the State from making any special provisions for women and children.
- ***Article 21 A***: State shall provide free and compulsory education to all children of the age of 6-14 years.
- ***Article 23***: Trafficking, beggary and other forms of forced labor are prohibited
- ***Article 24***: No child <14 year age shall be employed in any factory or mine or hazardous employment.

71. Ans. (d) Neural tube defects

Ref: K Park, 24th ed. p 613

Congenital anomaly is a "disease that is substantially determined before or during birth and is recognizable in early life"

- Incidence of congenital anomaly in infants is approximately 1 in 33.
- Most common congenital defects are heart defects, neural tube defects and downs syndrome.

Also Know......................

- In North India, Neural tube defects or spina bifida is most common
- In rest of India, musculoskeletal disorders e.g. clubfoot are most common.

Prevention

- Discouraging reproduction after the birth of a malformed child (Frequency of malformations in subsequent pregnancies is increased by about 10 times)
- Avoidance of pregnancy in conditions with high risk of malformations e.g., advanced maternal age, Down's syndrome
- Identification and removal of teratogens –
  - Drugs (e.g., Thalidomide, Steroid hormone, Folate antagonists, anticonvulsants)
  - Infective agents (e.g., rubella, CMV, herpes simplex virus, varicella zoster virus, Toxoplasma)
  - Physical agents (X-rays and irradiation)

72. Ans. (d) 18 years

Ref: K Park, 24th ed. p 622

National Plan of Action for Children (NPAC), 2005

NPAC, 2005 has 4 sections; *(i) Child Survival, (ii) Child Development (iii) Child Protection (iv) Child Participation*

Key Result Areas of the National Plan of Action for Children 2005

- Reducing Infant Mortality Rate [<30 per 1000 live birth by 2010], Child Mortality Rate [<31 per 1000 live births by 2010], Neonatal Mortality Rate [<18 per 1000 live births by 2010] and Maternal Mortality Rate.
- Reducing Malnutrition among children.
- Achieving 100% civil registration of births.
- Universalization of early childhood care and development and quality education.
- Complete abolition of female feticide, female infanticide and child marriage.
- Improving Water and Sanitation coverage both in rural and urban areas.
- Addressing and upholding the rights of children in difficult circumstances.
- Legal and social protection from all kinds of abuse exploitation and neglect.
- Complete abolition of child labor
- Monitoring, Review and Reform of policies, programs and laws
- Ensuring child participation and choice. Health insurance coverage for all children.

73. Ans. (b) Remuneration

Ref: K Park, 24th ed. p 625

5 Components of the **Ujjwala Scheme** *to combat child trafficking in India are:*

- Prevention
- Rescue of victims

- Rehabilitation of victims
- Reintegration of victims
- Repatriation of victims

74. Ans. (b) 2 and 3

Ref: K Park, 24th ed. p 587

As per the **United Nations declaration of Child Rights** adopted on 20th November 1959, Children have the following rights:

- Right to develop in an atmosphere of affection and security
- Right to enjoy social security
- Right to free education
- Right to free opportunity for play and recreation
- Right to name and nationality
- Right to special care
- Right to be among first to receive protection in time of disaster
- Right to learn to be useful member of society.
- Right to be brought up in a spirit of understanding. Tolerance.
- Right to enjoy these rights, regardless of race, color, sex, religion, national or social origin.

75. Ans. (b) Kerala

Ref: K Park, 24th ed. p 23

76. Ans. (b) Child trafficking

Ref: K. Park, 24th ed. p 625-66

Ujjwala Scheme was launched by the Ministry of Women and child development on 4th December 2007

- It is a *comprehensive scheme to combat child trafficking in India*
- It is being implemented by NGOs.

77. Ans. (c) Remand home

Ref: K. Park, 24th ed. p 626

Remand Home

- A child is put under care of doctors, psychiatrists, trained personnel to improve his/her mental and physical wellbeing
- Elementary schooling, Recreational activities (arts, crafts, games etc.) are conducted

Foster Home

- Rearing a child in more or less temporary placement away from natural family.
- A good foster home offers a child security, love and affection.

Orphanages

- Children who are homeless or could not be cared for by their parents are placed in orphanages.
- Warmth and intimacy of family life is lagging.

Borstal

- Difficult to handle boys >16 years of age or having done any misconduct are sent to Borstal usually for 3 years for training and reformation.
- It falls in between a certified school and an adult prison.
- Borstals come under the administration of State Inspector General of Prisons. It is not covered under the child act
- About 6 Borstals for boys are operational in India (None for girls).

78. Ans. (c) 46

- Article 24 – no child to be employed for age < 14 years
- Article 39: appropriate work for children of tender age, Health and strength of workers and tender age of children must not be abused.
- Article 45 – free primary and compulsory education for all children upto 14 years of age
- Article 46: The State shall promote, with special care, the education and economic interests of the weaker sections of the people, and, in particular of the Scheduled Castes and Scheduled Tribes, and shall protect them from social injustice and all forms of social exploitation hence, the child pertaining rights are safeguarded under article 24, 39 and 45 of the Indian Constitution

79. Ans. (c) Diarrhoeal diseases

Rashtriya Bal Swasthya Karyakram (RBSK) is an important initiative aiming at early identification and early intervention for children from birth to 18 years to cover 4 'D's viz. Defects at birth, Deficiencies, Diseases, Development delays including disability.

Health conditions to be screened Child Health Screening and Early Intervention Services under RBSK envisages to cover 30 selected health conditions for Screening, early detection and free management. States and UTs may also include diseases namely hypothyroidism, Sickle cell anaemia and Beta Thalassemia based on epidemiological situation and availability of testing and specialized support facilities within State and UTs.

Selected Health Conditions for Child Health Screening & Early Intervention Services

Defects at Birth	Deficiencies
▪ Neural tube defect	▪ Anaemia especially Severe anaemia
▪ Down's Syndrome	▪ Vitamin A deficiency (Bitot spot)
▪ Cleft Lip & Palate/Cleft palate alone #	▪ Vitamin D Deficiency, (Rickets)
▪ Talipes (club foot)	▪ Severe Acute Malnutrition
▪ Developmental dysplasia of the hip	▪ Goiter
▪ Congenital cataract	
▪ Congenital deafness	
▪ Congenital heart diseases	
▪ Retinopathy of Prematurity	

Contd...

Diseases of Childhood	Developmental delays and Disabilities
▪ Skin conditions (Scabies, fungal infection and Eczema)	▪ Vision Impairment
▪ Otitis Media	▪ Hearing Impairment
▪ Rheumatic heart disease	▪ Neuro-motor Impairment
▪ Reactive airway disease	▪ Motor delay
▪ 19.Dental conditions	▪ Cognitive delay
	▪ Language delay
Convulsive disorders	Behaviour disorder (Autism) Learning disorder Attention deficit hyperactivity disorder
Congenital hypothyroidism, sickle cell anemia, Beta thalassemia (Optional)	

80. Ans. (c) 9

Aiming for a single digit Neonatal mortality rate and still birth rate is the Target for INAP – India New Born Action Plan INAP:

India Newborn Action Plan (INAP)

- Together with NHM – will work for mother and child care
- Aims at attaining Single Digit Neonatal Mortality Rate by 2030, five years ahead of the global plan
- Prioritizes those babies that are born too soon, too small, or sick—as they account for majority of all newborn deaths
- Defines six pillars of interventions:
  - Pre-conception and antenatal care;
  - Care during labour and child birth;
  - Immediate newborn care;
  - Care of healthy newborn;
  - Care of small and sick newborn; and
  - Care beyond newborn survival

81. Ans. (c) Rashtriya Bal Swasthya Karyakram

RBSK – Rashtriya Bal swaasthya Karyakram
It evaluates for Defects, diseases, Deficiencies, Developmental delays

Defects at birth	Deficiencies
▪ Neural tube defect ▪ Down's syndrome ▪ Cleft lip and palate/cleft palate alone ▪ Talipes (club foot) ▪ Developmental dysplasia of the hip ▪ Congenital cataract ▪ Congenital deafness ▪ Congenital heart diseases ▪ Retinopathy of prematurity	▪ Anemia especially severe anemia ▪ Vitamin A deficiency (Bitot spot) ▪ Vitamin D deficiency, (Rickets) ▪ Severe acute malnutrition ▪ Goiter
Diseases of childhood	**Developmental delays and disabilities**
▪ Skin conditions (scabies, fungal infection and eczema) ▪ Otitis media ▪ Rheumatic heart disease ▪ Reactive airway disease ▪ Dental conditions	▪ Vision impairment ▪ Hearing impairment ▪ Neuro-motor impairment ▪ Motor delay ▪ Cognitive delay ▪ Language delay

Defects at birth	Deficiencies
▪ Neural tube defect ▪ Down's syndrome ▪ Cleft lip and palate/cleft palate alone ▪ Talipes (club foot) ▪ Developmental dysplasia of the hip ▪ Congenital cataract ▪ Congenital deafness ▪ Congenital heart diseases ▪ Retinopathy of prematurity	▪ Anemia especially severe anemia ▪ Vitamin A deficiency (Bitot spot) ▪ Vitamin D deficiency, (Rickets) ▪ Severe acute malnutrition ▪ Goiter
Diseases of childhood	**Developmental delays and disabilities**
▪ Skin conditions (scabies, fungal infection and eczema) ▪ Otitis media ▪ Rheumatic heart disease ▪ Reactive airway disease ▪ Dental conditions	▪ Vision impairment ▪ Hearing impairment ▪ Neuro-motor impairment ▪ Motor delay ▪ Cognitive delay ▪ Language delay
▪ Convulsive disorders	▪ Behaviour disorder (Autism) ▪ Learning disorder ▪ Attention deficit hyperactivity disorder
Congenital hypothyroidism, sickle cell anemia, Beta thalassemia (Optional)	

82. Ans. (b) 50

Ref: Park 25th Ed. Pg 183

Age and Criteria for Fast Breathing

- < 2 months – RR > 60 breaths/min
- 2 months – 12 months – RR > 50 breaths/min
- > 1 year – 5 years – RR > 40 breaths/min

83. Ans. (c) 2 lakh IU on days 0,1,14

Ref: Park 25th Ed. Pg 493

For all cases of SAM (Severe Acute Malnutrition)

- The dose for Vit A is:
  < 6 months 50,000 IU
  6-12 months or weight < 8kg 100,000 IU
  > 12 months 200,000 IU
- In case of clinical deficiency, same dose is given on day 1,2,14
- In children age > 12 moths, but weight < 8 kg – the dose is 100,000 IU Vit A irrespective of age

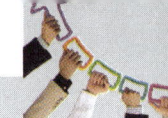

- Other micronutrients for SAM are:
  - Multivitamin (Vit B,C,D,E) supplement – twice the recommended dose
  - Folic acid – 5 mg on day 1, then 1mg / day
  - Elemental Iron: 3 mg/kg/day
  - Elemental zinc – 2 mg/kg/day
  - Copper: 0.3 mg/kg/day

84. Ans. (b) Weight for age < 3 standard deviation

Ref: Park 25th Ed. Pg 599

Criteria for malnourishment with the ICDS growth chart

- Undernutrition is below -2SD
- Severe underweight is below -3SD
- Flattening of curve initial sign of growth failure

Growth Chart for Girls

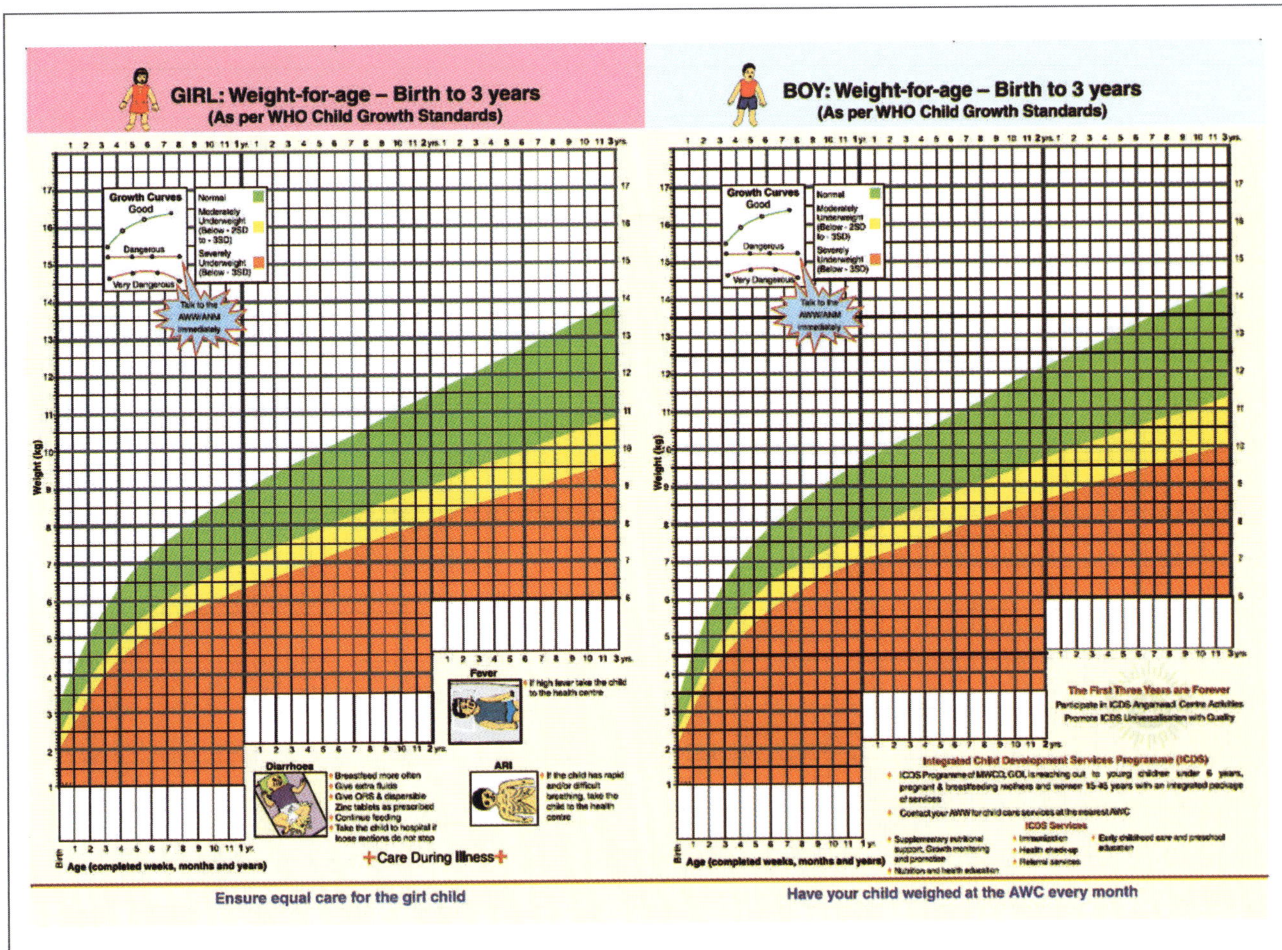

NOTES

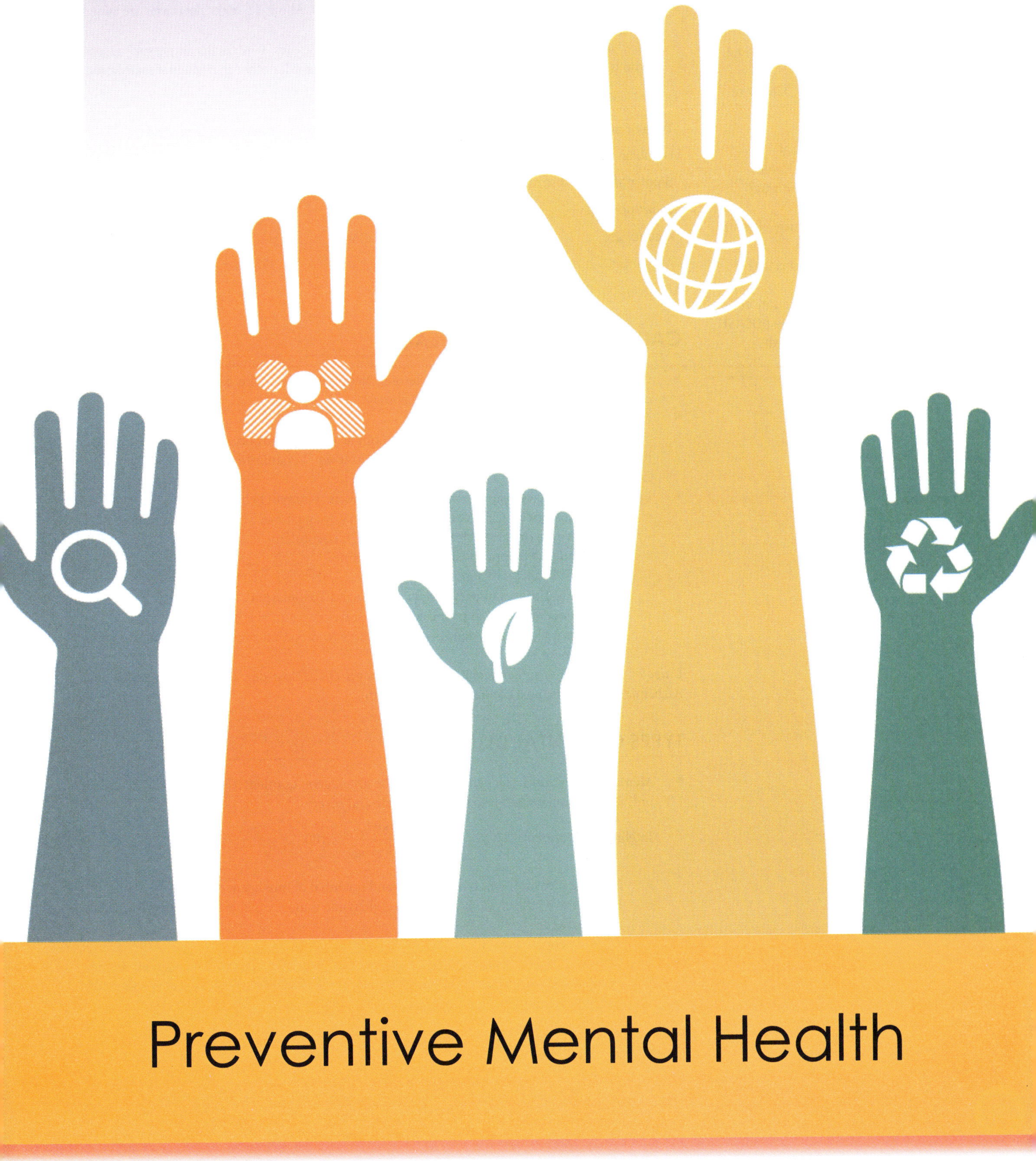

Preventive Mental Health

Chapter Outline

BURDEN OF MENTAL HEALTH DISORDERS

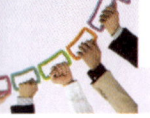

- Global point prevalence of neuropsychiatric disorder in adults (WHO, Global burden of disease, 2000) is 10%.
- Mental morbidity across India is about 18–20 per 1000. About 2.5 lakhs new cases are added per year.
- *Mental Health Act, 1987* (Applicable all over India) defines a "Mentally ill person" as one who is in need of treatment by reason of any mental disorder other than mental retardation.

Table 1: Statistical analysis of neuropsychiatric disorder

Type of neuropsychiatric disorder	DALY's lost	Deaths (in thousands)
Unipolar depressive disorder (Maximum)	64963	0
Bipolar affective disorder	13645	4
Schizophrenia	15686	17
Alcohol use	18469	84
Alzheimer & other dementia	12464	276 (Maximum)Q

Abbreviation: DALY, advisability-adjusted life year

CAUSES OF MENTAL ILL HEALTH

- *Organic condition*: Cerebral arteriosclerosis, Neoplasm, Metabolic/Neurological/Endocrine disease and Chronic diseases (i.e. TB, Leprosy)
- *Hereditary factors*: Family history
- *Sociopathological*: Worry, Anxieties, Emotional stress, Tension, Frustration, Unhappy marriage, Broken homes, Poverty, Industrialization, Urbanization, Population mobility, Economic insecurity, cruelty, rejection, neglect, etc.
- Environmental factors capable of producing abnormal human behavior are:
  - **Toxic substances:** Carbon disulfide, Mercury, Manganese, Tin, Lead compounds, etc.
  - **Psychotropic drugs:** Barbiturates, Alcohol, Griseofulvin
  - **Nutritional deficiency:** Thiamine, Pyridoxine.
  - **Minerals:** Iodine deficiency.
  - **Infectious diseases in pregnancy:** Rubella and Toxoplasma
  - **Trauma/accident:** Road traffic accidents and occupational accidents
  - **Radiation:** Nervous system is most sensitive to radiation during the period of neural development.

Unipolar Depressive Disorder result in the maximum DALY lost due to mental ill health and Alzheimer's disease is most common cause of death.

TYPES OF MENTAL DISORDERS

- **Mental Retardation**- Depending upon the intelligent quotient (IQ), mentally retarded individuals are classified into mild, moderate and severe.

$$\text{Intelligence Quotient}^{Q}\text{: (IQ)} = \frac{\text{Mental age}}{\text{Chronological age}} \times 100$$

  - IQ is the measurement of the quality and potential of intelligence
  - Higher the IQ the more "brilliant" the child is and is more capable of higher performance at school age Q.
  - 80 % of people have an IQ of or near 100Q.
  - IQ scores assume that intelligence distribution in general population follows normal distribution, with a mean of 100. (50% of general population achieve scores above 100 and 50% below).

WHO Classification of Mental Retardation[Q]

- Mild mental retardation: IQ—50–70
- Moderate mental retardation: IQ—35–49
- Severe mental retardation: IQ—20–34
- Profound mental retardation: IQ — <20

Table 2: Levels of intelligence and respective IQ range

Levels of intelligence[Q]	IQ Range
Idiot	0–24
Imbecile	25–49
Moron	50–69
Border line	70–79
Low normal	80–89
Normal	90–109
Superior	110–119
Very superior	120–139
Near genius	140 and over

- **Behavioral disorders:** Manifested as bed-wetting, tantrums, stealing, telling lies, aggressiveness, anti-social behavior, etc.
- **Mental diseases**: Acute (Delirium, Alcohol intoxication), chronic (Alzheimer's), psychotic disorders, neurotic disorders and personality disorders.
- Psychosomatic disorders.

Must Remember

DSM–V is the Diagnostic and Statistical Manual of Mental Disorders, 5th edition.

MAJOR CHANGES FROM DSM IV TO DSM V CLASSIFICATION

- Autism spectrum disorders—now encompasses various syndromes as - autism, Asperger's, childhood disintegrative disorder, and pervasive developmental disorder
- Childhood bipolar disorder is replaced with disruptive mood dysregulation disorder (DMDD)
- ADHD diagnostic criteria also includes adult onset ADHD
- Post-traumatic stress disorder (PTSD) includes child PTSD symptoms as arousal, avoidance, flashbacks, negative impacts on thought patterns and mood
- Dementia and the category of memory/learning difficulties called amnestic disorders have been subsumed into a new category—"Neurocognitive Disorders"
- "Mental retardation" are now classified as "intellectual disability"
- Diagnoses of somatization disorder, hypochondriasis, pain disorder, and undifferentiated somatoform disorder have been removed and somatoform disorders are now referred to as somatic symptom and related disorders

For further reading, it is recommended to look through the psychiatry subject textbooks or visit the web link: https://doi.org/10.1176/appi.books.9780890425596 - Diagnostic And Statistical Manual Of Mental Disorders, Fifth Edition.

SUBSTANCE ABUSE

Drugs commonly used:

- Amphetamine
  - These are similar to adrenaline and are used to treat medical conditions as obesity, depression and other behavioral disorders
  - Commonly known as "superman" drugs.
- Cocaine
  - Derived from coca plant and is used in medical practice as potent anesthetic.
  - Abuse of cocaine causes excitement, distorted awareness and hallucinations.
  - There is more psychological addiction (tiredness, increased sleep, irritability) than physical.

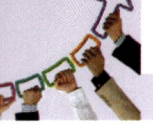

- Barbiturates
  - These medicines sedate.
  - Addiction causes severe physical and psychological dependence.
- Cannabis
  - Also known as bhang, hashish, charas, marijuana, ganja.
  - Most common symptom is development of dreamy state of altered consciousness, euphoria, relaxation and appreciation of colors and sounds.
  - Psychological dependence occurs.
- Heroine, codeine, morphine, methadone
  - These are narcotic analgesics.
  - Lead to severe psychological dependence.
  - Tolerance develops rapidly.
- Lysergic acid diethylamide (LSD)
  - Potent psychotogenic agent
  - Effect may start with a low dose of 20 mcg whereas 250 mcg can cause intense depersonalization.
  - Lethal dose is not known.
  - Intoxication symptoms include—intensification of color and auditory perception, body image distortion, illusions and fantasies.
  - Physical dependence is usually not seen.
- Alcohol
  - The maximum concentration in blood reaches after an hour of consumption.
  - Alcohol dependence in India is 20–30%.
- Tobacco
  - World No Tobacco Day is on May 31st each year.
  - Apart from documented side effects of tobacco, there is increased chances of osteoporosis and IUGR in pregnant female
- Volatile solvents
  - Glue, petrol, diethyl ether, correction fluids, paint, thinner, fevicol
  - Cause initial euphoria, followed by confusion, disorientation and ataxia.
- Caffeine
  - Most commonly used and abused substance worldwide.
  - Caffeine contents (per cup – 180 mL)
    - Brewed coffee 80–140 mg
    - Instant coffee 60–100 mg
    - Decaffeinated 1–6 mg
    - Tea 30–80 mg
    - Cola drink 30–65 mg
  - Symptoms of caffeinism occur when consumption increases more than 500 mg/day—anxiety, agitation, restless, insomnia
  - Withdrawal – headache, irritability, lethargy.

Must Remember

10th October is observed as the World Mental Health Day

Table 3: Substance abuse

Intoxication	HR	BP	RR	Temp	Pupils	Bowel sounds	Diaphoresis	Other
Sympathomimetic ▪ Epinephrine, cocaine, amphetamines	↑	↑	↑	↑	↑dilated	↑	↑	Nausea/vomiting, hallucinations, ↑reflexes
Anticholinergic ▪ Antipsychotics (TCA), oxybutynin, ipratropium	↑	↑		↑	↑dilated	↓	↓	Mad as a hatter, red as a beet, blind as a bat, hot as a hare, dry as a bone
Cholinergics ▪ ACh receptor antagonist					↓ pinpoint	↑	↑	
Sedatives ▪ Benzo, antihistamines	↓	↓	↓	↓		↓	↓	Nystagmus, ataxia
Opioids	↓	↓	↓	↓	↓ pinpoint	↓	↓	

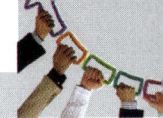

PREVENTION AND CONTROL

Primary Prevention

- Use of iodized salt to prevent cretinism and mental retardation
- Industrial safety measures to prevent chemical intoxication
- Prevention of infections like syphilis, rubella, encephalitis and HIV
- Prevention of nutritional deficiencies like pellagra, beriberi, and anemia
- Promoting security, love and affection among children
- Personality development

Secondary Prevention

- Early diagnosis and treatment of mental illness with specific drug therapy, general measures and electroconvulsive therapy.

Tertiary Prevention

- *Day care Program:* helping the patients in learning social skills for living
- *Half way home:* comes under social rehabilitation. It serves as a short stay homes between hospital and patient's family. Patients with unequivocal recovery or those who need support or guidance and not active medical or nursing care are admitted here for brief periods (few weeks to months).
- *Community psychiatry:* To have psychiatry beds as a part of a general hospital under the care of department of psychiatry. Earlier policy to set up mental asylum is no longer followed
- *Rehabilitation in Family:* encouraging the home care for the mentally ill persons in the comfort of his/her own family members. Families are motivated to accept the patient and aid in rehabilitation.

177 *High Yield Points*

Prevention level	Based on	Objective
Primary prevention	Done On community basis	Improving social, emotional and physical well-being of people
Secondary prevention	Via ▪ Screening programs ▪ Family based health services ▪ Individual counseling methods	Early diagnosis of mental illness and social/emotional disturbances
Tertiary prevention	Works at all levels	To reduce duration or the impact of mental illness at family/community level.

INITIATIVES ON MENTAL HEALTH

World Health Day- 7 April *(Theme for 2017: "Depression: let's talk")*

- Priority: Adolescents and young adults, women of childbearing age (particularly following childbirth), and Older adults (over 60s).
- Women are more affected by depression than men.
- By 2020, depression will be the second leading disability worldwide.
- 5% of India's population suffers from common mental disorders, such as depression and anxiety.
- WHO recommends interpersonal therapy (IPT) as a possible first line treatment for depression.

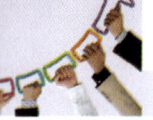

WHO's Mental Health Gap Action Program (MHGAP)

- It is scaling up of services for mental, neurological and substance use disorders, especially in low- and middle- income countries
- It focuses on a limited number of conditions and includes both pharmacological and non-pharmacological first-line treatment options for depression, including interpersonal therapy (IPT).
- Problem management plus (PM+) is a scalable psychological intervention called for adults impaired by distress in communities who are exposed to adversity.

WHO's Comprehensive Mental Health Action Plan 2013–2020

Goal is to *promote mental well-being*, *prevent mental disorders*, provide care, enhance recovery, promote human rights and reduce the mortality, morbidity and disability for persons with mental disorders.

Objectives

- Strengthen effective leadership and governance for mental health
- Provide comprehensive, integrated and responsive mental health and social care services in community-based settings
- Implement strategies for promotion and prevention in mental health
- Strengthen information systems, evidence and research for mental health

The Rights of Persons with Disabilities Bill - 2016

- It replaces the existing Persons with Disabilities (PWD) Act, 1995
- Types of disabilities have been increased from existing 7 to 21
- Speech and Language Disability and Specific Learning Disability have been added
- Acid Attack Victims have been included
- Dwarfism, muscular dystrophy is indicated as separate class of specified disability
- 3 Blood disorders: Thalassemia, Hemophilia and Sickle Cell disease are included
- Central Govt. has power to add more types of disabilities, notify any other category of specified disability
- *Responsibility*: Governments have to take effective measures to ensure that the persons with disabilities enjoy their rights equally with others
- Additional benefits: Reservation in higher education, government jobs (4%), reservation in allocation of land, poverty alleviation schemes, etc. have been provided for persons with benchmark disabilities and those with high support needs.
- Every child with benchmark disability between 6–18 years has the right to free education
- Government funded/recognized educational institutions will have to provide inclusive education to the children with disabilities
- Prime Minister's Accessible India Campaign: Stress has been given to ensure accessibility in public buildings (Govt. and Private) in a prescribed timeframe.
- Bill provides for grant of guardianship by District Court under which there will be joint decision making between the guardian and the persons with disabilities
- Central and State Advisory Boards on Disability are to be set up to serve as apex policy making bodies at the Central and State level
- Chief Commissioner of Persons with Disabilities is now to be assisted by 2 Commissioners and an Advisory Committee of not more than 11 members drawn from experts in various disabilities
- State Commissioners of Disabilities, is to be assisted by an Advisory Committee comprising of not more than 5 members drawn from experts in various disabilities
- Bill provides for penalties for offences committed against persons with disabilities and also violation of the provisions of the new law
- Special Courts will be designated in each district to handle cases concerning violation of rights of PWDs.

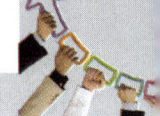

Indian Disability Evaluation and Assessment Scale (IDEAS)

- It is an assessment tool for measuring and certifying Disability developed by Committee of Indian Psychiatric Society in 2002.
- It is to be used only on out patients and those living in the community. Not appropriate for in- patients
- Trained social workers, psychologist or occupational therapists can administer IDEAS
- Only the Psychiatrist can do the diagnosis and certification. Frequency of re-certification is every 2 years.

Items

- Self -care: Body hygiene, grooming, bathing, toileting, eating, etc.
- Interpersonal Activities / Social Relationship
- Communication and Understanding
- Work performance in Employment/ House work/ Education
- Economic productivity and Absenteeism from job
- Scores for Each Item: (Total Disability score - is sum of scores in all 4 items ranges from 0-20).
  - 0 – No Disability, 1 - Mild Disability, 2 -Moderate Disability, 3 – Severe Disability, 4 – Profound Disability
  - Total Duration of illness should be at least 2 years. For scoring, number of months the patient was symptomatic in the last two years (MI2Y) is determined
  - MI2Y < 6 months → Add a score of 1, MI2Y = 7-12 month → add 2 MI2Y = 13-18 month → add 3, MI2Y > 18 month → add 4.
  - Total disability score + MI 2Y score = Global Disability Score (range 1-20).

Global Disability Score

- Score of 0 → No disability = 0%
- 1-7 → Mild Disability ≤ 40%,
- 8 and above (8-13 moderate disability; 14-19 Severe Disability; 20 Profound Disability) > 40%
- Patients with Schizophrenia, Bipolar Disorder, Dementia and Obsessive Compulsive Disorder only (as per ICD or DSM criteria) are eligible for disability benefits.

National Mental Health Program (1982)

- Integrate mental health services with Primary health care set up
- Utilise existing infrastructure of health services and deliver minimum mental health services
- Link mental health services with community development programs like ICDS and education.

Organization

- Tertiary care institutions:
  - These are National Institute of Mental Health and Neurosciences (NIMHANS), Bengaluru,
  - Central Institute of Psychiatry, Ranchi, and
  - Institute of Human Behavior and Allied Sciences, New Delhi.
- Mental Hospitals
- Supportive organizations:
  - Central Mental Health Authority oversees the implementation of Mental Health Act, 1987, which protects the mentally sick patients from stigmatization and discrimination,
  - The National Human Rights Commission monitors the structure and functions of the mental health hospitals in states.

> Nodal ministry for implementation of program of deaddiction and substance abuse– Ministry of Social Justice and Empowerment.

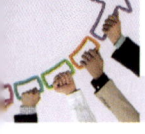

Multiple Choice Questions

1. **An IQ of 55 comes in which category:** *(Recent Question 2015)*
   a. Profound b. Mild
   c. Moderate d. Idiot

INTERNATIONAL CLASSIFICATION OF DISEASE

2. **In ICD-10 Mental and behavioral disorders are classified in chapter:** *(Recent Question 2015)*
   a. I b. III
   c. V d. X

MISCELLANEOUS

3. **National Mental Health Policy of India was launched in:**
   a. 1982 b. 1987
   c. 1994 d. 2014
4. **Not included in National Mental Health Programme 1982:**
   a. Minimum mental health care for all
   b. Application of mental health knowledge in general health care
   c. Human rights of mentally ill
   d. Community participation in mental health service development
5. **True about National mental health programme of India is:** *(Recent Question 2014)*
   a. Excludes OPD services
   b. Excludes neurological disorders
   c. Launched in 1982
   d. Excludes community participation and self help
6. **Mental health act was passed in:** *(Recent Question 2015)*
   a. 1982 b. 1987
   c. 1971 d. 1950
7. **Which of the following is NOT included in Mental Health Care Act 2011:**
   a. Promotion of mental health and prevention of mental illness
   b. Integration of mental health care system into all levels of health care
   c. Fundamental rights of mentally retarded
   d. Minimum mental health care for all
8. **Recent mental health act in India is designated as:**
   a. The Mental Health Act
   b. The Mental Health Care Act
   c. The Mental Health Care and Rehabilitation Act
   d. The Mental Health Treatment and Rehabilitation Act
9. **Mental health programme was started in:** *(Recent Question 2014)*
   a. 1982
   b. 1987
   c. 1990
   d. 1995
10. **The reading and writing skills of a moderately mental retarded child is:** *(Recent Question 2013)*
    a. Reasonable
    b. Minimal
    c. Basic
    d. None of the above
11. **Which of the following is true for mental retardation**
    a. Profound mental retardation is IQ < 40
    b. Mild mental retardation is IQ < 90
    c. Moron is in range of IQ 50-70
    d. Mental retardation is now classified as intellectual disability
12. **Which of the following score is/are not included in mild mental retardation?** *(PGI Pattern)*
    a. 85
    b. 50
    c. 45
    d. 75
    e. 65
13. **IDEAS scoring scale is used for:**
    a. Out-patient assessment for mental/intellectual disability
    b. In-Patient assessment for mental/intellectual disability
    c. Assess the mental age of patient
    d. Assess for alcohol overdose

Ans.
1. b
2. c
3. d
4. c
5. c
6. b
7. c
8. b
9. a
10. c
11. c
12. a, c, d
13. a

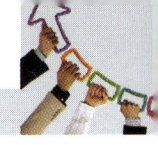

Answers with Explanations

1. Ans. (b) Mild

Ref: K. Park, 23rd ed. p 582

INTERNATIONAL CLASSIFICATION OF DISEASE

2. Ans. (c) V

Ref: K. Park, 24th ed. p 54

ICD 10 has 21 Major chapters

Chapter Number	Diseases Covered	Range of Codes
I	Certain Infectious and Parasitic Diseases	A00-B99
II	Neoplasms	C00-D48
III	Diseases of the Blood and Blood-forming Organs and Certain Disorders involving the Immune Mechanism	D50-D89
IV	Endocrine, Nutritional and Metabolic Diseases	E00-E90
V	Mental and Behavioral Disorders	F00-F99
VI	Diseases of the Nervous System	G00-G99
VII	Diseases of the Eye and Adnexa	H00-H59
VIII	Diseases of the Ear and Mastoid Process	H60-H95
IX	Diseases of the Circulatory System	I00-I99
X	Diseases of the Respiratory System	J00-J99
XI	Diseases of the Digestive System	K00-K93
XII	Diseases of the Skin and Subcutaneous Tissue	L00-L99
XIII	Diseases of the Musculoskeletal System and Connective Tissue	M00-M99
XIV	Diseases of the Genitourinary System	N00-N99
XV	Pregnancy, Childbirth and the Puerperium	O00-O99
XVI	Certain Conditions Originating in the Perinatal Period	P00-P96
XVII	Congenital Malformations, Deformations and Chromosomal Abnormalities	Q00-Q99
XVIII	Symptoms, Signs and Abnormal Clinical and Laboratory Findings, Not Elsewhere Classified	R00-R99
XIX	Injury, Poisoning and Certain Other Consequences of External Causes	S00-T98
XX	External Causes of Morbidity and Mortality	V01-Y98
XXI	Factors Influencing Health Status and Contact with Health Services	Z00-Z99
XXII	Codes for special purposes	U00-U99

Contd...

Also Know......................

- London Bills of Mortality by John Graunt in 17th Century and Nosologia Methodica by Sauvages in 18th century were the first systematic classification of diseases.

MISCELLANEOUS

3. Ans. (d) 2014

Ref: New Pathways New Hope, National Mental Health Policy of India-2014, MOHFW

National Mental Health Policy of India-2014

- **Goals**
  - To reduce distress, disability, exclusion morbidity and premature mortality associated with mental health problems across life-span of the person
  - To enhances understanding of mental health in the country.
  - To strengthen the leadership in the mental health sector at the national, state, and district levels.
- **Objectives**
  - To provide universal access to mental health care.
  - To increase access to and utilization of comprehensive mental health services (including prevention services, treatment and care and support services) by persons with mental health problems.
  - To increase access to mental health services for vulnerable groups including homeless person(s), person(s) in remote areas, difficult terrains, educationally/socially/economically deprived sections.
  - To reduce prevalence and impact of risk factors associated with mental health problems.
  - To reduce risk and incidence of suicide and attempted suicide.

- To ensure respect for rights and protection from harm of person(s) with mental health problems.
- To reduce stigma associated with mental health problems.
- To enhance availability and equitable distribution of skilled human resources for mental health.
- To progressively enhance financial allocation and improve utilization for mental health promotion and care.
- To identify and address the social, biological and psychological determinants of mental health problems and to provide appropriate interventions.

4. Ans. (c) Human rights of mentally ill

National Mental Health Programme, 1982

Objectives

- To ensure availability and accessibility of minimum mental health care for all in the foreseeable future (Specially to underprivileged and most vulnerable population)
- To encourage application of mental health knowledge in general health care and social development
- To promote community participation in mental health services development and stimulate self-help in community

Strategy

- Integration of mental health with Primary Health Care
- Tertiary care institutes for treatment of mental disorder
- Eradicate stigmatization of mentally ill persons and protecting their rights via regulatory bodies – Central/ State Mental Health Authority

5. Ans (c) Launched in 1982

Ref: K. Park, 24th ed. p 496

6. Ans. (b) 1987

Ref: J Kishore, National Health Programmes of India, 11th ed. p-849

The Mental Health Act (1987) replaces the Indian Lunacy Act, 1912 and Lunacy act 1977 (J and K) covers whole of India.

- Mentally ill person has been defined as "A person who is in need of treatment by reason of any mental disorder other than mental retardation"

7. Ans. (c) Fundamental rights of mentally retarded

Ref: Mental Health Care Bill, 2011, MOHFW

8. Ans. (b) The Mental Health Care Act

Ref: Mental Health Care Bill, 2011, MOHFW

9. Ans. (a) 1982

Ref: K. Park, 24th ed. p 496

10. Ans. (c) Basic

Ref: ICD-10 Guide for Mental Retardation, World Health Organization 1996

Classification of Mental Retardation

Moderate MR: Individuals are slow in developing comprehension and use of language and eventual achievement is limited. Achievement of self-care and motor skills is also retarded. Progress in school work is limited, but a proportion of these individuals learn the basic skills needed for reading, writing, and counting.

Mild MR: Individuals can have reasonable Reading and writing skills. They can be greatly helped by education designed to develop their skills and compensate for their handicaps.

Severe/Profound MR: Individuals have limited ability to understand or comply with requests or instructions. Most such individuals are immobile or severely restricted in mobility, incontinent, and capable at most of only very rudimentary forms of nonverbal communication

11. Ans. (c) Moron is in range of IQ 50-70

12. Ans. (a) 85; c. 45; d. 75

Intellectual disability (ID), once called mental retardation, is characterized by below-average intelligence or mental ability and a lack of skills necessary for day-to-day living. People with intellectual disabilities can and do learn new skills, but they learn them more slowly. A person with intellectual disability has limitations in two areas. These areas are:

- Intellectual functioning. Also known as IQ, this refers to a person's ability to learn, reason, make decisions, and solve problems.
- Adaptive behaviors. These are skills necessary for day-to-day life, such as being able to communicate effectively, interact with others, and take care of oneself.

The average IQ is 100. Individuals with IQs of less than 70-75 are considered Intellectually Disabled.

Mild ID	IQ 50–69
Moderate ID	IQ 35–49
Severe ID	IQ 20–34
Profound ID	IQ 19 or below

13. Ans. (a) Out-patient assessment for mental/intellectual disability

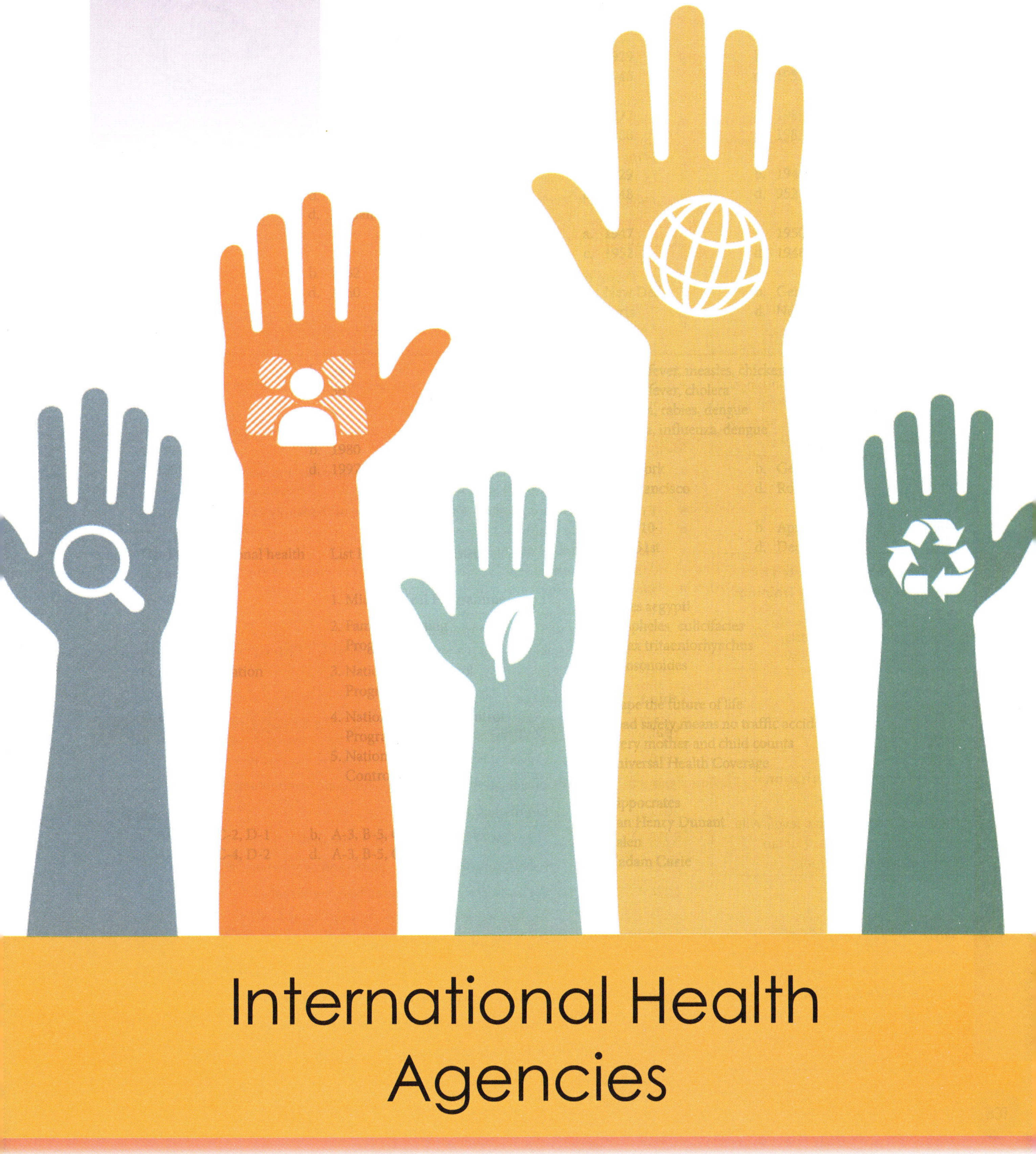

International Health Agencies

Chapter Outline

- World Health Organization
- UNICEF
- Other International Health Agencies
  - World Bank
  - Red Cross and Others
- Biological Weapons
- Medical Tourism
  - Travel during Pregnancy

WORLD HEALTH ORGANIZATION (WHO)

- WHO Constitution came into force on 7th April, 1948
- It is a specialized agency of United Nations (UN) with Headquarters at Geneva, Switzerland[Q].
- It has its own constitution, governing body, membership and budget.
- It is part of, but not subordinate to the UN[Q]
- Membership is open to all countries. *(Switzerland is a member of WHO, but not of the UN)*

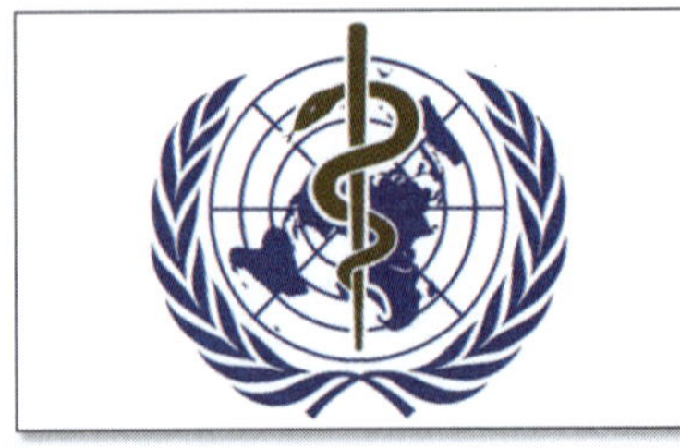

Fig. 1: World health organization (WHO) emblem

- In 1948, WHO had 56 members, presently there are 194 members and 2 Associate Members.
- *India became member of WHO in 1948.*

Structural Organization of WHO

Three Principal Organs

- **World Health Assembly** (supreme governing body)
- **Executive Board:** It has 31 members, 3 elected from each WHO region. 1/3rd members renewed every year.
  Executive Board takes decisions, formulates policies.
- **Secretariat:** Provides technical and managerial support to member countries for their national health programs.

Roles and Responsibilities of WHO

- Prevention and control of specific diseases communicable and noncommunicable.
- Development of comprehensive health services.
- **Family health:** Improvement of the quality of life of the family as a unit
- Environmental health
- **Health statistics:** Weekly Epidemiological Record, World Health Statistics (Quarterly and Annually), International Classification of Diseases (updated every 10th year)
- **Bio-medical research:** (Grants and Coordination)
- Health literature and information
- Cooperation with other organizations

World health day—celebrated each year on 7th April with a theme pertaining to public health importance

Table 1: Themes of last years World Health Day

Year	Theme
2019	Universal Health Coverage: Everyone, everywhere
2018	Universal Health Coverage: Everyone, everywhere
2017	Depression: Let's Talk
2016	Stay Super-Halt the Rise –BEAT the Diabetes
2015	Food safety, from farm to plate (and everywhere in between)
2014	Vector-borne diseases: Small bite, big threat
2013	Healthy heart beat, Healthy blood pressure
2012	Good health adds life to years
2011	Antimicrobial resistance: No action today no cure tomorrow
2010	Urbanization and health- 1000 cities –1000 lives
2009	Save lives. Make hospitals safe in emergencies
2008	Protecting health from climate change (60th anniversary of WHO)

178 *High Yield Points*

Members of South East Asia Region:

India, Bhutan, Bangladesh, Indonesia, Korea (Democratic Peoples Republic), Maldives, Myanmar, Nepal, Sri Lanka, Thailand and Timor-Leste.[Q]

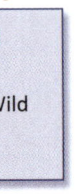

179 *High Yield Points*

Tropical diseases targeted by WHO for Research and Training:

Malaria, Schistosomiasis, Trypanosomiasis, Filariasis, Leishmaniasis and Leprosy

180 *High Yield Points*

Diseases under International Health Regulations:

Cholera, Plague, Yellow fever, Wild polio, SARS, Smallpox, Human influenza (new subtype)

181 *High Yield Points*

Diseases under International Surveillance by WHO:

Louse borne Typhus fever, Relapsing fever, Polio, Human influenza, SARS, Smallpox, Ebola

WHO Regional Organizations

Region	Headquarters
South East Asia	New Delhi (India)
Africa	Brazzaville Congo
The Americas	Washington D.C. (USA)
Europe	Copenhagen (Denmark)
Eastern Mediterranean	Alexandria (Egypt)
Western Pacific	Manila (Philippines)

UNITED NATIONS INTERNATIONAL CHILDREN'S EMERGENCY FUND (UNICEF)

- Specialized UN agency, established in 1946 to deal with rehabilitation of children in war ravaged countries.
- In 1953, renamed as "U.N. Children's Fund" but the initials, UNICEF was retained.
- *Regional office* of South Central Asian Region- [Afghanistan, Sri Lanka, India, Maldives, Mongolia and Nepal] is in New Delhi.[Q]
- Headquarters of the UNICEF is at United Nations, New York.[Q]
- Services rendered are Child health, Child Nutrition, Family and Child Welfare and Education - formal and non-formal.
- UNICEF is promoting campaign "GOBI-FFF" to encourage 4 strategies for child health revolution:
  - G-Growth Chart for monitoring child development
  - O- Oral rehydration for treating mild and moderate dehydration
  - B- Breastfeeding
  - I- Immunization against measles, diphtheria, polio, pertussis, tetanus and tuberculosis.
  - F- Family Planning
  - F- Female Literacy
  - F- Ferrum (iron) and Folic acid supplementation
- Thus, UNICEF promotes the concept of 'whole child', for their long-term development-personnel as well as those of countries in which they live. This approach is also known as 'Country Health Programming'.[Q]

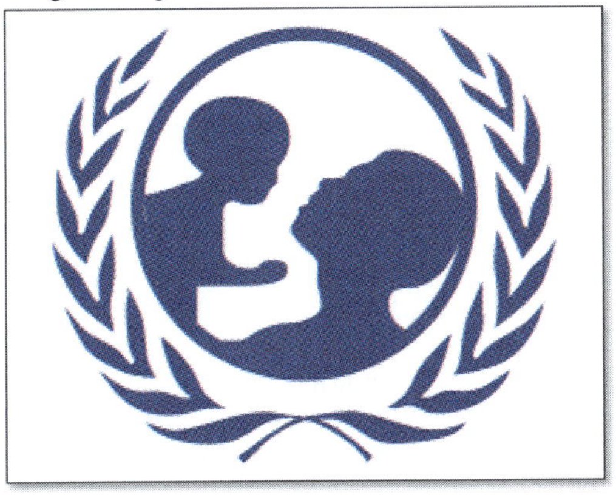

Fig. 2: Emblem of UNICEF

Must Remember

***SAARC [South Asian Association for Regional Cooperation*.** Established 1985]

India, Pakistan, Nepal, Sri Lanka, Bangladesh, Bhutan and Maldives are members.

OTHER INTERNATIONAL HEALTH AGENCIES INVOLVED IN GLOBAL HEALTH

Food and Agriculture Organization (FAO)

- Established in 1945 with headquarters in Rome.[Q]
- Prime concern is to increase production of food to keep pace with the growing world population.

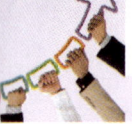

- Aims to help nations raise living standards, to improve nutrition of the people, to increase the efficiency of farming, forestry and fisheries, to improve the condition of rural people and to widen opportunity for all people for productive work.

United Nations Development Program (UNDP)

- Established in 1966.
- **Objective:** Help poorer nations to develop their human and natural resources.
- UNDP projects cover economic and social sector - agriculture, industry, education and science, health, social welfare, etc.

International Labor Organization (ILO)

- It was established in 1919, to improve working and living conditions of working population all over the world.[Q]
- Headquarters of ILO is in Geneva, Switzerland.
- ILO contributes to establishment of lasting peace by promoting social justice.
- Improvement by international action of labor conditions and living standards.
- Promotion of economic and social stability.

World Bank

- It is a specialized UN agency, to help less developed countries to raise their living standards.
- Provides loan for projects concerned with electric power, roads, railways, agriculture, water supply, education, family planning, etc. that will lead to economic growth.

United States Agency for International Development (USAID)

- US Government extends aid to India via 3 agencies:
  - USAID
  - Public Law 480 (Food for Peace) Program
  - US Export-Import Bank.
- USAID was established in 1961
  - It is assisting in Malaria eradication, Medical and nursing education, Health education, Water supply and sanitation, Control of communicable diseases, Nutrition and Family planning.

International Red Cross

- It is a nonpolitical, nonofficial international humanitarian organization devoted to the service of mankind in peace and war.
- Founded by Henry Dunant in 1864.
- In 1919, League of the Red Cross Society was created with headquarters in Geneva.
- **Role:**
  - Initially was humanitarian service to war victims.
  - Later extended to—service to armed forces and war veterans, disaster service, first aid and nursing, health education and maternity and child welfare services.

Indian Red Cross

- Red Cross Society of India was established in 1920.[Q]
- **Objective:** Improvement of health, prevention of disease and mitigation of suffering.
- In peacetime, provides military hospitals with amenities as newspapers, periodicals, musical instruments.
- Red Cross Home at Bengaluru for disabled ex-servicemen is one of the pioneer institutions in Asia.
- Disaster services comprise distribution of milk, medicines, vitamin tablets, cod liver oil and hundred other items to the famine stricken people and to those who have been hit by the floods.

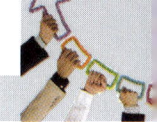

Rockefeller Foundation

- It is a philanthropic organization endowed by *Mr. John D. Rockefeller* (Started in 1913).
- It is active in public health, medical education and advancement of life sciences, social sciences, humanities and agricultural sciences.
- Work in India began in 1920 with a scheme for control of hookworm disease in the Madras Presidency.
- Established All India Institute of Hygiene and Public Health at Kolkata.

Functions

- Training of competent teachers and research workers [Via fellowships/travel grants]
- Sponsoring visits of medical specialists from USA
- Grants-in-aid to select institutions for research and development.

Ford Foundation

- Active in the development of rural health services and family planning.
- Ford Foundation has helped India in the following projects:
  - Rural health
  - Rural environment and sanitation
  - Establishment of National Institute of Health Administration and Education (NIHAE) at Delhi
  - Kolkata water supply and drainage scheme
  - Supporting research in reproductive biology and in family planning fellowship programs.

Bill and Melinda Gates Foundation

- Largest private foundation in the world based in Seattle, Washington
- Aims are:
  - To enhance healthcare and reduce extreme poverty globally and in America
  - To expand educational opportunities and access to information technology.
- Major assistance in polio eradication, global alliance for vaccine and immunization (GAVI), Vaccine program for JE, TB vaccine, HIV and Visceral Leishmaniasis research.

Swedish International Development Agency (SIDA)

Assisting National TB Control Program since 1979.

Danish International Development Agency (DANIDA)

Assistance in *DANLEP [Leprosy], DANTB [TB]* and *DANPCB [National Blindness Control Program]*.

World Food Program

It is the world's largest international food aid organization.

- *Beneficiaries:* Poor women and children at risk, poor forest dependent population.
- *Indiamix* – 40% Maize, 40% wheat and 20% full fat soya bean fortified with micronutrients [Iron, Calcium and vitamin A] distributed through Integrated Child Development Services (ICDS) project was developed under World Food Program (WFP).

Aga Khan Foundation

Focuses on Health systems, Education (including early childhood care and development), rural development and income generation to alleviate poverty and NGO enhancement.

Oxfam

Confederation of autonomous NGO committed to fight poverty and injustice in world.

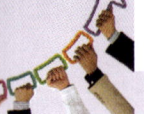

United Nations High Commission for Refugees (UNHCR)

It protects refugees and helps them restart their lives in normal environment.

United Nations Industrial Development Organization (UNIDO)

It helps developing countries in fight against marginalization in today's globalized world.

Department for International Development (DFID)

- Channelizes British government assistance.
- Focused in 4 states in India – MP, Andhra Pradesh, Orissa and West Bengal.
- Assisting Reproductive health, Control of HIV/AIDS, TB control, community eye care and polio eradication.
- **Objective:** Global effort to eliminate world poverty in 21st century.

Cooperative for Assistance and Relief Everywhere (CARE)

- Founded in North America in 1945.
- It is an independent, nonprofit, nonsectarian international relief and development organization.
- Provides emergency aid and long-term development assistance.
- CARE began its operation in India in 1950.
- *CARE-India* works in partnership with the Government of India, State Governments, NGOs etc.
- Aids in:
  - Integrated Nutrition and Health Project;
  - Anemia Control Project;
  - Improving Women's Health Project;
  - Improved Health Care for Adolescent Girl's Project;
  - Child Survival Project;
  - Improving Women's Reproductive Health and Family Spacing Project;
  - Konkan Integrated Development Project etc.

Table 2: UN agencies/NGO headquarters

UN agencies	Headquarters
WHO	Geneva, Switzerland
UNICEF	New York, USA
UNDP	New York, USA
Food and agricultural organization (FAO)	Rome, Italy
ILO	Geneva, Switzerland
International Red Cross	Geneva, Switzerland

International Decades

2011–2020—United Nations Decade of Action for Road Safety.
2003–2012—United Nations Literacy Decade: Education for All
2005–2014—United Nations Decade of Education for Sustainable Development
2005–2015—International Decade for Action, 'Water for Life'

BIOLOGICAL WEAPONS

"Poor man's atomic bomb" are microorganisms (Natural, Wild or Genetically engineered) that infect and grow in target hosts (humans, livestock and crops) to produce a clinical disease.

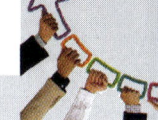

Table 3: Agents of bioterrorism

Category of bioterrorism agent	Characteristics	Disease
Category A (High-priority)	▪ Easily disseminated/ Transmitted ▪ High mortality ▪ Result Panic and Social disruption ▪ Special action needed for public health preparedness.	▪ Anthrax ▪ Botulism ▪ Plague ▪ Smallpox ▪ Tularemia ▪ Viral hemorrhagic fevers (Ebola, Marburg, Lassa)
Category B (Second highest priority)	▪ Moderately easy to disseminate ▪ Moderate morbidity and Low mortality ▪ Need enhanced diagnostic capacity and disease surveillance	▪ Brucellosis ▪ Epsilon toxin of Clostridium perfringens ▪ Food safety threat (Salmonella, E. coli O157:H7, Shigella) ▪ Glanders ▪ Melioidosis ▪ Psittacosis ▪ Q fever ▪ Ricin toxin (Castor Beans) ▪ Staphylococcal enterotoxin B ▪ Typhus fever ▪ Viral encephalitis (Venezuelan equine encephalitis) ▪ Water safety threats (e.g. vibrio cholerae Cryptosporidium parvum)
Category C (Third highest priority-Future Threats)	▪ Easily available ▪ Ease to produce and disseminate ▪ High morbidity and mortality	▪ Nipah virus ▪ Hanta virus

MEDICAL TOURISM (HEALTH TOURISM)

It is a term used to describe the rapidly-growing practice of traveling across international borders to obtain health care. It also refers to practice of health care providers traveling internationally to deliver health care.

Travel during Pregnancy

- Most commercial airlines allow pregnant travelers to *fly until 36 weeks* gestation—for domestic travel up to 36 weeks and for international travel up to 32 weeks of gestation.
- Risks of air travel include potential exposure to communicable disease, immobility and discomforts of flying.
- Cruise ship restricts travel beyond 28 weeks of pregnancy (some as early as 24 weeks).

Image-Based Questions

1. Identify the symbol in figure:

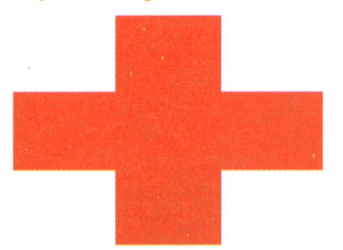

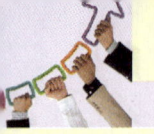

a. International Red Cross
b. International Peace Keeping Force
c. Indian Medical Association
d. Indian Veterinary Association

2. Headquarters of the international health agency shown in figure is at?

a. Rome
b. New York
c. Paris
d. Geneva

3. Identify the agency depicted by logo in figure?

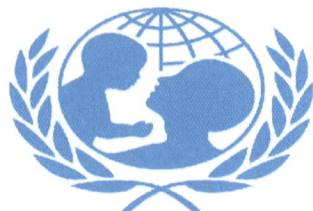

a. WHO
b. UNICEF
c. UNDP
d. WABA

4. Headquarter of the agency depicted by logo in figure in South East Asia is in:

a. New Delhi
b. Colombo
c. Dhaka
d. Bangalore

5. Headquarter of the agency depicted by logo in figure in South East Asia is in?

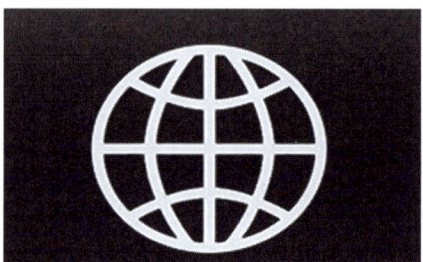

a. UNAIDS
b. UNDP
c. World Bank
d. DFID

6. The symbol shown in figure is of?

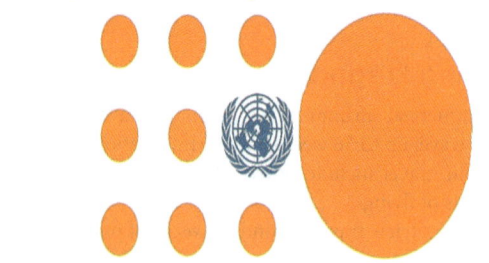

a. UNESCO
b. DFID
c. WHO
d. UNFPA

Answers of Image-Based Questions

1. **Ans. (a)** International Red Cross
2. **Ans. (a)** Rome
3. **Ans. (b)** UNICEF
4. **Ans. (a)** New Delhi
5. **Ans. (c)** World Bank
6. **Ans. (d)** UNFPA

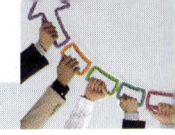

Multiple Choice Questions

1. **First country to introduce compulsory sickness insurance** *(Recent Question 2015)*
   a. Russia b. India
   c. Germany d. England
2. **Emporiatrics is a science dealing with:**
   a. Health of travelers b. Occupational health
   c. Making new drugs d. Genetic disease frequency
3. **The earliest public health law was promulgated in:**
   a. Germany b. Russia
   c. China d. England
4. **United Nations General Assembly established "UNICEF" in the year**
   a. 1946 b. 1952
   c. 1958 d. 1960
5. **According to International Health Regulations (IHR) Act, a pregnant woman, with the following duration of pregnancy (in weeks), cannot travel by air to other country**
   a. 20 b. 28
   c. 32 d. 36
6. **In which year, did WHO conceive the idea of Safe Motherhood initiative at a conference in Nairobi, Kenya**
   a. 1987 b. 1980
   c. 1990 d. 1997
7. **Match list I (International health organization) with list II (Program assisted) and select the correct answer using the codes given below:**

List I (International health organization)	List II (Program assisted)
A. SIDA	1. Midday Meal Programme
B. DANIDA	2. Family Planning Programme
C. Ford Foundation	3. National TB Control Programme
D. CARE	4. National Leprosy Control Programme
	5. National Blindness Control Programme

   Codes:
   a. A-5, B-3, C-2, D-1 b. A-3, B-5, C-4, D-2
   c. A-5, B-3, C-4, D-2 d. A-3, B-5, C-2, D-1
8. **The UNICEF was established in:**
   a. 1929 b. 1946
   c. 1948 d. 1952
9. **World was declared free of small pox by WHO in:**
   a. 1977 b. 1989
   c. 1980 d. 1985
10. **The WHO was set up in:**
    a. 1929 b. 1946
    c. 1948 d. 952
11. **The constitution of WHO came into force in:**
    a. 1947 b. 1950
    c. 1952 d. 1948
12. **The head quarter of UNESCO is located in:**
    a. New Delhi b. Geneva
    c. Paris d. New York
13. **Which of the following diseases are included under International Health Regulation by WHO:**
    a. Yellow fever, measles, chicken pox
    b. Yellow fever, cholera
    c. Cholera, rabies, dengue
    d. Malaria, influenza, dengue
14. **Headquarters of FAO is at:**
    a. New York b. Geneva
    c. San Francisco d. Rome
15. **WHO day is celebrated on:**
    a. April 10 b. April 7th
    c. May 31st d. Dec 1st
16. **Which of the following mosquito is important regarding the international travel?**
    a. Aedes aegypti
    b. Anopheles culicifacies
    c. Culex tritaeniorhynchus
    d. Mansonoides
17. **WHO theme for year 2019 is:**
    a. Shape the future of life
    b. Road safety means no traffic accidents
    c. Every mother and child counts
    d. Universal Health Coverage
18. **Red Cross was founded by:**
    a. Hippocrates
    b. Jean Henry Dunant
    c. Galen
    d. Madam Curie

Ans.

1. c
2. a
3. d
4. a
5. c
6. a
7. d
8. b
9. c
10. c
11. d
12. c
13. b
14. d
15. b
16. a
17. d
18. b

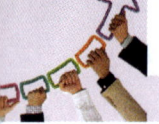

Answers with Explanations

1. Ans. (c) Germany

Ref: K. Park, 24th p-10

- Germany was the 1st country to introduce compulsory sickness insurance.
- Homeopathy also originated in Germany

2. Ans. (a) Health of travelers

Ref: Handbook of Community Medicine, Mangala Subramaniam p-136

Travel medicine or Emporiatrics is a branch of medicine that deals with prevention and management of health problems of international travelers.

3. Ans. (d) England

Ref: K. Park, 24th ed. p 5

The "Great sanitary awakening" led to enactment of the Public Health Act, 1848 in England.

4. Ans. (a) 1946

- ILO—founded in 1919
- WHO—origin—April, 1945, in Geneva. Constitution was drawn up at "International health conference" New York 1946, rectification were secured by April, 1948, constitution came into force on April 7, 1948 (World Health Day).
- FAO—1945
- UNICEF—1946
- Colombo Plan—1950
- CARE (in India)—1950

5. Ans. (c) (32)

- Domestic air travel is permitted until 36 weeks.
- International air travel is permitted until 32 weeks.

6. Ans. (a) 1987

WHO in the year 1987 conceived the idea of Safe Motherhood initiative at a conference in Nairobi, Kenya

7. Ans. (d) (A-3, B-5, C-2, D-1)

8. Ans. (b) 1946

- UNICEF [United Nation's International Children's Emergency Fund] is one of the specialized agencies of the United Nations. It was established in 1946 by the United Nation's General Assembly to deal with rehabilitation of children in war ravaged countries. In 1953, when the emergency functions were over, the general assembly gave it a new name "UN children's Fund", but retained the initials UNICEF.

9. Ans. (c) 1980

- World was declared free of small pox by WHO on 8th May, 1980.
- India was free of small pox in April, 1977,

10. Ans. (c) 1948

- World Health Organization (WHO), is a specialized agency of the United Nations (UN). Its headquarters is situated in Geneva, Switzerland. WHO was established in 1948. According to its constitution it is "the directing and coordinating authority on international health work" and is responsible for helping all people to attain "the highest possible levels of health".

11. Ans. (d) 1948

- In 1946, the constitution of the World Health Organization was drafted by the "Technical Preparatory Committee" under the chairmanship of Rene Sand and was approved in the same year by an International Health Conference of 51 nations in New York. The constitution came into force on 7TH APRIL, 1948 which is celebrated every year as "WORLD HEALTH DAY".

12. Ans. (c) Paris

- United nations educational, scientific and cultural organization (UNESCO), was established in 1946 to encourage collaboration among nation in the areas of science, culture, and communication. Its headquarter is located in PARIS, France.

13. Ans. (b) Yellow fever, cholera

- At the international level, the following diseases are notifiable to WHO under the International Health Regulation:
  - Cholera
  - Plague
  - Yellow fever
  - Poliomyelitis

14. Ans. (d) Rome

- Food and Agriculture Organization (FAO), is a specialized United Nations agency whose main goal is to afford freedom from hunger on a world scale. The FAO originated at a conference called by President Franklin D. Roosevelt in Hot Springs, Virginia, in May 1943. In October 1945 the first session of the FAO was held in Quebec. At present the organization has 161 members; it is headed by a director general. Main headquarters is in Rome.

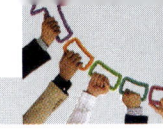

15. Ans. (b) April 7th

- In 1946, the constitution of the World Health Organization was drafted by the "Technical Preparatory Committee" under the chairmanship of Rene Sand and was approved in the same year by an International Health Conference of 51 nations in New York. The constitution came into force on 7th April 1948, which is celebrated every year as "World Health Day".

16. Ans. (a) Aedes aegypti

- It is important from prevention of yellow fever epidemic. Under the international health regulations. The policy for prevention of yellow fever is known as EYE strategy. (EYE – Elimination of Yellow fever Epidemics) which involves vector surveillance and control and prevention of spread of yellow fever.

Notifiable diseases under the International Health Regulations

- Cholera
- Plague
- Yellow fever
- Small pox
- Relapsing fever
- Salmonellosis
- Poliomyelitis
- Influenza
- SARS
- Rabies
- Louse born typhus fever

17. Ans. (d) Universal Health Coverage

18. Ans. (b) Jean Henry Dunant

- Red Cross was founded by JEAN HENRI DUNANT. He was a Swiss philanthropist. In 1863 an International Conference was held in Geneva, and the Geneva Convention of 1864 established the permanent International Red Cross. In 1901, Dunant shared the first Nobel Peace Prize with the French statesman Frederick Passy.

NOTES

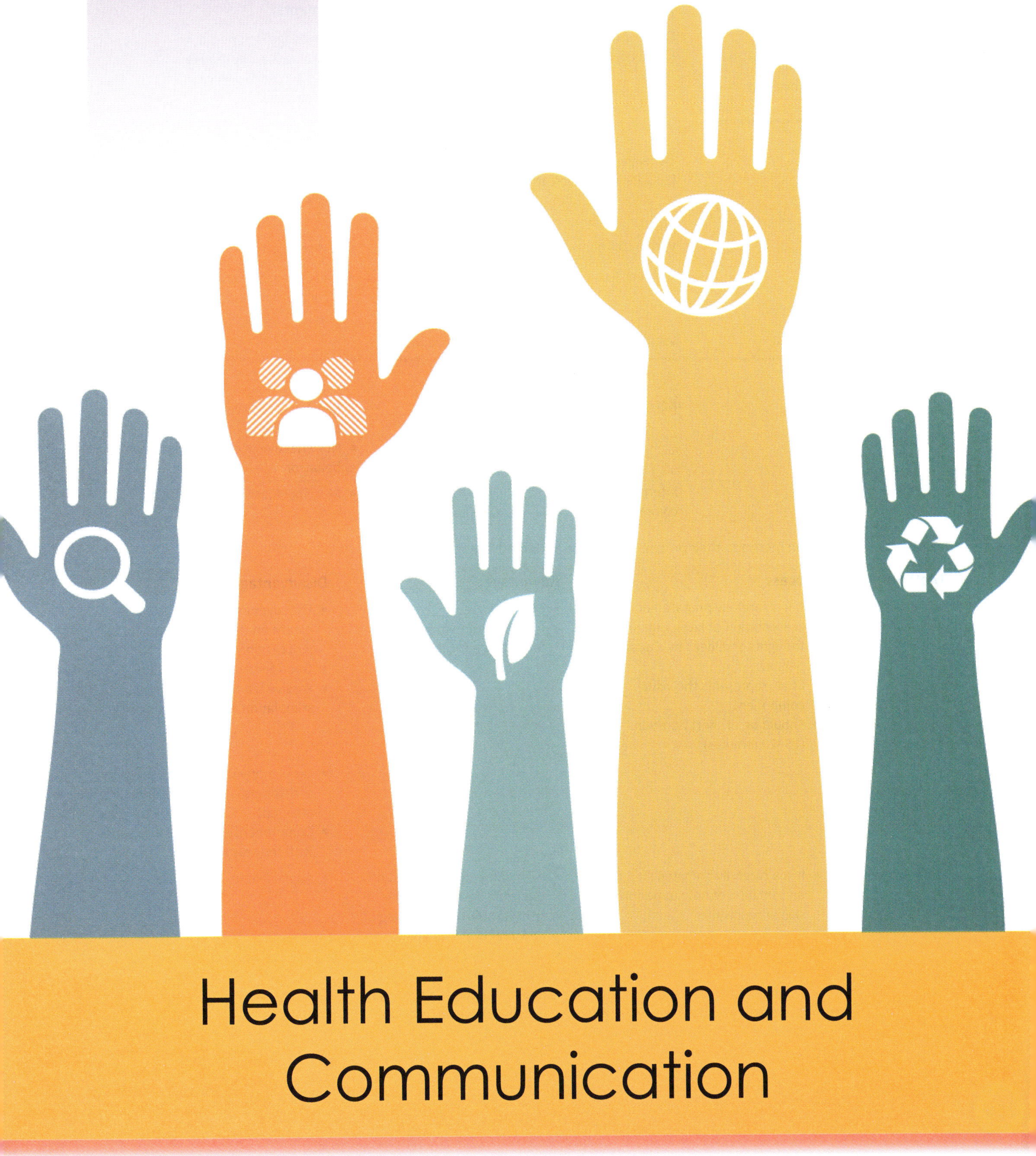

Health Education and Communication

Chapter Outline

COMMUNICATION—TYPES AND INTRODUCTION

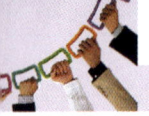

Table 1: Types of communication

Types	Examples	Comments
One – way (Didactic) communication	Lecture, TV, Radio, Newspaper	▪ Knowledge is imposed ▪ Learning is authoritative ▪ Little audience participation ▪ No feedback ▪ Does not influence human behavior or remove misconceptions
Two-way (Socratic) communication	Focus Group Discussion, Symposium, Panel discussion	▪ Learning is active, participatory and "democratic" ▪ More likely to influence behavior
Verbal communication	By word of mouth	▪ It is persuasive
Nonverbal communication	Body movements, Postures, Gestures, Facial expressions	▪ It can speak louder than words ▪ Stronger than verbal communication
Visual communication	Charts, Graphs, Pictograms, Tables, Maps, Posters	
Mass communication	Radio, TV and Internet	▪ Reaches a relatively larger and remote population in a short time ▪ Not effective in changing established behavior
Interpersonal communication	Face-to-face talk, Discussion	▪ More persuasive and effective

Table 2: Communication methods, their process, advantage and disadvantage

Method	Process	Advantage	Disadvantage
Lecture (Chalk and Talk)	▪ It is a carefully prepared oral presentation of facts, organized thoughts and ideas by a qualified person ▪ Chalk represents the visual component ▪ Should be of short duration (15–20 minutes)	▪ Economical ▪ Most common mode of imparting education	▪ Effectiveness depends to a large extent on the speaker's ability to write legibly and to draw ▪ Good for small groups (≤30) ▪ Passive learning (No thought stimulation or problem solving)
			▪ Lacks motivation (health behavior of listeners is not necessarily affected) ▪ Comprehension of a lecture varies with the student
Demonstration	▪ It is a carefully prepared step-by-step presentation of how to perform a skill or procedure ▪ It involves the audience in discussion, arouses interest and persuades them to adopt recommended practices ▪ It upholds the principle of "Seeing is believing" and "learning by doing"	▪ High motivational value and can bring desired changes in behavior pertaining to use of new practice ▪ It is of immense value in public health programs like environmental sanitation (e.g. installation of a hand pump, construction of a sanitary latrine)	▪ Applicable to small group

Contd...

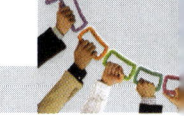

Method	Process	Advantage	Disadvantage
Group discussion	▪ 6–12 members sit in a circle fully visible to each other ▪ Group leader initiates the topic, facilitates discussion, prevents side-conversations, encourages everyone to participate and sums up the discussion in end ▪ Members interact among themselves and free exchange knowledge, ideas and opinions occurs ▪ "Recorder" prepares a report on issues discussed and agreements reached. *Rules* ▪ Ideas to be expressed clearly and concisely ▪ Listen to other and do not interrupt when other person is speaking ▪ Make only relevant remarks ▪ Accept criticism gracefully ▪ Help to reach conclusions	▪ Very effective where long-term compliance or change in attitude/behavior is desired	▪ Unequal participation ▪ Deviation and irrelevant discussion
Panel discussion	▪ Panel comprises a chairman and 4–8 qualified speakers, who discuss on a topic in front of an audience ▪ Chairman introduces the topic briefly and invites the panel speakers to present their points of view ▪ No specific agenda, no order of speaking and no set speeches ▪ Success depends on chairman who has to keep the discussion going on and develop the train of thoughts ▪ After the main aspects of the subject are explored by panel speakers, audience is invited to take part. ▪ If panel members are unacquainted with the method, they may have a preliminary meeting, prepare material on the subject and decide upon the method and plan of presentation	▪ Audience involvement, ▪ Flexible, spontaneous	▪ Needs through planning and advance preparation
Symposium	▪ It comprises a series of speeches by experts on different aspects of a selected subject ▪ Audience may raise questions in the end ▪ Chairman presents a comprehensive summary in end	▪ Scope for integrated teaching ▪ Not monotonous, as speakers change ▪ All aspects related to a topic covered in time	▪ No discussion is permitted during the symposium
Workshop	▪ Comprises a series of meetings usually ≥4 ▪ Emphasis is on individual work within small group ▪ Facilitators/consultants guide the group work	▪ Each participant has an opportunity to improve his effectiveness as a professional worker via group work	▪ Limited number of participants, ▪ Skilled facilitators needed ▪ Lot of baseline preparation is required

Contd...

Method	Process	Advantage	Disadvantage
Role play	▪ Situation is dramatized ▪ Role playing is followed by a discussion of the problem	▪ Audience active involvement (pay attention to what is going on, suggest alternative solutions) ▪ Useful when change in attitude behavior is desired	▪ Applicable to small group
Conference and seminar	▪ 1½ day to 1 week in length ▪ Cover a single topic in depth or broadly comprehensive ▪ A variety of formats are used to aid learning (Self-instruction, multimedia etc.)	▪ Helps to get recent updates ▪ Social interaction and long term bonding/associations	▪ Can be expensive

Communication is a two-way process of exchanging or shaping ideas, feelings and information. It leads to cognitive (knowledge, behavior and attitudes and psychomotor (new skills) changes

COMMUNICATION PROCESS

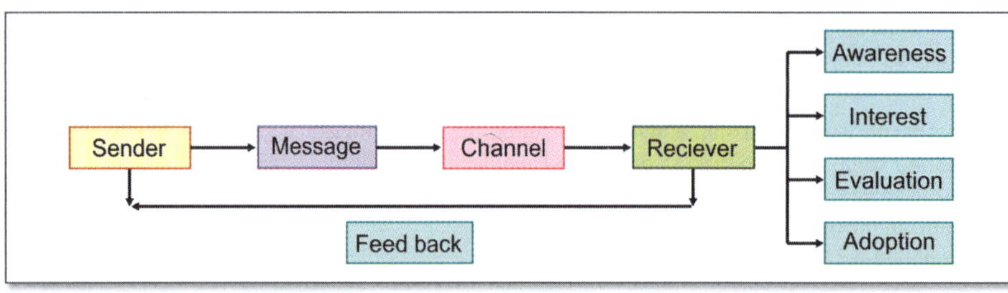

BARRIERS OF COMMUNICATION

- **Physiological:** Difficulties in hearing, expression.
- **Psychological:** Emotional disturbances, neurosis, levels of intelligence, language or comprehension difficulty.
- **Environmental:** Noise, invisibility, congestion.
- **Cultural:** Illiteracy, levels of knowledge/understanding, customs, beliefs, religion, socioeconomic class

HEALTH COMMUNICATION

Table 3: Methods in health communication

Mass approach	Individual approach	Group approach
▪ TV ▪ Radio ▪ Newspaper and print material ▪ Posters ▪ Direct mailing ▪ Internet ▪ Folk method ▪ Health museum and exhibition	▪ Personal contact ▪ Home visit ▪ Personal Letters	▪ Lecture ▪ Demonstration ▪ Discussion method

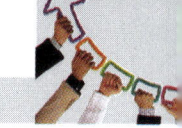

Table 4: Differences between mass media and personal communication

Mass media	Personal communication (interpersonal and group)
▪ Reaches a wider population (remote areas) in short time ▪ Gets public attention ▪ More effective among those with above average educational level ▪ Gives greater support for concentrated programs such as those for a week or month e.g. Pulse polio, Bal Swasthya Poshan Maah (BSPM)	▪ Capitalizes on warmth and understanding and knowledge of communication. *Reach is restricted*[Q] ▪ Provides opportunity for involvement, for asking questions, expressing fears, and learning more ▪ *Gets people to make changes in personal habits more readily*[Q] ▪ More influential among those with average and below average educational level

Functions of Health Communication

Information, education, motivation, persuasion, counseling, raising morals, health development and organization

- **Information:** Providing scientific knowledge or information to people about health problems, maintenance & promotion of health.
- **Health education** is a process by which individuals and group of people learn to behave in a manner conducive to promotion, restoration or maintenance of health (John M Last)
  - *Principles of health education* are credibility, interest, participation, motivation, comprehension, reinforcement, learning by doing, known to unknown, setting an example, good human relations, feedback and leaders.
- **Motivation:** Aims to help people to translate the health education into their personal behavior and lifestyle. It also aims to help people to evaluate and take decisions pertaining to their health status.
- **Persuasion** is a conscious attempt by one individual to change or influence the general beliefs, understanding, values and behavior of another individual or group of individuals in some desired way.
- **Propaganda** or *"brain washing"* is when persuasive communication is deliberately employed to manipulate feelings, attitudes and beliefs. Knowledge is instilled (Thought is not stimulated) and behavior is reflexive. It appeals to emotion, whereas health education appeals to reason.
- **Counseling** is a face to face communication that helps a client to make informed decision. (It is not same as advice)

ELEMENTS OF COUNSELING

Gather Approach

G- Greet the client (make them comfortable, give attention).
A - Ask/ascertain needs/problems or reason for coming
T- Tell different options/choices/methods to solve the problem
H- Help client to make voluntary decisions
E- Explain fully the chosen decision/options/action/methods to solve the problem
R- Return for follow-up.

Qualities of a Counselor

- Good communicator gain the trust of the people
- Sympathetic and patient.
- Understanding (Empathizes other's feeling and responds)
- Helps reduce or resolve problems and develop positive attitude

METHODS OF COMMUNICATION

Important Ways of Communication

- **Snowballing (Pyramidal group method)** is a method of group discussion, where every person of the group is involved in discussion. First it is discussed in pairs, then pairs join to make group of four, then group of four join to form group of eight and so on. Groups discuss and come to a common conclusion.

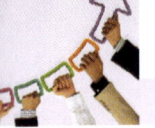

- **Colloquy:** Comprises a number of sessions, each session to find out answer to a particular question from the set of questions related to the topic. Each session is in charge of a leader known as 'interlocutor'.
- **Delphi method** is a systematic method of obtaining consensus forecasts from a panel of experts (without direct physical presence)
  - Questions are generated by researcher, but may sometimes be sought from panel members. 1st round does not always involve development of questionnaire.
  - It may be done of groups of experts to seek their reviews.
  - Usually the objective is to attain the best possible answer (or solution or result) for a complex problem (or activity or event)

Advantages

- Anonymity and lack of direct contact reduce interpersonal influence on opinions
- Cost effective
- Participants have time to consider their response (Revise, Supplement and even retract)

Disadvantages

- Level of consensus considered acceptable may be arbitrary
- Conducting a number of rounds can be time consuming

Flowchart 1: Ways of communication

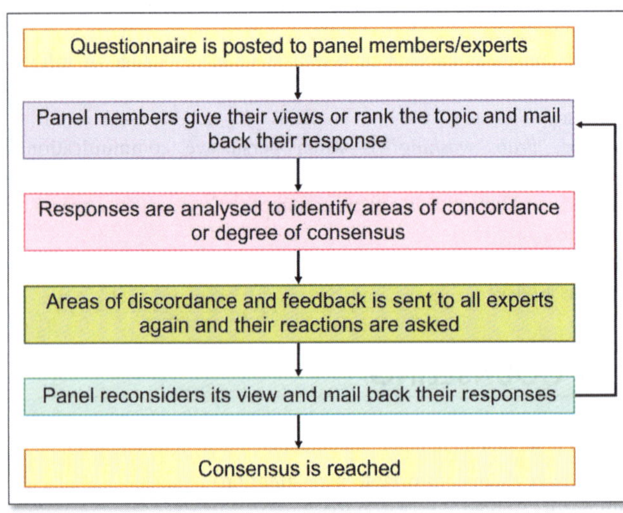

Attributes of a Leader

- Understand needs and demands of the community
- Takes initiative (leads from front) and provides proper guidance
- Receptive to views and suggestions
- Identifies himself with the community and is easily accessible to the people
- Self-less, honest, impartial, considerate and sincere
- Able to control and compromise various factions in the community
- Eliciting cooperation and coordination.
- Lead Model
  - L → Lead with clear purpose
  - E → Empower to participate
  - A → Aim for consensus
  - D → Direct the process

Flip Charts

- Comprise a series of charts (25 cm × 30 cm or more, each with an illustration pertaining to the talk.

114 Good to Remember

Central Health Education Bureau (CHEB), Delhi (under DGHS, Ministry of Health and Family Welfare, Government of India) is the apex institution for health education and health promotion in India.

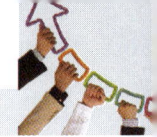

- Each chart is "flashed" or displayed before a group one after another as the talk is being given. Message on charts is brief, to the point and designed to hold attention of group and help lecture proceed.

Flannelgraph

- Cut-out pictures, graphs, drawings and other illustrations are displayed on a piece of rough flannel or khadi fixed over a wooden board.
- It is cheap, easy to transport and promotes thought and criticism.

HEALTH EDUCATION

- By John M Last, it is the process by which individuals and groups of people learn to behave in a manner conducive to the promotion, maintenance or restoration of health.
- It is a process aimed at encouraging people to want to be healthy, to know how to stay healthy, to do what they can individually and collectively to maintain health and seek help when needed.

182 High Yield Points

To educate means to cause or facilitate learning whereas *propaganda* means to spread particular systemized doctrine.

Table 5: Health education and propaganda

Education	Propaganda or publicity
Knowledge and skills actively acquired	Knowledge instilled in the minds of people
Makes people think for themselves	Prevents or discourages thinking by ready made slogans
Disciplines primitive desires	Arouses and stimulates primitive desires
Develops reflective behavior. Trains people to use judgement before acting	Develops reflexive behavior; aims at impulsive actions
Appeals to reason	Appeals to emotion
Develops individuality, personality and self-expression	Develops a standard pattern of attitudes and behaviors according to the mould used
Knowledge acquired through self-reliant activity	Knowledge is spoon-fed and passively received
The process is behavior-centered. Aims at developing favorable attitudes, habits and skills	The process is information centered. No change of attitude or behavior designed.

Multiple Choice Questions

1. **In interview, first stage is:** *(Recent Question 2017)*
   a. Establish contact
   b. Starting interview
   c. Establishing rapport
   d. Probe questions
2. **False about informed consent is:** *(Recent Question 2017)*
   a. All information must be given, except expected complications, as the patient may get frightened
   b. All information must be given regarding treatment options
   c. Information must be given, regarding any treatment options better than the treatment option being provided
   d. All disclosures must be in patient's own language
3. **Which of the following is NOT an approach of health education?**
   a. Regulatory b. Primary health care
   c. Service d. Management
4. **Which of the below is an example of affective learning?**
   a. Measuring pulse rate
   b Enumerating causes of obesity
   c. Motivating a person for blood donation
   d. Arriving at differential diagnosis
5. **Which is not a type of Interview?** *(Recent Question 2016)*
   a. Structured b. Nondirective
   c. Repetitive d. Nonrepetitive
6. **Method of health communication, involving 4 to 8 qualified persons discussing a given problem in front of a large group or audience, is called as**
   a. Symposium
   b. Panel discussion
   c. Workshop
   d. Seminar
7. **Group health education approach comprise all except-**
   a. Documentary
   b. Demonstration
   c. Role play
   d. Lecture
8. **Which of the following is/are didactic methods of health communication?** *(Recent Question 2016)*
   a. Group discussion
   b. Workshop
   c. Demonstration
   d. Lecture
   e. Panel discussion
9. **Best method of teaching an urban slum about ORS is**
   a. Lecture *(Recent Question 2015)*
   b. Role play
   c. Demonstration
   d. Flash card
10. **All are true about panel discussion except:**
    a. Panel of 4-8 experts discuss a health topic
    b. Audience is present
    c. Specific order, set speeches
    d. Audience can take part
11. **A group of 8 experts discussing and interaction about a topic in front of large audience is:** *(Recent Question 2014)*
    a. Workshop b. Symposium
    c. Seminar d. Panel discussion
12. **Socratic method of education consist of all except:**
    a. Lecture b. Group discussion
    c. Seminar d. Panel discussion
13. **"Internalization" occurs in which model of health education:** *(Recent Question 2014)*
    a. Medical model
    b. Social environmental model
    c. Service model
    d. Motivation model
14. **First requisite before conducting an interview is**
    a. Securing rapport
    b. Probe questions
    c. Establishing rapport
    d. Guiding the interview
15. **Workshop is:** *(Recent Question 2013)*
    a. Discussion of 4-8 experts in front of audience
    b. Discussion between 6-12 members
    c. Series of four or more meetings
    d. Series of speeches on given subject
16. **Total communication means:** *(Recent Question 2013)*
    a. Use of all methods of communication for advertisement
    b. Use of all methods of communication for school teaching
    c. Use of all methods of communication for community participation
    d. Using every communication option to teach deaf child
17. **Following is an example of one way communication**
    a. Visual communication b. Telemedicine
    c. Didactic method d. Socratic method

Ans.

1. a
2. a
3. d
4. c
5. d
6. b
7. a
8. c,d
9. c
10. c
11. d
12. a
13. d
14. c
15. c
16. d
17. c

Answers with Explanations

1. Ans. (a) Establish contact

Ref: K. Park, 24th ed. p 732

2. Ans. (a) All information must be given, except expected complications, as the patient may get frightened

Ref: Ethical Guidelines for Biomedical Research on Human Participants. ICMR 2006

Informed Consent of Participants

- In all biomedical research involving human participants, informed consent of participant or legal guardian (in case participant is not capable of giving informed consent) is must.
- Adequate information on the research in a simple and easily understandable unambiguous language is given in the Informed Consent Form with Participant/Patient Information Sheet containing the following information
- Nature and purpose of study
- Duration of participation with number of participants
- Procedures to be followed
- Investigations, if any, to be performed
- Foreseeable risks and discomforts whether project involves more than minimal risk
- Benefits to participant, community or medical profession
- Policy on compensation
- Availability of medical treatment for such injuries or risk management
- Alternative treatments if available
- Steps being taken for ensuring confidentiality
- No loss of benefits on withdrawal
- Benefit sharing in the event of commercialization
- Contact details of PI or local PI in multicentric study
- Contact details of Chairman of the IEC for appeal against violation of rights
- Voluntary participation
- For genetic studies and HIV, counseling for consent for testing must be given as per national guidelines
- Storage period of biological sample and related data with choice offered to participant regarding future use of sample, refusal for storage and receipt of its results

A copy of the participant/patient information sheet is to be given to the participant for her/his record.

3. Ans. (d) Management

Ref: K. Park, 24th ed. p 895-96

APPROACH TO HEALTH EDUCATION

Regulatory Approach (Managed Prevention)

- Government Intervention/Law (prohibition or imprisonment) is enacted to seek change in health behavior.
- Useful in times of emergency, control of an epidemic or management of fairs and festivals.
- Law enforcement needs a vast administrative infrastructure and expenditure
- Example, The Child Marriage Restraint Act, Compulsory seat belts while driving.

Disadvantage

- Cause of disease (medical or social) cannot be eradicated by legislation.
- In areas of personal choice (e.g., diet, exercise, smoking) no government can force people by law.

Service Approach

- Health services needed by people are provided at their door steps assuming they would use them. (E.g. Basic Health Services, 1960's).
- It is a failure, because it is not based on the felt-needs of the people. E.g. water-seal latrines provided free of cost by government in rural areas were not utilized because it was not a habit to use latrines.

Health Education Approach

- People are informed, educated, encouraged to make their own choice for a healthy life (Slow, but enduring)
- Mass media/social organizations are mobilized to introduce new attitudes and habits
- Emphasis is on youth, as attitudes and behavior are formed early in life.

Primary Health Care Approach

- Emphasizes on community participation and involvement in planning and delivery of health services.
- Seeks to make people self-reliant in identifying health problems and finding workable solutions.

Health education	Propaganda
Knowledge and skills are actively acquired	Knowledge is instilled in the minds
Encourages the thought process	Discourages thought process
Disciplines primitive desires	Arouses and stimulates primitive desires
Helps develop reflective behavior (Using Judgment before action)	Develops reflexive behavior (Impulsive actions)
Appeals to reasoning	Appeals to emotions
Knowledge is actively acquired (self-reliant activity)	Knowledge is acquired passively (Spoon fed)
It is behavior centered (Seeks to develop favorable attitudes, habits and skills)	It is information centered (Does not seek to change of attitude or behavior)
Develops individuality, personality and self-expression	Develops a set pattern of attitude and behavior

4. Ans. (c) Motivating a person for blood donation

Ref: Gowrishankar Kasilingam, Assessment of learning domains to improve student's learning in higher education. Journal of Young Pharmacists Vol. 6. Issue 4 Jan-Mar 2014

Bloom's taxonomy divides the educational objectives into three domains

- **Cognitive domain:** It focuses on intellectual skills.
- **Psychomotor domain:** It focuses on performing sequences of motor activities to a specified level of accuracy, smoothness, rapidity, or force.
- **Affective domain:** It causes on attitude, motivation, willingness to participate, valuing what is being learned and ultimately incorporating the discipline values into real life.

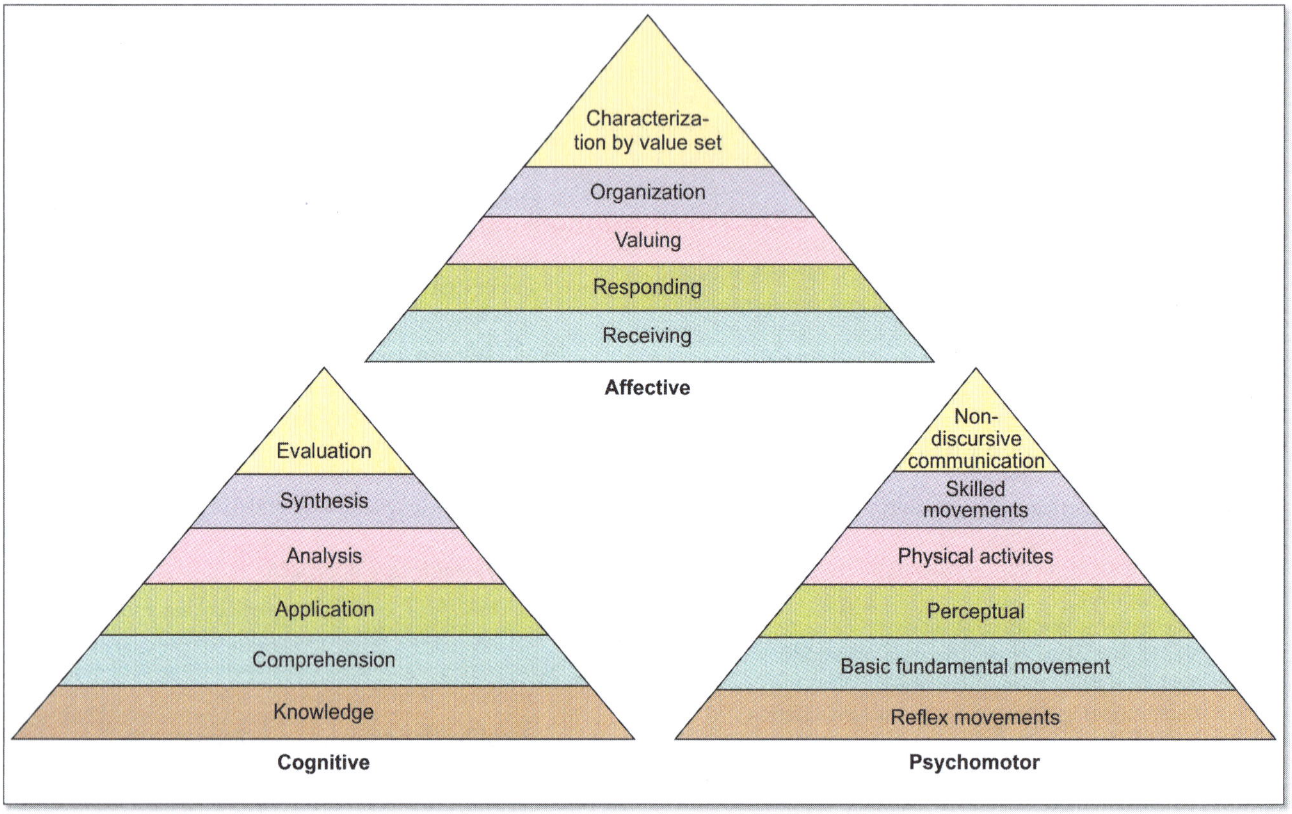

5. Ans. (d) Non-repetitive

Ref: K. Park, 24th ed. p 732

Types of Interview

- ***Direct or Structured:*** A schedule containing a set of predetermined questions is prepared.
- ***Nondirective or Unstructured:*** No predetermined questions. Researcher collects information by free discussion.
- ***Focused Interview***: To study social and psychological effects of mass communication, e.g., reaction of a film show or radio program.
- **Repetitive Interview:** To study the gradual influence of some social or psychological process.

6. Ans. (b) Panel discussion

Ref: K. Park, 24th ed, p 902

Refer to theory

7. Ans. (a) Documentary

Ref: K. Park, 24th ed. p 900

8. Ans. (c) Demonstration; (d) Lecture

Ref: K. Park, 24th ed. p 892

Didactic method of communication involves one-way communication

- Knowledge is imposed and learning is authoritative
- There is little audience participation
- No feedback is received by the communicator
- It does not influence human behavior

9. Ans. (c) Demonstration

Ref: K. Park, 24th ed. p 901

Refer to theory

10. Ans. (c) Specific order, set speeches

Ref: K. Park, 24th ed. p 902

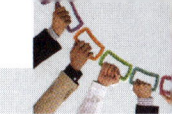

11. Ans. (d) Panel discussion

Ref: K. Park, 24th ed. p 902

12. Ans. (a) Lecture

Ref: K. Park, 24th ed. p 892

Also Know........................

Socratic Method of communication involves **two-way communication**

- Learning is *active, participatory and "democratic".* [Q] Both communicator and audience take part.
- Audiences raise questions and add to their own information, ideas and opinions on the subject.
- *More likely to influence behavior than one - way communication* [Q].
- E.g. Focus Group Discussion, Symposium, Panel discussion.

Lecture, Films, Exhibition, TV, Radio, Newspaper are all one way (Didactic) communication.

13. Ans. (d) Motivation model

Ref: K. Park, 23rd ed. p 859-60

Adoption process [Q]:

Phase I (*Awareness → Interest*) →**Phase II** (*Evaluation → Trial*) → **Phase III** (*Adoption and Dissemination*).

Motivation Model of Health Education– Emphasizes on "motivation" as the main force to translate health information into desired health action.

Motivation includes the stages of interest, evaluation and decision making.

Also Know........................

Other Models of Health Education

- **Medical Model-**Involves recognition and treatment of disease and technological advances to facilitate the process. It is concerned with disease (as defined by doctor) or opposed to illness (as defined by client).
- **Social Intervention Model-**Social environment shapes the behavior of individual and the community. Group support helps reaching the decisions and taking action.

14. Ans. (c) Establishing rapport

Ref: K. Park, 24th ed. p 732

Steps for Conducting a Interview

- Establishing contact: Prior appointment and fixing of time and place of interview.
- Starting an interview
- Securing rapport
- Recall
- Probe questions
- Encouragement
- Guiding the interview
- Recording
- Closing
- Report

15. Ans. (c) Series of four or more meetings

Ref: K. Park, 24th ed. p 902

Advantage: Each participant has an opportunity to improve his effectiveness as a professional worker via group work

Disadvantage: Limited number of participants, skilled facilitators needed and a lot of baseline preparation is required

16. Ans. (d) Using every communication option to teach deaf child

Ref: Hearing in Children. Jerry L. Northern, Marion P. Downs p 366

Total Communication is a philosophy that requires the incorporation of appropriate aural, manual, oral modes of communication to ensure effective communication with and among hearing impaired persons.

17. Ans. (c) Didactic method

Ref: K. Park, 24th ed p 892

Also Know........................

Nomogram/Sociogram is a graphical representation of interaction among participants in a FGD

NOTES

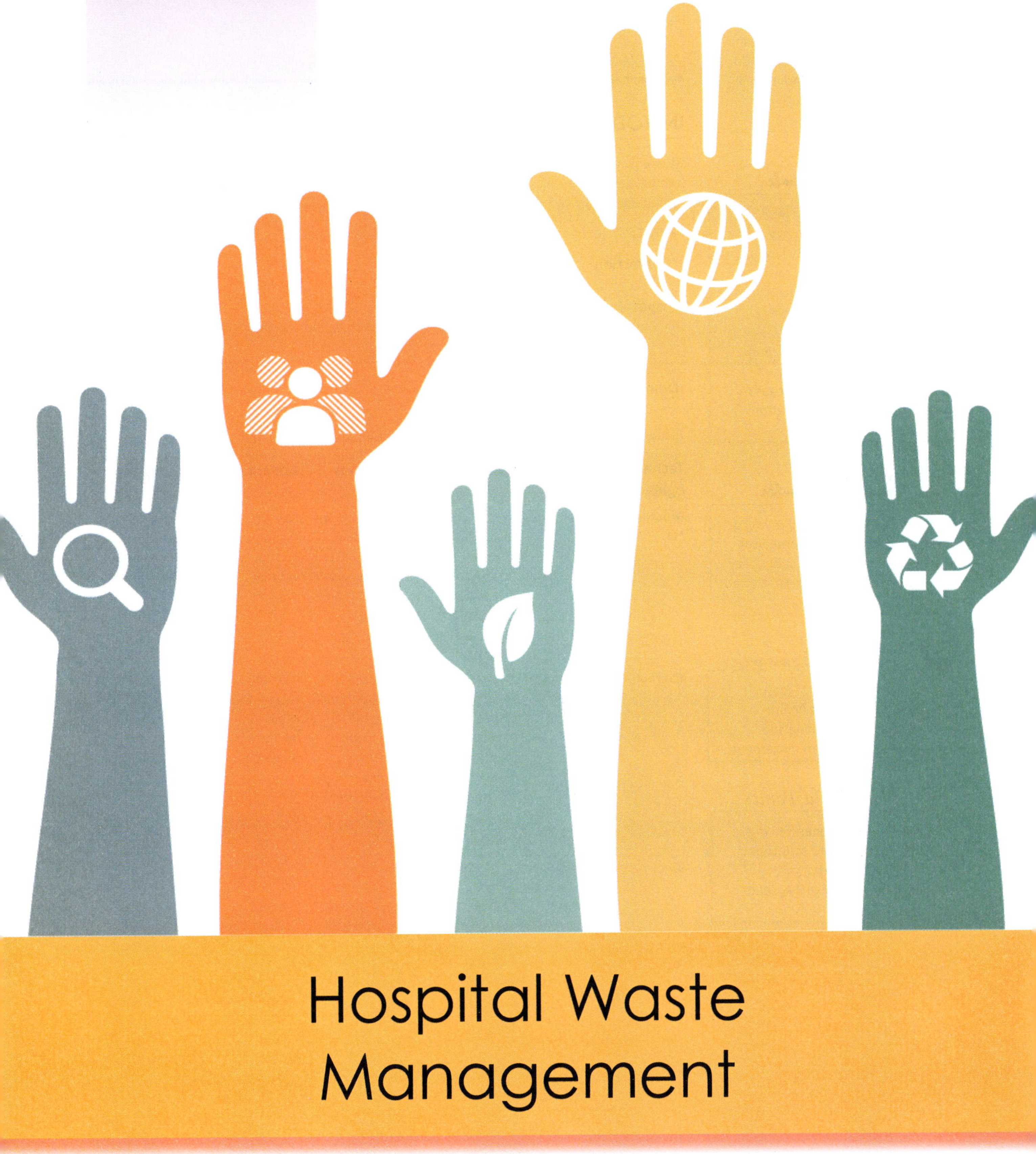

Hospital Waste Management

115 **Good to Remember**

Ministry of Environment, Forest and Climate Change, Government of India is assigned with the duty of Making Policies, Financial assistance for training/setting up of common biomedical waste treatment facility, Operational research, Notify standards or operating parameters.

116 **Good to Remember**

Central/State Ministry of Health and Family Welfare, Ministry for Animal Husbandry and Veterinary is assigned with the duty of Grant of license to health-care facilities or nursing homes or veterinary establishments, Monitoring, Refusal or Cancellation of license, Publication of list of registered health care facilities with regard to biomedical waste generation, treatment and disposal.

117 **Good to Remember**

Central Pollution Control Board- to prepare guidelines on biomedical waste management and submit to Ministry of Environment, Forest and Climate Change.

112 **Must Remember**

Waste audit is survey of waste generated in different health-care settings for planning and implementing waste management.

183 **High Yield Points**

Quantity of waste generated in a hospital, in developed countries is about 1–5 kg/bed/day.
In India, it is about *1 to 2 kg*/bed/day.

113 **Must Remember**

Recycling is a process by which a waste material is transformed into a new product in a manner that the original product loses its identity.

Chapter Outline

- Introduction
- Incineration and Autoclave
- Common Medical Waste Treatment Facilities
- BMW Rules, 2016
- Standards for Liquid Waste
- Labeling for Hospital and Biomedical Waste

INTRODUCTION

Biomedical waste (BMW) is defined as "Any waste generated during diagnosis, treatment, immunization of human beings or animals and research activities pertaining thereto or in the production or testing of biologicals".

Table 1: Objective of treatment of hospital/biomedical waste

Disinfection	▪ To render the waste nonhazardous or less hazardous ▪ To reduce volume
Disposal	▪ To prevent misuse or abuse ▪ To ensure occupational safety and health ▪ To maintain aesthetic surroundings ▪ To reuse or recycle waste to the extent possible
Drainage	▪ Liquid waste need chemical disinfection and discharge into drains

Table 2: Treatment and disposal technologies for biomedical waste

Technologies	Principles	Applicable for	Methods	Advantages	Disadvantages
Mechanical	Change in physical form and characteristics	Needle, syringes, tubes, catheters (Recyclable Plastics/Metal) Pharmaceutical waste and Incineration ash heavy metal content	Compacting, Shredding, Landfill (Open/ Sanitary), Encapsulation, Inertization, Pulverization	Relatively Inexpensive, Reduce volume	Need to be combined with other methods before final waste disposal
Thermal	Wet (Steam) Treatment	Sterilization of linen, dressings, gloves, syringes, Reusable instruments, Culture media and stock solution	Autoclave (Temperature: 121-149°C, Pressure: 15-51 psi, Time: -60–30 min)	Cost effective and No/ Minimum environmental emissions	Not suitable for anatomical, pharmaceutical, Pathologic, Chemical and Cytotoxic waste
	Dry Treatment	Infectious waste and sharp	Screw Feed Technology	Reduction in volume (80%) and weight (20%-35%)	Not suitable for Pathologic, Cytotoxic or Radioactive waste
	Microwave (Heat up waste from inside)	Needle, syringes, tubings, catheters (Recyclable Plastics/ Metal)	Exposure to microwaves 2450 MHz and Wave length 12.24 cm	Efficient, Environmentally sound, drastic volume reduction	High investment and operating cost
	Plasma arc (6000°C)	Nonrecyclable matter	Plasma torch	Reduction in volume (Plasma – Ionized gas)	High investment

Contd...

Technologies	Principles	Applicable for	Methods	Advantages	Disadvantages
Chemical	Destroy pathogens from inanimate objects Contact period (30 min-1 hour)	Sharps and Instruments contaminated with blood/ body fluid Contaminated floors/surfaces/ clothes/beds/ beddings/ bed pans Wet mopping-ICU/OT/ Wards Liquid waste - blood, urine, stools or hospital sewage	Sodium Hypochlorite (1-5%) Calcium Hypochlorite (70%) Chloramine (20%) Tincture of Iodine/Povidone Iodine (2.5%) Ethyl/Isopropyl alcohol (70%) Glutaraldehyde (2%) Formaldehyde (40%) Cresol (2.5% /5%)	Easily available, Effective and Cheap	High skilled operation Uses hazardous substance that needs safety measures Inadequate for pharmaceutical, Chemical and some infectious waste (Culture, sharps, etc)
Biological	Compost is a mixture of decaying organic matter like dead leaves, excreta, etc.)	Suitable for biodegradable waste Good for soil building (fertilizing land)	Composting, Vermicomposting	Yields manure and fuel (methane/ gobar gas)	Not suitable for non biodegradable waste Hazards involved in handling human excreta and Fly breeding in compost heap

- Effectiveness of thermal sterilization is checked by Bacillus stearothermophilus test and chemical sterilization by Bacillus subtilis test.

INCINERATION AND AUTOCLAVE

- ***Incineration (Mass burn technology)*** is a high temperature dry oxidation process that reduces organic and combustible waste to inorganic incombustible matter.

Advantages

- Reduction of waste-volume (85–95%) and weight (30%).
- No pretreatment is needed
- It has zero occupational hazard

Incineration is *not* suitable for:
- Pressurized gas containers
- Reactive chemicals (Large amounts) and cytotoxic drugs
- Silver salts and photographic/radiographic waste
- Halogenated plastics (PVC)
- Waste with high mercury (Broken thermometers) or Cadmium content (used batteries, lead-lined wooden panels, etc)
- Sealed ampoules containing heavy metals
- Sharps.

184 ***High Yield Points***

Incineration is suitable for :
Wastes that cannot be Recycled, Reused or Disposed of in a land fill[Q]

118 **Good to Remember**

Types of Incinerators:

- *Double Chamber Pyrolytic Incinerator*- especially designed for infectious health-care waste.
- *Single Chamber Furnaces with Static Grate*- used only if pyrolytic incinerator are not affordable.
- Rotary kilns operating at high temperature- Genotoxic substances and heat-resistant chemicals

185 **High Yield Points**

Inertization: Process of mixing cement with waste material before disposal.

Objective: To minimize the risk of toxic substances in the waste material.

Example:

- 65% pharmaceutical waste
- 15% lime with
- 15% cement and
- 5% water

Later the mixture is transported to a safe site for using

Operating Standards for Incinerator

- Combustion efficiency (CE) of at least 99.00%. The combustion efficiency is computed as follows:

  C.E = [% CO/(% CO + % CO)] × 100
- Temperature of primary chamber- 800°C.
- Temperature of secondary chamber- 1050 ± 50°C, Gas residence time at least 2 seconds, Oxygen in stack gas a minimum of 3%.
- Temperature of waste gas leaving secondary chamber brought down immediately to 230°C.

Incinerator Emission Standards: Concentration (mg/Nm^3)

- Particulate matter- 50
- Nitrogen oxides (NO and NO_2)- 400
- HCl- 50
- Total Dioxins and Furans- 0.1 ng TEQ/Nm^3 (at 11% O_2)
- Hg and its compounds- 0.05
- Minimum stack height of 30 meter above ground Fuel used in incinerator- low sulfur fuel like LDO/LSHS/Diesel/Compressed Natural Gas/Liquefied Natural Gas or Liquefied Petroleum Gas.

Operating Standards for Disposal by Plasma Pyrolysis or Gasification

- Combustion Efficiency (CE) shall be at least 99.99%.
- The temperature of the combustion chamber after plasma gasification shall be 1050 ± 50°C with gas residence time of at least 2 seconds, with minimum 3% Oxygen in the stack gas.
- The stack height should be minimum of 30 m above ground level.

Operating Standards for Autoclaving of Biomedical Waste

Gravity Flow Autoclave

Table 3: Operating standards for gravity flow autoclave

Temperature	Pressure	Time
Not less than 121°C	15 pounds per square inch (psi)	60 minutes
Not less than 135°C	31 pounds per square inch (psi)	45 minutes
Not less than 149°C	52 pounds per square inch (psi)	30 minutes

Vacuum Autoclave

BMW is subjected to pre-vacuum pulse (minimum 3) to purge the autoclave of all air. The air removed is decontaminated by HEPA and activated carbon filtration, steam treatment or any other method to prevent release of pathogen.

Table 4: Operating standards for vacuum autoclave

Temperature	Pressure	Time
Not less than 121°C	15 pounds per square inch (psi)	45 minutes
Not less than 135°C	31 pounds per square inch (psi)	30 minutes

Hydroclave

It is an advanced autoclave with consistently high sterility and much more even heat penetration.

- It is ideal for treating all infectious waste (except anatomical and cytotoxic waste) even bulk liquid and pathological
- There is complete dehydration of the waste and volume of waste is reduced by 70%.
- There is no harmful emission and operating cost is also very low. Steam used for sterilization is recycled

Level III disinfection: Decontamination of wastes to destroy spores of Bacillus subtilis at a concentration of 104 per mL

114 **Must Remember**

"3 R" or Green approach is the best solution for waste management.
It comprises of Reduce, Reuse and Recycle

COMMON MEDICAL WASTE TREATMENT FACILITIES (CTF)

It ensures safe collection, transportation, treatment and disposal of biomedical waste by an entrepreneur, a cooperative or the government on a pay-and-use basis

- Location: Reasonably away from residential and sensitive areas and near to area of its operation.
- Land Requirement: Minimum 1 acre.
- Coverage area: 10,000 beds or within radius of 150 km

Green purchasing or EPP (Environmentally Preferable Purchasing) aims to reduce harm to human health and environment by integrating environmental considerations into all stages of the purchasing process.

E.g. Substituting mercury thermometers with digital alternatives

Cradle to grave approach analyses the environmental impact of a product or service throughout its life cycle. Eco-labels are based on this approach – E.g. European label -"the flower", Scandinavian label -"the Nordic swan".

119 **Good to Remember**

Zero Waste means designing, managing products and processes to systematically avoid and eliminate the volume and toxicity of wastes, conserve and recover all resources. Implementing Zero Waste will eliminate all discharges to land, water or air that are a threat to human, animal or plant health.

BIOMEDICAL WASTE (MANAGEMENT AND HANDLING) RULES, 2016

- It applies to all those who generate, collect, receive, store, transport, dispose, treat or handle biomedical waste in any form.

  Biomedical Waste (Management and Handling) Rules, 2016 is ***not*** applicable to:
- Radioactive wastes covered under the Atomic Energy Act, 1962
- Hazardous chemicals covered under the Manufacture, Storage and Import of Hazardous Chemicals Rules, 1989
- Solid wastes covered under the Municipal Solid Waste (Management and Handling) Rules, 2000
- Lead acid batteries covered under the Batteries (Management and Handling) Rules, 2001
- Hazardous wastes covered under the Hazardous Wastes (Management, Handling and Transboundary Movement) Rules, 2008
- E-Waste covered under the e-Waste (Management and Handling) Rules, 2011
- Hazardous microorganisms, genetically engineered microorganisms and cells covered under the Manufacture, Use, Import, Export and Storage of Hazardous Microorganisms, Genetically Engineered Microorganisms or Cells Rules, 1989

The salient features of BMW Management Rules, 2016 include:

- The ambit of the rules has been expanded to include vaccination camps, blood donation camps, surgical camps or any other healthcare activity.
- Phase-out the use of chlorinated plastic bags, gloves and blood bags within two years.
- Pretreatment of the laboratory waste, microbiological waste, blood samples and blood bags through disinfection or sterilization on-site in the manner as prescribed by WHO or NACO.
- Provide training to all its health care workers and immunize all health workers regularly.
- Establish a Bar-Code System for bags or containers containing biomedical waste for disposal.
- Report major accidents.

- Existing incinerators to achieve the standards for retention time in secondary chamber and Dioxin and Furans within two years.
- Biomedical waste has been classified into 4 categories instead 10 to improve the segregation of waste at source.
- Procedure to get authorization simplified. Automatic authorization for bedded hospitals. The validity of authorization synchronized with validity of consent orders for Bedded HCFs. One time authorization for nonbedded HCFs.
- The new rules prescribe more stringent standards for incinerator to reduce the emission of pollutants in environment.
- Inclusion of emissions limits for Dioxin and furans.
- State Government to provide land for setting up common bio-medical waste treatment and disposal facility.
- No occupier shall establish on-site treatment and disposal facility, if a service of common biomedical waste treatment facility is available at a distance of seventy-five kilometer.
- Operator of a common biomedical waste treatment and disposal facility to ensure the timely collection of bio-medical waste from the HCFs and assist the HCFs in conduct of training.
- To immunize all its health care workers and others involved in handling of biomedical waste for protection against diseases including Hepatitis B and Tetanus that are likely to be transmitted by handling of biomedical waste.

Note: The quantum of waste generated in India is estimated to be 1–2 kg/day/bed in a hospital and 600 g/day/bed in a clinic.

Table 5: Biomedical waste management rules 2016

Categories	Waste types	Includes	Types of bag or containers	Treatment and disposal
Yellow	Human anatomical waste	Human tissues, organs, body parts, fetus	Yellow non-chlorinated plastic bags	Incineration or Plasma Pyrolysis or Deep burial*
	Animal waste	Animal tissues, body parts, organs, carcasses, fluids, blood	Yellow non-chlorinated plastic bags	Incineration or Plasma Pyrolysis or Deep burial*
	Soiled waste	Items contaminated with blood, and fluids, including cotton, dressing, soiled plaster casts, linen, beddings	Yellow non-chlorinated plastic bags	Incineration or Plasma Pyrolysis or Deep burial* In absence of above facilities Autoclaving or Microwaving/ Hydroclaving followed by shredding or mutilation and Energy Recovery from treated waste
	Expired or Discarded medicines and Cytotoxic drugs	Outdated contaminated and discarded medicine	Yellow non-chlorinated plastic bags or Container	Cytotoxic waste or items contaminated with cytotoxic drug to be returned to manufacturer/ common BMW treatment facility for incineration at >1200°C or Encapsulation or plasma pyrolysis at 1200°C Other medicines returned to manufacturer or Incinerated
	Chemicals	Chemical used in disinfection (insecticides) or in production of biologicals	Yellow containers or non-chlorinated plastic bags	Incineration or encapsulation or plasma pyrolysis

Contd...

Categories	Waste types	Includes	Types of bag or containers	Treatment and disposal
	Chemical Liquid waste	Waste from lab and washing, cleaning, housekeeping and disinfecting activities	Separate collection system leading to effluent treatment system	Resource recovery followed by pretreatment and discharge into drains
	Discarded linen, mat- tresses, beddings contaminated with blood or body fluid		Yellow non-chlorinated bags or suitable packing material	Nonchlorinated chemical disinfection followed by Incineration or Plasma Pyrolysis or Energy recovery. In absence of above facilities, shredding or mutilation or combination of sterilization and shredding. Treated waste to be sent for energy recovery or incineration or plasma pyrolysis
	Microbiology and Biotechnology waste	Waste from lab cultures, stocks, specimens of microorganisms, live and attenuated vaccines, Waste from the production of biologicals and toxins	Autoclave safe plastic bags or containers	Pretreat to sterilize with nonchlorinated chemicals on-site as per NACO or WHO guidelines thereafter Incineration
Red	Contaminated Waste (Recyclable)	Tubing, Bottles, IV tubes and sets, Catheters, Urine bags, Syringes (without needles and *fixed needle syringes*) and vacutainers with needle cut and gloves	Red non-chlorinated plastic bags or Container	Autoclaving or Micro-waving/ Hydroclaving followed by shredding or mutilation and waste sent to registered recyclers or for energy recovery/road making Plastic waste should not be sent to landfill sites
White (Translucent)	Waste sharps	Needles, syringes, blades, scalpels, glass	Puncture Proof, Leak proof, tamper proof containers	Autoclaving or Dry Heat Sterilization followed by shredding or mutilation or encapsulation in metal container or cement concrete Or sent for final disposal to iron foundries or sanitary landfill or designated concrete waste sharp pit
Blue	Glassware Metallic Body Implants	Broken or discarded and contaminated	Cardboard boxes with blue colored marking	Disinfection (cleaning with detergent and soaking in Sodium Hypochlorite) or Autoclaving or Microwaving or Hydroclaving and then sent for recycling

*Deep burial is permitted only in rural or remote areas where there is no access to common biomedical waste treatment facility

Features

- Chemical treatment using at least 1% hypochlorite solution or any other equivalent chemical reagent. It must be ensured that chemical solution has adequate strength to disinfect all the time during the chemical treatment.
- There will be no chemical pretreatment before incineration. Chlorinated plastics/bags shall not be incinerated.
- Disposal of biomedical waste by deep burial shall be prohibited in Towns and Cities. Disposal by deep burial is permitted only in rural areas where there is no access to common biomedical waste treatment facility, with prior approval from the prescribed authority. The deep burial facility shall be located as per provisions and guidelines issued by Central Pollution Control Board from time to time.
- Liquid waste generated from laboratory, washing, cleaning, housekeeping and disinfecting activities shall be treated along with other effluent generated from premises of the occupier or the facility operator so as to meet the discharge standards stipulated under these rules.

186 *High Yield Points*

As per Schedule I of the Biomedical Waste Management Rules, 2016 following color coding and type of container/bags is needed to be used by the HCFs for segregation and collection of generated Biomedical Waste from the facility

Table 6: Categories as per BMW 2016 and types of container

S. No	Category	Type of waste	Color and type of container
1.	Yellow	▪ Human anatomical waste ▪ Animal anatomical waste ▪ Soiled waste ▪ Discarded or expired medicine ▪ Microbiology, biotechnology and other clinical laboratory waste ▪ Chemical waste ▪ Chemical liquid waste	Yellow colored nonchlorinated plastic bags (having thickness equal to more than 50 μ) or containers 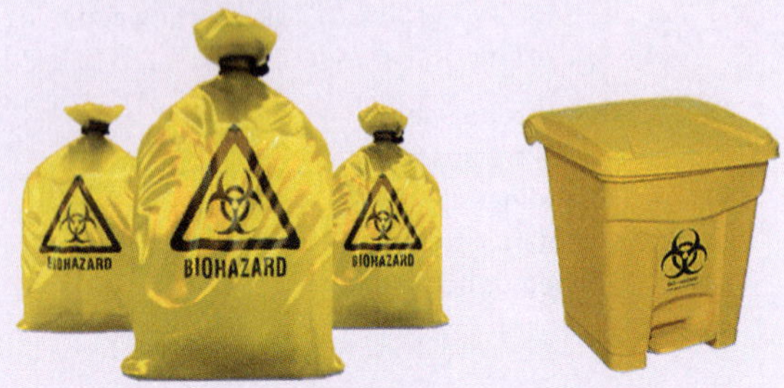 **Note** ▪ Chemical liquid waste such as spent hypo of X-ray should be stored in yellow container and sold to recycler authorized by SPCD/PCC ▪ Infected secretions, aspired body fluids etc. from laboratory should be disinfected before mixing with other wastewater from hospital ▪ Liquid chemical wastes should be pretreated/neutralized before mixing with other wastewater from hospital.
2.	Red	Contaminated waste (Recyclable)	Red colored nonchlorinated plastic bags (having thickness equal to more than 50 μ) and containers 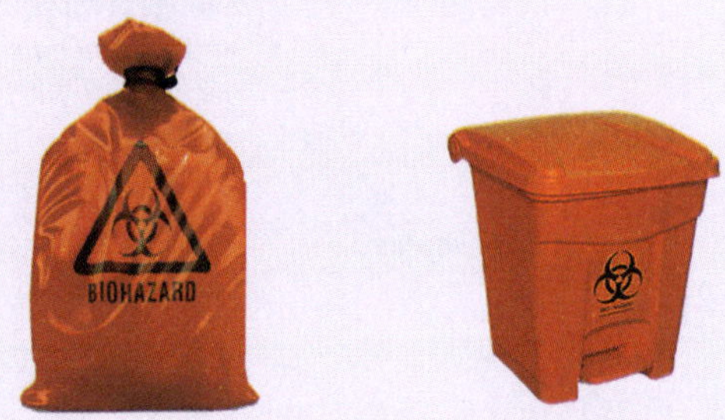
3.	White	Waste sharps including metals	White colored translucent, puncture proof, leak proof, temper proof containers 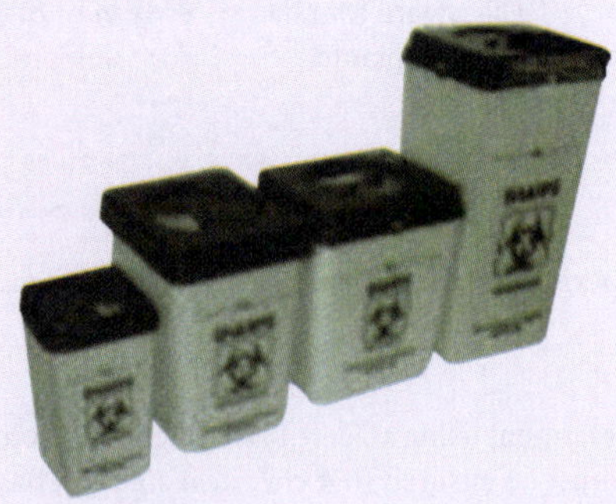
4.	Blue	▪ Glassware ▪ Metallic body implants	Cardboard boxes with blue colored marking or blue colored puncture proof, temper proof containers 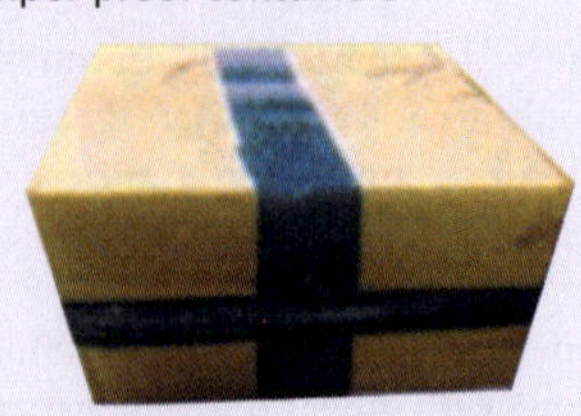 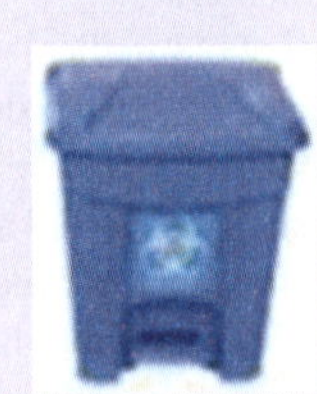 Cardboard box with blue marking

Effluent Treatment Plant

Effluent treatment plant should be provided in every HCF to treat the wastewater generated from the hospital in order to comply with the effluent standards prescribed under the BMWM Rules, 2016.

STANDARDS FOR LIQUID WASTE

The effluent generated or treated from the premises of occupier or operator of a common biomedical waste treatment facility, before discharge should conform to the following limits:

Table 7: Parameters and permissible limits for liquid waste

Parameters	Permissible limits
pH	6.5–9.0
Suspended solids	100 mg/L
Oil and grease	10 mg/L
BOD	30 mg/L
COD	250 mg/L
Bio-assay test	90% survival of fish after 96 hours in 100% effluent

187 *High Yield Points*

Guidelines for Sharps Disposal in Health Facility without BMW Treatment Facility

Health care facilities located where no CBWTF is available at a distance of 75 km and also not within the feasible coverage area of any nearby CBWTF, the treatment and disposal of BMW can be carried out in secured deep burial pits and sharp pits as per the authorization of SPCBs/PCCs

- Sharp pit must be a 1 mt × 1 mt × 1 mt concrete lined protected pit with a cemented lid
- Disposal of the sharp containers need to be done by discarding the containers in entirety into the sharp pits

The effluent treatment plant is given below:

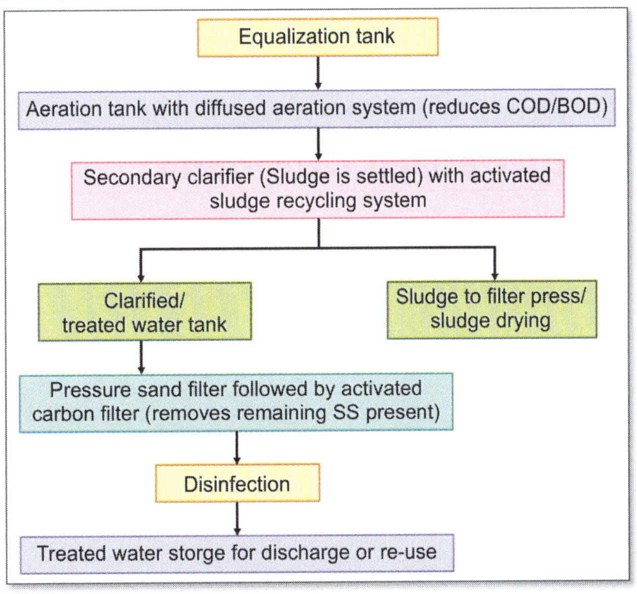

Fig. 1: Effluent treatment plant

LABELING FOR HOSPITAL AND BIOMEDICAL WASTE

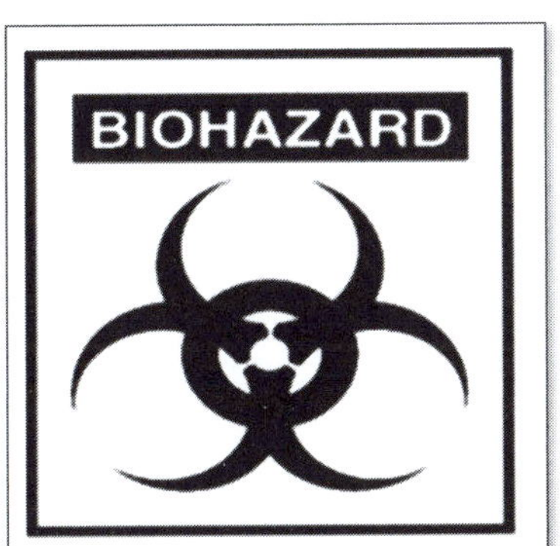

Fig. 2: Biohazard label

Fig. 3: Cytotoxic label

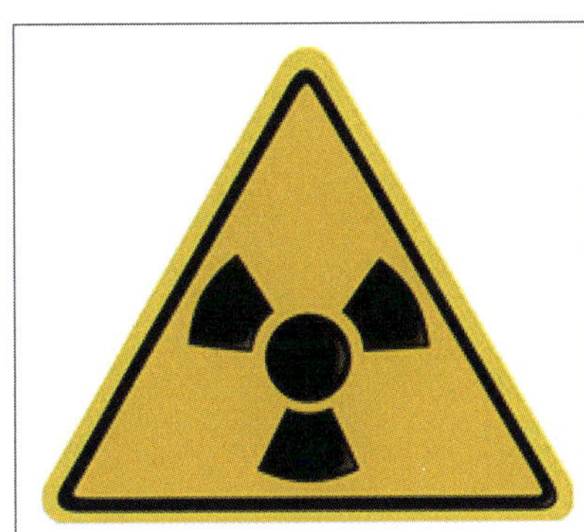

Fig. 4: Radiation hazard symbol

Image-Based Questions

1. Symbol shown in figure is used for:

a. Cytotoxic substance
b. Biohazardous substance
c. Radioactive substance
d. Carcinogenic substance

2. Identify the instrument in figure shown in:

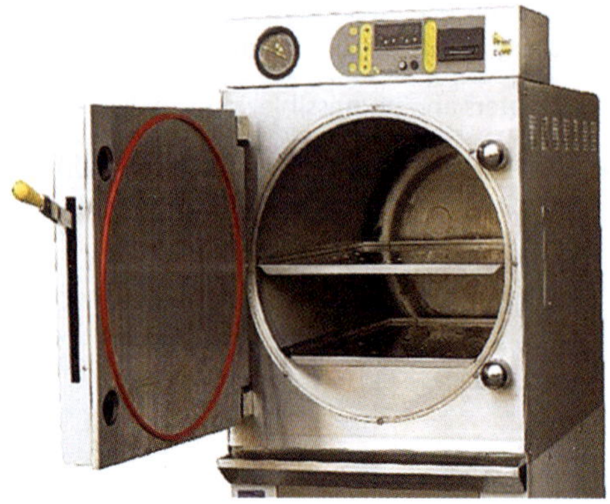

a. Autoclave
b. Incinerator
c. Microwave
d. Hot air oven

Answers of Image-Based Questions

1. **Ans. (b) Biohazardous substance**

2. **Ans. (a) Autoclave**

Multiple Choice Questions

1. **Cytotoxic and expired drug disposal is done by which method?** *(Recent Question 2018)*
   a. Dumping
   b. Autoclave
   c. Landfill
   d. Burning
2. **Which of the following wastes are disposed in the bag shown below:** *(AIIMS May 2017)*

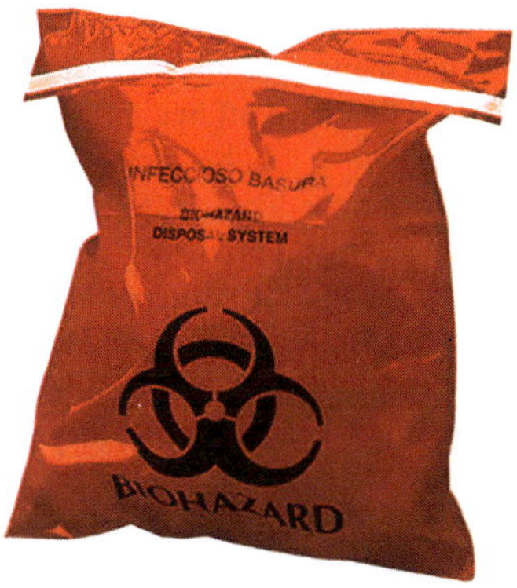

   a. Discarded catheter b. Empty blood bags
   c. Empty urine bags d. Waste needles
3. **Human anatomical waste is disposed of by:**
   a. Deep burial
   b. Incineration
   c. Chemical treatment
   d. Destruction and shredding

DISINFECTION

4. **Glass is sterilized by:** *(Recent Question 2017)*
   a. Incineration at 105°C for 5–10 minutes
   b. Autoclaving at 121°C for 30–60 minutes
   c. Hot air oven 160°C for 30–60 minutes
   d. Hot air oven 121°C for 30–60 minutes
5. **Which of the following is an Anti-viral agent?** *(Recent Question 2017)*
   a. Chlorhexidine
   b. Betapropionolactone
   c. Hypochlorite
   d. Phenol
6. **All of the following are Dry heat sterilization methods, except:**
   a. Flaming
   b. Incineration
   c. Hot air oven
   d. Autoclaving
7. **Fibreoptic scopes are sterilized by:**
   a. Glutaraldehyde
   b. Ethylene oxide
   c. Alcohol
   d. Autoclave
8. **The amount of bleaching powder necessary to disinfect cholera stools is:** *(Recent Question 2017)*
   a. 50 g/L
   b. 75 g/L
   c. 90 g/L
   d. 100 g/L
9. **Disinfection of urine is which type of disinfection:**
   a. Precurrent b. Concurrent
   c. Preconcurrent d. Terminal
10. **Oils and powders are sterilized by:**
    a. Autoclaving
    b. Microwave
    c. Hydroclave
    d. Hot air oven
11. **Sputum can be disinfected by all except:**
    a. Autoclaving
    b. Boiling
    c. Cresol
    d. Chlorhexidine
12. **Which is false regarding Spaulding's criteria?**
    a. Noncritical items require only decontamination
    b. Semicritical items are those which come in contact with mucous membranes or nonintact skin
    c. Semi critical items need low level disinfection
    d. Cardiac catheters are example of critical items
13. **There is an outbreak of MRSA in the hospital wards. Which of the following is the appropriate mode of containing the spread of infection?** *(Recent Question 2016)*
    a. Vancomycin given empirically to all patients
    b. Proper hand washing by all medical staff before and after attending patients
    c. Hospital staff wear masks
    d. Fumigating the ward frequently
14. **Savlon contains:** *(Recent Question 2015)*
    a. Cetrimide + Chlorhexidine
    b. Cetrimide + Chlorhexidine + Butyl alcohol
    c. Cetrimide + Butyl alcohol
    d. Cetrimide + Cetavlon
15. **Sterilization and disinfection of blood spills is done by:**
    a. Formaldehyde
    b. Sodium hypochloridte
    c. Tincture iodine
    d. Phenols

Ans.

1.	c
2.	c
3.	b
4.	c
5.	b
6.	d
7.	a
8.	a
9.	b
10.	d
11.	d
12.	c
13.	b
14.	a
15.	b

Most Recent Questions of 2019-18 are given at the end of MCQs

GENERAL VACCINE

16. Syringes and glassware are sterilized by:
a. Irradiation b. Autoclave
c. Hot air oven d. Glutaraldehyde

TREATMENT AND DISPOSAL TECHNOLOGIES

17. Brick incinerator is used for: *(Recent Question 2015)*
a. Waste sharp b. Discarded medicine
c. Infectious waste d. Disposable items

18. In hospitals, noninfectious human wastes are thrown in which colored bag:
a. Black b. Green
c. Yellow d. Red

19. All are true about inertization, except:
a. Mixing biomedical waste with cement
b. Used for pharmaceutical waste
c. Contaminates water sources
d. Not useful for infectious waste

20. All are true regarding screw-feed technology of waste disposal, except: *(Recent Question 2015)*
a. A method of dry thermal disinfection process
b. Waste reduced by 80% in volume and 20–35% in weight
c. Not suitable for treating infectious wastes and sharps
d. Should not be used for pathological, radioactive or cytotoxic wastes

21. Not true about screw feed technique is:
a. 80% volume reduction
b. Pathological waste are removed
c. Weight is decreased by 20–30%
d. Based on nonburn thermal treatment

22. Non true regarding incineration:
a. Pre-treatment with appropriate chemical needed for optimum results
b. Double chamber pyrolytic incinerators-to burn infectious health-care waste
c. Combustible matter > 60%
d. Moisture content <30%

23. The following waste is suitable for incineration:
a. Low heating volume
b. Pressurized gas containers
c. Reactive chemical wastes
d. Chlorinated plastics

24. Incineration is done for: *(Recent Question 2015)*
a. Waste sharps b. Human anatomical waste
c. Radiographic waste d. Used batteries

25. Good for soil building is:
a. Incineration b. Controlled tipping
c. Composting d. Dumping

26. Placental waste generated after delivery is disposed of by
a. Autoclave
b. Incineration
c. Microwave
d. Disposal in blue bags

27. Disposal of placenta at PHC is done by:
a. Dry burning
b. Deep burial
c. Boiling
d. Treat with bleaching powder and burial

28. Disinfection followed by Mutilation-Shredding is the method of choice for disposal of: *(Recent Question 2014)*
a. Sharps waste b. Solid waste
c. Biotechnology waste d. Human anatomical waste

29. Incineration is not done for: *(Recent Question 2014)*
a. Anatomical waste
b. Sharp waste
c. Cytotoxic waste
d. Radioactive waste
e. Animal waste

30. True about incinerator is/are:
a. Red bag can be incinerated
b. No pretreatment required
c. Yellow bag must be incinerated
d. Sharps must not be incinerated
e. Combustible matter must be above 30%

31. Animal waste is disposed off by:
a. Autoclaving b. Incineration
c. Chemical treatment d. Microwave

32. A known HIV positive patient is admitted in an isolation ward after an abdominal surgery following an accident. The resident doctor who changed his dressing the next day found it to be soaked in blood. Which of the following would be the right method of choice of discarding the dressing: *(Recent Question 2013)*
a. Pour 1% hypochlorite on the dressing material and send it for incineration in an appropriate bag
b. Pour 5% hypochlorite on the dressing material and send it for incineration in an appropriate bag
c. Put the dressing material directly in an appropriate bag and send for incineration
d. Pour 2% Lysol on the dressing material and send it for incineration in an appropriate bag

33. Incineration is not done for:
a. Cytotoxic waste
b. Waste Sharp
c. Human Anatomical Waste
d. Cotton contaminated by blood

34. Safe disposal of mercury is by: *(Recent Question 2013)*
a. Collect carefully and recycle
b. Controlled combustion
c. Chemical treatment
d. Deep burial

CATEGORIES OF BMW

35. Category 5 of biomedical waste indicates:
a. Waste sharps *(Recent Question 2013)*
b. Cytotoxic waste
c. Human anatomical waste
d. Biotechnology waste

36. Waste sharps belong to which category of biomedical waste:
a. 1 b. 2
c. 3 d. 4

37. Category 7 of biomedical waste in India includes:
a. Solid waste
b. Liquid waste
c. Microbiological waste
d. Discarded medicines

Ans.

16. c
17. c
18. a
19. c
20. c
21. b
22. a
23. a
24. b
25. c
26. b
27. b
28. b
29. b,c d
30. b,d
31. b
32. c
33. b
34. a
35. b
36. d
37. a

Most Recent Questions of 2019-18 are given at the end of MCQs

38. Category 7 on biomedical waste management contains:
a. Soiled waste b. Solid waste
c. Liquid waste d. Incineration waste

39. Amount of infectious waste among hospital waste is:
a. 1.5% b. 4.5%
c. 25% d. 12%

COLOR CODED SEGREGATION

40. Category 2 wastes are disposed in which bag:
a. Yellow b. Red
c. Black d. Blue

41. Incinerated is method of choice for all, except: *(Recent Question 2014)*
a. Human anatomical waste
b. Infected solid waste
c. Animal waste
d. Broken thermometers

42. Waste sharps are discarded in which color bin:
a. Yellow b. Red
c. Blue/white translucent d. Black

43. Color coding of container for disposal of human anatomical waste is: *(Recent Question 2014)*
a. Yellow b. Red
c. Blue d. Black

44. Waste sharp should be disposed in:
a. Black bag b. Yellow bag
c. White bag d. Red bag

45. Disposal mechanism for black color coded biomedical waste bag is: *(Recent Question 2013)*
a. Incineration b. Dumping
c. Shredding d. Landfill

46. Discarded and expired medicines are to be thrown into:
a. Blue bag b. Black bag
c. Yellow bag d. Red bag

47. Discarded cytotoxic medicines should be disposed in:
a. Blue bag
b. Black bag
c. Red bag
d. Yellow bag

48. Biomedical waste to be discarded in yellow bag is:
a. Human anatomical waste
b. Animal waste
c. Microbiological waste
d. Waste sharps
e. Soiled waste

49. Plastic cover of syringes is disposed in:
a. Red bag
b. Yellow bag
c. Black bag
d. Blue bag

50. All of the following regarding BMW management are true, except: *(Recent Question 2013)*
a. Human anatomical waste is thrown in yellow bag
b. Blue bag waste is disposed by landfill
c. Incineration ash is disposed in black bag
d. Materials in red bag can be a source of contamination

51. Color coded bag not to be incinerated as it contains Cadmium is:
a. Black bag
b. Yellow bag
c. Blue bag
d. Red bag

52. Yellow plastic bags containing biomedical wastes are treated by: *(Recent Question 2013)*
a. Autoclaving
b. Incineration
c. Microwaving
. Shredding

Most Recent Questions (2019–2018)

53. Following blood transfusion, blood bags are disposed which colour coded bin: *(AIIMS Nov 2018)*
a. Red b. Yellow
c. Blue d. White

54. The depicted image below represents: *(AIIMS Nov 2018)*

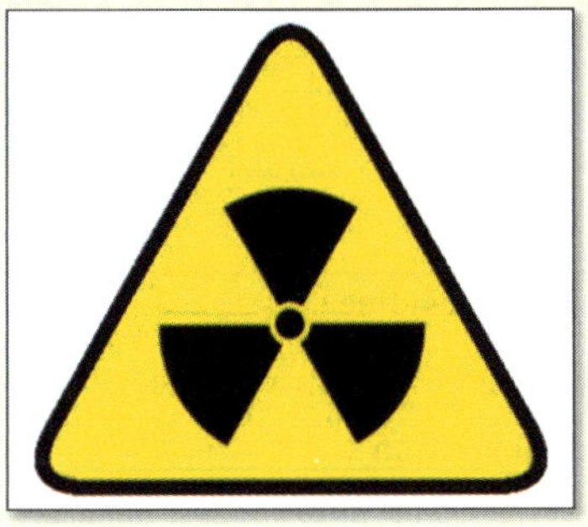

a. Biomedical waste b. Cytotoxic waste
c. Radiation hazard d. Bioterrorism

55. Biomedical waste management in Match the following: *(AIIMS May 2019)*

Correct Match is

a. Yellow	1. Glassware
b. Red	2. Scalpel
c. Blue	3. Cytotoxic waste
d. White	4. Gloves
	5. Syringe Wrapper

Ans.

38. b
39. a
40. a
41. d
42. c
43. a
44. c
45. d
46. b
47. d
48. a, b, c, e
49. c
50. b
51. c
52. b
53. b
54. c
55. a-3, b-4, c-1, d-2

Answers with Explanations

1. Ans. (c) Landfill

Ref: K. Park, 24th ed. p 830

2. Ans. (c) Empty urine bags

Ref: K. Park, 24th ed. p 830

3. Ans. (b) Incineration

DISINFECTION

4. Ans. (c) Hot air oven 160°C for 30-60 minutes

Ref: K. Park, 24th ed. p 129

Hot air oven is used for sterilizing articles such as glassware, syringes, swabs, dressing, oils and sharp instruments.

- It lacks penetrating power and is therefore not suitable for disinfection of bulky articles such as mattresses.
- A high temperature of about 160–180°C is maintained for at least one hour to kill spores.
- Heat generated can destroy plastic, rubber and other delicate substances, so not used for such items

5. Ans. (b) Betapropionolactone

Ref: Van der Groen G. Use of betapropionolactone inactivated Ebola, Marburg and Lassa intracellular antigens in immunofluorescent antibody assay. Ann SocBelg Med Trop. 1982 Mar; 62(1):49-54

Betapropionolactone is an antiviral agent and is used in inactivation of Ebola, Marburg and Lassa intracellular antigens in immunofluorescent antibody assay.

6. Ans. (d) Autoclaving

Ref: Textbook of Microbiology and Immunology. Subhash Chandra Parija,p-25

Heat Sterilization

Dry heat →Red heat, Flaming, Incineration, Hot air oven
Moist heat

- Sterilization at <100°C – Pasteurization,
- Sterilization at 100°C – Boiling, Steam sterilizer at 100°C (Koch and Arnold Steamer)
- Sterilization at >100°C–Autoclave, Intermittent Sterilization (Tyndallisation)

Also Know......................

- Efficiency of Hot air oven is tested by Bacillus Subtilis and Autoclave by Geobacillus Stearothermophilus.

7. Ans. (a) Glutaraldehyde

Ref: CDC Guideline for Disinfection and Sterilization in Healthcare Facilities, 2008

Fibreoptic scopes are heat-sensitive medical devices hence cannot be autoclaved.

Chemical sterilants and high-level disinfectants that have been cleared by FDA and marketed include:

- ≥2.4% Glutaraldehyde,
- 0.55% Ortho-phthalaldehyde (OPA)
- 0.95% Glutaraldehyde with 1.64% phenol/phenate
- 7.35% hydrogen peroxide with 0.23% peracetic acid
- 1.0% hydrogen peroxide with 0.08% peracetic acid 7.5% hydrogen peroxide

8. Ans. (a) 50 gm/L

Ref: K. Park, 24th ed. p 138

Disinfection of cholera stool is concurrent and terminal

- *Most effective disinfectant* is→A coal- tar disinfectant with a Rideal-Walker (RW) coefficient of ≥10 e.g. Cresol. A disinfectant with a RW coefficient <5 should not be used.
- Bedpans/Urinals should ideally be steam disinfected or disinfected with 2.5% cresol for an hour after cleaning.
- Bleaching powder (50 g/L -5%), Crude phenol (100 ml/L-10%), Cresol (50 ml/L-5%), Formalin (100 ml/L-10%) are suitable for **disinfection of Feces and Urine**

If none is available → Equal amount of quicklime or freshly prepared milk of lime may be added, mixed and left for 2 hours.

Or

A bucket of boiling water may be added to the feces which is then covered and allowed to stand until cool.

9. Ans. (b) Concurrent

Ref: K. Park, 24th ed. p 136-37

Disinfection kills infectious agents outside the body by direct exposure to chemical or physical agents.

- ***Concurrent disinfection*** is application of disinfective measures to kill disease agent as soon as it is released from body. E.g. Disinfection of urine, feces, vomit, contaminated linen, clothes etc throughout course of illness.
- ***Terminal disinfection*** is application of disinfective measures after the patient has been removed by death or has ceased to be a source of infection or hospital isolation practices have been discontinued. It is scarcely practiced
- ***Precurrent (prophylactic) disinfection*** is disinfection of water by chlorine, pasteurization of milk and handwashing

10. Ans. (d) Hot air oven

Ref: K. Park, 24th ed. p 137

Hot air oven is used for sterilizing glassware, syringes, swabs, dressing, oils and sharp instruments

11. Ans. (d) Chlorhexidine

Ref: K. Park, 24th ed. p 137-38

Sputum Disinfection

- *Sputum received in gauze or paper handkerchiefs are burnt.*
- *If the amount is large it is disinfected by boiling or autoclaving for 20 minutes at 20 lbs pressure.*

- *Patient is asked to spit in a sputum cup half filled with 5% cresol. When full, the cup is allowed to stand for an hour and then disposed of.*

12. Ans. (c) Semi critical items need low level disinfection

Ref:http://www.cdc.gov/hicpac/Disinfection_Sterilization/2_approach.html

Spaulding's criteria→Spaulding divided hospital usable into 3 categories:

- **Critical items**→ Items which enter sterile body tissue or vascular system.
  - Example → Surgical instruments, Cardiac and urinary catheters, Implants and Ultrasound probes used in sterile body cavities.
  - Such items should be bought sterile or sterilized with steam or chemical sterilants with strict guideline adherence.
- **Semi-critical items**→ Items which come in contact with intact mucous membrane or non-intact skin
  - Example → Respiratory therapy and anesthesia equipment, Endoscopes, Laryngoscope blades, Oesophageal manometry probes, Cystoscopes, Anorectal manometry catheters and diaphragm fitting rings.
  - Such items need minimal high level disinfection or intermediate level disinfection
- **Non-critical items** → Items which come in contact with intact skin but not with mucous membrane.
  - Example → Bedpans, Blood pressure cuffs, Crutches and Computers.
  - Such items need just decontamination using low level disinfectants.

13. Ans. (b) Proper hand washing by all medical staff before and after attending patients

Ref: http://www.goapic.org/MRSA.htm

Infection control measures for MRSA include:

- *Hand washing,*
- *Gloving*
- *Linen handling*
- *Environmental cleaning.*

Also Know.......................

- *Hand washing is the single most important factor in preventing the spread of MRSA*

14. Ans. (a) Cetrimide + chlorhexidine

Ref: K. Park, 24th ed. p 138

Savlon is a combination of Cetavlon (Cetrimide) and Hibitane (Chlorhexidine).

- Plastic appliances (e.g. Lippes loop) may be disinfected by keeping them in normal strength Savlon for 20 minutes.
- Savlon 1 in 6 in spirit is more effective than Savlon 1 in 20 aqueous solutions.
- Clinical thermometers are best disinfected in Savlon 1 in 6 in spirit in 3 minutes.

Dettol (Chloroxylenol) is a relatively nontoxic antiseptic.

- It is active against streptococci, but worthless against some gram-negative bacteria.
- Dettol (5%) is suitable for disinfection of instruments and plastic equipment
- A contact of at least 15 minutes is required for disinfection

15. Ans. (b) Sodium hypochlorite

Ref: CDC Guideline for Disinfection and Sterilization in Healthcare Facilities, 2008

Hypochlorites are widely used in healthcare facilities in a variety of settings.

- A 1:10–1:100 dilution of 5.25%–6.15% sodium hypochlorite (household bleach) or an EPA-registered tuberculocidal disinfectant has been recommended for decontaminating blood spills.
- Small spills of blood (i.e. drops) on noncritical surfaces can be disinfected with a 1:100 dilution of 5.25%-6.15% sodium hypochlorite or an EPA-registered tuberculocidal disinfectant.
- Large spills of blood → Surface must be cleaned before an EPA-registered disinfectant or a 1:10 solution of household bleach is applied.

GENERAL VACCINE

16. Ans. (c) Hot air oven

Ref: K. Park, 24th ed. p 137

TREATMENT AND DISPOSAL TECHNOLOGIES

17. Ans. (c) Infectious waste

Ref: K. Park, 24th ed p-830

18. Ans. (a) Black

Ref: K. Park, 23rd ed. p 793-94

Wrapper of surgical syringe constitute noninfectious waste for municipal dump → hence, discarded in Black bag

Noninfectious wastes are disposed of in black bags (Municipal waste)

19. Ans. (c) Contaminates water sources

Ref: K. Park, 24th ed. p 828

Inertization is mixing of biomedical waste with cement *and lime* to form a homogenous mass, that is made into cubes/pellets and transported to suitable storage site

- It minimizes risk of toxic substances contained in the wastes migrating into the surface water or ground water.

Also Know.......................

- *A typical proportion of the mixture is: 65% pharmaceutical waste, 15% lime, 15% cement and 5% water.*

Advantage: Relatively inexpensive
Disadvantage: Not applicable to infectious waste

20. Ans. (c) Not suitable for treating infectious...

Ref: K. Park, 24th ed. p 828

Screw-Feed Technology

- It is a non burn, dry thermal disinfection process (waste is shredded and heated in a rotating auger).
- **Advantage:** Reduction in volume (80%) and weight (20%-35%).
- **Suitable for:** Infectious waste, sharps
- Not suitable for-pathological, cytotoxic and radioactive waste.

21. Ans. (b) Pathological waste are removed

Ref: K. Park, 24th ed. p 828

22. Ans. (a) Pretreatment with appropriate...

Ref: K. Park, 24th ed. p 827

Also Know........................

Characteristics of waste suitable for incineration
- Low heating volume → Single chamber incinerators (>2000 kcal/kg) and Pyrolytic double-chamber incinerators. (>3500 kcal/kg)
- Content of combustible matter above 60%
- Content of non-combustible solids below 5% and non-combustible fines below 20%
- Moisture content below 30%

23. Ans. (a) Low heating volume

Ref: K. Park, 24th ed. p 827

24. Ans. (b) Human anatomical waste

Ref: K. Park, 24th ed. p 827

25. Ans. (c) Composting

Ref: Mahajan and Gupta, Textbook of Preventive and Social Medicine. 4th ed. p-72

Composting is a method of disposal of refuse, alone or in combination with human or animal excreta.
- End product is compost (A organic manure)
- It is good for soil building (fertilizing land) and quite hygienic and paying if done properly.
- Disadvantage - Health hazards involved in handling human excreta and Fly breeding
- It is suitable for communities with population between 5000-100,000.

Also Know........................

Methods of composting:
- Aerobic method- Indore method (Standardized by Sir Albert Howard)
- Anaerobic method- Bangalore method (Indian Institute of Science, Bengaluru and ICAR)
- Some countries like Israel, Switzerland, Germany and Holland use mechanical composting, using aerobic technique

26. Ans. (b) Incineration

Ref: K. Park, 23rd ed. p 793; Refer Annexure 1

As per BMW Management and Handling Rules – 2016, Human anatomical waste falls in Yellow Category

Refer to Annexure

27. Ans. (b) Deep burial

Ref: K. Park, 24th ed. p 830

Human anatomical waste is disposed of by either deep burial or Incineration

Deep burial is ideal for towns with a population less than 5 lakh and in rural areas.
- A pit/ trench about 2 meters deep is dug and covered with galvanized iron/wire mashes.
- Waste is put in the pit and is covered with a 10 cm layer of soil.
- When half filled with waste, it is covered with lime within 50 cm of the surface.

28. Ans. (b) Solid waste

Ref: K. Park, 23rd ed. p 793; Refer Annexure -13.1

Refer to Annexure

29. Ans. (b) Sharp waste; (c) Cytotoxic waste; (d) Radioactive waste

Ref: K. Park, 24th ed. p 827

30. Ans. (b) No pretreatment... (d) Sharps must...

Ref: K. Park, 24th ed. p 828

Incineration is a high temperature dry oxidation process that requires no pre-treatment.
- Red bag is used to segregate category 3, 6, 7 waste – Treated by Chemical disinfection/ Autoclaving/ Microwaving
- Yellow bag is used to segregate category 1, 2, 3 and 6 waste and treated by Incineration.

31. Ans. (b) Incineration

Ref: K. Park, 24th ed. p 827

32. Ans. (c) Put the dressing material directly...

Ref: K. Park, 24th ed. p 830

Also Know........................

- Chlorinated compounds/plastics on incineration release dioxins (human carcinogen) linked to cancer, immune disorders, birth defects, diabetes and disrupted sexual development.
- BMW is the 3rd major source of dioxins in Air.

33. Ans. (b) Waste Sharp

Ref: K. Park, 24th ed. p 827

34. Ans. (a) Collect carefully and recycle

Ref: Biomedical waste management self-learning document for Doctors, superintendents and administrators, EPTRI, Hyderabad

Steps to be followed in case of spillage of mercury:

Do's

- Remove everyone from the area that has been contaminated with mercury.
- Keep the heat below 20°C and ventilate the area if possible.
- Put on personal protective equipment (rubber gloves, goggles/face shield, clothing).

- Remove all jewelry so that mercury cannot combine (amalgamate) with precious metals.
- Locate all mercury beads and collect carefully using a cardboard sheet in a container with some water
- *Dispose of at a hazardous waste facility or Give to a mercury based equipment manufacturer for recycling*

Dont's

- *Never use a broom or vacuum cleaner. Not to be swept into the drain.*

Also Know......................

- **Mercury Spill Cleanup Kit -** Comprises of Gloves (2 pairs), Eye protection, Eye dropper or a syringe, 2 stiff pieces of paper or cardboard, 2 plastic bags, Large tray or box, Duct tape or packing tape, Flashlight and Wide mouth container.
- Any tools used for cleanup should be considered contaminated and disposed of with the mercury.

CATEGORIES OF BMW

35. Ans. (b) Cytotoxic waste (As per BMW Management and Handling...

Ref: K. Park, 24th ed. p 830

- As per biomedical waste (Management and Handling)
- Rules, 2016 – There are only 4 Categories –Yellow, Blue, Red and White. The waste earlier in category 5 (i.e. **Cytotoxic waste**) now falls in Yellow Category

36. Ans. (d) 4 (As per BMW Management and...

Ref: KDT 7th/e p. 604 K. Park, 24th ed. p 830

- As per BMW Management and Handling Rules – 2016, Waste
- Sharps (Previous Category 4) falls in White Category

37. Ans. (a) Solid Waste (As per BMW...

Ref: K. Park, 23rd ed. p 793)

38. Ans. (b) Solid waste

Ref: K. Park, 24th ed. p 830

- As per Schedule 1 (Biomedical Waste Management and Handling Rules, 1998) Category 7 comprises Solid waste
- As per Biomedical waste (Management and Handling)
- Rules, 2016 – There are only 4 Categories –Yellow, Blue, Red and White. The waste earlier in category 7 now falls in Red Category

39. Ans. (a) 1.5%

Ref: K. Park, 24th ed. p 826

Average Composition of Hospital Waste in India
Paper → 15%
Plastics → 10%
Rags→15 %
Metal (sharps etc.) → 1%
Infectious waste →1.5%
Glass → 4%
General waste (food waste, sweepings from hospital premises etc.) → 53.5%

Also Know......................

Health care waste generated in Middle and Low income countries is lower than High income countries
Health care waste generation in developing country (Used for preliminary planning):

- General health-care waste → 80%
- Pathological and infectious waste → 15%
- Sharps waste → 1%
- Chemical and pharmacological waste → 3 %
- Radioactive/Cytotoxic waste, pressurized containers, broken thermometers, used batteries → <1%

COLOR CODED SEGREGATION

40. Ans. (a) Yellow

Ref: Biomedical Waste Management and Handling Rules 2016; 24th ed p-830

Category 2 waste – As per: Biomedical Waste Management and Handling Rules 2016 comprised of Animal Waste and is collected in Yellow bag to be incinerated

41. Ans. (d) Broken thermometers

Ref: K. Park, 24th ed p-827

Refer to notes

42. Ans. (c) Blue/White transluscent (As per...

Ref: K. Park, 24th ed. p 830

As per BMW Management and Handling Rules – 2016 in Puncture Proof , Leak proof, tamper proof containers

43. Ans. (a) Yellow

Ref: K. Park, 24th ed. p 830

44. Ans. (c) White bag (As per BMW Management and Handling Rules -1998)

Ref: K. Park, 24th ed. p 830

As per BMW Management and Handling Rules – 2016, Waste sharps falls in White Category should be disposed of in Puncture Proof, Leak proof, tamper proof containers

45. Ans. (d) Landfill (As per BMW Manage...

Ref: K. Park, 23rd ed. p 794)

Earlier, Category 5 (Discarded medicines or Cytotoxic drug), 9 (Incineration Ash) and 10 (Chemicals used in production of biologicals) were discarded in black plastic bags and disposed of by secured landfill (Bags were not opened up, but pushed as such into landfill).

Sanitary (or Secured) Landfills

- *Result geological isolation of waste from the environment* (Away from residential area)

- *Need appropriate engineering preparation.* (Double lined impermeable clay and pebble base, graded base and stored earth for covering at end of each disposal)
- *Need a onsite staff to control operations*
- *There is organized deposit and daily coverage of waste* (to avoid stray animals)
- *Spray of insecticide is done frequently*

Also Know......................

- Hospital with 100 beds may need a landfill site of 500–600 cu ft.

46. Ans. (b) Black bag (As per BMW Manage...

Ref: K. Park, 24th ed. p 830

As per BMW Management and Handling Rules – 2016, discarded and expired medicines are to be segregated in Yellow non-chlorinated plastic bags or Container

47. Ans. (d) Yellow bag (As per BMW Manage...

Ref: K. Park, 24th ed. p 830

48. Ans. (a) Human anatomical waste; (b) Animal waste; (c) Microbiological waste; (e) Soiled waste

Ref: BMW Management and Handling Rules – 2016

49. Ans. (c) Black bag

Ref: K. Park, 23rd ed. p 793-94

Wrapper of surgical syringe constitute noninfectious for municipal dump → hence, discarded in Black bag

50. Ans. (b) Blue bag waste is disposed by landfill

Ref: K. Park, 23rd ed. p 793-94

51. Ans. (c) Blue bag (As per BMW Management and Handling Rules -1998)

Ref: K. Park, 23rd ed. p 793-94

52. Ans. (b) Incineration

Ref: K. Park, 24th ed. p 830

53. Ans. (b) Yellow

Yellow bin – Blood transfusion bags, infectious waste (not rubber, plastic or tubes)
Red category: Rubber, plastic or tubes – catheters, disposable syringes, IV sets, gloves, urine bags
White category: Sharps and Metals
Blue Category: Glass and Metallic Implants

54. Ans. (c) Radiation hazard

55. Ans. a-3, b-4, c-1, d-2

Ref: Park 25th ed. Pg 849, 853

Waste categories are:
Yellow – infectious waste
Red – rubber, tubes, plastic – non incinerable waste
White – sharps and metals
Blue – glass and metallic ortho implants
Note: Mercury containing waste is secured safely, categorized as yellow e-chemical waste and will be sent back to manufacturer for reuse or recycle or treated as per Hospital waste management rules 2008.

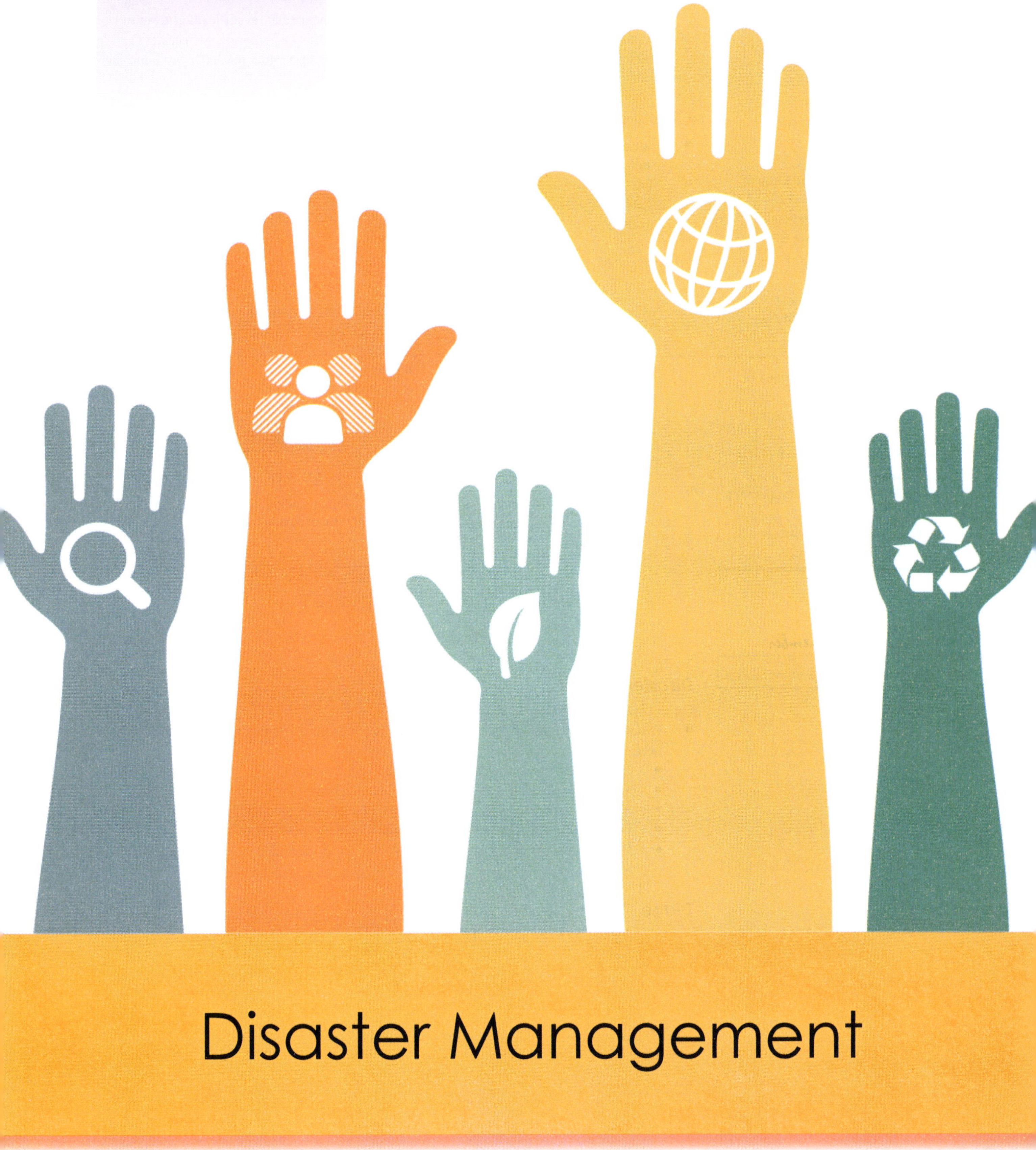

Disaster Management

Chapter Outline

120 **Good to Remember**

Disaster Risk = Hazard × Vulnerability

DISASTERS—TYPES, PHASES AND RESPONSE

Disaster is any occurrence that causes damage, ecological disruption, loss of human life or deterioration of health and health services on a scale sufficient to warrant an extraordinary response from outside the affected community or area. (WHO)

As per Colin Grant, Disaster is "Occurrence of an unexpected event leading to injury or illness simultaneously to at least 30 people who will require hospital emergency treatment".

Hazard is any phenomenon with potential to cause disruption or damage to people and their environment.

Classification of Disasters

- **Natural disasters:** Earthquake, Tsunami, Volcanic eruptions, Landslides or Avalanches, Hurricanes or Cyclones, Snow storms, Floods or Draughts
- **Man-made disasters:** Either caused by warfare (Nuclear, Biological or chemical) or Accidents (Road Traffic Accidents, Air/Rail accidents, Building collapse, Explosions, Massive fires or Poisonings)

Disaster Management Cycle

It comprises of:

Disaster impact, response, rehabilitation, reconstruction, mitigation and preparedness

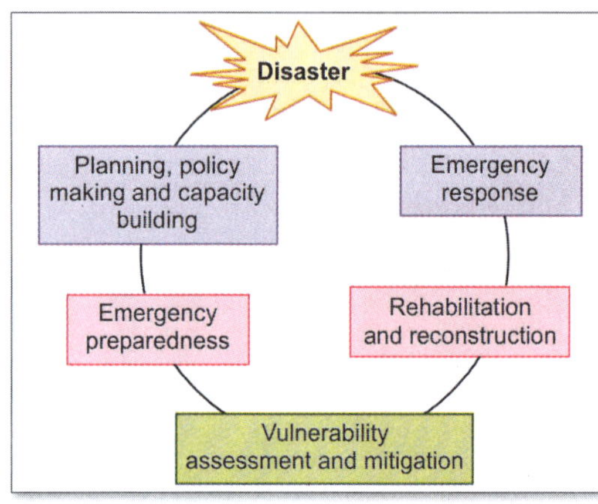

Fig. 1: Disaster management cycle

Disaster Impact

Let us Discuss the Disaster Management Cycle:

- **Disaster impact:** In a disaster the casualties occur as mass numbers, so the following steps need to be taken:
  - Rescue uninjured survivors and provide them first aid.
  - People are provided with food, shelter, medical help etc.
  - An enquiry center is established to respond to enquiries pertaining to victims.
  - Dead victims are identified and adequate mortuary space provided.
  - Due to limited number of resources, the victims are classified by **TRIAGE approach** on *basis* of severity of injury and likelihood of survival with prompt medical care.

Triage

The **Internationally Accepted** ***4 color code Triage system is as follows:***

Red → (*High priority*)[Q] → Immediate resuscitation or life/limb saving surgery in next 6 hours

Yellow (*Medium priority*)[Q] → Possible resuscitation or life/limb saving surgery in next 24 hours

Green (*Low priority*)[Q] → Ambulatory patients (minor or moderate injuries—treated at their own homes

Black (Least priority)[Q] → Dead or moribund patients (Require more attention, with questionable benefit)

Disaster Response and Rehabilitation

- **Response:** It involves:
  - Prevention of occurrence of epidemics.
  - Arrangements to provide food, clothes, shelter and drugs.

Relief phase begins when assistance from outside starts to reach the disaster area.

Primary phase (0–6 hours following a disaster) is most critical. First aid and treatment of victims is utmost priority.

Secondary phase (6–24 hours): Transport, sanitation and prevention of spread of communicable disease assume priority.

Tertiary phase (>24 hours -2 months): Food, blankets, clothing, shelter, sanitary engineering and construction are priority.

- **Rehabilitation:** Efforts are made to restore the normal living conditions as soon as possible by-
  - Ensuring water quality is 1st priority.
    - Chlorination of all water bodies (Residual chlorine >1 mg/L), high water pressure, cleaning and disinfection of repaired mains/reservoirs, protection of existing water sources (Restricting access to people and animals).
    - Use of chlorine tablet – 2.5 g for 225 L, 0.5 g for 20 L, 0.125 g for 1 L water, Bleaching powder – 2 g (35% chlorine) for 5 L water.
    - Sufficient water of low quality is better than little water of high quality, in disaster scenarios.
    - One tap per 200–250 people and 15 L/person/day is recommended by the United Nations High Commissioner for Refugees (UNHCR)
  - Gastroenteritis is the most common disease reported in the post disaster phase
  - Hygienic food supply
  - Safe sanitation services/provisions
  - Control of vectors
  - Re-integration of survivors into society through social workers & NGOs

Disaster Mitigation and Preparedness

Mitigation

- ***Disaster mitigation*** refers to measures designed to prevent hazards from causing emergency or lessen impact of emergencies.
  - It includes flood mitigation works, appropriate land-use planning, improved building codes and reduction or protection of vulnerable population and structures.
  - Mitigation complements the disaster preparedness and disaster response activities. It reduces vulnerability to hazards. Mitigation is essentially an effort to watch for the sequence of the events and materials to be used – when, how, what to be done during the disaster

Preparedness and Capacity Building

- ***Disaster or emergency preparedness*** is a long-term development activity to strengthen overall capacity and capability of a country to manage efficiently all types of emergency. It is a series of planning of activities involving – collection of the resources – material, manpower, financial, administrative and technical elements to be in place in an unfortunate event of disaster. It is a continuous, on-going multisectoral activity.

188 High Yield Points

Mean energy requirement per person per day at times of disasters is 2100 Kcal.[Q]

Most common Vitamin deficiency in disasters is Vitamin A (Measles, respiratory infections, diarrhea and poor relief diet are predisposing factors)

International Agencies for Disaster Response

The International Agencies that provide humanitarian assistance to the disaster struck areas are:

- Office for the Co-ordination of Humanitarian Affairs (OCHA)
- World Health Organization (WHO)
- UNICEF
- World Food Program (WFP)
- Food and Agriculture Organization (FAO)

Non-Governmental Organizations (NGOs) are:

- Co-operative American Relief Everywhere (CARE)
- International Committee of Red Cross
- International Council of Voluntary Agencies (ICVA)
- International Federation of Red Cross and Red Crescent Societies (IFRC), etc.

115 **Must Remember**

Guidelines for Residual Chlorine in Water Sources in Disasters

Water source	Residual chlorine after treatment
Clear piped water	1 mg/L
Protected tube wells, ring wells, clear rain water	2 mg/L
Unprotected wells and cloudy water (filtered before purifying)	5 mg/L
Water known to have fecal contamination (filtered before purifying)	10 mg/L

116 **Must Remember**

Tetanus and Hepatitis B vaccines are recommended for health workers but not for routine use in endemic areas.

Basic Sanitation and Personal Hygiene

- Sanitary disposal of excreta (Emergency latrines). Washing, cleaning and bathing facilities need to be ensured.
- Intensive vector control especially in endemic areas
- Method of choice for controlling mosquitoes and sand flies in disaster is Indoor residual spray[Q]
- Mass vaccination against Measles[Q] in children
- Reintegrate disaster survivors into the society via institutional program coordinated by ministries of health and family welfare, social welfare, education, and NGOs.
- In general vaccination for mass prophylaxis is not recommended, selective vaccine for emergency responders may be planned - for tetanus and hepatitis B prophylaxis
- Maximum risk for gastrointestinal disease - enteritis outbreak is there especially after natural disaster as earthquakes or floods

Table 1: Guidelines for accommodation of displaced in disaster (in temporary camps)

Area per person for collective activities	30 m^2
Shelter space per person	3.4 m^2 (4.5–5.5 m^2 in cold climates)
Distance between shelters	2 m (minimum)
Area for support services	7.5 m^2/person
Number of people per water point and distance to water point	250 and 150 m maximum
Number of people per latrine and distance to latrine	20 and 30 m
Distance between water point and latrine	100 m
Firebreaks	75 m length every 300 m

DISASTER MANAGEMENT IN INDIA

Disaster Management Act, 2005

Disaster Management Act came into force in 2005.

2nd Wednesday of October is observed as World Disaster Reduction Day[Q].

Morbidities from a disaster are—Injuries, Emotional stress, Epidemic of disease and Increase in indigenous diseases

Relative number of injuries and deaths depend on:

- Type of disaster
- Density and distribution of population
- Condition of the environment
- Degree of the preparedness and opportunity of the warning.
- Injuries exceed death in explosions, earthquakes, typhoons, hurricanes, fires, tornadoes etc.
- Death exceeds injuries in landslides, avalanches, volcanic eruptions, tidal waves, floods etc.

Levels of Disaster

Table 2: Levels of disasters

L0	Normal period It should be utilized for disaster risk reduction
L1	Manageable within capabilities and resources at District level State authorities need to be ready to provide assistance if needed
L2	It requires assistance and active mobilization of resources at state level and deployment of state level agencies for disaster management The central agencies must remain vigilant for immediate deployment if required by the State
L3	It is a nearly catastrophic situation or a very large-scale disaster that overwhelms the State and District authorities

Earthquake Seismic Zones in India

(Revised in 2000, Zone I was merged in Zone II by BIS Seismic Zoning Committee.)

- **Zone V (Very High Damage Risk Zone):** Seismic intensity IX and above on Modified Mercalli Intensity Scale. North eastern states, Bihar, Andaman and Nicobar, Himachal Pradesh
- **Zone IV (High Damage Risk Zone):** Seismic intensity MM VIII. Delhi, Chandigarh, Sikkim, Himachal Pradesh
- **Zone III (Moderate Damage Risk Zone):** Seismic intensity MM VII.
- **Zone II (Low Damage Risk Zone):** Seismic intensity MM VI.

Nodal Ministry for Disaster Response in India

Ministry of Home Affairs, Government of India is the national agency responsible for disaster management. (Earlier it was Ministry of Agriculture).

State governments are responsible for execution of relief work[Q]. Government of India has a supportive role.[Q]

Calamity Relief Fund has been constituted in each State (Contributions from Union and State Government are in ratio of 3:1)

Table 3: Nodal ministry for various disasters

Disaster	Nodal Ministry/Department
Biological	Ministry of Health and Family Welfare (MoHFW)
Chemical and industrial	Ministry of Environment, Forest and Climate Change (MoEFCC)
Civil aviation accidents	Ministry of Civil Aviation (MoCA)
Cyclone/Tornado	Ministry of Earth Sciences (MoES)
Tsunami	Ministry of Earth Sciences (MoES)
Drought/Hailstorm/cold wave and frost/pest attack	Ministry of Agriculture and Farmers Welfare (MoAFW)
Earthquake	Ministry of Earth Sciences (MoES)
Flood	Ministry of Water Resources (MoWR)
Forest fire	Ministry of Environment, forests, and Climate Change
Landslides	Ministry of Mines (MoM)
Avalanche	Ministry of Defence (MoD)
Nuclear and radiological emergencies	Department of Atomic Energy (DAE)
Rail accidents	Ministry of Railways (MoR)
Road accidents	Ministry of Road Transport and Highways (MoRth)
Urban floods	Ministry of Urban development (MoUD)

Table 4: Central agencies designated for natural hazard-specific early warnings

Hazard	Agencies
Avalanches	Snow and Avalanche Study Establishment (SASE)
Cyclone	India Meteorological Department (IMD)
Drought	Ministry of Agriculture and Farmers Welfare (MoAFW)
Earthquake	India Meteorological Department (IMD)
Epidemics	Ministry of Health and Family Welfare (MoHFW)
Floods	Central Water Commission (CWC)
Landslides	Geological Survey of India (GSI)
Tsunami	India National Center for Oceanic Information Services (INCOIS)

189 *High Yield Points*

Triage*—Rapidly classifying the injured on basis of severity of injury and likelihood of survival with prompt medical care*

Highest priority is given to victims whose immediate or long-term prognosis can be dramatically improved by simple care

Lowest priority is given to dead or moribund patients who require more attention, with questionable benefit.

Categorization of Alerts/Early Warning

- **Red (Severe):** PMO and Cabinet Secretariat to be updated every 3 hours on developing situation
- **Orange (Moderate):** PMO and Cabinet Secretariat to be updated every 12 hours
- **Yellow (Low):** PMO and Cabinet Secretariat to be updated through speed post.

National Disaster Management Plan (NDMP)–2016

- **Aim:** To make India disaster resilient and significantly reduce the loss of lives and assets.
- It is based on the four priority themes of the "**Sendai Framework**," for Disaster Risk Reduction 2015-2030
- Understanding disaster risk
- Improving disaster risk governance
- Investing in disaster risk reduction for resilience (structural and nonstructural measures)
- Enhancing disaster preparedness for effective response and "Building back better" in recovery, rehabilitation and reconstruction

Salient Features

- Covers all phases of disaster management: Prevention, mitigation, response and recovery
- Provides for horizontal and vertical integration among all agencies and departments
- Spells out roles and responsibilities of all levels of Government up to Panchayat and Urban Local Body level in a matrix format
- It has a regional approach for disaster management and planning
- It can be implemented in a scalable manner in all phases of disaster management
- It identifies major activities such as early warning, information dissemination, medical care, fuel, transportation, search and rescue, evacuation, etc. to serve as a checklist for agencies responding to a disaster
- Provides a generalized framework for recovery and offers flexibility to assess a situation and build back better
- To prepare communities to cope with disasters, it emphasizes on a greater need for information, education and communication activities

Objectives

- Improve the understanding of disaster risk, hazards, and vulnerabilities
- Strengthen disaster risk governance at all levels from local to center
- Invest in disaster risk reduction for resilience through structural, non-structural and financial measures, as well as comprehensive capacity development
- Enhance disaster preparedness for effective response
- Promote "Build Back Better" in recovery, rehabilitation and reconstruction
- Prevent disasters and achieve substantial reduction of disaster risk and losses in lives, livelihoods, health, and assets
- Increase resilience and prevent the emergence of new disaster risks and reduce the existing risks
- Promote the implementation of integrated and inclusive economic, structural, legal, social, health, cultural, educational, environmental, technological, political and institutional measures to prevent and reduce hazard exposure and vulnerabilities to disaster
- Empower both local authorities and communities as partners to reduce and manage disaster risks
- Strengthen scientific and technical capabilities in all aspects of disaster management
- Capacity development at all levels to effectively respond to multiple hazards and for community-based disaster management
- Provide clarity on roles and responsibilities of various Ministries and Departments involved in different aspects of disaster management
- Promote the culture of disaster risk prevention and mitigation at all levels
- Facilitate the mainstreaming of disaster management concerns into the developmental planning and processes

Organization for Disaster Management in India

Table 5: Organizational structure for disaster management in India

Institutions	Roles in disaster management
National Disaster Management Authority (NDMA)–Apex body headed by Prime Minister	▪ To lay down policies, plans and guidelines for disaster management and approve national disaster management plans of the central ministries/departments ▪ To oversee provision and application of funds for mitigation and preparedness ▪ To authorize concerned departments/authorities, to make emergency procurement of provisions or materials for rescue and relief in a disaster ▪ General superintendence, direction and control of national disaster response force ▪ Formulate guidelines and facilitate training and preparedness in respect of Chemical, Biological, Radiological and Nuclear (CBRN) emergencies
National Crisis Management Committee	Handle emergencies requiring close *involvement of security forces and/or intelligence agencies* such as terrorism, law and order situation, hijacking etc.

Contd...

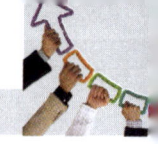

Institutions	Roles in disaster management
National Executive Committee (NEC)	▪ To monitor implementation of guidelines issued by NDMA and ensure compliance of the directions issued by the Central Government ▪ Coordinate the response in event of any threatening disaster situation ▪ Prepare national plan for disaster management
State Disaster Management Authority	To lay down policies and plans for DM in State and approve State plan
State Executive Committee (SEC)	To assist SDMA in the performance of its functions and to coordinate and monitor the implementation of National Policy, the National Plan and the State Plan
District Disaster Management Authority	Planning, coordinating and implementing DM (prevention, mitigation, preparedness and response measures) at district level as per guidelines
Local Authorities—Panchayati Raj Institutions	▪ Ensure capacity building of officers and employees for managing disasters, carry out relief, rehabilitation and reconstruction activities in the affected areas ▪ Prepare DM plans in consonance with guidelines of NDMA, SDMAs and DDMAs
National Institute of Disaster Management	Capacity development along with training, research, documentation and development of a national level information base
National Disaster Response Force (10 battalions)	Specialized response to disasters (Chemical, Biological, Radiological and Nuclear) and basic training to all stakeholders identified by State Governments
Cabinet Committee on Management of Natural Calamities (CCMNC) and Cabinet Committee on Security (CCS)	Assessment of situation and identification of measures to reduce impact, monitor and suggest long-term measures for prevention of such calamities, formulate and recommend program for public awareness and building up society's resilience CCS deals with issues related to defence, law and order and internal security
High level committee (HLC)	Assessment of damage caused by calamity and quantum of assistance to be given to states from the National Calamity Contingency Fund (NCCF) and its approval
Armed forces	Assist civil administration in communication, search and rescue operations (Air lift), health and medical facilities and transportation
Central Ministries and Departments (Nodal Agencies)	**Floods:** CWC, ministry of Water Resources **Cyclones and Earthquakes:** Indian Meteorological Directorate **Epidemics:** Ministry of Health and Family Welfare **Chemical Disasters:** Ministry of Environment and Forests **Industrial Disasters:** Ministry of Labor **Rail accidents:** Ministry of Railways **Air accidents:** Ministry of **Civil Aviation** **Fire;** Ministry of home Affairs **Nuclear accidents:** Department of Atomic Energy **Mine disasters:** Department of mines

Multiple Choice Questions

TRIAGE

1. **Triage refers to a** *(Recent Question 2017)*
   a. Concept in trauma
   b. Method of breast lump diagnosis
   c. Investigation for duodenum and pancreas
   d. Management of old age health problems
2. **In triage, yellow color indicates**
   a. High priority b. Medium priority
   c. Ambulatory patients d. Dead patients
3. **Triage is:** *(Recent Question 2017)*
   a. Treating mentally ill patients
   b. Giving priority to serious cases
   c. Treating patients with better prognosis on priority
   d. Treating only occupational injuries
4. **In disaster management, patients who need surgery within 24 hours, are categorized under which color category of Triage:** *(Recent Question 2017)*
   a. Red b. Green
   c. Yellow d. Black
5. **Black color in triage is for** *(Recent Question 2016)*
   a. Ambulatory patients b. Low priority patients
   c. Dead patients d. High priority patients
6. **Triage is done for**
   a. Treating the most serious cases
   b. Categorization of the patients and treating them according to the available resource
   c. Giving emergency services to all patients
   d. Treating mentally ill patients
7. **True about Triage is**
   a. Yellow least priority b. Red morbidity
   c. Green ambulatory d. Blue ambulatory
8. **Which color code is given first preference in disaster:**
   a. Red b. Black
   c. Yellow d. Green
9. **Black color in triage refers to:** *(Recent Question 2016)*
   a. Death
   b. Transfer
   c. High priority
   d. Low priority
10. **As per the most common classification of Triage system that is internationally accepted, color code that indicates high priority treatment or transfer is:**
    a. Black b. Yellow
    c. Red d. Blue
11. **Triage has how many colors:** *(Recent Question 2016)*
    a. 2
    b. 3
    c. 4
    d. 5
12. **Black color code in Triage is used in disaster for management of:**
    a. High priority patients b. Low priority patients
    c. Ambulatory patients d. Dead/moribund patients

DISASTER CYCLE AND MANAGEMENT

13. **World disaster reduction day is on?**
    a. 2nd Wednesday of October
    b. 3rd Wednesday of October
    c. 4th Wednesday of October
    d. 1st Wednesday of November
14. **Not true regarding disease control after a disaster**
    a. Gastroenteritis is the most commonly reported disease in the post-disaster period
    b. Vector borne diseases will not appear immediately, but take several weeks for an epidemic
    c. Displacement of domesticated and wild animals increases the risk of transmission of zoonoses
    d. WHO recommends typhoid and cholera vaccines in routine use in endemic areas
15. **Epidemic that does not occur post disaster is?**
    a. Leptospirosis b. Leishmania
    c. ARTI d. Rickettsia
16. **Most common disease after disaster**
    a. Tetanus b. Leptospirosis
    c. Malaria d. Gastroenteritis
17. **During disaster what should be done first**
    a. Search and rescue, first aid *(Recent Question 2015)*
    b. Triage
    c. Stabilization of victims
    d. Hospital treatment and redistribution of patients to hospital if necessary
18. **Which of the following is NOT included as fundamental aspects of disaster management?**
    a. Disaster prevention b. Disaster response
    c. Disaster preparedness d. Disaster mitigation
19. **In disaster management which of the following is not practiced?** *(Recent Question 2015)*
    a. Rehabilitation b. Mass vaccination
    c. Triage d. Disaster response
20. **All of the following with regards to disaster management are true except:** *(Recent Question 2014)*
    a. Response is done in predisaster phase
    b. Gastroenteritis is most common infection post disaster
    c. Yellow color in triage is for medium priority
    d. Mitigation is done in predisaster phase
21. **All vaccines are NOT given in disaster, except**
    a. Cholera b. Tetanus
    c. Measles d. Typhoid
22. **Nodal center in case of disaster management**
    a. PHC b. Sub center
    c. CHC d. District
23. **Which of the following is the nodal center for disaster management ?** *(Recent Question 2013)*
    a. PHC b. CHC
    c. Police Control room d. District
24. **Which is the calamity with most amount of damage?**
    a. Flood b. Earthquake
    c. Landslides d. Volcanoes

Ans.

1. a
2. b
3. c
4. c
5. c
6. b
7. c
8. a
9. a
10. c
11. c
12. d
13. a
14. d
15. b
16. d
17. a
18. a
19. b
20. a
21. c
22. d
23. d
24. a

Most Recent Questions of 2019-18 are given at the end of MCQs

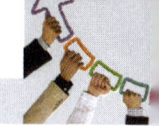

25. Natural disaster causing maximum death:
a. Hydrological
b. Meterological
c. Geological
d. Fires

26. The gas responsible for Bhopal gas tragedy is
a. Methyl Isocyanate
b. Potassium thiocyanate
c. Sodium thiocyanate
d. Ethyl thiocyanate

27. Triage is used in
a. All mass casualties
b. Warfare
c. Bomb blast
d. Suicide injuries

28. In "Triage" injured patients are classified according to basis of *(PGI Pattern)*
a. Severity of their injuries
b. Likelihood of their survival with prompt medical intervention
c. First come, first treated
d. Bed availability
e. Associated comorbidities

29. Microorganism used as weapon in biological terrorism is:
a. Small pox virus
b. Rabies virus
c. Ebola virus
d. Influenza C virus
e. Human parvovirus

30. Triage is:
a. Treating the most serious cases
b. Treating mentally ill patients
c. Categorization of patients and treating them according to the available resources
d. Treating terminally ill patients

31. According to colour code system of Triage, green colour indicates-
a. High priority patients
b. Medium priority patients
c. Ambulatory patient
d. Dead or moribund patients

32. Which of the following is not a fundamental aspect of disaster management: *(PGI Pattern)*
a. Disaster response
b. Disaster preparedness
c. Disaster mitigation
d. Disaster compensation
e. Disaster prevention

Most Recent Questions (2019–2018)

33. Which immunization is useful in post-disaster relief phase: *(AIIMS May 2019)*
a. Measles
b. Typhoid
c. Cholera
d. Polio

34. Following disaster green colour of triage used for which patients: *(Recent Question 2019)*
a. Dead
b. Medium priority
c. High priority
d. Ambulatory

Ans.

25. a
26. a
27. a
28. a,b,e
29. a
30. c
31. c
32. d,e
33. a
34. d

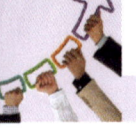

Answers with Explanations

TRIAGE

1. Ans. (a) Concept in trauma

Ref: K. Park, 24th ed. p 833

Triage[Q] means *rapidly classifying the injured on basis of severity of injury and likelihood of survival with prompt medical care*

- Highest Priority is given to victims whose immediate or long term prognosis can be dramatically improved by simple care
- Lowest priority is given to dead or moribund patients who require more attention, with questionable benefit

2. Ans. (b) Medium Priority

Ref: K. Park, 24th ed. p 833

Internationally Accepted ***4 color code Triage system.***

Red → (*High priority*)[Q] → Immediate resuscitation or life/limb saving surgery in next 6 hours

Yellow (*Medium priority*)[Q]→Possible resuscitation or life/limb saving surgery in next 24 hours

Green (*Low priority*)[Q] → Ambulatory patients (minor or moderate injuries- treated at their own homes

Black (*Least priority*)[Q]→ Dead or moribund patients (Require more attention, with questionable benefit)

3. Ans. (c) Treating patients with better prognosis on priority

Ref: K. Park, 24th ed p-833

4. Ans. (c) Yellow

Ref: K. Park, 24th ed. p 833

Also Know......................

- Triage is done at the site of disaster using locally available skills to determine transportation and treatment priority. It aims to provide maximum benefit to greatest number of injured in a major disaster situation.

5. Ans. (c) Dead patients

Ref: K. Park, 24th ed p-833

6. Ans. (b) Categorization of the patients and...

Ref: K. Park, 24th ed p-833

7. Ans. (c) Green ambulatory

Ref: K. Park, 24th ed. p 833

Also Know......................

- **Reverse triage→** Existing regular non-critical patients are triaged and those who do not need immediate care are discharged early post disaster to accommodate a greater number of new critical patients
- **Under triage** is underestimating the severity of an illness or injury (Acceptable rates 5% or less).

8. Ans. (a) Red

Ref: K. Park, 24th ed. p 833

9. Ans. (a) Death

Ref: K. Park, 24th ed. p 833

10. Ans. (c) Red

Ref: K. Park, 24th ed. p 833

11. Ans. (c) 4

Ref: K. Park, 24th ed. p 833

12. Ans. (d) Dead / moribund patients

Ref: K. Park, 24th ed. p 833

DISASTER CYCLE AND MANAGEMENT

13. Ans. (a) 2nd Wednesday of October

Ref: K. Park, 24th ed. p 839

14. Ans. (d) WHO recommends typhoid and...

Ref: K. Park, 24th ed. p 834

Also Know......................

- Gastroenteritis is the most commonly reported disease in the post-disaster period
- Vector-borne diseases take several weeks to reach epidemic levels.
- Typhoid and cholera vaccines are recommended for health workers but not for routine use in endemic areas.

Reasons for Increase in Transmission of Communicable Diseases Post Disaster are

- Overcrowding and poor sanitation in temporary resettlements
- Exposure of susceptible population (migrant or indigenous) to communicable diseases
- Disruption and contamination of water supply, damage to sewerage system and power systems
- Disruption of routine control programs (Diversion of funds and personnel for relief work)
- Ecological changes favoring breeding of vectors and increase in vector density
- Displacement of animals leading to increased risk of zoonosis (Domestic -Leptospirosis, rickettsiosis and Wild -equine encephalitis, rabies)
- Emergency food, water and shelter from different/new source may be a source of infection.

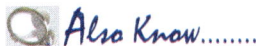

Also Know...................

Principals of prevention and control

- Immediate implementation of public health measures (safe drinking water, proper disposal of excreta) is the most practical and effective strategy[Q]
- Setting up a reliable disease reporting system to identify outbreaks and to initiate control measures
- Rapid investigation of all reported disease outbreaks

15. Ans. (b) Leishmania

Ref: K. Park, 24th ed. p 839 John T. Watson, Michelle Gayer, Maire A. Connolly. Epidemics after Natural Disasters Emerging Infectious Diseases Vol. 13, No. 1, January 2007

Post Disaster Epidemics

- Water related-
  - Diarrheal diseases-*V. cholerae* (O1 Ogawa and O1 Inaba) and enterotoxigenic *Escherichia coli, Salmonella* Paratyphi A (Paratyphoid fever)
  - Hepatitis A and E, Poliomyelitis
- Overcrowding related- Measles, *Neisseria meningitidis* (Meningitis), Acute Respiratory Infection(ARI), Epidemic typhus (Rickettsiae)
- Vector Borne- Malaria, Dengue, Filaria
- Other Diseases-Tetanus, Coccidioidomycosis. Rabies, Equine encephalitis
- Lack of personal hygiene-Skin diseases/Eye diseases

16. Ans. (d) Gastroenteritis

Ref: K. Park, 24th ed p-833

17. Ans. (a) Search and rescue, first aid

Ref: K. Park, 24th ed. p 833

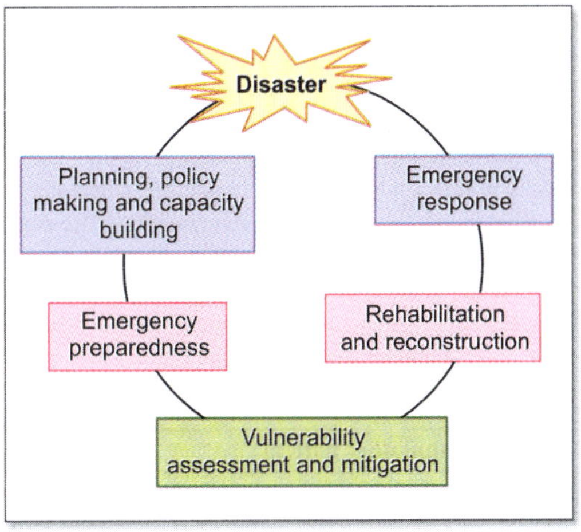

Post disaster-Emergency response is the first step. It comprises :

- Search/ Rescue and First aid
- Triage and Tagging
- Stabilization of victims
- Hospital treatment and redistribution of patients to other hospitals if necessary

18. Ans. (a) Disaster prevention

Ref: K. Park, 24th ed. p 833

Disaster Management Comprises

- Mitigation and Preparedness (Pre-disaster phase)
- Response/Relief, Rehabilitation and Reconstruction (Post-disaster phase).

19. Ans. (b) Mass vaccination

Ref: K. Park, 24th ed p-834

Reason for not recommending Mass vaccination in disaster:

- Multidose vaccines have poor compliance.
- Not yet proven effective, as a large-scale public health measure.
- Requires large number of health workers
- Supervision of sterilization and injection techniques may be impossible.
- May lead to false sense of security on risk of disease and neglect of effective control measures.

20. Ans. (a) Response is done in predisaster phase

Ref: K. Park, 24th ed p-833

21. Ans. (c) Measles

Ref: K. Park, 24th ed. p 834

WHO does not recommend mass vaccination of population against Tetanus, Typhoid and Cholera in endemic areas. These vaccinations are recommended only for health workers

- ***Post disaster highest priority vaccination for children*** is Measles [Q].

22. Ans. (d) District

Ref: S Lal, Textbook of Community Medicine, 3rd ed. p 723.J. Kishore, National Health Programs in India, 9thed. p -457

Districts headed by District Magistrate/Collector is the focal point for directing, supervising and monitoring relief measures in disaster and preparation of district level plans

23. Ans. (d) District

Ref: S Lal, Textbook of Community Medicine, 3rd ed. p 723. J. Kishore, National Health Programs in India, 9th ed. p -457

24. Ans. (a) Flood

Ref: Disaster management in India, Ministry of Home Affairs Government of India 2011

World Meteorological Organization (WMO), data of major natural disasters worldwide (1963-2002), indicates that floods and droughts cause the maximum damage.

- Damage caused by natural calamities → Flood (32%) Tropical Cyclone (30 %) Drought (22%) Earthquake (10%), Other disasters (6%)
- 85% of deaths during disasters are of women and children
- Economic loss of about 2% of the GDP is accounted for due to disasters.

Super cyclone — wind speed > 221 Km/Hour or > 119 Knots

Also Know........................

- **India is one of the ten worst disaster prone countries of the world. Out of 35 states and UT in the country, 27 are disaster prone.**
- Almost 58.6% of the landmass is prone to earthquakes of moderate to very high intensity
- Over 40 million hectares (12% of land) are prone to floods and river erosion
- Of the 7,516 km long coastline, close to 5,700 km is prone to cyclones and tsunamis
- 68% of the cultivable area is vulnerable to drought
- Hilly areas are at risk from landslides and avalanches.

25. Ans. (a) Hydrological

Ref: Disaster management in India, Ministry of Home Affairs Government of India 2011

Type of disaster	Example	Percentage
Hydro meteorological (water and climate related)	Floods, Cyclones, Tornadoes and hurricanes, Hailstorm, Cloud burst, Heat wave and cold wave, Snow avalanches, Droughts, Sea erosion, Thunder and Lightning, Tsunami	78.4
Geological	Landslides, Mudflows, Earthquakes, Dam failures/ Dam bursts, Minor fires	12.1
Biological	Epidemics, Pest attacks, Cattle epidemics, Food poisoning	11.3

- 78.4% of the disaster events between 1990-2009 were hydro meteorological and accounted for maximum deaths

Also Know........................

- Indian Meteorological Department (IMD) with centers in Kolkata, Bhubaneswar, Vishakhapatnam, Chennai and Mumbai issues forewarning of disaster.
- Snow and Avalanche Study Establishment (SASE), Manali issues forewarning on avalanches.

26. Ans. (a) Methyl Isocyanate

Ref: K. Park, 24th ed. p 838

Major manmade disasters	Cause	Impact
Bhopal Gas Tragedy (India - 3rd Dec, 1984 Union Carbide Pesticide Plant)	Leakage of Methyl Isocyanate gas	2 million people were exposed to gas and about 20,000 persons have died so far.
Chernobyl Nuclear Power Station (Soviet Union) Accident on 26th April 1986	Largest reported accidental release of radioactive material. (*Level 7* on International Nuclear Event Scale for nuclear accidents)	More than 7 million curies of I 131, Cs 134, Cs 137, Strontium 90 etc. deposited throughout northern hemisphere.

Public Health Measures against Manmade Disaster Comprise

- Tighter regulations of chemical plants/hazardous facilities.
- Engineering and technological measures (building codes, dam designs, containment of toxic materials)
- Early warning and protection against human errors.

27. Ans. (a) All mass casualties

- TRIAGE consists of rapidly classifying the injured on the basis of the severity of their injuries & the likelihood of their survival with prompt medical intervention. Triage should be carried out at the site of disaster and is the first phase of disaster cycle.

28. Ans. (a) Severity of their injuries; (b) Likelihood of their survival with prompt medical intervention; (e) Associated co morbidities

- Triage - it consists of rapidly classifying the injured on the basis of the severity of their injuries and the likelihood of their survival with prompt medical interventions.
- The principle of "first come, first treated" is not followed in mass emergencies.
- Internationally accepted four colour code system
  - Red—High priority treatment or transfer
  - Yellow—Medium priority patients
  - Green—Ambulatory patient
  - Black—Dead or moribund patient

29. Ans. (a) Small pox virus

30. Ans. (c) Categorization of patients and treating them according to the available resources

- *TRIAGE* is the screening and classification of sick or injured persons during war or other disasters to determine priority needs for the efficient use of medical personnel, equipment, and facilities. It is also done in emergency rooms and in acute care clinics to determine priority of treatment.
- The use of triage is necessary if the *maximum* number of lives is to be saved during an emergency situation that produces many more sick and wounded individuals than the available medical care facilities and personnel can handle.
- It is important to provide a quick and convenient method of noting the condition of each casualty. This can be done by attaching a color-coded tag to the body of the patient or labeling untraumatized skin with a marking pen. The classification is then upgraded or downgraded as indicated by the improvement or deterioration of the general condition of the patient.

31. Ans. (c) Ambulatory patient

- Triage - it consists of rapidly classifying the injured on the basis of the severity of their injuries and the likelihood of their survival with prompt medical interventions. The principle of first come, first treated' is not followed in mass emergencies.

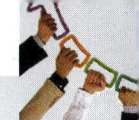

32. Ans. (d) Disaster compensation; (e) disaster prevention

- Disaster is any occurrence that causes damage, ecological disruption, loss of human life or deterioration of health and health services on a scale sufficient to warrant an extraordinary response from outside the affected community or area. All the choices except disaster compensation and disaster prevention form fundamental aspects of disaster management.

33. Ans. (a) Measles

Ref: https://www.who.int/immunization/sage/meetings/2012/april/2_SAGE_WGVHE_SG1__Lit_Review_CaseStudies.pdf; https://www.who.int/bulletin/volumes/91/12/12-117044/en/; Park 25th ed.; 858

Typhoid & Cholera

WHO does not recommend typhoid and cholera vaccine in routine use in postdisaster relief phase for endemic areas. Higher vaccination required more supervision and established logistics, which is often a big issue in postdisaster phase.

Also, a higher sense of security from the diseases along with media stress may lead to neglect of the effective control measures.

Tetanus: Mass vaccination is usually unnecessary. It is not a prerequisite, but health care providers are recommended to get vaccinated if they have not been

Vaccination recommendation by WHO—Special action group on vaccination for humanitarian emergencies:

- Measles is most often recommended and is well accepted as a priority health intervention in emergencies.
- Simultaneous introduction with other antigens is not generally recommended, but campaigns can include:
  - Polio vaccination where outbreaks or threats to eradication programs exist and
  - Tetanus vaccination for all those with open wounds or pregnant women.
- Vitamin A supplementation is almost universally recommended for implementation during a measles vaccination campaign.
- Where measles is recommended, vaccine coverage or needs assessments are also recommended to determine specific age ranges for targeting. Coverage rates of less than 90% for those under 15 years old are given as a qualifying criteria for recommendation of immediate mass immunization

For Emergency Responders, there is no Indication for:

- Hepatitis A vaccine (low probability of exposure). Vaccine will take at least one to two weeks to provide substantial immunity.
- Typhoid vaccine (low probability of exposure)
- Cholera vaccine (low probability of exposure, no licensed cholera vaccine available)
- Meningococcal vaccine (no expectation of increased risk of meningococcal disease among emergency responders).
- Rabies vaccine series (the full series is required for protection). evaluation as per case basis

34. Ans. (d) Ambulatory

Ref: Park 25th Ed. Pg 857; Suryakantha 3rd edition. 883

NOTES

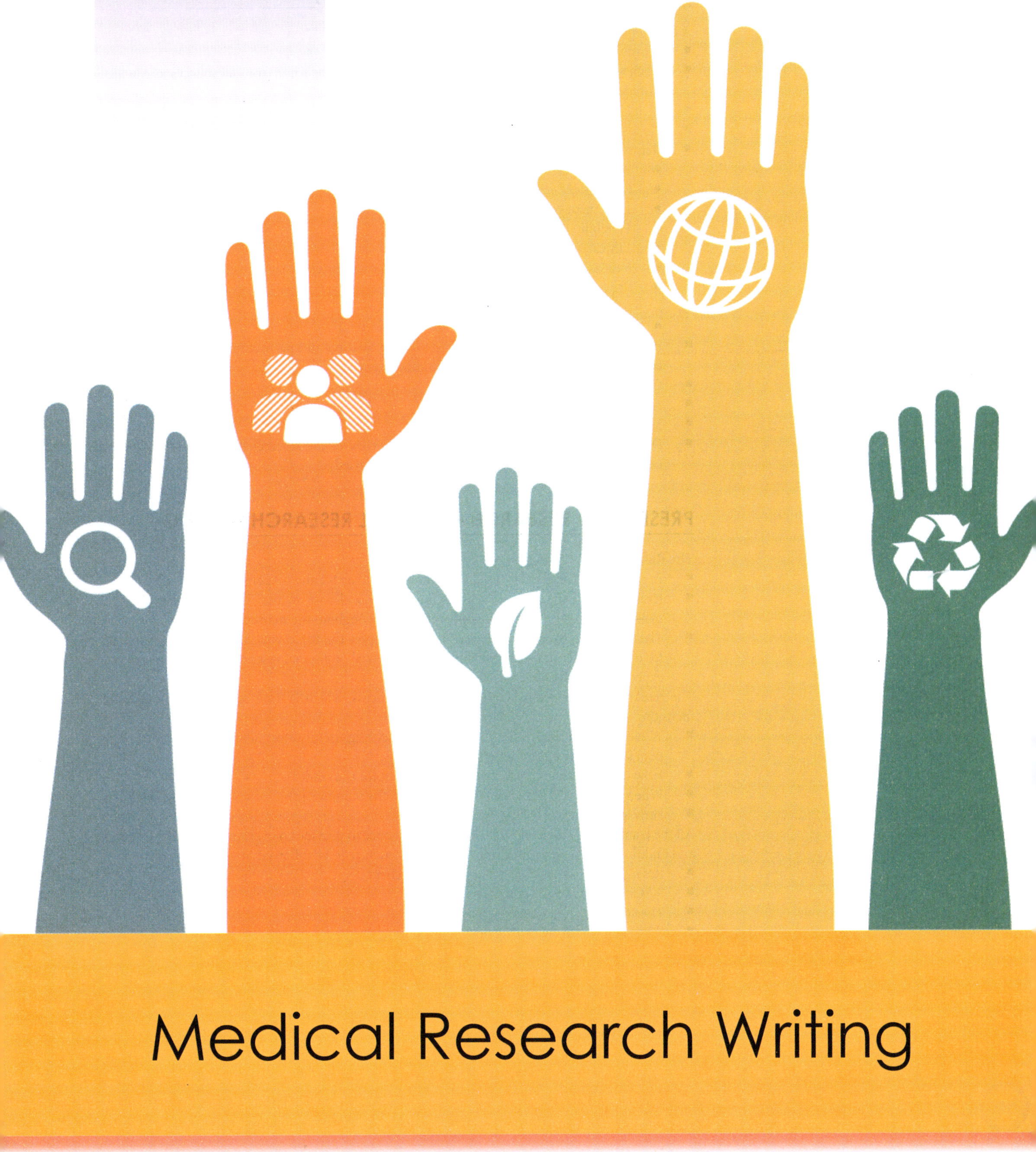

Medical Research Writing

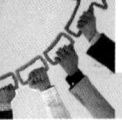

Chapter Outline

- Conducting Research (Re-Search)
- Presenting Research – Medical Research Writing

The rule of Thumb is:

"If you can't explain something simply, you don't understand it well enough"

CONDUCTING RESEARCH (RE-SEARCH)

A few steps to be adopted are:

- Formulate the research question
- Review the literature/research available on same/similar topic from all sources as Medline, PubMed, Cochrane, NHS and other established sources.
- Plan for gross materials and methods – Style, Design of research to be conducted
- Conduct a feasibility test
- ***R****eassess,* ***R****econfirm the* ***Research Checklist***:
    - Research question
    - Style, study design, outcome of the study
    - Data management & Statistical plan for research
    - Feasibility of the research
    - Ethical issues and clearance
    - Validated, pre-tested questionnaire, informed consent
    - Sequence of activites and estimated time for the research – evaluate the time using critical path approach and PERT methods
    - Funding and monetary aspects of the research
- Plan and prepare for Protocol writing for submission and permission to conduct research from regulatory authorities and/or funding agencies
- Conduct the research
- Medical writing
- Submission of the research
- Dissemination of the research and critical review of the research for formulating further research questions and evolution of medical knowledge

PRESENTING RESEARCH – MEDICAL RESEARCH WRITING

The **Rule** is:

- In scientific writing everything should be done to avoid any suspense or mystery
- Irrespective of the style of referencing that you choose to use, it is important that you maintain consistency by using only one style throughout the manuscript.
- The quality of your research work depends upon the topic you choose, whether you opt for a purely scientific experiment or a clinical trial or a social research study addressing the experiences of the patients, etc.

The research writing is absolutely an ongoing process, which is time consuming and requires focus on

- What to write (plan of the manuscript, presenting useful information to the reader rather than simple data and numbers)
- How much to write (what content is sufficient for the reader)
- When to write (placement of the contents in the manuscript)
- How to write (what style to be adopted)

All the components will be discussed here in sequence to provide an overview for medical writing and building better communication skills. The structure to be followed in general is same for:

- Research articles by students and/or researchers
- Systematic reviews of evidence available
- Thesis writing for masters programs
- Dissertation writing during doctoral programs
- Medical journalisms/Editorial
- Publications and presentations
- Regulatory documents, formulating standard protocols/Guidelines for Medical Education

(All the variants of medical writing will be referred to as *manuscript* for further reading)

A step-by-step approach for medical research writing, dissertation writing in general is as follows:

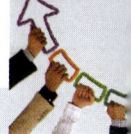

Step 1: Title

Start your manuscript with a suitable 'Title'

- Use: Attract readers interested in this field of study
- The title is an introduction to the content of the manuscript. An ideal title should be within 65 characters (5-15 words), without any abbreviations and grammatical mistakes, and not contain stop words like 'a', 'an', 'the', 'of', 'but', etc.
- A good title should contain:
  - The purpose of the research (topic of research)
  - The type of research method (study design)
  - Geographical/Temporal scope of the study (defined area or time of study)

Step 2: Introduction

Next, write your manuscript 'Introduction'

- Use: It tells the readers why you conducted the particular study.
- Essential components on introduction are:
  - Why this study is undertaken – what problems the author is trying to address
  - What has already been done in the field, what were the gaps, and how you fill those gaps with your study?
- The end of introduction usually contains a statement for "Aims and Objectives" of the research. It is a brief statement describing the study outcomes, how the work contributes to better understanding of the disease condition or research topic or unanswered questions

Step 3: Review of Literature (RoL)

This is usually the most time and effort consuming section.

- Use: RoL represents the literature that provides background information on your topic and shows a correspondence between those writings and your research question.
- RoL is essential for research writing as it:
  - Explains the background of research on a topic.
  - Demonstrates why a topic is significant to a subject area.
  - Discovers relationships between research studies/ideas.
  - Identifies major themes, concepts, and researchers on a topic.
  - Identifies critical gaps and points of disagreement.
  - Discusses further research questions that logically come out of the previous studies.

The research articles to be cited may be placed in the manuscript according to

- Temporal distribution: Chronologically sequencing of articles by event/trend/publishing of the article – usually adopted and accepted method
- Geographical distribution – Studies from various parts of world are listed followed by studies from specific continent/country or region specific researches.
- Based on methodology adopted by different researches.

Usual accepted and most followed way is using a chronological sequence of all previous researches with subclassifying the literature based on geographical and methodology distribution

Step 4: Material and Methods (M&M)

This section follows after Introduction.

- **Use:**
  - To enable the readers to evaluate the study design. Nothing should be kept as 'presumed' The author should try to write every detail of the methods used to conduct the study
  - To allow the reader/researcher to replicate the study using same methodology for future researches.
- **The outlay** of "*materials and methods*" is
  - Setting—the environmental conditions in which you conducted your research
  - Sample—what materials were used in research and details about the participants in the study.
    - Type of study
    - Sample size calculation, sampling methodology used for collecting data
    - Inclusion and exclusion criteria – what factors were considered to include or exclude any participant in the study

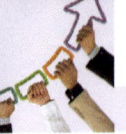

- **Measurement tools**—Discrete, elaborate description of all variable and methods used should be done. It may include all or some of the following:
  - Details about the methods and equipment used to measure the outcomes of the study. Include description of the instruments, devices used (manufacturer, quality control, year, and other specific descriptions) if any
  - Specifying the critical variables for that type of work, for example, how long the samples were incubated, how many minutes subjects were allowed to work on a task, or what strain of laboratory media was used or any other details.
  - Questionnaire used for establishing a condition, the source, reliability, consistency and validity of the questionnaire.
- **Independent and Dependent variables**—what were the factors you controlled or changed during the experiment and what you measured as the outcome
- **Statistical plan for research**—elaborate on the tests of significance used, measures for confidence limits, cut off for power of study, allowable statistical error in interpretation of the research, software used during analysis of the study

Step 5: Results and Observations

- **Use:** To present the data, useful and meaningful interpretation of the data
- A good research writing should include presentation using appropriate Text, Tables, figure, graphs and other statistical presentation methods
- **The general rule is**—the results represented as tables or graphs should contain:
  - Title—describing the table/graph
  - Number (separate for tables and graphs/presentations)
  - Table should have header for columns and rows
  - Data presented should always show the units of data measured
  - Legend for the graphs, curves or other statistical presentations
  - Graph, curves should be readable and understandable
  - Data Labels on graphs, curves indicating the data value and format (absolute number or percentage)
  - The tables should be presented as variables in rows/columns with row total and column total on sides
  - Statistical analysis tables (summary tables) should contain the cut-off for p-values, with the confidence limits set for the research

Step 5: Discussion

It is the most crucial step where you include the '**Discussion**' of your results. An ideal discussion should include:

- The principal findings of your study
- Strengths and weaknesses of your study in relation to other studies in the field
- A take-home message for the clinicians and policymakers
- Questions that your study can't answer to propagate further research

Step 6: Follow the discussion with the 'Limitations of your study'

Step 7: References

At the end of your thesis, include your 'References'. Track all your references so you don't miss out on anyone.

Common Terms

A **bibliography** is a list of sources that the writer recommends for further reading.
A '**works cited list**' or a '**reference list**' is a list of sources that were included in the author's writing.

Referencing, Citation Styles

The most commonly used referencing and citation styles are as follows:

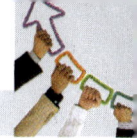

Vancouver Style

The Vancouver Style is formally known as Recommendations for the Conduct, Reporting, Editing and Publication of Scholarly Work in Medical Journals (ICMJE Recommendations). It was developed in Vancouver in 1978 by editors of medical journals and well over 1,000 medical journals (including ICMJE members BMJ, CMAJ, JAMA & NEJM) use this style

On the references page

- The last page of your paper is entitled references.
  - References are single spaced, with double-spacing between references.
- **Numbering:** List all references in order by number, not alphabetically.
  - Each reference is listed once only, since the same number is used throughout the paper.
- **Authors:**
  - List each author's last name followed by a space and then initials without any periods; there is a comma and space between authors and a period at the end of the last author.
  - If the number of authors exceeds six, give the first six followed by "et al."
  - For edited books, place the editors' names in the author position and follow the last editor with a comma and the word editor (or editors). For edited books with chapters written by individual authors, list the authors of the chapter first, then the chapter title, followed by "In:", the editors' names, and the book title.
- **Title:** Capitalize the first letter of the first word in the title. The rest of the title is in lower-case, with the exception of proper names. Do not underline the title; do not use italics. If there is an edition for a book, it appears after the title, abbreviated and followed by a period, for example: 8th ed.
- **Publication information:**
  - **Books**: After the title (and edition if applicable), place a period and space, then enter the city. Give the year of publication followed by a period. If no date of publication can be found, but the publication contains a date of copyright, use the date of copyright preceded by the letter "c", e.g. c2015.
  - **Journals**: List the abbreviated journal title, place a period and a space, year, (and abbreviated month and day if applicable), semi-colon, volume, issue number in parentheses, colon, page range, and a period.
- **Online sources:**
  - Include the same information and style as for print sources
  - Add the retrieval information for location by the reader of the manuscript
    - Place word [Internet] in square brackets after the book title or abbreviated journal title
    - Indicate date of retrieval, preceded by the word "cited", in square brackets after the date of publication
    - Add retrieval information at the end of the citation using the full URL.
    - If a DOI exists, it is optional to add it after the retrieval information

Example

- Mukhmohit S et al, COPD - Prevalence and risk study among females of rural area, District Ambala, Haryana, India. JEMDS. Apr 2014;3(16):4183-4191
- Edward Seferian, Bekele Afessa. Demographic and clinical variation of adult intensive care unit utilization from a geographically defined population. Crit Care Med. 2006 Aug;34(8):2113-9. PubMed PMID: 16763514
- Eat right [Internet]. Chicago: Academy of Nutrition and Dietetics; c2016 [cited 01 May 2019]. Available from: https://www.eatright.org/.
- Nipah Virus [Internet] World Health Organisation. May 2018 [cited 01 May 2019]. Available from: https://www.who.int/news-room/fact-sheets/detail/nipah-virus

Some other Referencing Styles are:

- **APA (American Psychological Association)**
  - Usually used for social sciences – for citing work from newspapers, articles, media, interviews and books
  - APA format structure:
    - Author, A. (Year of Publication). Title of work. Publisher City, State: Publisher

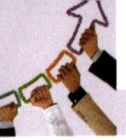

- **MLA:**
  - MLA format is often used for literature, language, liberal arts, and other humanities subjects.
  - It has separate section for bibliography and work cited
- **Harvard style**
  - AGPS (Australian) style
  - Usually used for legal documentations, citations, precedence and rulebook formulations

Step 8: Abstract

Purpose: To provide a brief summary of the paper. This is a crucial component of research article writing. After reading the title, the reader usually reads the abstract and will decide if they wish to read the rest of the research article. commonly the abstract is structured for 150-300 words

Content: The abstract is written as a mini-article, i.e., it contains the following information in this order:

- **Introduction:** A few sentences to provide background information on the problem investigated
- **Methods:** Methodology and tools used during research
- **Results:** The major results presented in the paper; provide quantitative information when possible.
- **Discussion:** The authors' interpretation of the results presented
- **Final summary:** The major conclusions and implication of the research. It should be understandable for a general readership and provide the use of research.

Principles for a good abstract:

- Give a brief background information about the topic
- State the importance of the problem and what is unknown about it
- Clearly state the objectives of your study
- A brief selected review of literature. Do not include duplicity of results or well known facts and results
- **Selected high yield information should be given in abstract for a very precise and to-the-point information**.

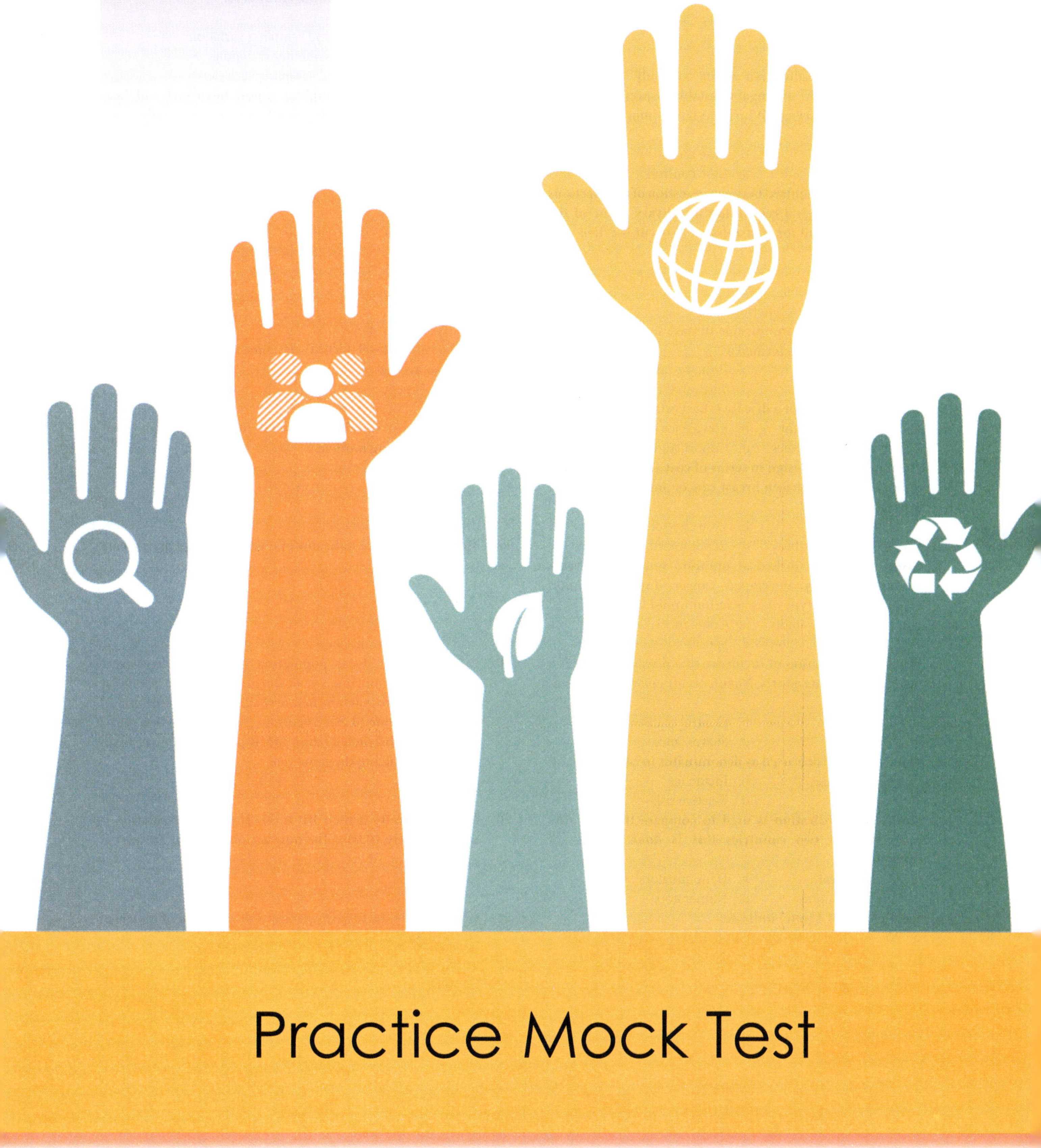

Practice Mock Test

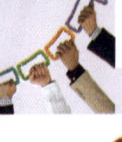

Multiple Choice Questions

1. **In case control study confounding bias can be prevented by:**
   a. Randomization b. Matching
   c. Double blinding d. Triple blinding
   e. Sampling
2. **A public health physician wants to study the load of hypertension in West Bengal to establish special screening and treatment service. Which design is more useful for this?**
   a. Cross sectional b. Case series
   c. Cohort d. Case control
3. **The time period required between ingestion of an infectious blood meal and viral replication in salivary tissue of the VECTOR sufficient for transmission to occur is called**
   a. Latent period
   b. Lead time
   c. Intrinsic incubation period
   d. Extrinsic incubation period
4. **The first case of communicable disease introduced into a defined population is termed as**
   a. Index case b. Primary case
   c. Secondary case d. Suspected case
5. **The natural history of a disease is best established by:**
   a. Morbidity indicator b. Prevalence studies
   c. Experimental studies d. Cohort studies
6. **The most feasible design in terms of cost and time to assess the relationship between breast cancer and risk factor can be established by:**
   a. Cohort study b. Case control study
   c. Cross sectional study d. Randomized trial
7. **Group of people worked at uranium mines for 5 years among them few developed cancer due to uranium exposure. Which type of association would it be?**
   a. Biological plausibility b. Coherence of association
   c. Temporal association d. Specificity of association
8. **Permanent reduction of incidence of a disease to zero as a result of deliberate efforts. No intervention is required now. It is:**
   a. Elimination of disease b. Control of disease
   c. Eradication d. Surveillance
9. **Population at risk is used as denominator in calculation of:**
   a. Mortality rate b. Incidence
   c. Prevalence d. Relative risk
10. **Direct standardization is used to compare the mortality rates between two countries this is done because of difference in:**
    a. Cause of death b. Denominators
    c. Age distribution d. Numerators
11. **Relative risk of 1 (one) indicate:**
    a. No association b. Highly positive association
    c. Positive association d. Negative association
    e. Highly negative association
12. **Recall bias mostly associated with which study design:**
    a. Case control study b. Cohort
    c. RCT d. Field trial
13. **The purpose of double blind study is to:**
    a. Avoid subject bias
    b. Avoid observer bias and sampling variation
    c. Reduce the effect of sampling variation
    d. Avoid subject bias and sampling variation
14. **Average number of daughter a new born girl will bear during life time assuming fixed age specific fertility and mortality is:**
    a. Gross reproductions rate
    b. Net reproduction rate
    c. Total fertility rate
    d. Total marital fertility rate
15. **The term 'family size' refers to:**
    a. Total number of female children born to women
    b. Total number of person in a family
    c. Total number of children a women has born at a point in time
    d. None of the above
16. **Replacement level fertility is considered to be achieved when an average**
    a. 3 birth per person b. 1 birth per person
    c. 2.1 birth person d. 2.5 birth person
17. **What is most suitable hormonal contraceptive for post-partum lactating mother:**
    a. Combined oral pills
    b. Nor-ethisterone enanthate (NET-EN)
    c. Antra
    d. Progesterone only pill
18. **The most sensitive indicator of obstetric and pediatric care is:**
    a. Still birth
    b. Post neonatal mortality rate
    c. Perinatal mortality rate (PMR)
    d. Under 5 mortality rate
19. **In city with midyear population of 1 lakh, there were 2500 live birth during a year, during same year, 5 females died due to postpartum hemorrhage, 1 due to toxemia of pregnancy, 1 due to electrocution, 2 due to abortion and 2 died due to obstructed labor. MMR per 100,000 lives birth for this city during the same year.**
    a. 400 b. 440
    c. 350 d. 300
20. **In a community if the CBR is 30. The town population is approximately 10,000. The number of pregnant females at given time for Td vaccination would be?**
    a. 150 b. 625
    c. 300 d. 330
21. **Which one of the following is not a direct cause of maternal mortality:**
    a. Cardiac disease b. Eclampsia
    c. Hemorrhage d. Abortion
22. **Multiload device contains:**
    a. Copper b. Progesterone
    c. Gold d. Silver

Ans.

1.	b
2.	a
3.	d
4.	b
5.	d
6.	b
7.	c
8.	c
9.	b
10.	c
11.	a
12.	a
13.	b
14.	b
15.	c
16.	c
17.	c
18.	c
19.	a
20.	d
21.	a
22.	a

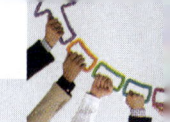

23. Contraindication of IUCD includes which of the following:
a. Pelvic inflammatory disease
b. Previous ectopic pregnancy
c. Cancer of cervix/uterus
d. All of the above

24. Failure rate of contraceptive method is determined by :
a. Sullivan's index
b. Number of accidental pregnancy
c. Pearl index
d. Half life

25. Height of group of 20 Boys aged 10 years was 140 ± 13 cm & 20 girl of same age was 135 cm ± 7 cm to test the statistical significance of difference in height test applicable is
a. chi square test b. Z test
c. T test paired d. T test unpaired

26. Which is true of cluster sampling
a. Every 10th cases is chosen for study,
b. Stratification of population done
c. A natural group is taken is sampling unit
d. Involves use of random number

27. Height for weight of boys in a classroom is
a. Correlation b. Association
c. Proportion d. Index

28. Sample size, in quantitative data is given by formula:
(P = prevalence, Q = 100-prevalence, L = allowable error, σ = standard deviation)
a. $N = 4\sigma^2/L^2$ b. $N = 4\ L2/\sigma^2$
c. $N = PQ/e$ d. $N = 4PQ/L^2$

29. If the sample size is increased 4 times, precision will:
a. Decrease 4 time b. Increase 4 time
c. Increase 2 time d. Decrease 2 time

30. A number of cases of malaria are collected over 10 years with extreme variation in data; best to calculate average is:
a. Arithmetic mean b. Mode
c. Geometric mean d. Median

31. Which of the following tests of significance can be used to compare unrelated variables when values are all binary?
a. t-test
b. Chi-square test
d. Correlation test
e. Regression test

32. If prevalence of diabetes is 10%, the probability that three people selected at random from the population will have diabetes is:
a. 0.01
b. 0.03
c. 0.001
d. 0.003

33. In respect of type I error, which one of the following is not correct?
a. It is also called alpha error
b. It is often assigned the value of 0.05 in studies
c. It is equal to 1- beta error
d. It is used to determine the sample size

34. Identify the logo:
a. Baby friendly hospital initiative
b. F-IMNCI
c. India new born action plan
d. Navjat Shishu Suraksha Karyakram

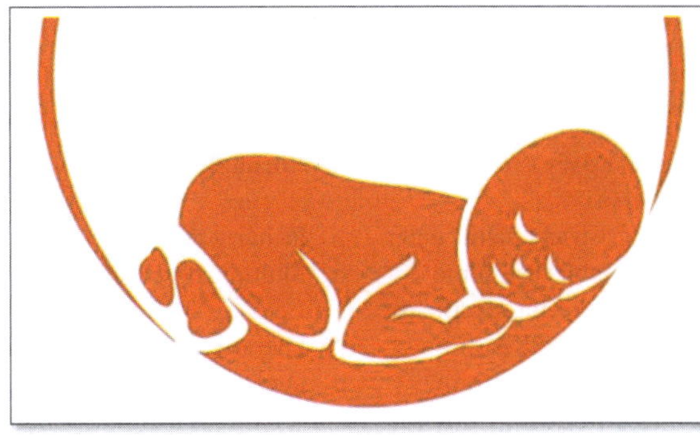

35. Sensitivity of a screening test 'X' is 80 % while its specificity is 80 %. Likelihood ratio for a positive test is -
a. 2.0 b. 4.0
c. 1.0 d. 0.1

36. In a normal distribution with mean 55 and standard deviation 10, the area to the right of 55 within 1 SD is approximately equal to:
a. 5% b. 34%
c. 95% d. 68%

37. Simple random sampling method is ideal for:
a. Heterogeneous population
b. Homogenous population
c. Vaccinated population
d. Different age structure population

38. Snowballing is:
a. Role plays
b. Group discussion
c. Mass Media approach
d. Management of metabolic syndrome

39. If the prevalence of mental depression in the elderly community is deemed to be 50%, calculate the minimum sample required for good statistical analysis at 95% Confidence level, a beta error (allowable relative error) of 10%.
a. 100 b. 200
c. 400 d. 1600

40. Calculate the 95% Confidence interval, if prevalence is 10% and the sample size of 100.
a. 9-11 b. 8-12
c. 6-14 d. 4-16

41. A child prolonged breast fed needs supplement of
a. Vitamin A b. Vitamin B
c. Calcium d. Vitamin C

42. Which of the following is rich in linoleic acid
a. Linseed oil b. Groundnut oil
c. Sunflower oil d. Soybean oil

43. Extend sickness benefit is payable for
a. 91 days b. 124 days
c. 2 years d. 1 year

44. The cholesterol 'HDL ratio that must be achieved to prevent CHD is less than:
a. 1 b. 2
c. 3.5 d. 4.5

45. Main risk factor for cerebral thrombosis is
a. Elevated blood lipids b. Diabetes
c. Hypertension d. Oral contraceptives

Ans.

23. d
24. c
25. d
26. c
27. a
28. d
29. d
30. d
31. b
32. c
33. c
34. c
35. b
36. b
37. b
38. b
39. c
40. d
41. c
42. c
43. c
44. a
45. c

46. **Prevention of recurrence of rheumatic fever by giving benzathine penicillin is:**
    a. Primordial prevention b. Primary prevention
    c. Secondary prevention d. Tertiary prevention
47. **Secondary eye care is provided through all of the following except:**
    a. District health center b. Primary health center
    c. Mobile eye clinic d. Multipurpose worker
48. **The varicella vaccine is:**
    a. Killed OKA strain b. Live attenuated OKA strain
    c. Killed VZ. strain d. Oral varicella vaccine
49. **80 Prevalence of disease in tuberculosis can be confirmed by:**
    a. Mass miniature radiograph
    b. Sputum microscopy
    c. Sputum culture
    d. Tuberculin test
50. **93 Vaccine associated paralytic polio is due to which virus in OPV:**
    a. Type I b. Type 2
    c. Type 3 d. All
51. **Children under 15 years of age constitute % of population in India:**
    a. 10 b. 17
    c. 22 d. 28
52. **FRU is important for:**
    a. Sick born neonates
    b. Still births
    c. Maternal mortality ratios
    d. Under five mortality rates
53. **Immunoglobulins may be used for all except:**
    a. Tetanus
    b. Rabies
    c. Hep A
    d. Hep B
54. **All are true about colostrum except:**
    a. Rich in proteins and minerals
    b. Rich in anti-infective factors
    c. Secreted for 3–6 days
    d. Rich in fats
55. **Which of the following infant is not at risk**
    a. Failure to gain weight during 2 successive months
    b. Spacing if less than 2 years
    c. 3rd birth order
    d. Working mother
56. **WHO criteria for metabolic syndrome is**
    a. WC > 102 in males and > 88 in females
    b. WC > 100 in males and > 85 in females
    c. WC > 88 in males and > 68 in females
    d. WC > 90 in males and > 72 in females
57. **ART should be initiated in all adults with HIV at ______ CD4 count**
    a. 200 b. 350
    c. 500 d. 100
58. **Delphi technique is:**
    a. Finance Management principle
    b. Human resource management principle
    c. Group discussion and IEC method
    d. Cluster sampling method
59. **Gather approach is used for:**
    a. Simple random sampling method
    b. Contraceptive use method
    c. Counseling method
    d. Census survey method
60. **Which of the following vaccine may be associated with TSS?**
    a. Measles vaccine b. MMR vaccine
    c. BCG vaccine d. Yellow fever vaccine
61. **Best indicator for nutritional status of the child is?**
    a. MAC
    b. Head circumference
    c. Rate of increase in height and weight
    d. Chest circumference
62. **Not a clinical manifestation of botulism?**
    a. Diplopia b. Diarrhea
    c. Urinary retension d. Apyrexia
63. **Which of the following is an indicator for operational efficacy?**
    a. API b. ABER
    c. AFI d. SPR
64. **In leprosy control programme, indicator of efficiency for early diagnosis of cases is:**
    a. Disability rate among newly diagnosed
    b. Lepromin +ve% among newly diagnosed
    c. Ratio of pauci/multi bacillary cases
    d. Any of the above
65. **Under RNTCP, a new case is one who has never had treatment for TB or has taken anti-TB drugs less than:**
    a. 2 weeks b. 4 weeks
    c. 6 weeks d. 8 weeks
66. **Most sensitive indicator of health and utilization of health facilities in a community is:**
    a. Maternal mortality rate b. Infant mortality rate
    c. Neonatal mortality rate d. Perinatal mortality rate
67. **Maternal mortality ratio in India is estimated to be:**
    a. 1/1000 live births b. 1.3/1000 live births
    c. 3.4/1000 live births d. 2.1/1000 live births
68. **Which of the following is not true about tetanus immunization during pregnancy**
    a. If mother is not immunized earlier, 2 doses of tetanus toxoid should be given
    b. The minimum interval between 2 doses should be 8 weeks
    c. Second dose preferably should be given one month before the expected date of delivery
    d. If pregnant woman is immunized 2 years back, then only one dose of tetanus toxoid is sufficient
69. **In AFP examination for residual paralysis should be done after:**
    a. 30 days
    b. 60 days
    c. 90 days
    d. 120 days
70. **Predominantly, for management of which one of the following resources is the critical path method (CPM) used as one of the health administration techniques?**
    a. Money
    b. Manpower
    c. Time
    d. Material

Ans.

46. b
47. d
48. d
49. b
50. c
51. d
52. c
53. c
54. c
55. d
56. a
57. c
58. c
59. c
60. a
61. a
62. b
63. b
64. a
65. b
66. d
67. b
68. b
69. b
70. c

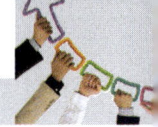

71. Strain used for JE Vaccine is:
a. Live vaccine, SA-14-14-2 strain
b. Killed Vaccine, SA 14-14-2 strain
c. Live Vaccine, RA 27 strain
d. Killed vaccine, RA 27 strain

72. Softening of water is indicated when the hardness reaches?
a. 200 mEq/L
b. 30 mEq/L
c. 3 nEq/L
d. 300 mEq/L

73. P4SR pertains to:
a. Air humidity
b. Thermal comfort zones
c. Water purification standards
d. Room ventilation standards

74. Micropolyspora faeni is the main cause for:
a. Byssinosis
b. Bagassosis
c. Anthracosis
d. Farmer's lung

75. Which of the following is true sequence of events?
a. Disease Disability Impairment Handicap
b. Disability Disease Impairment Handicap
c. Disease Impairment Handicap Disability
d. Disease Impairment Disability Handicap

76. Which is the best index for burden of disease?
a. Case fatality rate
b. Disability adjusted life years
c. Dependence rate
d. Morbidity data

77. Sullivan's index pertains to:
a. Obesity rates
b. Socio economic status
c. Dengue indices
d. Disability Index

78. SDG number of goals are:
a. 11
b. 14
c. 17
d. 32

79. Polio switch Day was on
a. 28 Oct 2015
b. 10 Feb 2016
c. 7 April 2016
d. 24 April 2016

80. Which is true regarding the Kolmogorov-2 Smirnov test
a. Used to find the spearman correlation between two variables
b. It is used to assess for equality of distribution of non-parametric data
c. It is to determine agreement between qualitative parameters
d. To find the significance between two ordinal grouped data set

Ans.
71. a
72. c
73. b
74. b
75. a
76. d
77. d
78. c
79. d
80. b

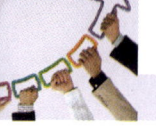

Answers with Explanations

1. Ans. (b) **Matching**

2. Ans. (a) **Cross sectional**

(Load of disease, burden of disease, prevalence of disease all carry same meaning and can be determined by cross sectional study)

3. Ans. (d) **Extrinsic incubation period**

4. Ans. (b) **Primary case**

And the First case came to the attention of the Investigator is called Index case

5. Ans. (d) **Cohort studies**

Cohort study is also called longitudinal study or incidence study

6. Ans. (b) **Case control study**

7. Ans. (c) **Temporal association**

8. Ans. (c) **Eradication**

9. Ans. (b) **Incidence**

10. Ans. (c) **Age distribution**

11. Ans. (a) **No association**

A relative risk of one means that the incidence of disease is equal in both the exposed and unexposed population. This would therefore imply no association

12. Ans. (a) **Case control study**

13. Ans. (b) **Avoid observer bias and sampling variation**

14. Ans. (b) **Net reproduction rate**

15. Ans. (c) **Total number of children a women has born at a point in time**

16. Ans. (c) **2.1 birth person**

17. Ans. (c) **Antra**

Antra is Medroxyprogesterone acetate

18. Ans. (c) **Perinatal mortality rate (PMR)**

Perinatal mortality includes both maternal care indicator and neonatal care indicator.

19. Ans. (a) **400**

Calculation: 5 + 1 + 2 + 2/2500 multiply by 100,000 = 400
Note: We do not take the death which occurs due to electrocution because they are not related to pregnancy, but it is accident al cause of death

20. Ans. (d) **330**

Number of mothers = number of pregnant females + pregnancy wastage (abortions) (10%)
Number of pregnant females = (total population * birth rate) /1000
= 10000*30/1000 = 300
Total number of mothers = number of pregnant females + pregnancy wastage
= 300 + (10% of 300) = 330

21. Ans. (a) **Cardiac disease**

22. Ans. (a) **Copper**

23. Ans. (d) **All of the above**

24. Ans. (c) **Pearl index**

25. Ans. (d) **T test unpaired**

26. Ans. (c) **A natural group is taken is sampling unit**

27. Ans. (a) **Correlation**

28. Ans. (d) **$N = 4PQ/L^2$**

29. Ans. (d) **Decrease 2 time**

30. Ans. (d) **Median**

31. Ans. (b) **Chi-square test**

32. Ans. (c) **0.001**

33. Ans. (c) **It is equal to 1- beta error**

34. Ans. (c) **India new born action plan**

35. Ans. (b) **4.0**

36. Ans. (b) **34%**

37. Ans. (b) **Homogenous population**

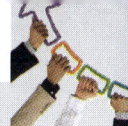

38. **Ans. (b) Group discussion**

39. **Ans. (c) 400**

Sample size is 4pq/L*L
p = prevalence = 50
q = 100-prev = 50
L = 10% of prev = 5
n = (4 * 50 * 50) / 5*5 = 400

40. **Ans. (d) 4-16**

We calculate the CI which corresponds to the SE
SE = sq rt (p*q)/n
P = 10
Q = 90 (100 – 10)
N = 100
SE = SqRt (10*90/100) = 3
So, The 95% CI = 2 SE,
Therefore 95 % CI = 2*3 = 6. i.e. 10 – 6 to 10 + 6 = 4 to 16
Hence ans d.

41. **Ans. (c) Calcium**

42. **Ans. (c) Sunflower oil**

43. **Ans. (c) 2 years**

44. **Ans. (c) 3.5**

45. **Ans. (c) Hypertension**

46. **Ans. (b) Primary prevention**

47. **Ans. (d) Multipurpose worker**

48. **Ans. (d) Oral varicella vaccine**

49. **Ans. (b) Sputum microscopy**

50. **Ans. (c) Type 3**

51. **Ans. (d) 28**

52. **Ans. (c) Maternal mortality ratios**

53. **Ans. (c) Hep A**

54. **Ans. (c) Secreted for 3–6 days**

55. **Ans. (d) Working mother**

56. **Ans. (a) WC > 102 in males and >88 n females**

57. **Ans. (c) 500**

58. **Ans. (c) Group discussion and IEC method**

59. **Ans. (c) Counseling method**

60. **Ans. (a) Measles vaccine**

61. **Ans. (a) MAC**

62. **Ans. (b) Diarrhea**

63. **Ans. (b) ABER**

64. **Ans. (a) Disability rate among newly diagnosed**

65. **Ans. (b) 4 weeks**

66. **Ans. (d) Perinatal mortality rate**

67. **Ans. (b) 1.3/1000 live births**

68. **Ans. (b) The minimum interval between 2 doses should be 8 weeks**

69. **Ans. (b) 60 days**

70. **Ans. (c) Time**

71. **Ans. (a) Live vaccine, SA-14-14-2 strain**

72. **Ans. (c) 3 MEq/L**

73. **Ans. (b) Thermal comfort zones**

74. **Ans. (b) Bagassosis**

75. **Ans. (a) Disease Disability Impairment Handicap**

76. **Ans. (d) Morbidity data**

77. **Ans. (d) Disability Index**

78. **Ans. (c) 17**

79. **Ans. (d) 24 April 2016**

80. **Ans. (b) It is used to assess for equality of distribution of non-parametric data**

Nonparametric **test** of the equality of continuous, one-dimensional probability distributions that can be used to compare a sample with a reference probability distribution (one-sample K–S **test**), or to compare two samples (two-sample K–S **test**).

NOTES